Biomarkers of the Tumor Microenvironment

Lars A. Akslen • Randolph S. Watnick

Editors

Biomarkers of the Tumor Microenvironment

Second Edition

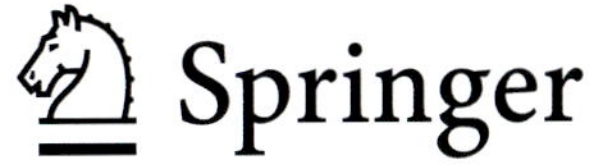
Springer

Editors
Lars A. Akslen
Centre for Cancer Biomarkers CCBIO
Department of Clinical Medicine
University of Bergen
Bergen, Norway

Randolph S. Watnick
Department of Surgery
Harvard Medical School
Vascular Biology Program
Boston Children's Hospital
Boston, USA

ISBN 978-3-030-98952-1   ISBN 978-3-030-98950-7   (eBook)
https://doi.org/10.1007/978-3-030-98950-7

This Springer imprint is published by the registered company Springer Nature Switzerland AG
The registered company address is: Gewerbestrasse 11, 6330 Cham, Switzerland

The editors would like to dedicate this book to the memory of the late Judah Folkman, who through his visionary research and mentoring inspired the concept that the tumor microenvironment is a critical component of tumor biology.

The editors would also like to express their deepest appreciation to their families for their continuous patience and support. Dr. Akslen specifically thanks his wife Åse, daughter Heidi, son Andreas, and in particular his grandson Hans, for constant joy and inspiration. Dr. Watnick thanks his wife Jing, daughter Audrey, son Eytan, and father David for their unconditional love and encouragement.

Foreword

Professor Lars A. Akslen (Director, Center for Cancer Biomarkers CCBIO, University of Bergen) and Professor Randolph S. Watnick (Boston Children's Hospital, Harvard University) have succeeded in the formidable task of assembling an extensively revisited book on the tumor microenvironment. This new edition deals with the most important aspects of the tumor microenvironment, providing an in-depth analysis of the interactions that take place between normal and malignant cell types. This new edition provides a rather exhaustive scrutiny of the phenotypes and organizations of components of the vascular systems, decoding the roles enacted by stromal fibroblasts, inflammatory cells, and immune cells and offers noteworthy insight into innervation within the tumor microenvironment. This book also provides in-depth insight into the clinical relevance of strategically important signaling systems. The advent of new technologies is also discussed, with a topical reflection on how these technologies are being engineered for the discovery of new biomarkers toward the optimization of clinical trials. Such technological improvements have also unveiled the advanced topological features of the tumor bed and, most importantly, identified a broad swathe of relevant biomarkers that will be instrumental in discriminating responders from non-responders and in monitoring the early acquisition of refractoriness. The new edition of this book presents new concepts that can be exploited for the design and thoughtful optimization of new therapeutic strategies. Particularly attractive are the model systems described in this book, which reflect the N-dimensional complexities of tumors. Personalized and precise treatment will likely ensue from these forms of adaptive therapy. Indeed, it is hoped that these objectives will be facilitated soon with advanced bioinformatics approaches supported by artificial intelligence algorithms.

Researching the tumor microenvironment is a daunting task: the array of disorganization allows for too many distinct topological organizations. Anatomists from the late 1800s and early 1900s were able to categorize most cell types and their three-dimensional organization within tissues and organs using the most rudimentary microscopes and staining techniques. The atlas of Mathias Duval of the chick embryo (Atlas d'embryologie (Masson, Paris, 1879)) has never been surpassed, and the remarkable treaties of the famous neurohistologist Santiago Ramon y Cajal cannot be matched today by even the most advanced imaging technologies (The cerebral cortex annotated translation of the complete writings DeFilipe and Jones, Oxford University Press, 1988). But these remarkable advances were only achievable in the early days because the analysis was performed on stereotyped structures. The latest studies seeking to revisit the anatomical organization and lineage tracing of such structures using single-cell sequencing have not revealed major new findings. Unlike such typical tissue architectures, the tumor microenvironment exhibits a formidable heterogeneity in terms of cell composition, phenotype, and 3D organization, with a complex extracellular matrix. Although clinical pathologists are able to recognize critical features that can distinguish tumor type and grade, the considerable variability in the organization of the tumor microenvironment is extremely challenging to describe in depth. How can we rationalize and conceptualize the tumor microenvironment to unravel the signaling networks and identify the Achille's heel of these tumors for effective targeting? We know that the communication systems mediated in part by cytokines and growth factors cannot be modeled easily because their distribution patterns cannot be predicted by the physical laws of diffusion. Similarly, drugs and antibodies delivered into the tumor bed are also largely affected by the strong local variation in stiffness and pressure. A tumor could be theoretically analyzed by soft matter physics; albeit, the heterogeneity of the tumor structure prevents the application of thermodynamic laws of polymers (Essentials of soft matter science CRC press, Brochard-Wyart, Nassoy and Puech, 2019). We hope that, to some extent, artificial intelligence will be able to rationalize these chaotic structures. Such a task, however, requires an international consortia to address the formidable issues we face. New mathematical models and algorithms will need to be developed, similar to those recently applied by particle physicists and cosmologists to decode the universe. What we need now is to identify another Jean Francois Champollion to decode this *new* Rosetta Stone.

Jean Paul Thiery
Guangzhou Regenerative Medicine and Health
Guangdong Laboratory, Guangzhou, China

Department of Clinical Medicine, Faculty of Medicine
University of Bergen, Bergen, Norway

CNRS UMR 7057, Matter and Complex Systems
University Paris Denis Diderot, Paris, France

Comprehensive Cancer Center Institut Gustave Roussy, Villejuif, France

Chief Scientific Consultant, Chair SAB Biosyngen Pte. Ltd., Singapore, Singapore

Scientific Founder and Chairman, BioCheetah Pte. Ltd., Singapore, Singapore

Preface

In 1889, Stephen Paget formally postulated his "seed and soil" hypothesis, building upon the previous observations of Ernst Fuchs. This seminal concept on tumor progression was based on the analogy that tumor cells were *seeds* and needed a proper *soil* to grow. However, the study of cancer for the next hundred years focused primarily on characterizing the morphologic and molecular aberrations unique to tumor cells. This field of study yielded remarkable insights into intrinsic tumor cell biology with dozens of oncogenes and tumor suppressors discovered. In contrast, very few papers dealt with the "tumor microenvironment" until the 1990s. However, the theory that tumors require a permissive environment or "tissue predisposition" to grow, both in the primary site and following dissemination to distant organs, is now commonly accepted.

That being said, our understanding of the basic composition of tumors has gradually transformed from a collection of tumor cells that grow in an uncontrolled fashion to miniature tissues or "organs" comprised of a neovasculature and complex stroma consisting of both resident and bone marrow-derived cells. This conceptual shift has been extended by the observations that tumor cells interact with their microenvironment and, in so doing, affect and are affected by the reciprocal intercellular signaling. These signaling events were recognized as critical by Judah Folkman, who postulated in the late 1960s that tumor growth and spread were linked to the ability to induce angiogenesis. By relentlessly pursuing the underlying biology behind these findings, he helped foster the notion that the tumor microenvironment was not a passive bystander but an active collaborator in tumor progression. Today, pathologists commonly use microvessel density or vascular proliferation as biomarkers for determining the aggressiveness of tumors. Moreover, the first identified angiogenic factor, VEGF, and its growth promoting receptor VEGFR2, are targets for anti-cancer therapeutic agents used widely in the treatment of cancer patients.

As the field matured, we discovered that many different cell types exist within the tumor microenvironment that possess both growth promoting and inhibitory roles in tumor progression. Among the most prominent cell types that affect tumor growth are immune cells. Harold Dvorak famously described tumors as "wounds that do not heal." This seemingly simple statement has profound implications not only on how tumors are studied and perceived, but also on the manner in which they are treated. Advancements in immunotherapy have led to the development of therapeutic agents that re-engage the adaptive immune response and enable the immune system to attack tumors. Immune checkpoint inhibitors that block PD-1, PD-L1, and CTLA-4 have been approved for multiple indications and have shown potent and durable responses in a subset of patients. Therapeutic agents targeting CD47, a "do not eat me" signal that represents an inflammatory checkpoint protein blocking macrophage phagocytosis, are in clinical trials.

It is now recognized that evasion of immune and inflammatory cells is not mediated solely by the expression of checkpoint inhibitors on the surface of tumor cells. Myeloid derived cells, including monocytes and macrophages, are potent suppressors of the immune and inflammatory response, as are cancer-associated fibroblasts (CAFs). Such cells might also repress the expression of thrombospondin-1, a potent anti-angiogenic, anti-inflammatory, and immunomodulatory protein. Recent findings have highlighted that angiogenesis and immune evasion are co-regulated, further underscoring the complexity and significance of these interactions between tumor cells and the microenvironment.

This textbook contains 34 chapters, divided in two main sections, that highlight the multi-dimensional and complex nature of the tumor microenvironment and its role in tumor progression, biomarker development, and therapeutic targeting. The first section deals with basic mechanisms and biomarkers of the tumor microenvironment (TME) and its various components. The second section delves into examples of organ directed biomarker studies and clinical applications. Following a masterful overview with integrated perspectives on this field by Robert Weinberg, Watnick (*Chap. 1*) sets the stage and focus on the importance of microenvironmental context in the regulation of tumor angiogenesis. It is argued that paracrine signaling should be considered in the search for tumor progression drivers and novel targets along with companion biomarkers of potential clinical importance. The identification of targets within the TME is envisioned to be complementary to the search for mutations and aberrant signaling in tumor cells. In *Chap. 2*, Akslen continues along the same theme to discuss how tissue-based markers of angiogenesis and vascular invasion can be defined and applied in studies of human cancers and how their aggressive behavior can be graded by such markers, while *Chaps. 3 and 4* see Milosevic et al. and Wagner & Wiig delve into the roles of vasculature and the lymphatic system in tumor growth and progression.

In *Chaps. 5 and 6*, Zeltz et al. and Legget & Nelson outline the dual functions of the extracellular matrix and tissue architecture as supportive or inhibitory with respect to cancer progression. Especially, the role of the insoluble extracellular matrix (ECM) is discussed, and how its components influence matrix remodeling, tumor metastasis, and even tumor heterogeneity. This theme is continued in *Chap. 7* as Dongre and Costea explore the roles of cancer-associated fibroblasts (CAFs), the major producers of ECM proteins in the TME, In *Chap. 8*, Strell and Östman describe the paracrine interactions between mesenchymal cells and epithelial or endothelial cells, with particular reference to the PDGF family of growth factors and receptors. By combining experimental and clinical studies, the PDGF signaling systems appear as critical regulators of tumor growth, metastasis, and drug efficacy. In *Chap. 9*, Gilligan et al. elaborate further on the function of lipid signaling and the dual role of inflammation in cancer. The complex interactions between various classes of immune cells and how these appear to be regulated by fatty acid-derived lipid mediators such as prostaglandin E2 are discussed.

Chapter 10 sees Kushekhar et al. delineate the multiple roles of lymphocytes in immunity and immune evasion. They explore mechanisms of immunoediting, immunosuppressive cytokines, and the multiple types of lymphocytes, their markers and function in tumor progression and treatment. In *Chap. 11*, Brekken and Wnuk-Lipinska discuss the regulation and relationship of epithelial plasticity (EMT programs) and immune escape mechanisms. The authors focus on molecules that can drive the immunosuppressive state in the tumor microenvironment and potentially serve as biomarkers for poor prognosis. Continuing on the role of the immune and inflammatory system in *Chap. 12*, Corthay and Haraldsen comment on a range of inflammatory biomarkers in cancer such as cytokines and interleukins converging on STAT3 signaling. In particular, this chapter discusses the biology of IL-33, the most recently identified member of the interleukin family. In *Chap. 13*, Floris et al. describe some tissue-based biomarkers of the immune response in solid tumors, such as tumor infiltrating lymphocytes (TILs) and tertiary lymphoid structures (TLSs), and how these can be recorded in human tumor tissues.

In *Chap. 14*, Ramchandani et al. explore the role of the bone marrow and bone marrow-derived cells on tumor progression and metastasis. They discuss how bone marrow-derived cells constitute a significant fraction of the primary tumor microenvironment and processes such as angiogenesis as well as metastasis and growth in distant sites. *Chapter 15* introduces the role of platelets in tumor progression. Guo et al. describe the intricate composition of platelets into multiple types of granules and the signals that elicit release of pro- and anti-tumorigenic proteins from these granules.

In *Chaps. 16 and 17,* Vethe et al. and Balasubbramanian et al. explore the nascent and exciting field of neurogenesis and neurogenic factors in tumors. Vethe et al. discuss the biology of nerve fiber infiltration in tumors and their role in influencing tumor growth and progression via specific tumor–nerve interactions. Balasubbramanian et al. focus on the roles of two proteins originally identified in neurogenesis, neuropilin 1 and 2. They outline the novel observations that these receptors are also expressed on tumor cells and discuss their functional role in tumor progression and as biomarkers.

In *Chap. 18,* Lotsberg et al. revisit epithelial plasticity and EMT, focusing on roles of the Axl receptor tyrosine kinase in tumor cell plasticity and tumor progress. In particular, the authors focus on the relationship between EMT programs, immune evasive phenotypes, and drug resistance, and how this suggests a potential for anti-Axl combination therapy in a range of aggressive cancers. Continuing the theme of advances in cancer treatment, in *Chap. 19,* Kleinmanns et al. provide an overview of the advances in patient-derived xenografts. They discuss their utility in modeling disease progression, identifying novel biomarkers, and testing clinical and pre-clinical stage therapeutic agents.

Herdlevær et al. provide an introduction to imaging mass cytometry as a method for deep interrogation of tissue biomarkers in *Chap. 20.* Specifically, they explain how this relatively new technique can assay up to 40 discrete biomarkers at once using metal affinity tagged antibodies. They discuss how researchers and clinicians are using this technology to gain unprecedented insights into the composition of the TME in naïve and treated tumors. To conclude *Section 1, Chap. 21* sees Pedersen et al. explore the exciting technology of artificial intelligence and how it is being implemented to discern molecular and pathological trends and patterns in malignant tumors.

Kicking off *Section 2,* which focuses on organ related studies and clinical applications of TME biomarkers, in *Chap. 22,* Moses et al. discuss the exploration of the TME for therapeutic targets. Specifically, they delineate the utility of the detection of biomarkers: exosomes, proteins, nucleic acids, lipids, miRNA, and cells in bodily fluids and how the modulation of these markers can be prognostic for disease outcome. In *Chap. 23,* Wik et al. explore the use of gene expression signatures of the tumor microenvironment in breast cancer. The authors discuss how composite signatures can be used as biomarkers and clinical tools to capture and reflect the complexity in human tumors that are not attainable using individual markers.

In *Chap. 24,* Kim and co-workers delineate the use of non-invasive magnetic resonance imaging (MRI) and spectroscopy (MRS) to measure dynamic biomarkers that can be used to characterize alterations in tumors during treatment and follow-up. Importantly, they discuss how contrast-enhanced MRI methods can aid in the evaluation of tumor vascularization and function. In *Chap. 25,* Jokela et al. propose a dominant role of the microenvironment in tumor progression. The authors explore the influence of tissue architecture on drug responses, by focusing on applications and analytic approaches used for functional cell-based exploration of combinatorial microenvironments using microarray technology.

In *Chap. 26,* Azeem et al. discuss the establishment of novel prostate cancer models, their applications, and their critical role in understanding disease progression and therapeutic strategies. Biomarkers of prostate cancer are further explored in *Chap. 27* by Magnussen and Mills. Specifically, they advocate for the use of biomarkers, and the necessity for informed patient consent, to monitor the progression of prostate cancer and explore LRG-1 as a promising marker.

In *Chap. 28,* Rogers draws insightful comparisons between the microenvironment of endometriosis and cancer and explores the idea that similar or analogous biological mechanisms and pathways may mediate both diseases. He proposes that rigorous experimental analysis of endometriosis is necessary for the field and that tools employed in cancer research can be utilized for this purpose. In *Chap. 29,* Ramnefjell and Akslen make the provocative case that angiogenesis and neovascularization are underutilized as biomarkers for non-small cell lung cancer (NSCLC). They further advocate that based on biomarker data and improved patient stratification, anti-angiogenic therapy might be more widely used to treat NSCLC patients.

In *Chap. 30*, Leiss and colleagues expound on the specific features of tumor–host interactions in malignant gliomas. They explore how interactions are shaped by the structural organization of the CNS and involve multiple cell types, extracellular matrix components, and host cell-derived soluble factors that are unique to the CNS. In *Chap. 31*, Dillekås et al. discuss the importance of tumor stress responses and the TME in progression of melanoma and other tumors to the metastatic stage. They focus on the dual nature of the melanoma TME as having both stimulatory and inhibitory properties, as well as the involvement of the immune system.

In *Chap. 32*, Wang and Dudley return to the brain tumor microenvironment to shed light on the exciting and still poorly understood field of vessel cooption. They first provide clinical evidence of vascular cooption and then explore experimental models. The authors postulate that the underlying biology of brain cancers and their often diffuse invasion patterns necessitate vessel cooption over neovascularization.

In *Chap. 33*, Jebsen and co-workers outline the most active pathways to therapy development: mutation driven drug development, immunomodulatory therapy, and evolution of conventional chemo- and radiotherapy. In this context, they promote the merits of personalized medicine and argue that successful implementation requires more precise biomarkers, not only to increase precision and enhance efficiency but also to avoid unnecessary toxicity for the patient, and costs for the society.

Section 2 and this text book conclude with a masterful treatise of the requirement for and development of novel biomarkers of the TME (*Chap. 34*). Sim et al. provide an overview of the myriad technologies and "omics" that can be marshalled to enhance the identification of new biomarkers and explain why they are needed. Finally, they advance the notion that "real-time" biomarkers are the next major development and their utility in monitoring both disease progression and treatment efficacy.

It would be impossible to provide an exhaustive and thorough analysis of this rapidly expanding field in a single volume. Still, we hope that readers find this second edition useful. As the field of identifying and utilizing biomarkers of the tumor microenvironment rushes forward at a breakneck pace, we will be presented with a myriad of exciting and novel treatment targets and companion biomarkers. We must remember, that as is the case with any rapidly growing field, the challenge is to integrate the newly generated knowledge into the evolving practice of medical oncology and precision medicine. This challenge demands that those whose work focuses on the basic sciences work diligently to translate their innovative approaches and discoveries with special focus on working closely with their colleagues in clinical practice and research to continually improve trial design and follow-up of patients.

Finally, we thank Springer Nature for allowing us the opportunity to work together *again* on this project. As longtime collaborators and friends who share a common passion for unlocking the mysteries and therapeutic potential of the tumor microenvironment, it has been truly awe inspiring to curate the remarkable advances made in this field. As is the case with any undertaking of this size and complexity, we, the editors, could not have successfully completed it without the help of several important contributors. We would like to thank the staff at Springer Nature, as well as our own staff, for their assistance and valuable advice.

Bergen, Norway
Boston, MA, USA

Lars A. Akslen
Randolph S. Watnick

Biomarkers of the Tumor Microenvironment—A Prologue

Until a quarter century ago, a powerful reductionist paradigm held sway in the field of cancer research: those interested in studying the mechanisms of cancer pathogenesis embraced the notion that the biology of tumors could be understood by analyzing the biology of the constituent cancer cells. Moreover, the biology and pathophysiology of individual cancer cells could be understood, in turn, by studying their genomes, more specifically cancer-associated somatically mutated genomes. This was, to be sure, a powerful model, in that it led to the discovery of the genetic determinants of cancer pathogenesis, including oncogenes, tumor suppressor genes, and yet other genes involved in DNA repair and apoptosis.

As useful as this paradigm was, it overlooked an important aspect of cancer pathogenesis: tumors are histologically complex structure composed of multiple distinct cell types, a reality recognized by pathologists for more than a century. Accordingly, beginning in the late 1990s, it became increasingly clear, even to the most committed reductionists, that tumors were functionally far more complex than aggregates of cancer cells. Thus, as tumors develop, it became apparent that neoplastic cells rely on recruited normal host cells for various types of cell-physiologic support. The latter cells had been termed stroma by the pathologists. More detailed characterization of the stroma revealed that it consists, at least in the case of common carcinomas, of a diverse collection of cells, virtually all of which are of mesenchymal origin. Included in the stroma are cells that often form its bulk, including fibroblasts and myofibroblasts, the latter often termed carcinoma-associated fibroblasts (CAFs). Interwoven among these stromal connective tissue cells are a variety of cells of hematopoietic origin, including endothelial cells, various subsets of lymphocytes, macrophages, and occasional granulocytes.

As carcinomas develop and progress to higher grades of malignancy, the stroma usually changes in lockstep, becoming increasingly "reactive" and thus assuming a biological state that exists only transiently in the wound sites within normal tissues that are in the midst of healing. Indeed, such reactive stroma increasingly resembles "wounds that do not heal." The coordinated changes of neoplastic cells together with adjacent stroma provided, on its own, a clear indication that the two groups of cells intercommunicate, doing so via processes that are often termed heterotypic signaling, i.e., communication between distinct types of cells.

In principle, this signaling might be unidirectional, in that, as an example, the neoplastic cells within a carcinoma might release signals that recruited a diverse array of stromal cells to the growing tumor and thereafter orchestrated their behavior. In truth, however, the heterotypic signaling is bidirectional, in that recruited stromal cells release signals that impinge reciprocally on the carcinoma cells that previously recruited them. Hence, the co-evolution of neoplastic cells and the co-opted host cells is enabled by bidirectional signaling. Importantly, while the neoplastic cells undergo both genetic and epigenetic evolution, the evidence to date indicates that the recruited stromal cells—which together form the "tumor microenvironment"—undergo phenotypic changes that are not driven by somatic mutations.

In fact, the histopathological appearance of islands of tumor cells is often strongly influenced by the signals that these cells receive from the tumor-associated stroma. Most prominent among the phenotypic changes experienced by carcinoma cells is the activation of a usually latent cell-biological program termed the epithelial–mesenchymal transition (EMT), which is normally operative during early embryogenesis, where it programs the interconversions of cell types that are destined to form distinct tissues and organs; in addition, the EMT program operates transiently during wound healing. In the case of carcinomas, the EMT-inducing signals received by carcinoma cells from their microenvironment drive the acquisition of a complex spectrum of cell-biological changes involving the shedding of preexisting epithelial traits (inherited from normal cells-of-origin) and the acquisition of mesenchymal traits, such as motility, invasiveness, an elevated resistance to various types of therapeutic intervention, and an ability to disseminate to anatomical sites distant from the primary tumor. The resulting secondary tumor colonies—metastases—are responsible for 90% of cancer-associated mortality.

These heterotypic signaling interactions between neoplastic cells and their stromal microenvironment are extremely complex. Each of the participating cell types releases a complex mixture of heterotypic signals that impinge upon and influence multiple other cell types. This multi-body problem dwarfs in its complexity the three-body problem that has thwarted the attempts by physicists to describe mathematically. As a consequence, we come to realize that the study of tumor microenvironments, which is already a highly active area of research, is still in its infancy, given the complexity of the cell–cell signaling networks that operate within the tumor-associated stroma and between this stroma and nearby cancer cells. The present volume lays out some of the more salient of these interactions. As complex as they are, the signaling networks described here still represent only a beginning. Thus, at present, the complexity of the signaling networks vastly outstrips our ability to understand them in their entirety, i.e., to understand how multiple heterotypic interactions conspire to create the complex biology of high-grade malignancies. Still, what is presented in this volume represents an interesting and exciting beginning! Enjoy what you read!

Robert A. Weinberg
Whitehead Institute for Biomedical Research
Ludwig/MIT Center for Integrative Cancer Research
MIT Department of Biology, Cambridge, MA, USA

Contents

Basic Studies: Tumor Mechanisms and Tissue Biomarkers

Randolph S. Watnick

Abstract

The tumor microenvironment plays a crucial role in cancer development and progression. Paracrine signaling between tumor cells and the normal cells that make up the microenvironment is a critical component influencing the progression of tumors from the in situ stage to metastatic disease. Despite the importance of these paracrine signaling mechanisms and factors, the vast majority of academic research and development in the pharmaceutical industry is still targeted toward mutations and aberrant signaling pathways within tumor cells. As a result, the intercellular signaling that between tumor cells and the microenvironment has not been as extensively studied with regard to the regulation of angiogenesis. In this chapter, we define the key players in the regulation of angiogenesis and examine how their expression is regulated in the microenvironment. The resulting analysis presents observations that at first glance may seem paradoxical. However, these nuances serve to underscore the complexity of these interactions and the need to better delineate and define the environmental context underlying these mechanisms.

Take-Home Lessons
- The cells in the tumor microenvironment (TME) play a major role in regulating angiogenesis.
- Non-tumor cells, such as fibroblasts, inflammatory cells, and immune cells, normally repress angiogenesis.
- Tumors secrete growth factors and cytokines that reprogram non-tumor cells in the TME to repress anti-angiogenic proteins and express pro-angiogenic proteins.
- Tumor-secreted modulators of the TME can act both locally via paracrine interactions and systemically to reprogram cells in both the primary tumor and potential sites of metastasis.

Introduction

In the earliest stages of cancer, carcinomas (tumors derived from epithelial cells), are physically confined within the epithelial compartment of the tissue from whence they arise. These early lesions (carcinomas in situ) are separated from the tissue parenchyma by the basement membrane [1]. Opposite the basement membrane are a myriad of cells consisting of fibroblasts, myofibroblasts, immune/inflammatory cells, and endothelial cells [2]. In addition to these cell types are extracellular matrix proteins, secreted largely by fibroblasts, which serve as a substrate for tumor cells to attach [2].

In order for tumors to progress to a clinically relevant and potentially lethal disease, they must, in a sequential manner, acquire the capacity to escape the epithelial compartment, invade the local parenchyma, and disseminate systemically. To enable this process, tumor cells must degrade, or induce the degradation of the basement membrane that separates the epithelial compartment from the parenchyma. Invasion of the tissue parenchyma by the tumor, or, conversely invasion of stromal cells into the tumor, initiates a phase of tumor progression in which tumor growth becomes dependent on non-cell autonomous processes regulated by paracrine and juxtacrine signaling interactions between the tumor and its microenvironment [3–5].

In other words, in order to expand in size beyond the diffusion limit of oxygen in tissue, a new vasculature must form

R. S. Watnick (✉)
Department of Surgery, Harvard Medical School,
Vascular Biology Program, Boston Children's Hospital,
Boston, USA
e-mail: Randy.watnick@childrens.harvard.edu

L. A. Akslen, R. S. Watnick (eds.), *Biomarkers of the Tumor Microenvironment*, https://doi.org/10.1007/978-3-030-98950-7_1

in and around the tumor. The ingrowth of this vasculature is driven by both soluble and matrix-bound growth factors and enzymes secreted by tumor cells and the stromal cells that comprise the microenvironment [6]. Strong evidence exists indicating that stromal cells play as central a role in matrix remodeling, invasion, and metastasis as the tumor cells themselves [7–9]. Critical to this process is the observation that carcinoma cells are able to reprogram and coopt the surrounding stromal cells to enhance tumor growth [10]. Specifically, tumor-stromal paracrine signaling pathways have been demonstrated to play a major role in the tumorigenesis and subsequent outgrowth of tumors in multiple sites [11–13]. For example, stromal fibroblasts from prostate tumors are able to stimulate tumor formation of immortal but non-transformed prostate epithelial cells when the mixture is injected orthotopically into nude mice [10].

As stated above, tumor angiogenesis is intricately linked to signaling between the tumor and microenvironment. In normal tissue architecture, the epithelial compartment is not vascularized as it is generally only 1–2 cell layers in thickness. The minimal thickness allows oxygen to diffuse readily across the basement membrane and nourish both epithelial cell layers. However, when tumors form and the lumen of epithelial ducts fills with tumor cells, the cells in the center become hypoxic due to their increased distance from existing blood vessels. Thus, in order for tumors to gain access to the vasculature, the basement membrane must be degraded allowing the blood vessels to grow into the epithelial compartment (Fig. 1.1). Degradation of the basement membrane

and ingrowth of blood vessels requires tumor cells to secrete pro-angiogenic growth factors, turn off production of anti-angiogenic factors. Further dissemination and metastasis require a recapitulation of that process in the distant metastatic microenvironment. Though a myriad of pro- and anti-angiogenic factors have been discovered and studied, the initial attempts to delineate their regulation were examined in a cell autonomous fashion, with most of the attention paid to vascular endothelial growth factor (VEGF) [14–18] and Thrombospondin-1 (Tsp-1) [19, 20], two of the major positive and negative regulators of angiogenesis. However, as the importance of the tumor microenvironment became more apparent the study of the regulation of angiogenic factors in stromal cells also increased.

Not only is the regulation of angiogenesis in the tumor microenvironment critical to primary tumor growth, but also for metastatic dissemination and growth in distant organs. It is well established that tumors arising in different sites preferentially metastasize to specific organs [21]. For example, prostate cancer metastasizes preferentially to bone and liver, while breast cancer metastasizes to brain, bone, and lung [22]. The ability of a tumor cell to survive and proliferate in a metastatic environment ultimately relies on its ability to augment the angiogenic output of its microenvironment. The tumor microenvironment can grossly be categorized into two types of cells: (1). Resident cells that are present in the tissue prior to tumor development and (2) Infiltrating cells that are recruited to the tumor from the circulation or bone marrow. The first group is mainly comprised of fibroblasts and endo-

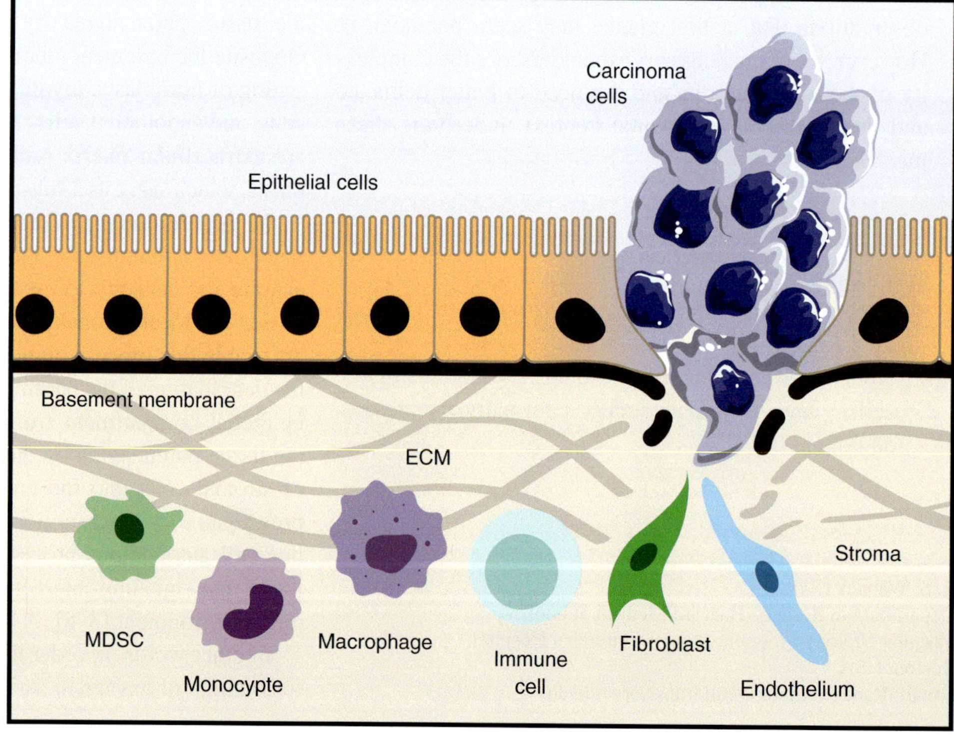

Fig. 1.1 Schematic diagram of tissue architecture with regard to the special distribution of normal epithelial and epithelial-derived carcinoma cells, extracellular components, as well as resident and infiltrating stromal cells

thelial cells. While the second is comprised of immune/inflammatory cells, which include B and T cells, neutrophils, mast cells, dendritic cells, and macrophages. In this chapter, we will explore the roles of these different cell types, as well as the growth factors and extracellular matrix proteins that contribute to tumor progression.

Cell Signaling Mechanisms and Factors Influencing Stromal Angiogenesis

To understand how resident and infiltrating cells contribute to tumor angiogenesis it is necessary to delineate and describe the major angiogenic factors that stimulate and inhibit vessel ingrowth. Distilled to the most basic principles, tumor cells secrete growth factors, cytokines, and enzymes that act on non-cancerous cells in the TME to induce the production of factors that stimulate blood vessel growth, i.e., angiogenesis (Fig. 1.2).

Basic Fibroblast Growth Factor (bFGF)

Basic fibroblast growth factor (bFGF, FGF2) was the first tumor-secreted pro-angiogenic factor to be isolated and purified [23]. It is one of the most potent pro-angiogenic growth factors [23–25]. One interesting oddity about bFGF is despite the presence of high affinity cell surface receptors [26] and the myriad of observations that bFGF stimulates endothelial cell proliferation and angiogenesis in vivo and in vitro, the protein lacks a signal sequence to direct its secretion [27, 28]. The paracrine regulation of bFGF in stromal cells and subsequent effect on tumor angiogenesis has been confounded by its ability to potently stimulate tumor cell proliferation through FGFR signaling via both autocrine and paracrine signaling [29–31]. Nevertheless, bFGF expression in the stroma of lung adenocarcinoma patients inversely correlates with disease progression and overall survival [32]. Additionally, bFGF production is stimulated by stem cell factor (SCF) and TGF-β in inflammatory cells, including macrophages, mast cells, and neutrophils [33]. The role of these cells in tumor angiogenesis will be detailed later in this chapter.

VEGF

Vascular endothelial growth factor (VEGF) is another tumor-secreted pro-angiogenic factor that was initially identified by its ability to induce vessel permeability, as such, it was first called vascular permeability factor or VPF [34, 35]. The regulation of VEGF in tumor cells has been exhaustively

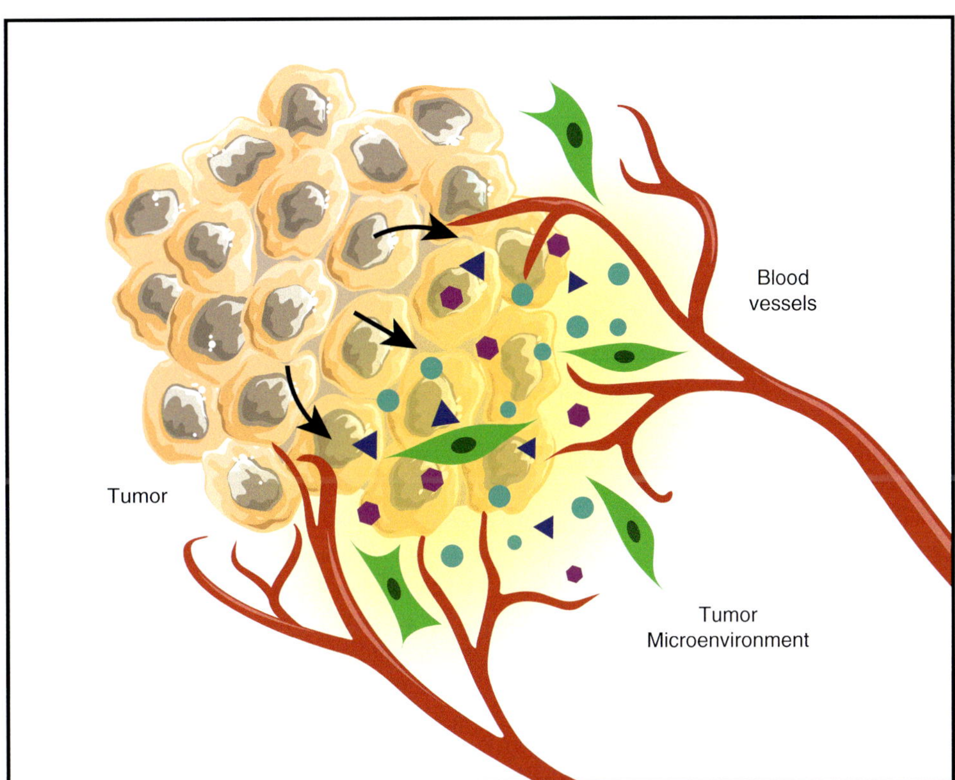

Fig. 1.2 Schematic diagram of the interaction between tumor cells and their microenvironment as mediated by tumor-secreted factors paracrine acting factors that modulate angiogenesis

studied. Signal transduction pathways leading from receptor tyrosine kinases or oncogenic Ras and PI3 kinase via the MAPK or Akt pathway lead to increased transcription of VEGF and its subsequent secretion into the extracellular matrix [16]. However, carcinoma cells also secrete proteins into the extracellular space, which do not act directly on endothelial cells but rather modulate VEGF production and secretion by stromal cells in the microenvironment, such as TGF-β, PDGF, and bFGF [36, 37].

Stromal VEGF expression was first demonstrated to be regulated by carcinoma cells in a transgenic mouse model in which GFP, driven by the VEGF promoter, was inserted into the mouse genome [38]. In this model, activation of the VEGF promoter results in the expression of GFP. Examination of tumor xenografts in these VEGF-GFP mice revealed, via fluorescence microscopy, that the stromal fibroblasts that had infiltrated the tumor fluoresced green, indicating that the VEGF promoter had been activated. Strikingly, in normal tissues there were no fluorescent cells, indicating the VEGF expression is not required for normal tissue homeostasis. These results indicated that tumors secrete factors that act on cells in the microenvironment to stimulate VEGF expression.

However, while it was clear from these experiments that VEGF expression was being stimulated, it was not evident whether this stimulation was required for tumor growth, supportive of tumor growth or merely a physiological reaction to local tumor growth. The evidence that stromally produced VEGF was critical for tumor growth was obtained from studies designed to test the efficacy of a human-specific anti-VEGF antibody, bevacizumab (Avastin). In these experiments, human tumor cells were injected into immunocompromised mice, which were subsequently treated with the human-specific VEGF antibody [39]. While the antibody was able to dramatically inhibit tumor growth the tumors still grew. The authors of the study hypothesized that the continued growth of the treated tumors was due to a residual angiogenic stimulus driven by VEGF produced and secreted from the murine tumor microenvironment, which could not be inhibited by the human-specific antibody. To test their hypothesis, human tumor xenografts were treated with human-specific VEGF antibodies as well as a soluble version of murine VEGFR1 (mFlt) fused to IgG, which acts as a decoy receptor for VEGF [40]. The combination of these two treatment modalities resulted in the complete blockage of tumor growth, demonstrating the importance of the contribution of stromal-produced VEGF.

PDGF

Another growth factor that possesses both pro- and anti-angiogenic characteristics is PDGF. In 1991, Goldsmith et al. demonstrated that PDGF was able to potently stimulate

bFGF in lung fibroblasts [41]. Additionally, in response to the results achieved with the human-specific VEGF antibody described above, it was demonstrated that stromal VEGF expression was stimulated by tumor-derived PDGF [42]. Within that context, inhibition of PDGF activity via a soluble version of PDGFR was able to block the stimulation of VEGF in the microenvironment and inhibit angiogenesis. Moreover, another member of the PDGF family, PDGF B is also able to upregulate VEGF expression in vascular smooth muscle cells [36]. These data indicated that tumor-derived PDGF is a potent inducer of VEGF expression in the microenvironment.

The most logical conclusion to be drawn from the above study is that PDGF promotes angiogenesis via the induction of stromal VEGF. However, somewhat analogous to TGF-β, the activities of PDGF is not as straightforward as these results would indicate. In addition to stimulating VEGF and bFGF, PDGF also stimulates Tsp-1 expression [43]. PDGF stimulation of Tsp-1 in fibroblasts is mediated by the Raf-MAPK pathway in a manner analogous to the stimulation of Tsp-1 by serum [44]. Intriguingly, the PDGF-mediated stimulation of VEGF is also mediated by the Raf-MAPK pathway [45]. Thus, whether PDGF acts as an anti-angiogenic factor or a pro-angiogenic factor is most likely dependent on complimentary or inhibitory orthogonal signals that act to inhibit or stimulate VEGF or Tsp-1.

TGF-β

One growth factor with perhaps the most paradoxical role in tumor growth and angiogenesis is TGF-β. TGF-β has been documented to have potent pro-angiogenic activity in vivo [46]. However, in vitro the effects of TGF-β on endothelial cells are in diametric opposition as in this context it is actually growth-inhibitory [47, 48]. These seemingly incongruous activities were resolved by the discovery that TGF-β stimulates the expression of VEGF in stromal fibroblasts, indicating that the pro-angiogenic effects of TGF-β were mediated by the induction of VEGF in the tumor microenvironment [36, 49]. Moreover, TFG-β potently stimulates the expression of bFGF in fibroblasts [41]. These results suggest that low levels of tumor-secreted TGF-β induce tumor-associated fibroblasts to express VEGF and bFGF thereby stimulating angiogenesis. Conversely, higher levels of TGF-β may act directly on endothelial cells inhibiting their proliferation thus having an anti-angiogenic effect.

Adding to the paradox of TGF-β's role in tumor angiogenesis is its ability to stimulate the expression of the anti-angiogenic protein Tsp-1 (which will be discussed in detail later in this chapter). In a classic example of a feed-forward loop, Tsp-1 then activates TGF-β from its latent form [50–54]. TGF-β is activated by two discrete processes: via proteases that cleave the latent associate peptide; and via undergoing a conformational change, that exposes the receptor-binding region. Tsp-1 activates TGF-β via the latter mechanism. Moreover, TGF-β expression in fibroblasts is induced by hypoxia, which is most often a result of a lack of tumor vascularization [55].

Matrix Metalloproteases

The ability of tumors to invade locally, across the basement membrane, is critical for tumor growth and ultimately metastasis. One of the most crucial steps in tumor invasion and migration is the remodeling of the extracellular matrix (ECM) by proteases. Some of the major players in this field are the matrix metalloproteases, or MMPs. For example, an experiment in which MCF7 breast cancer cells and fibroblasts were co-injected into mice resulted in the significant acceleration of tumor growth [56]. Moreover, in a parallel experiment in which fibroblasts were engineered to ectopically express an inhibitor of MMP activity, TIMP-2 (tissue inhibitor of metalloprotease 2), the tumor stimulating activity of the co-injected fibroblasts was abrogated [57]. Analogously, administration of a broad spectrum MMP inhibitor, batimastat, also abrogated the ability of fibroblasts to stimulate tumor formation by MCF7 cells [57].

The matrix remodeling mediated by MMPs not only facilitates tumor cell migration into the surrounding microenvironment but also stimulates the migration of endothelial cells into the tumor by facilitating the formation of the leading edge of new blood vessels. MMPs also liberate growth factors such as VEGF and bFGF that would otherwise be sequestered in the ECM. The ability of MMPs to stimulate angiogenesis was established in an elegant genetic experiment in which tumor prone RIP-TAG2 mice were crossed with various matrix protease knockout mice [58]. By crossing the RIP-TAG mice with MMP2 knockout mice the authors demonstrated that tumor growth was impaired but not due to any defect in angiogenesis [58]. Conversely, MMP9⁻/⁻ RIP-TAG mice displayed delayed tumor growth kinetics and defective angiogenesis [58]. The conclusion drawn from these observations was that in addition to cleaving matrix proteins, MMP9 also cleaves the latent associated peptide from TGF-β, converting it to the active form, and thereby stimulating tumor growth in a mammary tumor model [59].

Hormones and Nuclear Receptors

The studies described above indicate that two of the most potent inducers of stromal VEGF and, consequently, angiogenesis also possess the seemingly counterproductive ability to stimulate Tsp-1. These divergent events downstream from TGF-β and PDGF ligation to their cognate receptors suggest that tumor-derived TGF-β and PDGF expression should have no net effect on angiogenesis. That being said, it has also been demonstrated that inhibition of PDGF activity inhibits tumor angiogenesis [42]. Also, as described above, despite its ability to stimulate Tsp-1, TGF-β is a potent stimulator of angiogenesis. One potential explanation for the observed pro-angiogenic activities of these two proteins is that the expression of Tsp-1 in the microenvironment is suppressed by an independent signaling mechanism. This suppression of Tsp-1 would result in the stimulation of only the pro-angiogenic factors VEGF and bFGF by these two growth factors and thus resolve the seemingly paradoxical observations.

Two candidates for such a Tsp-1 repressing factor are the hormones estrogen and androgen, which have both been demonstrated to repress Tsp-1 expression [60, 61]. While these hormones both repress Tsp-1 expression the mechanisms utilized are different between them. Estrogen-mediated inhibition of Tsp-1 is achieved via activation of ERK1/2 and JNK [60]. Additionally, Tsp-1 repression by estrogen is mediated via inhibition of both transcription and protein secretion. Conversely, androgen-mediated repression of Tsp-1 is solely mediated by inhibition of transcription, via an androgen responsive element (ARE) in the Tsp-1 promoter [61].

While hormone-mediated effects on tumor growth have been largely studied through their actions on hormone-responsive tumor cells, it has also been demonstrated that estrogen can regulate angiogenesis on a systemic level [62]. This elegant study revealed that estrogen receptor (ER) positive stromal cells stimulate angiogenesis and promote tumor growth in response to estrogen even when the tumor cells were ER-negative.

It has also been demonstrated that another nuclear receptor family, the peroxisome proliferator-activator receptors (PPAR), can regulate both VEGF and Tsp-1 expression. Specifically, it has been demonstrated that when normal tumor are cells injected into PPARα⁻/⁻ mice they remain dormant for a prolonged period of time [63]. Moreover, the dormancy of these tumors was found to be the result of increased Tsp-1 expression in the host stroma. Surprisingly, it was later determined that fenofibrate and WY14643, two agonists of PPARα, also stimulated the expression of Tsp-1 [64]. These seemingly discordant results suggest that in the absence of PPARα, another member or the PPAR family, perhaps, may compensate and stimulate the expression of Tsp-1. Of note, PPARγ also stimulates the expression of CD36 [65], a receptor for Tsp-1. In keeping with these observations, it was demonstrated that the PPARγ agonists rosiglitazone and pioglitazone inhibit bFGF- and VEGF-mediated angiogenesis [66].

Thrombospondin-1

While much of the attention in the field of angiogenesis has been given to the identification and characterization of pro-angiogenic factors, the studies detailing the role of one of the most potent anti-angiogenic proteins, Tsp-1, should not be overlooked. Thrombospondin-1 (Tsp-1) is an endogenous anti-angiogenic protein that functions via a multimodal approach. Tsp-1 binds to cell surface receptors CD36 and CD47 on the endothelial cell surface and renders the cells insensitive to both VEGF and bFGF. Tsp-1 also induces caspase-dependent apoptosis mediated by Src-family kinase Fyn signaling downstream from CD36 [67–70]. Tsp-1 also binds to MMP-9 and functionally inactivates it [71, 72]. In tumor cells, Tsp-1 expression is repressed via a signal transduction cascade emanating from PI3-kinase via Rho GTPase to ROCK to Myc, which represses Tsp-1 in a phosphorylation-dependent manner [73]. The Rho-Rock pathway has been shown to be active in several human breast cancer cell lines in which Tsp-1 expression was virtually silenced [73]. Accordingly, this pathway represents the first biochemical elucidation of a cell autonomous "angiogenic switch."

While the expression of VEGF in the tumor-associated stroma is widely accepted to have a positive correlation with tumor progression [38, 74, 75], the role of Thrombospondin-1 (Tsp-1) expression in the tumor-associated stroma is unclear. Tsp-1 expression by epithelial tumor cells is observed infrequently and ectopic expression of Tsp-1 is inhibitory to tumor growth [19, 73, 76]. Stromal Tsp-1, meanwhile, has been correlated with a desmoplastic response and increased invasiveness in a subset of breast cancers [74, 77, 78], while it has been demonstrated to be inhibitory to early stage breast cancers [79]. Expression of Tsp-1 by stromal fibroblasts has been shown to be inhibitory to tumor formation and growth [80]. Intriguingly, the same report demonstrated that tumors that arose in an environment high in Tsp-1 eventually overcame the inhibitory effects of this protein by increasing their production of VEGF. Thus, the complex interrelationship between these two proteins and their relative expression levels in the tumor-associated stroma plays a critical role in the induction and maintenance of angiogenesis in human tumors.

The work described above demonstrated that VEGF expression in the stroma is a critical component in tumor-mediated angiogenesis. Conversely, Tsp-1 expression in the tumor-associated stroma can be a potent inhibitor of tumor angiogenesis and growth. The question that arises then is how do tumors stimulate the expression of VEGF in the stroma while concomitantly repressing the expression of Tsp-1?

Nonprotein Mediators of Angiogenesis

One largely understudied signaling mechanism in the regulation of tumor angiogenesis is lipid and phospholipid signaling. Significantly, two landmark studies demonstrated that these molecules could regulate the expression of Tsp-1. These independent studies showed that the generation of phospholipids and the resultant signaling pathways potently repress Tsp-1 expression in stromal fibroblasts. The first study demonstrated that platelet-mediated generation of phospholipids, specifically sphingosine 1 phosphate (S1P), downregulated Tsp-1 expression in dermal fibroblasts by activating the G_i-protein coupled S1P receptors [81].

The second study also implicated S1P as a repressor of Tsp-1 by demonstrating that secretion of a low molecular weight molecule (<3kD) was upregulated in Ras-transformed cells, and that it repressed Tsp-1 in dermal fibroblasts in an S1P-dependent manner [82]. These two reports indicate that tumor cells augment the angiogenic output of their microenvironment by secreting lipid signaling molecules that repress Tsp-1 in the surrounding stromal cells.

Carcinoma-associated Fibroblasts

Tumor progression is intricately regulated by the interactions between tumor cells and fibroblasts present in the tumor microenvironment [83]. Fibroblasts in the tumor microenvironment are referred to as carcinoma-associated fibroblasts (CAFs) [84]. Based on the epigenetic and transcriptomic analysis, CAFs are very similar, virtually identical, to activated fibroblasts found in the stroma of damaged or wounded tissue [85–88]. Specifically, both express smooth muscle actin, EGF [89, 90], HGF [91–95], IGF-I and -2 [96–98] as well as matrix metalloproteases (MMPs) [57, 99–108].

Strikingly, underscoring the importance of their contribution to tumor progression, some carcinomas are comprised of up to 90% fibroblasts [109]. While the paracrine signaling mechanisms that convert normal fibroblasts to CAFs have not been completely delineated, in vitro studies have demonstrated that TGF-β can induce CAF-like properties in normal fibroblasts [110]. Moreover, human carcinoma cells have been shown to be able to convert normal fibroblasts into CAFs in a mouse xenograft model [111]. The CAF phenotype is also very stable as they can be cultured in the absence of carcinoma cells in culture until they undergo senescence [112]

When carcinomas progress to the invasive state the basement membrane is degraded and stromal cells, including CAFs, inflammatory cells, and newly formed capillaries, come into contact with the tumor cells [1]. CAFs in the stroma of invasive carcinomas continue depositing large amounts of ECM, including tenascin C in some cases [113, 114]. It has been demonstrated that the expression of tenascin C in breast and bladder carcinomas correlates with increased tumor invasiveness [115, 116]. The accumulation of ECM in tumors contributes to increased interstitial fluid pressure that hinders oxygen and nutrient diffusion [117, 118]. Thus, CAF-mediated hypoxia could lead to the expression of HIF-1α and the induction of VEGF thereby providing a mechanism by which CAFs can promote angiogenesis in tumors.

An elegant study utilizing both in vivo and in vitro models demonstrated that injecting human breast cancer cells mixed with CAFs into the mouse mammary gland resulted in tumors that grew faster and were more angiogenic than mixtures of tumor cells with normal fibroblasts [112]. The increased tumor growth was mediated by the production and secretion of stromal cell-derived factor 1 (SDF1) by CAFs which, in turn, bound to and activated its cognate receptor, CXCR4, on the surface of tumor cells. Moreover, the study found that CAF-secreted SDF1 stimulated angiogenesis by recruiting endothelial progenitor cells (EPCs) to the tumor.

Another study demonstrating the tumor-promoting activity of CAFs utilized a genetically engineered mouse model in which the Mts1 gene, which stimulates tumor metastasis, was knocked out. When otherwise metastatic breast cancer cells were injected into these mice they were unable to form metastases [119]. However, when tumor cells were mixed with Mts1-expressing fibroblasts and injected into *mts1* knockout mice, the metastatic potential of these tumors was partially restored.

Bone Marrow-derived Cells

In addition to fibroblasts, the tumor microenvironment is made up of several other nonresidents that migrate to tumor tissue. Most prominent among these cells are bone marrow-derived cells: mesenchymal stem cells, macrophages, neutrophils, mast cells, and T cells. These cells migrate to tumors in response to the growing tumor mas and by the secretion of discrete growth factors and chemokines produced by the tumor cells, which create a wound-like environment.

Macrophages

By far, the most prevalent nonresident cell present in tumors are tumor associate macrophages (TAMs) [120]. Activated macrophages, those recruited to sites of inflammation, are generally categorized into two types: M1 and M2 [121–123]. M1 macrophages are effector cells that are able to potently kill microorganisms as well as tumor cells [121]. They also secrete high levels of proinflammatory cytokines [121]. M2 macrophages scavenge debris and stimulate angiogenesis as well as tissue remodeling and repair [121, 124–127]. TAMs are most similar to M2 macrophages.

TAMs have been shown to stimulate the growth and progression of carcinomas in cancer patients and experimental tumor models [128]. TAMs are also preferentially recruited to sites of hypoxia, which, in non-tumorigenic contexts is symptomatic of damaged or inflamed tissue [128]. Hypoxia stimulates the activity of the transcription factor HIF-1, which activates the expression of the pro-angiogenic growth factors VEGF, bFGF, TNFα, and CXCL8 [128].

While TAMs normally stimulate tumor growth, they can also inhibit tumor growth. For example, CSF has been shown to stimulate the production and secretion of metalloelastase by macrophages [129, 130]. Metalloelastase is an extracellular protease that cleaves plasminogen into multiple fragments, one of which is the anti-angiogenic protein angiostatin [131]. Thus, the effects of macrophage recruitment on tumor growth are highly context-dependent.

Neutrophils

While TAMS are the most prevalent and common leukocyte present in the tumor microenvironment, neutrophils are the most abundant leukocyte in the circulation in cancer patients [132]. Neutrophil recruitment from the bone marrow is mediated, in part, by the chemokine CXCL12 (SDF-1) as its cognate receptor, CXCR4, is expressed at high levels on the cell surface of neutrophils [133]. There are two types of neutrophils present in the circulation: circulating neutrophils, which, as their name suggests, are freely circulating and are recruited to tumors [134, 135]; and marginated neutrophils, which are bound to the endothelium of capillaries [132]. The marginated pool can be mobilized into the circulating pool by cytokines such as IL-6 [136, 137].

Elevated levels of neutrophils are associated with multiple human tumors, including colon, lung, melanoma, myxoid fibrosarcoma, and gastric carcinoma [138–141]. In addition to CXCL12, one of the most potent chemoattractants of neutrophils is CXCL8, which is expressed by both tumor and stromal cells in many types of tumors [138, 142]. Once recruited to tumors, neutrophils stimulate angiogenesis by secreting VEGF and matrix metalloproteases, which release angiogenic growth factors from sequestration in the extracellular matrix [143, 144].

In a genetic murine model of squamous cell skin carcinoma, it was observed that the source of MMP9 was not the tumors themselves but rather neutrophils. Specifically, MMP9 produced and secreted by neutrophils was required for the angiogenic switch [145]. These results have since been recapitulated using anti-GR1 antibody-mediated neutrophil ablation in the RIP-TAG2 islet cell tumor model as well as a human ovarian cancer xenograft model in MMP9 deficient mice [146, 147].

Analogous to observations related to macrophages and mast cells, neutrophils also possess anti-tumor activity. For example, in 1975 it was observed that neutrophils could kill tumor cells [148]. The original conclusion was that the killing was mediated exclusively by myeloperoxidase. However, it was later shown that neutrophils kill tumor cells via multiple mechanisms: secreting proteases, membrane perforating agents, reactive oxygen species, and cytokines such as TNFα and IL-1β [149]. Additionally, neutrophils can inhibit angiogenesis via two distinct mechanisms, mediated by the same protease—neutrophil elastase. The first mechanism is characterized by neutrophil elastase degradation of VEGF and bFGF [150]. Secondly, neutrophil elastase also cleaves plasminogen into angiostatin, which inhibits VEGF- and bFGF-mediated angiogenesis [151]. These findings underscore the complexity of the role of the tumor microenvironment in tumor angiogenesis and progression, and serve as an example that analysis of any cell type of biomarker requires a more complete understanding of the contextual signals within the tumor microenvironment.

Mast Cells

Mast cells are multifunctional secretory cells, characterized by numerous large electron-dense granules comprised of proteoglycans, predominantly heparin [152]. Mast cells are the progeny of pluripotent bone marrow progenitor cells, which are characterized as positive for CD34, c-kit, and CD13 [153]. In the circulation mast cells are progenitor-like cells that differentiate/mature after being recruited to sites of inflammation or infection. Mast cells express and secrete a myriad of proteases, most notably chymases, tryptases, and matrix metalloproteases, which are stored in secretory granules [152]. These proteases, specifically MMP2 and 9, are crucial for mast cell-mediated tissue repair and remodeling [154]. Additionally, mast cell secretory granules are depots for cytokines and growth factors, including VEGF, bFGF, TNF-α, GM-CSF, SCF, EGF, PDGF, and IFN-gamma, multiple interleukins, and chemokines, such as MIP-1-α and MCP-1[152].

The release of proteases, cytokines, and growth factors stored in the secretory granules of macrophages can be triggered by multiple cytokines, including IL-1, IL-3, and GM-CSF, Platelet factor 4, IL-8, SCF, (MCP)-1, and MIP-1-alpha [132]. Moreover, mast cells also produce and secrete matrix metalloproteases (MMPs) 2 and 9, which have been

shown to promote angiogenesis by liberating VEGF and bFGF from the extracellular matrix [145, 155]. Interestingly, mast cells are recruited to tumors by VEGF, bFGF, and TGF-β [156, 157]. Thus, conditions within a tumor that necessitate the growth of new blood vessels recruit mast cells, which, in turn, further stimulate angiogenesis.

Experimental evidence for the functional role of mast cells in angiogenesis and tumor growth was provided by an elegant murine genetic model in which Myc expression in β cells was driven via fusion to a mutant form of the estrogen receptor [158]. In this model, it was demonstrated that Myc activation by systemic administration of 4-hydroxy tamoxifen, induced β cell tumors characterized by blood vessel infiltration accompanied by mast cell recruitment. These findings indicated that mast cells are required for angiogenesis at the onset of tumorigenesis and for maintenance of angiogenesis during tumor growth and progression.

Mesenchymal stem cells

Mesenchymal stem cells (MSCs) are bone marrow-derived cells that have the ability to differentiate into a myriad of cells of mesenchymal lineage including fibroblasts, osteoblasts, chondrocytes, adipocytes, pericytes, and muscle cells. MSCs are an extremely rare cell type within the bone marrow, comprising between 0.01% and 0.001% of the mononuclear cells [159, 160]. Human MSCs are defined by the expression of CD44 adhesion molecule (HCAM), CD73, CD90, CD105 (endoglin), CD106 (VCAM-1), and STRO-1 [161].

MSCs have been shown to be recruited to sites of wounding or inflammation, as well as to tumors [162]. MSCs are recruited to tumors by multiple different growth factors and cytokines, including VEGF, bFGF, IL-8, EGF, HGF, and PDGF as well as CCL2, CCL7, and CXCL12 (SDF-1) [163–167]. Following recruitment to the tumor MSCs have been shown to secrete VEGF to stimulate angiogenesis [168]. Moreover, in melanoma a correlation has been demonstrated between MSCs and angiogenesis [169].

In addition to correlation and expression studies, MSCs have been demonstrated to stimulate angiogenesis in in vitro models as well as in murine pancreatic xenografts [170]. In that study, tumors that formed subsequent to the injection of wild-type MSCs had twice as many blood vessels as control tumors. Conversely, tumors in mice injected with MSCs, in which VEGF had been silenced by lentiviral shRNA, had comparable numbers of blood vessels to control tumors [170]. Thus, the ability of MSCs to home to tumors and secrete VEGF stimulates tumor growth via enhanced angiogenesis.

Concluding Remarks/Summary

Angiogenesis is a complex process that is stimulated by a myriad of growth factors and cytokines and inhibited by an equally diverse cohort of proteins. Accordingly, the regulation of angiogenesis by the tumor-microenvironment is an extremely complex phenomenon. Underscoring this complexity is the fact that signaling molecules secreted by tumors that act on stromal cells can often have different, and even opposite, activities with respect to the production of pro- and anti-angiogenic factors. Therefore, the composition of the tumor microenvironment, as well as the stage of the tumor, have profound effects on whether the tumor microenvironment is pro-angiogenic or anti-angiogenic. The complex signaling mechanisms described in this chapter constitute multiple potential, and largely untapped, targets for therapeutic intervention to inhibit tumor growth in patients. Ultimately, the strategy of targeting molecules that mediate processes, such as angiogenesis, via tumor-stromal interactions may prove to be hugely successful as the genomic instability and high mutational burden in tumor cells is t exceedingly rare in the non-tumorous cells that make up the TME. The hope, then is that anti-angiogenic therapy targeting the tumor microenvironment will result in lower rates and incidences of acquired resistance than traditional therapeutic strategies.

References

1. Hanahan D, Weinberg RA. The hallmarks of cancer. Cell. 2000;100(1):57–70.
2. Ronnov-Jessen L, Petersen OW, Bissell MJ. Cellular changes involved in conversion of normal to malignant breast: importance of the stromal reaction. Physiol Rev. 1996;76(1):69–125.
3. Chung LW, Davies R. Prostate epithelial differentiation is dictated by its surrounding stroma. Mol Biol Rep. 1996;23(1):13–9.
4. Tuxhorn JA, Ayala GE, Rowley DR. Reactive stroma in prostate cancer progression. J Urol. 2001;166(6):2472–83.
5. Henshall SM, et al. Altered expression of androgen receptor in the malignant epithelium and adjacent stroma is associated with early relapse in prostate cancer. Cancer Research. 2001;61(2):423–7.
6. Hanahan D, Folkman J. Patterns and emerging mechanisms of the angiogenic switch during tumorigenesis. Cell. 1996;86(3):353–64.
7. Camps JL, et al. Fibroblast-mediated acceleration of human epithelial tumor growth in vivo. Proc Natl Acad Sci U S A. 1990;87(1):75–9.
8. Grey AM, et al. Purification of the migration stimulating factor produced by fetal and breast cancer patient fibroblasts. Proc Natl Acad Sci U S A. 1989;86(7):2438–42.
9. Picard O, Rolland Y, Poupon MF. Fibroblast-dependent tumorigenicity of cells in nude mice: implication for implantation of metastases. Cancer Res. 1986;46(7):3290–4.
10. Olumi AF, et al. Carcinoma-associated fibroblasts direct tumor progression of initiated human prostatic epithelium. Cancer Res. 1999;59(19):5002–11.
11. Hom YK, et al. Uterine and vaginal organ growth requires epidermal growth factor receptor signaling from stroma. Endocrinology. 1998;139(3):913–21.
12. Donjacour AA, Cunha GR. Stromal regulation of epithelial function. Cancer Treat Res. 1991;53:335–64.
13. Cunha GR, et al. Stromal-epithelial interactions in adult organs. Cell Differ. 1985;17(3):137–48.
14. Akiyama H, et al. Induction of VEGF gene expression by retinoic acid through Sp1-binding sites in retinoblastoma Y79 cells. Investig Ophthalmol Vis Sci. 2002;43(5):1367–74.
15. Damert A, Ikeda E, Risau W. Activator-protein-1 binding potentiates the hypoxia-inducible factor-1-mediated hypoxia-induced transcriptional activation of vascular-endothelial growth factor expression in C6 glioma cells. Biochem J. 1997;327(Pt 2):419–23.
16. Rak J, et al. Mutant ras oncogenes upregulate VEGF/VPF expression: implications for induction and inhibition of tumor angiogenesis. Cancer Res. 1995;55(20):4575–80.
17. Wojta J, et al. Hepatocyte growth factor increases expression of vascular endothelial growth factor and plasminogen activator inhibitor-1 in human keratinocytes and the vascular endothelial growth factor receptor flk-1 in human endothelial cells. Lab Investig. 1999;79(4):427–38.
18. Xiong S, et al. Up-regulation of vascular endothelial growth factor in breast cancer cells by the heregulin-beta 1-activated p38 signaling pathway enhances endothelial cell migration. Cancer Res. 2001;61(4):1727–32.
19. Watnick R, et al. Ras modulates Myc activity to repress thrombospondin-1 expression and increase tumor angiogenesis. Cancer Cell. 2003;3(3):219–31.
20. Rak J, et al. Oncogenes and tumor angiogenesis: differential modes of vascular endothelial growth factor up-regulation in ras-transformed epithelial cells and fibroblasts. Cancer Res. 2000;60(2):490–8.
21. Chambers AF, Groom AC, MacDonald IC. Dissemination and growth of cancer cells in metastatic sites. Nat Rev Cancer. 2002;2(8):563–72.
22. Pettaway CA, et al. Selection of highly metastatic variants of different human prostatic carcinomas using orthotopic implantation in nude mice. Clin Cancer Res: An Official Journal of the American Association For Cancer Research. 1996;2(9):1627–36.
23. Shing Y, et al. Heparin affinity: purification of a tumor-derived capillary endothelial cell growth factor. Science. 1984;223(4642):1296–9.
24. Folkman J, Klagsbrun M. Angiogenic factors. Science. 1987;235(4787):442–7.
25. Klagsbrun M, et al. Human tumor cells synthesize an endothelial cell growth factor that is structurally related to basic fibroblast growth factor. Proc Natl Acad Sci U S A. 1986;83(8):2448–52.
26. Dionne CA, et al. Cloning and expression of two distinct high-affinity receptors cross-reacting with acidic and basic fibroblast growth factors. EMBO J. 1990;9(9):2685–92.
27. Abraham JA, et al. Human basic fibroblast growth factor: nucleotide sequence and genomic organization. EMBO J. 1986;5(10):2523–8.
28. Abraham JA, et al. Nucleotide sequence of a bovine clone encoding the angiogenic protein, basic fibroblast growth factor. Science. 1986;233(4763):545–8.
29. Rogelj S, et al. Characterization of tumors produced by signal peptide-basic fibroblast growth factor-transformed cells. J Cell Biochem. 1989;39(1):13–23.
30. Rogelj S, et al. Basic fibroblast growth factor fused to a signal peptide transforms cells. Nature. 1988;331(6152):173–5.
31. Gleave M, et al. Acceleration of human prostate cancer growth in vivo by factors produced by prostate and bone fibroblasts. Cancer Res. 1991;51(14):3753–61.

32. Guddo F, et al. The expression of basic fibroblast growth factor (bFGF) in tumor-associated stromal cells and vessels is inversely correlated with non-small cell lung cancer progression. Hum Pathol. 1999;30(7):788–94.

33. Qu Z, et al. Synthesis of basic fibroblast growth factor by murine mast cells. Regulation by transforming growth factor beta, tumor necrosis factor alpha, and stem cell factor. Int Arch Allergy Immunol. 1998;115(1):47–54.

34. Leung DW, et al. Vascular endothelial growth factor is a secreted angiogenic mitogen. Science. 1989;246(4935):1306–9.

35. Senger DR, et al. Tumor cells secrete a vascular permeability factor that promotes accumulation of ascites fluid. Science. 1983;219(4587):983–5.

36. Brogi E, et al. Indirect angiogenic cytokines upregulate VEGF and bFGF gene expression in vascular smooth muscle cells, whereas hypoxia upregulates VEGF expression only. Circulation. 1994;90(2):649–52.

37. Tsai JC, Goldman CK, Gillespie GY. Vascular endothelial growth factor in human glioma cell lines: induced secretion by EGF, PDGF-BB, and bFGF. J Neurosurg. 1995;82(5):864–73.

38. Fukumura D, et al. Tumor induction of VEGF promoter activity in stromal cells. Cell. 1998;94(6):715–25.

39. Kim KJ, et al. Inhibition of vascular endothelial growth factor-induced angiogenesis suppresses tumour growth in vivo. Nature. 1993;362(6423):841–4.

40. Gerber HP, et al. Complete inhibition of rhabdomyosarcoma xenograft growth and neovascularization requires blockade of both tumor and host vascular endothelial growth factor. Cancer Res. 2000;60(22):6253–8.

41. Goldsmith KT, Gammon RB, Garver RI Jr. Modulation of bFGF in lung fibroblasts by TGF-beta and PDGF. Am J Physiol. 1991;261(6 Pt 1):L378–85.

42. Dong J, et al. VEGF-null cells require PDGFR alpha signaling-mediated stromal fibroblast recruitment for tumorigenesis. Embo J. 2004;23(14):2800–10.

43. Majack RA, Mildbrandt J, Dixit VM. Induction of thrombospondin messenger RNA levels occurs as an immediate primary response to platelet-derived growth factor. J Biol Chem. 1987;262(18):8821–5.

44. Majack RA, Cook SC, Bornstein P. Platelet-derived growth factor and heparin-like glycosaminoglycans regulate thrombospondin synthesis and deposition in the matrix by smooth muscle cells. J Cell Biol. 1985;101(3):1059–70.

45. Chang HJ, et al. Extracellular signal-regulated kinases and AP-1 mediate the up-regulation of vascular endothelial growth factor by PDGF in human vascular smooth muscle cells. Int J Oncol. 2006;28(1):135–41.

46. Roberts AB, et al. Transforming growth factor type beta: rapid induction of fibrosis and angiogenesis in vivo and stimulation of collagen formation in vitro. Proc Natl Acad Sci U S A. 1986;83(12):4167–71.

47. Baird A, Durkin T. Inhibition of endothelial cell proliferation by type beta-transforming growth factor: interactions with acidic and basic fibroblast growth factors. Biochem Biophys Res Commun. 1986;138(1):476–82.

48. Frater-Schroder M, et al. Transforming growth factor-beta inhibits endothelial cell proliferation. Biochem Biophys Res Commun. 1986;137(1):295–302.

49. Pertovaara L, et al. Vascular endothelial growth factor is induced in response to transforming growth factor-beta in fibroblastic and epithelial cells. J Biol Chem. 1994;269(9):6271–4.

50. Murphy-Ullrich JE, Schultz-Cherry S, Hook M. Transforming growth factor-beta complexes with thrombospondin. Mol Biol Cell. 1992;3(2):181–8.

51. Penttinen RP, Kobayashi S, Bornstein P. Transforming growth factor beta increases mRNA for matrix proteins both in the presence and in the absence of changes in mRNA stability. Proc Natl Acad Sci U S A. 1988;85(4):1105–8.

52. Schultz-Cherry S, Lawler J, Murphy-Ullrich JE. The type 1 repeats of thrombospondin 1 activate latent transforming growth factor-beta. J Biol Chem. 1994;269(43):26783–8.

53. Schultz-Cherry S, Murphy-Ullrich JE. Thrombospondin causes activation of latent transforming growth factor-beta secreted by endothelial cells by a novel mechanism. J Cell Biol. 1993;122(4):923–32.

54. Schultz-Cherry S, et al. Thrombospondin binds and activates the small and large forms of latent transforming growth factor-beta in a chemically defined system. J Biol Chem. 1994;269(43):26775–82.

55. Falanga V, et al. Hypoxia upregulates the synthesis of TGF-beta 1 by human dermal fibroblasts. J Invest Dermatol. 1991;97(4):634–7.

56. Noel A, et al. Enhancement of tumorigenicity of human breast adenocarcinoma cells in nude mice by matrigel and fibroblasts. Br J Cancer. 1993;68(5):909–15.

57. Noel A, et al. Inhibition of stromal matrix metalloproteases: effects on breast-tumor promotion by fibroblasts. Int J Cancer. 1998;76(2):267–73.

58. Bergers G, et al. Matrix metalloproteinase-9 triggers the angiogenic switch during carcinogenesis. Nat Cell Biol. 2000;2(10):737–44.

59. Yu Q, Stamenkovic I. Cell surface-localized matrix metalloproteinase-9 proteolytically activates TGF-beta and promotes tumor invasion and angiogenesis. Genes Dev. 2000;14(2):163–76.

60. Sengupta K, et al. Thrombospondin-1 disrupts estrogen-induced endothelial cell proliferation and migration and its expression is suppressed by estradiol. Mol Cancer Res. 2004;2(3):150–8.

61. Colombel M, et al. Androgens repress the expression of the angiogenesis inhibitor thrombospondin-1 in normal and neoplastic prostate. Cancer Res. 2005;65(1):300–8.

62. Gupta PB, et al. Systemic stromal effects of estrogen promote the growth of estrogen receptor-negative cancers. Cancer Res. 2007;67(5):2062–71.

63. Kaipainen A, et al. PPARalpha deficiency in inflammatory cells suppresses tumor growth. PLoS ONE. 2007;2(2):e260.

64. Panigrahy D, et al. PPARalpha agonist fenofibrate suppresses tumor growth through direct and indirect angiogenesis inhibition. Proc Natl Acad Sci U S A. 2008;105(3):985–90.

65. Han J, et al. Transforming growth factor-beta1 (TGF-beta1) and TGF-beta2 decrease expression of CD36, the type B scavenger receptor, through mitogen-activated protein kinase phosphorylation of peroxisome proliferator-activated receptor-gamma. J Biol Chem. 2000;275(2):1241–6.

66. Aljada A, et al. PPAR gamma ligands, rosiglitazone and pioglitazone, inhibit bFGF- and VEGF-mediated angiogenesis. Angiogenesis. 2008;11(4):361–7.

67. Dawson DW, et al. CD36 mediates the In vitro inhibitory effects of thrombospondin-1 on endothelial cells. J Cell Biol. 1997;138(3):707–17.

68. Saumet A, et al. Type 3 repeat/C-terminal domain of thrombospondin-1 triggers caspase-independent cell death through CD47/alphavbeta3 in promyelocytic leukemia NB4 cells. Blood. 2005;106(2):658–67.

69. Lamy L, et al. Interactions between CD47 and thrombospondin reduce inflammation. J Immunol. 2007;178(9):5930–9.

70. Henkin J, Volpert OV. Therapies using anti-angiogenic peptide mimetics of thrombospondin-1. Expert Opin Ther Targets. 2011;15(12):1369–86.

71. Bergers G, et al. Matrix metalloproteinase-9 triggers the angiogenic switch during carcinogenesis. Nature Cell Biol. 2000;2(10):737–44.

72. Rodriguez-Manzaneque JC, et al. Thrombospondin-1 suppresses spontaneous tumor growth and inhibits activation of matrix metalloproteinase-9 and mobilization of vascular endothelial growth factor. Proc Natl Acad Sci U S A. 2001;98(22):12485–90.

73. Watnick RS, et al. Thrombospondin-1 repression is mediated via distinct mechanisms in fibroblasts and epithelial cells. Oncogene. 2015;34(22):2823–35.

74. Brown LF, et al. Vascular stroma formation in carcinoma in situ, invasive carcinoma, and metastatic carcinoma of the breast. Clin Cancer Res. 1999;5(5):1041–56.

75. Mueller MM, Fusenig NE. Tumor-stroma interactions directing phenotype and progression of epithelial skin tumor cells. Differentiation. 2002;70(9–10):486–97. Research in Biological Diversity

76. Streit M, et al. Overexpression of thrombospondin-1 decreases angiogenesis and inhibits the growth of human cutaneous squamous cell carcinomas. Am J Pathol. 1999;155(2):441–52.

77. Wong SY, Purdie AT, Han P. Thrombospondin and other possible related matrix proteins in malignant and benign breast disease. An immunohistochemical study. Am J Pathol. 1992;140(6):1473–82.

78. Bertin N, et al. Thrombospondin-1 and -2 messenger RNA expression in normal, benign, and neoplastic human breast tissues: correlation with prognostic factors, tumor angiogenesis, and fibroblastic desmoplasia. Cancer Res. 1997;57(3):396–9.

79. Clezardin P, et al. Expression of thrombospondin (TSP1) and its receptors (CD36 and CD51) in normal, hyperplastic, and neoplastic human breast. Cancer Res. 1993;53(6):1421–30.

80. Filleur S, et al. In vivo mechanisms by which tumors producing thrombospondin 1 bypass its inhibitory effects. Genes Dev. 2001;15(11):1373–82.

81. Kalas W, Klement P, Rak J. Downregulation of the angiogenesis inhibitor thrombospondin 1 in fibroblasts exposed to platelets and their related phospholipids. Biochem Biophys Res Commun. 2005;334(2):549–54.

82. Kalas W, et al. Oncogenes and Angiogenesis: down-regulation of thrombospondin-1 in normal fibroblasts exposed to factors from cancer cells harboring mutant ras. Cancer Res. 2005;65(19):8878–86.

83. Elenbaas B, Weinberg RA. Heterotypic signaling between epithelial tumor cells and fibroblasts in carcinoma formation. Exp Cell Res. 2001;264(1):169–84.

84. Olumi AF, et al. Carcinoma-associated fibroblasts direct tumor progression of initiated human prostatic epithelium. Cancer Res. 1999;59(19):5002–11.

85. Durning P, Schor SL, Sellwood RA. Fibroblasts from patients with breast cancer show abnormal migratory behaviour in vitro. Lancet. 1984;2(8408):890–2.

86. Schor SL, et al. Foetal and cancer patient fibroblasts produce an autocrine migration-stimulating factor not made by normal adult cells. J Cell Sci. 1988;90(Pt 3):391–9.

87. Schor SL, Schor AM, Rushton G. Fibroblasts from cancer patients display a mixture of both foetal and adult-like phenotypic characteristics. J Cell Sci. 1988;90(Pt 3):401–7.

88. Tsukada T, et al. HHF35, a muscle actin-specific monoclonal antibody. II. Reactivity in normal, reactive, and neoplastic human tissues. Am J Pathol. 1987;127(2):389–402.

89. Normanno N, et al. Expression of messenger RNA for amphiregulin, heregulin, and cripto-1, three new members of the epidermal growth factor family, in human breast carcinomas. Breast Cancer Res Treat. 1995;35(3):293–7.

90. Panico L, et al. Differential immunohistochemical detection of transforming growth factor alpha, amphiregulin and CRIPTO in human normal and malignant breast tissues. Int J Cancer. 1996;65(1):51–6.

91. Jin L, et al. Expression of scatter factor and c-met receptor in benign and malignant breast tissue. Cancer. 1997;79(4):749–60.

92. Montesano R, Schaller G, Orci L. Induction of epithelial tubular morphogenesis in vitro by fibroblast-derived soluble factors. Cell. 1991;66(4):697–711.

93. Seslar SP, Nakamura T, Byers SW. Regulation of fibroblast hepatocyte growth factor/scatter factor expression by human breast carcinoma cell lines and peptide growth factors. Cancer Res. 1993;53(6):1233–8.

94. To CT, Tsao MS. The roles of hepatocyte growth factor/scatter factor and met receptor in human cancers (Review). Oncol Rep. 1998;5(5):1013–24.

95. Vande Woude GF, et al. Met-HGF/SF: tumorigenesis, invasion and metastasis. Ciba Found Symp. 1997;212:119–30. discussion 130-2, 148-54

96. Cullen KJ, et al. Insulin-like growth factor expression in breast cancer epithelium and stroma. Breast Cancer Res Treat. 1992;22(1):21–9.

97. Ellis MJ, et al. Insulin-like growth factor mediated stromal-epithelial interactions in human breast cancer. Breast Cancer Res Treat. 1994;31(2-3):249–61.

98. Yee D, et al. Analysis of insulin-like growth factor I gene expression in malignancy: evidence for a paracrine role in human breast cancer. Mol Endocrinol. 1989;3(3):509–17.

99. Basset P, et al. A novel metalloproteinase gene specifically expressed in stromal cells of breast carcinomas. Nature. 1990;348(6303):699–704.

100. Basset P, et al. Stromelysin-3 in stromal tissue as a control factor in breast cancer behavior. Cancer. 1994;74(3 Suppl):1045–9.

101. Chambers AF, Matrisian LM. Changing views of the role of matrix metalloproteinases in metastasis. J Natl Cancer Inst. 1997;89(17):1260–70.

102. Engel G, et al. Correlation between stromelysin-3 mRNA level and outcome of human breast cancer. Int J Cancer. 1994;58(6):830–5.

103. Heppner KJ, et al. Expression of most matrix metalloproteinase family members in breast cancer represents a tumor-induced host response. Am J Pathol. 1996;149(1):273–82.

104. Lochter A, et al. The significance of matrix metalloproteinases during early stages of tumor progression. Ann N Y Acad Sci. 1998;857:180–93.

105. Masson R, et al. In vivo evidence that the stromelysin-3 metalloproteinase contributes in a paracrine manner to epithelial cell malignancy. J Cell Biol. 1998;140(6):1535–41.

106. McCawley LJ, Matrisian LM. Matrix metalloproteinases: multifunctional contributors to tumor progression. Mol Med Today. 2000;6(4):149–56.

107. Newell KJ, et al. Expression and localization of matrix-degrading metalloproteinases during colorectal tumorigenesis. Mol Carcinog. 1994;10(4):199–206.

108. Wolf C, et al. Stromelysin 3 belongs to a subgroup of proteinases expressed in breast carcinoma fibroblastic cells and possibly implicated in tumor progression. Proc Natl Acad Sci U S A. 1993;90(5):1843–7.

109. Sappino AP, et al. Smooth-muscle differentiation in stromal cells of malignant and non-malignant breast tissues. Int J Cancer. 1988;41(5):707–12.

110. Ronnov-Jessen L, Petersen OW. Induction of alpha-smooth muscle actin by transforming growth factor-beta 1 in quiescent human breast gland fibroblasts. Implications for myofibroblast generation in breast neoplasia. Lab Invest. 1993;68(6):696–707.

111. Orimo A, Weinberg RA. Stromal fibroblasts in cancer: a novel tumor-promoting cell type. Cell Cycle. 2006;5(15):1597–601.

112. Orimo A, et al. Stromal fibroblasts present in invasive human breast carcinomas promote tumor growth and angiogenesis through elevated SDF-1/CXCL12 secretion. Cell. 2005;121(3):335–48.

113. Chiquet-Ehrismann R, et al. Tenascin: an extracellular matrix protein involved in tissue interactions during fetal development and oncogenesis. Cell. 1986;47(1):131–9.

114. Inaguma Y, et al. Epithelial induction of stromal tenascin in the mouse mammary gland: from embryogenesis to carcinogenesis. Dev Biol. 1988;128(2):245–55.

115. Brunner A, et al. Prognostic significance of tenascin-C expression in superficial and invasive bladder cancer. J Clin Pathol. 2004;57(9):927–31.

116. Mackie EJ, et al. Tenascin is a stromal marker for epithelial malignancy in the mammary gland. Proc Natl Acad Sci U S A. 1987;84(13):4621–5.

117. Brown EB, et al. Measurement of macromolecular diffusion coefficients in human tumors. Microvasc Res. 2004;67(3):231–6.

118. Netti PA, et al. Role of extracellular matrix assembly in interstitial transport in solid tumors. Cancer Res. 2000;60(9):2497–503.

119. Grum-Schwensen B, et al. Suppression of tumor development and metastasis formation in mice lacking the S100A4(mts1) gene. Cancer Res. 2005;65(9):3772–80.

120. Balkwill F, Mantovani A. Inflammation and cancer: back to Virchow? Lancet. 2001;357(9255):539–45.

121. Balkwill F, Charles KA, Mantovani A. Smoldering and polarized inflammation in the initiation and promotion of malignant disease. Cancer Cell. 2005;7(3):211–7.

122. Mantovani A, et al. The chemokine system in diverse forms of macrophage activation and polarization. Trends Immunol. 2004;25(12):677–86.

123. Sher A, Pearce E, Kaye P. Shaping the immune response to parasites: role of dendritic cells. Curr Opin Immunol. 2003;15(4):421–9.

124. Goerdt S, Orfanos CE. Other functions, other genes: alternative activation of antigen-presenting cells. Immunity. 1999;10(2):137–42.

125. Gordon S. Alternative activation of macrophages. Nat Rev Immunol. 2003;3(1):23–35.

126. Mantovani A, et al. Macrophage polarization: tumor-associated macrophages as a paradigm for polarized M2 mononuclear phagocytes. Trends Immunol. 2002;23(11):549–55.

127. Mosser DM. The many faces of macrophage activation. J Leukoc Biol. 2003;73(2):209–12.

128. Crowther M, et al. Microenvironmental influence on macrophage regulation of angiogenesis in wounds and malignant tumors. J Leukoc Biol. 2001;70(4):478–90.

129. Dong Z, et al. Angiostatin-mediated suppression of cancer metastases by primary neoplasms engineered to produce granulocyte/macrophage colony-stimulating factor. J Exp Med. 1998;188(4):755–63.

130. Dong Z, et al. Macrophage-derived metalloelastase is responsible for the generation of angiostatin in Lewis lung carcinoma. Cell. 1997;88(6):801–10.

131. O'Reilly MS, et al. Angiostatin: a novel angiogenesis inhibitor that mediates the suppression of metastases by a Lewis lung carcinoma. Cell. 1994;79(2):315–28.

132. Tazzyman S, Lewis CE, Murdoch C. Neutrophils: key mediators of tumour angiogenesis. Int J Exp Pathol. 2009;90(3):222–31.

133. Suratt BT, et al. Role of the CXCR4/SDF-1 chemokine axis in circulating neutrophil homeostasis. Blood. 2004;104(2):565–71.

134. Friedman AD. Transcriptional regulation of granulocyte and monocyte development. Oncogene. 2002;21(21):3377–90.

135. Kanwar VS, Cairo MS. Neonatal neutrophil maturation, kinetics, and function. In: Abramson JS, Wheeler JG, editors. The neutrophil. New York: Oxford University Press; 1993. p. 1–16.

136. Steele RW, et al. Functional capacity of marginated and bone marrow reserve granulocytes. Infect Immun. 1987;55(10):2359–63.

137. Suwa T, et al. Interleukin-6 induces demargination of intravascular neutrophils and shortens their transit in marrow. Am J Physiol Heart Circ Physiol. 2000;279(6):H2954–60.

138. Bellocq A, et al. Neutrophil alveolitis in bronchioloalveolar carcinoma: induction by tumor-derived interleukin-8 and relation to clinical outcome. Am J Pathol. 1998;152(1):83–92.

139. Mentzel T, et al. The association between tumour progression and vascularity in myxofibrosarcoma and myxoid/round cell liposarcoma. Virchows Arch. 2001;438(1):13–22.

140. Mhawech-Fauceglia P, et al. The source of APRIL up-regulation in human solid tumor lesions. J Leukoc Biol. 2006;80(4):697–704.

141. Nielsen BS, et al. 92 kDa type IV collagenase (MMP-9) is expressed in neutrophils and macrophages but not in malignant epithelial cells in human colon cancer. Int J Cancer. 1996;65(1):57–62.

142. Xie K. Interleukin-8 and human cancer biology. Cytokine Growth Factor Rev. 2001;12(4):375–91.

143. Coussens LM, Werb Z. Matrix metalloproteinases and the development of cancer. Chem Biol. 1996;3(11):895–904.

144. Gaudry M, et al. Intracellular pool of vascular endothelial growth factor in human neutrophils. Blood. 1997;90(10):4153–61.

145. Coussens LM, et al. MMP-9 supplied by bone marrow-derived cells contributes to skin carcinogenesis. Cell. 2000;103(3):481–90.

146. Huang S, et al. Contributions of stromal metalloproteinase-9 to angiogenesis and growth of human ovarian carcinoma in mice. J Natl Cancer Inst. 2002;94(15):1134–42.

147. Nozawa H, Chiu C, Hanahan D. Infiltrating neutrophils mediate the initial angiogenic switch in a mouse model of multistage carcinogenesis. Proc Natl Acad Sci U S A. 2006;103(33):12493–8.

148. Clark RA, Klebanoff SJ. Neutrophil-mediated tumor cell cytotoxicity: role of the peroxidase system. J Exp Med. 1975;141(6):1442–7.

149. Di Carlo E, et al. The intriguing role of polymorphonuclear neutrophils in antitumor reactions. Blood. 2001;97(2):339–45.

150. Ai S, et al. Angiogenic activity of bFGF and VEGF suppressed by proteolytic cleavage by neutrophil elastase. Biochem Biophys Res Commun. 2007;364(2):395–401.

151. Scapini P, et al. Generation of biologically active angiostatin kringle 1-3 by activated human neutrophils. J Immunol. 2002;168(11):5798–804.

152. Norrby K. Mast cells and angiogenesis. APMIS. 2002;110(5):355–71.

153. Kirshenbaum AS, et al. Demonstration that human mast cells arise from a progenitor cell population that is CD34(+), c-kit(+), and expresses aminopeptidase N (CD13). Blood. 1999;94(7):2333–42.

154. Matrisian LM. Metalloproteinases and their inhibitors in matrix remodeling. Trends Genet. 1990;6(4):121–5.

155. Coussens LM, et al. Inflammatory mast cells up-regulate angiogenesis during squamous epithelial carcinogenesis. Genes Dev. 1999;13(11):1382–97.

156. Gruber BL, Marchese MJ, Kew R. Angiogenic factors stimulate mast-cell migration. Blood. 1995;86(7):2488–93.

157. Gruber BL, Marchese MJ, Kew RR. Transforming growth factor-beta 1 mediates mast cell chemotaxis. J Immunol. 1994;152(12):5860–7.

158. Soucek L, et al. Mast cells are required for angiogenesis and macroscopic expansion of Myc-induced pancreatic islet tumors. Nat Med. 2007;13(10):1211–8.

159. Pittenger MF, et al. Multilineage potential of adult human mesenchymal stem cells. Science. 1999;284(5411):143–7.

160. Civin CI, et al. Highly purified CD34-positive cells reconstitute hematopoiesis. J Clin Oncol. 1996;14(8):2224–33.

161. Dennis JE, Charbord P. Origin and differentiation of human and murine stroma. Stem Cells. 2002;20(3):205–14.

162. Hall B, Andreeff M, Marini F. The participation of mesenchymal stem cells in tumor stroma formation and their application as targeted-gene delivery vehicles. Handb Exp Pharmacol. 2007;180:263–83.

163. Schichor C, et al. Vascular endothelial growth factor A contributes to glioma-induced migration of human marrow stromal cells (hMSC). Exp Neurol. 2006;199(2):301–10.

164. Birnbaum T, et al. Malignant gliomas actively recruit bone marrow stromal cells by secreting angiogenic cytokines. J Neurooncol. 2007;83(3):241–7.
165. Kidd S, et al. The (in) auspicious role of mesenchymal stromal cells in cancer: be it friend or foe. Cytotherapy. 2008;10(7):657–67.
166. Spaeth E, et al. Inflammation and tumor microenvironments: defining the migratory itinerary of mesenchymal stem cells. Gene Ther. 2008;15(10):730–8.
167. Dwyer RM, et al. Monocyte chemotactic protein-1 secreted by primary breast tumors stimulates migration of mesenchymal stem cells. Clin Cancer Res. 2007;13(17):5020–7.
168. Coffelt SB, et al. The pro-inflammatory peptide LL-37 promotes ovarian tumor progression through recruitment of multipotent mesenchymal stromal cells. Proc Natl Acad Sci U S A. 2009;106(10):3806–11.
169. Sun B, et al. Correlation between melanoma angiogenesis and the mesenchymal stem cells and endothelial progenitor cells derived from bone marrow. Stem Cells Dev. 2005;14(3):292–8.
170. Beckermann BM, et al. VEGF expression by mesenchymal stem cells contributes to angiogenesis in pancreatic carcinoma. Br J Cancer. 2008;99(4):622–31.

Tissue-Based Biomarkers of Tumor-Vascular Interactions

2

Lars A. Akslen

Abstract

The vascular systems are key components of the tumor microenvironment and angiogenesis is recognized as a hallmark of cancer. Although studies have indicated that the prognosis of certain cancer patients might be improved by targeting tumor-associated blood vessels, there is a lack of markers that can predict the clinical response to such anti-tumor therapy and thereby stratify patients for optimal management. Microvessel density (MVD) and other angiogenesis markers are known to be effective prognostic factors, but information on response prediction is virtually lacking. In addition to the use of novel endothelial proteins and markers for improved tumor imaging and targeting strategies, the potential practical value of selected histologic indicators for better stratification and predictive purposes needs to be more deeply explored and validated in future studies.

L. A. Akslen (✉)
Centre for Cancer Biomarkers CCBIO, Department of Clinical Medicine, University of Bergen, Bergen, Norway
e-mail: lars.akslen@uib.no

© The Author(s), under exclusive license to Springer Nature Switzerland AG 2022
L. A. Akslen, R. S. Watnick (eds.), *Biomarkers of the Tumor Microenvironment*, https://doi.org/10.1007/978-3-030-98950-7_2

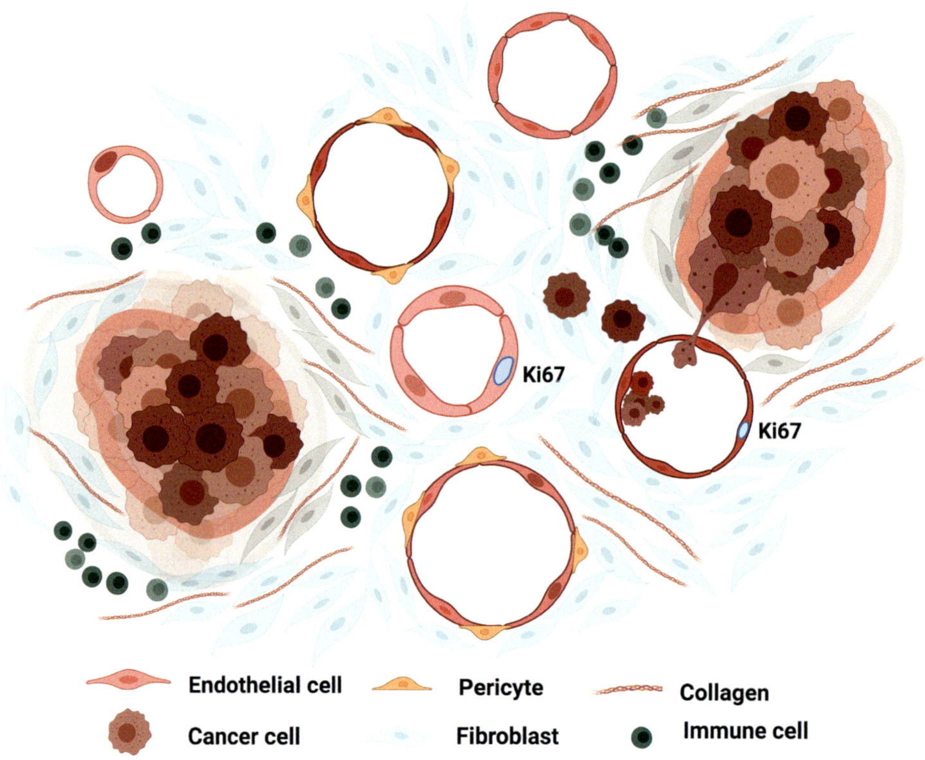

Tumor-associated vessels are unevenly distributed with variation in diameter and shape. They show increased endothelial proliferation (e.g., by Ki67 expression) and are more immature with decreased pericyte coverage. These atypical vessels are more prone to invasion by tumor cells as an early marker of vascular dissemination

Take-Home Lessons
- Tumor-associated blood vessels are different from normal vessels
- Angiogenesis in malignant tumors is most often associated with increased endothelial proliferation and less pericyte coverage
- Vascular proliferation is frequently a stronger prognostic factor than standard microvessel density
- There is no clear association between vascular markers and response to neoadjuvant or adjuvant treatment
- Glomeruloid microvascular proliferation (GMP) is a form of aberrant vascular phenotype with increased occurrence in malignant tumors, being associated with decreased survival in several cancer types

Introduction

In 1971, Folkman suggested that the growth of malignant tumors is dependent on the process of angiogenesis and that tumors can be treated by attacking their blood supply [1]. Since then, mechanisms of angiogenesis have been explored [2–5], and multiple cell types and regulatory pathways have been shown to interact in this complex process, e.g., tumor cells, endothelial cells, perivascular cells, tumor fibroblasts, inflammatory cells, and circulating endothelial progenitor cells from the bone marrow [2, 6, 7]. Studies have indicated an effect of anti-angiogenesis treatment on certain human cancers, such as metastatic colorectal carcinoma, breast cancer, and other tumors [8–10]. A few attempts have been made to identify predictors of response to anti-angiogenesis treatment or traditional chemotherapy [11–15]. Although identification of predictive factors would be important for individual patients and for cost-effective clinical practice, this search has not been convincing in the angiogenesis field [16], in contrast to the reported value of various angiogenesis markers as significant prognostic factors.

Notably, is it possible to classify or grade the vascular response in malignant tumors on a routine basis, so that this information can be used for improved prognostication as well as for response prediction? Histologic grading of tumor-associated angiogenesis was suggested by Brem et al. in 1972 [17] and was later modified by Weidner and Folkman with the introduction of microvessel density (MVD) as a prognostic indicator for breast cancer [18]. Although MVD has later been shown to predict patient prognosis in multiple clinical studies, this marker has some limitations [19]. Hlatky et al. stated that microvessel density is not a simple measure of the angiogenic dependence of tumors, but is rather a reflection of the metabolic burden of the supported tumor cells. The authors proposed that there would be no direct relationship between microvessel density and the tumor response to anti-angiogenesis therapy.

More recently, other prognostic features of angiogenesis have been reported such as vascular proliferation [20–24] and vascular maturation status [24–26]. Also, architectural patterns like vascular nesting or glomeruloid microvascular proliferation (GMP) have been focused and studied in relation to the diversity of tumor-associated angiogenesis and aggressive tumor features including reduced survival in human cancers [27–29].

In addition to markers of tumor-associated angiogenesis, studies have also reported the frequency and impact of vascular invasion, i.e., the ability of tumor cells to enter blood vessels or lymphatic vasculature, and the different influence of these characteristics on tumor progress in various organs [30–33].

Since there is limited data on the prediction of response to anti-angiogenic treatment or standard chemotherapy using histology-based markers of tumor angiogenesis, this needs to be further explored and validated in translational studies of clinical trials, with respect to response prediction in the era of precision treatment and cost-effective medical practice.

It should be mentioned, although not reviewed here, that the process of angiogenesis in solid tumors is not only a local process, but systemic aspects have gained increasing attention [3]. Thus, it has been shown that populations of circulating bone marrow-derived endothelial progenitor cells can differentiate into mature endothelial cells and contribute to pathological neovascularization. These cells can be detected in tissue sections by immunohistochemistry. However, the relative contribution and role of circulating endothelial progenitor cells to tumor neovascularization in humans is not well understood.

Further, the premetastatic niche concept represents an important part of the systemic interactions and regulatory cross-talk between primary tumors, bone marrow and distant tissues that can be influenced to receive or resist metastatic cells. From a diagnostic point of view, circulating cells, e.g., tumor cells, endothelial precursor cells, or other classes of cells, have also received much attention lately as representing a key part of the "liquid biopsy" concept [34]. These diagnostic modalities will likely supplement the tissue-based assessment of primary and metastatic lesions in the future.

Markers of Angiogenesis

Microvessel Density

In 1972, Brem, Cotran, and Folkman suggested criteria for histologic grading of tumor-associated angiogenesis [17], based on the combined assessment of vasoproliferation (number of microvessels within a microscopic field), endothelial cell hyperplasia (number of endothelial cells lining the cross section of a capillary), and endothelial cytology (nuclear changes in proliferating endothelium). In 1988, Srivastava et al. showed in a small study that histologic quantification of microvessels provided significant prognostic information in melanoma [35]. In 1991, Weidner and Folkman reported criteria for microvessel density (MVD) and demonstrated prognostic value in breast cancer [18, 36]. After highlighting the vessels or individual endothelial cells by pan-endothelial markers like Factor VIII (von Willebrand's factor) or CD31, microvessels were counted in the most active area of the tumors, i.e., within hot-spots (Fig. 2.1). Subsequently, after these important papers, MVD has been widely studied for prognostication in several types of malignant tumors, like breast cancer [18, 36], endometrial cancer

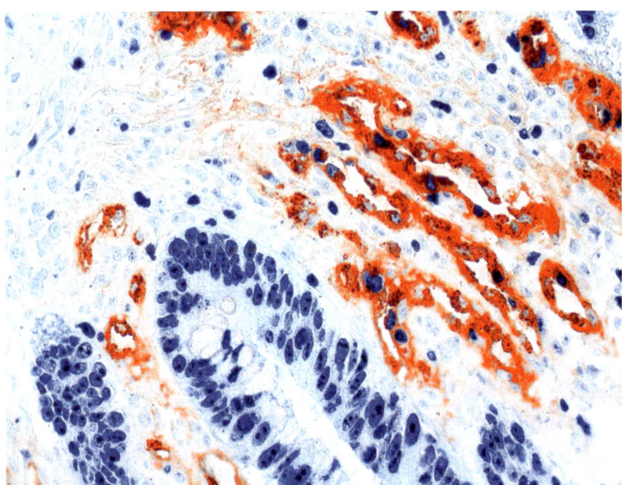

Fig. 2.1 Microvascular proliferation: Microvessels in red (Factor VIII) with some dividing endothelial cells in blue (Ki67). Tumor cells (to the left) show a high degree of proliferation (Ki67 positive nuclei)

[37], lung cancer [23], malignant melanoma [35, 38], and prostate cancer [39, 40]. MVD has been a significant prognostic factor in a majority of studies reported, although some have been negative [41]. In a large meta-analysis of breast cancer [42], including 43 studies and almost 9000 patients, MVD was a significant but rather weak prognostic factor. The conclusions implied that other angiogenic markers might potentially add prognostic information and should be studied.

Modifications of this method have been reported, by using Chalkley counts or image analysis and morphometric measurements based on random area selection [43–45]. The Chalkley counts, giving a relative area estimate of immunostained vessels, may increase the reproducibility of counts within a given hot spot [42]. Tissue sampling is important since there is considerable heterogeneity within individual tumors [46]. However, these methods have not increased the practical value of microvessel counts.

Whereas most studies suggest that microvessel density is a significant prognostic factor, data on response prediction are very limited. Paulsen et al. reported in 1997 that clinical response to neoadjuvant doxorubicin monotherapy for locally advanced breast cancer could not be predicted by MVD [11]. Similar conclusions were reached by others [12]. Further, Jubb et al. [13] concluded that MVD, in addition to VEGF and TSP-1 expression, did not correlate with treatment response or patient outcome in the series of metastatic colorectal carcinoma for which the effect of bevacizumab was first shown [8].

In a study by Tolaney et al. in 2015 [47], a trial of preoperative bevacizumab treatment followed by a combination of bevacizumab and chemotherapy in HER2-negative breast cancer patients was performed to determine how vessel morphology and function was influenced by bevacizumab. The clinical response appeared to reflect the process of vascular normalization primarily in patients with high baseline tumor microvessel density, especially among triple negative breast cancers. In a recent clinical trial study from 2021 of locally advanced or large breast cancer, Krüger et al. examined tissue-based angiogenesis markers for their potential predictive value and found that high baseline MVD significantly predicted response to neoadjuvant bevacizumab treatment [48]. In contrast, microvessel proliferation and the GMP vascular phenotype did not predict response but were instead associated with aggressive tumor features, including basal-like and triple negative tumor phenotypes. Taken together, more data on the predictive value of different tissue-based and other angiogenesis markers is clearly needed. Recently, the introduction of more refined analysis algorithms have been presented [26, 49]. In the latter study, Mezheyeuski et al. reported that the use of novel digitally scored vessel-density-related metrics might identify stroma-normalized microvessel density in the invasive margin as a candidate marker for benefit of adjuvant 5-FU-based chemotherapy in colon cancer. Also, in a study by Corvigno et al., vessel distribution and high "vessel distance" were found to be significantly associated with poor survival in both renal cell and colorectal cancers [50].

Vascular Proliferation

There is limited knowledge of endothelial cell proliferation in human cancers (Fig. 2.1), and its prognostic or predictive importance is not well described in most tumor types. A few studies of breast, lung, prostate, and colorectal tumors have reported a vascular proliferation rate ranging from 0.15% to 17% [20–23, 25, 51–53]. Eberhard et al. studied endothelial cell proliferation in six types of human tumors and found a range from 2.0% (prostate) to 9.6% (glioblastomas) within vascular hot spots [25]. Fox et al. showed a mean labeling index for endothelial cell proliferation in breast cancer of 2.2%, being highest in the tumor periphery [51]. Notably, there was no correlation between endothelial cell proliferation and microvessel density in any of these studies, similar to what others have reported [53]. In a study of 21 colorectal carcinomas, Vermeulen et al. found an average endothelial proliferation labeling index of 9.9%, compared to 21% in vascular hot spots [21]. In a recent study of lung cancer, Ramnefjell et al. found a value of 2.9% in lung cancer [23].

In the early studies, there was no information on the importance of vascular proliferation for patient prognosis. In 2006, Stefansson et al. showed for the first time that vascular proliferation (i.e., proliferating microvessel density, pMVD; microvessel proliferation, MVP) was an independent prognostic factor, shown in endometrial cancer, and pMVD was superior to microvessel density by multivariate analysis [24]. In this study, the median vascular proliferation index (VPI), i.e., the percentage of microvessels, within hot spot areas, with evidence of proliferating endothelial cells by Ki67 staining, was 3.9%, with a range of 0–21% within the tumor tissue. Microvessel proliferation (MVP) was found to be increased in cases with presence of tumor necrosis, and with high tumor stage (by FIGO categories). In the same study, vascular proliferation was an independent prognostic factor by multivariate analysis in addition to histologic grade, vascular invasion by tumor cells, and tumor stage.

In subsequent studies of breast cancer, using three independent cohorts including 499 patients, Arnes et al. found that median vascular proliferation ranged from 0.95% to 1.95% and was associated with estrogen receptor negative tumors and reduced patient survival, whereas microvessel density was not significant [54]. It was further shown by Nalwoga et al., in two breast cancer cohorts including 431 cases, that vascular proliferation was significantly increased in estrogen receptor negative cases and in tumors with a basal-like or triple negative phenotype [55]. In 2021, Krüger et al. found a median vascular proliferation of 5.2% among 128 patients with locally advanced breast cancer, being associated with basal-like and triple negative phenotypes [48]. Increased vascular proliferation in basal-like compared to luminal breast cancer was recently shown by Kraby et al. [56]. The mechanism for such a relationship in breast cancer is not known. It was found that basal-like and triple negative cancers were associated with VEGF expression [57], a key regulator of breast cancer angiogenesis [58], and VEGF-driven angiogenesis might contribute to the increased vascular proliferation that we found among basal-like tumors. Notably, in a study of locally advanced breast cancer, response to anti-VEGF therapy by bevacizumab was predicted by overall MVD although not by microvessel proliferation [48].

It was reported in 2009 by Gravdal et al. that when combining Ki-67 for endothelial proliferation with a marker of immature endothelium, Nestin, the prognostic sensitivity was increased [59]. By studying prostate cancer, Nestin/Ki67 co-expression, as a marker of vascular proliferation, was four to fivefold higher in castration-resistant cancers and metastases compared with localized tumors and prostatic hyperplasias. Still, even among localized cancers, high vascular proliferation was a strong and independent predictor of biochemical failure, clinical recurrence, and time to skeletal metastasis by multivariate analysis. In castration-resistant cancers, vascular proliferation was associated with reduced patient survival. In a more recent study of prostate cancer, vascular proliferation was found to be associated with EMT factors Twist and Snail [60]. In breast cancer, by Nestin/Ki67 co-expression, a median vascular proliferation of 2.7% was found by Krüger et al. [61]. There were significant associations with estrogen receptor negative tumors as well as basal-like and triple negative phenotypes. In this study, vascular proliferation was an independent predictor of death from breast cancer. In lung cancer, the median vascular proliferation (by Nestin/Ki67) was 2.9% [23].

Interestingly, in a study by Haldorsen et al., microvascular proliferation in endometrial cancers was compared with imaging parameters obtained from preoperative dynamic contrast-enhanced magnetic resonance imaging (DCE-MRI) and diffusion-weighted imaging (DWI) to explore the relationship between these markers and their potential ability to identify patients with poor outcome [62]. Notably, microvessel proliferation was found to be negatively correlated to tumor blood flow by MRI, possibly reflecting an abnormal and reduced functionality in newly formed tumor-associated vasculature. In this study, vascular proliferation was significantly associated with reduced patient survival, similar to what was previously found [24].

In a study by Stefansson et al. in 2015, a 32-gene expression signature was found to separate tumors with high versus low microvascular proliferation [63]. This 32-gene signature associated with high-grade tumor features and reduced survival by independent cohorts. Interestingly, copy number studies revealed a strong association between microvessel proliferation and 6p21 amplification. VEGF-A is known to be located in the 6p21 chromosomal region [64], and integrated analyses demonstrated significant associations between increased vascular proliferation and VEGF-A mRNA expression, pointing to a possible angiogenesis driver mechanism in endometrial cancer. In a previous study of endometrial cancer, VEGF-A was significantly associated with vascular proliferation and reduced patient survival [24]. In locally advanced breast cancer, this 32-gene angiogenesis signature was associated with vascular proliferation and a basal-like tumor phenotype, although not with response to anti-VEGF therapy by bevacizumab [48].

Vascular Maturation

The structural integrity and maturation status of blood vessels, i.e., the degree of coverage by cells like pericytes, has been reported [3, 65], and several factors are known to contribute to pericyte recruitment [66, 67]. Reduced maturation appears to accompany the atypical structure of vessels in malignant tumors [27, 68]. Also, tumor-associated pericytes are often abnormal when present [69]. Vascular maturation, as estimated by pericyte coverage, appears to be a dynamic process. In prostate cancer, androgen ablation therapy may induce a downregulation of intra-tumoral VEGF followed by selective regression of immature tumor microvessels by apoptosis of endothelial cells not covered by pericytes [70]. The authors suggested that vessel maturation status of individual tumors might predict the efficacy of anti-VEGF tumor treatment. In 2001, Jain proposed that anti-angiogenic therapy might lead to improved maturation and normalization of the tumor vasculature thereby increasing the efficacy of combined treatment including chemotherapy or radiation [71, 72]. In a clinical study, injection of anti-VEGF was followed by increased maturation of tumor-associated vessels [73], as has also been reported in experimental studies [74, 75]. It was shown that anti-VEGFR2 treatment creates a "normalization window" of the vasculature for increased efficacy of additional radiation treatment by upregulation of Ang1 and degradation of the basement membrane by MMP activation [76]. In a trial of preoperative bevacizumab followed by a combination of bevacizumab and chemotherapy in HER2-negative breast cancer, Tolaney et al. reported that the tumor response appeared to reflect vascular normalization, primarily in patients with high tumor microvessel density [47].

Data on human tumors are limited with respect to clinical correlates and outcomes. In early clinical studies of this marker, Eberhard et al. reported vascular maturation in six human tumor types and found a wide range in pericyte coverage index from 13% (glioblastoma) to 67% (breast cancer) [25], although no clinical or prognostic evaluation was presented. In a study of lung cancer [77], a better outcome was found for tumors with high vascular maturation. The mean vascular maturation index (VMI) was 46%, and high VMI was associated with low microvessel density and absence of nodal metastases. In contrast, a report on breast cancer showed no prognostic impact of VMI [78]. In both studies, the basement membrane antibody LH39 was used as a maturation marker. The authors concluded that differences between various tissues in vascular proliferation and maturation might be relevant for the suitability of anti-angiogenic treatment. In a study of endometrial cancer in 2006, Stefansson et al. showed that median pericyte coverage, as estimated by the α-SMA coverage index (SMAI), was 35%, and lower SMAI was significantly associated with increased vascular invasion by tumor cells and impaired patient prognosis [24].

In a study of colorectal cancer from 2016, semi-quantitative and digital image analyses-based scoring identified significant associations between low expression of perivascular PDGFR and shorter overall survival. Notably, perivascular PDGFR-α and PDGFR-β remained independent factors for survival by multivariate analyses [26].

Glomeruloid Microvascular Proliferation

Although tumor vessels frequently have abnormal structure, architectural and cytologic atypia might be difficult to assess, and there is no consensus on how to report vascular morphology in a reproducible way. Some studies have suggested pattern-based angiogenesis markers, such as glomeruloid microvascular proliferations (GMP) (Fig. 2.2). GMP, also called "microvascular nests" or "glomeruloid bodies," are focal proliferative buddings of a mixture of vascular cells (primarily multilayered endothelial cells in addition to pericytes and macrophages) that superficially resemble renal glomeruli [79–82]. In standard tissue sections, GMPs generally consist of 15–100 cells; one or more vascular lumens are usually present, especially in more mature GMPs.

GMPs represent a defining histologic feature of glioblastoma multiforme [79, 80] and have been associated with increased aggressiveness in brain tumors [83, 84]. GMP-like patterns have also been sporadically reported in other tumors, including gastrointestinal carcinomas, thymomas, and different vascular tumors [81, 85–89]. However, until quite recently, human tumors have not been studied systematically.

In animal studies, Dvorak and coworkers induced the formation of "glomeruloid bodies" from preexisting microves-

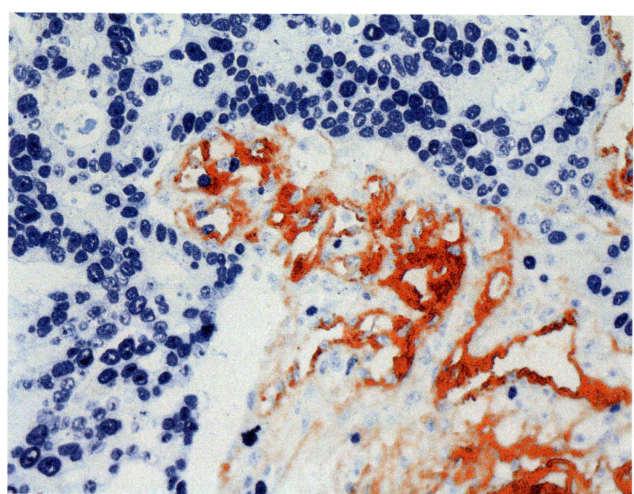

Fig. 2.2 Glomeruloid microvascular proliferation (GMP) (red vessels, Factor VIII), with a few dividing endothelial cells in blue (Ki67), and marked proliferation in tumor cells (Ki67)

sels in mouse skin, through the injection of an adenoviral vector expressing VEGF-A$_{164}$, indicating that the formation of the GMP phenotype might represent a VEGF-A dependent and dysregulated angiogenic response [90]. The formation of new blood vessels through several steps, each with a distinctive morphology, was described in detail; these include *mother vessels* (MOV), *glomeruloid microvascular proliferation* (GMP), and *arterio-venous malformations* (AVM) [27, 81, 82, 91]. The GMP phenotype was dependent on the continued presence of VEGF-A$_{164}$, and as VEGF-A$_{164}$ expression declined, GMPs underwent apoptosis and progressively devolved into smaller, more normal-appearing microvessels [82]. Thus, the GMP generated in this model also required exogenous VEGF-A$_{164}$ for their maintenance, and this finding is likely relevant to GMP in human tumors. All of the tumor types known to form GMP also express VEGF-A. Another human parallel appears to be the POEMS syndrome, where increased VEGF-A levels are associated with glomeruloid vascular proliferations in the skin, i.e., glomeruloid hemangioma [85].

In a study by Straume et al. in 2002 of more than 700 human cancers (breast, endometrial, prostate, melanoma), approximately 20% of the cases were considered GMP positive (range 13–23%). Presence of GMP was significantly related to poor prognosis [29], and this has been confirmed in studies of non-small cell lung cancer [92] and pancreatic cancer [93]. This angiogenic phenotype was found to be a better predictor of outcome than microvessel density [16].

In the series of nodular melanomas [29], 23% were GMP positive, and the presence of GMP was significantly associated with aggressive tumor features like increasing lesion thickness (a.m. Breslow) and ulceration. In survival analysis, GMP was an independent prognostic factor along with Clark's level of tumor invasion and ulceration, and GMP was of greater value in this regard than standard microvessel density. To extend these studies, the presence of GMP in relation to the expression of several different angiogenic factors and their receptors in melanoma was evaluated [94]. GMP was associated with increased endothelial cell expression of VEGF receptor-1 (FLT-1), VEGF receptor-2 (KDR), and Neuropilin-1. The expression of VEGF-A protein in tumor or endothelial cells was not associated with the presence of GMP, whereas VEGF-A expression was significantly stronger in GMP endothelium compared with non-GMP endothelium within the tumors. There was a significant association between lack of Tie-2 expression in tumor-associated endothelial cells and the presence of GMP, whereas there was no association with the expression of angiopoietin-1 (Ang-1) [94]. Taken together, our findings indicate that increased expression of VEGF receptors on the endothelium in melanomas was associated with presence of GMP, whereas the opposite was found for Tie-2, a receptor that has been linked to vessel maturation [10]. Expression of bFGF was decreased in GMP endothelium, and this has been associated with a less mature vasculature [29].

In our initial study [29], 17% of breast carcinomas were GMP positive, and presence of GMP was related to the ductal histotype, high grade, estrogen receptor negativity, and HER2 expression. Regarding prognosis, GMP was found to be an independent prognostic indicator by multivariate analysis, providing additional information beyond basic variables such as tumor size, histologic grade, and lymph node metastases. Notably, GMP was not correlated with microvessel density (MVD) which was not prognostic in this patient cohort. These findings indicate that GMP may provide a novel prognostic marker, indicative of a more aggressive vascular phenotype.

Further studies on breast cancer indicated that GMP is associated with multiple markers of aggressive tumors like estrogen receptor negativity and a basal-like phenotype [95], and the GMP vascular phenotype has been associated with presence of *BRCA1* germline mutations and p53 alterations [96]. *BRCA1*-related breast cancers have a distinct profile on microarray analysis [97] and also a characteristic spectrum of *TP53* mutations [98]. Our data suggest that *BRCA1* mutations might induce a genetic profile of which GMP is an important manifestation and part of the tumor phenotype. Of relevance, BRCA1 protein has been associated with inhibition of VEGF transcription and secretion in breast cancer cells [99].

We previously found a significant association between GMP and pathologic expression of p53 protein [96], whereas p53 overexpression was not associated with increased microvessel density. The relationship between p53 and angiogenesis could involve several different mechanisms: 1. p53 is known to suppress the expression of VEGF [100] and interacts with the transcription factor Sp1

[101]; 2. p53 degrades hypoxia inducible factor 1 [102]; 3. p53 downregulates the expression of bFGF binding protein [103]; and 4. p53 upregulates thrombospondin-1 expression [104].

In a study of locally advanced breast cancer, treated with standard chemotherapy, Akslen et al. found that the presence of GMP, occurring in 21% of the cases, was significantly associated with high-grade tumors and *TP53* mutations in addition to basal-like and HER2 positive subtypes of breast cancer as defined by gene expression data [15]. The GMP phenotype was significantly associated with a lack of treatment response and progressive disease, indicating a potential predictive value. In these tumors, GMP was also correlated to a gene expression signature for tumor hypoxia response, pointing to a possible mechanistic relationship. In a randomized clinical trial of neoadjuvant bevacizumab treatment of locally advanced breast cancer, GMP was associated with aggressive tumor features, although not with treatment response, which was predicted by baseline microvessel density [48].

In a study of metastatic melanoma, GMP in primary tumors (25%) or metastatic tissue (12%) did not predict the response to bevacizumab monotherapy, although limited tissue from metastatic lesions could decrease sensitivity [105].

In endometrial cancer, GMPs were found to be significantly associated with increasing histologic grade, diffusely invasive growth pattern, presence of necrosis, vascular invasion, deep myometrial invasion, and high clinical stage [24]. This study also indicated an association between GMP formation and increased vascular proliferation, by Factor VIII/Ki67 co-expression. The findings provide further evidence that GMP is an angiogenic marker of high-grade and aggressive tumors.

In prostate cancer, GMP was present in 13% of cases [29] and was associated with high preoperative levels of serum PSA. The GMP phenotype was an independent predictor of time to biochemical failure as determined by multivariate analysis.

In other tumor types, GMP was a significant prognostic factor in a study of non-small cell lung cancer [92]. A total of 25% of these tumors were GMP positive, and the frequency of GMP was not associated with basic factors such as histologic grade or clinical stage. Similar to our findings [29], there was no association between GMP status and microvessel density in these lung cancers. There was no correlation between VEGF-A expression and the frequency of GMP, although this phenotype was more often seen in Ang-1 positive tumors. Multivariate analysis indicated that GMP was a significant and independent prognostic factor, whereas microvessel density was not. Taken together, these data support our initial observation that GMP might be a novel and significant tissue-based angiogenesis marker for potential clinical use.

Other Vascular Patterns

There has been some additional focus on architectural patterns of angiogenesis in malignant tumors [106]. It seem that qualitative features, rather than quantitative metrics of microvessel density and other markers, may provide some prognostic relevance in certain tumor types, like glioblastomas of the brain, and ocular melanomas. Some studies have focused on the distribution pattern of microvessels within tumors. The EDVIN concept ("edge versus inner") suggests that comparing vessel counts at the edge of the tumor with the inner area might give a better picture of the angiogenic activity and patient survival. The prognostic value of EDVIN was shown in studies of breast and colorectal cancers [107].

Quantification of vascular pattern by image analysis has shown increased prognostic impact by use of syntactic structure analysis [108]. Studies of pheochromocytomas, which are highly vascular tumors of the adrenal medulla, have shown that complex and irregular vascular patterns are associated with malignant behavior [109].

Vascular Molecular Phenotypes

Can certain vascular immunomarkers discriminate between endothelial cells in benign tissues and "activated" tumor-associated endothelium? If so, these markers could be applied in tumor imaging and therapeutic targeting, in addition to response prediction and prognostication. This field is very promising but not well developed, and it is not the primary topic of this chapter. Chi et al. reported expression differences between endothelial cells from various sites of the vascular system [110]. Also, proteins are differentially expressed in tumor-associated endothelium [111, 112], and such endothelial markers might provide "zip codes" or "maps" for homing of anti-tumor peptides like LyP1 [113]. St. Croix et al. showed multiple novel antigens being expressed selectively in tumor endothelium from colorectal cancers, some of them associated with the cell membrane (TEM1, TEM7, TEM8), or extracellular matrix [114]. In the same setting, studies from our team indicate that when using the marker Nestin for immature endothelium, in addition to Ki67 as a proliferation marker, enhanced and significant prognostic information can be obtained from tissue sections [59, 61].

Pan-endothelial markers, such as Von Willebrand's Factor (Factor VIII), CD31, and CD34, are frequently used to visualize endothelial cells by immunohistochemistry when estimating microvessel density. Some reports suggest that CD105/endoglin, a TGF-β receptor involved in vascular development and remodeling, might be suitable as a marker of active angiogenesis in malignant tumors, as well as a therapeutic target on tumor-associated vessels [115]. Microvessel density by CD105 was superior and independent as a prognostic factor in breast cancer [116]. Similar results were presented for lung cancer [117] and prostate cancer [118], whereas no advantage of CD105 was found in studies of endometrial cancer [119] and malignant melanoma [120].

VEGF and its receptors may be present on tumor cells and vessels and might represent targets for imaging and treatment [121]. It was shown that activated microvessel density (aMVD), as estimated by VEGF/KDR staining on endothelial cells, was highest in the tumor periphery and superior to standard microvessel density (sMVD) as a prognostic factor evaluated by multivariate survival analysis of non-small cell lung cancer [122].

Expression of bFGF on tumor-associated endothelial cells was inversely associated with lymph node metastases and pathological stage of non-small cell lung cancer [123]. Similar findings, together with a prognostic role, have been found for prostate cancer [124] and malignant melanoma [125]. These findings further support the diversity of tumor-associated vessels.

Other angiogenesis markers have been explored, like the expression of tumor-specific endothelial (TEM) antigens [126–128]. Expression of certain integrins, like $\alpha v\beta 3$, has been associated with tumor vasculature [129], and this marker might also be applied for imaging [130] and treatment strategies [131]. The main challenge will be to validate such proteins in further studies. It is not clear whether simple histology-based tissue markers will prove effective in comparison with other classes of angiogenic markers, like circulating endothelial cells. Taken together, studies of vascular markers are important for our understanding of tumor-associated angiogenesis, vascular imaging techniques, and the development of therapeutic modalities. Whether gene expression signatures might capture the complexity of malignant tumors and better reflect their angiogenesis capacity should be studied in more detail.

Markers of Vascular Invasion

One important hallmark of cancer progression is the ability of tumor cells to migrate into vascular channels, i.e., blood vessels or lymphatic vasculature, as an early step of metastatic spread [132]. In breast tumors, vascular invasion is usually considered to be lymphatic vessel involvement (LVI) more often than blood vascular invasion (BVI) [31], but there are few studies in this field. Vascular invasion, as observed on standard tissue sections, is associated with an increased risk of tumor recurrence, metastasis, and death from disease [31, 133]. Lymphatic invasion is particularly important as a prognostic factor in early stage breast cancer [134, 135]. Gujam et al. highlighted that immunohistochemistry discriminates better between BVI and LVI, and this distinction improves the prognostic value of vascular invasion compared to standard sections [32, 33, 136–138].

A potentially different impact of blood vessel invasion as compared with lymphatic involvement has not been well established, for example, in relation to the molecular subtypes of breast cancer. This might be due to the lack of firm criteria to separate blood vessel and lymphatic invasion. Usually, CD31 staining for blood vessel endothelium and D2-40 for lymphatic vessels are applied, although overlapping staining patterns exist. Still, D2-40 expression is considered to be specific for lymphatic endothelium. In a breast cancer study by Klingen et al., blood vessel invasion, present in 15% of the cases, showed strong associations with non-luminal tumors such as the basal-like, triple negative, and HER2 positive subgroups [32]. In survival analysis, BVI was significantly associated with recurrence-free and breast cancer-specific survival, whereas LVI was not. When adjusting for basic factors, BVI was an independent prognostic marker, indicating that this feature might be recorded in breast cancer diagnostics, although more studies need to confirm these findings. Development of even more specific markers for blood vessels would be desirable in a routine setting to identify patients at a higher risk for early systemic spread. The potential use of such diagnostic approaches for improved therapy among cases with blood vessel invasion should be considered.

We previously reported that basal-like breast cancers appear to have increased angiogenesis with more microvessel proliferation and higher frequency of the glomeruloid microvascular pattern (GMP) when compared with other breast cancer subtypes [54, 55]. These findings suggest a possible relationship between increased angiogenesis and blood vessel invasion among basal-like breast cancers. The relationships between vascular proliferation, immature vessels, and vascular invasion have also been shown in endometrial cancer [24].

Notably, studies of disseminated tumor cells from the bone marrow, as well as expression profiles of primary tumor cells, suggest that hematogenous spread is often an early event in tumor progression [139]. Early systemic dissemination of breast cancer cells is associated with a specific expression signature, and the molecular pathways associated with primary hematogenous spread and lymphatic dissemination appear to be different [140]. The present data suggest that blood vessel invasion by tumor cells is strongly associated with aggressive tumor subtypes (basal-like, triple negative, HER2 positive). Blood vessel invasion has also been related to interval breast cancer presentation compared with screen-detected tumors [32]. Based on such findings, it might be of practical importance to examine the presence of blood vascular invasion in breast cancers.

It has been suggested that the basal-like phenotype of breast cancer may be related to non-lymphatic spread [141], and findings indicate a reduced risk of axillary lymphatic spread in triple negative breast cancer [142]. Although the presence of metastases in axillary lymph nodes predicts the development of distant metastases, 20–30% of patients with node-negative breast cancer develop metastatic spread at distant sites [143]. Early systemic dissemination of breast cancer cells is associated with a specific gene expression signature [140].

In a large study of endometrial cancer, 18% of the tumors showed blood vessel invasion, whereas 31% of the tumors revealed lymphatic involvement [30]. Both BVI and LVI were associated with features such as high histologic grade and diffuse tumor growth. Patients without vascular invasion had the best prognosis and those with BVI (with or without LVI) had the worst outcome, whereas patients with LVI had an intermediate survival by univariate analysis. Both BVI and LVI had independent prognostic importance. Such findings support the biological importance of vascular spread through the haematogenic and lymphatic routes in endometrial cancer. The significant correlation found with clinical phenotype indicates that these markers may be relevant for patient management.

In further studies of endometrial cancer, certain gene expression patterns were associated with vascular invasion by tumor cells as examined in standard sections [144]. Thus, a vascular invasion signature of 18 genes was significantly associated with patient survival and clinicopathologic phenotype. Vascular involvement was related to gene sets for epithelial-mesenchymal transition, wound response, endothelial cells, and vascular endothelial growth factor (VEGF) activity. Further, expression of Collagen 8 and MMP3 were associated with vascular invasion, and ANGPTL4 and IL-8 showed a relationship to patient survival. These findings indicate that vascular involvement within primary tumors is associated with gene expression profiles related to angiogenesis and epithelial-mesenchymal transition. This 18-gene expression signature was furthermore studied in multiple cohorts of breast cancer and found to associate with aggressive features like high tumor grade, hormone receptor negativity, HER2 positivity, a basal-like phenotype, reduced patient survival, and response to neoadjuvant chemotherapy [145]. The 18-gene vascular invasion signature was associated with several other gene expression profiles related to vascular biology and tumor progression, including the Oncotype DX breast cancer recurrence signature. Taken together, the findings indicate that markers for vascular invasion by tumor cells in the primary tumor, including gene expression patterns, might provide information that indicates an increased risk of metastatic spread.

Concluding Remarks/Summary

It has become increasingly evident that some malignant tumors can be treated by attacking their blood supply. At the same time, both experimental and clinical data have demonstrated that tumor-associated angiogenesis is more complex than reflected simply by the number of microvessels on tissue sections. In the era of targeted therapy, companion biomarkers are becoming crucial to increase treatment efficacy by defining subgroups of patients with high probability of response to the treatment [13, 16], similar to the role of HER2 in breast cancer management. Whereas this is a "hallmark of tailored treatment," such markers have not yet been successfully established in the field of anti-angiogenesis therapy. In the case of anti-VEGF regimens, there is no simple relationship between presence of the target (VEGF) and treatment response [13], and no reliable association with the "end-point" of angiogenic stimulation, i.e., microvessel density, has been found. At the same time, there is a relative lack of translational studies of human tumors, and tissue-based angiogenesis markers should therefore be further studied and validated. Markers reflecting the angiogenic response in primary tumors, such as vascular proliferation and vascular maturation status, need to be examined across different tumor types to increase the evidence of their potential utility, especially as predictive factors. The presence of glomeruloid microvascular proliferation (GMP), reflecting some of the increased irregularity and complexity of tumor-associated angiogenesis, and a marker of VEGF-driven angiogenesis, should be considered. Furthermore, a refined immunophenotypic profiling of the tumor vasculature might improve the basis and indications for novel imaging techniques and treatment targets. Complementary systemic biomarkers, such as circulating endothelial progenitor cells, are likely to gain increased importance. Different markers might be combined into profiles to obtain a balance between high-technology methods and simpler cost-effective techniques.

References

 1. Folkman J. Tumor angiogenesis: therapeutic implications. N Engl J Med. 1971;285(21):1182–6.
 2. Carmeliet P. Angiogenesis in health and disease. Nat Med. 2003;9(6):653–60.
 3. Carmeliet P. Molecular mechanisms and clinical applications of angiogenesis. Nature. 2011;473(7347):298–307.
 4. Kerbel RS. Tumor angiogenesis. N Engl J Med. 2008;358(19):2039–49.
 5. Yancopoulos GD, Gale NW, Rudge JS, Wiegand SJ, Holash J. Vascular specific growth factors and blood vessel formation. Nature. 2000;407(6801):242–8.
 6. Lyden D, Dias S, Costa C, Blaikie P, Butros L. Impaired recruitment of bone marrow derived endothelial and hematopoietic precursor cells blocks tumor angiogenesis and growth. Nat Med. 2001;7(11):1194–201.
 7. Kaplan RN, Zacharoulis S, Bramley AH, Vincent L, Costa C. VEGFR1-positive haematopoietic bone marrow progenitors initiate the pre-metastatic niche. Nature. 2005;438(7069):820–7.
 8. Hurwitz H, Novotny W, Cartwright T, Hainsworth J, Heim W. Bevacizumab plus irinotecan, fluorouracil, and leucovorin for metastatic colorectal cancer. N Engl J Med. 2004;350(23):2335–42.
 9. Jain RK, Clark JW, Loeffler JS. Lessons from phase III clinical trials on anti-VEGF therapy for cancer. Nat Clin Pract Oncol. 2006;3(1):24–40.
10. Potente M, Carmeliet P. Basic and therapeutic aspects of angiogenesis. Cell. 2011;146(6):873–87.
11. Paulsen T, Borresen AL, Varhaug JE, Lonning PE, Akslen LA. Angiogenesis does not predict clinical response to doxorubicin monotherapy in patients with locally advanced breast cancer. Int J Cancer. 1997;74(1):138–40.
12. Tynninen O, von Boguslawski K, Bengtsson NO, Heikkila R, Malmstrom P. Tumor microvessel density as predictor of chemotherapy response in breast cancer patients. Br J Cancer. 2002;86(12):1905–8.
13. Jubb AM, Hurwitz HI, Bai W, Holmgren EB, Tobin P, Guerrero AS, et al. Impact of vascular endothelial growth factor-A expression, thrombospondin-2 expression, and microvessel density on the treatment effect of bevacizumab in metastatic colorectal cancer. J Clin Oncol. 2006;24(2):217–27.
14. Lambrechts D, Lenz HJ, de Haas S, Carmeliet P, Scherer SJ. Markers of response for the antiangiogenic agent bevacizumab. J Clin Oncol. 2013;31(9):1219–30.
15. Akslen LA, Straume O, Geisler S, Sorlie T, Chi JT, Aas T, et al. Glomeruloid microvascular proliferation is associated with lack of response to chemotherapy in breast cancer. Br J Cancer. 2011;105(1):9–12.
16. Bergsland EK. When does the presence of the target predict response to the targeted agent? J Clin Oncol. 2006;24(2):213–6.
17. Brem S, Cotran R, Folkman J. Tumor angiogenesis: a quantitative method for histologic grading. J Natl Cancer Inst. 1972;48(2):347–56.
18. Weidner N, Semple JP, Welch WR, Folkman J. Tumor angiogenesis and metastasis--correlation in invasive breast carcinoma. N Engl J Med. 1991;324(1):1–8.
19. Hlatky L, Hahnfeldt P, Folkman J. Clinical application of antiangiogenic therapy: microvessel density, what it does and doesn't tell us. J Natl Cancer Inst. 2002;94(12):883–93.
20. Vartanian RK, Weidner N. Correlation of intratumoral endothelial cell proliferation with microvessel density (tumor angiogenesis) and tumor cell proliferation in breast carcinoma. Am J Pathol. 1994;144(6):1188–94.
21. Vermeulen PB, Verhoeven D, Hubens G, Van Marck E, Goovaerts G, Huyghe M, et al. Microvessel density, endothelial cell proliferation and tumour cell proliferation in human colorectal adenocarcinomas. Ann Oncol. 1995;6(1):59–64.
22. Prall F, Gringmuth U, Nizze H, Barten M. Microvessel densities and microvascular architecture in colorectal carcinomas and their liver metastases: significant correlation of high microvessel densities with better survival. Histopathology. 2003;42(5):482–91.
23. Ramnefjell M, Aamelfot C, Aziz S, Helgeland L, Akslen LA. Microvascular proliferation is associated with aggressive tumour features and reduced survival in lung adenocarcinoma. J Pathol Clin Res. 2017;3(4):249–57.
24. Stefansson IM, Salvesen HB, Akslen LA. Vascular proliferation is important for clinical progress of endometrial cancer. Cancer Res. 2006;66(6):3303–9.
25. Eberhard A, Kahlert S, Goede V, Hemmerlein B, Plate KH, Augustin HG. Heterogeneity of angiogenesis and blood vessel maturation in human tumors: implications for antiangiogenic tumor therapies. Cancer Res. 2000;60(5):1388–93.
26. Mezheyeuski A, Bradic Lindh M, Guren TK, Dragomir A, Pfeiffer P, Kure EH, et al. Survival-associated heterogeneity of

marker-defined perivascular cells in colorectal cancer. Oncotarget. 2016;7(27):41948–58.

27. Dvorak HF. Rous-Whipple Award Lecture. How tumors make bad blood vessels and stroma. Am J Pathol. 2003;162(6):1747–57.

28. Dvorak HF. Tumor Stroma, Tumor Blood Vessels, and Antiangiogenesis Therapy. Cancer J. 2015;21(4):237–43.

29. Straume O, Chappuis PO, Salvesen HB, Halvorsen OJ, Haukaas SA, Goffin JR, et al. Prognostic importance of glomeruloid microvascular proliferation indicates an aggressive angiogenic phenotype in human cancers. Cancer Res. 2002;62(23):6808–11.

30. Mannelqvist M, Stefansson I, Salvesen HB, Akslen LA. Importance of tumour cell invasion in blood and lymphatic vasculature among patients with endometrial carcinoma. Histopathology. 2009;54(2):174–83.

31. Mohammed RA, Ellis IO, Mahmmod AM, Hawkes EC, Green AR, Rakha EA, et al. Lymphatic and blood vessels in basal and triple-negative breast cancers: characteristics and prognostic significance. Mod Pathol. 2011;24(6):774–85.

32. Klingen TA, Chen Y, Stefansson IM, Knutsvik G, Collett K, Abrahamsen AL, et al. Tumour cell invasion into blood vessels is significantly related to breast cancer subtypes and decreased survival. J Clin Pathol. 2017;70(4):313–9.

33. Ramnefjell M, Aamelfot C, Helgeland L, Akslen LA. Vascular invasion is an adverse prognostic factor in resected non-small-cell lung cancer. APMIS. 2017;125(3):197–206.

34. Mohme M, Riethdorf S, Pantel K. Circulating and disseminated tumour cells - mechanisms of immune surveillance and escape. Nat Rev Clin Oncol. 2017;14(3):155–67.

35. Srivastava A, Laidler P, Davies RP, Horgan K, Hughes LE. The prognostic significance of tumor vascularity in intermediate-thickness (0.76-4.0 mm thick) skin melanoma. A quantitative histologic study. Am J Pathol. 1988;133(2):419–23.

36. Weidner N, Folkman J, Pozza F, Bevilacqua P, Allred EN, Moore DH, et al. Tumor angiogenesis: a new significant and independent prognostic indicator in early-stage breast carcinoma. J Natl Cancer Inst. 1992;84(24):1875–87.

37. Salvesen HB, Iversen OE, Akslen LA. Independent prognostic importance of microvessel density in endometrial carcinoma. Br J Cancer. 1998;77(7):1140–4.

38. Straume O, Salvesen HB, Akslen LA. Angiogenesis is prognostically important in vertical growth phase melanomas. Int J Oncol. 1999;15(3):595–9.

39. Weidner N, Carroll PR, Flax J, Blumenfeld W, Folkman J. Tumor angiogenesis correlates with metastasis in invasive prostate carcinoma. Am J Pathol. 1993;143(2):401–9.

40. Halvorsen OJ, Haukaas S, Hoisaeter PA, Akslen LA. Independent prognostic importance of microvessel density in clinically localized prostate cancer. Anticancer Res. 2000;20(5C):3791–9.

41. Axelsson K, Ljung BM, Moore DH 2nd, Thor AD, Chew KL, Edgerton SM, et al. Tumor angiogenesis as a prognostic assay for invasive ductal breast carcinoma. J Natl Cancer Inst. 1995;87(13):997–1008.

42. Uzzan B, Nicolas P, Cucherat M, Perret GY. Microvessel density as a prognostic factor in women with breast cancer: a systematic review of the literature and meta-analysis. Cancer Res. 2004;64(9):2941–55.

43. Belien JA, Somi S, de Jong JS, van Diest PJ, Baak JP. Fully automated microvessel counting and hot spot selection by image processing of whole tumour sections in invasive breast cancer. J Clin Pathol. 1999;52(3):184–92.

44. Vermeulen PB, Gasparini G, Fox SB, Colpaert C, Marson LP, Gion M, et al. Second international consensus on the methodology and criteria of evaluation of angiogenesis quantification in solid human tumours. Eur J Cancer. 2002;38(12):1564–79.

45. Fox SB, Harris AL. Histological quantitation of tumour angiogenesis. APMIS. 2004;112(7-8):413–30.

46. de Jong JS, van Diest PJ, Baak JP. Heterogeneity and reproducibility of microvessel counts in breast cancer. Lab Invest. 1995;73(6):922–6.

47. Tolaney SM, Boucher Y, Duda DG, Martin JD, Seano G, Ancukiewicz M, et al. Role of vascular density and normalization in response to neoadjuvant bevacizumab and chemotherapy in breast cancer patients. Proc Natl Acad Sci U S A. 2015;112(46):14325–30.

48. Kruger K, Silwal-Pandit L, Wik E, Straume O, Stefansson IM, Borgen E, et al. Baseline microvessel density predicts response to neoadjuvant bevacizumab treatment of locally advanced breast cancer. Sci Rep. 2021;11(1):3388.

49. Mezheyeuski A, Hrynchyk I, Herrera M, Karlberg M, Osterman E, Ragnhammar P, et al. Stroma-normalised vessel density predicts benefit from adjuvant fluorouracil-based chemotherapy in patients with stage II/III colon cancer. Br J Cancer. 2019;121(4):303–11.

50. Corvigno S, Frodin M, Wisman GBA, Nijman HW, Van der Zee AG, Jirstrom K, et al. Multi-parametric profiling of renal cell, colorectal, and ovarian cancer identifies tumour-type-specific stroma phenotypes and a novel vascular biomarker. J Pathol Clin Res. 2017;3(3):214–24.

51. Fox SB, Gatter KC, Bicknell R, Going JJ, Stanton P, Cooke TG, et al. Relationship of endothelial cell proliferation to tumor vascularity in human breast cancer. Cancer Res. 1993;53(18):4161–3.

52. Vartanian RK, Weidner N. Endothelial cell proliferation in prostatic carcinoma and prostatic hyperplasia: correlation with Gleason's score, microvessel density, and epithelial cell proliferation. Lab Invest. 1995;73(6):844–50.

53. Colpaert CG, Vermeulen PB, Benoy I, Soubry A, van Roy F, van Beest P, et al. Inflammatory breast cancer shows angiogenesis with high endothelial proliferation rate and strong E-cadherin expression. Br J Cancer. 2003;88(5):718–25.

54. Arnes JB, Stefansson IM, Straume O, Baak JP, Lonning PE, Foulkes WD, et al. Vascular proliferation is a prognostic factor in breast cancer. Breast Cancer Res Treat. 2012;133(2):501–10.

55. Nalwoga H, Arnes JB, Stefansson IM, Wabinga H, Foulkes WD, Akslen LA. Vascular proliferation is increased in basal-like breast cancer. Breast Cancer Res Treat. 2011;130(3):1063–71.

56. Kraby MR, Kruger K, Opdahl S, Vatten LJ, Akslen LA, Bofin AM. Microvascular proliferation in luminal A and basal-like breast cancer subtypes. J Clin Pathol. 2015;68(11):891–7.

57. Ribeiro-Silva A, Ribeiro do Vale F, Zucoloto S. Vascular endothelial growth factor expression in the basal subtype of breast carcinoma. Am J Clin Pathol. 2006;125(4):512–8.

58. Morabito A, Sarmiento R, Bonginelli P, Gasparini G. Antiangiogenic strategies, compounds, and early clinical results in breast cancer. Crit Rev Oncol Hematol. 2004;49(2):91–107.

59. Gravdal K, Halvorsen OJ, Haukaas SA, Akslen LA. Proliferation of immature tumor vessels is a novel marker of clinical progression in prostate cancer. Cancer Res. 2009;69(11):4708–15.

60. Borretzen A, Gravdal K, Haukaas SA, Mannelqvist M, Beisland C, Akslen LA, et al. The epithelial-mesenchymal transition regulators Twist, Slug, and Snail are associated with aggressive tumour features and poor outcome in prostate cancer patients. J Pathol Clin Res. 2021;7(3):253–70.

61. Kruger K, Stefansson IM, Collett K, Arnes JB, Aas T, Akslen LA. Microvessel proliferation by co-expression of endothelial nestin and Ki-67 is associated with a basal-like phenotype and aggressive features in breast cancer. Breast. 2013;22(3):282–8.

62. Haldorsen IS, Stefansson I, Gruner R, Husby JA, Magnussen IJ, Werner HM, et al. Increased microvascular proliferation is negatively correlated to tumour blood flow and is associated with unfavourable outcome in endometrial carcinomas. Br J Cancer. 2014;110(1):107–14.

63. Stefansson IM, Raeder M, Wik E, Mannelqvist M, Kusonmano K, Knutsvik G, et al. Increased angiogenesis is associated with a

32-gene expression signature and 6p21 amplification in aggressive endometrial cancer. Oncotarget. 2015;6(12):10634–45.

64. Vincenti V, Cassano C, Rocchi M, Persico G. Assignment of the vascular endothelial growth factor gene to human chromosome 6p21.3. Circulation. 1996;93(8):1493–5.

65. Jain RK. Molecular regulation of vessel maturation. Nat Med. 2003;9(6):685–93.

66. Lindblom P, Gerhardt H, Liebner S, Abramsson A, Enge M, Hellstrom M, et al. Endothelial PDGF-B retention is required for proper investment of pericytes in the microvessel wall. Genes Dev. 2003;17(15):1835–40.

67. Gerhardt H, Betsholtz C. Endothelial-pericyte interactions in angiogenesis. Cell Tissue Res. 2003;314(1):15–23.

68. Dvorak HF. Tumors: wounds that do not heal. Similarities between tumor stroma generation and wound healing. N Engl J Med. 1986;315(26):1650–9.

69. Morikawa S, Baluk P, Kaidoh T, Haskell A, Jain RK, McDonald DM. Abnormalities in pericytes on blood vessels and endothelial sprouts in tumors. Am J Pathol. 2002;160(3):985–1000.

70. Benjamin LE, Golijanin D, Itin A, Pode D, Keshet E. Selective ablation of immature blood vessels in established human tumors follows vascular endothelial growth factor withdrawal. J Clin Invest. 1999;103(2):159–65.

71. Jain RK. Normalizing tumor vasculature with anti-angiogenic therapy: a new paradigm for combination therapy. Nat Med. 2001;7(9):987–9.

72. Jain RK. Normalization of tumor vasculature: an emerging concept in antiangiogenic therapy. Science. 2005;307(5706):58–62.

73. Willett CG, Boucher Y, di Tomaso E, Duda DG, Munn LL, Tong RT, et al. Direct evidence that the VEGF-specific antibody bevacizumab has antivascular effects in human rectal cancer. Nat Med. 2004;10(2):145–7.

74. Gee MS, Procopio WN, Makonnen S, Feldman MD, Yeilding NM, Lee WM. Tumor vessel development and maturation impose limits on the effectiveness of anti-vascular therapy. Am J Pathol. 2003;162(1):183–93.

75. Baluk P, Hashizume H, McDonald DM. Cellular abnormalities of blood vessels as targets in cancer. Curr Opin Genet Dev. 2005;15(1):102–11.

76. Winkler F, Kozin SV, Tong RT, Chae SS, Booth MF, Garkavtsev I, et al. Kinetics of vascular normalization by VEGFR2 blockade governs brain tumor response to radiation: role of oxygenation, angiopoietin-1, and matrix metalloproteinases. Cancer Cell. 2004;6(6):553–63.

77. Kakolyris S, Giatromanolaki A, Koukourakis M, Leigh IM, Georgoulias V, Kanavaros P, et al. Assessment of vascular maturation in non-small cell lung cancer using a novel basement membrane component, LH39: correlation with p53 and angiogenic factor expression. Cancer Res. 1999;59(21):5602–7.

78. Kakolyris S, Fox SB, Koukourakis M, Giatromanolaki A, Brown N, Leek RD, et al. Relationship of vascular maturation in breast cancer blood vessels to vascular density and metastasis, assessed by expression of a novel basement membrane component, LH39. Br J Cancer. 2000;82(4):844–51.

79. Wesseling P, Vandersteenhoven JJ, Downey BT, Ruiter DJ, Burger PC. Cellular components of microvascular proliferation in human glial and metastatic brain neoplasms. A light microscopic and immunohistochemical study of formalin-fixed, routinely processed material. Acta Neuropathol. 1993;85(5):508–14.

80. Rojiani AM, Dorovini-Zis K. Glomeruloid vascular structures in glioblastoma multiforme: an immunohistochemical and ultrastructural study. J Neurosurg. 1996;85(6):1078–84.

81. Pettersson A, Nagy JA, Brown LF, Sundberg C, Morgan E, Jungles S, et al. Heterogeneity of the angiogenic response induced in different normal adult tissues by vascular permeability factor/vascular endothelial growth factor. Lab Invest. 2000;80(1):99–115.

82. Sundberg C, Nagy JA, Brown LF, Feng D, Eckelhoefer IA, Manseau EJ, et al. Glomeruloid microvascular proliferation follows adenoviral vascular permeability factor/vascular endothelial growth factor-164 gene delivery. Am J Pathol. 2001;158(3):1145–60.

83. Brat DJ, Van Meir EG. Glomeruloid microvascular proliferation orchestrated by VPF/VEGF: a new world of angiogenesis research. Am J Pathol. 2001;158(3):789–96.

84. Schiffer D, Bosone I, Dutto A, Di Vito N, Chio A. The prognostic role of vessel productive changes and vessel density in oligodendroglioma. J Neurooncol. 1999;44(2):99–107.

85. Tsai CY, Lai CH, Chan HL, Kuo T. Glomeruloid hemangioma--a specific cutaneous marker of POEMS syndrome. Int J Dermatol. 2001;40(6):403–6.

86. Ohtani H. Glomeruloid structures as vascular reaction in human gastrointestinal carcinoma. Jpn J Cancer Res. 1992;83(12):1334–40.

87. Blaker H, Dragoje S, Laissue JA, Otto HF. Pericardial involvement by thymomas. Entirely intrapericardial thymoma and a pericardial metastasis of thymoma with glomeruloid vascular proliferations. Pathol Oncol Res. 1999;5(2):160–3.

88. Dargent JL, Lespagnard L, Verdebout JM, Bourgeois P, Munck D. Glomeruloid microvascular proliferation in angiomyomatous hamartoma of the lymph node. Virchows Arch. 2004;445(3):320–2.

89. Lyons LL, North PE, Mac-Moune Lai F, Stoler MH, Folpe AL, Weiss SW. Kaposiform hemangioendothelioma: a study of 33 cases emphasizing its pathologic, immunophenotypic, and biologic uniqueness from juvenile hemangioma. Am J Surg Pathol. 2004;28(5):559–68.

90. Brat DJ, Castellano-Sanchez A, Kaur B, Van Meir EG. Genetic and biologic progression in astrocytomas and their relation to angiogenic dysregulation. Adv Anat Pathol. 2002;9(1):24–36.

91. Dvorak HF. Vascular permeability factor/vascular endothelial growth factor: a critical cytokine in tumor angiogenesis and a potential target for diagnosis and therapy. J Clin Oncol. 2002;20(21):4368–80.

92. Tanaka F, Oyanagi H, Takenaka K, Ishikawa S, Yanagihara K, Miyahara R, et al. Glomeruloid microvascular proliferation is superior to intratumoral microvessel density as a prognostic marker in non-small cell lung cancer. Cancer Res. 2003;63(20):6791–4.

93. Hoem D, Straume O, Immervoll H, Akslen LA, Molven A. Vascular proliferation is associated with survival in pancreatic ductal adenocarcinoma. APMIS. 2013;121(11):1037–46.

94. Straume O, Akslen LA. Increased expression of VEGF-receptors (FLT-1, KDR, NRP-1) and thrombospondin-1 is associated with glomeruloid microvascular proliferation, an aggressive angiogenic phenotype, in malignant melanoma. Angiogenesis. 2003;6(4):295–301.

95. Foulkes WD, Brunet JS, Stefansson IM, Straume O, Chappuis PO, Begin LR, et al. The prognostic implication of the basal-like (cyclin E high/p27 low/p53+/glomeruloid-microvascular-proliferation+) phenotype of BRCA1-related breast cancer. Cancer Res. 2004;64(3):830–5.

96. Goffin JR, Straume O, Chappuis PO, Brunet JS, Begin LR, Hamel N, et al. Glomeruloid microvascular proliferation is associated with p53 expression, germline BRCA1 mutations and an adverse outcome following breast cancer. Br J Cancer. 2003;89(6):1031–4.

97. van't Veer LJ, Dai H, van de Vijver MJ, He YD, Hart AA, Mao M, et al. Gene expression profiling predicts clinical outcome of breast cancer. Nature. 2002;415(6871):530–6.

98. Greenblatt MS, Chappuis PO, Bond JP, Hamel N, Foulkes WD. TP53 mutations in breast cancer associated with BRCA1 or BRCA2 germ-line mutations: distinctive spectrum and structural distribution. Cancer Res. 2001;61(10):4092–7.

99. Kawai H, Li H, Chun P, Avraham S, Avraham HK. Direct interaction between BRCA1 and the estrogen receptor regulates vascular endothelial growth factor (VEGF) transcription and secretion in breast cancer cells. Oncogene. 2002;21(50):7730–9.

100. Zhang L, Yu D, Hu M, Xiong S, Lang A, Ellis LM, et al. Wild-type p53 suppresses angiogenesis in human leiomyosarcoma and synovial sarcoma by transcriptional suppression of vascular endothelial growth factor expression. Cancer Res. 2000;60(13):3655–61.

101. Pore N, Liu S, Shu HK, Li B, Haas-Kogan D, Stokoe D, et al. Sp1 is involved in Akt-mediated induction of VEGF expression through an HIF-1-independent mechanism. Mol Biol Cell. 2004;15(11):4841–53.

102. Ravi R, Mookerjee B, Bhujwalla ZM, Sutter CH, Artemov D, Zeng Q, et al. Regulation of tumor angiogenesis by p53-induced degradation of hypoxia-inducible factor 1alpha. Genes Dev. 2000;14(1):34–44.

103. Sherif ZA, Nakai S, Pirollo KF, Rait A, Chang EH. Downmodulation of bFGF-binding protein expression following restoration of p53 function. Cancer Gene Ther. 2001;8(10):771–82.

104. Dameron KM, Volpert OV, Tainsky MA, Bouck N. Control of angiogenesis in fibroblasts by p53 regulation of thrombospondin-1. Science. 1994;265(5178):1582–4.

105. Schuster C, Akslen LA, Straume O. Expression of Heat Shock Protein 27 in Melanoma Metastases Is Associated with Overall Response to Bevacizumab Monotherapy: Analyses of Predictive Markers in a Clinical Phase II Study. PLoS One. 2016;11(5):e0155242.

106. Sharma S, Sharma MC, Sarkar C. Morphology of angiogenesis in human cancer: a conceptual overview, histoprognostic perspective and significance of neoangiogenesis. Histopathology. 2005;46(5):481–9.

107. Giatromanolaki A, Sivridis E, Koukourakis MI. Tumour angiogenesis: vascular growth and survival. APMIS. 2004;112(7-8):431–40.

108. Weyn B, Tjalma WA, Vermeylen P, van Daele A, Van Marck E, Jacob W. Determination of tumour prognosis based on angiogenesis-related vascular patterns measured by fractal and syntactic structure analysis. Clin Oncol (R Coll Radiol). 2004;16(4):307–16.

109. Favier J, Plouin PF, Corvol P, Gasc JM. Angiogenesis and vascular architecture in pheochromocytomas: distinctive traits in malignant tumors. Am J Pathol. 2002;161(4):1235–46.

110. Chi JT, Chang HY, Haraldsen G, Jahnsen FL, Troyanskaya OG, Chang DS, et al. Endothelial cell diversity revealed by global expression profiling. Proc Natl Acad Sci U S A. 2003;100(19):10623–8.

111. Ruoslahti E. Targeting tumor vasculature with homing peptides from phage display. Semin Cancer Biol. 2000;10(6):435–42.

112. Ruoslahti E. Vascular zip codes in angiogenesis and metastasis. Biochem Soc Trans. 2004;32(Pt3):397–402.

113. Laakkonen P, Akerman ME, Biliran H, Yang M, Ferrer F, Karpanen T, et al. Antitumor activity of a homing peptide that targets tumor lymphatics and tumor cells. Proc Natl Acad Sci U S A. 2004;101(25):9381–6.

114. St Croix B, Rago C, Velculescu V, Traverso G, Romans KE, Montgomery E, et al. Genes expressed in human tumor endothelium. Science. 2000;289(5482):1197–202.

115. Fonsatti E, Altomonte M, Nicotra MR, Natali PG, Maio M. Endoglin (CD105): a powerful therapeutic target on tumor-associated angiogenetic blood vessels. Oncogene. 2003;22(42):6557–63.

116. Kumar S, Ghellal A, Li C, Byrne G, Haboubi N, Wang JM, et al. Breast carcinoma: vascular density determined using CD105 antibody correlates with tumor prognosis. Cancer Res. 1999;59(4):856–61.

117. Tanaka F, Otake Y, Yanagihara K, Kawano Y, Miyahara R, Li M, et al. Evaluation of angiogenesis in non-small cell lung cancer: comparison between anti-CD34 antibody and anti-CD105 antibody. Clin Cancer Res. 2001;7(11):3410–5.

118. Wikstrom P, Lissbrant IF, Stattin P, Egevad L, Bergh A. Endoglin (CD105) is expressed on immature blood vessels and is a marker for survival in prostate cancer. Prostate. 2002;51(4):268–75.

119. Salvesen HB, Gulluoglu MG, Stefansson I, Akslen LA. Significance of CD 105 expression for tumour angiogenesis and prognosis in endometrial carcinomas. APMIS. 2003;111(11):1011–8.

120. Straume O, Akslen LA. Expression of vascular endothelial growth factor, its receptors (FLT-1, KDR) and TSP-1 related to microvessel density and patient outcome in vertical growth phase melanomas. Am J Pathol. 2001;159(1):223–35.

121. Brekken RA, Huang X, King SW, Thorpe PE. Vascular endothelial growth factor as a marker of tumor endothelium. Cancer Res. 1998;58(9):1952–9.

122. Koukourakis MI, Giatromanolaki A, Thorpe PE, Brekken RA, Sivridis E, Kakolyris S, et al. Vascular endothelial growth factor/KDR activated microvessel density versus CD31 standard microvessel density in non-small cell lung cancer. Cancer Res. 2000;60(11):3088–95.

123. Guddo F, Fontanini G, Reina C, Vignola AM, Angeletti A, Bonsignore G. The expression of basic fibroblast growth factor (bFGF) in tumor-associated stromal cells and vessels is inversely correlated with non-small cell lung cancer progression. Hum Pathol. 1999;30(7):788–94.

124. Gravdal K, Halvorsen OJ, Haukaas SA, Akslen LA. Expression of bFGF/FGFR-1 and vascular proliferation related to clinicopathologic features and tumor progress in localized prostate cancer. Virchows Arch. 2006;448(1):68–74.

125. Straume O, Akslen LA. Importance of vascular phenotype by basic fibroblast growth factor, and influence of the angiogenic factors basic fibroblast growth factor/fibroblast growth factor receptor-1 and ephrin-A1/EphA2 on melanoma progression. Am J Pathol. 2002;160(3):1009–19.

126. Davies G, Cunnick GH, Mansel RE, Mason MD, Jiang WG. Levels of expression of endothelial markers specific to tumour-associated endothelial cells and their correlation with prognosis in patients with breast cancer. Clin Exp Metastasis. 2004;21(1):31–7.

127. Rmali KA, Puntis MC, Jiang WG. Prognostic values of tumor endothelial markers in patients with colorectal cancer. World J Gastroenterol. 2005;11(9):1283–6.

128. Rmali KA, Watkins G, Harrison G, Parr C, Puntis MC, Jiang WG. Tumour endothelial marker 8 (TEM-8) in human colon cancer and its association with tumour progression. Eur J Surg Oncol. 2004;30(9):948–53.

129. Neri D, Bicknell R. Tumour vascular targeting. Nat Rev Cancer. 2005;5(6):436–46.

130. Sipkins DA, Cheresh DA, Kazemi MR, Nevin LM, Bednarski MD, Li KC. Detection of tumor angiogenesis in vivo by alphaVbeta3-targeted magnetic resonance imaging. Nat Med. 1998;4(5):623–6.

131. Hood JD, Cheresh DA. Targeted delivery of mutant Raf kinase to neovessels causes tumor regression. Cold Spring Harb Symp Quant Biol. 2002;67:285–91.

132. van Zijl F, Krupitza G, Mikulits W. Initial steps of metastasis: cell invasion and endothelial transmigration. Mutat Res. 2011;728(1-2):23–34.

133. Rakha EA, Martin S, Lee AH, Morgan D, Pharoah PD, Hodi Z, et al. The prognostic significance of lymphovascular invasion in invasive breast carcinoma. Cancer. 2012;118(15):3670–80.

134. Arnaout-Alkarain A, Kahn HJ, Narod SA, Sun PA, Marks AN. Significance of lymph vessel invasion identified by the endothelial lymphatic marker D2-40 in node negative breast cancer. Mod Pathol. 2007;20(2):183–91.

135. Roses DF, Bell DA, Flotte TJ, Taylor R, Ratech H, Dubin N. Pathologic predictors of recurrence in stage 1 (TINOMO) breast cancer. Am J Clin Pathol. 1982;78(6):817–20.

136. Gujam FJ, Going JJ, Mohammed ZM, Orange C, Edwards J, McMillan DC. Immunohistochemical detection improves the

prognostic value of lymphatic and blood vessel invasion in primary ductal breast cancer. BMC Cancer. 2014;14:676.

137. Chen Y, Klingen TA, Aas H, Wik E, Akslen LA. Tumor-associated lymphocytes and macrophages are related to stromal elastosis and vascular invasion in breast cancer. J Pathol Clin Res. 2021;7(5):517–27.

138. Klingen TA, Chen Y, Aas H, Wik E, Akslen LA. Tumor-associated macrophages are strongly related to vascular invasion, non-luminal subtypes, and interval breast cancer. Hum Pathol. 2017;69:72–80.

139. Pantel K, Brakenhoff RH, Brandt B. Detection, clinical relevance and specific biological properties of disseminating tumour cells. Nat Rev Cancer. 2008;8(5):329–40.

140. Woelfle U, Cloos J, Sauter G, Riethdorf L, Janicke F, van Diest P, et al. Molecular signature associated with bone marrow micrometastasis in human breast cancer. Cancer Res. 2003;63(18):5679–84.

141. Foulkes WD, Grainge MJ, Rakha EA, Green AR, Ellis IO. Tumor size is an unreliable predictor of prognosis in basal-like breast cancers and does not correlate closely with lymph node status. Breast Cancer Res Treat. 2009;117(1):199–204.

142. Holm-Rasmussen EV, Jensen MB, Balslev E, Kroman N, Tvedskov TF. Reduced risk of axillary lymphatic spread in triple-negative breast cancer. Breast Cancer Res Treat. 2015;149(1):229–36.

143. Braun S, Pantel K, Muller P, Janni W, Hepp F, Kentenich CR, et al. Cytokeratin-positive cells in the bone marrow and survival of patients with stage I, II, or III breast cancer. N Engl J Med. 2000;342(8):525–33.

144. Mannelqvist M, Stefansson IM, Bredholt G, Hellem Bo T, Oyan AM, Jonassen I, et al. Gene expression patterns related to vascular invasion and aggressive features in endometrial cancer. Am J Pathol. 2011;178(2):861–71.

145. Mannelqvist M, Wik E, Stefansson IM, Akslen LA. An 18-gene signature for vascular invasion is associated with aggressive features and reduced survival in breast cancer. PLoS One. 2014;9(6):e98787.

Molecular Phenotypes of Endothelial Cells in Malignant Tumors

3

Vladan Milosevic, Reidunn J. Edelmann,
Johanna Hol Fosse, Arne Östman, and Lars A. Akslen

Abstract

Angiogenesis is an essential process for tumor growth, progression, and metastasis, and it is one of the *hallmarks of cancer.* In addition to being structurally atypical, tumor blood vessels exhibit distinctly abnormal molecular phenotypes compared to their normal counterparts. As noticed by Aird: "The phenotypes of endothelial cells vary in structure and function, in space and time, and health and disease." The palette of tumor endothelial phenotypes results from the specific conditions that guide the formation of these vessels, including activation of specific signaling pathways and a range of environmental pressures.

The focus of this chapter is to outline the roles endothelial cells play in basic physiological and pathological processes, to provide an overview of the mechanisms of dysregulated tumor angiogenesis, and to point out well-established and some novel molecular markers and phenotypes of tumor endothelial cells. We list key experimental and clinical studies that discuss the clinical relevance of specific molecular markers in predicting prognosis and therapy response, supporting the importance of tumor-associated angiogenesis in pathological processes such as metastasis. In addition to this, we discuss novel therapeutic approaches based on exploiting the molecular specificity of tumor endothelial cells to provide selective and efficient therapies.

V. Milosevic (✉) · R. J. Edelmann · A. Östman
Department of Clinical Medicine, Centre for Cancer Biomarkers
CCBIO, University of Bergen, Bergen, Norway

Department of Oncology and Pathology, Karolinska Institutet,
Stockholm, Sweden
e-mail: v.milosevic@uib.no; reidunn.edelmann@uib.no;
arne.ostman@ki.se

J. H. Fosse
Norwegian Veterinary Institute, Ås, Norway
e-mail: johanna.hol.fosse@vetinst.no

L. A. Akslen
Centre for Cancer Biomarkers CCBIO, Department of Clinical
Medicine, University of Bergen, Bergen, Norway
e-mail: lars.akslen@uib.no

© The Author(s), under exclusive license to Springer Nature Switzerland AG 2022
L. A. Akslen, R. S. Watnick (eds.), *Biomarkers of the Tumor Microenvironment*, https://doi.org/10.1007/978-3-030-98950-7_3

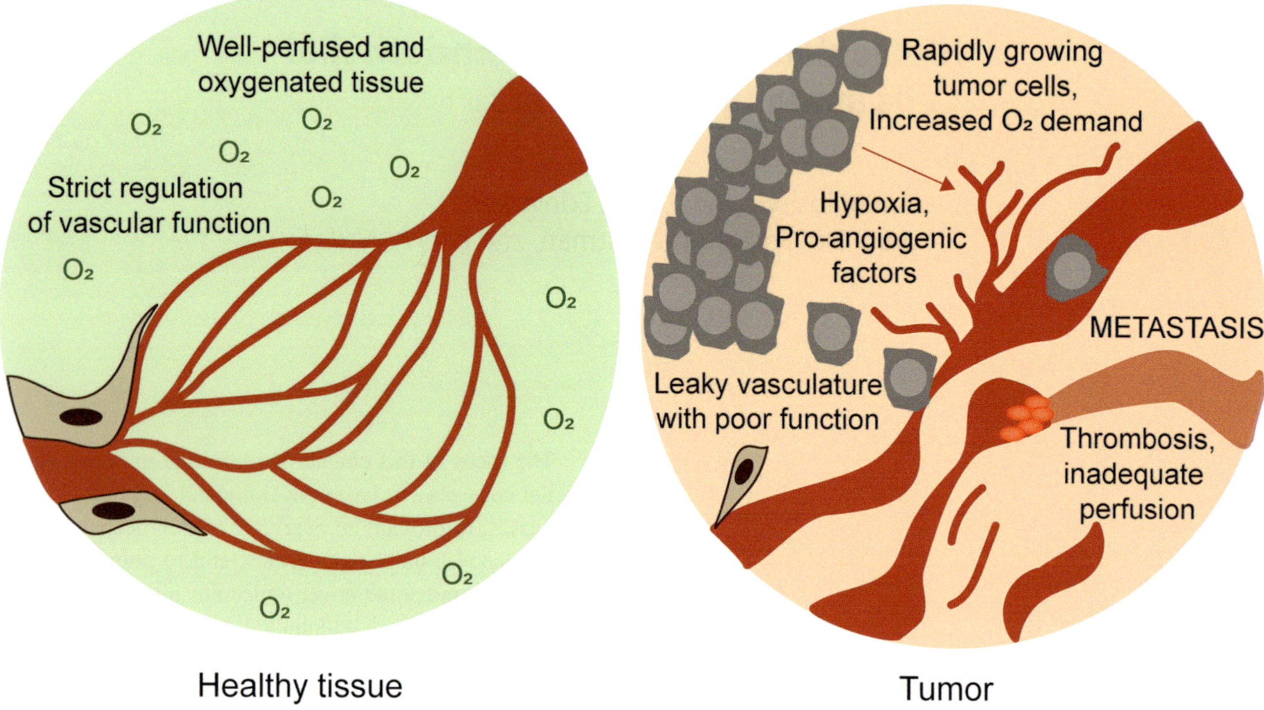

Pathological stimulation of endothelial cells in tumors induces abnormal vascular phenotypes with altered function. Molecular markers of tumor endothelial cells can aid in predicting prognosis and response to therapy in cancer

Take-Home Lessons
- Endothelial cells actively control the function of specific organs, acting as "gatekeepers" of their microenvironment
- Blood vessel formation in physiological processes results in the formation of mature and fully functional vessels
- Initiation of angiogenesis is an important requirement for tumor growth and progression
- Tumor vessels are morphologically and molecularly abnormal with significant heterogeneity

Introduction

Tumor blood vessels display markedly abnormal phenotypes and are molecularly distinct from normal blood vessels. Under healthy conditions, endothelial cells act as gatekeepers of tissue homeostasis. They line the inner surface of all blood and lymphatic vessels, where they create a semipermeable barrier between blood or lymph and its surrounding tissues. This single cell layer is a highly metabolically active organ, and dynamic endothelial cell phenotypes constantly shift in response to cues within the extracellular environment, governing the needs of the tissues they serve. Thus, signals generated during homeostasis, hypoxia, inflammation, and repair are pivotal for the endothelial cell capacity to maintain blood fluidity, regulate blood flow and control trans-endothelial extravasation of solutes, macromolecules, hormones, and circulating immune cells. Accordingly, a growing body of evidence suggests that tumor cells and their microenvironment induce characteristic phenotypic changes in the surrounding tumor vasculature, reflected in unique gene expression profiles when compared to normal endothelial cells. However, different tumor types and stages of progression, show diverse patterns of altered gene expression, and no unique tumor endothelial marker has so far been proven to be suitable as a durable target for anticancer therapy. In recent years, novel tools have made it possible to analyze the tumor microenvironment at a much higher resolution, providing hope that the near future may bring improved prediction of therapy response and perhaps better patient outcomes.

Healthy Endothelial Cells Are Gatekeepers of Tissue Homeostasis

Endothelial Cell Phenotype Vary Across Vascular Beds, Branches, and Activation Status

The vascular network, often referred to as the vascular tree, forms a highly branched closed circulation that extends into all organs, nourishes every tissue, and provides a gateway for extravasation of fluids, solutes, macromolecules, hormones, and circulating immune cells. Microvascular beds, composed of arterioles, capillaries and postcapillary venules, make up the greatest surface of the vascular circulation. This is also where most physiological processes brought on by the endothelium occur [1], and, accordingly, where tumor-induced vascular pathology most commonly manifests.

Endothelial phenotypes change along the vascular tree, in line with the functionality of the vascular segments. Briefly, the arterial segment of the circulation is responsible for delivering nutrients and oxygen, the venous segment predominantly takes part in waste management, and the thin-walled capillary network represents the main site for exchange of gases and molecules between blood and tissues. To accommodate the different requirements imposed by these functional differences, arterial, venous, and capillary endothelial cells differ both on the structural and molecular levels [2].

The tissue microenvironment drives endothelial heterogeneity by two distinct mechanisms. Firstly, cell-derived, biochemical and biomechanical signals contribute to activation of specific genes and signaling pathways, in turn producing tissue-specific phenotypes. For example, blood pressure, blood flow, shear stress, blood-gas concentration, pH, and plasma components of arterial and venous blood are very different, all providing input that contributes to the heterogeneity of endothelial cells (EC) lining the different vascular segments. Secondly, specific traits of the microenvironment may induce epigenetic modifications in endothelial cells that cause site-specific heterogeneity [3]. Such epigenetic signatures, like those contributing to arterial or venous endothelial profiles, are generally more robust than those imposed by dynamic signals.

Structural heterogeneity can be examined by light and electron microscopy and includes variations in cellular morphology, thickness, nuclear orientation, size, surface properties, and the types of cell junctions present [2, 4]. The thickness of endothelial cells varies between 0.1 μm in capillaries and 1 μm in the aorta. Moreover, while commonly flat, endothelial cells in the high endothelial venules of secondary lymphoid organs take on a cuboidal morphology [1]. Endothelial cells tend to be larger in big veins compared to big arteries. Nuclei of endothelial cells lining big arterial vessels, like the aorta, are positioned downstream related to the blood flow, opposite from big vein vessels where endothelial nuclei are positioned upstream relative to the middle cell axis [1].

It has been already discussed that the phenotype of the endothelial cells can vary significantly between different tissue types, allowing tissue-specific endothelial cells to exert their specific functions [5, 6]. Depending on the tissue type they are isolated from, EC has been shown to respond differently to different signaling molecules. Endothelial cells isolated from different segments of the vascular tree display specific metabolic signatures and vary in their response to stimulation. In one study, endothelial cells isolated from coronary arteries, coronary veins, and the capillary network showed different capabilities to produce prostaglandins [2, 7]. Another study from Johnson et al. [2, 8] found significantly higher angiotensin converting enzyme activity in endothelial cells isolated from the arterial wall than in venous endothelial cells. Conversely, endothelial cells isolated from large veins produced significantly more tissue plasminogen activator (t-PA) compared to endothelial cells from arteries. Differences have been noted in the endothelial response to vasoactive molecules and inflammatory cytokines [2], with a more intense response being observed in postcapillary venules, in line with their prominent function in tissue leukocyte recruitment.

In addition to the variation found along the vascular tree, endothelial phenotypes also vary between different tissues to accommodate tissue-specific vascular functions [5, 6]. Tissue-based heterogeneity is most pronounced in the capillary segment [9], and microvascular endothelial cells isolated from different anatomical sites demonstrate distinct gene expression profiles [10]. While endothelial cells in some organs, like brain, liver, and kidney, express unique sets of genes, endothelial cells in other organs, like heart and aorta, display a more generalized endothelial signature [11].

The interaction between endothelial cells and their tissue-specific microenvironment starts during development and continues throughout life in a two-way process. First, endothelial cells actively contribute to specific organ function, acting as "gatekeepers of their microenvironment" [5, 12]. Endothelial cells take active part in guiding and controlling tissue development, during the embryonic stage and postnatally, before proceeding to control tissue homeostasis and regeneration in adulthood. For example, during brain development, endothelial cells contribute to regulation of neuronal differentiation [13, 14], while in adulthood they take part in maintaining the blood–brain barrier. On the other hand, the microenvironment also provides input that shapes the colorful range of EC phenotypes.

Hence, it is not surprising that endothelial cells also differ in their response to signaling molecules, depending on their tissue of origin. For example, lung endothelial cells are highly specialized in gas exchange and at the same time assist in providing a prompt immune response, in line with their proximity to the external environment [15]. Moreover, endothelial cells in the heart muscle specialize in providing a prompt and regular supply of fatty acids required for proper cardiomyocyte metabolism [6]. In order to investigate and further understand the nature and molecular origin of tissue-specific endothelial heterogeneity, Jambusaria et al. performed a study using the RiboTag transgenic mouse model that enables direct isolation of tissue-specific ribosome-associated mRNAs from complex tissues without cell dissociation [5]. This study provided surprising insight into the molecular milieu responsible for shaping tissue-specific EC phenotypes. The analyses revealed that genes responsible for physiological processes typical for neuronal cells, such as neurotransmitter transport and axon development, were highly expressed by endothelial cells of the brain. Similarly, endothelial-enriched genes in lung tissue were related to immune function and endothelial-enriched genes in the myocardium to myofiber assembly, muscle tissue development, and myocardial contraction [5]. These findings are intriguing, because they suggest that a certain level of plasticity exists between endothelial cells and surrounding tissue-specific cell types. Another study, based on analysis of 100,000 single cells from the Tabula Muris study, also detected transcripts of hepatocyte and cardiomyocyte genes in endothelial cells of the respective organs, but found no evidence for endothelial expression of neuronal, kidney, or lung transcripts [11].

Endothelial Cells Are Essential Regulators of Vascular Function

Under physiological conditions, one of the main functions of endothelium is to form a tightly regulated barrier at the interface between the blood and the surrounding tissue. The position of endothelial cells is optimal for allowing them to respond to physical and chemical signals, either carried in the blood from distant anatomical sites or produced locally by tissue-resident cells. Activated endothelial cells produce a wide range of factors that in turn regulate vascular tone, cellular adhesion, blood fluidity, smooth muscle cell proliferation, and vessel wall inflammation and remodeling [16]. Moreover, in inflammation, endothelial cells take an active part in regulating vascular permeability and blood flow, the development of tissue edema and hyperemia, as well as tissue leukocyte recruitment [17] (Fig. 3.1).

Endothelial cells regulate blood flow in close crosstalk with vascular smooth muscle cells [18]. Importantly, they produce and secrete the vasodilators nitric oxide (NO) and

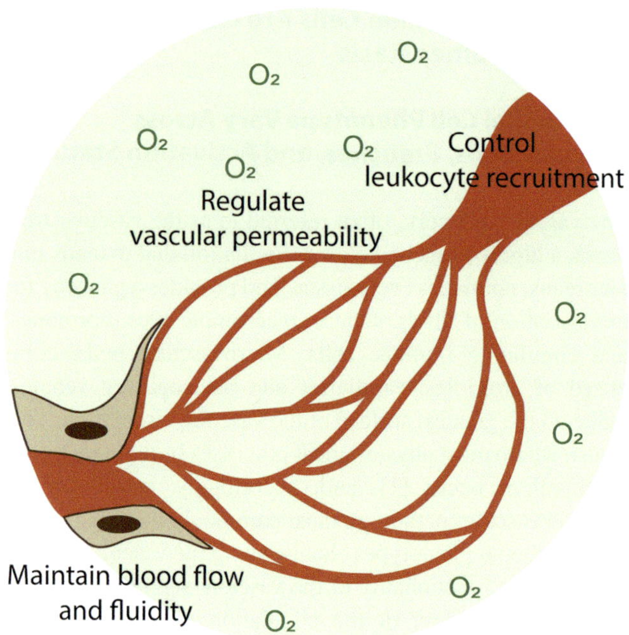

Fig. 3.1 Normal endothelial cells maintain a healthy tissue microenvironment by regulating blood flow, preventing coagulation and exerting strict control over the movement of substances and cells between blood and tissues

prostacyclin (PGI2) [19–21]. NO is released after stimulation of EC with a number of molecules, including bradykinin, angiotensin II, histamine, acetylcholine, adenine nucleotides, and arachidonic acid [22]. Apart from NO, EC also produce and secrete PGI2 that also causes relaxation of underlying smooth muscle cells [23]. In addition to mediating vasodilation, EC also play an active role in the opposing process of vasoconstriction through the synthesis of molecules with vasoconstrictor activity, including angiotensin II, endothelins, prostaglandin H2, thromboxane A2, and reactive oxygen species [24–26].

Endothelial cells also secrete a number of molecules, including NO and PGI2, that contribute to maintaining the balance between coagulation and anticoagulation. Both NO and PGI2 are major anticoagulatory signaling factors that exert their function by increasing cAMP levels in platelets to prevent their aggregation [27, 28]. Another anticoagulatory pathway supported by endothelial cells is the protein C/protein S pathway, initiated by the interaction between thrombomodulin (receptor on the surface of EC) and thrombin with the consequent activation of protein C. Protein C consequently inactivates coagulation factors VIIIa and Va [29].

Healthy endothelial cells also contribute to innate immune responses that protect the body from invading microorganisms and tissue damage. Inflammatory activated endothelial cells mount an efficient response that facilitates elimination of the underlying cause of inflammation. For example, stimulation by hypoxia activated thrombocytes or histamine induces the release of endothelial Weibel Palade bodies. These storage granules contain preformed von Willebrand factor (VWF) that induces a pro-coagulant state, as well as membrane-bound P-selectin and platelet activating factor that allows neutrophils recruitment within minutes [30, 31]. Furthermore, inflammatory signaling molecules and pathogen-associated molecules, such as inflammatory cytokines and endotoxin, induce and upregulate the expression of inflammatory molecules that further drives the endothelial phenotype toward efficient leukocyte recruitment, vascular leakiness and thrombus formation. Additionally, with production and secretion of the chemokines, endothelial cells play an important roles in trafficking dendritic cells and T cells. Namely, endothelial cells are capable of producing and secreting CCL5, also known by the acronym RANTES (Regulated on Activation, Normal T Expressed and Secreted), which is a very powerful T cell attractant [32, 33]. Additionally, activated endothelial cells are capable of synthetizing and secreting CCL21 which directly stimulates chemotactic migration of dendritic cells [33, 34]. Heparin sulfate is another molecule produced by endothelial cells which contributes to trafficking of both dendritic and T cells [33]. Activated endothelial cells express on their surface adhesion molecules, such as E-selectin, vascular cell-adhesion molecule 1 (VCAM1), and intercellular adhesion molecule 1 (ICAM1), well-known for their importance in binding and redirecting of immune cells [35]. This pro-inflammatory state facilitates the efficient elimination of invading microbes and damaged cells and tissues. However, if excessive or prolonged, it may detrimentally affect tissue function. Hence, endothelial cells have also developed mechanisms to limit inflammation and promote resolution. For example, in viral infections, endothelial sphingosine-1-phosphate-receptor signaling protects against cytokine storm and related mortality [36]. Endothelial cells also take part in crosstalk with other cell types and influence their response to stimuli. For example, in ischemia, endothelial cells secrete factors that stimulate macrophage polarization toward a phenotype that promotes tissue repair rather than inflammation [37].

Tumor Vasculature Is Dysfunctional and Contributes to Pathological Conditions

Tumor Blood Vessels Display Abnormal Phenotypes and Are Structurally Different from Normal Vessels

As a distorted reflection of their functions in maintaining tissue homeostasis in health and during infections, endothelial cells also play an important role in malignant processes. The vasculature in solid tumors is morphologically and physiologically abnormal, and this contributes to cancer cell extravasation and metastatic processes [38] (Fig. 3.2).

Fig. 3.2 Tumor endothelial cells are dysfunctional and contribute to microenvironment that affects tumor growth

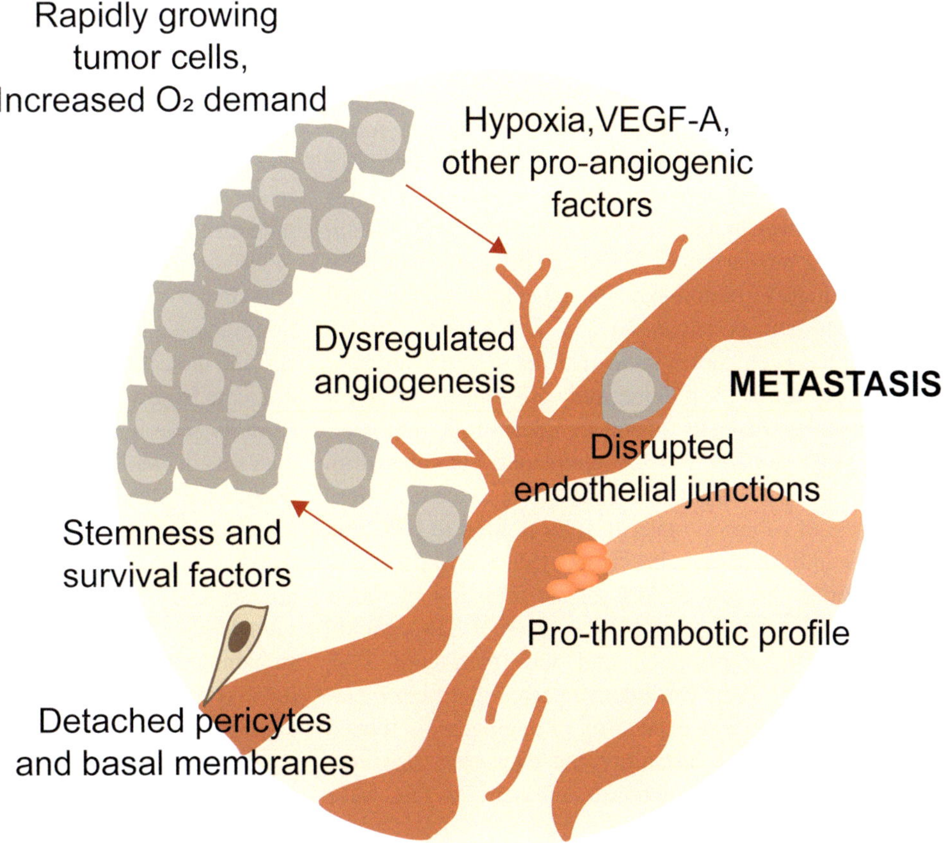

Blood vessel formation in physiological processes, such as embryonic development, growth, and wound healing, is a strictly controlled physiological process, which results in the formation of mature and fully functional vessels. This fine-tuned regulatory machinery is disrupted in tumors, due to the persisting presence of proangiogenic factors. One of these is VEGFA, a key driver of the abnormal tumor endothelial phenotype [39]. In this context, excessive VEGF signaling loosens the tight junctions between endothelial cells, inducing dysfunctional activation and vascular leakiness. Over time, the strong proangiogenic profile of the tumor microenvironment leads to the formation of aberrant and immature vasculature. Newly formed tumor vessels may fail to mature, and the clear distinction between arterioles, capillaries, and venules might be lost. Because of this dysregulation, tumor vessels are typically tortuous and branch irregularly in a dysfunctional network, often with the consequence of disordered blood flow [40–42]. This again results in poor perfusion and hypoxic areas within the tumor mass [43–46]. Although most tumors are densely vascularized, the malfunctional vasculature means that they are also usually hypoxic and nutrient-deprived [47], resulting in a vicious cycle that reinforces the proangiogenic microenvironment.

Tumor vasculature is morphologically and physiologically abnormal which contributes to cancer cell extravasation and metastatic process [38]. What is being observed in the tumor vasculature is that VEGF signaling causes loosening of the tight junctions between EC and makes such blood vessel prone to leakage. With addition of high interstitial fluid pressure and lack of pericyte lining, cancer cells are easily shad in the vasculature [48]. In addition to these mechanical shading mechanisms, it has been shown that EC can actively promote metastasis by secreting specific molecules and activating specific molecular pathways [38]. For example, it has been demonstrated that activation of Notch signaling pathway in tumor endothelial cells (TEC) contributes to inducing stemness in cancer cells together with inducing higher tumorogenicity, chemoresistance, and higher metastatic potential [49–55]. TEC secrete chemokines that has been known to be involved in tumor progression and metastasis [38]. In the study of Yadav et al. [56], it has been shown that TEC play a significant role in protecting CTC from anoikis. Namely, circulating TEC present in the cancer patients' circulation have been reported to express high levels of adhesion molecules which bind to CTC and protect them from undergoing anoikis [56–58]. Maishi et al. have reported the role of TEC in the initiation of tumor metastasis [59]. They isolated two types of TEC, highly metastatic TEC (HM-TEC) and low metastatic TEC (LM-TEC) [60]. Their work demonstrated that high metastatic TEC have higher expression of angiogenesis related genes, higher genetic instability and they exert stem-like properties. They further demonstrated that HM-TEC have higher ability to attract and adhere to CTC when compared to LM-TEC and normal EC. HM-TEC had upregulated biglycan which has been suggested as a key molecule on TEC, that is enabling tumor cells to get through the vessel barrier into the circulation. In addition, biglicans are proved to be capable of binding to the toll-like receptor 2 (TLR2) and toll-like receptor 4 (TLR4) on tumor cells causing activation of NF-κB and ERK signaling and consequently unleashing their migratory potential [38]. In another study of Branco-Price et al. from 2012, it has been discussed the importance of hypoxia inducible transcription factors in regulation of metastatic processes. They concluded that the loss of HIF-1α in endothelial cells leads to reduction of NO synthesis, which consequently suppresses the migration of tumor cells through the endothelium and prevents metastasis. In the contrary of the loss of HIF-2α which has an opposite effect thus supporting the metastatic process [61].

Molecular Signatures of Tumor Endothelial Cells

Molecular Signatures and Markers of Tumor Endothelial Cells Are Heterogeneous

The structural differences between normal and tumor endothelial cells are reflected by distinct molecular characteristics [62–67]. As discussed in the previous section, both the tumor microenvironment and the range of mechanisms used by tumors to satisfy their needs for nutrients and oxygen exert pressure on endothelial cells. This influences endothelial gene expression and induces a range of variations from the normal endothelial profile. Furthermore, the transcriptional and molecular signatures of tumor endothelial cells differ in relation to tumor type, anatomical localization, different pathohistological stages, and even between different blood vessels in the same tumor [68, 69]. As stated by Aird: "the phenotypes of endothelial cells vary in structure and function, in space and time, and in health and disease" [3]. The specific molecular traits that make up this heterogeneity may either be triggered by the pathological process itself or arise from its underlying cause [70]. In this section, we will discuss specific molecular markers arising from different tumor endothelial phenotypes. Many of these molecular markers are also expressed by normal endothelial cells, where they take part in physiological processes, including development, angiogenesis, survival, and extracellular matrix (ECM) remodeling. Other markers suggest the presence of specific subpopulations, like endothelial progenitors or tumor cells involved in vascular mimicry. Finally, the expression level of pan-endothelial marker genes can be measured to indicate the fraction of endothelial cells and therefore the vascular density of a tumor [71].

Over the past few decades, many different methods have been used to discover and validate novel tumor endothelial markers. The range of tools includes histological studies, targeted techniques like immunostaining, flow cytometry and cell sorting by flow-assisted and magnetic techniques, experiments in cell culture and unbiased transcriptomic and proteomic analyses, including serial analysis of gene expression and, more recently, single cell transcriptomics. In the case of antibody-based imaging, the introduction of digital image analysis and digital scoring methods have improved quantitation and eliminated the subjectivity of manual analyses [72]. In this section, we will discuss a range of studies undertaken to reveal specific tumor endothelial signatures that could be used as prognostic and predictive markers.

Markers of Endothelial Progenitor Cells

Tumors are capable of recruiting the endothelial progenitor cells (EPC) from the bone marrow and guide their differentiation into mature endothelial cells [69]. The first identification of putative EPC was in 1997 by Asahara et al. [73]. Using two antigens (CD34 and the VEGF receptor Flk-1) shared between angioblasts and hematopoietic stem cells, the authors isolated putative angioblasts from peripheral blood. Both C34 and Flk-1 are expressed by all hematopoietic stem cells but are lost during differentiation of the hematopoietic lineages while remaining present in most adult EC. CD34+/Flk-1+ cells were isolated from the human peripheral blood using antibody-coated magnetic beads and then cultured in vitro using collagen and fibronectin-coated dishes [73]. Following this, further characterization of EPC was done by other authors. Yin et al. in 1997 in their study were using peripheral and umbilical cord blood, fetal liver and fetal and adult bone marrow from which they isolated CD34 positive cells and performed in vitro colony assays and in vivo engraftment assays. They recognized AC133 as a novel hematopoietic stem cell marker present on EPC but not on mature EC [74]. This was in concordance with Peichev et al., who demonstrated that a small subpopulation of CD34 cells isolated from umbilical cord blood and fetal liver using MACS immunomagnetic technique, express both AC133 and VEGFR-2. When they cultured these cells in the presence of VEGF, FGF-2, and collagen, EPC cells differentiated into AC133-/VEGFR-2+ mature EC [75]. In more recent years, the study by Romagnani et al. used CD14+ cells isolated from peripheral blood, and by using highly sensitive antibody-conjugated magnetofluorescent liposomes (ACMFL) technique, the authors concluded that almost all CD14+ cell from the bone marrow were also CD34low cells.

These double positive CD14+/CD34low cells express other embryonic stemness markers such as Nanog and Oct-4 [76]. The idea of EPC generated in the bone marrow, being capable of entering circulation and taking part in neovascularization, was confirmed in human, dog, and mouse transplantation model studies of Shi et al; Asahara et al.; Lin et al.; and Kalka et al. [77–81]. Therefore, EPCs are usually characterized by the expression of vascular markers such as CD14, CD34, CD133, VEGFR1, Tie-2 (endothelial tyrosine kinase receptor), but also Oct-4 and Nanog. Additionally, they are characterized by the ability to uptake low-density lipoproteins and to bind ulex-lectin [69, 76, 82]. EPC's role in tumor vascularization has been confirmed in a study by Asahara et al. from 1999, where the authors used mice that were subjected to bone marrow transplantation from transgenic mice constitutively expressing β- galactosidase gene regulated by an EC specific promoter. These mice were then inoculated with murine colon cancer cells and 3 weeks later, histological examination of the developed tumors has shown Lac-Z positive cells both in the tumor mass and integrated into the endothelium layer of tumor vessels [77, 78]. In years to come, there were multiple efforts to use circulating endothelial cells (CEC) as markers [83]. This idea was supported by numerous studies discussed in Bertolini et al. [84] where a number of approaches have been suggested (flow cytometry, positive enrichment using immunobeads, etc.) in order to follow the kinetics, number, and viability of CEC and CEP. These parameters have been recognized to correlate with the clinical outcome and prognosis in cancer patients receiving anti-angiogenic therapy [84]. Because there is still no perfect single marker identified as being suitable for this purpose, multiparametric single cell analysis is needed at this point. In 2010, the predictive value of CEC in colorectal cancer patients, undergoing bevacizumab-based combination therapy, has been confirmed in a study by Ronzoni et al. [85], where CEC levels in circulation correlated with the therapy response. In a study by Mehran et al. from 2014, an attempt has been made to identify the tumor specific CEC by observing tumor specific endothelial markers on their surface (TEM7/8), first in preclinical cancer models and afterwards in patients with esophageal and non-small cell lung cancer. They observed that CEC levels decreased after tumor resection [86]. Following this, there was another study from 2016 by Cima et al., where they reported identification of tumor-derived circulating endothelial cell clusters in early stage colorectal cancer patients, suggesting their use as non-invasive screening for colorectal cancer [87]. A study from 2017 by Rahbari et al. suggested that CEC are of higher prognostic value when detected in blood of patients suffering from metastatic colorectal cancer than detection of CTC [88] (Fig. 3.3).

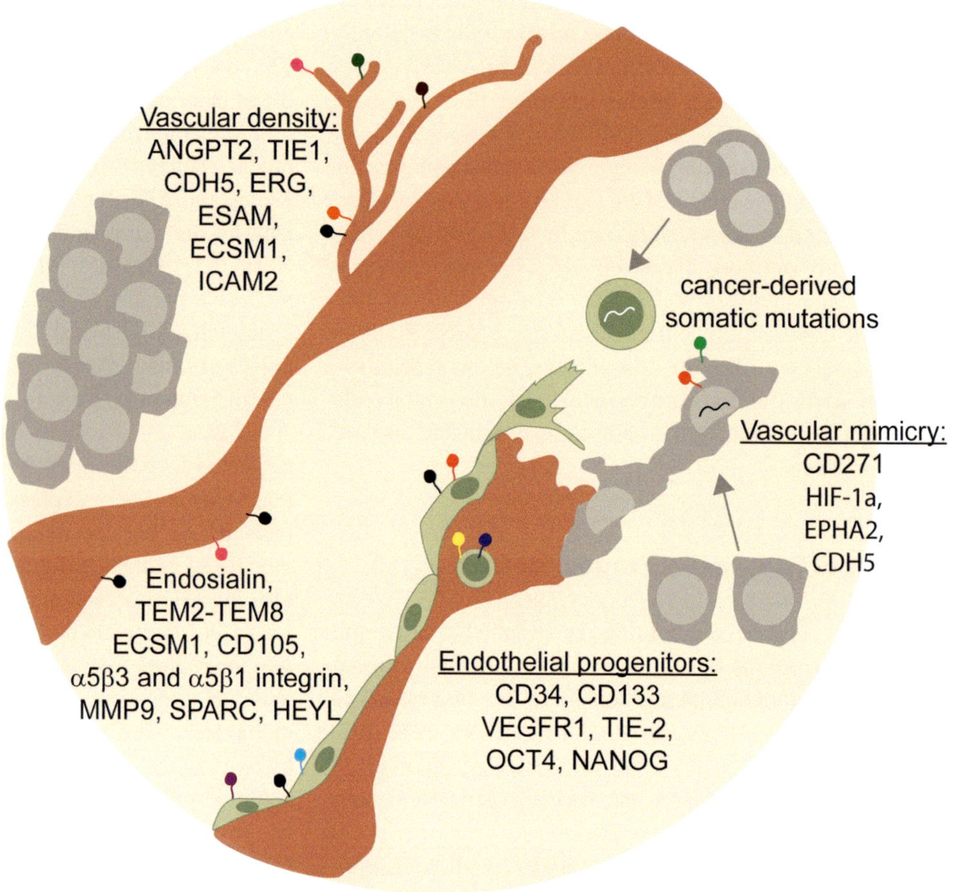

Fig. 3.3 Tumor endothelial cells display a range of molecular markers that can be used to characterize the tumor and predict prognosis and therapy response (endothelial cells in green, tumor cells in grey)

Markers of Vascular Mimicry

Vascular mimicry (VM) is a strategy mostly used by highly aggressive tumors [69, 89, 90]. In this case, tumor cells driven by hypoxia create vascular channels made of endothelial-like cancer stem cells (CSC) [89] which are capable of delivering oxygen and nutrients to the tumor tissue. There is a number of potential mechanisms that support the formation and occurrence of VM. For example, the role of EMT in VM forming cancer cells has been discussed [91]. It has been known that cells undergoing EMT lose some of the epithelial markers including α-catenin, E-cadherin, and zonula occludins-1, and at the same time they upregulated some of the mesenchymal markers, such as fibronectin, cadherin-2, vimentin, and VE-cadherin. VE-cadherin is proven to be crucial for VM formation [91]. The first identification of the vascular mimicry process goes back to 1999 by Maniotis et al. where they used tissue sections of uveal and melanoma origin to identify functional vascular-like channels, which were not giving staining for known vascular markers. They examined tissue samples histologically, using various microscopy techniques, including light and TEM microscopy for visualization of these, matrix embedded channels; and IHC panel for endothelial cell markers to confirm their phenotype as CD31, CD34, Flk-1, factor VIII, and

ulex eurapeus I lectin negative cells [92]. Further molecular characterization revealed that these specific cells express CD271 (Low-affinity Nerve Growth Factor Receptor) also known as mesenchymal stem cell marker and they often lack expression of CD31 and VWf [89, 93]. Using the Crispr/CAS9 method, the importance of VE-Cadherin in the occurrence of VM has been supported [94]. Additionally, it has been revealed that in breast cancer, these endothelial-like cells overexpress HIF1α, EphA2, and VE-cadherin [89]. Aside from this, CSC characterized by the CD44+/CD24- profile and high expression of ALDH1 has been kept accountable for regulation of vascular mimicry in triple negative breast cancer [89]. In a meta-analysis from 2013, including 22 clinical studies, Cao et al. evaluated VM as a prognostic marker in 3062 patients and across 15 malignancies, including metastatic conditions of sarcoma, liver, lung, melanoma, and colon cancers. They concluded that VM+ cancers give a poor 5-year overall survival rate when compared to VM cancers [95]. Subsequently, there were other studies where VM has been investigated from the ground of cancer differentiation and metastatic potential [96] and as an unfavorable prognostic indicator in breast cancer [97]. In 2019, Zhang et al. performed a meta-analysis study to define a prognostic value of vascular mimicry in advanced melanoma patients. The authors found a significant association between VM and poor prognosis in melanoma patients [98]. They concluded that VM status can be relied on as an accurate prognostic biomarker when diagnosed using CD31-/Pas+ IHC staining, which gives a relatively accurate VM diagnostic value of 75% sensitivity and 70% specificity, compared to the less accurate CD34-/PAS+ staining or PAS+ staining alone [98].

Markers of Endothelial Trans-differentiation

Trans-differentiation of CSC to endothelial and smooth muscle-like cells has been confirmed in many different tumor types [99–103]. These cells often carry similar somatic mutations as the accompanying tumor epithelia confirming their malignant origin [103, 104]. In an example, this process has been confirmed in glioma CD133+ stem cells cultured in endothelial promoting media. As a result glioma cancer stem cells were forming tubular structures expressing VWF, CD34, CD144, CD31, Tie-2, endothelial NOS, and VEGFR2 [104, 105]. In the study by Bussolati et al., it has been demonstrated that CD105+ cells isolated from renal carcinomas have the possibility to differentiate into VWF/KDR/VEGFR3/CD31 positive endothelial cells in vitro and in murine models [106]. CD105 showed high correlation with other prognostic factors in breast cancer when used as a neovascularization marker [107]. In the study from 2014, CD105 has been evaluated and confirmed as a potential independent predictive marker in patients with clear-cell renal cell carcinoma after resection [108]. Aomatsu et al., in the study from 2012, demonstrated the predictive value of CD133 for neoadjuvant chemotherapy in breast cancer patients [109]. In addition, Kim et al. in 2015 published a study where they evaluated the potential predictive value of CD133 and ALDH1 in breast cancer patients [110].

General Tumor Endothelial Markers

The first observation of molecular heterogeneity in TEC was in 1992 when endosialin, also known as tumor endothelial marker (TEM) 1 or CD248, has been identified by Rettig et al. [111]. This discovery has been followed by the identification of prostate-specific membrane antigen on the membrane of TEC (normally not present on the surface of normal endothelial cells) [112]. Similar studies have revealed other TEC markers such as endothelial-specific molecule 1 (ESM1), endoglin (CD105), $\alpha v \beta 3$ and $\alpha 5 \beta 1$ integrin [113–116]. Some other reports concluded that a number of genes appear to be downregulated in TEC, like intercellular adhesion molecule 1 (ICAM-1) and CD34 [117, 118].

Using the SAGE method (serial analysis of gene expression) on endothelial cells isolated from colorectal cancer and compared with normal colon tissue as a control, St. Croix et al. in 2000 have identified a total number of 46 transcripts that are more than tenfold upregulated in TECs compared to normal colon endothelial cells. This study yielded eight new TEMs [63]. TEMs have been extensively exploited as vascular prognostic markers in various tumor tissues [119–121]. For example, high expression of TEM7 has been related to metastasis and poor survival of osteogenic sarcoma patients [122]. Even though TEM markers have been defined as specific and reliable, additional studies showed that some of these newly identified markers, even in the beginning believed to be TEC specific [111], are not specific for TEC. TEM1 (endosialin) has been proven to be expressed in some fibroblasts, perivascular cells, and developing tissues [123, 124]. Additionally, TEM7 has been identified in the brain and sarcoma cell lines [125, 126] and TEM8 has been known to be present in the vessels of developing corpus luteum [63].

Nevertheless, the importance of TEM markers and their clinical relevance has been confirmed in the following years. In a study from 2015, Zhang et al. reported TEM7 as a key prognostic marker in resectable gastric cancer [127] and in the study from 2018, Czekierdowski et al. reported a prognostic significance of TEM7 and nestin in high grade serous ovarian cancer [128]. Further, TEM8 has been reported as a relevant prognostic marker in a number of studies. Gutwein et al. discussed the relevance of TEM8 as a marker in triple negative breast cancer being consistently expressed in significantly higher amounts in tumor tissue compared to healthy controls as well as in metastatic sites. Notably, TEM8 was not heavily expressed in the tumor-associated endothelium as confirmed by dual IHC, where the TEM8-positive cells did not show co-expression with SMA, calponin, CD31, or CD34 [129]. An interesting diagnostic approach using anti-TEM8 antibody labeled with ^{89}Zr and immune-PET imaging was described by Kuo et al. in 2014 in a murine model [130]. The authors suggested that TEM8 targeted PET imaging could improve the diagnostic of angiogenic tumors, which might be susceptible to anti-TEM8 therapy. This type of PET imaging can also help in defining an appropriate therapeutic dose needed for optimal tumor uptake [130]. In the more recent study from 2020, Pietrzyk et al. concluded that TEM8 is a superior prognostic marker than the routinely used Ca 19–9 marker, exerting higher sensitivity and specificity. They were measuring serum levels of TEM8 pointing to its potential as an early diagnostic marker as well as a clinical predictor of progression and prognosis in patients suffering from colorectal cancers [131]. In addition to these studies, endoglin (CD105), another TEM marker, has been confirmed as a prognostic factor related to poor prognosis, metastasis and tumor recurrence in various cancers [132–135].

Microvascular mural cells (MMC) take part in the building of the microvasculature three together with endothelial cells. They consist of rather heterogeneous cell populations of pericytes, vascular smooth muscle cells, and intermediate cell types which are still not fully characterized [136]. These cells take part in the regulation of many biological functions but also play a major role in tumor pathology. Namely, it has been known that specific mural cells can have a particular effect on cancer therapy response and overall prognosis, the metastatic potential of the tumor and immune surveillance. Better characterization of these cells in the last few years conducted on murine metastasis models gave insights into the specific molecules and signaling pathways that can be related to "bad" versus "good" mural cell phenotypes. In an example, it has been known that mural microvascular cells expressing endosialin/CD248, KLF4, or having CD45-/VLA-1 bright phenotype are related to a higher risk of metastasis [136]. In addition to this, some studies pointed to the importance of MMC in premetastatic niches where metastasis supportive perivascular cells expressing *KLF4* gene promoted metastasis by inducing fibronectin rich microenvironment [137, 138]. Expression of PDGFRb and NG2 are suggested as markers of "good" MMC phenotypes as they have been related to increased chemosensitivity and drug efficiency, better lymphocyte infiltration and better response to immunotherapy, and being antimetastatic [139–145]. On the other side MMC expressing desmin, Rgs5 and a-SMA are correlated to higher resistance to chemotherapy, loss of immunosurveillance and resistance to angiogenic therapy. In addition to this, a-SMA together with PDGFRb has been correlated with worse prognosis in a number of different studies [72, 137, 146–150].

The SAGE method has been used in studies on many other tumors such as breast cancer, ovarian cancer, and gliomas [62, 151–154]. These studies concluded that most of the overexpressed genes were tumor specific, or they were specific to high invasiveness and higher tumor grade, and a few of them were shared between different tumor types. For example, MMP9 has been connected to both ovary cancers and breast cancers. SPARC was shared between breast, colon, and brain tumors and HEYL between breast and colon cancers [3, 155]. Nevertheless, HEYL was particularly distinct to invasive breast cancer TEC, indicating stage and tumor type specificity of TEC molecular signature [3, 155]. In one glioma study, 14 endothelial markers have been identified in the malignant brain compared to a healthy brain, further confirming the existence of a TEC-specific transcriptional profile, different from the physiological signature. This has been supplemented by demonstrating that plasmalemmal vesicle associated protein 1 (PV-1), which is usually suppressed in the blood–brain barrier (BBB), is highly expressed in high grade gliomas and that this expression pattern is governed by glioma cells implying the high specificity and importance as a novel brain TEC marker [152, 156]. In a study conducted by Seaman et al., on healthy and tumor

affected liver tissues, 13 genes were identified which were at least tenfold upregulated in malignant tissues compared to controls. Furthermore, additional studies on colorectal carcinoma, breast and ovarian cancers, confirmed the position of TEC molecular signatures being highly specific and distinct from the normal endothelial cells signature [153, 157–159].

All previous studies were generally facing the same limitations by being performed on the cell bulk which enabled discoveries of only a limited number of endothelial cell phenotypes [160–163]. Introducing robust single cell transcriptomic methods in endothelial cell studies allowed more detailed understanding of EC phenotypes and changed the perspective on tumor endothelial cells. In a study from 2020, Goveia et al. [68] described 16 previously unknown endothelial cell phenotypes in a lung tumor. The authors identified 2 novel capillary phenotypes that could be induced by cancer-derived cytokines and which were named scavenging capillaries, being characterized by upregulation of scavenging receptors (CD52, CD68) and genes related to macrophages and antigen presenting. They identified two distinct alveolar capillary EC phenotypes they named type I and type II. Type I was characterized by overexpression of endomucin (*EMCN*) and lower expression of von Willebrand factor (*VWF*) compared to type II, together with high expression of *EDNRB* and *IL1RL1*. Compared to all other clusters they identified, capillary EC expressed a signature of genes characteristic to MHC II antigen presenting cells, although they were lacking costimulatory molecules CD80 and CD86 [68]. Further, in the tumor endothelial cells, they identified tip EC (expressing high levels of tip cell marker CXCR4 and low expression of CD36, CA4, and HLA-II—capillary markers) that were expressing genes associated with migration, matrix remodeling, and VEGF signaling. Along with this, immature TEC phenotypes have been identified, similar to tip cells but characterized by overexpression of genes involved in vessel barrier integrity, vessel maturation, and Notch signaling, resembling stalk-like cells. TECs exert a specific phenotype of postcapillary veins EC (ACKR1high/VWF high) which upregulated immunomodulatory factors and ribosomal proteins corresponding to high endothelial venules in inflamed tissues including CCL14. By using CyTOF, the authors generally confirmed increased levels of capillary EC markers HLA-II and CD36 in normal EC but being downregulated in TEC [68]. The study gave some novel prognostic implications, suggesting that patients expressing high levels of gene signatures associated with angiogenic tip TEC, immature, activated postcapillary TEC or lymphatic TEC indicated worse prognosis and shorter overall survival.

Recently, in a study from 2021, Kahn et al. [71] designed a classifier for estimation of tumor vascularity that was named endothelial index (EI). In their approach, the authors used computer algorithms to correlate histological VD with mRNA expression data. The list of seven genes appearing as endothelial classifiers can quite precisely predict the VD, as confirmed in 31 different human malignancies. Genes used for this endothelial index (EI) consisted of angiopoietin 2 (*ANGPT2*), cadherin 5 (*CDH5*), ETS-related gene (*ERG*), endothelial cell selective adhesion molecule (*ESAM*), endothelial cell specific molecule 1 (*ESM1*), intracellular adhesion molecule 2 (*ICAM2*), and tyrosine kinase with immunoglobulin like domains 1 (*TIE1*). Although the EI score was very precise in estimating VD, it failed to deliver accurate prognostic information. As the authors suggest, one of the possible reasons for this is that in their study the observed 95% confidence interval (CI) was very wide when calculating the hazard ratio (HR) in relation to EI and overall survival. This observation was still in concordance with a study that pointed out the limitations of using VD alone in predicting response to anti-angiogenesis therapy [164]. Following this, the authors attempted in identifying specific signaling pathways related to variations in tumor vascularity and they focused on genes overexpressed in high EI tumors (EI score > 0.9—hypervascular tumors) and compared them with low EI tumors (EI score < 0.1—hypovascular tumors). Using EI score to stratify tumors as hyper/hypo vascularized, they concluded that VEGFA/VEGFR2 signaling is correlated to higher EI score but was not the only pathway that was strongly correlated with higher vascularization. Stratification on high versus low EI enabled them to the identification of multiple alternative signaling pathways which correlated strongly with high EI. This led to the identification of 24 hub genes in total, representing in the best manner the signaling networks of hypervascularized tumors. Using this information, the authors were able to group all tumor types they examined into six distinct vascular microenvironment signatures with specific signaling patterns. This vascular microenvironment approach was able to provide additional prognostic value beyond the use of VD and EI alone as it was based on a more robust metric of tumor–vessel signaling and mirrors comprehensive molecular and cellular interactions which are responsible for driving tumor vascularization. In the long run, this novel approach could enable more patient-oriented anti-vascular cancer therapy, with better therapy response prediction, promising the best possible results and therapy outcomes.

Tumor Endothelial-Specific Molecular Signatures and Signaling Pathways as Potential Therapeutic Targets

The Emergence of the Anti-angiogenic Therapy Concept

Cancer cells, being highly metabolically active, demand a high input of oxygen and nutrients from the blood and need to be in close proximity to the vasculature [69]. Led by this reasoning, Judah Folkman proposed the theory that the initiation of angiogenesis constitutes an important requirement for tumor growth and progression. Initial findings showed that more aggressive and quickly growing tumors are highly vascularized in comparison with less aggressive and slowly growing tumors [165]. This led Folkman to identify and isolate a tumor-derived angiogenic factor. His findings suggested that modulation of angiogenic signaling pathways to block tumor vessel formation could be a strategy to suppress tumor growth by starvation. In the following years, his work inspired many studies committed to identify and isolate tumor-derived angiogenic factors and describe their signaling pathways [166, 167]. The approval of this new family of anticancer drugs is undoubtedly one of the most important advances in the clinical oncology therapeutic approaches. Although, the high expectations has been given, these therapies often endure significant drawbacks. The first to prove the existence of VEGF independent tumors in 2003 was a study by Viloria-Petit et al. [168]. There is a number of molecules that are known to be secreted by the tumor mass and are able to promote angiogenesis. These molecules are VEGF, FGF2, angiopoietins, apelin, PDGF, and a variety of chemokines [69]. Many of these have important roles in physiological conditions. As in the beginning targeting VEGF gave promise and hope to the patients suffering from malignant diseases, very often the anti-angiogenic therapy failed to give expecting therapeutic results due to the number of mechanism tumor tissue avoid the therapeutic effect of the drugs, either by recruiting alternative ways of angiogenesis or by developing mechanism of resistance to the therapy.

As discussed above, a tumor can recruit additional tactics to fulfill its hunger for nutrients, which is even more evident when one of the angiogenesis pathways has been targeted. In addition to this, many times it is not perfectly clear if a patient expresses the specific drug target, or whether drug-target interaction will yield the desired therapeutic effect. Due to the high cost, of both drugs in use and the valuable reaction time patients and physicians have, it is of crucial importance to select and classify the patients according to their molecular signatures and identify the most fruitful molecular pathways which could be targeted. Although recent clinical trials data clearly point the value of anti-angiogenic drugs in prolonging the survival of patients, there are still challenges to meet when development of alternative therapeutic targets and their preclinical and clinical validations comes into focus [84].

VEGFR-Directed Therapies

As previously mentioned, VEGF is a well-known angiogenesis and vasculogenesis promotor both in cancer and physiological conditions. In a tumor, VEGF is often related to increased vessel density (VD), higher invasiveness and tumor progression, metastasis, and recurrence [69, 169]. VEGF is upregulated in hypoxic tumor conditions and regulates vessel formation by activation of VEGFR2 on endothelial cells [69, 170]. Activation of VEGFR2 causes the cascade of responses by various signaling pathways such as ERK and PI3K/Akt that as a consequence have endothelial cell proliferation, migration, invasion, and survival [69, 171, 172]. Endothelial invasion is regulated by expression of MMP-2, MMP-9, and urokinase plasmin activator which are helping in dissolving the basal membrane and ECM facilitating the formation of capillary sprouts [171, 173]. Dysregulated VEGF might as well play a significant role in metastasis by taking part in junctional remodeling, vascular hyperpermeability, and increased interstitial pressure which all together can allow the escape of tumor cells into the bloodstream [69, 174]. As previously mentioned, VEGF pathway has been very early recognized as an important regulator of tumor angiogenesis, and therefore efforts has been made to exploit it as antiangiogenic therapeutic target. Targeting this pathway has been looked upon as an effective approach, especially in solid tumors, as confirmed by numbers of preclinical and clinical studies [175]. This led to the development of multiple strategies to target this pathway which consists of

molecules preventing VEGF binding to the receptors (bevacizumab, pegaptanib, VEGF trap) [176–180], antibodies against VEGFR-2 (ramucirumab) [181], and molecules which can inhibit the kinase activity of VEGFR-2 consequentially blocking the VEGF signaling pathway (sunitinib, pazapanib and sorafenib) [182–187]. There are 11 different drugs approved for targeting VEGF [188]. The whole complexity of the tumor angiogenic process is still not completely understood and there are alternative pathways involved; therefore, the main difficulty in anti VEGF-VEGFR therapy is that it is not the only angiogenic pathway active in tumors (Fig. 3.4).

Other Candidate Pathways for Anti-angiogenic Drugs

FGF2, also known as basic FGF (bFGF), exerts its function by binding to FGFR and has an important role in the regulation of many physiological functions. In tumors, it can increase cell proliferation and resistance to apoptosis. By increasing invasiveness and motility of cancer cells, regulating CSC as well as governing angiogenesis, it promotes metastasis [69, 189, 190]. FGF signals in a paracrine manner. After its release into the ECM, it induces secretion of matrix

Fig. 3.4 Tumors can adapt alternative strategies to overcome insufficient perfusion and oxygenation. These include recruitment of endothelial progenitor cells from the bone marrow, vascular mimicry, and endothelial transdifferentiation of cancer stem cells. (endothelial cells in green, tumor cells in grey)

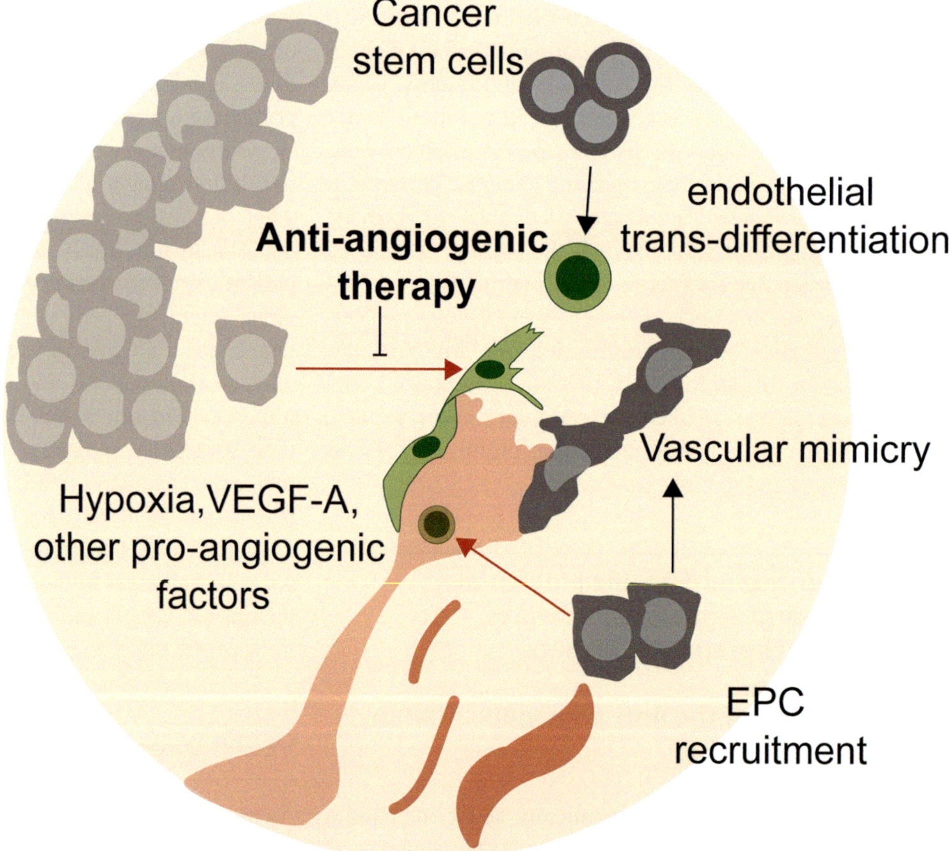

metalloproteinases (MMPs) and collagenases that cause ECM degradation. FGF also regulates endothelial metabolism through Myc-dependent glycolysis, which is proven to be essential for endothelial proliferation, sprouting, and migration [190, 191]. FGF2 can act as an alternative to VEGF orchestrated angiogenesis and a possible reason why VEGF therapies fail to give expected results, as suggested by a study where downregulation of FGF receptor restored tumor sensitivity to anti-VEGF therapies in a murine model [192] making FGF2-FGFR2 a potential therapeutic target targeting both angiogenesis and CSC [189, 193, 194]. Studies in mice were showing promising results in using combined ANGPT-2/VEGFR2 blockage, which in return slowed down the tumor growth, induced vessel normalization, and blocked macrophage recruitment consequently prolonging survival in glioma, breast cancer colorectal cancer, and renal cancer mouse models [69, 195, 196].

Ephrin signaling contributes to embryogenesis, tissue organization, cell migration, and vasculogenesis [69, 197–199]. In addition to its physiological roles, ephrin signaling has important roles in cancer angiogenesis, tumor progression, and metastasis. Dysregulation of ephrin signaling has been identified in a variety of cancers including breast, liver, brain, colon, melanoma, and prostate cancer [200–202]. The EphB2–ephB4 signaling axis was shown essential for tumor angiogenesis and progression in glioma, by altering vascular morphology, pericyte vessel coverage, and the resistance to antiangiogenic therapy [69, 203, 204]. Additionally, EphB2 signaling has been recognized as an important factor for proliferation and perivascular invasion of glioblastoma stem cells [205]. Ephrins A1/2 have been recognized as important markers of blood vessels in preclinical models of Kaposi sarcoma and breast carcinoma [201]. Their functional role and potential therapeutic target were proven by utilizing soluble EphA receptors that were able to induce a decrease of VD, reduce tumor volume, and cell proliferation [206–208].

Apelin—apelin receptor signaling increases in both endothelial cells and tumors in many malignancies. Increased expression of apelin has been shown to be a good predictor of disease progression and overall poor outcome [209–216]. Apelin expression is driven by tissue hypoxia and is known to promote tumor growth by direct stimulation of the tumor cell migration and metastasis [69, 211, 217–220]. Apelin pathway is an attractive therapeutic target, and some studies have shown usefulness in targeting apelin pathway in breast, glioma, and lung cancer, where it showed reduced tumor growth, reducing metastatic potential and improved vessel structure and function [221–223]. The study undertaken on renal cell carcinoma APLNR receptor overexpression in a group of patients was correlated with lower PD-L1 expression indicating its role in cancer immunomodulation [215].

Angiopoietins, aside from their physiological role in vasculogenesis, angiogenesis, and blood vessel remodeling, also have functions in tumor angiogenesis and tumor growth. The angiopoietin signaling pathway consists of three ligands, ANGPT-1, ANGPT-2, and ANGPT-4, which bind endothelial receptor tyrosine kinases, including TIE-1 and TIE-2 [69]. TIE-2 has an important role in both physiological and tumor processes, and its function depends on the ligand. Levels of ANGPT-2 in tumor-associated vessels increase in response to hypoxia and VEGF. Excessive ANGPT-2 has been also shown to cause decreased efficiency of anti-VEGF therapy in glioblastoma [69, 224, 225].

Tumors also adopt strategies that are not commonly part of physiological angiogenic processes to afford their increased oxygen and nutrient demands. Many tumors are capable of recruiting endothelial progenitor cells (EPC) from the bone marrow and guide their differentiation into mature endothelial cells [69]. Vascular mimicry (VM) is another tactic where the tumor cells take on the role of endothelial cells and line vascular channels [89]. Progressing along this line, cancer stem cells (CSC) can also trans-differentiate into endothelial cells and thereby take part in new vessel formation and tumor vascularization [69, 102, 226]. In addition to providing mechanisms for tumor escape from anti-angiogenic therapy, these mechanisms also add to the high endothelial molecular heterogeneity in tumors and the complexity of the molecular processes involved in tumor angiogenesis.

Vascular mimicry, aside from being an indicator of bad prognosis and bad survival, can also be exploited as a therapeutic target. Many attempts have been made to target the VM process specifically in malignant tumors. Specific therapy targeting CSC, using oncolytic measles viruses toward CD133, showed useful effects in mouse models, having potential both against vascular mimicry and endothelial trans-differentiation [227]. It has been discussed that the use of vincristine in combination with a specific inhibitor of the sarcoma family kinases could have a positive effect on inhibition of vascular mimicry. In addition to this, some other compounds have been suggested to have a positive effect on inhibition of VM, such as brucine (exerting its effect by modifying the structure of actin and tubulin), hinokitiol (governs EGFR proteasome degradation), and 6′-bis (2.3-dimethoxybenzoyl)- α,α-D-trehalose (DMBT) a derivative of brartemicin [89]. Brucin has been also reported to have a negative effect on expression of some key mediators of metastasis and VM formation such as MMP-2, MMP-9, and EpHhA2 in triple negative breast cancer cell line MDA-MB-231 [228]. In the study of Serwe et al. from 2012 has been reported the effect of flavone isoxanthohumol which was capable of decreasing the formation of VM in triple negative breast cancer cell line MDA-MB-231 cultured in Matrigel by blocking IL-4, IL-6, and IFN-γ-dependent Jak/Stat pathway [229]. Furthermore, in 2019 a study conducted by Kumar et al. on potential effect of tivantinib on VM in melanoma cell lines was presented [230]. It has been known that tivantinib targets MET and microtubule construction by affecting proteins such as vinculin and RhoC. In their study they suggest that tivantinib could target VM in melanoma, aside its already known effects on MET [230]. Specific therapeutic approach targeting VM has been undergoing clinical trials (NCT03582618). In this trial, a specific molecular compound named CVM-1118 has been used. This chemical is classified as a phenyl-quinoline derivate with reported anti-mutagenic and anti-neoplastic properties [231]. Another approach is to target the activity of FAK/y658 VE-cadherin with PF-271 which can consequently repress genes involved in VM promotion [232]. In addition to this, inhibition of VE-PTP/Tie-2 with AKB-9778 has been discussed as a way to control the VM forming capacity of pseudo endothelial cells [231, 233]. An approach for targeting pericytes has been proposed as well, where PDGFb axis is being targeted using STI-571 which has been proven efficient in vitro and in vivo in murine models [234–236].

Targeting chemokine pathways might have the potential as an anti-angiogenic treatment. It has been known that certain chemokines, such as CXCL1, CXCL2, CXCL3, CXCL5, CXCL6, CXCL7 and CXCL8, have proangiogenic effects when bound to CXCR2 receptor on TEC [237, 238]. It has been known that this effect of the CXCR2 receptor comes from the increased expression of VEGF in ovarian cancer [239]. Inhibition of this receptor has been shown to cause inhibition of angiogenesis and tumor growth in a murine model of pancreatic ductal adenocarcinoma [240]. CXCR4 is shown to be highly expressed in tumor vasculature and to promote endothelial cell sprouting [241]. IL8 or CXCL8 has been proven as a very important regulator of tumor angiogenesis, chemoresistance, and cancer stemness [242–245]. It is able to promote angiogenesis by inducing proangiogenic factors, namely VEGF, MMP-2, and MMP-9, and by governing endothelial survival [69, 246, 247]. CCL2 has been described to govern endothelial permeability and higher metastatic potential when bound to CCR2 receptor on endothelial cells [248]. Furthermore, endothelial cells expressing CCR2 can be recruited by tumor secretion of CCL2. Blocking the function of CCR2 by using its antagonist CCX872 has shown to increase the survival in Her2/neu mice models [249].

It has been demonstrated that annexin A1 and aminopeptidase—P are highly expressed in the lung cancer vasculature and therefore might be potential therapeutic targets. Furthermore, it has been demonstrated that ^{125}I labeled anti-annexin A1 antibodies accumulate in the lung tumor tissue in rats, destroying the tumor and prolonging the survival [250].

In recent years, knowledge accumulated on molecular characteristics of tumor vasculature was exploited for designing vaccines targeting specific proangiogenic antigens. This anti-angiogenic vaccination program is suggested to be undertaken along with the immunotherapy and chemotherapy. A number of antigens has been proposed to be used for the development of vaccines. VEGF being an important factor in vasculogenesis has tried to been exploited first in 2001 as reported by Wei et al. [251]. In their study they used a *Xenopus levis* VEGF DNA vaccine that showed promising results in several murine models. The first clinical trials came in 2014 as reported by Gavilondo et al. [252] where they reported a phase I clinical study (CENTAURO) on 30 patients with advanced solid tumors, using CIGB-247 vaccine which was consisting of human VEGF variant molecule together with bacterial adjuvant. This study revealed some very promising data. Namely, after 8 weeks after subcutaneous immunization and after revaccination on week 12, this vaccine showed immunogenicity in three sequential analyses of the patients' serum and neither physiological parameters have been altered by vaccination nor it has triggered the autoimmune response, giving high promises as a novel therapeutic strategy. Along with VEGF, VEGFR2 (FLK-1) has been as well exploited as a potential vaccine antigen giving promising results as reported in a number of studies [253–260]. There has been a number of attempts to exploit bFGF (FGF-2) and FGFR (CD331) in anti-angiogenic vaccine development. Recombinant protein vaccines, xenogeneic plasmid DNA vaccines, peptide vaccines with adjuvants, and liposome-based peptide vaccines have been tested in preclinical murine models [261–264]. In the study from 2004 by Plum et al. using liposome based peptide vaccine against (FGF-2), anti-angiogenic response has been reported without any adverse physiological effects [265]. In a study from 2005, McNeel et al. reported a successfully completed phase I clinical trial of monoclonal anti- αvβ3 antibody for the treatment of advanced solid tumors named MEDI-522 [266]. Endoglin, being highly expressed on the surface of TEC, has been used as a potential vaccine as an antigen on bacterial surface or oral DNA vaccine [267, 268]. There was a number of monoclonal antibodies and vaccines developed to target EGFR. Many of these are already in clinical use including monoclonal antibodies cetuximab, panitumumab, and nimotuzumab, and the small tyrosine kinase molecules erlotinib and gefitinib. A vaccine based on EGF bounded to a carrier protein from *Neisseria meningitidis*, CIMAvax® has been proven beneficial in patients with non-small-cell lung cancer and there were no adverse effects noted in postoperative wound healing [269, 270].

Concluding Remarks/Summary

With this chapter, we tried to bring closer to the reader a complex topic of molecular diversity of tumor endothelium, and a possibility to exploit specific molecular markers and signatures as prognostic and predictive indicators and therapeutic targets. It has been known that one of the hallmarks of cancer is angiogenesis. Tumors, having high metabolic demands, use angiogenesis to meet their increasing needs for oxygen and nutrients. Tumor angiogenesis leads to aberrant vessel formation and aberrant endothelial phenotypes and functions. Here, various studies have been discussed, undertaken in order to reveal specific tumor endothelial signatures, with a possibility for prognostic and predictive use. Because there is no perfect single marker that would be suitable for providing robust information on prognosis and prediction, multiparametric single cell analysis might be necessary, and some single cell studies have been discussed in this chapter. Focus has also been given to experimental and clinical studies, which all clearly point to the fact that tumor related angiogenesis is different from physiological vasculogenesis and that through all of its challenging complexity there is a possibility to exploit its diagnostic and therapeutic value. In the era of precision therapies, there is an increased importance for specific companion biomarkers in order to sort out the patients into subgroups with an aim to define responders, better select the therapeutic strategy, and increase the efficiency of treatment. Biomarkers reflecting the anti-angiogenic therapy response are of high importance. Based on specific molecular pathways, many novel therapeutic approaches have been suggested. In addition, novel vaccines have been designed targeting specific TEM proteins and have been shown to be successful in reducing tumor angiogenesis and preventing the occurrence of metastasis, while being successful in avoiding autoimmune response against normal vessels. With the development of more powerful single cell and imaging methods, we can expect to map the tumor microenvironment at a higher resolution, possibly yielding better biomarkers and better therapeutic options in the near future.

References

1. Aird WC. Phenotypic heterogeneity of the endothelium: I. Structure, function, and mechanisms. Circ Res. 2007;100(2):158–73. https://doi.org/10.1161/01.RES.0000255691.76142.4a.
2. Krüger-Genge A, et al. Vascular endothelial cell biology: an update. Int J Mol Sci. 2019;20(18):4411. https://doi.org/10.3390/ijms20184411.
3. Aird WC. Molecular heterogeneity of tumor endothelium. Cell Tissue Res. 2009;335:271–81. https://doi.org/10.1007/s00441-008-0672-y.
4. Aird WC. Endothelial cell heterogeneity. Crit Care Med. 2003;31(4 Suppl):S221–30. https://doi.org/10.1097/01.CCM.0000057847.32590.C1.
5. Jambusaria A, et al. Endothelial heterogeneity across distinct vascular beds during homeostasis and inflammation. eLife. 2020;9:e51413. https://doi.org/10.7554/eLife.51413.
6. Potente M, Mäkinen T. Vascular heterogeneity and specialization in development and disease. Nat Rev Mol Cell Biol. 2017;18(8):477–94. https://doi.org/10.1038/nrm.2017.36.
7. Gerritsen ME, Printz MP. Sites of prostaglandin synthesis in the bovine heart and isolated bovine coronary microvessels. Circ Res. 1981;49(5):1152–63. https://doi.org/10.1161/01.res.49.5.1152.
8. Johnson AR. Human pulmonary endothelial cells in culture. Activities of cells from arteries and cells from veins. J Clin Invest. 1980;65(4):841–50. https://doi.org/10.1172/JCI109736.
9. Kalucka J, et al. Single-cell transcriptome atlas of murine endothelial cells. Cell. 2020;180(4):764–779.e20. https://doi.org/10.1016/j.cell.2020.01.015.
10. Chi JT, et al. Endothelial cell diversity revealed by global expression profiling. Proc Natl Acad Sci U S A. 2003;100(19):10623–8. https://doi.org/10.1073/pnas.1434429100.
11. Paik DT, et al. Single-cell RNA sequencing unveils unique transcriptomic signatures of organ-specific endothelial cells. Circulation. 2020;142(19):1848–62. https://doi.org/10.1161/CIRCULATIONAHA.119.041433.
12. Augustin HG, Koh GY. Organotypic vasculature: from descriptive heterogeneity to functional pathophysiology. Science (New York, NY). 2017;357(6353):eaal2379. https://doi.org/10.1126/science.aal2379.
13. Bussmann J, Wolfe SA, Siekmann AF. Arterial-venous network formation during brain vascularization involves hemodynamic regulation of chemokine signaling. Development. 2011;138(9):1717–26. https://doi.org/10.1242/dev.059881.
14. Matsuoka H, et al. The retinoic acid receptor-related orphan receptor α positively regulates tight junction protein claudin domain-containing 1 mRNA expression in human brain endothelial cells. J Biochem. 2017;161(5):441–50. https://doi.org/10.1093/jb/mvw092.
15. Gillich A, et al. Capillary cell-type specialization in the alveolus. Nature. 2020;586(7831):785–9. https://doi.org/10.1038/s41586-020-2822-7.
16. Deanfield JE, Halcox JP, Rabelink TJ. Endothelial function and dysfunction: testing and clinical relevance. Circulation. 2007;115(10):1285–95. https://doi.org/10.1161/CIRCULATIONAHA.106.652859.
17. Pober JS, Sessa WC. Inflammation and the blood microvascular system. Cold Spring Harb Perspect Biol. 2014;7(1):a016345. https://doi.org/10.1101/cshperspect.a016345.
18. Michiels C. Endothelial cell functions. J Cell Physiol. 2003;196(3):430–43. https://doi.org/10.1002/jcp.10333.
19. Gori T. Endothelial function: a short guide for the interventional cardiologist. Int J Mol Sci. 2018;19(12):3838. https://doi.org/10.3390/ijms19123838.
20. Miura H, Gutterman DD. Human coronary arteriolar dilation to arachidonic acid depends on cytochrome P-450 monooxygenase and Ca2+-activated K+ channels. Circ Res. 1998;83(5):501–7. https://doi.org/10.1161/01.res.83.5.501.
21. Palmer RM, Ferrige AG, Moncada S. Nitric oxide release accounts for the biological activity of endothelium-derived relaxing factor. Nature. 1987;327(6122):524–6. https://doi.org/10.1038/327524a0.
22. Loh YC, et al. Overview of the microenvironment of vasculature in vascular tone regulation. Int J Mol Sci. 2018;19(1):120. https://doi.org/10.3390/ijms19010120.
23. Moncada S, Higgs EA, Vane JR. Human arterial and venous tissues generate prostacyclin (prostaglandin x), a potent inhibitor of platelet aggregation. Lancet. 1977;1(8001):18–20. https://doi.org/10.1016/s0140-6736(77)91655-5.
24. Chien S. Effects of disturbed flow on endothelial cells. Ann Biomed Eng. 2008;36(4):554–62. https://doi.org/10.1007/s10439-007-9426-3.
25. Garland CJ, Dora KA. EDH: endothelium-dependent hyperpolarization and microvascular signalling. Acta Physiol (Oxf). 2017;219(1):152–61. https://doi.org/10.1111/apha.12649.

26. Yanagisawa M, et al. A novel potent vasoconstrictor peptide produced by vascular endothelial cells. Nature. 1988;332(6163):411–5. https://doi.org/10.1038/332411a0.

27. Cines DB, et al. Endothelial cells in physiology and in the pathophysiology of vascular disorders. Blood. 1998;91(10):3527–61.

28. de Graaf JC, et al. Nitric oxide functions as an inhibitor of platelet adhesion under flow conditions. Circulation. 1992;85(6):2284–90. https://doi.org/10.1161/01.cir.85.6.2284.

29. Sadler JE. Thrombomodulin structure and function. Thromb Haemost. 1997;78(1):392–5.

30. Denis CV, et al. Defect in regulated secretion of P-selectin affects leukocyte recruitment in von Willebrand factor-deficient mice. Proc Natl Acad Sci U S A. 2001;98(7):4072–7. https://doi.org/10.1073/pnas.061307098.

31. Eppihimer MJ, et al. Heterogeneity of expression of E- and P-selectins in vivo. Circ Res. 1996;79(3):560–9. https://doi.org/10.1161/01.res.79.3.560.

32. Salsman VS, et al. Crosstalk between medulloblastoma cells and endothelium triggers a strong chemotactic signal recruiting T lymphocytes to the tumor microenvironment. PLoS One. 2011;6(5):e20267. https://doi.org/10.1371/journal.pone.0020267.

33. Young MR. Endothelial cells in the eyes of an immunologist. Cancer Immunol Immunother. 2012;61(10):1609–16. https://doi.org/10.1007/s00262-012-1335-0.

34. Johnson LA, Jackson DG. Inflammation-induced secretion of CCL21 in lymphatic endothelium is a key regulator of integrin-mediated dendritic cell transmigration. Int Immunol. 2010;22(10):839–49. https://doi.org/10.1093/intimm/dxq435.

35. Pober JS, Sessa WC. Evolving functions of endothelial cells in inflammation. Nat Rev Immunol. 2007;7(10):803–15. https://doi.org/10.1038/nri2171.

36. Teijaro JR, et al. Endothelial cells are central orchestrators of cytokine amplification during influenza virus infection. Cell. 2011;146(6):980–91. https://doi.org/10.1016/j.cell.2011.08.015.

37. Zhang J, et al. Endothelial lactate controls muscle regeneration from ischemia by inducing M2-like macrophage polarization. Cell Metab. 2020;31(6):1136–1153.e7. https://doi.org/10.1016/j.cmet.2020.05.004.

38. Maishi N, Hida K. Tumor endothelial cells accelerate tumor metastasis. Cancer Sci. 2017;108(10):1921–6. https://doi.org/10.1111/cas.13336.

39. Geindreau M, Ghiringhelli F, Bruchard M. Vascular endothelial growth factor, a key modulator of the anti-tumor immune response. Int J Mol Sci. 2021;22(9):4871. https://doi.org/10.3390/ijms22094871.

40. Brat DJ, Van Meir EG. Glomeruloid microvascular proliferation orchestrated by VPF/VEGF: a new world of angiogenesis research. Am J Pathol. 2001;158(3):789–96. https://doi.org/10.1016/S0002-9440(10)64025-4.

41. Nagy JA, et al. Heterogeneity of the tumor vasculature. Semin Thromb Hemost. 2010;36(3):321–31. https://doi.org/10.1055/s-0030-1253454.

42. Pettersson A, et al. Heterogeneity of the angiogenic response induced in different normal adult tissues by vascular permeability factor/vascular endothelial growth factor. Lab Invest. 2000;80(1):99–115. https://doi.org/10.1038/labinvest.3780013.

43. Baluk P, Hashizume H, McDonald DM. Cellular abnormalities of blood vessels as targets in cancer. Curr Opin Genet Dev. 2005;15(1):102–11. https://doi.org/10.1016/j.gde.2004.12.005.

44. Bennewith KL, Durand RE. Quantifying transient hypoxia in human tumor xenografts by flow cytometry. Cancer Res. 2004;64(17):6183–9. https://doi.org/10.1158/0008-5472.CAN-04-0289.

45. Kimura H, et al. Fluctuations in red cell flux in tumor microvessels can lead to transient hypoxia and reoxygenation in tumor parenchyma. Cancer Res. 1996;56(23):5522–8.

46. McDonald DM, Baluk P. Imaging of angiogenesis in inflamed airways and tumors: newly formed blood vessels are not alike and may be wildly abnormal: Parker B. Francis lecture. Chest. 2005;128(6 Suppl):602S–8S. https://doi.org/10.1378/chest.128.6_suppl.602S-a.

47. Carmeliet P, Jain RK. Molecular mechanisms and clinical applications of angiogenesis. Nature. 2011;473(7347):298–307. https://doi.org/10.1038/nature10144.

48. Chang YS, et al. Mosaic blood vessels in tumors: frequency of cancer cells in contact with flowing blood. Proc Natl Acad Sci U S A. 2000;97(26):14608–13. https://doi.org/10.1073/pnas.97.26.14608.

49. Cao Z, et al. Angiocrine factors deployed by tumor vascular niche induce B cell lymphoma invasiveness and chemoresistance. Cancer Cell. 2014;25(3):350–65. https://doi.org/10.1016/j.ccr.2014.02.005.

50. Cao Z, et al. Molecular checkpoint decisions made by subverted vascular niche transform indolent tumor cells into chemoresistant cancer stem cells. Cancer Cell. 2017;31(1):110–26. https://doi.org/10.1016/j.ccell.2016.11.010.

51. Ghiabi P, et al. Endothelial cells provide a notch-dependent pro-tumoral niche for enhancing breast cancer survival, stemness and pro-metastatic properties. PLoS One. 2014;9(11):e112424. https://doi.org/10.1371/journal.pone.0112424.

52. Lu J, et al. Endothelial cells promote the colorectal cancer stem cell phenotype through a soluble form of Jagged-1. Cancer Cell. 2013;23(2):171–85. https://doi.org/10.1016/j.ccr.2012.12.021.

53. Pedrosa AR, et al. Endothelial Jagged1 promotes solid tumor growth through both pro-angiogenic and angiocrine functions. Oncotarget. 2015;6(27):24404–23. https://doi.org/10.18632/oncotarget.4380.

54. Wieland E, et al. Endothelial Notch1 Activity facilitates metastasis. Cancer Cell. 2017;31(3):355–67. https://doi.org/10.1016/j.ccell.2017.01.007.

55. Zhu TS, et al. Endothelial cells create a stem cell niche in glioblastoma by providing NOTCH ligands that nurture self-renewal of cancer stem-like cells. Cancer Res. 2011;71(18):6061–72. https://doi.org/10.1158/0008-5472.CAN-10-4269.

56. Yadav A, et al. Tumor-associated endothelial cells promote tumor metastasis by chaperoning circulating tumor cells and protecting them from anoikis. PLoS One. 2015;10(10):e0141602. https://doi.org/10.1371/journal.pone.0141602.

57. Beerepoot LV, et al. Increased levels of viable circulating endothelial cells are an indicator of progressive disease in cancer patients. Ann Oncol. 2004;15(1):139–45. https://doi.org/10.1093/annonc/mdh017.

58. Mancuso P, et al. Resting and activated endothelial cells are increased in the peripheral blood of cancer patients. Blood. 2001;97(11):3658–61. https://doi.org/10.1182/blood.v97.11.3658.

59. Maishi N, et al. Tumour endothelial cells in high metastatic tumours promote metastasis via epigenetic dysregulation of biglycan. Sci Rep. 2016;6:28039. https://doi.org/10.1038/srep28039.

60. Ohga N, et al. Heterogeneity of tumor endothelial cells: comparison between tumor endothelial cells isolated from high- and low-metastatic tumors. Am J Pathol. 2012;180(3):1294–307. https://doi.org/10.1016/j.ajpath.2011.11.035.

61. Branco-Price C, et al. Endothelial cell HIF-1α and HIF-2α differentially regulate metastatic success. Cancer Cell. 2012;21(1):52–65. https://doi.org/10.1016/j.ccr.2011.11.017.

62. Buckanovich RJ, et al. Tumor vascular proteins as biomarkers in ovarian cancer. J Clin Oncol. 2007;25(7):852–61. https://doi.org/10.1200/JCO.2006.08.8583.

63. St. Croix B, et al. Genes expressed in human tumor endothelium. Science. 2000;289(5482):1197–202. https://doi.org/10.1126/science.289.5482.1197.

64. Dieterich LC, et al. Transcriptional profiling of human glioblastoma vessels indicates a key role of VEGF-A and TGFβ2 in vascular abnormalization. J Pathol. 2012;228(3):378–90. https://doi.org/10.1002/path.4072.

65. Roudnicky F, et al. Endocan is upregulated on tumor vessels in invasive bladder cancer where it mediates VEGF-A-induced angiogenesis. Cancer Res. 2013;73(3):1097–106. https://doi.org/10.1158/0008-5472.CAN-12-1855.

66. Zhang L, et al. Tumor-derived vascular endothelial growth factor up-regulates angiopoietin-2 in host endothelium and destabilizes host vasculature, supporting angiogenesis in ovarian cancer. Cancer Res. 2003;63(12):3403–12.

67. Zhao Q, et al. Single-cell transcriptome analyses reveal endothelial cell heterogeneity in tumors and changes following antiangiogenic treatment. Cancer Res. 2018;78(9):2370–82. https://doi.org/10.1158/0008-5472.CAN-17-2728.

68. Goveia J, et al. An integrated gene expression landscape profiling approach to identify lung tumor endothelial cell heterogeneity and angiogenic candidates. Cancer Cell. 2020;37(1):21–36.e13. https://doi.org/10.1016/j.ccell.2019.12.001.

69. Lugano R, Ramachandran M, Dimberg A. Tumor angiogenesis: causes, consequences, challenges and opportunities. Cell Mol Life Sci. 2020;77(9):1745–70. https://doi.org/10.1007/s00018-019-03351-7.

70. Hwa C, Sebastian A, Aird WC. Endothelial biomedicine: its status as an interdisciplinary field, its progress as a basic science, and its translational bench-to-bedside gap. Endothelium. 2005;12(3):139–51. https://doi.org/10.1080/10623320500192016.

71. Kahn BM, et al. The vascular landscape of human cancer. J Clin Invest. 2021;131(2):e136655. https://doi.org/10.1172/JCI136655.

72. Mezheyeuski A, et al. Survival-associated heterogeneity of marker-defined perivascular cells in colorectal cancer. Oncotarget. 2016;7(27):41948–58. https://doi.org/10.18632/oncotarget.9632.

73. Asahara T, et al. Isolation of putative progenitor endothelial cells for angiogenesis. Science. 1997;275(5302):964–7. https://doi.org/10.1126/science.275.5302.964.

74. Yin AH, et al. AC133, a novel marker for human hematopoietic stem and progenitor cells. Blood. 1997;90(12):5002–12. https://doi.org/10.1182/blood.v90.12.5002.

75. Peichev M, et al. Expression of VEGFR-2 and AC133 by circulating human CD34+ cells identifies a population of functional endothelial precursors. Blood. 2000;95(3):952–8. https://doi.org/10.1182/blood.v95.3.952.003k27_952_958.

76. Romagnani P, et al. CD14+CD34low cells with stem cell phenotypic and functional features are the major source of circulating endothelial progenitors. Circ Res. 2005;97(4):314–22. https://doi.org/10.1161/01.RES.0000177670.72216.9b.

77. Asahara T, et al. Bone marrow origin of endothelial progenitor cells responsible for postnatal vasculogenesis in physiological and pathological neovascularization. Circ Res. 1999a;85(3):221–8. https://doi.org/10.1161/01.RES.85.3.221.

78. Asahara T, et al. VEGF contributes to postnatal neovascularization by mobilizing bone marrow-derived endothelial progenitor cells. EMBO J. 1999b;18(14):3964–72. https://doi.org/10.1093/emboj/18.14.3964.

79. Kalka C, et al. Transplantation of ex vivo expanded endothelial progenitor cells for therapeutic neovascularization. Proc Natl Acad Sci. 2000;97(7):3422–7. https://doi.org/10.1073/pnas.97.7.3422.

80. Lin Y, et al. Origins of circulating endothelial cells and endothelial outgrowth from blood. J Clin Investig. 2000;105(1):71–7. https://doi.org/10.1172/JCI8071.

81. Shi Q, et al. Evidence for circulating bone marrow-derived endothelial cells. Blood. 1998;92(2):362–7. https://doi.org/10.1182/blood.v92.2.362.

82. Shin JW, et al. Isolation of endothelial progenitor cells from cord blood and induction of differentiation by Ex Vivo expansion. Yonsei Med J. 2005;46(2):260–7. https://doi.org/10.3349/ymj.2005.46.2.260.

83. Blann AD, et al. Circulating endothelial cells. Biomarker of vascular disease. Thromb Haemost. 2005;93(2):228–35. https://doi.org/10.1160/TH04-09-0578.

84. Bertolini F, et al. The multifaceted circulating endothelial cell in cancer: towards marker and target identification. Nat Rev Cancer. 2006;6(11):835–45. https://doi.org/10.1038/nrc1971.

85. Ronzoni M, et al. Circulating endothelial cells and endothelial progenitors as predictive markers of clinical response to bevacizumab-based first-line treatment in advanced colorectal cancer patients. Ann Oncol. 2010;21(12):2382–9. https://doi.org/10.1093/annonc/mdq261.

86. Mehran R, et al. Tumor endothelial markers define novel subsets of cancer-specific circulating endothelial cells associated with antitumor efficacy. Cancer Res. 2014;74(10):2731–41. https://doi.org/10.1158/0008-5472.CAN-13-2044.

87. Cima I, et al. Tumor-derived circulating endothelial cell clusters in colorectal cancer. Sci Transl Med. 2016;8(345):345ra89. https://doi.org/10.1126/scitranslmed.aad7369.

88. Rahbari NN, et al. Prognostic value of circulating endothelial cells in metastatic colorectal cancer. Oncotarget. 2017;8(23):37491–501. https://doi.org/10.18632/oncotarget.16397.

89. Andonegui-Elguera MA, et al. An overview of vasculogenic mimicry in breast cancer. Front Oncol. 2020;10(February):1–8. https://doi.org/10.3389/fonc.2020.00220.

90. Lizárraga-Verdugo E, et al. Cancer stem cells and its role in angiogenesis and vasculogenic mimicry in gastrointestinal cancers. Front Oncol. 2020;10(March):1–8. https://doi.org/10.3389/fonc.2020.00413.

91. Luo Q, et al. Vasculogenic mimicry in carcinogenesis and clinical applications. J Hematol Oncol. 2020;13(1):1–15. https://doi.org/10.1186/s13045-020-00858-6.

92. Maniotis AJ, et al. Vascular channel formation by human melanoma cells in vivo and in vitro: vasculogenic mimicry. Am J Pathol. 1999;155(3):739–52. https://doi.org/10.1016/S0002-9440(10)65173-5.

93. Álvarez-Viejo M, et al. CD271 as a marker to identify mesenchymal stem cells from diverse sources before culture. World J Stem Cells. 2015;7(2):470–6. https://doi.org/10.4252/wjsc.v7.i2.470.

94. Delgado-Bellido D, et al. VE-cadherin promotes vasculogenic mimicry by modulating kaiso-dependent gene expression. Cell Death Differ. 2019;26(2):348–61. https://doi.org/10.1038/s41418-018-0125-4.

95. Cao Z, et al. Tumour vasculogenic mimicry is associated with poor prognosis of human cancer patients: a systemic review and meta-analysis. Eur J Cancer. 2013b;49(18):3914–23. https://doi.org/10.1016/j.ejca.2013.07.148.

96. Yang JP, et al. Tumor vasculogenic mimicry predicts poor prognosis in cancer patients: a meta-analysis. Angiogenesis. 2016;19(2):191–200. https://doi.org/10.1007/s10456-016-9500-2.

97. Shen Y, et al. Tumor vasculogenic mimicry formation as an unfavorable prognostic indicator in patients with breast cancer. Oncotarget. 2017;8(34):56408–16. https://doi.org/10.18632/oncotarget.16919.

98. Zhang Z, et al. The role of vascular mimicry as a biomarker in malignant melanoma: a systematic review and meta-analysis. BMC Cancer. 2019;19(1):1–12. https://doi.org/10.1186/s12885-019-6350-5.

99. Alvero AB, et al. Stem-like ovarian cancer cells can serve as tumor vascular progenitors. Stem Cells. 2009;27(10):2405–13. https://doi.org/10.5949/liverpool/9780853236788.003.0003.

100. Bussolati B, et al. Endothelial cell differentiation of human breast tumour stem/progenitor cells. J Cell Mol Med. 2009;13(2):309–19. https://doi.org/10.1111/j.1582-4934.2008.00338.x.

101. Li F, Xu J, Liu S. Cancer stem cells and neovascularization. Cells. 2021;10(5):1070. https://doi.org/10.3390/cells10051070.

102. Mei X, et al. Glioblastoma stem cell differentiation into endothelial cells evidenced through live-cell imaging. Neuro-Oncology. 2017;19(8):1109–18. https://doi.org/10.1093/neuonc/nox016.

103. Wang R, et al. Glioblastoma stem-like cells give rise to tumour endothelium. Nature. 2010;468(7325):829–33. https://doi.org/10.1038/nature09624.

104. Ricci-Vitiani L, et al. Tumour vascularization via endothelial differentiation of glioblastoma stem-like cells. Nature. 2010;468(7325):824–30. https://doi.org/10.1038/nature09557.

105. Zhao Y, et al. Endothelial cell transdifferentiation of human glioma stem progenitor cells in vitro. Brain Res Bull. 2010;82(5–6):308–12. https://doi.org/10.1016/j.brainresbull.2010.06.006.

106. Bussolati B, et al. Identification of a tumor-initiating stem cell population in human renal carcinomas. FASEB J. 2008;22(10):3696–705. https://doi.org/10.1096/fj.08-102590.

107. Rau K-M, et al. Neovascularization evaluated by CD105 correlates well with prognostic factors in breast cancers. Exp Ther Med. 2012;4(2):231–6. https://doi.org/10.3892/etm.2012.594.

108. Saroufim A, et al. Tumoral CD105 is a novel independent prognostic marker for prognosis in clear-cell renal cell carcinoma. Br J Cancer. 2014;110(7):1778–84. https://doi.org/10.1038/bjc.2014.71.

109. Aomatsu N, et al. CD133 is a useful surrogate marker for predicting chemosensitivity to neoadjuvant chemotherapy in breast cancer. PLoS One. 2012;7(9):e45865. https://doi.org/10.1371/journal.pone.0045865.

110. Kim SJ, et al. Prognostic impact and clinicopathological correlation of CD133 and ALDH1 expression in invasive breast cancer. J Breast Cancer. 2015;18(4):347–55. https://doi.org/10.4048/jbc.2015.18.4.347.

111. Rettig WJ, et al. Identification of endosialin, a cell surface glycoprotein of vascular endothelial cells in human cancer. Proc Natl Acad Sci U S A. 1992;89(22):10832–6. https://doi.org/10.1073/pnas.89.22.10832.

112. Chang SS, et al. Prostate-specific membrane antigen is produced in tumor-associated neovasculature. Clinical Cancer Res. 1999;5(10):2674–81.

113. Abid MR, et al. Vascular endocan is preferentially expressed in tumor endothelium. Microvasc Res. 2006;72(3):136–45. https://doi.org/10.1016/j.mvr.2006.05.010.

114. Burrows FJ, et al. Up-regulation of endoglin on vascular endothelial cells in human solid tumors: implications for diagnosis and therapy. Clin Cancer Res. 1995;1(12):1623–34.

115. Gasparini G, et al. Vascular integrin alpha(v)beta3: a new prognostic indicator in breast cancer. Clin Res. 1998;4(11):2625–34.

116. Kim S, et al. Regulation of angiogenesis in vivo by ligation of integrin alpha5beta1 with the central cell-binding domain of fibronectin. Am J Pathol. 2000;156(4):1345–62. https://doi.org/10.1016/s0002-9440(10)65005-5.

117. Griffioen AW, et al. Endothelial intercellular adhesion molecule-1 expression is suppressed in human malignancies: the role of angiogenic factors. Cancer Res. 1996;56(5):1111–7.

118. Hellwig SMM, et al. Endothelial CD34 is suppressed in human malignancies: role of angiogenic factors. Cancer Lett. 1997;120(2):203–11. https://doi.org/10.1016/S0304-3835(97)00310-8.

119. Davies G, et al. Levels of expression of endothelial markers specific to tumour-associated endothelial cells and their correlation with prognosis in patients with breast cancer. Clin Exp Metastasis. 2004;21(1):31–7. https://doi.org/10.1023/b:clin.0000017168.83616.d0.

120. Rmali KA, et al. Tumour endothelial marker 8 (TEM-8) in human colon cancer and its association with tumour progression. Eur J Surg Oncol. 2004;30(9):948–53. https://doi.org/10.1016/j.ejso.2004.07.023.

121. Rmali KA, Puntis MCA, Jiang WG. Prognostic values of tumor endothelial markers in patients with colorectal cancer. World J Gastroenterol. 2005;11(9):1283–6. https://doi.org/10.3748/wjg.v11.i9.1283.

122. Fuchs B, et al. High expression of tumor endothelial marker 7 is associated with metastasis and poor survival of patients with osteogenic sarcoma. Gene. 2007;399(2):137–43. https://doi.org/10.1016/j.gene.2007.05.003.

123. MacFadyen J, et al. Endosialin is expressed on stromal fibroblasts and CNS pericytes in mouse embryos and is downregulated during development. Gene Expr Patterns. 2007;7(3):363–9. https://doi.org/10.1016/j.modgep.2006.07.006.

124. Opavsky R, et al. Molecular characterization of the mouse Tem1/endosialin gene regulated by cell density in vitro and expressed in normal tissues in vivo. J Biol Chem. 2001;276(42):38795–807. https://doi.org/10.1074/jbc.M105241200.

125. Halder C, et al. Preferential expression of the secreted and membrane forms of tumor endothelial marker 7 transcripts in osteosarcoma. Anticancer Res. 2009;29(11):4317–22.

126. Lee HK, et al. Cloning, characterization and neuronal expression profiles of tumor endothelial marker 7 in the rat brain. Brain Res Mol Brain Res. 2005a;136(1–2):189–98. https://doi.org/10.1016/j.molbrainres.2005.02.010.

127. Zhang ZZ, et al. TEM7 (PLXDC1), a key prognostic predictor for resectable gastric cancer, promotes cancer cell migration and invasion. Am J Cancer Res. 2015;5(2):772–81.

128. Czekierdowski A, et al. Prognostic significance of TEM7 and nestin expression in women with advanced high grade serous ovarian cancer. Ginekol Pol. 2018;89(3):135–41. https://doi.org/10.5603/GP.a2018.0023.

129. Gutwein LG, et al. Tumor endothelial marker 8 expression in triple-negative breast cancer. Anticancer Res. 2011;31(10):3417–22. Available at: https://ar.iiarjournals.org/content/31/10/3417

130. Kuo F, et al. Immuno-PET imaging of tumor endothelial Marker 8 (TEM8). Mol Pharm. 2014;11(11):3996–4006. https://doi.org/10.1021/mp500056d.

131. Pietrzyk Ł, et al. Clinical value of detecting tumor endothelial marker 8 (Antxr1) as a biomarker in the diagnosis and prognosis of colorectal cancer. Cancer Manag Res. 2021;13:3113–22. https://doi.org/10.2147/CMAR.S298165.

132. Basilio-de-Oliveira RP, Pannain VLN. Prognostic angiogenic markers (endoglin, VEGF, CD31) and tumor cell proliferation (Ki67) for gastrointestinal stromal tumors. World J Gastroenterol. 2015;21(22):6924–30. https://doi.org/10.3748/wjg.v21.i22.6924.

133. Salvesen HB, et al. Significance of CD 105 expression for tumour angiogenesis and prognosis in endometrial carcinomas. APMIS. 2003;111(11):1011–8. https://doi.org/10.1111/j.1600-0463.2003.apm1111103.x.

134. Straume O, Akslen LA. Expression of vascular endothelial growth factor, its receptors (FLT-1, KDR) and TSP-1 related to microvessel density and patient outcome in vertical growth phase melanomas. Am J Pathol. 2001;159(1):223–35. https://doi.org/10.1016/S0002-9440(10)61688-4.

135. Svatek RS, et al. Preoperative plasma endoglin levels predict biochemical progression after radical prostatectomy. Clin Cancer Res. 2008;14(11):3362–6. https://doi.org/10.1158/1078-0432.CCR-07-4707.

136. Östman A, Corvigno S. Microvascular mural cells in cancer. Trends Cancer. 2018;4(12):838–48. https://doi.org/10.1016/j.trecan.2018.10.004.

137. Sinha D, et al. Pericytes promote malignant ovarian cancer progression in mice and predict poor prognosis in serous ovarian cancer patients. Clin Cancer Res. 2016;22(7):1813–24. https://doi.org/10.1158/1078-0432.CCR-15-1931.

138. Viski C, et al. Endosialin-expressing pericytes promote metastatic dissemination. Cancer Res. 2016;76(18):5313–25. https://doi.org/10.1158/0008-5472.CAN-16-0932.

139. Cantelmo AR, et al. Inhibition of the glycolytic activator PFKFB3 in endothelium induces tumor vessel normalization, impairs metastasis, and improves chemotherapy. Cancer Cell. 2016;30(6):968–85. https://doi.org/10.1016/j.ccell.2016.10.006.

140. Cooke VG, et al. Pericyte depletion results in hypoxia-associated epithelial-to-mesenchymal transition and metastasis mediated by met signaling pathway. Cancer cell. 2012;21(1):66–81. https://doi.org/10.1016/j.ccr.2011.11.024.

141. Hamzah J, et al. Vascular normalization in Rgs5-deficient tumours promotes immune destruction. Nature. 2008;453(7193):410–4. https://doi.org/10.1038/nature06868.

142. Hong J, et al. Role of tumor pericytes in the recruitment of myeloid-derived suppressor cells. J Natl Cancer Inst. 2015;107(10):djv209. https://doi.org/10.1093/jnci/djv209.

143. Lyle LT, et al. Alterations in pericyte subpopulations are associated with elevated blood-tumor barrier permeability in experimental brain metastasis of breast cancer. Clin Cancer Res. 2016;22(21):5287–99. https://doi.org/10.1158/1078-0432.CCR-15-1836.

144. Nisancioglu MH, Betsholtz C, Genové G. The absence of pericytes does not increase the sensitivity of tumor vasculature to vascular endothelial growth factor-A blockade. Cancer Res. 2010;70(12):5109–15. https://doi.org/10.1158/0008-5472.CAN-09-4245.

145. Xian X, et al. Pericytes limit tumor cell metastasis. J Clin Invest. 2006;116(3):642–51. https://doi.org/10.1172/JCI25705.

146. Cao Y, et al. Pericyte coverage of differentiated vessels inside tumor vasculature is an independent unfavorable prognostic factor for patients with clear cell renal cell carcinoma. Cancer. 2013a;119(2):313–24. https://doi.org/10.1002/cncr.27746.

147. Corvigno S, et al. Markers of fibroblast-rich tumor stroma and perivascular cells in serous ovarian cancer: inter- and intra-patient heterogeneity and impact on survival. Oncotarget. 2016;7(14):18573–84. https://doi.org/10.18632/oncotarget.7613.

148. Frödin M, et al. Perivascular PDGFR-β is an independent marker for prognosis in renal cell carcinoma. Br J Cancer. 2017;116(2):195–201. https://doi.org/10.1038/bjc.2016.407.

149. Tolaney SM, et al. Role of vascular density and normalization in response to neoadjuvant bevacizumab and chemotherapy in breast cancer patients. Proc Natl Acad Sci U S A. 2015;112(46):14325–30. https://doi.org/10.1073/pnas.1518808112.

150. Zhou W, et al. Targeting glioma stem cell-derived pericytes disrupts the blood-tumor barrier and improves chemotherapeutic efficacy. Cell Stem Cell. 2017;21(5):591–603.e4. https://doi.org/10.1016/j.stem.2017.10.002.

151. Bhati R, et al. Molecular characterization of human breast tumor vascular cells. Am J Pathol. 2008;172(5):1381–90. https://doi.org/10.2353/ajpath.2008.070988.

152. Madden SL, et al. Vascular gene expression in nonneoplastic and malignant brain. Am J Pathol. 2004;165(2):601–8. https://doi.org/10.1016/s0002-9440(10)63324-x.

153. Parker BS, et al. Alterations in vascular gene expression in invasive breast carcinoma. Cancer Res. 2004;64(21):7857–66. https://doi.org/10.1158/0008-5472.CAN-04-1976.

154. Pen A, et al. Molecular markers of extracellular matrix remodeling in glioblastoma vessels: microarray study of laser-captured glioblastoma vessels. Glia. 2007;55(6):559–72. https://doi.org/10.1002/glia.20481.

155. Dudley AC. Tumor endothelial cells. Cold Spring Harb Perspect Med. 2012;2(3):1–18. https://doi.org/10.1101/cshperspect.a006536.

156. Carson-Walter EB, et al. Plasmalemmal vesicle associated protein-1 is a novel marker implicated in brain tumor angiogenesis. Clinical Cancer Res. 2005;11(21):7643–50. https://doi.org/10.1158/1078-0432.CCR-05-1099.

157. van Beijnum JR, et al. Gene expression of tumor angiogenesis dissected: specific targeting of colon cancer angiogenic vasculature. Blood. 2006;108(7):2339–48. https://doi.org/10.1182/blood-2006-02-004291.

158. Hoda MA, et al. Temsirolimus inhibits malignant pleural mesothelioma growth in vitro and in vivo: synergism with chemotherapy. J Thorac Oncol. 2011;6(5):852–63. https://doi.org/10.1097/JTO.0b013e31820e1a25.

159. Lu C, et al. Gene alterations identified by expression profiling in tumor-associated endothelial cells from invasive ovarian carcinoma. Cancer Res. 2007;67(4):1757–68. https://doi.org/10.1158/0008-5472.CAN-06-3700.

160. Coppiello G, et al. Meox2/Tcf15 heterodimers program the heart capillary endothelium for cardiac fatty acid uptake. Circulation. 2015;131(9):815–26. https://doi.org/10.1161/CIRCULATIONAHA.114.013721.

161. Marcu R, et al. Human organ-specific endothelial cell heterogeneity. iScience. 2018;4:20–35. https://doi.org/10.1016/j.isci.2018.05.003.

162. Nolan DJ, et al. Molecular signatures of tissue-specific microvascular endothelial cell heterogeneity in organ maintenance and regeneration. Dev Cell. 2013;26(2):204–19. https://doi.org/10.1016/j.devcel.2013.06.017.Molecular.

163. Sabbagh MF, et al. Transcriptional and epigenomic landscapes of CNS and non-CNS vascular endothelial cells. eLife. 2018;7:e36187. https://doi.org/10.7554/eLife.36187.

164. Tewari KS, et al. Final overall survival of a randomized trial of bevacizumab for primary treatment of ovarian cancer. J Clin Oncol. 2019;37(26):2317–28. https://doi.org/10.1200/JCO.19.01009.

165. Folkman J. Tumor angiogenesis: therapeutic implications. N Engl J Med. 1971;285(21):1182–6. https://doi.org/10.1056/NEJM197111182852108.

166. Cao Y, et al. Forty-year journey of angiogenesis translational research. Sci Transl Med. 2011;3(114):114rv3. https://doi.org/10.1126/scitranslmed.3003149.

167. Folkman J, et al. Isolation of a tumor factor responsible for angiogenesis. J Exp Med. 1971;133(2):275–88. https://doi.org/10.1084/jem.133.2.275.

168. Viloria-Petit A, et al. Contrasting effects of VEGF gene disruption in embryonic stem cell-derived versus oncogene-induced tumors. EMBO J. 2003;22(16):4091–102. https://doi.org/10.1093/emboj/cdg408.

169. Apte RS, Chen DS, Ferrara N. VEGF in signaling and disease: beyond discovery and development. Cell. 2019;176(6):1248–64. https://doi.org/10.1016/j.cell.2019.01.021.

170. Ferrara N. Vascular endothelial growth factor: basic science and clinical progress. Endocr Rev. 2004;25(4):581–611. https://doi.org/10.1210/er.2003-0027.

171. Jiang BH, Liu LZ. Chapter 2 PI3K/PTEN signaling in angiogenesis and tumorigenesis. Adv Cancer Res. 2009;102(09):19–65. https://doi.org/10.1016/S0065-230X(09)02002-8.

172. Takahashi T, et al. A single autophosphorylation site on KDR/Flk-1 is essential for VEGF-A-dependent activation of PLC-γ and DNA synthesis in vascular endothelial cells. EMBO J. 2001;20(11):2768–78. https://doi.org/10.1093/emboj/20.11.2768.

173. van Hinsbergh VWM, Koolwijk P. Endothelial sprouting and angiogenesis: matrix metalloproteinases in the lead. Cardiovasc Res. 2008;78(2):203–12. https://doi.org/10.1093/cvr/cvm102.

174. Weis S, et al. Endothelial barrier disruption by VEGF-mediated Src activity potentiates tumor cell extravasation and metastasis. J Cell Biol. 2004;167(2):223–9. https://doi.org/10.1083/jcb.200408130.

175. Niu G, Chen X. Vascular endothelial growth factor as an anti-angiogenic target for cancer therapy.

Curr Drug Targets. 2010;11(8):1000–17. https://doi.org/10.2174/138945010791591395.

176. Bell C, et al. Oligonucleotide NX1838 inhibits VEGF165-mediated cellular responses in vitro. In Vitro cell Dev Biol Anim. 1999;35(9):533–42. https://doi.org/10.1007/s11626-999-0064-y.

177. Lee JH, et al. A therapeutic aptamer inhibits angiogenesis by specifically targeting the heparin binding domain of VEGF165. Proc Natl Acad Sci. 2005b;102(52):18902–7. https://doi.org/10.1073/pnas.0509069102.

178. Lin YS, et al. Preclinical pharmacokinetics, interspecies scaling, and tissue distribution of a humanized monoclonal antibody against vascular endothelial growth factor. J Pharmacol Exp Ther. 1999;288(1):371–8.

179. Lockhart AC, et al. Phase I study of intravenous vascular endothelial growth factor trap, aflibercept, in patients with advanced solid tumors. J Clin Oncol. 2010;28(2):207–14. https://doi.org/10.1200/JCO.2009.22.9237.

180. Zhou B, Wang B. Pegaptanib for the treatment of age-related macular degeneration. Exp Eye Res. 2006;83(3):615–9. https://doi.org/10.1016/j.exer.2006.02.010.

181. Spratlin JL, et al. Phase I pharmacologic and biologic study of ramucirumab (IMC-1121B), a fully human immunoglobulin G1 monoclonal antibody targeting the vascular endothelial growth factor receptor-2. J Clin Oncol. 2010;28(5):780–7. https://doi.org/10.1200/JCO.2009.23.7537.

182. Faivre S, et al. Safety, pharmacokinetic, and antitumor activity of SU11248, a novel oral multitarget tyrosine kinase inhibitor, in patients with cancer. J Clin Oncol. 2006;24(1):25–35. https://doi.org/10.1200/JCO.2005.02.2194.

183. Hutson TE, et al. Efficacy and safety of pazopanib in patients with metastatic renal cell carcinoma. J Clin Oncol. 2010;28(3):475–80. https://doi.org/10.1200/JCO.2008.21.6994.

184. Iwamoto FM, et al. Phase II trial of pazopanib (GW786034), an oral multi-targeted angiogenesis inhibitor, for adults with recurrent glioblastoma (North American Brain Tumor Consortium Study 06-02). Neuro-Oncology. 2010;12(8):855–61. https://doi.org/10.1093/neuonc/noq025.

185. Sloan B, Scheinfeld NS. Pazopanib, a VEGF receptor tyrosine kinase inhibitor for cancer therapy. Curr Opin Investig Drugs. 2008;9(12):1324–35.

186. Strumberg D, et al. Phase I clinical and pharmacokinetic study of the Novel Raf kinase and vascular endothelial growth factor receptor inhibitor BAY 43-9006 in patients with advanced refractory solid tumors. J Clin Oncol. 2005;23(5):965–72. https://doi.org/10.1200/JCO.2005.06.124.

187. Wilhelm SM, et al. BAY 43-9006 exhibits broad spectrum oral antitumor activity and targets the RAF/MEK/ERK pathway and receptor tyrosine kinases involved in tumor progression and angiogenesis. Cancer Res. 2004;64(19):7099–109. https://doi.org/10.1158/0008-5472.CAN-04-1443.

188. Zirlik K, Duyster J. Anti-angiogenics: current situation and future perspectives. Oncol Res Treat. 2018;41(4):166–71. https://doi.org/10.1159/000488087.

189. Jimenez-Pascual A, et al. FGF2: a novel druggable target for glioblastoma? Expert Opin Ther Targets. 2020;24(4):311–8. https://doi.org/10.1080/14728222.2020.1736558.

190. Turner N, Grose R. Fibroblast growth factor signalling: from development to cancer. Nat Rev Cancer. 2010;10(2):116–29. https://doi.org/10.1038/nrc2780.

191. Yu P, et al. FGF-dependent metabolic control of vascular development. Nature. 2017;545(7653):224–8. https://doi.org/10.1038/nature22322.

192. Incio J, et al. Obesity promotes resistance to anti-VEGF therapy in breast cancer by up-regulating IL-6 and potentially FGF-2. Sci Transl Med. 2018;10(432):eaag0945. https://doi.org/10.1126/scitranslmed.aag0945.

193. Brady N, et al. The FGF/FGFR axis as a therapeutic target in breast cancer. Expert Rev Endocrinol Metab. 2013;8(4):391–402. https://doi.org/10.1586/17446651.2013.811910.

194. Jain VK, Turner NC. Challenges and opportunities in the targeting of fibroblast growth factor receptors in breast cancer. Breast Cancer Res. 2012;14(3):208. https://doi.org/10.1186/bcr3139.

195. Kloepper J, et al. Ang-2/VEGF bispecific antibody reprograms macrophages and resident microglia to anti-tumor phenotype and prolongs glioblastoma survival. Proc Natl Acad Sci U S A. 2016;113(16):4476–81. https://doi.org/10.1073/pnas.1525360113.

196. Peterson TE, et al. Dual inhibition of Ang-2 and VEGF receptors normalizes tumor vasculature and prolongs survival in glioblastoma by altering macrophages. Proc Natl Acad Sci U S A. 2016;113(16):4470–5. https://doi.org/10.1073/pnas.1525349113.

197. Adams RH, Klein R. Eph receptors and ephrin ligands. Essential mediators of vascular development. Trends Cardiovasc Med. 2000;10(5):183–8. https://doi.org/10.1016/s1050-1738(00)00046-3.

198. Holder N, Klein R. Eph receptors and ephrins: effectors of morphogenesis. Development. 1999;126(10):2033–44.

199. Kullander K, Klein R. Mechanisms and functions of Eph and ephrin signalling. Nat Rev Mol Cell Biol. 2002;3(7):475–86. https://doi.org/10.1038/nrm856.

200. Dodelet VC, Pasquale EB. Eph receptors and ephrin ligands: embryogenesis to tumorigenesis. Oncogene. 2000;19(49):5614–9. https://doi.org/10.1038/sj.onc.1203856.

201. Ogawa K, et al. The ephrin-A1 ligand and its receptor, EphA2, are expressed during tumor neovascularization. Oncogene. 2000;19(52):6043–52. https://doi.org/10.1038/sj.onc.1204004.

202. Surawska H, Ma PC, Salgia R. The role of ephrins and Eph receptors in cancer. Cytokine Growth Factor Rev. 2004;15(6):419–33. https://doi.org/10.1016/j.cytogfr.2004.09.002.

203. Noren NK, et al. Interplay between EphB4 on tumor cells and vascular ephrin-B2 regulates tumor growth. Proc Natl Acad Sci U S A. 2004;101(15):5583–8. https://doi.org/10.1073/pnas.0401381101.

204. Uhl C, et al. EphB4 mediates resistance to antiangiogenic therapy in experimental glioma. Angiogenesis. 2018;21(4):873–81. https://doi.org/10.1007/s10456-018-9633-6.

205. Krusche B, et al. EphrinB2 drives perivascular invasion and proliferation of glioblastoma stem-like cells. elife. 2016;5:1–32. https://doi.org/10.7554/elife.14845.

206. Brantley DM, et al. Soluble Eph A receptors inhibit tumor angiogenesis and progression in vivo. Oncogene. 2002;21(46):7011–26. https://doi.org/10.1038/sj.onc.1205679.

207. Cheng N, et al. Inhibition of VEGF-dependent multistage carcinogenesis by soluble EphA receptors. Neoplasia. 2003;5(5):445–56. https://doi.org/10.1016/s1476-5586(03)80047-7.

208. Dobrzanski P, et al. Antiangiogenic and antitumor efficacy of EphA2 receptor antagonist. Cancer Res. 2004;64(3):910–9. https://doi.org/10.1158/0008-5472.can-3430-2.

209. Berta J, et al. Apelin expression in human non-small cell lung cancer: role in angiogenesis and prognosis. J Thorac Oncol. 2010;5(8):1120–9. https://doi.org/10.1097/JTO.0b013e3181e2c1ff.

210. Feng M, et al. Tumor apelin, not serum apelin, is associated with the clinical features and prognosis of gastric cancer. BMC Cancer. 2016;16(1):1–8. https://doi.org/10.1186/s12885-016-2815-y.

211. Heo K, et al. Hypoxia-induced up-regulation of apelin is associated with a poor prognosis in oral squamous cell carcinoma patients. Oral Oncol. 2012;48(6):500–6. https://doi.org/10.1016/j.oraloncology.2011.12.015.

212. Kälin RE, et al. Paracrine and autocrine mechanisms of apelin signaling govern embryonic and tumor angiogenesis. Dev Biol. 2007;305(2):599–614. https://doi.org/10.1016/j.ydbio.2007.03.004.

213. Lacquaniti A, et al. Apelin beyond kidney failure and hyponatremia: a useful biomarker for cancer disease progression evaluation. Clin Exp Med. 2015;15(1):97–105. https://doi.org/10.1007/s10238-014-0272-y.

214. Seaman S, et al. Genes that distinguish physiological and pathological angiogenesis. Cancer Cell. 2007;11(6):539–54. https://doi.org/10.1016/j.ccr.2007.04.017.

215. Tolkach Y, et al. Apelin and apelin receptor expression in renal cell carcinoma. Br J Cancer. 2019;120(6):633–9. https://doi.org/10.1038/s41416-019-0396-7.

216. Wysocka MB, Pietraszek-Gremplewicz K, Nowak D. The role of apelin in cardiovascular diseases, obesity and cancer. Front Physiol. 2018;9:557. https://doi.org/10.3389/fphys.2018.00557.

217. Berta J, et al. Apelin promotes lymphangiogenesis and lymph node metastasis. Oncotarget. 2014;5(12):4426–37. https://doi.org/10.18632/oncotarget.2032.

218. Hall C, et al. Inhibition of the apelin/apelin receptor axis decreases cholangiocarcinoma growth. Cancer Lett. 2017;386:179–88. https://doi.org/10.1016/j.canlet.2016.11.025.

219. Lv D, et al. PAK1-cofilin phosphorylation mediates human lung adenocarcinoma cells migration induced by apelin-13. Clin Exp Pharmacol Physiol. 2016;43(5):569–79. https://doi.org/10.1111/1440-1681.12563.

220. Macaluso NJM, et al. Discovery of a competitive apelin receptor (APJ) antagonist. ChemMedChem. 2011;6(6):1017–23. https://doi.org/10.1002/cmdc.201100069.

221. Harford-Wright E, et al. Pharmacological targeting of apelin impairs glioblastoma growth. Brain. 2017;140(11):2939–54. https://doi.org/10.1093/brain/awx253.

222. Mastrella G, et al. Targeting APLN/APLNR improves antiangiogenic efficiency and blunts proinvasive side effects of VEGFA/VEGFR2 blockade in glioblastoma. Cancer Res. 2019;79(9):2298–313. https://doi.org/10.1158/0008-5472.CAN-18-0881.

223. Uribesalgo I, et al. Apelin inhibition prevents resistance and metastasis associated with anti-angiogenic therapy. EMBO Mol Med. 2019;11(8):e9266. https://doi.org/10.15252/emmm.201809266.

224. Chae S, et al. Angiopoietin-2 interferes with anti-VEGFR2-induced vessel normalization and survival benefit in mice bearing gliomas. Clin Cancer Res. 2010;16(14):3618–27. https://doi.org/10.1158/1078-0432.CCR-09-3073.Angiopoietin-2.

225. Shim WSN, Ho IAW, Wong PEH. Angiopoietin: a TIE(d) balance in tumor angiogenesis. Mol Cancer Res. 2007;5(7):655–65. https://doi.org/10.1158/1541-7786.MCR-07-0072.

226. Ping YF, Bian XW. Consice review: contribution of cancer stem cells to neovascularization. Stem Cells. 2011;29(6):888–94. https://doi.org/10.1002/stem.650.

227. Bach P, et al. Specific elimination of CD133+ tumor cells with targeted oncolytic measles virus. Cancer Res. 2013;73(2):865–74. https://doi.org/10.1158/0008-5472.CAN-12-2221.

228. Xu MR, et al. Brucine suppresses vasculogenic mimicry in human triple-negative breast cancer cell line MDA-MB-231. In: W.-L. Lu, Editor. Biomed Res Int. 2019;2019:6543230. https://doi.org/10.1155/2019/6543230.

229. Serwe A, et al. Inhibition of TGF-β signaling, vasculogenic mimicry and proinflammatory gene expression by isoxanthohumol. Investig New Drugs. 2012;30(3):898–915. https://doi.org/10.1007/s10637-011-9643-3.

230. Kumar SR, et al. Molecular targets for tivantinib (ARQ 197) and vasculogenic mimicry in human melanoma cells. Eur J Pharmacol. 2019;853:316–24. https://doi.org/10.1016/j.ejphar.2019.04.010.

231. Fernández-Cortés M, Delgado-Bellido D, Javier Oliver F. Vasculogenic mimicry: become an endothelial cell "But not so much". Front Oncol. 2019;9(AUG):1–6. https://doi.org/10.3389/fonc.2019.00803.

232. Jean C, et al. Inhibition of endothelial FAK activity prevents tumor metastasis by enhancing barrier function. J Cell Biol. 2014;204(2):247–63. https://doi.org/10.1083/jcb.201307067.

233. Goel S, et al. Effects of vascular-endothelial protein tyrosine phosphatase inhibition on breast cancer vasculature and metastatic progression. J Natl Cancer Inst. 2013;105(16):1188–201. https://doi.org/10.1093/jnci/djt164.

234. George D. Platelet-derived growth factor receptors: a therapeutic target in solid tumors. Semin Oncol. 2001;28:27–33. https://doi.org/10.1016/S0093-7754(01)90100-9.

235. Thijssen VL, et al. Targeting PDGF-mediated recruitment of pericytes blocks vascular mimicry and tumor growth. J Pathol. 2018;246(4):447–58. https://doi.org/10.1002/path.5152.

236. Uehara H, et al. Effects of blocking platelet-derived growth factor-receptor signaling in a mouse model of experimental prostate cancer bone metastases. J Natl Cancer Inst. 2003;95(6):458–70. https://doi.org/10.1093/jnci/95.6.458.

237. Heidemann J, et al. Angiogenic effects of interleukin 8 (CXCL8) in human intestinal microvascular endothelial cells are mediated by CXCR2. J Biol Chem. 2003;278(10):8508–15. https://doi.org/10.1074/jbc.M208231200.

238. Kitadai Y, et al. Regulation of disease-progression genes in human gastric carcinoma cells by interleukin 8. Clin Cancer Res. 2000;6(7):2735–40.

239. Yang G, et al. CXCR2 promotes ovarian cancer growth through dysregulated cell cycle, diminished apoptosis, and enhanced angiogenesis. Clin Cancer Res. 2010;16(15):3875–86. https://doi.org/10.1158/1078-0432.CCR-10-0483.

240. Ijichi H, et al. Inhibiting Cxcr2 disrupts tumor-stromal interactions and improves survival in a mouse model of pancreatic ductal adenocarcinoma. J Clin Invest. 2011;121(10):4106–17. https://doi.org/10.1172/JCI42754.

241. Xu J, et al. Vascular CXCR4 expression promotes vessel sprouting and sensitivity to sorafenib treatment in hepatocellular carcinoma. Clin Cancer Res. 2017;23(15):4482–92. https://doi.org/10.1158/1078-0432.ccr-16-2131.

242. Chen L, et al. The IL-8/CXCR1 axis is associated with cancer stem cell-like properties and correlates with clinical prognosis in human pancreatic cancer cases. Sci Rep. 2014;4:1–7. https://doi.org/10.1038/srep05911.

243. Ha H, Debnath B, Neamati N. Role of the CXCL8-CXCR1/2 axis in cancer and inflammatory diseases. Theranostics. 2017;7(6):1543–88. https://doi.org/10.7150/thno.15625.

244. Milosevic V, et al. Wnt/IL- 1β/IL -8 autocrine circuitries control chemoresistance in mesothelioma initiating cells by inducing ABCB5. Int J Cancer. 2020;146(1):192–207. https://doi.org/10.1002/ijc.32419.

245. Smith DR, et al. Inhibition of interleukin 8 attenuates angiogenesis in bronchogenic carcinoma. J Exp Med. 1994;179(5):1409–15. https://doi.org/10.1084/jem.179.5.1409.

246. Martin D, Galisteo R, Gutkind JS. CXCL8/IL8 stimulates vascular endothelial growth factor (VEGF) expression and the autocrine activation of VEGFR2 in endothelial cells by activating NFkappaB through the CBM (Carma3/Bcl10/Malt1) complex. J Biol Chem. 2009;284(10):6038–42. https://doi.org/10.1074/jbc.C800207200.

247. Scapini P, et al. CXCL1/macrophage inflammatory protein-2-induced angiogenesis in vivo is mediated by neutrophil-derived vascular endothelial growth factor-A. J Immunol. 2004;172(8):5034–40. https://doi.org/10.4049/jimmunol.172.8.5034.

248. Wolf MJ, et al. Endothelial CCR2 signaling induced by colon carcinoma cells enables extravasation via the JAK2-Stat5 and p38MAPK pathway. Cancer Cell. 2012;22(1):91–105. https://doi.org/10.1016/j.ccr.2012.05.023.

249. Chen X, et al. CCL2/CCR2 regulates the tumor microenvironment in HER-2/neu-driven mammary carcinomas in mice. PLoS

One. 2016;11(11):e0165595. https://doi.org/10.1371/journal. pone.0165595.

250. Oh P, et al. Subtractive proteomic mapping of the endothelial surface in lung and solid tumours for tissue-specific therapy. Nature. 2004;429(6992):629–35. https://doi.org/10.1038/nature02580.

251. Wei YQ, et al. Immunogene therapy of tumors with vaccine based on Xenopus homologous vascular endothelial growth factor as a model antigen. Proc Natl Acad Sci U S A. 2001;98(20):11545–50. https://doi.org/10.1073/pnas.191112198.

252. Gavilondo JV, et al. Specific active immunotherapy with a VEGF vaccine in patients with advanced solid tumors. results of the CENTAURO antigen dose escalation phase I clinical trial. Vaccine. 2014;32(19):2241–50. https://doi.org/10.1016/j. vaccine.2013.11.102.

253. Chen R, et al. Anti-metastatic effects of DNA vaccine encoding single-chain trimer composed of MHC I and vascular endothelial growth factor receptor 2 peptide. Oncol Rep. 2015;33(5):2269–76. https://doi.org/10.3892/or.2015.3820.

254. Ishizaki H, et al. Inhibition of tumor growth with antiangiogenic cancer vaccine using epitope peptides derived from human vascular endothelial growth factor receptor 1. Clin Cancer Res. 2006;12(19):5841–9. https://doi.org/10.1158/1078-0432. CCR-06-0750.

255. Liang P, et al. Construction of a DNA vaccine encoding Flk-1 extracellular domain and C3d fusion gene and investigation of its suppressing effect on tumor growth. Cancer Immunol Immunother. 2010;59(1):93–101. https://doi.org/10.1007/s00262-009-0727-2.

256. Liu JY, et al. Immunotherapy of tumors with vaccine based on quail homologous vascular endothelial growth factor receptor-2. Blood. 2003;102(5):1815–23. https://doi.org/10.1182/ blood-2002-12-3772.

257. McKinney KA, et al. Effect of a novel DNA vaccine on angiogenesis and tumor growth in vivo. Arch Otolaryngol. 2010;136(9):859–64. https://doi.org/10.1001/archoto.2010.139.

258. Wada S, et al. Rationale for antiangiogenic cancer therapy with vaccination using epitope peptides derived from human vascular endothelial growth factor receptor 2. Cancer Res. 2005;65(11):4939–46. https://doi.org/10.1158/0008-5472. CAN-04-3759.

259. Xie K, et al. Anti-tumor effects of a human VEGFR-2-based DNA vaccine in mouse models. Genet Vaccines Ther. 2009;7:10. https:// doi.org/10.1186/1479-0556-7-10.

260. Zuo SG, et al. Orally administered DNA vaccine delivery by attenuated Salmonella typhimurium targeting fetal liver kinase 1 inhibits murine Lewis lung carcinoma growth and metastasis.

Biol Pharm Bull. 2010;33(2):174–82. https://doi.org/10.1248/ bpb.33.174.

261. He Q, et al. Inhibition of tumor growth with a vaccine based on xenogeneic homologous fibroblast growth factor receptor-1 in mice. J Biol Chem. 2003;278(24):21831–6. https://doi. org/10.1074/jbc.M300880200.

262. Li M, et al. bFGF peptide combined with the pVAX-8CpG plasmid as adjuvant is a novel anticancer vaccine inducing effective immune responses against Lewis lung carcinoma. Mol Med Rep. 2012;5(3):625–30. https://doi.org/10.3892/mmr.2011.725.

263. Plum SM, et al. Administration of a liposomal FGF-2 peptide vaccine leads to abrogation of FGF-2-mediated angiogenesis and tumor development. Vaccine. 2000;19(9–10):1294–303. https:// doi.org/10.1016/s0264-410x(00)00210-3.

264. Zheng SJ, et al. Synergistic anti-tumor effect of recombinant chicken fibroblast growth factor receptor-1-mediated anti-angiogenesis and low-dose gemcitabine in a mouse colon adenocarcinoma model. World J Gastroenterol. 2007;13(17):2484–9. https://doi.org/10.3748/wjg.v13.i17.2484.

265. Plum SM, et al. Generation of a specific immunological response to FGF-2 does not affect wound healing or reproduction. Immunopharmacol Immunotoxicol. 2004;26(1):29–41. https:// doi.org/10.1081/iph-120029942.

266. McNeel DG, et al. Phase I trial of a monoclonal antibody specific for alphavbeta3 integrin (MEDI-522) in patients with advanced malignancies, including an assessment of effect on tumor perfusion. Clin Cancer Res. 2005;11(21):7851–60. https://doi. org/10.1158/1078-0432.CCR-05-0262.

267. Huang FY, et al. Bacterial surface display of endoglin by antigen 43 induces antitumor effectiveness via bypassing immunotolerance and inhibition of angiogenesis. Int J Cancer. 2014;134(8):1981–90. https://doi.org/10.1002/ijc.28511.

268. Jarosz M, et al. Therapeutic antitumor potential of endoglin-based DNA vaccine combined with immunomodulatory agents. Gene Ther. 2013;20(3):262–73. https://doi.org/10.1038/gt.2012.28.

269. Fernández Lorente A, et al. Effect of blockade of the EGF system on wound healing in patients vaccinated with CIMAvax® EGF. World J Surg Oncol. 2013;11:275. https://doi. org/10.1186/1477-7819-11-275.

270. García B, et al. Effective inhibition of the epidermal growth factor/epidermal growth factor receptor binding by anti-epidermal growth factor antibodies is related to better survival in advanced non-small-cell lung cancer patients treated with the epidermal growth factor. Clin Cancer Res. 2008;14(3):840–6. https://doi. org/10.1158/1078-0432.CCR-07-1050.

Lymphatics in Malignant Tumors

4

Marek Wagner and Helge Wiig

Abstract

The lymphatic system constitutes a one-way conduit returning filtered interstitial fluid back to the blood circulation and also performing immunosurveillance. As most other tissues, solid tumors have lymphatics, and inherent and draining lymphatics influence solid tumor development and progression. Tumor lymphatics are also associated with metastasis to regional lymph nodes and dissemination to distant organs. Recent insights indicate that the tumor-associated lymphatic vasculature does not merely serve as a passive conduit for metastasis but also shapes the immune microenvironment in various tumors. It is reasonable to expect that modulating the lymphatic vasculature in combination with immunotherapeutic strategies will improve treatment efficacy. There are studies implying that the development of new lymphatic vessels might be associated with resolution of an immune response and induction of an immune tolerance, which may explain why high lymphatic vessel density is often associated with poor prognosis. Therefore, it is likely that lymphatic vessels play multiple complex roles at different stages of cancer development, and that the research on the impact of lymphatics on cancer will continue to increase.

Take-Home Lessons
- The role of the lymphatic vascular system, in the setting of cancer, is relatively understudied compared to the blood vascular system.
- Tumor-associated lymphatic vasculature does not merely serve as a passive conduit for metastasis but also shapes immune microenvironment in various tumors.
- Modulating the lymphatic vasculature in combination with the immunotherapeutic strategies might improve treatment efficacy.
- Development of new lymphatic vessels might be associated with resolution of an immune response and induction of an immune tolerance, and thus explain why high lymph vessel density is often associated with poor prognosis.
- It is likely that lymphatic vessels play multiple complex roles at different stages of cancer development.

Introduction

In mammals, there are two circulatory systems, the blood vessels that form a closed circulatory system and the lymphatic vessels. The latter, which is the topic of this chapter, constitutes a one-way conduit returning filtered interstitial fluid (i.e., the fluid phase that baths and surrounds cells in the tissues) and leukocytes back to the blood circulation. Although parts of the lymphatic system were recognized in the early seventeenth century, it was not until the eighteenth century that William Hunter concluded that "lymphatic vessels are the absorbing vessels all over the body … they constitute one great and general system dispersed throughout the whole body for absorption" [1]. The lymphatic system has three main functions: (1) fluid balance preservation by returning capillary ultrafiltrate and escaped plasma proteins to the blood circulation, (2) absorption of digested fat via intestinal lymphatics, and (3) defense function. Filtered interstitial fluid contains foreign material such as antigens, which is transported to lymph nodes as part of the body's

M. Wagner · H. Wiig (✉)
Department of Biomedicine, University of Bergen, Bergen, Norway
e-mail: helge.wiig@uib.no

L. A. Akslen, R. S. Watnick (eds.), *Biomarkers of the Tumor Microenvironment*, https://doi.org/10.1007/978-3-030-98950-7_4

immunosurveillance. As most other tissues, solid tumors have lymphatics. The function of inherent and draining lymphatics has particular relevance in as much as solid tumor progression is associated with metastasis to regional lymph nodes and dissemination to distant organs. Moreover, because the immune system and immunosurveillance via lymphatics can be assumed to take part in control of tumor progression, it is of interest to discuss here. Importantly, lymphatic vessels represent a route for tumor cells to escape from the primary tumor and metastasize. In the present chapter, we will discuss the tumor interstitium (microenvironment) where the lymph originates, and lymphatics embedded in interstitium, their role in fluid transport and cancer cell dissemination, and finally place the regulation of tumor immune microenvironments by lymphatics in a translational perspective by considering the implications for immunotherapy. The biological functions of lymphatic vessels and their role in disease, notably those of solid tumors, have been extensively reviewed elsewhere, including papers from pioneers in the field, e.g., [2–4].

Tumor Interstitium (Microenvironment) and Lymphatics Embedded in Interstitium

Tumor lymph originates from the tumor interstitium or in the fluid phase of the extracellular matrix (ECM) where it is produced by filtration and thereafter finds its way to draining lymphatic vessels [5]. Because the interstitium represents the tumor microenvironment and is one of the determinants of lymph formation also hosting immune cells, which serves as a central element in this chapter, we will first briefly consider the interstitial structure and lymph formation in tumors. Normal interstitial tissue, as well as that of tumors, consists of a collagen fiber framework, a gel phase of glycosaminoglycans (GAGs), a salt solution, and plasma proteins [6]. The structure and composition of the tumor interstitium/stroma have been covered in many extensive reviews, e.g., Ref. [7–11], and therefore only salient features of particular relevance are discussed here. A schematic picture of the tumor interstitium is shown in Fig. 4.1. As described by Lu et al. [8], the ECM directly or indirectly regulates most cellular behavior and consequently also draining lymph composi-

tion. Notwithstanding the fact that the tumor interstitium consists of the same components as that of normal tissues as outlined in Fig. 4.1a, it has special features of relevance here. One of these is the stroma's "reactive" character [7], involving an increased number of inflammatory cells, endothelial cells, and fibroblasts, which evolve with and provide support to tumor cells during the transition to malignancy [13].

Among inflammatory cells, macrophages are probably the most abundant innate immune cells in the tumor microenvironment of most solid tumors. Macrophages are also, perhaps, the most plastic cells with tumor-associated macrophages (TAMs) serving as an example for their functional polarization. TAMs stimulate angiogenesis and enhance tumor invasion, and metastasis by secreting angiogenic and lymphangiogenic molecules (e.g., vascular endothelial growth factor (VEGF)-A and VEGF-C, respectively) as well as proteases, including cathepsins and matrix metalloproteinases (MMPs). Therefore, an abundance of TAMs in the tumor interstitium often portends a poor prognosis in numerous malignancies as revealed by pre-clinical and clinical data [5]. Importantly, some of the signaling molecules involved in macrophage polarization have already been defined in vitro. For example, classically activated (or M1) macrophages, which generally exert antitumoral functions, are induced following the stimulation with IFNγ alone or together with lipopolysaccharide (LPS), or TNF-α and granulocyte-macrophage colony-stimulating factor (GM-CSF). On the other hand, IL-4, IL-13, and macrophage colony-stimulating factor (M-CSF) trigger an alternative (or M2) form of macrophage activation, which normally elicits tumor-promoting functions. In solid tumors, the crosstalk between macrophages and components of the tumor interstitium forges their phenotype. In response to numerous tumor- and stroma-derived signals, TAMs acquire an activation state that resembles a signature feature of M2 macrophages [5]. In contrast to macrophages, strong lymphocytic infiltration, particularly that of CD8+ T cells correlates with good prognosis and is often associated with the presence of functional lymphatic vasculature [5], which will be discussed later in this chapter.

In the tumor interstitium there is an increased number of fibroblasts termed cancer-associated fibroblasts (CAFs) that have a profound role with respect to tumor ECM composition and function [8]. CAFs produce increased amounts of

Fig. 4.1 Schematic overview of the interstitium with some of its major extracellular matrix components in normal tissue and tumors. (**a**) Fluid containing plasma proteins and other solutes is filtered from the capillary percolates through the interstitium and is absorbed and thus returned to the circulation by lymph. In addition to proteins and solutes, immune cells migrate into lymphatic vessels and are transported to lymph nodes where they may initiate an immune response. Reproduced from Wiig et al. [12] with permission. (**b**) Role of the extracellular matrix and microenvironment in lymphan-

giogenesis in tumors. Growth factors and cytokines produced by tumor cells and stroma are transported by fluid flow and down a diffusion gradient to lymphatics and blood capillaries. Tumor and immune cells (expressing CCR7) are chemoattracted to and enter peritumoral initial lymphatics expressing CCL19/21. + (plus) and − (minus) denote stimulating and inhibiting lymphangiogenesis, respectively. *x-collagen* crosslinked collagen, P_{if} interstitial fluid pressure, *CAF* cancer-associated fibroblast. Reproduced from Wiig et al. [12] with permission

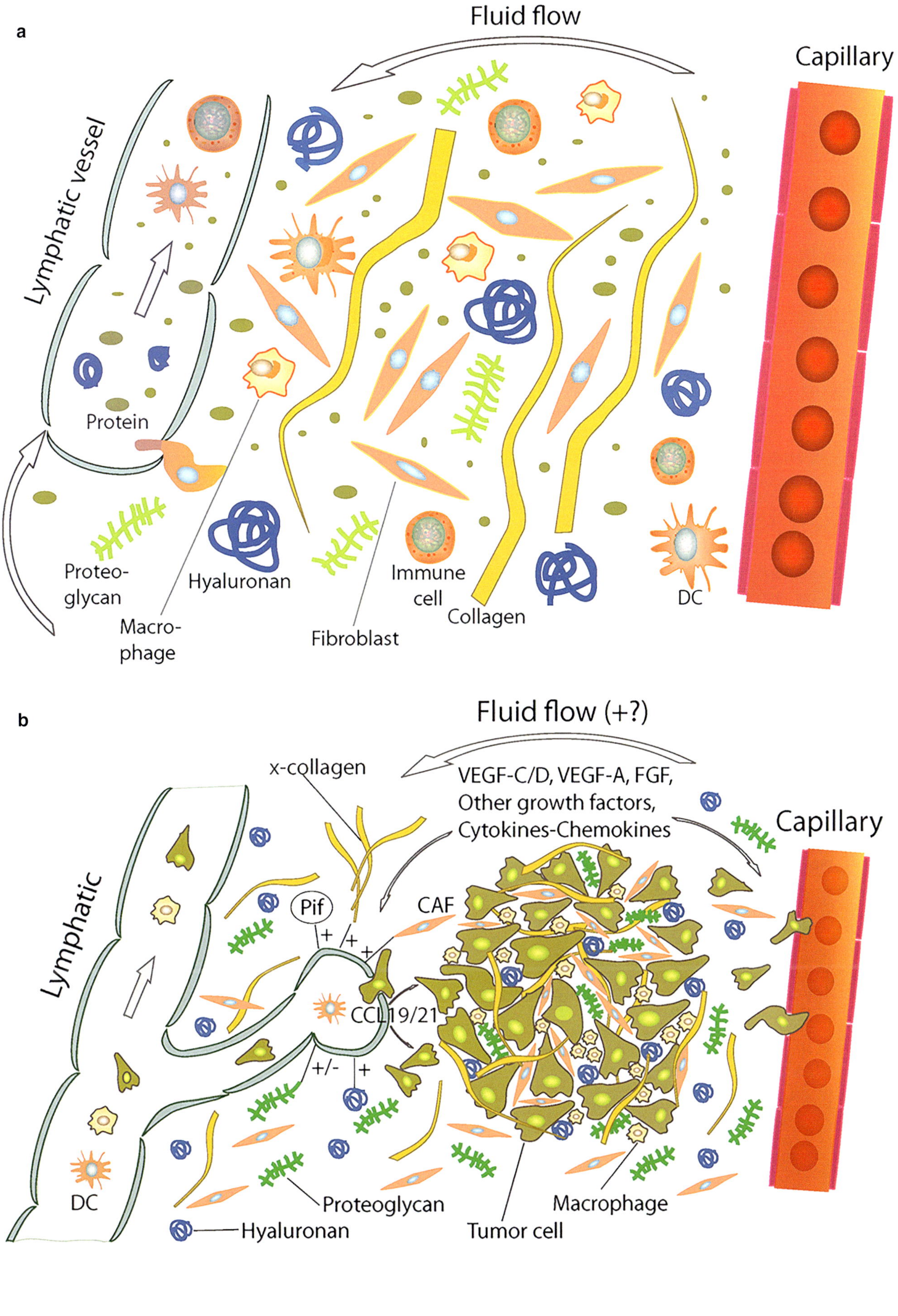

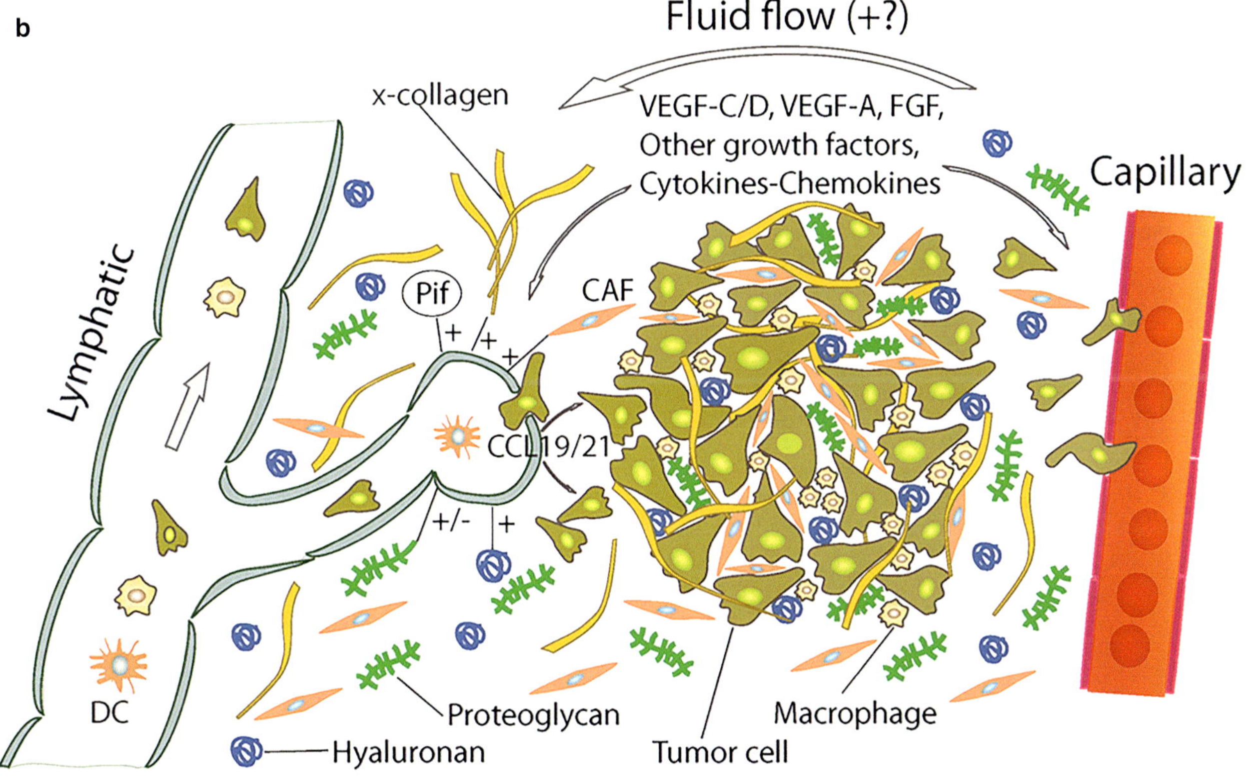
a
Fluid flow
Capillary
Lymphatic vessel
Protein
Proteo-
glycan
Hyaluronan
Macro-
phage
Immune
cell
Fibroblast
Collagen
DC
b
Fluid flow (+?)
x-collagen
VEGF-C/D, VEGF-A, FGF,
Other growth factors,
Cytokines-Chemokines
Capillary
Lymphatic
Pif
+
+
+
CAF
CCL19/21
+/-
+
DC
Proteoglycan
Hyaluronan
Tumor cell
Macrophage

collagen, proteoglycans, and GAGs, in particular hyaluronan and chondroitin sulfate [14]: For such reactive stroma formation, VEGF-A secreted by multiple cells of the tumor is a critical factor [15]. The resulting high levels of VEGF-A in tumors induce high-microvascular permeability, again resulting in extravasation of plasma proteins like fibrin, followed by attraction of fibroblasts, inflammatory cells, and endothelial cells [16]. Whereas it is well established that stromal cells and fibroblasts secrete angiogenetic factors [17], lymphangiogenic factors have received less attention. Secretion of such factors does take place, and immune as well as tumor cells are important sources for lymphangiogenic factors, notably VEGF-C and VEGF-D [18] that modulate the tumor stroma structure and function (Fig. 4.1b).

Although lymph vessels were described early in the seventeenth century, growth factors and molecular markers for such vessels have only been identified in the past two decades. In this time period, lymphatic vascular biology in all areas, including that of tumors, has advanced rapidly through the discovery of lymphangiogenic factors, identification of lymphatic vascular markers, isolation of lymphatic endothelial cells, and the development of animal models to study lymphangiogenesis [3, 4]. These lymphatic vessel markers, which can be used to distinguish lymphatic from blood vessels, have been instrumental for recent progress in understanding tumor lymphatic biology.

There are several growth factors that induce growth of lymphatic vessels, although most important are VEGF-C and VEGF-D [2], which both bind to VEGFR-3 (flt-4) on lymphatic endothelial cells and result in downstream signaling as illustrated in Fig. 4.2. Many of the lymphangiogenic factors are also angiogenic factors, due to the common embry-

onic origins of lymphatic and blood vessels [2]. Tumors overexpressing these factors induce sprouting of lymphatic vessels, enlargement of collecting vessels, and lymph node lymphangiogenesis in the draining lymph nodes, apparently making the primary tumor more prone to developing lymph node metastases [2]. There are several other lymphatic growth factors such as VEGF, fibroblast growth factors, platelet derived growth factor-B, hepatocyte growth factor, and insulin-like growth factor-1 that can induce lymphangiogenesis and metastasis, but then via more indirect pathways like inflammation and induction of VEGF-C and VEGF-D expression [2].

Lymphangiogenesis induced by VEGF-C secreted by stromal and tumor cells affects the tumor formation process in several ways. One might think that tumor growth would increase lymphatic drainage or lead to lymph flow in collaterals if the lymphatics are impinged upon by the expanding tumor. Whereas tumor lymphangiogenesis has been extensively studied, there are comparatively fewer studies in which lymphatic function is experimentally assessed. In a classical study addressing this issue, Padera et al. [19] investigated whether intratumoral lymphatic vessels generated by overexpression of VEGF-C in mice were functional. They found that although VEGF-C overexpression increased the lymphatic vessel surface area in the tumor margin and lymphatic metastasis, these tumors contained no functional vessels as evaluated by several independent assays. Their data suggested that intratumoral transport of injected (and thereby also filtered) fluid did not occur through lymphatic vessels but rather through preferential channels in the tumor interstitium. As an explanation for the lack of lymphatic vessel function they suggested that this could be due to: a lack of valve structure in newly formed lymphatics; mechanical forces such as an elevated interstitial fluid pressure could collapse the lymphatic vessels rendering them nonfunctional; or that invading tumor cells could destroy the lymphatic network. Lymphatics in the tumor margin were, however, functional and sufficient for lymphatic metastasis [19]. These studies should remind us that increased tumor lymphangiogenesis does not necessarily lead to increased lymphatic function.

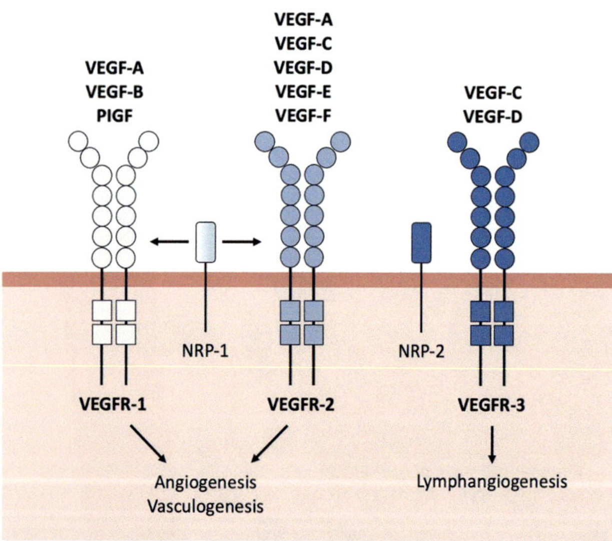

Fig. 4.2 Lymphangiogenesis. The formation of new lymphatic vessels is triggered by the binding of VEGF-C and VEGF-D to the VEGFR3 that is present on the surface of lymphatic endothelial cells

Tumor Lymphatics in Fluid Transport and Cancer Cell Dissemination

Interstitial fluid that percolates the tumor tissue and eventually enters initial lymphatics to become lymph is formed in a similar manner as in normal tissues. Such formation is determined by properties of the capillary wall, hydrostatic pressures, and protein concentrations in the blood and interstitium according to basic principles for fluid exchange described by Starling more than a century ago. Starling proposed, based on his own experiments, that capillaries are semipermeable membranes, and that transcapillary fluid filtration is determined by the imbalance between oncotic (colloid osmotic) exerted by proteins in plasma (COP_p) and interstitium (COP_{if}) and the hydrostatic pressures in the capillaries (P_c) and the interstitial fluid (P_{if}).

Although similar in many ways to normal tissue like skin and muscle, solid tumors have special features. In particular, this applies to P_{if} that is elevated compared with normal tissues [20]. Skin and muscle P_{if} are slightly subatmospheric, whereas tumor P_{if} is above atmospheric pressure in experimental animals as well as in humans, observed to be the range of 10–40 mm Hg in humans [20]. The high intratumoral P_{if} represents a counterpressure against filtration from capillaries and thus affects the formation of tumor interstitial fluid and thereby lymph per se. It may also negatively influence the transport of therapeutic substances from blood to the tumor [21], thereby acting as a potential target in tumor therapy.

The high tumor P_{if} counteracting lymph production is a result of several specific features of the tumor microenvironment, notably its vasculature [20]. Because of the increased production of angiogenetic factors, notably VEGF-A, tumor vessels are convoluted, irregular, and highly permeable [22]. These vascular changes result in low restriction of protein and transcapillary water transport and tissue "counterpressure" equal to P_{if} [21]. An additional effect of the permeable tumor vessels is an increased transcapillary protein transport that will result in an increased interstitial fluid colloid osmotic pressure again contributing the high tumor P_{if}. Additionally, direct effects of growth factors such as VEGF-A, PDGF, and TGF-β may also drive tumor P_{if} upwards [20]. Knowledge of interstitial fluid and lymph formation is critical when attempting to overcome microenvironmental obstacles in therapy and to improve drug delivery to solid tumors [21].

The lymphatic system consists of lymphatic vessels and lymphoid organs. With the exception of avascular tissues such as epidermis, cartilage, and cornea and a few vascularized organs like the retina and brain (proper), all organs have blind-ended lymphatic capillaries [12]. These are known as initial lymphatics and transport lymph to larger collecting lymphatic vessels, again returning lymph to the general circulation in lymphatic-vascular junctions in the cervical area [2–4].

Before entering into the blood stream, lymph passes through the following conduits with increasing size, lymph capillaries (also called initial lymphatics), collecting vessels, lymph nodes, trunks, and ducts [3]. Accordingly, lymphatics are a transport route where metastatic cells can reach the blood circulation. The initial lymphatics are thin-walled, relatively large vessels compared with blood capillaries composed by a single layer of endothelial cells. These vessels are not ensheathed by pericytes and smooth muscle cells, have little or no basement membrane, and are the site of interstitial fluid absorption. From the initial lymphatics, lymph moves centrally via collecting lymphatics lined with smooth muscle propelled by spontaneous contractions. Moving centrally, lymph in collecting vessels passes through lymph nodes, and is accordingly classified as prenodal or postnodal (or afferent or efferent) depending on whether lymph is carried to or from the nodes, respectively. Importantly, the lymph composition as well as immune cells can be affected by the passage through the lymph nodes [23]. Moreover, the lymph nodes may determine whether disseminating tumor cells enter the blood via high endothelial venules or through the lymph system and thus whether there is lymphatic or hematogenic metastasis as will be discussed below. Eventually, the lymph enters the blood circulation through the thoracic duct that connects to the subclavian vein.

Tumor Dissemination via Lymphatic Vessels

The role of tumor lymphatics in relation to cancer progression and metastasis is an area of ongoing research. One might imagine that tumor cells could disseminate via lymphatics, and this was actually shown by Skobe et al. [24]. They found that lymphatic vessels support metastasis and interpreted their findings to suggest that the lymphatic vessels support the development of a route for the tumor cells to escape from the primary tumor to enter the lymph node and beyond. Moreover, lymphatic vessel density at the tumor margin has been demonstrated to correlate with poor prognosis of patients with melanoma, breast, colorectal, and lung cancer [25]. Presence of lymphatic vessels at the tumor margin, using mouse melanoma as a model, is shown in Fig. 4.3. However, it has been found that removal of sentinel lymph nodes only incrementally improves patient prognosis [25]. Moreover, for colorectal cancer metastases, different sites of metastases arise from different clones in the primary tumor and 65% of lymph node metastases are unrelated to distal metastases [26]. The lack of correlation between lymph node and distal metastases suggests that the role of lymphatic vasculature and associated lymph nodes in distal metastasis is not straightforward. This notwithstanding, one third of liver and lymph node metastases arise from tumors having passed lymph nodes [26]. Metastatic tumor cells escape the tumor via afferent lymphatic vessels led into lymph node subcapsular sinus. From there, the tumor cells can invade the lymph node stroma and enter the blood circulation via high endothelial venules or alternatively pass through a series of lymph nodes and enter the thoracic duct feeding into the subclavian vein and thereby the systemic circulation [27, 28]. As reviewed by Oliver et al. [4], the great concern that lymphat-

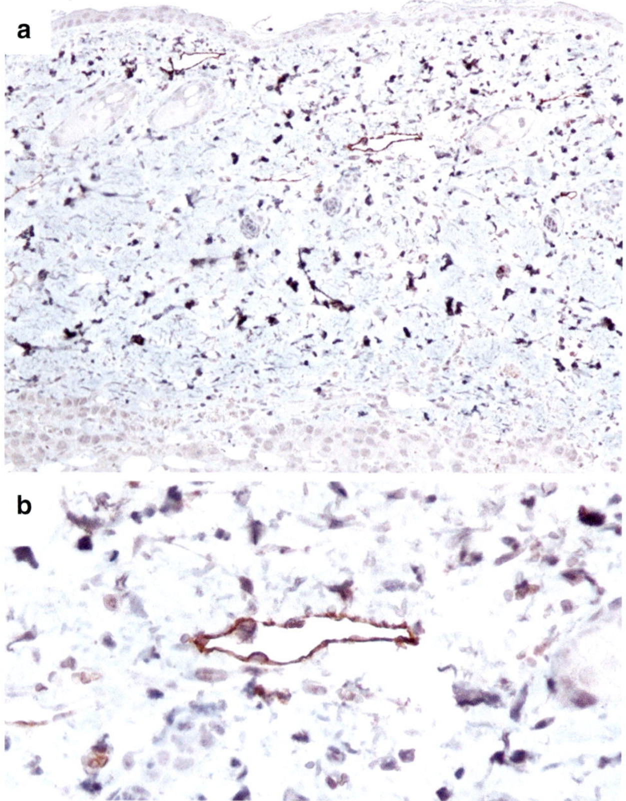

Fig. 4.3 Presence of lymphatic vessels in the peritumoral tissue. Analysis of a section of mouse melanoma (B16F10; skin cancer) reveals (via specific anti-LYVE1 antibody staining) that lymphatic vessels (arrows and asterisks) are present in the normal tissue above the tumor tissue (dotted line) but are absent within the tumor tissue itself. Size bars: 100 µm (**a**) and 50 µm (**b**)

ics might promote cancer progression solely via enhanced metastasis is now shifting toward a view that induction of lymphangiogenesis might modulate the tumor immune microenvironment. As discussed below, inhibition of lymphangiogenesis together with T cell-mediated immunotherapy may be efficacious for treating cancer patients without increasing the risk of metastasis.

Immune Microenvironment and Tumor Progression

Apart from serving as a route for tumor cells to escape from the primary tumor, lymphatic vessels together with lymphoid organs (e.g., lymph nodes) along with tissues in mucous layers of the body provide the structural basis for the proper function of the immune system. The field of cancer immunology has been faced with a number of challenges and controversies. The idea that the immune system plays a role in controlling the development of tumors or shaping the nature of the diseases has been a long-term debate that continued

throughout the past century. Paul Ehrlich, in the early nineteenth century, was the first to propose the concept that "cancer would be quite common in long-lived organisms, if it was for a properly functioning or a fully competent immune system" [29]. However, at that time, there was little known about the components of the immune system and their function and thus no effective way of validating or testing this hypothesis. The idea of cancer immunosurveillance re-emerged five decades later due to the work of Lewis Thomas [30] and Macfarlane Burnet [31]. They proposed that the immune system, particularly an adaptive immune system, might play an important role in protecting against the development of cancer. However, a number of research groups argued against the hypothesis of cancer immunosurveillance. Instead, they suggested that tumor cells would not present signals that would alert the immune system to their presence. It was proposed that tumors (which arise from the self-tissue) would likely present antigens that induce self-tolerance. Further to that, it was also suggested that chronic inflammation, which usually precedes tumor growth, is able to promote malignant transformation, thus prohibiting the protective mechanism of the immune system in controlling cancer development.

With the development of a wide array of immunodeficient mouse models on a very specific genetic background, the idea of cancer immunosurveillance re-emerged. Indeed, it has been found that mice deficient of particular components of the adaptive immune system such as T and B cells or mice that lack the production of immune-modulatory cytokines such as IFNγ are more prone or susceptible to the spontaneous development of carcinogen-induced tumors as well as spontaneous tumor growth. The idea that the immune system has the capacity to act as an extrinsic tumor suppressor mechanism is now well established. There is substantial amount of evidence to support the concept that an adaptive immune system plays an important role along with an innate immune system in protecting the host against cancer and also influencing the evolution of the disease. However, in order to develop an effective immune response that can kill cancer cells, the immune response has to go through a series of steps, which requires functional lymphatic vasculature.

The lymphatic vessels transport fluid and cells from basically all tissues in the body into lymph nodes and other lymphoid organs, making the lymphatic system ideally suited for immunosurveillance [32]. This role specifically applies to soluble antigens that are sequestered by antigen-presenting cells resident to the lymph node [33] as well as antigens that are displayed by dendritic cells moving to the lymph node after phagocytosis [34]. However, the mechanism of this action, which is fundamental for the initiation and propagation of an immune response, is not yet completely understood, but seems to require chemokines such as chemokine (C-C motif) ligand 21 (CCL21), CCL 19, and CCL 12 secreted by lymphatic endothelial cells that bind to the receptors CCR7 and CXCR4 that are present on the surface of mature dendritic cells to induce migration, vessel entry, and trafficking (reviewed in [23]).

Regulation of Tumor Immune Microenvironment by Lymphatics

In fact, a positive correlation between lymphatic density and immune cell infiltration has been revealed in a mouse model of melanoma [35]. This model utilized K14-VEGFR3-Ig mice that lack dermal lymphatics due to the constitutive expression of soluble vascular endothelial growth factor receptor (VEGFR) 3-Ig in the skin, which scavenges VEGF-C and VEGF-D. It was found that syngeneic B16F10 melanomas in these mice expressed decreased levels of pro-inflammatory molecules. Moreover, these melanomas had reduced infiltration of T and B cells as well as proinflammatory myeloid cells [35]. Similar observations were made using Chy mice, which harbor a heterozygous inactivating mutation of VEGFR-3 that leads to impaired dermal lymphangiogenesis. Syngeneic C3HBA breast adenocarcinomas were characterized by decreased leukocytic infiltration in Chy mice compared with wild type littermates, coinciding with reduced peritumoral lymphangiogenesis [35, 36]. Altogether, these results suggest that lymphatic vessels are indeed indispensable for the induction of an immune response in cancer.

Lymphatic vessels have also been shown to accelerate tumor antigen-loaded dendritic cell trafficking and priming of T cell immunity in a CCR7-dependent manner [37]. Additionally, decreased levels of tumor antigens and reduced number of cytotoxic CD8 T cells have been found in the tumor-draining lymph nodes of B16F10 melanoma-bearing kCYC mice, which demonstrate severe lymphatic dysfunction due to the expression of the Kaposi's sarcoma-associated herpesvirus latent-cycle gene, k-cyclin, under the control of the VEGFR-3 promoter [38].

Subsequently, a clinical study demonstrated that the assessment of the immune status in human colorectal cancer might serve as a stronger predictor of patient's survival, since distant metastases occurred more frequently in tumors with diminished immune cytotoxicity profile [39]. Additionally, tumors with decreased density of peritumoral lymphatics have been observed to metastasize more frequently, suggesting a positive correlation between lymphatic vascular density and immune cytotoxicity profile [39]. Collectively, this clinical study demonstrated that the lymphatic vasculature facilitates an antitumor immune response and shapes tumor immune microenvironment [39].

However, one of the most prominent steps in impeding the generation of an effective antitumor immune response is the development of a strong immunosuppressive tumor microenvironment. There are a number of factors that might contribute to this process, but certainly one of the most important is the recruitment of regulatory or immunosuppressive immune cells into the tumor microenvironment. Lymphatic structures are often found embedded in adipose tissue. However, the impact of lymphangiogenesis on tumor-associated adipose tissue has only recently been investigated, despite the fact though many tumors grow in close proximity to or physically interact with adipocytes or metastasize to lymph nodes that are shrouded by adipocytes [40–42]. For example, an increased number of macrophages, enriched particularly with an alternatively activated (or M2) population, have been found in tumor-associated adipose tissue from B16F10 melanoma-bearing K14-VEGFR3-Ig mice [43]. This observation suggests that the blockade of pathways regulating the formation of lymphatic vessels influences an inflammatory response within tumor-associated adipose tissue by enhancing the development of the microenvironment that facilitates tumor growth and progression.

The development of antitumor immunity primarily occurs in the tumor-draining lymph nodes. The formation of new lymphatic vessels provides a route for the delivery of tumor antigens to the draining lymph nodes in order to initiate priming of T cells [44]. The lymph may deliver tumor-derived antigens directly to dendritic cells or B cells residing in the tumor-draining lymph nodes [44]. Additionally, dendritic cells that are patrolling peripheral tissues may also take up tumor antigens, invade lymphatic vasculature, and enter tumor-draining lymph nodes [44]. Antigen-loaded dendritic cells subsequently prime T cells, in order to induce antigen-specific antitumor immunity. It is also worth mentioning that the local microenvironment has the potential to influence the quality of the immune response (i.e., immune activation or induction of tolerance) during antigen presentation [44]. Additionally, the architecture and function of the tumor-draining lymph nodes may be distantly modulated by the lymphatic vasculature through the delivery of extracellular mediators (e.g., exosomes) derived from the primary tumor microenvironment [45].

To test the hypothesis that tumor-draining lymph nodes promote antitumor immunity, an adjuvant therapy specifically targeting dendritic cells in the tumor-draining lymph nodes of mice bearing B16F10 melanomas was performed via delivery of CpG oligodeoxynucleotide (CpG). In this model, treatment with CpG significantly inhibited the growth of implanted B16F10 melanomas. Additionally, alterations in immune cell repertoires such as increased frequencies of mature dendritic cells within the tumor-draining lymph nodes as well as increases in tumor antigen-specific CD8 T cells in the tumor tissue have been observed [46]. An enhanced antitumor immunity illustrated by increased cytotoxic CD8 T cell responses, has also been obtained via therapeutic vaccination using lymph node-targeting nanoparticle-conjugate vaccines, leading to increased tumor regression and survival [47]. Additionally, ectopic expression of CCL3, which orchestrates T cell-antigen-presenting cell encounters in the lymph nodes, in CT26 colon tumor cells resulted in reduced tumor growth, most likely by enhanced homing of dendritic cells to the tumor-draining lymph nodes and increased antitumor immunity [48]. Also of significant importance is the fact that effective checkpoint inhibition therapy requires functional tumor-draining lymph nodes [49]. Taken together, these studies suggest that tumor-draining lymph nodes are not only important for the initiation of antitumor immune response but are also critical to achieve optimal immunotherapeutic efficacy.

However, lymph nodes, apart from their function in immune activation, also appear to play an important role in the maintenance of self-tolerance [50]. The lymphatic vasculature regulates self-tolerance by generating a conduit for antigen transportation and orchestrating the structural organization of the draining lymph nodes [44]. Therefore, the lymphatic system not only triggers antitumor immune response but also promotes tolerance [51].

An increasing body of evidence suggests that lymphatic endothelial cells, under both physiological and pathological conditions, participate in the induction of peripheral tolerance through various mechanisms [52]. Lymphatic endothelial cells express peripheral tissue antigens as well as major histocompatibility complex (MHC) molecules. Accordingly, they are able to recognize and inhibit T cell activation when expression levels of inhibitory receptors are high and the expression levels of co-stimulatory molecules are low [53]. Interestingly, IFNγ has been found to strongly induce the expression level of programmed death-ligand 1 (PD-L1) in lymphatic endothelial cells [54]. Consequently, specific deletion of IFNγ receptor (IFNγR) in lymphatic endothelial cells resulted in dampened immune suppression and increased tumor immunity [55]. Thus, the induction of PD-L1 expression by IFNγ appears to constitute a feedback mechanism utilized by the immune system to achieve equilibrium. Lymphatic endothelial cells themselves also secrete immunosuppressive molecules such as nitric oxide (NO), TGF-β, and indoleamine-2,3-dioxygenase (IDO) in order to induce tolerant dendritic cells and inhibit T cell function [56, 57]. Accordingly, the lymphatics in the tumor microenvironment not only induce an active immune response characterized via immune cell infiltration, but also directly promote the formation of an immunosuppressive microenvironment through an increased expression of IDO, arginase-1, and inducible nitric oxide synthase (iNOS) by lymphatic endothelial cells [58]. The lymphatic system can also suppress the activity of CD8+ T cells by directly presenting tumor-derived antigens [59]. In summary, these findings suggest that tumor lymphatics regulate both immune activation and tolerance.

Consequently, the identification of mechanisms that link lymphatics to cancer progression and/or the possibility to regulate their tumor-suppressing effects is fundamental for designing effective therapeutic strategies.

Concluding Remarks/Summary

The role of the lymphatic vascular system, in the setting of cancer, is still relatively understudied compared to the blood vascular system. Nevertheless, the research over the past few decades has established a fundamental knowledge of how the lymphatic vascular system develops, matures, and functions. Recent insights indicate that the tumor-associated lymphatic vasculature does not merely serve as a passive conduit for metastasis but also shapes the immune microenvironment in various tumors. Given the current successes in cancer immunotherapy, it is reasonable to expect that modulating the lymphatic vasculature in combination with immunotherapeutic strategies will improve treatment efficacy. Research on this topic is only in the beginning stages, and obviously much more work is needed to verify the role of lymphatics in tumor development and progression. Further confounding the issue are studies implying that the development of new lymphatic vessels might be associated with resolution of an immune response and induction of immune tolerance, which may explain why high lymphatic vessel density is often associated with poor prognosis. Therefore, it is likely that lymphatic vessels play multiple complex roles at different stages of cancer development, and that research on the impact of lymphatics on cancer will continue to increase our knowledge and understanding of the field.

References

1. Levick JR. An introduction to cardiovascular physiology. 5th ed. Boca Raton: CRC Press, Taylor and Francis Group; 2010.
2. Alitalo K. The lymphatic vasculature in disease. Nat Med. 2011;17(11):1371–80.
3. Petrova TV, Koh GY. Biological functions of lymphatic vessels. Science. 2020;369(6500):eaax4063.
4. Oliver G, Kipnis J, Randolph GJ, Harvey NL. The lymphatic vasculature in the 21(st) century: novel functional roles in homeostasis and disease. Cell. 2020;182(2):270–96.
5. Wagner M, Wiig H. Tumor interstitial fluid formation, characterization, and clinical implications. Front Oncol. 2015;5:115.
6. Wiig H, Swartz MA. Interstitial fluid and lymph formation and transport: physiological regulation and roles in inflammation and cancer. Physiol Rev. 2012;92(3):1005–60.
7. Kalluri R, Zeisberg M. Fibroblasts in cancer. Nat Rev Cancer. 2006;6(5):392–401.
8. Lu P, Weaver VM, Werb Z. The extracellular matrix: a dynamic niche in cancer progression. J Cell Biol. 2012;196(4):395–406.
9. Eble JA, Niland S. The extracellular matrix in tumor progression and metastasis. Clin Exp Metastasis. 2019;36(3):171–98.

10. Rigoglio NN, Rabelo ACS, Borghesi J, de Sa Schiavo Matias G, Fratini P, Prazeres P, et al. The tumor microenvironment: focus on extracellular matrix. Adv Exp Med Biol. 2020;1245:1–38.

11. Cox TR. The matrix in cancer. Nat Rev Cancer. 2021;21(4):217–38.

12. Wiig H, Keskin D, Kalluri R. Interaction between the extracellular matrix and lymphatics: consequences for lymphangiogenesis and lymphatic function. Matrix Biol. 2010;29(8):645–56.

13. Junttila MR, de Sauvage FJ. Influence of tumour microenvironment heterogeneity on therapeutic response. Nature. 2013;501(7467):346–54.

14. Ronnov-Jessen L, Petersen OW, Bissell MJ. Cellular changes involved in conversion of normal to malignant breast: importance of the stromal reaction. Physiol Rev. 1996;76(1):69–125.

15. Brown LF, Guidi AJ, Schnitt SJ, Van De Water L, Iruela-Arispe ML, Yeo TK, et al. Vascular stroma formation in carcinoma in situ, invasive carcinoma, and metastatic carcinoma of the breast. Clin Cancer Res. 1999;5(5):1041–56.

16. Senger DR, Galli SJ, Dvorak AM, Perruzzi CA, Harvey VS, Dvorak HF. Tumor cells secrete a vascular permeability factor that promotes accumulation of ascites fluid. Science. 1983;219(4587):983–5.

17. Fukumura D, Xavier R, Sugiura T, Chen Y, Park EC, Lu N, et al. Tumor induction of VEGF promoter activity in stromal cells. Cell. 1998;94(6):715–25.

18. Christiansen A, Detmar M. Lymphangiogenesis and cancer. Genes Cancer. 2011;2(12):1146–58.

19. Padera TP, Kadambi A, di Tomaso E, Carreira CM, Brown EB, Boucher Y, et al. Lymphatic metastasis in the absence of functional intratumor lymphatics. Science. 2002;296(5574):1883–6.

20. Heldin CH, Rubin K, Pietras K, Ostman A. High interstitial fluid pressure—an obstacle in cancer therapy. Nat Rev Cancer. 2004;4(10):806–13.

21. Goel S, Duda DG, Xu L, Munn LL, Boucher Y, Fukumura D, et al. Normalization of the vasculature for treatment of cancer and other diseases. Physiol Rev. 2011;91(3):1071–121.

22. Dvorak HF. Vascular permeability factor/vascular endothelial growth factor: a critical cytokine in tumor angiogenesis and a potential target for diagnosis and therapy. J Clin Oncol. 2002;20(21):4368–80.

23. Randolph GJ, Angeli V, Swartz MA. Dendritic-cell trafficking to lymph nodes through lymphatic vessels. Nat Rev Immunol. 2005;5(8):617–28.

24. Skobe M, Hawighorst T, Jackson DG, Prevo R, Janes L, Velasco P, et al. Induction of tumor lymphangiogenesis by VEGF-C promotes breast cancer metastasis. Nat Med. 2001;7(2):192–8.

25. Vaahtomeri K, Alitalo K. Lymphatic Vessels in Tumor Dissemination versus Immunotherapy. Cancer Res. 2020;80(17):3463–5.

26. Naxerova K, Reiter JG, Brachtel E, Lennerz JK, van de Wetering M, Rowan A, et al. Origins of lymphatic and distant metastases in human colorectal cancer. Science. 2017;357(6346):55–60.

27. Pereira ER, Kedrin D, Seano G, Gautier O, Meijer EFJ, Jones D, et al. Lymph node metastases can invade local blood vessels, exit the node, and colonize distant organs in mice. Science. 2018;359(6382):1403–7.

28. Brown M, Assen FP, Leithner A, Abe J, Schachner H, Asfour G, et al. Lymph node blood vessels provide exit routes for metastatic tumor cell dissemination in mice. Science. 2018;359(6382):1408–11.

29. Ehrlich P. In: Himmelweit F, editor. The collected papers of Paul Ehrlich. 2nd ed. London: Pergamon Press; 1957.

30. Thomas L. In: Lawrence HS, editor. Cellular and humoral aspects of hypersensitivity. New York: Hoeber-Harper; 1959.

31. Burnet FM. Cancer—a biological approach. 1. The process of control. Br Med J. 1957;1:779–82.

32. Swartz MA, Hubbell JA, Reddy ST. Lymphatic drainage function and its immunological implications: from dendritic cell homing to vaccine design. Semin Immunol. 2008;20(2):147–56.

33. Junt T, Moseman EA, Iannacone M, Massberg S, Lang PA, Boes M, et al. Subcapsular sinus macrophages in lymph nodes clear lymph-borne viruses and present them to antiviral B cells. Nature. 2007;450(7166):110–4.

34. Randolph GJ, Ochando J, Partida-Sanchez S. Migration of dendritic cell subsets and their precursors. Annu Rev Immunol. 2008;26:293–316.

35. Lund AW, Wagner M, Fankhauser M, Steinskog ES, Broggi MA, Spranger S, et al. Lymphatic vessels regulate immune microenvironments in human and murine melanoma. J Clin Invest. 2016;126(9):3389–402.

36. Steinskog ES, Sagstad SJ, Wagner M, Karlsen TV, Yang N, Markhus CE, et al. Impaired lymphatic function accelerates cancer growth. Oncotarget. 2016;7(29):45789–802.

37. Roberts EW, Broz ML, Binnewies M, Headley MB, Nelson AE, Wolf DM, et al. Critical role for CD103(+)/CD141(+) dendritic cells bearing CCR7 for tumor antigen trafficking and priming of T cell immunity in melanoma. Cancer Cell. 2016;30(2):324–36.

38. Kimura T, Sugaya M, Oka T, Blauvelt A, Okochi H, Sato S. Lymphatic dysfunction attenuates tumor immunity through impaired antigen presentation. Oncotarget. 2015;6(20):18081–93.

39. Mlecnik B, Bindea G, Kirilovsky A, Angell HK, Obenauf AC, Tosolini M, et al. The tumor microenvironment and Immunoscore are critical determinants of dissemination to distant metastasis. Sci Transl Med. 2016;8(327):327ra26.

40. Wagner M, Bjerkvig R, Wiig H, Dudley AC. Loss of adipocyte specification and necrosis augment tumor-associated inflammation. Adipocyte. 2013;2(3):176–83.

41. Wagner M, Bjerkvig R, Wiig H, Melero-Martin JM, Lin RZ, Klagsbrun M, et al. Inflamed tumor-associated adipose tissue is a depot for macrophages that stimulate tumor growth and angiogenesis. Angiogenesis. 2012;15(3):481–95.

42. Wagner M, Dudley AC. A three-party alliance in solid tumors: adipocytes, macrophages and vascular endothelial cells. Adipocyte. 2013;2(2):67–73.

43. Wagner M, Steinskog ES, Wiig H. Blockade of Lymphangiogenesis Shapes Tumor-Promoting Adipose Tissue Inflammation. Am J Pathol. 2019;189(10):2102–14.

44. Thomas SN, Rohner NA, Edwards EE. Implications of lymphatic transport to lymph nodes in immunity and immunotherapy. Annu Rev Biomed Eng. 2016;18:207–33.

45. Rohner NA, McClain J, Tuell SL, Warner A, Smith B, Yun Y, et al. Lymph node biophysical remodeling is associated with melanoma lymphatic drainage. FASEB J. 2015;29(11):4512–22.

46. Thomas SN, Vokali E, Lund AW, Hubbell JA, Swartz MA. Targeting the tumor-draining lymph node with adjuvanted nanoparticles reshapes the anti-tumor immune response. Biomaterials. 2014;35(2):814–24.

47. Jeanbart L, Ballester M, de Titta A, Corthesy P, Romero P, Hubbell JA, et al. Enhancing efficacy of anticancer vaccines by targeted delivery to tumor-draining lymph nodes. Cancer Immunol Res. 2014;2(5):436–47.

48. Allen F, Rauhe P, Askew D, Tong AA, Nthale J, Eid S, et al. CCL3 enhances antitumor immune priming in the lymph node via IFNgamma with dependency on natural killer cells. Front Immunol. 2017;8:1390.

49. Fransen MF, Schoonderwoerd M, Knopf P, Camps MG, Hawinkels LJ, Kneilling M, et al. Tumor-draining lymph nodes are pivotal in PD-1/PD-L1 checkpoint therapy. JCI Insight. 2018;3(23):e124507.

50. Forster R, Davalos-Misslitz AC, Rot A. CCR7 and its ligands: balancing immunity and tolerance. Nat Rev Immunol. 2008;8(5):362–71.

51. Chen DS, Mellman I. Elements of cancer immunity and the cancer-immune set point. Nature. 2017;541(7637):321–30.

52. Randolph GJ, Ivanov S, Zinselmeyer BH, Scallan JP. The lymphatic system: integral roles in immunity. Annu Rev Immunol. 2016;35:31–52.

53. Tewalt EF, Cohen JN, Rouhani SJ, Guidi CJ, Qiao H, Fahl SP, et al. Lymphatic endothelial cells induce tolerance via PD-L1 and lack of costimulation leading to high-level PD-1 expression on CD8 T cells. Blood. 2012;120(24):4772–82.

54. Dieterich LC, Ikenberg K, Cetintas T, Kapaklikaya K, Hutmacher C, Detmar M. Tumor-associated lymphatic vessels upregulate PDL1 to inhibit T-cell activation. Front Immunol. 2017;8:66.

55. Lane RS, Femel J, Breazeale AP, Loo CP, Thibault G, Kaempf A, et al. IFNgamma-activated dermal lymphatic vessels inhibit cytotoxic T cells in melanoma and inflamed skin. J Exp Med. 2018;215(12):3057–74.

56. Christiansen AJ, Dieterich LC, Ohs I, Bachmann SB, Bianchi R, Proulx ST, et al. Lymphatic endothelial cells attenuate inflammation via suppression of dendritic cell maturation. Oncotarget. 2016;7(26):39421–35.

57. Lukacs-Kornek V, Malhotra D, Fletcher AL, Acton SE, Elpek KG, Tayalia P, et al. Regulated release of nitric oxide by nonhematopoietic stroma controls expansion of the activated T cell pool in lymph nodes. Nat Immunol. 2011;12(11):1096–104.

58. Bordry N, Broggi MAS, de Jonge K, Schaeuble K, Gannon PO, Foukas PG, et al. Lymphatic vessel density is associated with CD8(+) T cell infiltration and immunosuppressive factors in human melanoma. Oncoimmunology. 2018;7(8):e1462878.

59. Lund AW, Duraes FV, Hirosue S, Raghavan VR, Nembrini C, Thomas SN, et al. VEGF-C promotes immune tolerance in B16 melanomas and cross-presentation of tumor antigen by lymph node lymphatics. Cell Rep. 2012;1(3):191–9.

Cédric Zeltz, Roya Navab, Ning Lu,
Marion Kusche-Gullberg, Ming-Sound Tsao,
and Donald Gullberg

Abstract

Extensive evidence exists to functionally implicate stromal cancer-associated fibroblasts in tumor progression. Data from experimental cancer models has questioned the exclusive tumor-supportive function of the tumor stroma and suggested that the stroma might also act as a barrier to inhibit tumor metastasis. With consideration of this shift in dogma, we discuss the role of a specific part of the tumor stroma, the insoluble extracellular matrix (ECM), in tumor growth and spread. We summarize data from experimental tumor models on the role of fibrillar collagens, the fibronectin EDA splice form, proteoglycans and the matricellular proteins, periostin and tenascins, which are all major components of the tumor stroma. In addition to the composition of the ECM being able to regulate tumorigenesis via integrin-mediated signaling, recent data indicate that the stiffness of the ECM also significantly impacts tumor growth and progression. These two properties add to the complexity of tumor-stroma interactions and have significant implications for gene regulation, matrix remodeling, and tumor metastasis. The role of the tumor stroma is thus extremely complex and highlights the importance of relating findings to tumor-type-, tissue-, and stage-specific effects in addition to considering inter-tumor and intra-tumor heterogeneity. Further work is needed to determine the relative contribution of different ECM proteins to the tumor-supporting and tumor-inhibiting roles of the tumor stroma.

Take-Home Lessons

- The extracellular matrix (**ECM**) is a meshwork of macromolecules which in the tumor microenvironment (**TME**) is present in **interstitial matrix** and **basement membranes**.
- Major producers of interstitial ECM rich in fibrillar collagens are the **cancer-associated fibroblasts** (**CAFs**) whereas tumor basement membranes are dependent on endothelial cells for production of the laminin and collagen IV networks which are major structural components in basement membranes.
- Except for **fibrillar collagens**, key ECM molecules in the interstitial TME include **EDA fibronectin** (tumor progression, TGF-β activation), **periostin** (metastatic niches, extravasation stage of metastasis), **tenascin-C** (metastasis, seeding stage of metastasis) and **proteoglycans** (inhibit or stimulate tumor growth, depending on proteoglycan type). Many of these effects are mediated via **integrins** or **toll-like receptors.**
- One controversial issue in the field concerns the role of the **ECM** in the **TME**. It is becoming clear that identical ECM molecules might have diametrically different functions in different tumor types at distinct stages of tumorigenesis. Except for a *structural support* of the tissue the interstitial **TME ECM** can develop into a *protective barrier* (prevent access of immune cells and therapeutic drugs), in other instances it can *lead the way for metastasizing tumor cells*, but also be involved in establishing the pre-metastatic niche.

C. Zeltz · N. Lu · M. Kusche-Gullberg · D. Gullberg (✉)
Department of Biomedicine, Centre for Cancer Biomarkers,
University of Bergen, Bergen, Norway
e-mail: donald.gullberg@uib.no

R. Navab · M.-S. Tsao
Princess Margaret Cancer Center, University Health Network,
Toronto, ON, Canada

© The Author(s), under exclusive license to Springer Nature Switzerland AG 2022
L. A. Akslen, R. S. Watnick (eds.), *Biomarkers of the Tumor Microenvironment*, https://doi.org/10.1007/978-3-030-98950-7_5

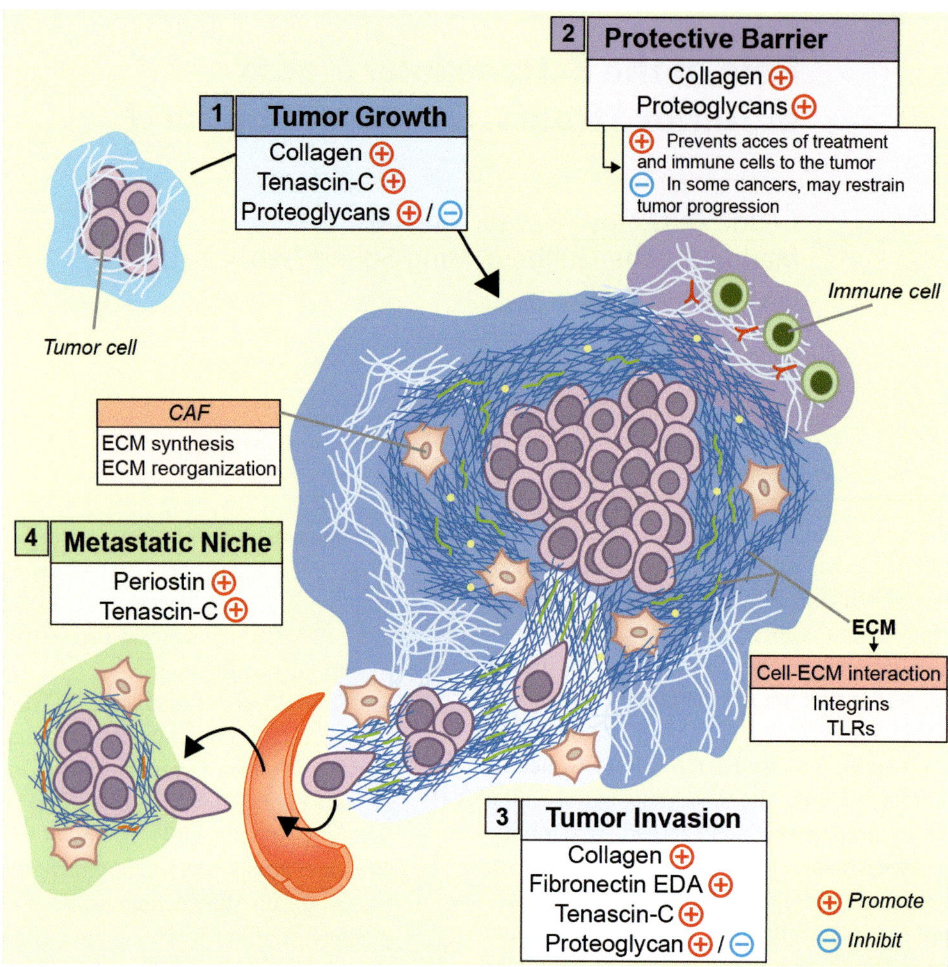

Schematic illustration of the role of extracellular matrix in the tumor microenvironment. The schematic summarizes some of the effects seen for extracellular matrix (ECM) molecules in different forms of cancer. Cancer-associated fibroblasts (CAFs) play a major role in ECM synthesis and ECM reorganization

Introduction

How one views a solid tumor depends on which "glasses" one uses. One can thus look at a tumor from a pathologist's point of view, from a cell biologist's point of view or from a molecular biologist's point of view. These different approaches provide different perspectives and information. A pathologist might note different aspects related to encapsulation, vascularization, and the amount of stroma. A cell biologist might distinguish signs of inflammation, degree of vascularization and choose to isolate cells to study their phenotypes in vitro. A molecular biologist aims to understand the molecular and genetic mechanisms involved in tumor pathogenesis, and designs experiments accordingly. No matter which "glasses" you have on, developments in the field of tumor cell-tumor stroma interactions highlight the importance of the tumor microenvironment (TME), and it is becoming increasingly clear that one needs to pay close attention to the tumor stroma when analyzing tumors.

The understanding that the tumor microenvironment influences tumor cell growth, also has implications for the design and interpretations of in vitro experiments. It has become clear that simple two-dimensional (2D) in vitro co-culture experiments are not sufficient to recapitulate the complex interactions that take place in the tumor in situ. Thus, in order to understand the cellular dynamics in the tumor, one needs to create model systems where the interactions between multiple types of cells as well as their three-dimensional (3D) compositions are incorporated. In molecular studies, inter-cellular communication, amount and properties of the extracellular matrix (ECM) and paracrine signaling, which all influence the signaling within cells, have to be taken into consideration when interpreting the data. New innovative strategies to study the influence of ECM in tumorigenesis are needed, heterospheroids [1, 2] and 3D organoid cultures are being recent methodological developments with great potential. 3D organoid cultures of patient tumors have recently generated great interest as novel in vitro cancer models that have several advantages over and are complementary to established cell lines and patient-derived mouse xenograft models [3]. Unlike cell lines, organoids are both genetically and phenotypically stable during prolonged periods of cell culture and maintain the genomic representation of high-frequency gene alterations found in primary tumors [4]. Organoid models have been successfully developed for multiple tumor types, including pancreas [5] and breast cancer [6].

When discussing different mechanisms in the tumor microenvironment, it is important to avoid generalizations and to always relate the findings to a certain tumor and to the specific experimental conditions. The reasons to avoid such generalizations are:

– The TME can vary greatly between different tumors. Part of this heterogeneity is due to the source and nature of the stromal fibroblasts [7–9].
– The composition of the TME varies with the dynamics in, and stage of, the tumor: initiation, growth, and metastasis phases, all contain a TME with specific characteristics (e.g., differences in amounts of immune cells, fibroblast activation states, proteolytic activity, and stiffness).
– Matrix stiffness is another critical feature for tumor growth and for tensional homeostasis in the tumor [7, 8, 10]. Matrix stiffness has been shown to be intimately linked to posttranslational modifications of the matrix proteins, such as glycation, citrullination [9] and cross-linking, but also to ECM organization, which will vary in different regions within the tumor. In addition to the complexity in the assembly and structure of the ECM, the finding that tumor-derived exosomes affect cellular interactions in the TME introduces yet another level of complexity. Provocative data have described roles for exosomes in chemoresistance, miRNA-directed effects on gene silencing, and even in mediating changes in integrin repertoire affecting metastasis of tumor cells [11, 12].

The function of collagen in the tumor stroma is tightly linked to stromal fibroblasts, which in the solid tumor context are called cancer-associated fibroblasts (CAFs) [13–16]. CAFs have multiple roles in the tumor stroma in addition to ECM-related functions discussed below, including paracrine signaling [13] and chemoresistance [17]. A major function of CAFs is to serve as producers of ECM proteins like fibrillar collagens, and act as mechano-sensitive cells performing integrin-mediated reorganization of the matrix, resulting in changes in stromal stiffness [8]. In order for CAFs to take on this contractile function, they need to become activated. A prime signal for CAF activation is TGF-β. Data has demonstrated that integrin αvβ6 on the tumor cells is involved in TGF-β activation by binding to an RGD sequence in the latency-associated peptide (LAP) of the TGF-β/LAP complex, resulting in increased TGF-β bioavailability. Activation of TGF-β results in CAF activation [18]. Moreover, antibodies

to αvβ6 in vivo have been shown to reduce growth and metastasis of the 4T1 murine breast cancer cell line [19]. Data in fibrosis and in vitro models further suggest that myofibroblasts themselves can play a vital role in activating TGF-β, by pre-straining the matrix and sensitizing latent TGF-β (LTGF-β) to activation [20–22]. In studies with dermal fibroblasts, the EDS fibronectin splice variant (EDA FN) has been shown to be induced by stiffness and to bind LTGF-β, in this way concentrating LTGF-β and enabling further activation by integrins. Integrin αvβ1 is increasingly becoming recognized for its role in TGF-β activation of myofibroblasts [23, 24].

Additionally, the finding that PDL-1/PD-1-based immunotherapy varies greatly between tumor types has resulted in an increased interest in alternative/supportive strategies that can abrogate immunosuppression [25]. In this context integrin αvβ8 has entered the spotlight. Whereas previous studies suggested that intestinal T-cells expressed αvβ8, and that this expression correlated with TGF-β activation [26], more recent studies suggest that most T-cell types lack detectable levels of αvβ8 and instead in most solid tumors the roles are reversed, i.e., tumor cells express high levels of αvβ8 and T-cells express inactive LTGF-β on their cell surface (anchored at cell surfaces via the membrane protein GARP) [27]. Further studies in mouse tumor models revealed that αvβ8 in this setting can activate TGF-β and by reducing immune cell activity help tumor cells evade host immunity. Interestingly, in this scenario, the activation of TGF-β appeared to occur independent of MMP-14. Later studies using cryo-EM confirmed the MMP-14 independency of the activation and instead demonstrated that in this context αvβ8 can bind to TGF-β while still bound to LTGF-β, without the release and diffusion of TGF-β to its receptor [28]. Another argument for considering αvβ8 as a cancer target comes from studies of pancreatic ductal adenocarcinoma where β8 was found to be over-expressed. When cultured human PDAC cells were irradiated, β8 expression protected cells from autophagy, which is also the major suggested mechanism for its radiochemoresistance effects [29].

At the stage of metastasis, CAFs have been reported to generate migratory paths in the stroma that facilitate collective cell invasion in an integrin-, caveolin-1-, RhoA-, Rab21-, and YAP-dependent manner [30, 31]. Interestingly, two highly cited reports have challenged the dogma that the tumor stroma plays a supportive role in tumor growth and metastasis [32, 33]. Both studies take advantage of advanced genetic techniques to ablate stromal cells in experimental models for pancreatic cancer after the tumors had formed. Contrary to what was expected, the tumors became more aggressive in the absence of the stroma. When analyzing these data, a number of caveats with these studies have been mentioned. However, a detailed update on the role of the tumor stroma in pancreatic ductal adenocarcinoma (PDA) using clinical patient PDA material as well as the use of transgenic mouse models, support a barrier role of the PDA

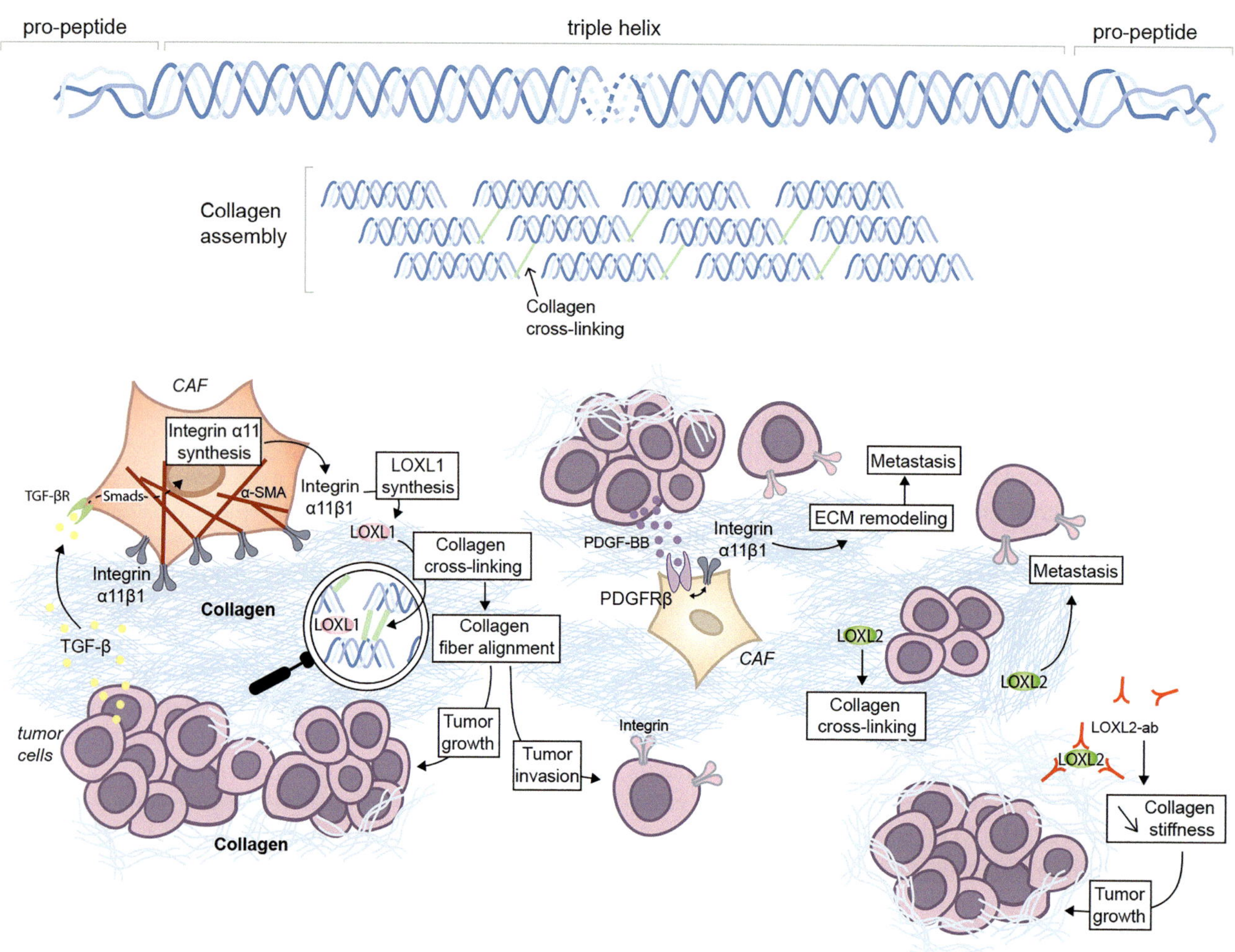

Fig. 5.1 Fibrillar collagen in cancer. Fibrillar collagens are composed of three chains that form a triple helix. The pro-peptides are cleaved for collagen assembly into fibrils. TGF-β signaling induces fibroblast differentiation into contractile myofibroblasts. The myofibroblasts express and deposit collagen, express α11β1 collagen-binding integrin, which mediates collagen remodelling. Integrin α11 induces LOXL1 expression in cancer-associated fibroblast (CAF). Secreted LOXL1 cross-links collagen fibers that enhances integrin-mediated collagen matrix reorganization and alignment of collagen fibers to support tumor growth and tumor invasion. Breast tumor cells releases PDGF-BB that activates PDGFRβ on CAFs. PDGFRβ interacts with integrin α11β1 to mediate metastasis. LOXL2, like LOXL1, mediates collagen cross-linking and is involved in metastasis of breast cancer. However, blocking LOXL2 activity using anti-LOXL2 antibody (ab) in pancreatic ductal adenocarcinoma reduces collagen stiffness that favors tumor aggressiveness and progression. This suggests that fibrillar collagens play different roles in different cancer types

stroma [34]. When the authors analyzed tumor-stromal density, patients with high tumor-stromal density enjoyed a longer survival and stromal content showed a negative correlation with overall survival. A PDA model in mouse where collagen content was modified by anti-Loxl2 monoclonal antibody (mAb) treatment confirmed that stromal depletion promoted, rather than inhibited, PDA development (Fig. 5.1). Interestingly, no striking changes in CAF subtypes, endothelial cell number, T-cell or myeloid cell infiltration were observed. In this transgenic mouse model, pharmacologic depletion of stroma thus decreased tissue ten-

sion and increased tumor aggressiveness [34]. The study suggests that the stroma has an important protective barrier role in PDA that outweighs any hypothetical pro-tumorigenic influence it may have in PDA tumor biology. The study highlights the need to firmly establish whether a fibrotic stroma in a particular tumor model is tumor promoting or tumor impeding and based on this to identify CAF subsets that are tumor promoting or tumor impeding.

Although the overall role of CAFs most likely differs between tumor types and CAF heterogeneity differs in different tumors, this does not mean that all fibroblast-targeted therapy approaches are doomed to fail in tumors, but it highlights the complexity of tumor-stroma interactions and points to the potential need to target specific subsets of fibroblasts or even specific signaling pathways in fibroblasts, which are central to the tumor-promoting aspect of the stroma. In summary, a global targeting of all CAFs may not be the best anti-stroma therapeutic strategy [16, 35] since both tumor-supportive CAFs and tumor-inhibitory CAFs appear to exist in the tumor stroma. Continued cell lineage tracing and RNA single-cell profiling will be critical to unravel these mechanisms and provide useful insight into new CAF-associated therapies for treating tumors.

The Extracellular Matrix of the Tumor Stroma

Fibrillar Collagens in the Stroma

Fibrillar Collagen Types in the Tumor Stroma

The collagen family is composed of 28 trimeric triple helical proteins [36, 37]. The most abundant collagens are the fibrillar collagens (collagens I, II, III, V, XI, XIV, and type XXVII), which together with a subset of fibril-associated collagens with interrupted triple helices (FACIT collagens) are present in interstitial tissues [37]. In interstitial tissues, collagen I dominates with lesser amounts of collagen III being present. Collagens I and III form heterotypic fibrils where the minor collagens collagen V and XI are present in the core of these heterotypic fibrils. Collagen V in some studies has been suggested to constitute less than 5% of interstitial matrices, whereas collagen XI is present only in specialized matrices under physiological conditions [36, 37]. In carcinomas, the fibrillar collagens I/III dominate, and relatively little information is available on the status or roles, if any, of collagens V and XI [38]. The tumor stroma has been likened to a *wound that does not heal*, representing the tumor stroma in a sense as a granulation tissue, which is rich in fibrillar collagens [39, 40]. In the granulation tissue, collagen III is replaced with collagen I as the wound heals [41], but in the tumor stroma, the ratio of collagen I and III is determined by tumor type as well as the stage of the tumor and tissue-specific factors.

Cells can adhere to collagen matrices, either directly or indirectly via proteins bound to collagens. Direct binding occurs via collagen receptors such as the integrins $\alpha1\beta1$, $\alpha2\beta1$, $\alpha10\beta1$ and $\alpha11\beta1$ [42, 43]. Indirect binding is mediated via collagen-integrin bridging molecules (COLINBRIs), which typically bind RGD-binding integrins like $\alpha5\beta1$, $\alpha\nu\beta1$, $\alpha\nu\beta3$ and $\alpha\nu\beta5$ [42, 44]. Interestingly, the discoidin domain receptors (DDRs) have been shown to affect the function of collagen-binding integrins by supporting integrin activation [45–47]. The role of fibrillar collagens in the tumor TME for tumor growth and metastasis is receiving increasing attention. Some of the most provocative studies have addressed the role

of collagen composition, processing, and posttranslational modifications including cross-linking in regulating stiffness, tumor growth, tumor invasion, and metastasis [48–52].

The ability of fibroblasts to produce and remodel the collagen matrix is in turn affected by interactions with other cell types in the TME such as the tumor cells themselves, different types of inflammatory and vascular cells [53]. Cell-mediated collagen remodeling can be mediated by direct binding of collagen-binding integrins and indirect binding of COLINBRI-binding integrins [44, 54]. The main integrin-collagen receptors for direct binding to the fibril form of fibrillar collagens are $\alpha2\beta1$ and $\alpha11\beta1$ [55]. These two integrins are both efficient in remodeling the collagen matrix, as assessed in collagen gel contraction assays [56]. Although in vitro experiments have largely failed to demonstrate a direct binding of $\alpha1\beta1$ to collagens fibrils, $\alpha1\beta1$ has been postulated to bind indirectly to the fibrillar forms of collagens I/III via FACIT collagens [57].

Integrin $\alpha11\beta1$ is a receptor for fibrillar collagens and is expressed on subsets of fibroblasts and mesenchymal stem cells [58–61]. In an $\alpha11$-positive subset of non-hematopoietic bone marrow-derived mesenchymal stem cells, $\alpha11$ expression correlated with osteogenic potential of these cells [62]. The potential role of $\alpha11$ bone marrow expression for leukemia development remains to be determined. Recent screening of tumor tissue array revealed expression of $\alpha11$ in CAFs in multiple solid tumors [63]. Importantly, studies using animals deficient in $\alpha11$ expression in the tumor stroma reveal a major attenuation of tumor growth and metastasis in non-small cell lung cancer and breast cancer in the absence of $\alpha11$ [64–66]. In the breast cancer model, we have shown that stromal integrin $\alpha11$ displays a pro-tumorigenic and pro-metastatic activity in breast cancer and strongly associates with a PDGFRβ+ CAF subset [64] (Fig. 5.1). Integrin $\alpha11$ expression is strongly upregulated in the stromal compartment during mammary tumor progression. Histological analyses revealed a strong association between integrin $\alpha11$ and PDGFRβ, both in clinical breast cancer samples and in the pre-clinical transgenic mouse MMTV-PyMT model. Among several tested stromal markers (PDGFRα, PDGFRβ, αSMA, FAP, FSP1, and NG2), this collagen-binding integrin was mostly associated with a PDGFRβ^+ CAF subpopulation at late stages of invasive tumors. Genetic ablation of integrin $\alpha11$ in the PyMT model drastically reduced not only tumor growth and metastasis, but also the desmoplastic reaction in these tumors, further highlighting the contribution of this specific $\alpha11^+$ CAF subset to tumor progression through ECM regulation. This is further supported by the fact that myofibroblastic CAFs (mCAFs) are thought to derive from resident fibroblasts, as well as from integrin $\alpha11$/PDGFRβ^+ CAFs. Mechanistically, this study revealed that integrin $\alpha11$/ PDGFRβ cross-talk in CAFs endows breast cancer tumor cells with pro-invasive features through the deposition of tenascin-C protein (TN-C) (Fig. 5.2). TN-C was strongly

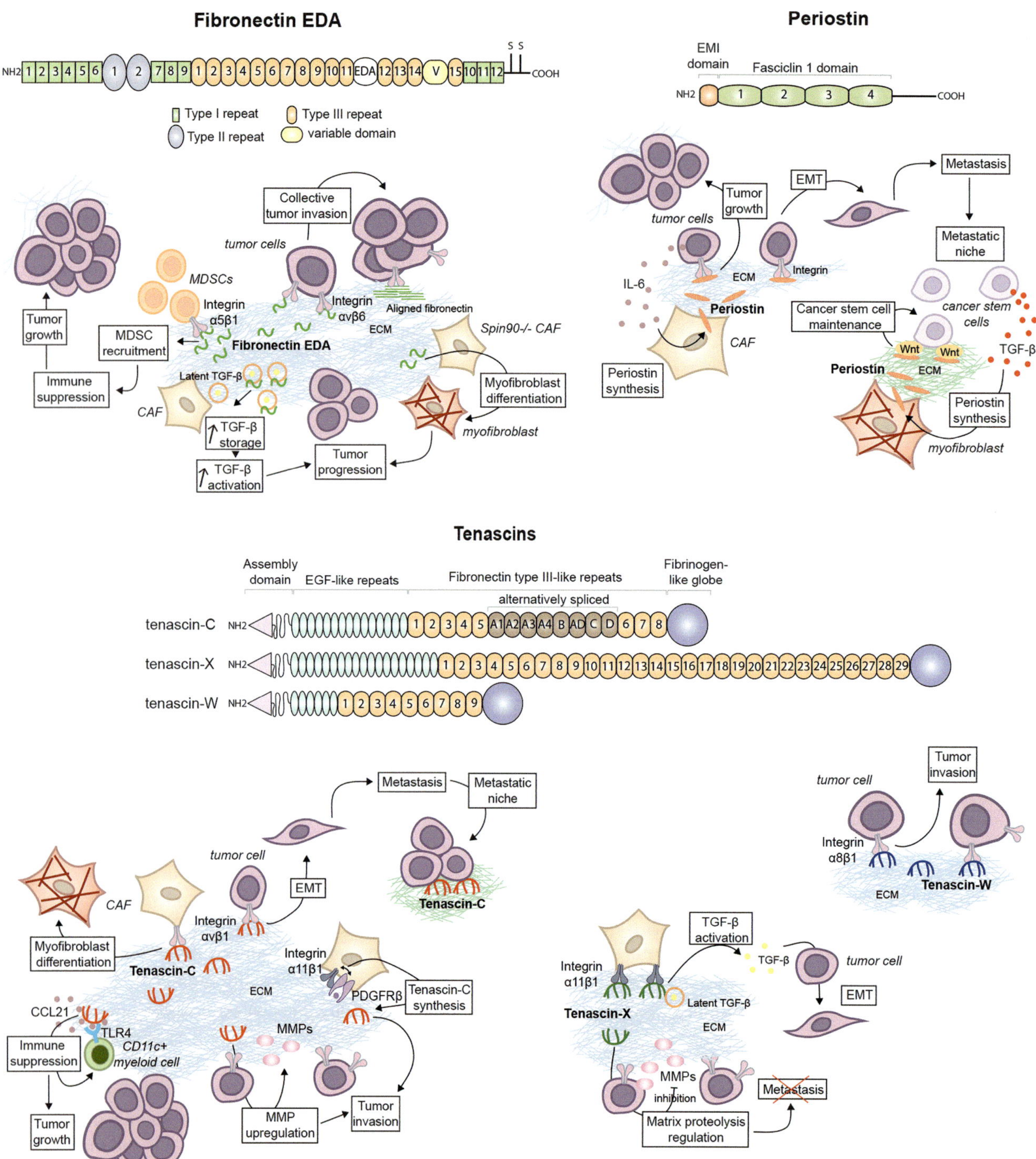

Fig. 5.2 Structure of EDA fibronectin, periostin and tenascins and their role in tumorigenesis. Fibronectin (FN) presents alternatively spliced domains, EDA and the variable domain. FN dimerizes through two disulfide bonds in the C-terminal part of the protein. EDA has been shown to reduce immune response in cancer models and to direct collective tumor cell migration. EDA FN increases recruitment and activation of the latent TGF-β in the fibroblast matrix. EDA FN induces myofibroblast differentiation of SPIN90-deficient fibroblasts to promote tumor progression. Periostin is composed of an EMI domain and four fasciclin 1 domains. Tumor cells induce periostin synthesis in CAF via IL-6. Periostin induces tumor growth and EMT. Periostin synthesis is stimulated in metastatic niches through secretion of TGF-β3 by cancer stem cells, where periostin is needed to support the metastatic colo-nization. Members of the tenascin family display an assembly domain at the N-terminal to form hexamers. Tenascin-C presents an alternatively spliced region within the fibronectin type III-like repeats. Tenascin-C has been shown to contribute to EMT through integrin αvβ1, promoting metastasis. Tenascin-C is required in metastatic niches to support the metastatic colonization. Tenascin-C also mediates immune suppression by immobilizing CD11c+ myeloid cell in the stroma, cancer cell invasion and myofibroblast differentiation of CAF. Tenascin-X activates TGF-β through interaction with α11β1 leading to EMT. In contrast, tenascin-X has been shown to reduce invasion and metastasis by inhibiting MMPs. Tenascin-W mediates cancer cell migration via interaction with α8β1 integrins. (For more details, please refer to the main text)

expressed by the same subset of CAFs expressing integrin α11 and PDGFRβ in the late-stage PyMT tumors, as well as in clinical samples of invasive breast cancer. Overall, this study discloses an example of a collaborative cross-talk between an integrin and a growth factor receptor in CAFs, which acts as a driver of tumor invasiveness in breast cancer. In support of a role for integrin α11 in human breast cancer, a careful analysis of α11 integrin levels in a larger cohort of breast cancer patients demonstrated that high α11 expression level was associated with aggressive breast cancer phenotypes [67]. In addition to the direct role of collagen-binding integrins in mechanotransduction to remodel the matrix, a role of matrix metalloproteinases (MMPs) to help and facilitate remodeling of the collagen matrix has also been demonstrated [68, 69]. This aspect is developed in a latter section of this chapter.

In the tumor context, the organization of the collagen matrix has been suggested to serve as an optical biomarker for metastatic propensity [70]. For this purpose, the term "Tumor associated collagen signatures (TACS)" has been introduced: TACS-1 (normal stage): anisotropic, wavy collagen fibrils, similar to normal quiescent tissue; TACS-2 (predisposed stage): prealigned collagen fibrils; TACS-3 (desmoplastic stage): aligned collagen fibrils [70]. It is important to remember that the tumor ECM is complex, and although collagen might align in specific patterns, cellular interactions during tumor spread might occur via many mechanisms, both collagen-dependent and collagen-independent. As such, the TACS signature may have to be combined with other biomarkers to be clinically useful.

Although there is some tendency to consider the biological effects of all stromal collagens to be equivalent, a recent study suggests that different fibrillar collagens have divergent functions. Whereas collagen I in the tumor stroma, according to the dogma, was considered to be pro-carcinogenic (increased density and increased stiffness, which promotes tumor growth and invasion), another independent study suggests that fibrillar collagen III has opposite effects [71]. In that study using collagen III heterozygous knockout mice (*Col3a1*$^{+/-}$ mice, $^{-/-}$ mice rarely survive perinatal age) it was demonstrated that mammary carcinomas grown in these mice were larger, more invasive and contained thicker, more organized and linearized collagen stroma. It is likely that in this model, several indirect mechanisms were operative, which need to be elucidated, including characterization of possible changes in integrin repertoire concomitant with collagen ratio switches. In the TME, the epithelial-derived carcinoma cells are, to varying degrees, surrounded by collagen IV containing basement membrane structures. As cells de-differentiate and go through epithelial-to-mesenchymal transition (EMT), they are exposed to fibrillar collagens in the tumor stroma. Multiple studies have highlighted the importance of collagens and the MMPs in this process [72–74].

Collagens Affecting Tumor Cell Growth

A number of studies have demonstrated that a collagen matrix promotes tumor growth. In the MMTV-PyMT breast tumor model, crossing the MMTV-PyMT mice with transgenic mice expressing a collagen α1 chain in which the collagenase cleavage site has been mutated, resulted in increased breast tumor growth and collagen accumulation at the tumor site [75]. In other experiments, collagen synthesis was blocked by inactivating certain enzyme isoforms, such as the intracellular enzymes prolyl 4- hydroxylase [76] and lysyl hydroxylase [77]. Blocking these enzymes in the stroma, resulted in reduced collagen accumulation and reduced collagen stiffness. These results are supported by data from tumor models inhibiting the collagen receptor α1β1, which implicate a role of cell-collagen interaction in non-small cell lung cancer and breast cancer growth and metastasis [64–66]. In these models, the decreased α11β1 function resulted in an attenuation of breast and lung tumor progression and metastasis, thus supporting a role of fibrillar collagens in supporting rather than restraining tumor growth. In yet other studies, fibrillar collagens have been shown to induce apoptosis of tumor cells [78]. In one study, MMP-14 was demonstrated to protect invading mammary carcinoma cells from collagen-induced apoptosis once they entered the fibrillar collagen I matrix [79, 80]. In experiments taking advantage of the model expressing collagen I with mutated collagenase cleavage site, pharmacologic depletion of stroma and decreased tissue tension increased tumor aggressiveness [34]. In summary, the disparate results on the varying roles of stromal collagens demonstrate the complexity of the stromal collagen interactions but probably also hint that the role of fibrillar collagens varies with the tumor type. It will be interesting to determine if the pancreatic desmoplastic tumors are the norm or the exception with regard to collagen function in the tumor stroma.

Collagens Affecting Cell Migration

Several studies have also reported MMP-dependent changes in collagen fibril diameters. In one study, MMTV-PyMT mice crossed with mice deficient in MMP-13 protein demonstrated no effect of MMP-13 depletion on breast tumor progression and lung metastasis [81]. Conversely, another study using a similar model observed a modest increase of lung metastasis in the absence of endogenous MMP-13 activity [82]. In the latter study, monitoring of breast tumors revealed that in the absence of MMP-13, the collagen content was not increased, but was comprised of thinner fibrillar collagen fibrils and a different organization of collagen at the tumor-stroma interface [82].

Two interesting explanations from the last study were proposed to explain the effects of the thinner fibrillar collagen structures. First, the normal cleavage of telopeptides from collagen I by MMP-13 may affect lateral fibril growth. Thus, if cleavage is reduced, fibrillar growth would be inhibited [83]. Alternatively, MMP-13 can also cleave collagen III, which acts to regulate fiber diameter, offering another possible mechanism for the observed thinner fibrils in the absence of MMP-13 [84]. Interestingly, a study of wound healing in zebrafish revealed that increased level of MMP-9 leads to larger fibril diameter. The authors suggest that this might be due to a switch in synthesis from collagen III to collagen I [85], offering more indications that MMP levels can have unpredictable effects on collagen fibril diameter. Although the effect of MMPs is complex due to multiple targets, the effects on fibril diameter are interesting and warrant further studies in the context of tumor growth and spread. Finally, in a study by Herchenhan et al., lysyl oxidase (LOX) inhibition in artificial tendon cultures also resulted in irregular fibril diameters, suggesting a role for LOX enzymes in regulating fibril diameter [86]. So far, corresponding effects have not been reported in the tumor context, but one might expect similar results in dense tumor matrices. The findings of different collagen fibril diameters might mainly be relevant for tumor cell migration. Previous elegant studies have demonstrated that cells can switch between protease-dependent and -independent migration, in 3D matrices, depending on the matrix pore diameter [87, 88]. A detailed study of collagen organization in aging tissues has revealed that collagen organization can also affect immune cell migration [89]. Studies of collagen in the aged skin paired with proteomic analysis of fibroblasts from young and aged individuals identified hyaluronan proteoglycan link protein 1 (HAPLN1) as a candidate protein involved in changed matrix collagen organization and increased collagen contractility of the aged cells. In the young ECM, HAPLN was suggested to take part in organizing collagen into an anisotropic basket weave structure, which could readily support T-cell migration. With regard to melanoma, the collagen organization in young skin was suggested to suppress invasion of melanoma cells, whereas in the aged skin (low HAPLN), an invasion-permissive microenvironment for melanoma cells was created, which was also characterized by a hampered immune cell infiltration.

Collagen Stiffness Regulating Tumor Growth

The stiffness of the tumor stroma has also been recognized as being able to influence tumor growth. Since collagens are major constituents of the tumor stroma, they might also play a major role in this regard. There are different mechanisms that can affect stiffness, including glycation [9]. A landmark paper in this area demonstrated that artificially forced expression of LOX in CAFs in a xenograft breast tumor model increased stiffness of the tumor with enhanced $\beta1$ integrin/FAK/ERK signaling in tumor cells, resulting in increased tumor growth [10]. It is worth noting that in non-experimental tumors, LOX is produced by different cell types, not only by CAFs [90]. Moreover, the role of LOX has also received considerable attention in relation to the metastatic niche and tumor metastasis [52, 91, 92]. These studies have demonstrated that LOX is deposited and crosslinks the basement membrane collagen IV at future sites of metastasis. In addition to collagens, other important ECM components of the metastatic niche stroma include periostin, fibronectin, EDA, and tenascin-C [93–95].

LOX expression has also been associated with poorer patient prognosis in lung adenocarcinoma [96]. For example, it has been shown that down-regulation of LOXL1, which belongs to the LOX family oxidases (LOXL 1–5), in xenograft tumors of both established and primary non-small cell lung cancer lines in integrin $\alpha11$ knockout in SCID background as compared to wild-type SCID mice leads to decreased tumor growth [97]. The decrease in tumor growth was closely associated with reduced organization and stiffness of fibrillar collagen matrices (Fig. 5.1) [66].

In summary, in some tumor types, collagen matrices that are rich in collagen I and comprised of large diameter fibrils seem to be required for optimal support of tumor growth and metastasis. Current data from pancreatic cancer models suggest a barrier function of fibrillar collagens. Furthermore, stiffer matrices comprised of linear fibrils around the tumor can provide routes for invasion. Stromal collagen organization is dependent on: (1) CAFs, which produce the majority of the ECM and express cell surface integrins able to reorganize the collagen matrix, (2) LOX enzymatic activity for matrix cross-linking and (3) MMPs to facilitate ECM reorganization.

As already mentioned, experiments using two different experimental model systems that severely restrict production of mouse pancreatic tumor stroma together with more recent studies in a mouse model where mAbs to LOXL2 was used to decrease collagen levels and stroma tension have demonstrated that global obliteration of the stroma can result in tumors becoming more aggressive (Fig. 5.1) [32–34]. One way of interpreting these data is that in desmoplastic pancreatic tumors, the stroma acts as a barrier, the removal of which facilitates tumor cell migration and invasion. In light of these findings, it becomes critical to reconcile the data suggesting that linearized fibrillar collagen acts as a highway for tumor invasion [70, 75] with the multiple studies suggesting that a stiff dense matrix promotes tumor growth and tumor metastasis [10, 76, 77, 98]. The most obvious explanation is that fibrillar collagens play different roles in different tumor types. These questions will need to be addressed in order to fully delineate, which pathways involved in collagen biosynthesis, posttranslational modifications or collagen remodeling, represent attractive future therapeutic targets in the tumor stroma.

Methods for Measuring Fibrillar Collagen Stiffness

Structural alterations of the ECM during tumor initiation and progression have been shown to occur in several epithelial tumors [99, 100]. As mentioned earlier, TACS signatures predict that collagen fibers in normal tissue are curly and non-oriented, which is different from the highly linearized fibers of intra-tumoral collagen [10, 66]. The fibrotic reaction observed in the stroma of many cancers, characterized by an excess accumulation of some fibrillar collagens (especially type I, III, V, XI) as a result of desmoplasia, is considered to be a hallmark of cancer [91, 101, 102]. There are multiple collagen receptors in addition to collagen-binding integrins, such as DDRs, leukocyte-associated Ig-like receptors (LAIRs), and glycoprotein VI [103]. These receptors are: (1) not necessarily expressed on tumor cells or stroma cells (LAIRs on immune cells, GPVI on platelets); and (2) unlike integrins their role as mechanoreceptors with the ability to reorganize collagen has not been established.

Since fibrillar collagen has a non-centrosymmetric structure, it can be readily visualized with second harmonic generation (SHG) two-photon confocal microscopy both in vivo and ex-vivo (i.e., histology sections) and its organization can be probed with SHG polarization measurement [104–106]. In SHG, an excitation wavelength of 840 nm is applied to a sample, the resultant SHG signal is then measured, which is exactly one-half of the excitation wavelength (i.e., 420 nm). SHG has multiple advantages such as it enables optical sectioning and 3D imaging. Also, SHG does not require staining and absorption for signal generation, therefore, sample photobleaching is reduced. Overall, the intensity and polarization of the SHG signal depends on the sample structure and organization. Polarimetric SHG microscopy (P-SHG) allows the structural details of collagen organization in the tissue to be studied. In the use of P-SHG, the orientation of incoming laser polarization relative to a set of outgoing SHG polarizations is measured (polarization-in, polarization-out (PIPO) SHG), revealing the second-order susceptibility component ratio in each pixel of the image. These measurements reflect the hierarchical organization of collagen in the tissue [107]. The SHG polarization measurement is influenced by several factors, including the amino acid composition and sequence of the collagen triple-helix, organization of the triple helices in the collagen fibrils, arrangement of these fibrils in the fibers and finally fiber orientation with respect to the tissue section plane [106]. In addition, The SHG analysis renders an average fiber orientation in each pixel of the image, and provides information on the orientation related to the helical pitch angle of the polypeptide chain of the collagen triple-helix in the tissue [108]. Hence, polarization SHG is a promising technique to detect collagen alterations in the ECM during cancer progression [109]. SHG enables pathologists to perform a live biopsy, for example, in the endoscopic setting, or provides a quick histopathology investigation possibility that does not require staining. SHG microscopy presents unique advantages compared to conventional optical techniques to investigate the 3D heterogeneous accumulation of fibrillar collagen during fibrotic pathologies [110]. Another way to analyze the fibril orientation distribution is to measure the degree of waviness or alignment and orientation of collagen by an Image J plug-in method [111]. In this way, the local collagen fiber orientation was derived from the angle of the oriented collagen structure. The shape of the distribution indicated the degree of alignment within the image, where wide and broad shapes suggested little coherence in alignment and tight peaks implied aligned structures. In another study, the collagen fiber arrangement in NSCLC tumor xenografts was measured by a novel relative linearity index [66]. The combination of SHG polarimetric analysis and texture analysis revealed significant differences in the collagen structure between NSCLC and normal lung tissue and could quantify the structural alteration of collagen in stage-I, -II, and III-NSCLC tissue (PMID: 32341852). Therefore, the combination of polarimetric SHG microscopy and histopathology may lead to more accurate cancer diagnostics and staging.

Another method of studying the collagen linearity on a nanometer scale is electron microscopy, which involves measuring how straight or "curly" an individual fiber is [66]. Accordingly, the linearity on this scale would correlate to the stiffness of individual fibers. The advantage of the SHG images is that they show collagen arrangement on a larger scale (the images are 0.5 mm × 0.5 mm), which is indicative of the stiffness or stretchiness of tissue on the micron-to-mm scale.

In a more advanced way, the self-assembly of the native collagen fibrils in vitro could be characterized by the use of atomic force microscopy (AFM) [112, 113]. AFM elasticity measurements are a powerful tool to directly assess mechanical stiffness on the level of individual, or groups of, fibers. In fact, AFM can be used as a microdissection tool to study the inner assembly of the collagen fibrils. The AFM technique is based on detection of forces acting between a sharp probe, known as AFM tip, and the sample's surface [114]. To determine the elastic properties of collagen fibrils, the tip of the AFM (cantilever) was used as a nanoindentor by recording force-displacement curves [115]. It has been shown that a new variant of AFM, which is called in situ atomic force indentation microscopy [116], is capable of measuring stiffness changes in mammary gland tissue as it evolves from normal to malignant with exquisite spatial detail. Based on this method, in a mouse model of human breast cancer that metastasizes to the lungs, the extracellular matrix at the tumor boundary turned out to be the stiffest of all the tumor's components. In this study, AFM was applied to measure the stiffness of the surrounding extracellular matrix as a prognostic indicator for tumor development and aggressiveness [117].

Another technique of interest for measuring ECM and tissue stiffness at the macroscopic level is shear rheology [118]. At its simplest, this approach provides high-resolution determination of the matrix and tissue elasticity by measurements of mechanical compression and nano-indentation [118]. Shear rheology is a commonly applied means of testing the mechanical properties of materials by indenting the test material with a diamond tip while measuring the force-displacement response [118]. Although the techniques described above provide accurate and useful quantitative data on the biomechanical properties of matrix and tissue, most are generally considered invasive and/or destructive methodologies [119]. Hence, there is a need to develop methods to measure elastic properties and stiffness of tissues and matrix in a non-invasive manner for clinical application. Magnetic resonance and ultrasound elastography are routinely used tools in the clinic that provides the image contrast of elastic properties of tissues [120]. Clinical in vivo imaging by elastography shows that malignant breast tumors tend to appear stiffer than benign breast tumors; in particular, the stiffer tissue is frequently observed at the tumor margin or the invasive edge of the tumor [120]. Newer technologies based on fluorescence resonance energy transfer (FRET) [121], magnetic resonance imaging (MRI), positron emission tomography (PET) and single-photon emission computed tomography (SPECT) [122] are being developed to image the dynamic status of ECM remodeling [123]. Advances in μ-ultrasound, optical coherence tomography (OCT), optical acoustic microscopy and scanning acoustic microscopy (SAM) [118] are under development to facilitate imaging and quantitative measurement of stiffness at the microscopic scale [124]. In addition, increasing the resolution of many of the above techniques will be possible with improved contrast agents, such as so-called "smart probes," which are MRI contrast agents that can be used to study ECM components [125–127]. More information on these techniques is available in other reviews and reference materials.

In summary, new techniques that image the dynamics of cell-ECM interactions to non-invasively quantify remodeling of the ECM at the sub-millimeter level will ultimately provide additional resources for basic research and in the clinic. Therefore, increased understanding of the molecular basis of mechanotransduction may lead to identification of an entirely new class of molecular targets for anticancer therapy.

Role of EDA Fibronectin in the Tumor Stroma

Fibronectin (FN) is a large modular extracellular matrix protein composed of type I, type II and type III repeats [128] (Fig. 5.2). FN RNA is alternatively spliced at three conserved regions EIIIA (EDA), EIIB (EDB) and V (CS-1). The FN gene structure and splicing have been described in detail elsewhere [129]. The EDA and EDB domains display 29% sequence identity, but are each highly conserved among vertebrates [129]. Whereas a number of receptors have been described for EDA (described later), the cellular receptor(s) for the EDB domain remains largely unknown. Therefore, most of the focus has been on the EDA isoform.

The EDA and EDB isoforms are both highly expressed during embryonic development, especially in developing blood vessels [130], but are almost absent in the adult organism, where vascularization and tissue reorganization are quiescent. During wound healing [131], fibrosis and in solid tumors [132], the EDA/EDB embryonic splice variants are re-expressed [133], leading to the term "oncofetal" splice variants. Some studies suggest that these embryonic splice forms in tumors are mainly expressed in neo-vasculature [134], whereas other studies demonstrated their presence in the fibrotic stroma associated with myofibroblasts [135, 136].

The EDA domain is composed of 7 antiparallel beta strands separated by loops [129]. Early studies suggested that the presence of EDA in intact FN indirectly influenced the exposure of the RGD sequence in the tenth FN type III repeat leading to higher binding affinity for integrin $\alpha5\beta1$ to FN EDA [137]. In later studies, it was demonstrated that integrin $\alpha9\beta1$ and $\alpha4\beta1$ bound directly to a cryptic loop region in an EDA containing fragment, but not to the intact FN EDA [138]. Binding of these integrins to the cryptic site would thus require proteolytic cleavage of fibronectin. $\alpha4\beta7$ integrin on lung fibroblasts has also been shown to bind directly to FN EDA [139]. Similarly, Toll-like receptor 4 (TLR4) has been reported to be activated upon binding to the isolated EDA fragment, but not upon binding to the intact fibronectin EDA [140]. Importantly, FN EDA enhances TLR4 response, which in turn has been reported to augment TGF-β signaling [141]. $\alpha9\beta1$ on basal keratinocytes co-localizes with EDA at the dermal-epidermal junction in skin wounds, but in dermal wounds, some dermal fibroblasts also express $\alpha9\beta1$ [131]. Endothelial cells on developing and adult lymphatic vessels also express $\alpha9\beta1$ [142]. Depending on the relative levels of different receptors, the effect of EDA FN is thus likely to vary.

Upon gross examination, mice deficient in either EDA or EDB appear normal, suggesting a redundancy for these splice forms during development [143, 144]. In contrast, mice lacking both isoforms die at E9–10, due to cardiovascular defects and leaky blood vessels [145]. Careful analysis of fibronectin EDA$^{-/-}$ mice reveals some mild phenotypes including a mild lymph vessel impairment, due to a transient role for α9β1/fibronectin EDA during lymphangiogenesis [142]. However, other data suggests that EMILIN1 might play a more prominent role than FN EDA as an α9β1 ligand during lymph vessel development, especially in mature lymph vessels [146]. Whereas the expression of FN EDA clearly is a marker for certain biological processes such as wound healing, fibrosis, and a reactive tumor stroma, the exact role of EDA in these events is more complex [53].

Function of EDA Fibronectin Domain in Wound Healing

The role of EDA in wound healing has been studied in great detail. In a much-cited study, an essential role of EDA in TGF-β stimulated myofibroblast differentiation of rat dermal fibroblasts in vitro was determined using neutralizing antibodies [147]. In another study, EDA induced a pro-fibrotic effect in in dermal fibroblasts via binding to α4β1-mediated without affecting myofibroblast differentiation [148]. Similarly, studies of wound healing in EDA knockout mice failed to detect any major myofibroblast differentiation defects in the granulation tissue, though reduced epithelial migration was observed at the epidermal-dermal border along with some defects in granulation tissue [144, 149]. A role for integrin α9 and EDA in keratinocyte migration was further supported by experiments where α9 was conditionally deleted on keratinocytes, resulting in epithelial thinning [149]. Independent studies using EDA blocking antibodies in vivo resulted in mild effects on granulation tissue. The authors of these studies suggest that the less dense granulation tissue observed in these experiments was due to defective migration of dermal fibroblasts into the wounds, rather than defective myofibroblast differentiation [150].

Function of EDA Fibronectin Domain in Fibrosis

In the last 5–10 years, the role of fibronectin and the EDA FN isoform have attracted considerable interest in fibroblasts biology and accumulating data now attest to the biologic importance of the EDA FN isoform in tissue and tumor pathology. An in vitro study suggests that integrin α4β7 on lung fibroblasts stimulates myofibroblast differentiation [139]. In a mouse model, EDA FN deficiency prevented bleomycin-induced lung fibrosis [151]. Mechanistic analyses suggested an effect related to TGF-β activation in the lungs in this fibrosis model. Studies of infarcted hearts have also revealed reduced cardiac fibrosis and myofibroblast differentiation in the absence of EDA FN [152].

More and more studies are being published on the role of non-integrin receptors taking part in mediating the effects of EDA FN. In dermal fibroblasts both α4β1 integrin and the non-integrin receptor TLR4 have been shown to cooperate to induce fibrotic gene expression [153]. In smooth muscle cells, both receptors cooperate to mediate phenotype switching in Akt/mTOR (TLR4- mediated) and FAK/ERK/NF-kB mediated Il-1β release (integrin α4β1-mediated) [154]. Given the finding in Jain et al. [154], it would be interesting to determine the role of TLR4 in collagen remodeling under conditions when EDA FN is present. It has been suggested that EDA FN associated with TLR4 may play a role in keloids to couple a fibrotic response with an inflammatory response in the skin [141].

In a detailed in vitro study using fibroblasts, the group of Boris Hinz has convincingly demonstrated that EDA FN is increasingly produced under stiff conditions and enhances the recruitment of latent TGF-β-binding protein-1 (LTBP-1) to the ECM matrix [155]. In the context of fibrosis, EDA FN is important in myofibroblast activation (suggested to occur via integrins α4β [148], α9β1 [156] and α4β7 [139] in different experimental systems), but prior to this careful study, the link between EDA FN and TGF-β activation/storage had been elusive. Although the study was performed using skin fibroblasts, the data is probably of high relevance to different forms of tissue- and tumor fibrosis.

Function of EDA Fibronectin Domain in Tumorigenesis

In the context of tumors, in vitro and in vivo experiments have suggested different roles for EDA FN (Fig. 5.2). For fibronectin fibrillogenesis, integrins α5β1 and αvβ3 seem to cooperate to assemble a fibrillar EDA FN matrix and to direct tumor cell migration [157, 158]. The appearance and organization of fibronectin are thus closely associated with the behavior of integrin fibronectin receptors in CAFs. Elegant studies have demonstrated a role for αvβ5 in regulating α5β1 endocytosis and function in CAFs [159]. In another study, CD93 was shown to promote integrin activation and fibronectin fibrillogenesis during tumor angiogenesis [160].

In one cancer-related study, it was suggested that EDA FN, indirectly, by increased binding of α5β1 to RGD and induction of arginase-1, inhibits the immune response in cancer [161]. The elaborate mechanism worked out in this study involved α5β1- mediated increase in myeloid differentiation followed by an arginase-1-mediated suppression of the immune response, in turn potentiating enhanced tumor growth and reduced fibrosis. In yet another study, a role for CAF-produced EDA FN in directing the collective migration of HNSCC was demonstrated to depend on both α9β1 and αvβ6 in HNSCC cells [162].

Studies in spheroids using MDA-MB-231 cells demonstrated that under stiff conditions (12kP), the actin modulatory protein Mena was upregulated to potentiate α5β1 integrin-mediated assembly of EDA FN, which in turn was found to further stimulate integrin α4β1-mediated EDA

FN-dependent invasion in this spheroid context [163]. The study is intriguing given that it was performed with homo-spheroids, composed only of tumor cells, and it will be compelling to determine if similar data can be obtained in heterospheroids containing co-cultures of tumor cells and CAFs, since CAFs are the main contributing producers of EDA FN in the TME.

A detailed study on the role of the SH3 and NCk-binding protein Spin90 in α4β1 integrin signaling in CAF-like MEF cells in vitro and in vivo experiments demonstrates a role of SPIN90 in regulating EDA FN synthesis and fibrillogenesis as well as myofibroblast activation, in turn regulating breast cancer cell proliferation, migration and invasion [164]. The increased EDA FN synthesis in the Spin90$^{-/-}$ CAF-like MEFS could be reversed in the *Spin90* rescued cells. Interestingly, in the studies of Kwon et al, α4β1-mediated binding to EDA FN is able to reorganize a collagen matrix in *Spin90*$^{-/-}$ cells, whereas wild-type MEF cells failed to demonstrate a contribution of a cell-fibronectin interaction to the collagen matrix remodeling. In addition to the intra-cellular protein SPIN90 being able to control the mechanism of collagen matrix remodeling under very specific gene deletion conditions, it is likely that the integrin repertoire is a more general determinant of collagen reorganization. In conditions of high levels of collagen-binding integrins (i.e., α2β1 and α11β1) and low fibronectin synthesis, collagen-binding integrins would dominate [55]. Whereas under conditions with low levels collagen-binding integrins, high levels of fibronectin synthesis, high levels of fibronectin-binding integrins (i.e., α4β1 or α5β1), fibronectin-binding integrins would mediate collagen reorganization. The study of Kwon et al demonstrates a role for α4β1/EDA FN in collagen remodeling in genetically modified cells, and it will be interesting to determine if this interaction also can be demonstrated under more physiological conditions and in the tumor TME.

In colon carcinoma, EDA FN sustained tumor cell proliferation and induced lymphangiogenesis through VEGF-C secretion in mouse xenograft models [165, 166]. EDA FN has also been shown to induce EMT in lung and colon carcinomas, thus promoting metastasis [167, 168]. In a radiotherapeutic aspect, the presence of EDA FN reduced radiation sensitivity in head and neck carcinoma by inhibiting apoptosis of tumor cells [169]. Despite these findings, the absence of either EDA or EDB did not affect tumor growth, tumor angiogenesis, α-SMA expression in the tumor stroma, or tumor metastasis in either the Rip1- Tag2 tumor model or a xenograft model [130].

In summary, EDA FN is highly expressed in granulation tissue, in fibrotic lesions and in the tumor stroma. Critical analysis in genetic models demonstrated a moderate effect of EDA FN in wound healing, but with new methods and more careful analyses in new experimental genetic models, impor-tant contributions to fibrosis and tumorigenesis are also increasingly being recorded.

Matricellular Proteins: Tenascins and Periostin

Matricellular proteins are secreted macromolecules that do not play a primary role in matrix structure, but are able to modulate cell interactions and functions [170]. In cancer, matricellular proteins are involved in different steps of tumorigenesis due to their ability to bind different cell receptors [171]. The matricellular protein family includes thrombospondins, tenascins, SPARC, periostin, osteopontin and CCN proteins. In this chapter, we focus on the role of tenascins and periostin in cancer progression (Fig. 5.2).

Tenascins

The tenascin family is composed of four members in vertebrates, expressed in different tissues with a common role in modulation of cell adhesion and spreading [172]. Although all tenascin isoforms are expressed in different cancer forms, TN-C has been studied the most. TN-C is absent or lowly expressed in adult tissues, in contrast to the strong expression observed in cancer. TN-C is dynamically expressed during embryogenesis and pathological disorders but mice carrying a null mutation in the *Tnc* gene display no phenotype [173]. A continued interest in this molecule has, however, indicated important biological roles for TN-C, which thus is a completely different scenario compared to the largely negative results obtained in these initial challenging experiments using *Tnc*$^{-/-}$ mice. Although TN-C is highly expressed in fibrotic conditions in tissues and the tumor stroma as well as tumor metastases, several studies failed to reveal a functional role of TN-C in these fibrotic matrices. This included studies of TN-C in the PyMT breast cancer model [174]. In contrast to data from the PyMT model in *Tnc*$^{-/-}$ genetic background which suggested a very mild phenotype with macrophage filled *Tnc*$^{-/-}$ stroma with little consequences for tumor cell proliferation or lung metastasis in the absence of TN-C, continued studies in a number of models have more recently confirmed a functional role of TN-C in specific fibrotic and tumorigenesis events (please see below for details).

Just as Toll-like receptor 4 (TLR4) has emerged as a receptor mediating pro-fibrotic signal for EDA FN, TLR4 has also emerged as a receptor for different tenascin isoforms. A detailed study focusing on different motifs in TN-C has identified a structure in fibrinogen-like globe domain (FBG) of TN-C that is predicted to be active in TLR4 binding also in tenascin R- and tenascin-W, but notably not in TN-X [175]. A number of studies suggest that tenascin-C effects are mediated by both integrins and TLR4 receptors, often creating a complex interaction network involving paracrine signaling. Experiments using cell cultures and experimental fibrosis in $Tnc^{-/-}$ mice have demonstrated a role for TLR4 in TN-C-dependent skin and lung fibrosis [176]. A recent study demonstrates an interesting role of TN-C in heart fibrosis following experimental myocardial infarction suggesting involvement of TIMP-3 in the reduced fibrosis observed in the absence of TN-C. In an independent study, the transcriptional regulators twist and paired-related homeobox1 (Prrx1) were identified in a positive feedback loop together with TN-C to be involved in regulating fibroblast activation both under physiological and fibrosis/wound healing responses [177]. Such fibrogenic niches composed of TN-C in has been shown to be active in kidney fibrosis [178].

Tenascin-C expression is induced in several solid tumors and is often associated with poor prognosis (for review, see [179]). It is now clear that TN-C promotes tumorigenesis, acting at different steps of this process, with the metastasis step probably being the most prominent step. TN-C can stimulate tumor growth by abolishing the cell proliferation-suppressing effect of fibronectin [180, 181]. TN-C has also been demonstrated to compete with fibronectin for syndecan-4 binding, thus weakening breast carcinoma cell adhesion and spreading on fibronectin [182]; this cell adhesion inhibition leads to cell rounding that enhances tumor cell proliferation. TN-C can reduce apoptosis of pancreatic cancer cells, by activating the anti-apoptotic Bcl-2 and Bcl-xl and inhibiting cleavage of caspase-3 [183]. Tenascin-C also stimulates EMT of breast cancer cells, in an $\alpha v\beta 1$- and $\alpha v\beta 6$- dependent manner [184, 185]. The Wnt/β-catenin signaling pathway, which is known to induce EMT [186], is enhanced in the presence of tenascin-C via the down-regulation of the Wnt inhibitor Dickkopf 1, which stabilizes β-catenin [181, 187]. It is interesting to note that the TNC gene was identified as a β-catenin signaling target in colorectal cancer, suggesting a feed-forward loop that could stabilize the EMT phenotype and influence invasion in this tumor type [188].

Furthermore, TN-C plays a role in tumor cell migration and invasion [189, 190]. In a study of invasive melanoma, tenascin-C was found to form, in addition to fibronectin and collagen I, tubular structures that were proposed to serve as channels for melanoma cell invasion [191]. Interestingly, TN-C can also up-regulate MMP-9 and MMP-13 expression in breast cancer, thus promoting cancer cell invasion [192, 193]. Knockdown of tenascin-C in the MDA-MB-435 melanoma cell line decreased the number of lung metastasis in nude mice, demonstrating that tenascin-C may stimulate metastatic progression [194]. Another publication demonstrated that in lung metastatic sites, TN-C is over-expressed by $S100A4^+$ stromal cells, most likely fibroblasts, supporting metastatic colonization [195]. In the same study, $Tnc^{-/-}$ mice injected with 4T1 murine breast cancer cells displayed fewer and smaller metastatic lung nodules [195]. Another interesting study initiated by Oskarsson et al. showed that TN-C

secretion by breast cancer cells is required to form a metastatic niche for the establishment of lung metastases [93].

A detailed careful study of ECM proteins induced in lung fibrosis, in lung cancer and in lung cancer metastases using mass spectrometry technology and various mouse models identified TN-C as being induced in all these conditions [196]. However, additional experiments in knockout models and in transgenic overexpressing mice revealed a functional role of Tn-C restricted to metastasis, which is still in stark contrast to the early experiments in PyMT mice, where no effects on lung metastasis were seen (Fig. 5.2). With regard to the cellular mechanisms, a study of human mammary fibroblasts, as a model of breast cancer CAFs, suggest that TN-C treatment increase collagen gel contraction and increased synthesis of TN-C and integrin $\alpha v\beta 1$, in turn leading to increased TGF-β activation [197]. This is suggested to be a mechanism promoting increased matrix stiffness. It will be interesting to pursue how actually TN-C mediates this effect on collagen gel contraction. Since this process ultimately depends on a stable link between cells and the collagen matrix, it is possible that the cell-TN-C interaction creates a stimulatory autocrine signal strengthening the link between collagen-binding integrins and the collagen matrix.

In a detailed study of a mouse model of head and neck cancer, TN-C was demonstrated to be present in tumor TME to contribute to shape an immunosuppressive pro-tumoral microenvironment [198]. When TN-C was depleted in this tumor model, tumor growth and lymph node invasion were affected. The observed TN-C effects were shown to be mediated by $\alpha 9\beta 1$ integrin on endothelial cells acting via CCL21 secretion and TLR4 on $CD11c+$ myeloid cells acting via CCR7. It will be interesting to determine if these immunosuppressive systemic effects also are operational in other tumor types.

Tenascin-W was the last tenascin member to be described, and relatively little is known about this tenascin family member. The expression of tenascin-W has been shown to be regulated by TGF-β [199], and was initially observed to be strongly upregulated in the tumor stroma of breast and colon cancer patients [200, 201]. In the context of breast cancer, tenascin-W has been shown to promote the migration of breast tumor cells through interaction with $\alpha 8\beta 1$ integrin [202]. In later studies, Brellier et al. determined that tenascin-W expression was also induced in melanoma and in pancreatic, kidney and lung carcinomas; the authors suggested that tenascin-W might be a useful cancer biomarker in several solid tumors [203].

Tenascin-X is expressed in several tissues, with high expression in skin and skeletal muscle [204]. Deficiency or mutation in tenascin-X gene leads to a form of Ehlers-Danlos syndrome, characterized by skin and joint hyperextensibility [205]. In contrast with other tenascins, tenascin-X was first predicted to be anti-tumorigenic: its expression was strongly decreased in malignant melanoma [206], and mice deficient in tenascin-X displayed increased melanoma invasion and metastasis [207]. This was explained by an induction of MMPs, including MMP-2, in the absence of tenascin-X through JNK signaling, indicating a role of this tenascin in matrix proteolysis regulation [208]. Alcaraz et al. have suggested a different role of tenascin-X in breast cancer progression. In their study, tenascin-X was curiously enough suggested to contribute to TGF-β activation via its interaction with α11β1 integrin, thus promoting EMT [209]. It will be interesting to determine if the binding of tenascin to α11β1 is direct, and if so, which part of integrin α11β1 binds to tenascin-X.

Periostin

Periostin is a matricellular protein, which is highly expressed in mesenchymal tissues during development [210]. Periostin is a homodimeric matricellular protein belonging to fasciclin family (Fig. 5.2). Like TN-C, periostin is induced in the tumor stroma. Detailed studies have revealed complex interactions with αv integrins (αvβ1, αvβ3, αvβ5) [211]. Genetic deletion of periostin leads to tooth defects and a periodontal-like disease, which result in dwarfism [210]. Wound healing studies suggest a promoting effect of periostin in dermal myofibroblast differentiation and collagen gel contraction [212]. A pro-fibrogenic role for periostin in cardiac and skeletal muscle fibrosis has also been reported [213, 214]. Interestingly, periostin has been observed to interact with fibrillar collagen and in the absence of periostin the collagen fibrillar diameter increases [215, 216].

In the tumor context, an early study reported reduced numbers of activated CAFs and less collagen in capsule and TME, leading to increased growth of grafted mouse tumor cell lines in postn$^{-/-}$ mice [217]. Later studies have focused on the presence of periostin in the tumor stroma of gastric cancer, melanoma, glioblastoma and in metastatic niches [218–220]. In one study, the ability of periostin to bind Wnt was suggested to be the mechanism underlying the ability of periostin to support cancer stem cell maintenance and tumor metastasis (Fig. 5.2) [94, 221]. Periostin was shown to induce EMT in cholangiocarcinoma through α5β1 integrin and the TWIST-2 axis [222]. In colorectal cancer, periostin secreted by stromal fibroblasts promotes YAP/TAZ activation and IL-6 expression in tumor cells, which in turn activates myofibroblasts and periostin synthesis to facilitate tumor progression [223]. In a study of B16F10 melanoma model, chemotherapy treatment with cisplatin was found to increase periostin levels, in turn suggested to contribute to liver metastasis by enhancing metastatic niche formation [224].

Stromal Proteoglycans

Proteoglycans (PGs), abundant at cell surfaces and in the extracellular matrix, belong to a group of glycoproteins in which the core protein is substituted with one or more polysaccharide chains (called glycosaminoglycans; GAGs). PGs play important roles during different aspects of cancer progression (for review, see [225–227]). Heparan sulfate (HS) PGs execute their function by binding to a variety of molecules including members of several growth factor families, chemokines, morphogens, serine protease inhibitors, and extracellular matrix proteins [228]. Protein binding is generally mediated by their sulfated GAG chains, but may in a few cases involve interaction with core proteins [229]. Examples of proteins that depend on binding to HSPGs for function include members of the FGF-family and their corresponding receptors, VEGF, members of the transforming growth factor-β family, Wnt proteins, pleotropin and the serin protease inhibitor antithrombin [230]. Depending on the molecule, the activity of the bound factors is mostly enhanced, although there are few examples of activities that are inhibited by the binding to HSPGs. The morphogen Wnt is sequestered by HS chains at the cell surface and becomes available for receptor activation only following enzyme-catalyzed release of specific sulfate groups from the HS chains [231].

In addition to the direct effect of HSPGs on growth factor signaling, the HSPG bound factors are protected from proteolytic degradation and can be released and activated under different physiological or pathological conditions like cancer [232]. Sequestration of chemokines and cytokines plays a critical role in regulating the shape of morphogen gradients and in inducing a signal for cell migration, a first step for invasion and metastasis [233, 234]. The major PGs are subclassified into three groups depending on their localization; intracellular PGs (serglycin), cell surface-associated PGs (syndecans, glypicans) and secreted PGs (hyalectans, small leucine-rich proteoglycans, perlecan) [235]. In this chapter, we focus on the stromal PGs the most characterized in the tumor context, shed syndecans and small leucine-rich proteins/proteoglycans (SLRPs) and summarize how their presence in tumor stroma influences cancer progression (Fig. 5.3).

Syndecans

Syndecans are transmembrane HSPGs with four members in vertebrates, syndecan-1 to -4. When present at the cell surface, they are formally not part of the tumor ECM, but since they can be shed into the ECM they are discussed in the context of TME, both for roles of unshed and shed forms. They are involved in diverse biological processes, such as regulating cell adhesion, cell migration and differentiation, as well

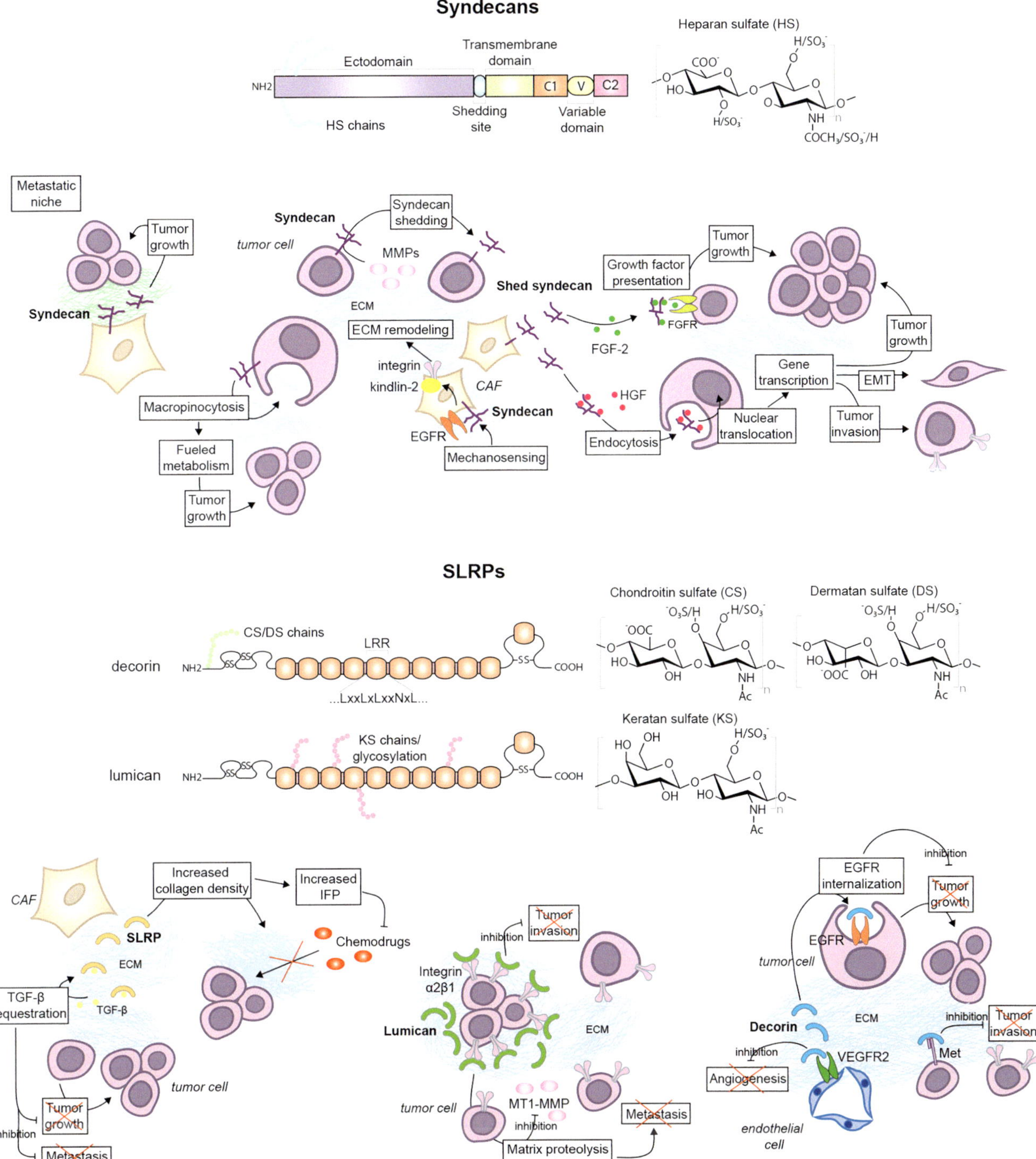

Fig. 5.3 Structure of stromal proteoglycans and their role in tumorigenesis. Syndecans is a family of four members that differ by the size of the ectodomain and the variable domain. All syndecans exhibit heparan sulfate (HS) chains, but only syndecan-1 and -3 have chondroitin sulfate (CS) chains in the ectodomain part close to the transmembrane domain. Syndecans at the cell surface can be shed by MMPs to induce its effect on cancer cells. Syndecans as co-factor for FGF receptor (FGFR) stimulate tumor growth by delivering FGF-2. Syndecan-1 could be endocytosed to deliver growth factors into the nucleus leading to increased gene transcription. Syndecan-1 can regulate macropinocytosis to fuel cancer cell growth. Syndecan-1 is also required in metastatic niches to support the metastatic colonization. Force on syndecan-4 induces activation of integrins involving kindlin-2 with the potential to reorganize the ECM. Small leucine-rich proteoglycans (SLRPs) are composed of leucine-rich repeats (LRR) that contain the LxxLxLxxNxL motif (L, leu-cine; N, asparagine; x, any amino acid). Decorin could exhibit one chain of chondroitin sulfate (CS) or dermatan sulfate (DS), whereas lumican could exhibit one to four keratan sulfate (KS) chains. HS, DS, CS, and KS chains are composed of repeats of disaccharide units that could be sulfated (SO_3^-) at different locations as indicated in the figure. As shown for fibromodulin, SLRPs could increase thickness of collagen fibers resulting in increased interstitial fluid pressure (IFP). Some SLRPs, such as asporin, have ability to bind and sequester TGF-β resulting in cancer growth and metastasis inhibition. Lumican has been shown to inhibit cancer cell migration by interaction through α2β1 integrin and by inhibiting MT1-MMP. Decorin has been shown to interact with tyrosine kinase receptors. Binding to EGF receptor (EGFR) leads to the receptor internalization and tumor growth inhibition. Binding to c-met inhibits cancer cell migration. Binding to VEGFR2 in endothelial cells inhibits angiogenesis. (For more details, please refer to the main text)

as participating in the organization of ECM and the cytoskeleton [236]. Syndecans can serve as co-receptors in various signaling pathways on the cell surface and also provide a link between the ECM and the cytoskeleton by directly interacting with the cytoskeleton or via other molecules [237]. In pancreatic cancer, localization of syndecan-1 at the cell surface of PDAC cells regulates macropinocytosis, which consists of uptaking proteins from the extracellular matrix to fuel cell metabolism, promoting tumor growth [238]. As described for tenascin-C and periostin (see above), stromal fibroblast-derived syndecan-1 is required in metastatic niche to promote metastases outgrowth. Syndecan-1-mediated lung metastases of breast carcinoma cells is a temperature-dependent process [239].

Syndecan-4 is ubiquitously expressed at low levels. Although integrins are the canonical mechanotransducing cell surface receptors, syndecans have also been regarded to take part in mechanosensing through their role as co-receptors for collagen- and fibronectin-binding integrins (Fig. 5.3) [240, 241]. Recent studies suggest that syndecan-4 rather than only being present with integrins in the same adhesion sites, also can generate signals in response to tension (at subcellular sites separate from integrin adhesions) that activates kindlin-2/β1 integrin/RhoA axis in a PI3K -dependent manner [242]. These new results have been obtained in an advanced experimental in vitro system using fibronectin- and collagen-coated magnetic beads. It will be interesting to see if the proposed model of syndecan-4 mechanosignaling activating integrins is also valid under more in vivo-like 3D conditions.

One interesting feature of syndecans is the shedding of the extracellular domain that enables syndecans to act as soluble factors [243], which plays an important role in tumorigenesis (Fig. 5.3). The shedding occurs next to the plasma membrane and is processed by different MMPs: MMP-7 is involved in syndecan-1 and -2 shedding, MMP-2 and -9 can cleave syndecan-1, -2 and -4, whereas MMP-14 can cleave syndecan-1 and -4 [244–246]. The shedding is regulated by different growth factors and cytokines present in the tumor microenvironment, such as FGF-2 and TNF-α [247, 248]. In addition, heparanase, an enzyme that cleaves the HS chains, regulates syndecan-1 expression and promotes syndecan-1 shedding, resulting in increased myeloma tumor growth [249].

In general, shed syndecans promote tumor progression and it was described earlier that highly soluble syndecan-1 was associated with poor outcome in non-small cell lung cancer [250]. This correlation was also observed in myeloma and bladder carcinoma [251, 252]. In breast carcinoma, shedding of syndecan-1 from CAFs stimulates tumor cell proliferation via FGF-2; shed syndecan-1 thus serving as a paracrine mediator [253, 254]. However, another study demonstrated an inhibitory effect of shed syndecan-1 on breast adenocarcinoma cell proliferation [255]. The study interestingly suggested the duality of membrane-bound and soluble syndecan-1. In a study by Nikolova et al., transmembrane syndecan-1 promoted cell proliferation and inhibited invasion, whereas shed syndecan-1 inhibited proliferation but increased invasiveness, suggesting that both syndecan forms contributed to breast cancer progression, but at different stages [255]. More recently, shed syndecan-2 has been shown to contribute to colorectal tumor growth and metastasis by up-regulating MMP-7, suggesting a positive regulatory loop between these two proteins [256].

Another study suggests that shed syndecan-1 translocates to the nucleus of tumor cells, indicating that syndecan-1 may deliver growth factors (e.g., HGF) to the nucleus, and also down-regulates histone acetylation, leading to increased gene transcription [252]. Nuclear translocation is believed to involve endocytosis of syndecan-1 growth factor complex from the cell surface and transport to the nucleus, but the exact mechanism of nuclear import has not been elucidated.

It has been reported that chemotherapeutic drugs, used in myeloma treatment, stimulate the shedding of syndecan-1, thus contributing to increased tumor growth [251]. Additionally, shed syndecan-1 contributes to chemotherapy resistance in colon cancer [257]. Targeting shed syndecans could be an effective strategy to control cancer progression; however better understanding of the molecular mechanisms of action is needed in order to avoid any potential adverse side effects.

Small Leucine-Rich Proteoglycans

SLRPs are extracellular matrix proteins rich in leucine-rich repeats, conferring a "banana" shape structure with a concave face involved in protein-protein interactions. Most SLRPs bind to fibrillar collagen and regulate collagen fibrillogenesis and matrix assembly [258]. Among the many biological processes regulated by SLRPs, tumor growth is one of the most well studied. The SLRP family encompasses 18 members, grouped into five classes (I–V) [235]. In this section, we will focus on the role of four SLRPs from classes I and II in tumor progression (Fig. 5.3).

Decorin is a chondroitin/dermatan sulfate SLRP that is expressed in several tissues. Although one study associated high expression of decorin with metastasis and poor survival in breast cancer [259], decorin is often described as having anti-tumor properties, as listed below. Decorin expression is down-regulated in bladder cancer [260], prostate cancer [261], lung cancer [262] and breast cancer [263, 264], where a reduced expression is associated with poor survival [265]. Consistent with these observations, liver carcinogenesis was promoted in decorin-null mice [266]. Moreover, overexpression of decorin was shown to inhibit metastasis of prostate cancer [267], inhibit proliferation of bladder tumor cells [260], and inhibit colorectal carcinoma cell growth and migration [268]. Systemic injection of decorin in MDA-231 triple negative breast carcinoma xenografts induced expression of cellular adhesion molecules and promoted tumor suppressor genes, whereas inflammatory and immune response genes were down-regulated [269].

From a mechanistic point of view, decorin can affect tumor progression via its interaction with tyrosine kinase receptors. It has been demonstrated that decorin can bind to the EGF receptor and mediate internalization and degradation of the receptor and induce expression of p21^{WAF}, an inhibitor of the cell cycle and apoptosis [270]. Decorin can also antagonize Met, a receptor for hepatocyte growth factor, via degradation of β-catenin, leading to reduced cell migration and invasion [271]. The decorin/Met axis appears to be required for the induction of an oncostatic mitochondrial protein, mitostatin [272]. In addition, decorin has been shown to bind and antagonize VEGFR2, inhibiting angiogenesis through endothelial cell autophagy [273, 274] and to bind IGF-IR to inhibit tumor cell migration and invasion [275].

Based on these observations, decorin is considered as a promising therapeutic protein in cancer progression treatment [267]. However, similar to syndecan-1, decorin has also been reported to induce resistance to some chemotherapeutics [276, 277]. Moreover, P-cadherin expression induces decorin secretion that is required to realigned collagen fibers to promote collective cell migration in breast tumor [239].

Biglycan, like decorin, is a chondroitin/dermatan sulfate proteoglycan, which belongs to the class I of SLRPs. Available data indicates that high expression levels of biglycan correlate with poor prognosis in pancreatic adenocarcinoma and esophageal carcinoma [278, 279]. Moreover, biglycan was shown to promote migration and invasion of gastric carcinoma through FAK signaling activation [280]. However, biglycan also displays anti-tumor activity, inhibiting bladder carcinoma and pancreatic carcinoma cell proliferation [281, 282].

Lumican is expressed as keratan sulfate PG in the cornea, but exists as a glycoprotein substituted by non- or low-sulfated polylactosamine chains in other tissues [275]. In tumor tissues, lumican is often over-expressed by stromal cells and/or tumor cells, and the correlation of its expression to malignancy is complex [283, 284]. In advanced colorectal cancer, Seya et al. have shown that lumican expression in tumor cells is associated with poor survival [285], whereas de Wit et al. have described a correlation with good survival in stage II patients [286]. In breast cancer, lumican expression was found to decrease with the progression of disease [287]. Consistent with this observation, high expression of lumican is associated with good survival in invasive stages of breast cancer [265]. Lumican upregulates the expression of α2β1 integrin but decreases integrin signaling in the highly metastatic MDA-MB-231 breast cancer cell line, inhibiting migratory cell morphology [288]. In pancreatic cancer,

patient outcome is dependent on the type of cells expressing lumican. Expression in tumor cells is associated with longer survival, whereas expression in pancreatic stromal cells is associated with poor outcome [289]. However, a recent study showed that lumican expression in pancreatic stroma was only correlated with good survival after surgery [290]. This correlation is also observed in lung adenocarcinoma patients, where patients with stromal lumican-positive tumors had longer survival than those expressing lumican in tumor cells [291]. We suggest that these differences could be related to the secretion of different glycosylated forms of lumican in different cellular contexts.

The anti-tumor properties of lumican have mainly been reported in melanoma, where lumican is expressed in the peritumoral stroma [292] and is suggested to serve as a biological barrier, controlling melanoma invasion. Lumican was shown to inhibit melanoma cell progression via interaction with α2β1 integrin and altering composition of focal adhesion complexes [293–295]. Lumican was defined as a new inhibitor of MT1-MMP in melanoma cells, thus inhibiting tumor environment proteolysis and invasiveness [296]. Anti-tumorigenic activities of lumican were also found in prostate cancer [297], in colon cancer by affecting tumor cell migration through up-regulation of gelsolin [298], and in pancreatic cancer, in which lumican reduced EGF receptor expression resulting in reduced Akt signaling and tumor cell growth inhibition [290].

Fibromodulin, like lumican, is a keratan sulfate SLRP that belongs to class II and is expressed in dense regular connective tissues. Although fibromodulin expression has been described in some types of cancer, its role has been poorly investigated. Oldberg et al. have shown that in experimental carcinomas, fibromodulin promotes the formation of a dense collagen matrix through the regulation of fibril diameter, leading to an increased interstitial fluid pressure (IFP), with possible adverse consequences for delivery of chemotherapeutics [299]. It is interesting to remember that other SLRPs also modulate collagen fibrillogenesis and could be thus involved in IFP regulation in different types of cancers, despite their anti-tumorigenic properties.

SLRPs also function to sequester TGF-β [300], a growth factor already described in this chapter, involved in EMT and fibroblast activation. A work by Maris et al. demonstrates that asporin, a member of the class I SLRPs, inhibits TGF-β activity resulting in reduced breast cancer growth and metastasis in NOD-SCID mice [301]. Interestingly, asporin expression is induced by TGF-β, thus asporin and TGF-β appear to regulate each other in an intricate feedback loop.

In summary, proteoglycans and matricellular proteins show different effects on tumorigenesis, sometimes with opposite effects in different tumor types. Table 5.1 summarizes the role of stromal proteins in tumorigenesis and the experiments we have mentioned in the text.

Table 5.1 Role of extracellular matrix proteins in the tumor microenvironment

ECM protein	Knockout phenotype mice	Potential ECM receptors in tumor stroma	Localization in tumors	Effects in tumor context
Collagen I	Embryonic lethal, severe structural defects in connective tissues [302–304]	α2β1, α11β1	Stroma	– Supports tumor growth [64–66] – Highway for metastasis [305] – Protective barrier role in pancreatic ductal adenocarcinoma [34]
Collagen III	Perinatal lethal [306]	α2β1, α11β1	Stroma	– Restricts tumor growth [71]
EDA Fibronectin	Normal, defective lymph vessels [130, 142]	α5β1 α4β1, α4β7 α9β1 TLR2/4	Stroma [130]	– No effect angiogenesis in Rip1-Tag2 model [130] – Reduces immune response in cancer models [161] – Stimulates breast cancer progression [164] – Direct collective cell migration of head and neck cancer cells [162] – Recruits latent TGF-β binding protein-1 to EDA FN fibrils [155]
Tenascin-C	Viable, subtle defects hair follicles [307, 308]	αvβ1, α4β1 [200], TLR4	Stroma	Minimal effect in pyMT model in TN-C$^{-/-}$ background, no effect on tumor growth, or metastasis [174] Stimulates metastasis in tumor models of melanoma, breast cancer and lung cancer 190, 193, 194] Role in metastatic niche formation in lung cancer [196] Role in shaping immunosuppressive TME in head and neck cancer models [198]
Periostin	Tooth eruption defect [309]	αv-integrins (αvβ1,αvβ3, αvβ5)	Stroma	– Breast cancer metastasis to lungs, concentrates Wnt in cancer stem cell niches [94, 220, 310, 311]
Decorin	Skin fragility [312]	Affect integrin expression indirectly via TGF-β pathway, TLR2/4 [313]	Stroma	– Inhibits tumor growth [314] – Affects inflammatory status of TME [315]
Lumican	Skin fragility, cornea opacity [316]	α2β1	Stroma, tumor cells	– Inhibits melanoma growth and invasion [295]
Syndecan-1	Normal	Cooperate with integrins on cell surface.	Tumor and stromal cells	– Shedding [254], increased angiogenesis [254, 317], affect tumor growth [318]
Syndecan-4	Normal	Co-receptor for certain β1 integrins	Stromal cells	– Co-receptor for integrins binding fibronectin and collagen [241, 319], cross-talks with integrins via intracellular signaling [242, 320]

Concluding Remarks/Summary

The tumor stroma is complex and dynamic during tumor growth and contains an ECM with changing composition. The exact function of the tumor stroma varies with the tumor type, the tumor stage, and it will be important to better elucidate the function of ECM molecules at different stages of tumor growth and metastasis. To determine if the tumor stroma acts as a fertile soil, providing a supportive ECM network rich in blood vessels, or if it acts as a stiff barrier, we have to consider additional components of the stroma. In this chapter, we have highlighted some aspects ascribed to the insoluble ECM of the stroma, but additional consideration of the integrated roles of the immune system, paracrine signaling and above all, intertumoral and intra-tumoral heterogeneity in tumor composition is necessary in order to fully address the central question: Tumor stroma—friend or foe? Barrier or support?

Acknowledgments We acknowledge the useful comments from Sandy Der (University Health Network, Toronto).

Supported by grants to DG from the Research Council of Norway (Norwegian Center of Excellence grant, grants 223250) and Nasjonalföreningen for folkhelsen (Project 16216).

References

1. Osterholm C, Lu N, Liden A, Karlsen TV, Gullberg D, Reed RK, et al. Fibroblast EXT1-levels influence tumor cell proliferation and migration in composite spheroids. PLoS One. 2012;7(7):e41334.
2. Lu N, Karlsen TV, Reed RK, Kusche-Gullberg M, Gullberg D. Fibroblast alpha11beta1 integrin regulates tensional homeostasis in fibroblast/A549 carcinoma heterospheroids. PLoS One. 2014;9(7):e103173.
3. Fatehullah A, Tan SH, Barker N. Organoids as an in vitro model of human development and disease. Nat Cell Biol. 2016;18(3):246–54.

4. Shi R, Radulovich N, Ng C, Liu N, Notsuda H, Cabanero M, et al. Organoid cultures as preclinical models of non-small cell lung cancer. Clin Cancer Res. 2020;26(5):1162–74.

5. Boj SF, Hwang CI, Baker LA, Chio II, Engle DD, Corbo V, et al. Organoid models of human and mouse ductal pancreatic cancer. Cell. 2015;160(1–2):324–38.

6. Sachs N, de Ligt J, Kopper O, Gogola E, Bounova G, Weeber F, et al. A living biobank of breast cancer organoids captures disease heterogeneity. Cell. 2018;172(1-2):373–86.e10.

7. Weaver VM. The microenvironment matters. Mol Biol Cell. 2014;25(21):3254–8.

8. Piersma B, Hayward MK, Weaver VM. Fibrosis and cancer: a strained relationship. Biochim Biophys Acta Rev Cancer. 2020;1873(2):188356.

9. Zeltz C, Gullberg D. Post-translational modifications of integrin ligands as pathogenic mechanisms in disease. Matrix Biol. 2014;40:5–9.

10. Levental KR, Yu H, Kass L, Lakins JN, Egeblad M, Erler JT, et al. Matrix crosslinking forces tumor progression by enhancing integrin signaling. Cell. 2009;139(5):891–906.

11. Azmi AS, Bao B, Sarkar FH. Exosomes in cancer development, metastasis, and drug resistance: a comprehensive review. Cancer Metastasis Rev. 2013;32(3-4):623–42.

12. Hoshino A, Costa-Silva B, Shen TL, Rodrigues G, Hashimoto A, Tesic Mark M, et al. Tumour exosome integrins determine organotropic metastasis. Nature. 2015;527(7578):329–35.

13. Östman A, Augsten M. Cancer-associated fibroblasts and tumor growth—bystanders turning into key players. Curr Opin Genet Dev. 2009;19(1):67–73.

14. Cirri P, Chiarugi P. Cancer associated fibroblasts: the dark side of the coin. Am J Cancer Res. 2011;1(4):482–97.

15. Ohlund D, Elyada E, Tuveson D. Fibroblast heterogeneity in the cancer wound. J Exp Med. 2014;211(8):1503–23.

16. Sahai E, Astsaturov I, Cukierman E, DeNardo DG, Egeblad M, Evans RM, et al. A framework for advancing our understanding of cancer-associated fibroblasts. Nat Rev Cancer. 2020;20(3):174–86.

17. Hu Y, Yan C, Mu L, Huang K, Li X, Tao D, et al. Fibroblast-Derived Exosomes Contribute to Chemoresistance through Priming Cancer Stem Cells in Colorectal Cancer. PLoS One. 2015;10(5):e0125625.

18. Eberlein C, Rooney C, Ross SJ, Farren M, Weir HM, Barry ST. E-Cadherin and EpCAM expression by NSCLC tumour cells associate with normal fibroblast activation through a pathway initiated by integrin alphavbeta6 and maintained through TGFbeta signalling. Oncogene. 2014;34(6):704–16.

19. Eberlein C, Kendrew J, McDaid K, Alfred A, Kang JS, Jacobs VN, et al. A human monoclonal antibody 264RAD targeting alphav-beta6 integrin reduces tumour growth and metastasis, and modulates key biomarkers in vivo. Oncogene. 2013;32(37):4406–16.

20. Klingberg F, Chow ML, Koehler A, Boo S, Buscemi L, Quinn TM, et al. Prestress in the extracellular matrix sensitizes latent TGF-beta1 for activation. J Cell Biol. 2014;207(2):283–97.

21. Hinz B. The extracellular matrix and transforming growth factor-beta1: tale of a strained relationship. Matrix Biol. 2015;47:54–65.

22. Henderson NC, Arnold TD, Katamura Y, Giacomini MM, Rodriguez JD, McCarty JH, et al. Targeting of alphav integrin identifies a core molecular pathway that regulates fibrosis in several organs. Nat Med. 2013;19(12):1617–24.

23. Reed NI, Jo H, Chen C, Tsujino K, Arnold TD, DeGrado WF, et al. The alphavbeta1 integrin plays a critical in vivo role in tissue fibrosis. Sci Transl Med. 2015;7(288):288ra79.

24. Lodyga M, Hinz B. TGF-beta1—a truly transforming growth factor in fibrosis and immunity. Semin Cell Dev Biol. 2020;101:123–39.

25. Jiang X, Wang J, Deng X, Xiong F, Ge J, Xiang B, et al. Role of the tumor microenvironment in PD-L1/PD-1-mediated tumor immune escape. Mol Cancer. 2019;18(1):10.

26. Stockis J, Lienart S, Colau D, Collignon A, Nishimura SL, Sheppard D, et al. Blocking immunosuppression by human Tregs in vivo with antibodies targeting integrin alphaVbeta8. Proc Natl Acad Sci U S A. 2017;114(47):E10161–E8.

27. Takasaka N, Seed RI, Cormier A, Bondesson AJ, Lou J, Elattma A, et al. Integrin alphavbeta8-expressing tumor cells evade host immunity by regulating TGF-beta activation in immune cells. JCI Insight. 2018;3(20):e122591.

28. Campbell MG, Cormier A, Ito S, Seed RI, Bondesson AJ, Lou J, et al. Cryo-EM reveals integrin-mediated TGF-beta activation without release from latent TGF-beta. Cell. 2020;180(3):490–501. e16.

29. Jin S, Lee WC, Aust D, Pilarsky C, Cordes N. beta8 integrin mediates pancreatic cancer cell radiochemoresistance. Mol Cancer Res. 2019;17(10):2126–38.

30. Gaggioli C, Hooper S, Hidalgo-Carcedo C, Grosse R, Marshall JF, Harrington K, et al. Fibroblast-led collective invasion of carcinoma cells with differing roles for RhoGTPases in leading and following cells. Nat Cell Biol. 2007;9(12):1392–400.

31. Sanz-Moreno V, Gaggioli C, Yeo M, Albrengues J, Wallberg F, Viros A, et al. ROCK and JAK1 signaling cooperate to control actomyosin contractility in tumor cells and stroma. Cancer Cell. 2011;20(2):229–45.

32. Ozdemir BC, Pentcheva-Hoang T, Carstens JL, Zheng X, Wu CC, Simpson TR, et al. Depletion of carcinoma-associated fibroblasts and fibrosis induces immunosuppression and accelerates pancreas cancer with reduced survival. Cancer Cell. 2014;25:719–34.

33. Rhim AD, Oberstein PE, Thomas DH, Mirek ET, Palermo CF, Sastra SA, et al. Stromal elements act to restrain, rather than support, pancreatic ductal adenocarcinoma. Cancer Cell. 2014;25(6):735–47.

34. Jiang H, Torphy RJ, Steiger K, Hongo H, Ritchie AJ, Kriegsmann M, et al. Pancreatic ductal adenocarcinoma progression is restrained by stromal matrix. J Clin Invest. 2020;130(9):4704–9.

35. Zeltz C, Primac I, Erusappan P, Alam J, Noel A, Gullberg D. Cancer-associated fibroblasts in desmoplastic tumors: emerging role of integrins. Semin Cancer Biol. 2020;62:166–81.

36. Rubashkin MG, Ou G, Weaver VM. Deconstructing signaling in three dimensions. Biochemistry. 2014;53(13):2078–90.

37. Ricard-Blum S. The collagen family. Cold Spring Harb Perspect Biol. 2011;3(1):a004978.

38. Egeblad M, Rasch MG, Weaver VM. Dynamic interplay between the collagen scaffold and tumor evolution. Curr Opin Cell Biol. 2010;22(5):697–706.

39. Dvorak HF. Tumors: wounds that do not heal. Similarities between tumor stroma generation and wound healing. N Engl J Med. 1986;315(26):1650–9.

40. Dvorak HF. Tumors: wounds that do not heal-redux. Cancer Immunol Res. 2015;3(1):1–11.

41. Merkel JR, DiPaolo BR, Hallock GG, Rice DC. Type I and type III collagen content of healing wounds in fetal and adult rats. Proc Soc Exp Biol Med. 1988;187(4):493–7.

42. Barczyk M, Carracedo S, Gullberg D. Integrins. Cell Tissue Res. 2010;339(1):269–80.

43. Zeltz C, Gullberg D. The integrin-collagen connection—a glue for tissue repair? J Cell Sci. 2016;129(4):653–64.

44. Zeltz C, Orgel J, Gullberg D. Molecular composition and function of integrin-based collagen glues-introducing COLINBRIs. Biochim Biophys Acta. 2014;1840(8):2533–48.

45. Staudinger LA, Spano SJ, Lee W, Coelho N, Rajshankar D, Bendeck MP, et al. Interactions between the discoidin domain receptor 1 and beta1 integrin regulate attachment to collagen. Biol Open. 2013;2(11):1148–59.

46. Xu H, Bihan D, Chang F, Huang PH, Farndale RW, Leitinger B. Discoidin domain receptors promote alpha1beta1- and alpha2beta1-integrin mediated cell adhesion to collagen by enhancing integrin activation. PLoS One. 2012;7(12):e52209.

47. Abbonante V, Gruppi C, Rubel D, Gross O, Moratti R, Balduini A. Discoidin domain receptor 1 protein is a novel modulator of megakaryocyte-collagen interactions. J Biol Chem. 2013;288(23):16738–46.

48. DuFort CC, Paszek MJ, Weaver VM. Balancing forces: architectural control of mechanotransduction. Nat Rev Mol Cell Biol. 2011;12(5):308–19.

49. Gilkes DM, Semenza GL, Wirtz D. Hypoxia and the extracellular matrix: drivers of tumour metastasis. Nat Rev Cancer. 2014;14(6):430–9.

50. Malik R, Lelkes PI, Cukierman E. Biomechanical and biochemical remodeling of stromal extracellular matrix in cancer. Trends Biotechnol. 2015;33(4):230–6.

51. Cox TR, Erler JT. Molecular pathways: connecting fibrosis and solid tumor metastasis. Clin Cancer Res. 2014;20(14):3637–43.

52. Miller BW, Morton JP, Pinese M, Saturno G, Jamieson NB, McGhee E, et al. Targeting the LOX/hypoxia axis reverses many of the features that make pancreatic cancer deadly: inhibition of LOX abrogates metastasis and enhances drug efficacy. EMBO Mol Med. 2015;7(8):1063–76.

53. Kalluri R, Zeisberg M. Fibroblasts in cancer. Nat Rev Cancer. 2006;6(5):392–401.

54. Cooke ME, Sakai T, Mosher DF. Contraction of collagen matrices mediated by a2b1A and avb3 integrins. J Cell Sci. 2000;113(Pt 13):2375–83.

55. Schulz JN, Zeltz C, Sorensen IW, Barczyk M, Carracedo S, Hallinger R, et al. Reduced granulation tissue and wound strength in the absence of alpha11beta1 integrin. J Invest Dermatol. 2015;135(5):1435–44.

56. Gullberg D, Tingstrom A, Thuresson AC, Olsson L, Terracio L, Borg TK, et al. b1 integrin-mediated collagen gel contraction is stimulated by PDGF. Exp Cell Res. 1990;186(2):264–72.

57. Jokinen J, Dadu E, Nykvist P, Kapyla J, White DJ, Ivaska J, et al. Integrin-mediated cell adhesion to type I collagen fibrils. J Biol Chem. 2004;279(30):31956–63.

58. Shen B, Vardy K, Hughes P, Tasdogan A, Zhao Z, Yue R, et al. Integrin alpha11 is an Osteolectin receptor and is required for the maintenance of adult skeletal bone mass. elife. 2019;8:e42274.

59. Velling T, Kusche-Gullberg M, Sejersen T, Gullberg D. cDNA cloning and chromosomal localization of human alpha(11) integrin. A collagen-binding, I domain-containing, beta(1)-associated integrin alpha-chain present in muscle tissues. J Biol Chem. 1999;274(36):25735–42.

60. Popova SN, Rodriguez-Sanchez B, Liden A, Betsholtz C, Van Den Bos T, Gullberg D. The mesenchymal alpha11beta1 integrin attenuates PDGF-BB-stimulated chemotaxis of embryonic fibroblasts on collagens. Dev Biol. 2004;270(2):427–42.

61. Popova SN, Barczyk M, Tiger CF, Beertsen W, Zigrino P, Aszodi A, et al. Alpha11 beta1 integrin-dependent regulation of periodontal ligament function in the erupting mouse incisor. Mol Cell Biol. 2007;27(12):4306–16.

62. Popov C, Radic T, Haasters F, Prall WC, Aszodi A, Gullberg D, et al. Integrins alpha2beta1 and alpha11beta1 regulate the survival of mesenchymal stem cells on collagen I. Cell Death Dis. 2011;2:e186.

63. Zeltz C, Alam J, Liu H, Erusappan PM, Hoschuetzky H, Molven A, et al. α11β1 integrin is induced in a subset of cancer-associated fibroblasts in desmoplastic tumor stroma and mediates in vitro cell migration. Cancers. 2019;11:765. https://doi.org/10.3390/cancers11060765.

64. Primac I, Maquoi E, Blacher S, Heljasvaara R, Van Deun J, Smeland HY, et al. Stromal integrin alpha11 regulates PDGFR-beta signaling and promotes breast cancer progression. J Clin Invest. 2019;130:4609–28.

65. Zhu CQ, Popova SN, Brown ER, Barsyte-Lovejoy D, Navab R, Shih W, et al. Integrin alpha11 regulates IGF2 expression in fibroblasts to enhance tumorigenicity of human non-small-cell lung cancer cells. Proc Natl Acad Sci U S A. 2007;104(28):11754–9.

66. Navab R, Strumpf D, To C, Pasko E, Kim KS, Park CJ, et al. Integrin alpha11beta1 regulates cancer stromal stiffness and promotes tumorigenicity and metastasis in non-small cell lung cancer. Oncogene. 2016;35(15):1899–908.

67. Smeland HY, Askeland C, Wik E, Knutsvik G, Molven A, Edelmann RJ, et al. Integrin alpha11beta1 is expressed in breast cancer stroma and associates with aggressive tumor phenotypes. J Pathol Clin Res. 2020;6(1):69–82.

68. Barczyk MM, Lu N, Popova SN, Bolstad AI, Gullberg D. alpha-11beta1 integrin-mediated MMP-13-dependent collagen lattice contraction by fibroblasts: evidence for integrin-coordinated collagen proteolysis. J Cell Physiol. 2013;228:1108–19.

69. Ravanti L, Heino J, Lopez-Otin C, Kahari VM. Induction of collagenase-3 (MMP-13) expression in human skin fibroblasts by three-dimensional collagen is mediated by p38 mitogen-activated protein kinase. J Biol Chem. 1999;274(4):2446–55.

70. Provenzano PP, Eliceiri KW, Keely PJ. Shining new light on 3D cell motility and the metastatic process. Trends Cell Biol. 2009;19(11):638–48.

71. Brisson BK, Mauldin EA, Lei W, Vogel LK, Power AM, Lo A, et al. Type III collagen directs stromal organization and limits metastasis in a murine model of breast cancer. Am J Pathol. 2015;185(5):1471–86.

72. Radisky D, Muschler J, Bissell MJ. Order and disorder: the role of extracellular matrix in epithelial cancer. Cancer Investig. 2002;20(1):139–53.

73. Nistico P, Bissell MJ, Radisky DC. Epithelial-mesenchymal transition: general principles and pathological relevance with special emphasis on the role of matrix metalloproteinases. Cold Spring Harb Perspect Biol. 2012;4(2):a011908.

74. Smith BN, Bhowmick NA. Role of EMT in metastasis and therapy resistance. J Clin Med. 2016;5(2):17.

75. Provenzano PP, Inman DR, Eliceiri KW, Knittel JG, Yan L, Rueden CT, et al. Collagen density promotes mammary tumor initiation and progression. BMC Med. 2008;6:11.

76. Xiong G, Deng L, Zhu J, Rychahou PG, Xu R. Prolyl-4-hydroxylase alpha subunit 2 promotes breast cancer progression and metastasis by regulating collagen deposition. BMC Cancer. 2014;14:1.

77. Chen Y, Terajima M, Yang Y, Sun L, Ahn YH, Pankova D, et al. Lysyl hydroxylase 2 induces a collagen cross-link switch in tumor stroma. J Clin Invest. 2015;125(3):1147–62.

78. Montgomery AM, Reisfeld RA, Cheresh DA. Integrin alpha v beta 3 rescues melanoma cells from apoptosis in three-dimensional dermal collagen. Proc Natl Acad Sci U S A. 1994;91(19):8856–60.

79. Maquoi E, Assent D, Detilleux J, Pequeux C, Foidart JM, Noël A. MT1-MMP protects breast carcinoma cells against type I collagen-induced apoptosis. Oncogene. 2011;31(4):480–93.

80. Assent D, Bourgot I, Hennuy B, Geurts P, Noel A, Foidart JM, et al. A membrane-type-1 matrix metalloproteinase (MT1-MMP)-discoidin domain receptor 1 axis regulates collagen-induced apoptosis in breast cancer cells. PLoS One. 2015;10(3):e0116006.

81. Nielsen BS, Egeblad M, Rank F, Askautrud HA, Pennington CJ, Pedersen TX, et al. Matrix metalloproteinase 13 is induced in fibroblasts in polyomavirus middle T antigen-driven mammary carcinoma without influencing tumor progression. PLoS One. 2008;3(8):e2959.

82. Perry SW, Schueckler JM, Burke K, Arcuri GL, Brown EB. Stromal matrix metalloprotease-13 knockout alters Collagen I structure at the tumor-host interface and increases lung metas-

tasis of C57BL/6 syngeneic E0771 mammary tumor cells. BMC Cancer. 2013;13:411.

83. Krane SM, Byrne MH, Lemaitre V, Henriet P, Jeffrey JJ, Witter JP, et al. Different collagenase gene products have different roles in degradation of type I collagen. J Biol Chem. 1996;271(45):28509–15.

84. Romanic AM, Adachi E, Kadler KE, Hojima Y, Prockop DJ. Copolymerization of pNcollagen III and collagen I. pNcollagen III decreases the rate of incorporation of collagen I into fibrils, the amount of collagen I incorporated, and the diameter of the fibrils formed. J Biol Chem. 1991;266(19):12703–9.

85. LeBert DC, Squirrell JM, Rindy J, Broadbridge E, Lui Y, Zakrzewska A, et al. Matrix metalloproteinase 9 modulates collagen matrices and wound repair. Development. 2015;142(12):2136–46.

86. Herchenhan A, Uhlenbrock F, Eliasson P, Weis M, Eyre D, Kadler KE, et al. Lysyl oxidase activity is required for ordered collagen fibrillogenesis by tendon cells. J Biol Chem. 2015;290(26):16440–50.

87. Sabeh F, Shimizu-Hirota R, Weiss SJ. Protease-dependent versus -independent cancer cell invasion programs: three-dimensional amoeboid movement revisited. J Cell Biol. 2009;185(1):11–9.

88. Wolf K, Te Lindert M, Krause M, Alexander S, Te Riet J, Willis AL, et al. Physical limits of cell migration: control by ECM space and nuclear deformation and tuning by proteolysis and traction force. J Cell Biol. 2013;201(7):1069–84.

89. Kaur A, Ecker BL, Douglass SM, Kugel CH 3rd, Webster MR, Almeida FV, et al. Remodeling of the collagen matrix in aging skin promotes melanoma metastasis and affects immune cell motility. Cancer Discov. 2019;9(1):64–81.

90. Nishioka T, Eustace A, West C. Lysyl oxidase: from basic science to future cancer treatment. Cell Struct Funct. 2012;37(1):75–80.

91. Cox TR, Erler JT. Remodeling and homeostasis of the extracellular matrix: implications for fibrotic diseases and cancer. Dis Model Mech. 2011;4(2):165–78.

92. Cox TR, Rumney RM, Schoof EM, Perryman L, Hoye AM, Agrawal A, et al. The hypoxic cancer secretome induces pre-metastatic bone lesions through lysyl oxidase. Nature. 2015;522(7554):106–10.

93. Oskarsson T, Acharyya S, Zhang XH, Vanharanta S, Tavazoie SF, Morris PG, et al. Breast cancer cells produce tenascin C as a metastatic niche component to colonize the lungs. Nat Med. 2011;17(7):867–74.

94. Oskarsson T, Massague J. Extracellular matrix players in metastatic niches. EMBO J. 2012;31(2):254–6.

95. Kaplan RN, Riba RD, Zacharoulis S, Bramley AH, Vincent L, Costa C, et al. VEGFR1-positive haematopoietic bone marrow progenitors initiate the pre-metastatic niche. Nature. 2005;438(7069):820–7.

96. Wilgus ML, Borczuk AC, Stoopler M, Ginsburg M, Gorenstein L, Sonett JR, et al. Lysyl oxidase: a lung adenocarcinoma biomarker of invasion and survival. Cancer. 2011;117(10):2186–91.

97. Zeltz C, Pasko E, Cox TR, Navab R, Tsao MS. LOXL1 Is regulated by integrin alpha11 and promotes non-small cell lung cancer tumorigenicity. Cancers (Basel). 2019;11(5):705.

98. Erler JT, Bennewith KL, Nicolau M, Dornhofer N, Kong C, Le QT, et al. Lysyl oxidase is essential for hypoxia-induced metastasis. Nature. 2006;440(7088):1222–6.

99. Pupa SM, Menard S, Forti S, Tagliabue E. New insights into the role of extracellular matrix during tumor onset and progression. J Cell Physiol. 2002;192(3):259–67.

100. Theret N, Musso O, Turlin B, Lotrian D, Bioulac-Sage P, Campion JP, et al. Increased extracellular matrix remodeling is associated with tumor progression in human hepatocellular carcinomas. Hepatology. 2001;34(1):82–8.

101. Ronnov-Jessen L, Petersen OW, Bissell MJ. Cellular changes involved in conversion of normal to malignant breast: importance of the stromal reaction. Physiol Rev. 1996;76(1):69–125.

102. Hanahan D, Weinberg RA. Hallmarks of cancer: the next generation. Cell. 2011;144(5):646–74.

103. Leitinger B, Hohenester E. Mammalian collagen receptors. Matrix Biol. 2007;26(3):146–55.

104. Chen X, Nadiarynkh O, Plotnikov S, Campagnola PJ. Second harmonic generation microscopy for quantitative analysis of collagen fibrillar structure. Nat Protoc. 2012;7(4):654–69.

105. Tuer A, Tokarz D, Prent N, Cisek R, Alami J, Dumont DJ, et al. Nonlinear multicontrast microscopy of hematoxylin-and-eosin-stained histological sections. J Biomed Opt. 2010;15(2):026018.

106. Tuer AE, Akens MK, Krouglov S, Sandkuijl D, Wilson BC, Whyne CM, et al. Hierarchical model of fibrillar collagen organization for interpreting the second-order susceptibility tensors in biological tissue. Biophys J. 2012;103(10):2093–105.

107. Tuer AE, Krouglov S, Prent N, Cisek R, Sandkuijl D, Yasufuku K, et al. Nonlinear optical properties of type I collagen fibers studied by polarization dependent second harmonic generation microscopy. J Phys Chem B. 2011;115(44):12759–69.

108. Amat-Roldan I, Psilodimitrakopoulos S, Loza-Alvarez P, Artigas D. Fast image analysis in polarization SHG microscopy. Opt Express. 2010;18(16):17209–19.

109. Golaraei A, Cisek R, Krouglov S, Navab R, Niu C, Sakashita S, et al. Characterization of collagen in non-small cell lung carcinoma with second harmonic polarization microscopy. Biomed Opt Express. 2014;5(10):3562–7.

110. Strupler M, Pena AM, Hernest M, Tharaux PL, Martin JL, Beaurepaire E, et al. Second harmonic imaging and scoring of collagen in fibrotic tissues. Opt Express. 2007;15(7):4054–65.

111. Rezakhaniha R, Agianniotis A, Schrauwen JT, Griffa A, Sage D, Bouten CV, et al. Experimental investigation of collagen waviness and orientation in the arterial adventitia using confocal laser scanning microscopy. Biomech Model Mechanobiol. 2012;11(3-4):461–73.

112. Zhang J, Wang YL, Gu L, Pan J. Atomic force microscopy of actin. Sheng Wu Hua Xue Yu Sheng Wu Wu Li Xue Bao (Shanghai). 2003;35(6):489–94.

113. Paige MF, Rainey JK, Goh MC. A study of fibrous long spacing collagen ultrastructure and assembly by atomic force microscopy. Micron. 2001;32(3):341–53.

114. Glatzel T, Holscher H, Schimmel T, Baykara MZ, Schwarz UD, Garcia R. Advanced atomic force microscopy techniques. Beilstein J Nanotechnol. 2012;3:893–4.

115. Strasser S, Zink A, Janko M, Heckl WM, Thalhammer S. Structural investigations on native collagen type I fibrils using AFM. Biochem Biophys Res Commun. 2007;354(1):27–32.

116. Lopez JI, Kang I, You WK, McDonald DM, Weaver VM. In situ force mapping of mammary gland transformation. Integr Biol (Camb). 2011;3(9):910–21.

117. Braet F, Vermijlen D, Bossuyt V, De Zanger R, Wisse E. Early detection of cytotoxic events between hepatic natural killer cells and colon carcinoma cells as probed with the atomic force microscope. Ultramicroscopy. 2001;89(4):265–73.

118. Akhtar R, Schwarzer N, Sherratt MJ, Watson RE, Graham HK, Trafford AW, et al. Nanoindentation of histological specimens: mapping the elastic properties of soft tissues. J Mater Res. 2009;24(3):638–46.

119. Gueta R, Barlam D, Shneck RZ, Rousso I. Measurement of the mechanical properties of isolated tectorial membrane using atomic force microscopy. Proc Natl Acad Sci U S A. 2006;103(40):14790–5.

120. Barbone PE, Bamber JC. Quantitative elasticity imaging: what can and cannot be inferred from strain images. Phys Med Biol. 2002;47(12):2147–64.

121. Jiang T, Olson ES, Nguyen QT, Roy M, Jennings PA, Tsien RY. Tumor imaging by means of proteolytic activation of cell-penetrating peptides. Proc Natl Acad Sci U S A. 2004;101(51):17867–72.

122. Scherer RL, VanSaun MN, McIntyre JO, Matrisian LM. Optical imaging of matrix metalloproteinase-7 activity in vivo using a proteolytic nanobeacon. Mol Imaging. 2008;7(3):118–31.

123. Littlepage LE, Sternlicht MD, Rougier N, Phillips J, Gallo E, Yu Y, et al. Matrix metalloproteinases contribute distinct roles in neuroendocrine prostate carcinogenesis, metastasis, and angiogenesis progression. Cancer Res. 2010;70(6):2224–34.

124. Low AF, Tearney GJ, Bouma BE, Jang IK. Technology Insight: optical coherence tomography—current status and future development. Nat Clin Pract Cardiovasc Med. 2006;3(3):154–62. quiz 72

125. Spuentrup E, Buecker A, Katoh M, Wiethoff AJ, Parsons EC Jr, Botnar RM, et al. Molecular magnetic resonance imaging of coronary thrombosis and pulmonary emboli with a novel fibrin-targeted contrast agent. Circulation. 2005;111(11):1377–82.

126. Stracke CP, Katoh M, Wiethoff AJ, Parsons EC, Spangenberg P, Spuntrup E. Molecular MRI of cerebral venous sinus thrombosis using a new fibrin-specific MR contrast agent. Stroke. 2007;38(5):1476–81.

127. Miserus RJ, Herias MV, Prinzen L, Lobbes MB, Van Suylen RJ, Dirksen A, et al. Molecular MRI of early thrombus formation using a bimodal alpha2-antiplasmin-based contrast agent. JACC Cardiovasc Imaging. 2009;2(8):987–96.

128. Hynes R. Molecular biology of fibronectin. Annu Rev Cell Biol. 1985;1:67–90.

129. White ES, Baralle FE, Muro AF. New insights into form and function of fibronectin splice variants. J Pathol. 2008;216(1):1–14.

130. Astrof S, Crowley D, George EL, Fukuda T, Sekiguchi K, Hanahan D, et al. Direct test of potential roles of EIIIA and EIIIB alternatively spliced segments of fibronectin in physiological and tumor angiogenesis. Mol Cell Biol. 2004;24(19):8662–70.

131. Singh P, Reimer CL, Peters JH, Stepp MA, Hynes RO, Van De Water L. The spatial and temporal expression patterns of integrin alpha9beta1 and one of its ligands, the EIIIA segment of fibronectin, in cutaneous wound healing. J Invest Dermatol. 2004;123(6):1176–81.

132. Bhattacharyya S, Tamaki Z, Wang W, Hinchcliff M, Hoover P, Getsios S, et al. FibronectinEDA promotes chronic cutaneous fibrosis through Toll-like receptor signaling. Sci Transl Med. 2014;6(232):232ra50.

133. Rybinski B, Franco-Barraza J, Cukierman E. The wound healing, chronic fibrosis, and cancer progression triad. Physiol Genomics. 2014;46(7):223–44.

134. Rybak JN, Roesli C, Kaspar M, Villa A, Neri D. The extra-domain A of fibronectin is a vascular marker of solid tumors and metastases. Cancer Res. 2007;67(22):10948–57.

135. Matsumoto E, Yoshida T, Kawarada Y, Sakakura T. Expression of fibronectin isoforms in human breast tissue: production of extra domain A+/extra domain B+ by cancer cells and extra domain A+ by stromal cells. Jpn J Cancer Res. 1999;90(3):320–5.

136. Pujuguet P, Hammann A, Moutet M, Samuel JL, Martin F, Martin M. Expression of fibronectin ED-A+ and ED-B+ isoforms by human and experimental colorectal cancer. Contribution of cancer cells and tumor-associated myofibroblasts. Am J Pathol. 1996;148(2):579–92.

137. Manabe R, Ohe N, Maeda T, Fukuda T, Sekiguchi K. Modulation of cell-adhesive activity of fibronectin by the alternatively spliced EDA segment. J Cell Biol. 1997;139(1):295–307.

138. Shinde AV, Bystroff C, Wang C, Vogelezang MG, Vincent PA, Hynes RO, et al. Identification of the peptide sequences within the EIIIA (EDA) segment of fibronectin that mediate integrin alpha9beta1-dependent cellular activities. J Biol Chem. 2008;283(5):2858–70.

139. Kohan M, Muro AF, White ES, Berkman N. EDA-containing cellular fibronectin induces fibroblast differentiation through binding to alpha4beta7 integrin receptor and MAPK/Erk 1/2-dependent signaling. FASEB J. 2010;24(11):4503–12.

140. Okamura Y, Watari M, Jerud ES, Young DW, Ishizaka ST, Rose J, et al. The extra domain A of fibronectin activates Toll-like receptor 4. J Biol Chem. 2001;276(13):10229–33.

141. Kelsh RM, McKeown-Longo PJ, Clark RA. EDA fibronectin in keloids create a vicious cycle of fibrotic tumor formation. J Invest Dermatol. 2015;135(7):1714–8.

142. Bazigou E, Xie S, Chen C, Weston A, Miura N, Sorokin L, et al. Integrin-alpha9 is required for fibronectin matrix assembly during lymphatic valve morphogenesis. Dev Cell. 2009;17(2):175–86.

143. Fukuda T, Yoshida N, Kataoka Y, Manabe R, Mizuno-Horikawa Y, Sato M, et al. Mice lacking the EDB segment of fibronectin develop normally but exhibit reduced cell growth and fibronectin matrix assembly in vitro. Cancer Res. 2002;62(19):5603–10.

144. Muro AF, Chauhan AK, Gajovic S, Iaconcig A, Porro F, Stanta G, et al. Regulated splicing of the fibronectin EDA exon is essential for proper skin wound healing and normal lifespan. J Cell Biol. 2003;162(1):149–60.

145. Astrof S, Crowley D, Hynes RO. Multiple cardiovascular defects caused by the absence of alternatively spliced segments of fibronectin. Dev Biol. 2007;311(1):11–24.

146. Danussi C, Del Bel BL, Pivetta E, Modica TM, Muro A, Wassermann B, et al. EMILIN1/alpha9beta1 integrin interaction is crucial in lymphatic valve formation and maintenance. Mol Cell Biol. 2013;33(22):4381–94.

147. Serini G, Bochaton-Piallat ML, Ropraz P, Geinoz A, Borsi L, Zardi L, et al. The fibronectin domain ED-A is crucial for myofibroblastic phenotype induction by transforming growth factor-beta1. J Cell Biol. 1998;142(3):873–81.

148. Shinde AV, Kelsh R, Peters JH, Sekiguchi K, Van De Water L, PJ MK-L. The alpha4beta1 integrin and the EDA domain of fibronectin regulate a profibrotic phenotype in dermal fibroblasts. Matrix Biol. 2015;41:26–35.

149. Singh P, Chen C, Pal-Ghosh S, Stepp MA, Sheppard D, Van De Water L. Loss of integrin alpha9beta1 results in defects in proliferation, causing poor re-epithelialization during cutaneous wound healing. J Invest Dermatol. 2009;129(1):217–28.

150. Nakayama Y, Kon S, Kurotaki D, Morimoto J, Matsui Y, Uede T. Blockade of interaction of alpha9 integrin with its ligands hinders the formation of granulation in cutaneous wound healing. Lab Investig. 2010;90(6):881–94.

151. Muro AF, Moretti FA, Moore BB, Yan M, Atrasz RG, Wilke CA, et al. An essential role for fibronectin extra type III domain A in pulmonary fibrosis. Am J Respir Crit Care Med. 2008;177(6):638–45.

152. Arslan F, Smeets MB, Riem Vis PW, Karper JC, Quax PH, Bongartz LG, et al. Lack of fibronectin-EDA promotes survival and prevents adverse remodeling and heart function deterioration after myocardial infarction. Circ Res. 2011;108(5):582–92.

153. Kelsh-Lasher RM, Ambesi A, Bertram C, McKeown-Longo PJ. Integrin alpha4beta1 and TLR4 Cooperate to Induce Fibrotic Gene Expression in Response to Fibronectin's EDA Domain. J Invest Dermatol. 2017;137(12):2505–12.

154. Jain M, Dhanesha N, Doddapattar P, Chorawala MR, Nayak MK, Cornelissen A, et al. Smooth muscle cell-specific fibronectin-EDA mediates phenotypic switching and neointimal hyperplasia. J Clin Invest. 2020;130(1):295–314.

155. Klingberg F, Chau G, Walraven M, Boo S, Koehler A, Chow ML, et al. The fibronectin ED-A domain enhances recruitment of latent TGF-beta-binding protein-1 to the fibroblast matrix. J Cell Sci. 2018;131(5):jcs201293.

156. Liao YF, Gotwals PJ, Koteliansky VE, Sheppard D, Van De Water L. The EIIIA segment of fibronectin is a ligand for integrins

alpha 9beta 1 and alpha 4beta 1 providing a novel mechanism for regulating cell adhesion by alternative splicing. J Biol Chem. 2002;277(17):14467–74.

157. Erdogan B, Ao M, White LM, Means AL, Brewer BM, Yang L, et al. Cancer-associated fibroblasts promote directional cancer cell migration by aligning fibronectin. J Cell Biol. 2017;216(11):3799–816.

158. Attieh Y, Clark AG, Grass C, Richon S, Pocard M, Mariani P, et al. Cancer-associated fibroblasts lead tumor invasion through integrin-beta3-dependent fibronectin assembly. J Cell Biol. 2017;216(11):3509–20.

159. Franco-Barraza J, Francescone R, Luong T, Shah N, Madhani R, Cukierman G, et al. Matrix-regulated integrin alphavbeta5 maintains alpha5beta1-dependent desmoplastic traits prognostic of neoplastic recurrence. elife. 2017;6:e20600.

160. Lugano R, Vemuri K, Yu D, Bergqvist M, Smits A, Essand M, et al. CD93 promotes beta1 integrin activation and fibronectin fibrillogenesis during tumor angiogenesis. J Clin Invest. 2018;128(8):3280–97.

161. Rossnagl S, Altrock E, Sens C, Kraft S, Rau K, Milsom MD, et al. EDA-fibronectin originating from osteoblasts inhibits the immune response against cancer. PLoS Biol. 2016;14(9):e1002562.

162. Gopal S, Veracini L, Grall D, Butori C, Schaub S, Audebert S, et al. Fibronectin-guided migration of carcinoma collectives. Nat Commun. 2017;8:14105.

163. Berger AJ, Renner CM, Hale I, Yang X, Ponik SM, Weisman PS, et al. Scaffold stiffness influences breast cancer cell invasion via EGFR-linked Mena upregulation and matrix remodeling. Matrix Biol. 2020;85–86:80–93.

164. Kwon A, Chae IH, You E, Kim SH, Ahn SY, Lee OJ, et al. Extra domain A-containing fibronectin expression in Spin90-deficient fibroblasts mediates cancer-stroma interaction and promotes breast cancer progression. J Cell Physiol. 2020;235(5):4494–507.

165. Ou J, Deng J, Wei X, Xie G, Zhou R, Yu L, et al. Fibronectin extra domain A (EDA) sustains CD133(+)/CD44(+) subpopulation of colorectal cancer cells. Stem Cell Res. 2013;11(2):820–33.

166. Xiang L, Xie G, Ou J, Wei X, Pan F, Liang H. The extra domain A of fibronectin increases VEGF-C expression in colorectal carcinoma involving the PI3K/AKT signaling pathway. PLoS One. 2012;7(4):e35378.

167. Sun X, Fa P, Cui Z, Xia Y, Sun L, Li Z, et al. The EDA-containing cellular fibronectin induces epithelial-mesenchymal transition in lung cancer cells through integrin alpha9beta1-mediated activation of PI3-K/AKT and Erk1/2. Carcinogenesis. 2014;35(1):184–91.

168. Ou J, Peng Y, Deng J, Miao H, Zhou J, Zha L, et al. Endothelial cell-derived fibronectin extra domain A promotes colorectal cancer metastasis via inducing epithelial-mesenchymal transition. Carcinogenesis. 2014;35(7):1661–70.

169. Ou J, Pan F, Geng P, Wei X, Xie G, Deng J, et al. Silencing fibronectin extra domain A enhances radiosensitivity in nasopharyngeal carcinomas involving an FAK/Akt/JNK pathway. Int J Radiat Oncol Biol Phys. 2012;82(4):e685–91.

170. Mosher DF, Adams JC. Adhesion-modulating/matricellular ECM protein families: a structural, functional and evolutionary appraisal. Matrix Biol. 2012;31(3):155–61.

171. Wong GS, Rustgi AK. Matricellular proteins: priming the tumour microenvironment for cancer development and metastasis. Br J Cancer. 2013;108(4):755–61.

172. Chiquet-Ehrismann R, Tucker RP. Tenascins and the importance of adhesion modulation. Cold Spring Harb Perspect Biol. 2011;3(5):a004960.

173. Forsberg E, Hirsch E, Frohlich L, Meyer M, Ekblom P, Aszodi A, et al. Skin wounds and severed nerves heal normally in mice lacking tenascin-C. Proc Natl Acad Sci U S A. 1996;93(13):6594–9.

174. Talts JF, Wirl G, Dictor M, Muller WJ, Fassler R. Tenascin-C modulates tumor stroma and monocyte/macrophage recruitment but not tumor growth or metastasis in a mouse strain with spontaneous mammary cancer. J Cell Sci. 1999;112(Pt 12):1855–64.

175. Zuliani-Alvarez L, Marzeda AM, Deligne C, Schwenzer A, McCann FE, Marsden BD, et al. Mapping tenascin-C interaction with toll-like receptor 4 reveals a new subset of endogenous inflammatory triggers. Nat Commun. 2017;8(1):1595.

176. Bhattacharyya S, Wang W, Morales-Nebreda L, Feng G, Wu M, Zhou X, et al. Tenascin-C drives persistence of organ fibrosis. Nat Commun. 2016;7:11703.

177. Yeo SY, Lee KW, Shin D, An S, Cho KH, Kim SH. A positive feedback loop bi-stably activates fibroblasts. Nat Commun. 2018;9(1):3016.

178. Fu H, Tian Y, Zhou L, Zhou D, Tan RJ, Stolz DB, et al. Tenascin-C is a major component of the fibrogenic niche in kidney fibrosis. J Am Soc Nephrol. 2017;28(3):785–801.

179. Orend G, Chiquet-Ehrismann R. Tenascin-C induced signaling in cancer. Cancer Lett. 2006;244(2):143–63.

180. Martin D, Brown-Luedi M, Chiquet-Ehrismann R. Tenascin-C signaling through induction of 14-3-3 tau. J Cell Biol. 2003;160(2):171–5.

181. Ruiz C, Huang W, Hegi ME, Lange K, Hamou MF, Fluri E, et al. Growth promoting signaling by tenascin-C [corrected]. Cancer Res. 2004;64(20):7377–85.

182. Huang W, Chiquet-Ehrismann R, Moyano JV, Garcia-Pardo A, Orend G. Interference of tenascin-C with syndecan-4 binding to fibronectin blocks cell adhesion and stimulates tumor cell proliferation. Cancer Res. 2001;61(23):8586–94.

183. Shi M, He X, Wei W, Wang J, Zhang T, Shen X. Tenascin-C induces resistance to apoptosis in pancreatic cancer cell through activation of ERK/NF-kappaB pathway. Apoptosis. 2015;20(6):843–57.

184. Nagaharu K, Zhang X, Yoshida T, Katoh D, Hanamura N, Kozuka Y, et al. Tenascin C induces epithelial-mesenchymal transition-like change accompanied by SRC activation and focal adhesion kinase phosphorylation in human breast cancer cells. Am J Pathol. 2011;178(2):754–63.

185. Katoh D, Nagaharu K, Shimojo N, Hanamura N, Yamashita M, Kozuka Y, et al. Binding of alphavbeta1 and alphavbeta6 integrins to tenascin-C induces epithelial-mesenchymal transition-like change of breast cancer cells. Oncogenesis. 2013;2:e65.

186. Ghahhari NM, Babashah S. Interplay between microRNAs and WNT/beta-catenin signalling pathway regulates epithelial-mesenchymal transition in cancer. Eur J Cancer. 2015;51(12):1638–49.

187. Saupe F, Schwenzer A, Jia Y, Gasser I, Spenle C, Langlois B, et al. Tenascin-C downregulates wnt inhibitor dickkopf-1, promoting tumorigenesis in a neuroendocrine tumor model. Cell Rep. 2013;5(2):482–92.

188. Beiter K, Hiendlmeyer E, Brabletz T, Hlubek F, Haynl A, Knoll C, et al. beta-Catenin regulates the expression of tenascin-C in human colorectal tumors. Oncogene. 2005;24(55):8200–4.

189. Nong Y, Wu D, Lin Y, Zhang Y, Bai L, Tang H. Tenascin-C expression is associated with poor prognosis in hepatocellular carcinoma (HCC) patients and the inflammatory cytokine TNF-alpha-induced TNC expression promotes migration in HCC cells. Am J Cancer Res. 2015;5(2):782–91.

190. Grahovac J, Becker D, Wells A. Melanoma cell invasiveness is promoted at least in part by the epidermal growth factor-like repeats of tenascin-C. J Invest Dermatol. 2013;133(1):210–20.

191. Kaariainen E, Nummela P, Soikkeli J, Yin M, Lukk M, Jahkola T, et al. Switch to an invasive growth phase in melanoma is associated with tenascin-C, fibronectin, and procollagen-I forming specific channel structures for invasion. J Pathol. 2006;210(2):181–91.

192. Kalembeyi I, Inada H, Nishiura R, Imanaka-Yoshida K, Sakakura T, Yoshida T. Tenascin-C upregulates matrix metalloproteinase-9 in breast cancer cells: direct and synergistic effects with transforming growth factor beta1. Int J Cancer. 2003;105(1):53–60.

193. Hancox RA, Allen MD, Holliday DL, Edwards DR, Pennington CJ, Guttery DS, et al. Tumour-associated tenascin-C isoforms promote breast cancer cell invasion and growth by matrix metalloproteinase-dependent and independent mechanisms. Breast Cancer Res. 2009;11(2):R24.

194. Calvo A, Catena R, Noble MS, Carbott D, Gil-Bazo I, Gonzalez-Moreno O, et al. Identification of VEGF-regulated genes associated with increased lung metastatic potential: functional involvement of tenascin-C in tumor growth and lung metastasis. Oncogene. 2008;27(40):5373–84.

195. O'Connell JT, Sugimoto H, Cooke VG, MacDonald BA, Mehta AI, LeBleu VS, et al. VEGF-A and Tenascin-C produced by S100A4+ stromal cells are important for metastatic colonization. Proc Natl Acad Sci U S A. 2011;108(38):16002–7.

196. Gocheva V, Naba A, Bhutkar A, Guardia T, Miller KM, Li CM, et al. Quantitative proteomics identify Tenascin-C as a promoter of lung cancer progression and contributor to a signature prognostic of patient survival. Proc Natl Acad Sci U S A. 2017;114(28):E5625–E34.

197. Katoh D, Kozuka Y, Noro A, Ogawa T, Imanaka-Yoshida K, Yoshida T. Tenascin-C induces phenotypic changes in fibroblasts to myofibroblasts with high contractility through the integrin alphavbeta1/TGF-beta/SMAD signaling axis in human breast cancer. Am J Pathol. 2020;190(10):2123–35.

198. Spenle C, Loustau T, Murdamoothoo D, Erne W, la Forest B-d, Divonne S, Veber R, et al. Tenascin-C orchestrates an immune-suppressive tumor microenvironment in oral squamous cell carcinoma. Cancer Immunol Res. 2020;8(9):1122–38.

199. Chiovaro F, Martina E, Bottos A, Scherberich A, Hynes NE, Chiquet-Ehrismann R. Transcriptional regulation of tenascin-W by TGF-beta signaling in the bone metastatic niche of breast cancer cells. Int J Cancer. 2015;137(8):1842–54.

200. Degen M, Brellier F, Kain R, Ruiz C, Terracciano L, Orend G, et al. Tenascin-W is a novel marker for activated tumor stroma in low-grade human breast cancer and influences cell behavior. Cancer Res. 2007;67(19):9169–79.

201. Degen M, Brellier F, Schenk S, Driscoll R, Zaman K, Stupp R, et al. Tenascin-W, a new marker of cancer stroma, is elevated in sera of colon and breast cancer patients. Int J Cancer. 2008;122(11):2454–61.

202. Scherberich A, Tucker RP, Degen M, Brown-Luedi M, Andres AC, Chiquet-Ehrismann R. Tenascin-W is found in malignant mammary tumors, promotes alpha8 integrin-dependent motility and requires p38MAPK activity for BMP-2 and TNF-alpha induced expression in vitro. Oncogene. 2005;24(9):1525–32.

203. Brellier F, Martina E, Degen M, Heuze-Vourc'h N, Petit A, Kryza T, et al. Tenascin-W is a better cancer biomarker than tenascin-C for most human solid tumors. BMC Clin Pathol. 2012;12:14.

204. Matsumoto K, Saga Y, Ikemura T, Sakakura T, Chiquet-Ehrismann R. The distribution of tenascin-X is distinct and often reciprocal to that of tenascin-C. J Cell Biol. 1994;125(2):483–93.

205. Chiquet-Ehrismann R, Chiquet M. Tenascins: regulation and putative functions during pathological stress. J Pathol. 2003;200(4):488–99.

206. Geffrotin C, Horak V, Crechet F, Tricaud Y, Lethias C, Vincent-Naulleau S, et al. Opposite regulation of tenascin-C and tenascin-X in MeLiM swine heritable cutaneous malignant melanoma. Biochim Biophys Acta. 2000;1524(2-3):196–202.

207. Matsumoto K, Takayama N, Ohnishi J, Ohnishi E, Shirayoshi Y, Nakatsuji N, et al. Tumour invasion and metastasis are promoted in mice deficient in tenascin-X. Genes Cells. 2001;6(12):1101–11.

208. Matsumoto K, Minamitani T, Orba Y, Sato M, Sawa H, Ariga H. Induction of matrix metalloproteinase-2 by tenascin-X deficiency is mediated through the c-Jun N-terminal kinase and protein tyrosine kinase phosphorylation pathway. Exp Cell Res. 2004;297(2):404–14.

209. Alcaraz LB, Exposito JY, Chuvin N, Pommier RM, Cluzel C, Martel S, et al. Tenascin-X promotes epithelial-to-mesenchymal transition by activating latent TGF-beta. J Cell Biol. 2014;205(3):409–28.

210. Rios H, Koushik SV, Wang H, Wang J, Zhou HM, Lindsley A, et al. periostin null mice exhibit dwarfism, incisor enamel defects, and an early-onset periodontal disease-like phenotype. Mol Cell Biol. 2005;25(24):11131–44.

211. Conway SJ, Izuhara K, Kudo Y, Litvin J, Markwald R, Ouyang G, et al. The role of periostin in tissue remodeling across health and disease. Cell Mol Life Sci. 2014;71(7):1279–88.

212. Elliott CG, Wang J, Guo X, Sw X, Eastwood M, Guan J, et al. Periostin modulates myofibroblast differentiation during full-thickness cutaneous wound repair. J Cell Sci. 2012;125(1):121–32.

213. Shimazaki M, Nakamura K, Kii I, Kashima T, Amizuka N, Li M, et al. Periostin is essential for cardiac healing after acute myocardial infarction. J Exp Med. 2008;205(2):295–303.

214. Lorts A, Schwanekamp JA, Baudino TA, McNally EM, Molkentin JD. Deletion of periostin reduces muscular dystrophy and fibrosis in mice by modulating the transforming growth factor-beta pathway. Proc Natl Acad Sci U S A. 2012;109(27):10978–83.

215. Norris RA, Damon B, Mironov V, Kasyanov V, Ramamurthi A, Moreno-Rodriguez R, et al. Periostin regulates collagen fibrillogenesis and the biomechanical properties of connective tissues. J Cell Biochem. 2007;101(3):695–711.

216. Egbert M, Ruetze M, Sattler M, Wenck H, Gallinat S, Lucius R, et al. The matricellular protein periostin contributes to proper collagen function and is downregulated during skin aging. J Dermatol Sci. 2014;73(1):40–8.

217. Shimazaki M, Kudo A. Impaired capsule formation of tumors in periostin-null mice. Biochem Biophys Res Commun. 2008;367(4):736–42.

218. Kikuchi Y, Kunita A, Iwata C, Komura D, Nishiyama T, Shimazu K, et al. The niche component periostin is produced by cancer-associated fibroblasts, supporting growth of gastric cancer through ERK activation. Am J Pathol. 2014;184(3):859–70.

219. Fukuda K, Sugihara E, Ohta S, Izuhara K, Funakoshi T, Amagai M, et al. Periostin is a key niche component for wound metastasis of melanoma. PLoS One. 2015;10(6):e0129704.

220. Zhou W, Ke SQ, Huang Z, Flavahan W, Fang X, Paul J, et al. Periostin secreted by glioblastoma stem cells recruits M2 tumour-associated macrophages and promotes malignant growth. Nat Cell Biol. 2015;17(2):170–82.

221. Malanchi I, Santamaria-Martinez A, Susanto E, Peng H, Lehr HA, Delaloye JF, et al. Interactions between cancer stem cells and their niche govern metastatic colonization. Nature. 2012;481(7379):85–9.

222. Sonongbua J, Siritungyong S, Thongchot S, Kamolhan T, Utispan K, Thuwajit P, et al. Periostin induces epithelialtomesenchymal transition via the integrin alpha5beta1/TWIST2 axis in cholangiocarcinoma. Oncol Rep. 2020;43(4):1147–58.

223. Ma H, Wang J, Zhao X, Wu T, Huang Z, Chen D, et al. Periostin promotes colorectal tumorigenesis through integrin-FAK-Src pathway-mediated YAP/TAZ activation. Cell Rep. 2020;30(3):793–806 e6.

224. Zenitani M, Nojiri T, Hosoda H, Kimura T, Uehara S, Miyazato M, et al. Chemotherapy can promote liver metastasis by enhancing metastatic niche formation in mice. J Surg Res. 2018;224:50–7.

225. Wegrowski Y, Maquart FX. Involvement of stromal proteoglycans in tumour progression. Crit Rev Oncol Hematol. 2004;49(3):259–68.

226. Theocharis AD, Skandalis SS, Tzanakakis GN, Karamanos NK. Proteoglycans in health and disease: novel roles for proteoglycans in malignancy and their pharmacological targeting. FEBS J. 2010;277(19):3904–23.

227. Iozzo RV, Sanderson RD. Proteoglycans in cancer biology, tumour microenvironment and angiogenesis. J Cell Mol Med. 2011;15(5):1013–31.

228. Sarrazin S, Lamanna WC, Esko JD. Heparan sulfate proteoglycans. Cold Spring Harb Perspect Biol. 2011;3(7):a004952.

229. Li JP, Kusche-Gullberg M. Heparan sulfate: biosynthesis, structure, and function. Int Rev Cell Mol Biol. 2016;325:215–73.

230. Bishop JR, Schuksz M, Esko JD. Heparan sulphate proteoglycans fine-tune mammalian physiology. Nature. 2007;446(7139):1030–7.

231. Ai X, Do AT, Lozynska O, Kusche-Gullberg M, Lindahl U, Emerson CP Jr. QSulf1 remodels the 6-O sulfation states of cell surface heparan sulfate proteoglycans to promote Wnt signaling. J Cell Biol. 2003;162(2):341–51.

232. Billings PC, Pacifici M. Interactions of signaling proteins, growth factors and other proteins with heparan sulfate: mechanisms and mysteries. Connect Tissue Res. 2015;56(4):272–80.

233. Lau EK, Paavola CD, Johnson Z, Gaudry JP, Geretti E, Borlat F, et al. Identification of the glycosaminoglycan binding site of the CC chemokine, MCP-1: implications for structure and function in vivo. J Biol Chem. 2004;279(21):22294–305.

234. Dowsland MH, Harvey JR, Lennard TW, Kirby JA, Ali S. Chemokines and breast cancer: a gateway to revolutionary targeted cancer treatments? Curr Med Chem. 2003;10(7):579–92.

235. Iozzo RV, Schaefer L. Proteoglycan form and function: a comprehensive nomenclature of proteoglycans. Matrix Biol. 2015;42:11–55.

236. Choi Y, Chung H, Jung H, Couchman JR, Oh ES. Syndecans as cell surface receptors: unique structure equates with functional diversity. Matrix Biol. 2011;30(2):93–9.

237. Couchman JR, Gopal S, Lim HC, Norgaard S, Multhaupt HA. Syndecans: from peripheral coreceptors to mainstream regulators of cell behaviour. Int J Exp Pathol. 2015;96(1):1–10.

238. Yao W, Rose JL, Wang W, Seth S, Jiang H, Taguchi A, et al. Syndecan 1 is a critical mediator of macropinocytosis in pancreatic cancer. Nature. 2019;568(7752):410–4.

239. Chute C, Yang X, Meyer K, Yang N, O'Neil K, Kasza I, et al. Syndecan-1 induction in lung microenvironment supports the establishment of breast tumor metastases. Breast Cancer Res. 2018;20(1):66.

240. Gondelaud F, Ricard-Blum S. Structures and interactions of syndecans. FEBS J. 2019;286(15):2994–3007.

241. Vuoriluoto K, Hognas G, Meller P, Lehti K, Ivaska J. Syndecan-1 and -4 differentially regulate oncogenic K-ras dependent cell invasion into collagen through alpha2beta1 integrin and MT1-MMP. Matrix Biol. 2011;30(3):207–17.

242. Chronopoulos A, Thorpe SD, Cortes E, Lachowski D, Rice AJ, Mykuliak VV, et al. Syndecan-4 tunes cell mechanics by activating the kindlin-integrin-RhoA pathway. Nat Mater. 2020;19(6):669–78.

243. Ihrcke NS, Platt JL. Shedding of heparan sulfate proteoglycan by stimulated endothelial cells: evidence for proteolysis of cell-surface molecules. J Cell Physiol. 1996;168(3):625–37.

244. Manon-Jensen T, Multhaupt HA, Couchman JR. Mapping of matrix metalloproteinase cleavage sites on syndecan-1 and syndecan-4 ectodomains. FEBS J. 2013;280(10):2320–31.

245. Choi S, Kim JY, Park JH, Lee ST, Han IO, Oh ES. The matrix metalloproteinase-7 regulates the extracellular shedding of syndecan-2 from colon cancer cells. Biochem Biophys Res Commun. 2012;417(4):1260–4.

246. Manon-Jensen T, Itoh Y, Couchman JR. Proteoglycans in health and disease: the multiple roles of syndecan shedding. FEBS J. 2010;277(19):3876–89.

247. Ding K, Lopez-Burks M, Sanchez-Duran JA, Korc M, Lander AD. Growth factor-induced shedding of syndecan-1 confers glypican-1 dependence on mitogenic responses of cancer cells. J Cell Biol. 2005;171(4):729–38.

248. Tan X, Khalil N, Tesarik C, Vanapalli K, Yaputra V, Alkhouri H, et al. Th1 cytokine-induced syndecan-4 shedding by airway smooth muscle cells is dependent on mitogen-activated protein kinases. Am J Physiol Lung Cell Mol Physiol. 2012;302(7):L700–10.

249. Yang Y, Macleod V, Miao HQ, Theus A, Zhan F, Shaughnessy JD Jr, et al. Heparanase enhances syndecan-1 shedding: a novel mechanism for stimulation of tumor growth and metastasis. J Biol Chem. 2007;282(18):13326–33.

250. Joensuu H, Anttonen A, Eriksson M, Makitaro R, Alfthan H, Kinnula V, et al. Soluble syndecan-1 and serum basic fibroblast growth factor are new prognostic factors in lung cancer. Cancer Res. 2002;62(18):5210–7.

251. Ramani VC, Sanderson RD. Chemotherapy stimulates syndecan-1 shedding: a potentially negative effect of treatment that may promote tumor relapse. Matrix Biol. 2014;35:215–22.

252. Stewart MD, Ramani VC, Sanderson RD. Shed syndecan-1 translocates to the nucleus of cells delivering growth factors and inhibiting histone acetylation: a novel mechanism of tumor-host cross-talk. J Biol Chem. 2015;290(2):941–9.

253. Su G, Blaine SA, Qiao D, Friedl A. Membrane type 1 matrix metalloproteinase-mediated stromal syndecan-1 shedding stimulates breast carcinoma cell proliferation. Cancer Res. 2008;68(22):9558–65.

254. Su G, Blaine SA, Qiao D, Friedl A. Shedding of syndecan-1 by stromal fibroblasts stimulates human breast cancer cell proliferation via FGF2 activation. J Biol Chem. 2007;282(20):14906–15.

255. Nikolova V, Koo CY, Ibrahim SA, Wang Z, Spillmann D, Dreier R, et al. Differential roles for membrane-bound and soluble syndecan-1 (CD138) in breast cancer progression. Carcinogenesis. 2009;30(3):397–407.

256. Choi S, Choi Y, Jun E, Kim IS, Kim SE, Jung SA, et al. Shed syndecan-2 enhances tumorigenic activities of colon cancer cells. Oncotarget. 2015;6(6):3874–86.

257. Wang X, Zuo D, Chen Y, Li W, Liu R, He Y, et al. Shed Syndecan-1 is involved in chemotherapy resistance via the EGFR pathway in colorectal cancer. Br J Cancer. 2014;111(10):1965–76.

258. Chen S, Birk DE. The regulatory roles of small leucine-rich proteoglycans in extracellular matrix assembly. FEBS J. 2013;280(10):2120–37.

259. Cawthorn TR, Moreno JC, Dharsee M, Tran-Thanh D, Ackloo S, Zhu PH, et al. Proteomic analyses reveal high expression of decorin and endoplasmin (HSP90B1) are associated with breast cancer metastasis and decreased survival. PLoS One. 2012;7(2):e30992.

260. Sainio A, Nyman M, Lund R, Vuorikoski S, Bostrom P, Laato M, et al. Lack of decorin expression by human bladder cancer cells offers new tools in the therapy of urothelial malignancies. PLoS One. 2013;8(10):e76190.

261. Henke A, Grace OC, Ashley GR, Stewart GD, Riddick AC, Yeun H, et al. Stromal expression of decorin, Semaphorin6D, SPARC, Sprouty1 and Tsukushi in developing prostate and decreased levels of decorin in prostate cancer. PLoS One. 2012;7(8):e42516.

262. Campioni M, Ambrogi V, Pompeo E, Citro G, Castelli M, Spugnini EP, et al. Identification of genes down-regulated during lung cancer progression: a cDNA array study. J Exp Clin Cancer Res. 2008;27:38.

263. Bostrom P, Sainio A, Kakko T, Savontaus M, Soderstrom M, Jarvelainen H. Localization of decorin gene expression in normal human breast tissue and in benign and malignant tumors of the human breast. Histochem Cell Biol. 2013;139(1):161–71.

264. Oda G, Sato T, Ishikawa T, Kawachi H, Nakagawa T, Kuwayama T, et al. Significance of stromal decorin expression during the progression of breast cancer. Oncol Rep. 2012;28(6):2003–8.

265. Troup S, Njue C, Kliewer EV, Parisien M, Roskelley C, Chakravarti S, et al. Reduced expression of the small leucine-rich proteoglycans, lumican, and decorin is associated with poor outcome in node-negative invasive breast cancer. Clin Cancer Res. 2003;9(1):207–14.

266. Horvath Z, Kovalszky I, Fullar A, Kiss K, Schaff Z, Iozzo RV, et al. Decorin deficiency promotes hepatic carcinogenesis. Matrix Biol. 2014;35:194–205.

267. Xu W, Neill T, Yang Y, Hu Z, Cleveland E, Wu Y, et al. The systemic delivery of an oncolytic adenovirus expressing decorin inhibits bone metastasis in a mouse model of human prostate cancer. Gene Ther. 2015;22(3):31–40.

268. Nyman MC, Sainio AO, Pennanen MM, Lund RJ, Vuorikoski S, Sundstrom JT, et al. Decorin in human colon cancer: localization in vivo and effect on cancer cell behavior in vitro. J Histochem Cytochem. 2015;63(9):710–20.

269. Buraschi S, Neill T, Owens RT, Iniguez LA, Purkins G, Vadigepalli R, et al. Decorin protein core affects the global gene expression profile of the tumor microenvironment in a triple-negative orthotopic breast carcinoma xenograft model. PLoS One. 2012;7(9):e45559.

270. Goldoni S, Iozzo RV. Tumor microenvironment: modulation by decorin and related molecules harboring leucine-rich tandem motifs. Int J Cancer. 2008;123(11):2473–9.

271. Buraschi S, Pal N, Tyler-Rubinstein N, Owens RT, Neill T, Iozzo RV. Decorin antagonizes Met receptor activity and down-regulates {beta}-catenin and Myc levels. J Biol Chem. 2010;285(53):42075–85.

272. Neill T, Torres A, Buraschi S, Owens RT, Hoek JB, Baffa R, et al. Decorin induces mitophagy in breast carcinoma cells via peroxisome proliferator-activated receptor gamma coactivator-1alpha (PGC-1alpha) and mitostatin. J Biol Chem. 2014;289(8):4952–68.

273. Neill T, Painter H, Buraschi S, Owens RT, Lisanti MP, Schaefer L, et al. Decorin antagonizes the angiogenic network: concurrent inhibition of Met, hypoxia inducible factor 1alpha, vascular endothelial growth factor A, and induction of thrombospondin-1 and TIMP3. J Biol Chem. 2012;287(8):5492–506.

274. Buraschi S, Neill T, Goyal A, Poluzzi C, Smythies J, Owens RT, et al. Decorin causes autophagy in endothelial cells via Peg3. Proc Natl Acad Sci U S A. 2013;110(28):E2582–91.

275. Morcavallo A, Buraschi S, Xu SQ, Belfiore A, Schaefer L, Iozzo RV, et al. Decorin differentially modulates the activity of insulin receptor isoform A ligands. Matrix Biol. 2014;35:82–90.

276. Koninger J, Giese NA, di Mola FF, Berberat P, Giese T, Esposito I, et al. Overexpressed decorin in pancreatic cancer: potential tumor growth inhibition and attenuation of chemotherapeutic action. Clin Cancer Res. 2004;10(14):4776–83.

277. Kasamatsu A, Uzawa K, Minakawa Y, Ishige S, Kasama H, Endo-Sakamoto Y, et al. Decorin in human oral cancer: a promising predictive biomarker of S-1 neoadjuvant chemosensitivity. Biochem Biophys Res Commun. 2015;457(1):71–6.

278. Zhu YH, Yang F, Zhang SS, Zeng TT, Xie X, Guan XY. High expression of biglycan is associated with poor prognosis in patients with esophageal squamous cell carcinoma. Int J Clin Exp Pathol. 2013;6(11):2497–505.

279. Aprile G, Avellini C, Reni M, Mazzer M, Foltran L, Rossi D, et al. Biglycan expression and clinical outcome in patients with pancreatic adenocarcinoma. Tumour Biol. 2013;34(1):131–7.

280. Hu L, Duan YT, Li JF, Su LP, Yan M, Zhu ZG, et al. Biglycan enhances gastric cancer invasion by activating FAK signaling pathway. Oncotarget. 2014;5(7):1885–96.

281. Niedworok C, Rock K, Kretschmer I, Freudenberger T, Nagy N, Szarvas T, et al. Inhibitory role of the small leucine-rich proteoglycan biglycan in bladder cancer. PLoS One. 2013;8(11):e80084.

282. Weber CK, Sommer G, Michl P, Fensterer H, Weimer M, Gansauge F, et al. Biglycan is overexpressed in pancreatic cancer and induces G1-arrest in pancreatic cancer cell lines. Gastroenterology. 2001;121(3):657–67.

283. Nikitovic D, Papoutsidakis A, Karamanos NK, Tzanakakis GN. Lumican affects tumor cell functions, tumor-ECM interactions, angiogenesis and inflammatory response. Matrix Biol. 2014;35:206–14.

284. Brezillon S, Pietraszek K, Maquart FX, Wegrowski Y. Lumican effects in the control of tumour progression and their links with metalloproteinases and integrins. FEBS J. 2013;280(10):2369–81.

285. Seya T, Tanaka N, Shinji S, Yokoi K, Koizumi M, Teranishi N, et al. Lumican expression in advanced colorectal cancer with nodal metastasis correlates with poor prognosis. Oncol Rep. 2006;16(6):1225–30.

286. de Wit M, Belt EJ, Delis-van Diemen PM, Carvalho B, Coupe VM, Stockmann HB, et al. Lumican and versican are associated with good outcome in stage II and III colon cancer. Ann Surg Oncol. 2013;20(Suppl 3):S348–59.

287. Panis C, Pizzatti L, Herrera AC, Cecchini R, Abdelhay E. Putative circulating markers of the early and advanced stages of breast cancer identified by high-resolution label-free proteomics. Cancer Lett. 2013;330(1):57–66.

288. Karamanou K, Franchi M, Onisto M, Passi A, Vynios DH, Brezillon S. Evaluation of lumican effects on morphology of invading breast cancer cells, expression of integrins and downstream signaling. FEBS J. 2020;287:4862–80.

289. Ishiwata T, Cho K, Kawahara K, Yamamoto T, Fujiwara Y, Uchida E, et al. Role of lumican in cancer cells and adjacent stromal tissues in human pancreatic cancer. Oncol Rep. 2007;18(3):537–43.

290. Li X, Truty MA, Kang Y, Chopin-Laly X, Zhang R, Roife D, et al. Extracellular lumican inhibits pancreatic cancer cell growth and is associated with prolonged survival after surgery. Clin Cancer Res. 2014;20(24):6529–40.

291. Matsuda Y, Yamamoto T, Kudo M, Kawahara K, Kawamoto M, Nakajima Y, et al. Expression and roles of lumican in lung adenocarcinoma and squamous cell carcinoma. Int J Oncol. 2008;33(6):1177–85.

292. Brezillon S, Venteo L, Ramont L, D'Onofrio MF, Perreau C, Pluot M, et al. Expression of lumican, a small leucine-rich proteoglycan with antitumour activity, in human malignant melanoma. Clin Exp Dermatol. 2007;32(4):405–16.

293. Brezillon S, Radwanska A, Zeltz C, Malkowski A, Ploton D, Bobichon H, et al. Lumican core protein inhibits melanoma cell migration via alterations of focal adhesion complexes. Cancer Lett. 2009;283(1):92–100.

294. Zeltz C, Brezillon S, Perreau C, Ramont L, Maquart FX, Wegrowski Y. Lumcorin: a leucine-rich repeat 9-derived peptide from human lumican inhibiting melanoma cell migration. FEBS Lett. 2009;583(18):3027–32.

295. Zeltz C, Brezillon S, Kapyla J, Eble JA, Bobichon H, Terryn C, et al. Lumican inhibits cell migration through alpha2beta1 integrin. Exp Cell Res. 2010;316(17):2922–31.

296. Pietraszek K, Chatron-Colliet A, Brezillon S, Perreau C, Jakubiak-Augustyn A, Krotkiewski H, et al. Lumican: a new inhibitor of matrix metalloproteinase-14 activity. FEBS Lett. 2014;588(23):4319–24.

297. Coulson-Thomas VJ, Coulson-Thomas YM, Gesteira TF, Andrade de Paula CA, Carneiro CR, Ortiz V, et al. Lumican expression, localization and antitumor activity in prostate cancer. Exp Cell Res. 2013;319(7):967–81.

298. Radwanska A, Litwin M, Nowak D, Baczynska D, Wegrowski Y, Maquart FX, et al. Overexpression of lumican affects the migration of human colon cancer cells through up-regulation of gelsolin and filamentous actin reorganization. Exp Cell Res. 2012;318(18):2312–23.

299. Oldberg A, Kalamajski S, Salnikov AV, Stuhr L, Morgelin M, Reed RK, et al. Collagen-binding proteoglycan fibro-

modulin can determine stroma matrix structure and fluid balance in experimental carcinoma. Proc Natl Acad Sci U S A. 2007;104(35):13966–71.

300. Hildebrand A, Romaris M, Rasmussen LM, Heinegard D, Twardzik DR, Border WA, et al. Interaction of the small interstitial proteoglycans biglycan, decorin and fibromodulin with transforming growth factor beta. Biochem J. 1994;302(Pt 2):527–34.

301. Maris P, Blomme A, Palacios AP, Costanza B, Bellahcene A, Bianchi E, et al. Asporin Is a Fibroblast-Derived TGF-beta1 Inhibitor and a Tumor Suppressor Associated with Good Prognosis in Breast Cancer. PLoS Med. 2015;12(9):e1001871.

302. Lohler J, Timpl R, Jaenisch R. Embryonic lethal mutation in mouse collagen I gene causes rupture of blood vessels and is associated with erythropoietic and mesenchymal cell death. Cell. 1984;38(2):597–607.

303. Andrikopoulos K, Liu X, Keene DR, Jaenisch R, Ramirez F. Targeted mutation in the col5a2 gene reveals a regulatory role for type V collagen during matrix assembly. Nat Genet. 1995;9(1):31–6.

304. Wenstrup RJ, Florer JB, Brunskill EW, Bell SM, Chervoneva I, Birk DE. Type V collagen controls the initiation of collagen fibril assembly. J Biol Chem. 2004;279(51):53331–7.

305. Provenzano PP, Eliceiri KW, Campbell JM, Inman DR, White JG, Keely PJ. Collagen reorganization at the tumor-stromal interface facilitates local invasion. BMC Med. 2006;4(1):38.

306. Liu X, Wu H, Byrne M, Krane S, Jaenisch R. Type III collagen is crucial for collagen I fibrillogenesis and for normal cardiovascular development. Proc Natl Acad Sci U S A. 1997;94(5):1852–6.

307. Saga Y, Yagi T, Ikawa Y, Sakakura T, Aizawa S. Mice develop normally without tenascin. Genes Dev. 1992;6:1821–31.

308. Hendaoui I, Tucker RP, Zingg D, Bichet S, Schittny J, Chiquet-Ehrismann R. Tenascin-C is required for normal Wnt/beta-catenin signaling in the whisker follicle stem cell niche. Matrix Biol. 2014;40:46–53.

309. Kii I, Amizuka N, Minqi L, Kitajima S, Saga Y, Kudo A. Periostin is an extracellular matrix protein required for eruption of incisors in mice. Biochem Biophys Res Commun. 2006;342(3):766–72.

310. Ontsuka K, Kotobuki Y, Shiraishi H, Serada S, Ohta S, Tanemura A, et al. Periostin, a matricellular protein, accelerates cutaneous wound repair by activating dermal fibroblasts. Exp Dermatol. 2012;21(5):331–6.

311. Ishiba T, Nagahara M, Nakagawa T, Sato T, Ishikawa T, Uetake H, et al. Periostin suppression induces decorin secretion leading to reduced breast cancer cell motility and invasion. Sci Rep. 2014;4:7069.

312. Danielson KG, Baribault H, Holmes DF, Graham H, Kadler KE, Iozzo RV. Targeted disruption of decorin leads to abnormal collagen fibril morphology and skin fragility. J Cell Biol. 1997;136(3):729–43.

313. Neill T, Schaefer L, Iozzo RV. Decorin: a guardian from the matrix. Am J Pathol. 2012;181(2):380–7.

314. Yamaguchi Y, Mann DM, Ruoslahti E. Negative regulation of transforming growth factor-beta by the proteoglycan decorin. Nature. 1990;346(6281):281–4.

315. Merline R, Moreth K, Beckmann J, Nastase MV, Zeng-Brouwers J, Tralhao JG, et al. Signaling by the matrix proteoglycan decorin controls inflammation and cancer through PDCD4 and MicroRNA-21. Sci Signal. 2011;4(199):ra75.

316. Chakravarti S, Magnuson T, Lass JH, Jepsen KJ, LaMantia C, Carroll H. Lumican regulates collagen fibril assembly: skin fragility and corneal opacity in the absence of lumican. J Cell Biol. 1998;141(5):1277–86.

317. Beauvais DM, Ell BJ, McWhorter AR, Rapraeger AC. Syndecan-1 regulates {alpha}v{beta}3 and {alpha}v{beta}5 integrin activation during angiogenesis and is blocked by synstatin, a novel peptide inhibitor. J Exp Med. 2009;16:691–705.

318. Theocharis AD, Karamanos NK. Proteoglycans remodeling in cancer: underlying molecular mechanisms. Matrix Biol. 2019;75-76:220–59.

319. Multhaupt HA, Leitinger B, Gullberg D, Couchman JR. Extracellular matrix component signaling in cancer. Adv Drug Deliv Rev. 2016;97:28–40.

320. Guilluy C, Dolega ME. Syndecan-4 forces integrins to cooperate. Nat Mater. 2020;19(6):587–8.

Tissue Architecture in Cancer Initiation and Progression

6

Susan E. Leggett and Celeste M. Nelson

Abstract

Tumors that originate from epithelial cells are referred to as carcinomas and represent the most frequently diagnosed cancers. Epithelial tissue is abundant throughout the body, where it lines organs to serve as a protective barrier against biological, chemical, and physical insults. As such, the maintenance of epithelial tissue architecture is critical for tissue homeostasis and healthy tissue functioning. The structure and function of epithelial tissues are largely influenced by the surrounding microenvironment, which is comprised of an acellular interstitial matrix and stromal cells. The makeup and architecture of this surrounding microenvironment are thus key players in cancer suppression, initiation, progression, and metastasis. Over the course of disease progression, the tumor microenvironment undergoes extensive extracellular matrix remodeling, while stromal cells infiltrate and undergo phenotypic switches to mediate tumor-suppressive and tumor-promoting roles. The detection of aberrant extracellular matrix and stromal cell infiltration and activation thus serve as important biomarkers of patient disease and may provide diagnostic and prognostic value. Consequently, a promising avenue for the future of personalized medicine is the development of targeted therapeutics aimed at normalizing the tumor microenvironment.

S. E. Leggett
Department of Chemical & Biological Engineering, Princeton University, Princeton, NJ, USA

C. M. Nelson (✉)
Department of Chemical & Biological Engineering, Princeton University, Princeton, NJ, USA

Department of Molecular Biology, Princeton University, Princeton, NJ, USA
e-mail: celesten@princeton.edu

L. A. Akslen, R. S. Watnick (eds.), *Biomarkers of the Tumor Microenvironment*, https://doi.org/10.1007/978-3-030-98950-7_6

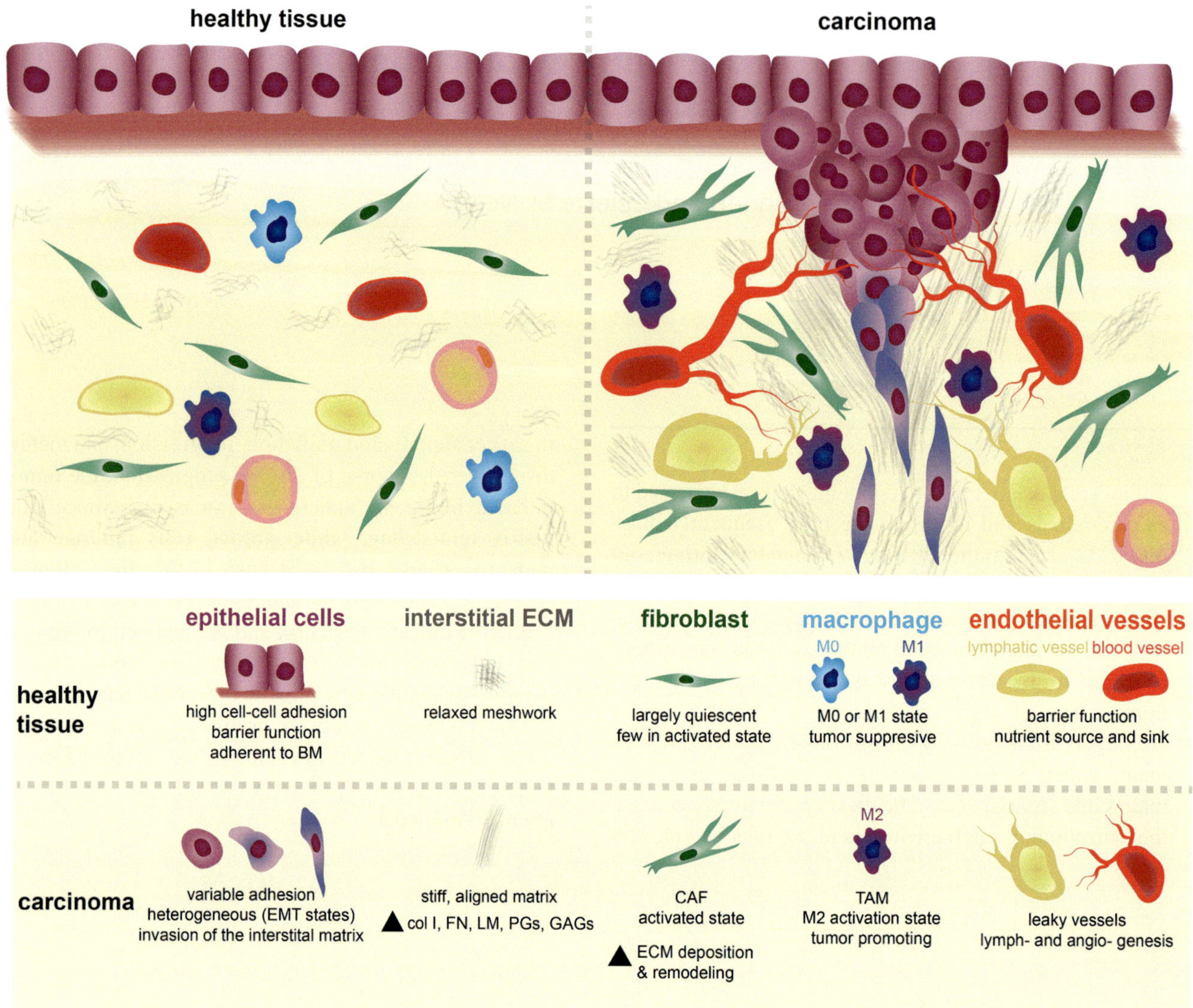

Carcinomas are malignant tumors that originate from cells in epithelial tissue. There, abnormal epithelial cells grow uncontrollably, breach the basement membrane, undergo cell-state transitions, invade into the underlying interstitial matrix, and subsequently disseminate to form distant metastases. Concomitantly, dramatic alterations of the tissue stroma contribute to the generation of a tumor-promoting microenvironment. Solid stress and interstitial fluid pressure are elevated in tumors, and the interstitial matrix becomes increasingly stiffened and aligned compared to that of healthy tissues. These physical changes are facilitated by dynamic processes, such as angiogenesis and the recruitment and activation of stromal cells. Further, tumor cells, cancer-associated fibroblasts, and tumor-associated macrophages drive matrix remodeling, which aids in the escape of tumor cells from the primary site. Overall, the tumor microenvironment plays a critical role in cancer initiation and progression. Thus, the tumor microenvironment may be viewed as a complex ecosystem that could be exploited to generate unconventional therapeutics for cancer treatment in the future.

Abbreviations

CAF	cancer-associated fibroblast
ECM	extracellular matrix
EMT	epithelial-mesenchymal transition
FAP	fibroblast activation protein
GAG	glycosaminoglycan
GF	growth factor
HLA	hyaluronic acid
IFP	interstitial fluid pressure
LOX	lysyl oxidase
MMP	matrix metalloproteinase
MET	mesenchymal-epithelial transition
3D	three-dimensional
TAM	tumor-associated macrophage
TME	tumor microenvironment
TGF-β	transforming growth factor-beta
VEGF	vascular endothelial growth factor

Take-Home Lessons

- In healthy tissues, epithelial cells are adherent to each other and anchored to a basement membrane, which separates them from the underlying connective tissue, or stroma, which contains an organized ECM and stromal cells
- Cancer is a complex disease state marked by abnormal cell growth, invasion of the stroma, and spread throughout the body, which mimics features of aberrant wound healing, including a persistent inflammatory response
- The stroma is initially tumor-suppressive in healthy tissues and early stages of malignancy, but switches to tumor-promoting as cancer progresses
- Cellular phenotypic transitions, activation, and stromal cell infiltration can lead to the production of an aberrant tumor stroma, which supports cancer progression and metastasis
- Alterations in the TME contribute to the transition from healthy to pro-tumorigenic stroma. These may include a denser, stiffer ECM with increased cross-linking and alignment of ECM proteins, infiltration of stromal cells, and leaky vasculature, which promotes tumor progression and decreases the efficacy of therapeutic approaches

Introduction

Cancer is an extremely complex group of diseases that have pervaded human history and perplexed scientists and physicians for centuries [1]. Indeed, the Greek physician and "father of medicine," Hippocrates (460–377 BC), is credited with the origin of the word cancer as a term to describe tumors, in which he recognized the great difficulty in treating the often fatal disease [2]. Advances in modern science and medicine have dramatically increased our understanding of the mechanisms of cancer initiation, progression, and metastasis. Despite this progress, cancer remains a global health problem and a leading cause of death. One reason for this persistence is that cancer therapeutics often fail to translate from preclinical to clinical trials and, in fact, demonstrate the lowest success rates of clinical trials for therapeutics across all major diseases [3]. This failure to translate may be attributed to inherent differences between humans and the classical model systems used to evaluate preclinical therapeutics (two-dimensional culture models, mouse models, etc.). On the other hand, a plausible alternative explanation is that traditional cancer therapies have attempted to target the wrong culprit—the cancer cell itself. The tumor cell-centric strategy was based on decades of research

that led to an incomplete description of the hallmarks of cancer at the dawn of the twenty-first century, which were centered around the attributes of cancer cells explicitly [4]. Since that time, the tumor cell-centric vision has been revisited to include additional enabling and emerging hallmarks of cancer, which serve to better recognize the complexity of tumors and the crucial role of the tumor microenvironment (TME) in malignant progression [5]. As such, the cellular and noncellular components of the microenvironment surrounding cancer cells are equally important to cancer initiation, progression, metastasis, and immune response. Continued investigations into the roles of tissue architecture and tumor-stroma interactions during the process of malignant progression will provide the crucial insight required to generate novel therapeutics targeted at "normalizing" the TME for cancer therapy.

In this chapter, we define the characteristics of the architecture of healthy epithelial tissues and the dysregulation of stroma that occurs during carcinogenesis and malignant progression. Specifically, we highlight the acellular and cellular components of the stroma in healthy tissue and in tumors. We define the hallmarks of cancer and illuminate the similarities between cancer progression and wound healing. We describe the tumor-inhibiting and tumor-supporting roles of the TME, as well as cellular state transitions that take place during cancer progression. We demonstrate how these ECM and stromal cell changes can be used as clinical biomarkers to aid in cancer diagnosis and inform clinical decision-making. Further, we discuss how the tumor stroma may be exploited for the development of novel targeted cancer therapeutics.

The Form and Function of Epithelial Tissue and the Extracellular Matrix

Composition and Architecture of Healthy Epithelial Tissues

Animals are comprised of four main tissue types: epithelial tissue, connective tissue, muscle tissue, and nerve tissue. Of these tissues, cancers most commonly originate from epithelial cells and are known as carcinomas. Epithelial tissues form tightly associated sheets of cells that line the external and internal surfaces of the body, including organs, cavities, vessels, and glands. The architecture of the epithelium is classified first by its apparent cell morphology and second by the number of epithelial cell layers in the tissue. Basic epithelial cell shapes include flat, boxy, and rectangular, which are referred to as "squamous," "cuboidal," and "columnar," respectively (Fig. 6.1a). Epithelial cells are arranged into single-layered "simple epithelium," multilayered "stratified epithelium," and single-layered "pseudostratified epithelium" with a multilayered appearance (Fig. 6.1b). In a simi-

lar fashion, exocrine glands are classified by their structure, which is broken down by the shape of the secretory portion of the duct (elongated/"tubular" or rounded/"acinar") and the number of ducts (single/"simple gland" or multiple branches/"compound gland") (Fig. 6.1c). The epithelium

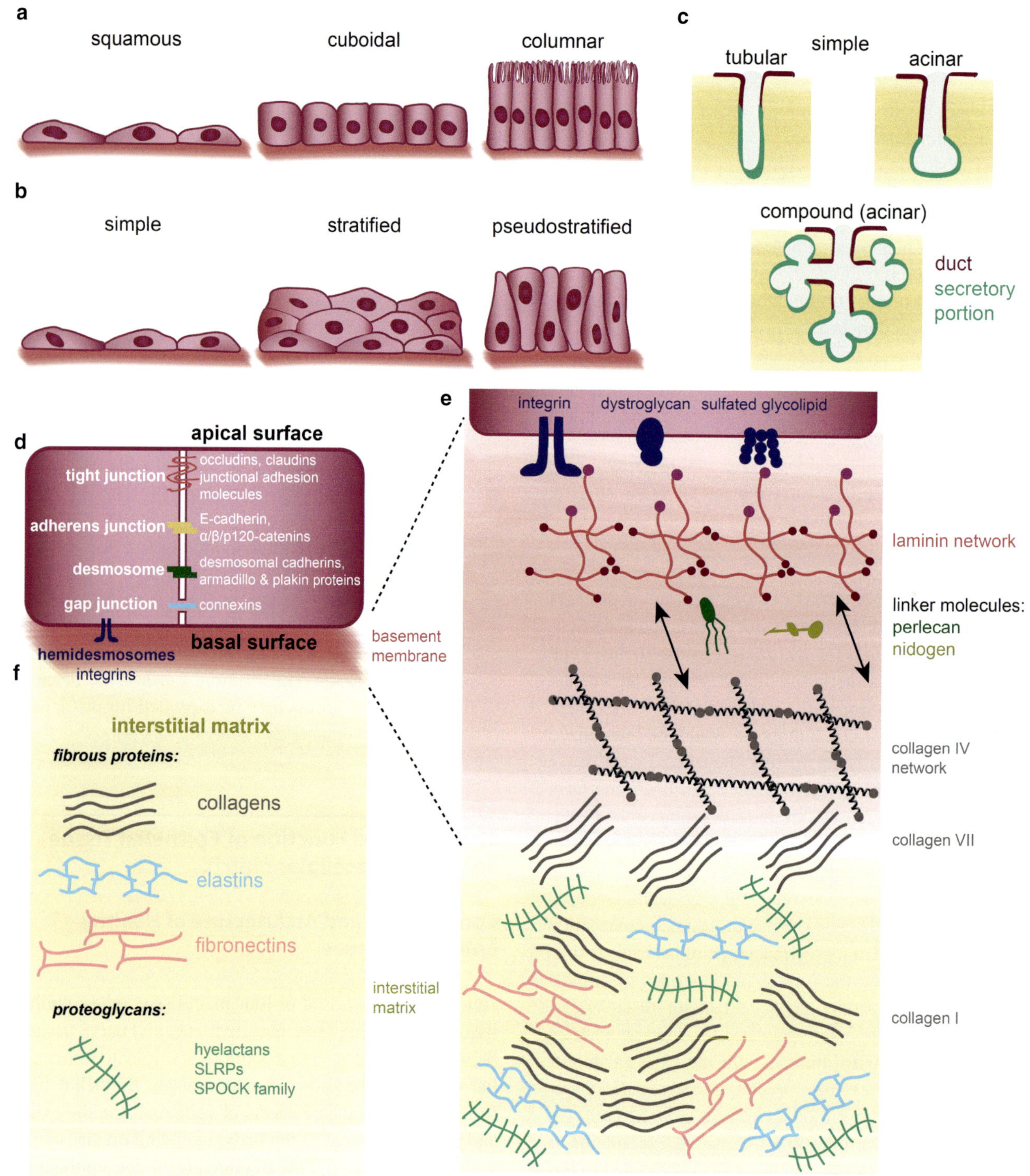

Fig. 6.1 Schematic of healthy epithelial tissue. (**a–b**) Cartoon of epithelial cell classification. (**c**) Cartoon of epithelial ductal structures. (**d**) Cartoon of cell-cell junction complexes. (**e**) Cartoon of the basement membrane: composition and structure. (**f**) Cartoon of the interstitial matrix: composition and structure

serves to provide a barrier against physical, chemical, and biological insults; performs critical roles in mediating the transport of substances across the tissue interface (e.g., by regulating secretion, absorption, diffusion, osmosis, and filtration); and thus supports tissue integrity and function. These functions depend on the establishment of apical-basal polarity and the preservation of strong cell-cell junctions that permit cohesion and communication between neighboring epithelial cells.

In general, a characteristic tripartite junctional complex exists between epithelial cells [6], which is comprised of the tight junction (zonula occludins; claudins; occludins) [7], adherens junction (zonula adherens; cadherins) [8], and the desmosome (macula adherens; desmosomal cadherins) [9]. The junctional complex contributes to the establishment and maintenance of apical-basal polarity of the epithelium, anchoring adjacent epithelial cells to one another and their respective cytoskeletons, and participates in intracellular signaling and mechanotransduction [10]. The gap junction (connexins) forms a channel that spans the membranes of adjacent cells, permitting direct cell-cell communication via the transmission of small molecules (<1 kDa) through the connected cytoplasms [11] (Fig. 6.1d). Further, the epithelium exhibits a remarkable capacity to dynamically respond to external stressors (e.g., during morphogenesis, tissue turnover/regeneration, and wound healing), owing in part to epithelial plasticity and fluid behavior, which are critical for the maintenance of tissue homeostasis [12]. Overall, the epithelium has robust mechanical strength and performs essential barrier and transport functions; however, this tissue does not perform these vital functions in isolation. Rather, the epithelium is responsive to its surrounding microenvironment, which is comprised of an acellular extracellular matrix (ECM) and cell-laden stroma that exists within the underlying connective tissue.

Composition of the Extracellular Matrix

The ECM is a composite of intricately entangled molecules (predominantly proteins and polysaccharides), which form a three-dimensional (3D) network. This complex mesh acts as a physical scaffold and plays a critical role in directing biochemical and biomechanical signaling of the surrounding cellular constituents [13]. Although the precise composition and structure of the ECM vary by tissue type, the core components are highly conserved and comprise the "adhesome" of tissues, the evolution of which dates back to the origin of multicellular organisms (*Metazoa*) [14]. In general, the ECM is formed by two groups of macromolecules, including proteoglycans and fibrous proteins (Fig. 6.1f). Proteoglycans are made up of a protein core that is covalently tethered to one or more glycosaminoglycan (GAG) chains. The proteoglycan

gene family consists of at least 43 members, which are classified into four distinct groups according to three main criteria: cellular/subcellular localization, gene/protein homology, and the protein module contained within the protein core. Extracellular proteoglycans represent the largest of these classes and are critical for ECM structure, function, and mediating biological functions. These include hyalectans (aggrecan, versican, neurocan, brevican), small leucine-rich proteoglycans (SLRPs; 5 classes), and the SPOCK family of proteoglycans. While proteoglycans are diverse in form and function, their general roles involve participating in a myriad of biological processes including cell adhesion, migration, the regulation of inflammation, and growth factor (GF) binding, as well as binding to the fibrous proteins in the ECM. Together, proteoglycans and fibrous proteins form a hydrated gel with force-resistant properties (load-bearing, compressive stress, tensile stress) [15]. The major fibrous proteins of the ECM include collagens, elastins, fibronectins, and laminins, which present with a diversity of structural architectures that enable these critical physical tissue properties and mediate cellular processes, which are described in the following sections. Critically, a subset of these ECM components make up a specialized form of ECM known as the basement membrane.

Structure and Function of the Basement Membrane

The epithelium is anchored to a specialized form of ECM, the basement membrane (BM), which protects the tissue from mechanical stress and serves as a physical barrier that separates the epithelium from its underlying connective tissue (Fig. 6.1d–e). The BM is a thin, dense, sheet-like structure that surrounds most tissues, including the epithelium. The BM structure is generated by two independent polymer networks, those of collagen IV and laminin, which self-assemble and are associated with each other by additional ECM proteins such as the nidogen glycoproteins and heparin sulfate proteoglycans (e.g., perlecan) (Fig. 6.1e) [16]. These molecules each have high affinity for both collagen IV and laminin and thus are key linkers within the BM, which increases the stability of the BM network and provides it with structural integrity [17]. Laminin is intricately linked to the cell surface through interactions with integrins, dystroglycan, and sulfated glycolipids, which is discussed in further detail in subsequent sections. The BM network thus plays a pivotal role in the maintenance of epithelial tissue structure and function.

The BM is critical in morphogenesis for establishing cell and tissue polarity. Throughout development and in adult tissues, the BM also serves as a reservoir for signaling molecules (e.g., GFs and ligands) that direct cellular signaling and downstream functions. The binding or uptake of these factors regulates several cellular processes including proliferation, polarization, survival, and migration. Thus, BM integrity is vital to tissue homeostasis and normal physiological functioning of the epithelium, while altered BM is associated with varied pathological states. Of note, breaching of the BM and dysregulation of BM components are frequently observed in cancer, whereby tumor and stromal cells can play an active role in BM remodeling [18], which is discussed in more detail below.

Composition and Architecture of the Tissue Microenvironment

Establishment and Maintenance of the Stroma

Epithelia are supported by an underlying tissue known as the stroma and, more specifically, loose connective tissue. The stroma is comprised predominantly of ECM, in which cells and ground substance fill the space between ECM fibers. The ground substance is largely formed by glycosaminoglycans, proteoglycans, and adhesive glycoproteins (e.g., laminin and fibronectin). In early development, BM and interstitial ECM components (e.g. collagen and elastin) are secreted by embryonic cells and are necessary for normal embryogenesis (Fig. 6.1f), as evidenced by the varied loss-of-function phenotypes such as abnormal development and embryonic lethality [19]. In more mature tissues, the primary cell type that directs the synthesis, secretion, and remodeling of the ECM is the resident fibroblast. Local ECM composition and structure direct the adhesion, migration, survival, differentiation, and proliferation of adjacent cells. Reciprocal interactions with cells that reside in the microenvironment further regulate the dynamic remodeling of the ECM in a spatiotemporal manner [20]. Establishment and homeostasis of the normal structure and function of the ECM components are critical for the maintenance of tissue architecture. Here, we first describe the supramolecular assembly of these fibrous molecules under normal physiological conditions.

Major Constituents of the ECM

Collagens

Collagen is the most abundant structural protein in mammals and is the predominant component of the ECM in humans. The collagen superfamily consists of 28 proteins that contain at least one triple-helical domain, which is comprised of three α polypeptide chains. These α polypeptide chains may be interspersed, as is the case for fibril-associated collagens with interrupted triple-helices, or assembled into a singular triple-helix, as is the case for fibrillar collagens. Collagens assemble into distinct architectures, which distinguish the different collagen subfamilies, including fibrils (collagens I, II, III, V, XI), beaded filaments (collagen VI), anchoring fibrils (collagen VII), and networks (collagen IV). For fibrillar collagens, three left-handed α polypeptide chains are twisted into a right-handed triple helix [21], which then laterally associates to form fibrils 20–500 nm in diameter and up to several micrometers long [22]. For a subset of collagens (collagens I and III), fibrils aggregate to form fibers and, for collagen I, fibers associate to form bundles. The supramolecular assembly provides marked tensile strength to the ECM and corresponding tissue. However, much diversity exists across different tissues, in which collagen family members have a triple-helical component ranging from 10% (collagen XI) to 96% (collagen I) of the protein structure. Further, collagens may be composed of homo- or hetero-trimers of the α polypeptide chains, which impart differences in structure and stability of the fibrous protein. For instance, the heterotrimer of collagen I ($[\alpha1(I)]_2 \alpha2(I)$) can be degraded by specialized matrix metalloproteinases (MMPs), known as collagenases, while the homotrimer ($[\alpha2(I)]_3$) is resistant to degradation due to high stability. The varying ability of different collagen isoforms to be degraded has important implications for matrix remodeling, which is prevalent in diseased states such as fibrosis and cancer. Further, collagens serve critical roles in directing cell phenotype through cell-matrix interactions. Collagens in the ECM interact with cells by serving as ligands for receptors on the cell surface, which include specialized integrins containing a $\beta1$ subunit and dimeric discoidin receptors (DDR1 and DDR2). These collagen receptor-ligand interactions can promote cell differentiation, growth, and migration [21]. Altogether, the supramolecular assembly of collagens provides physical properties that protect against external stresses by imparting mechanical stability, strength, and toughness to the ECM and serves an important role in preserving tissue integrity and directing biological functions.

Elastin

Elastin is a critical ECM component that affords resilience and elasticity to vertebrate tissues [23] and is particularly prevalent in tissue layers within the aorta, ligaments, vasculature, lungs, tendons, and skin, which rely on high elasticity for normal functionality. Elastin is predominantly synthesized during embryonic development rather than in adulthood. In healthy tissue, elastin is highly stable and insoluble, with a half-life of 70 years and minimal turnover. Elastin fiber formation involves the association of tropoelastin monomers with microfibrillar proteins and subsequent cross-linking of the soluble precursor to insoluble elastin by lysyl oxidase (LOX). Cross-linking of elastin fibers leads to the formation of an extensive network, which can expand and contract. Uniquely, the elastic properties of elastin are thought to be driven by entropy whereby, in response to stretch of the elastin polymer, the return to maximal entropy is mediated by recoil [24]. In addition to its critical functions in imparting tissue elasticity, elastin is involved in direct and indirect cell signaling to regulate a variety of vital functions. Elastin-binding protein (EBP) is a peripheral membrane protein that, when associated with the extracellular surface of the cell, binds to elastin and transduces intracellular signaling based on the sequence and conformation of the bound elastin motif [25]. In addition, integrin $\alpha_5\beta_3$ binds to tropoelastin by recognizing a non-RGD site within the protein, the RKRK sequence (amino acid sequences: RGD, Arginine-Glycine-Aspartate; RKRK, Arginine-Lysine-Arginine-Lysine) [26]. Cells may also interact with elastin indirectly by associating with glycosaminoglycans (GAGs). Cell-elastin interactions elicit a variety of biological functions such as adhesion, migration and chemotaxis, growth, protease production, and morphogenesis [27]. Overall, elastin serves critical roles in mediating tissue mechanics (elasticity) and cellular functions.

Fibronectin

Fibronectin (FN) is an extracellular glycoprotein that is both an abundant and a universal component of the ECM. FN plays a critical role in many physiological processes, including embryogenesis, morphogenesis, and wound healing. FN is present in insoluble form in the ECM, while soluble FN is present in bodily fluids. FN is secreted as a dimer in which two monomers are joined by a disulfide bond. Further, FN is a mosaic protein incorporating three main modules (FN1, FN2, FN3), each of which contains binding domains for other ECM proteins, cell-surface receptors, and GAGs such as collagen, integrins, and heparin, respectively [28]. Secreted FN assembles into a mature fibrillar network in the ECM through cell-mediated interactions. FN binding to cell-surface receptors at RGD domains, primarily through integrin $\alpha_5\beta_1$, initiates integrin clustering and FN matrix assembly. Specifically, FN-integrin binding results in subsequent FN-FN interactions, which promote additional FN interactions to form an insoluble FN matrix. Receptor clustering induced by FN-integrin binding results in the recruitment of proteins (e.g., focal adhesion kinase, paxillin, and Src) to form a focal complex. The focal complex is important for initiating interactions with the actin cytoskeleton and transducing cellular signaling. In addition, reciprocal interactions between the actin cytoskeleton and integrin-FN binding are critical for the maintenance of the FN matrix. For example, local depolymerization or rearrangement of actin will result in the loss of FN matrix. As such, FN matrix assembly and matrix turnover are dynamic processes [29]. However, these processes must be tightly controlled for normal physiological functions. For instance, high levels of FN are associated with cell survival, proliferation, and robust cell-ECM adhesions, and excessive deposition is linked to organ fibrosis.

Low levels of FN may be associated with cell migration in pathological settings such as cancer cell invasion and metastasis. Altogether, FN is a key ECM component and scaffolding protein, which plays a role in the maintenance of tissue architecture and directs cellular processes [30].

Laminins

Laminins are predominantly present in the BM and are critical for its structure and function. Laminins represent a family of glycoproteins, in which each member consists of a heterotrimer of α, β, and γ chain subunits. In theory, these subunits could assemble into 45 distinct isomers; however, only 18 laminin isoforms have been described [31]. Whereas diversity in structure and size exists across laminin family members, the conserved structural elements of laminin include globular, rod-like, and coiled-coil domains assembled in parallel to form a cross-shaped molecule. This cross-shaped morphology correspondingly presents with one long arm and either two or three short arms. Laminin heterotrimers self-assemble into a mesh-like polymer and bind to other ECM components (e.g., nidogen and collagen IV) to form a network (Fig. 6.1e). Laminin deposition is regulated, at least in part, by cell-surface receptor signaling, including those downstream of integrins (e.g., integrins $\alpha_3\beta_1$ and $\alpha_6\beta_1$), dystroglycan, and syndecans. Further, laminin deposition and matrix stabilization may be modulated by non-receptor molecules, such as nidogen, heparan sulfate proteoglycans, netrins, and collagen VII. As such, the deposition, assembly, and stabilization of laminin matrices is a complex process in which cell-surface receptors and laminin-associated matrix proteins serve coregulatory roles [32].

Stromal Cell Components of the Tissue Microenvironment

Epithelial-stromal interactions play an essential role in regulating tissue form and function. The connective tissue underlying the epithelium contains several stromal cell types (Fig. 6.2). Each cell type performs distinct functions and critical reciprocal interactions occur between stromal cells, the local ECM, and epithelial cells. Whereas the specific origin of stromal cells varies by cell type, the principal origin of these cells is the mesenchyme. The two major overarching categories of stromal cell origin include undifferentiated mesenchymal cells and hematopoietic stem cells. Further, stromal cells may include those that are permanent tissue-resident cells and those that are recruited to the stroma to perform specialized functions for short-term periods. As such, the stroma can undergo dynamic changes in response to cell signaling and stressors, which influence development, wound healing, aging, and diseased states such as fibrosis and cancer.

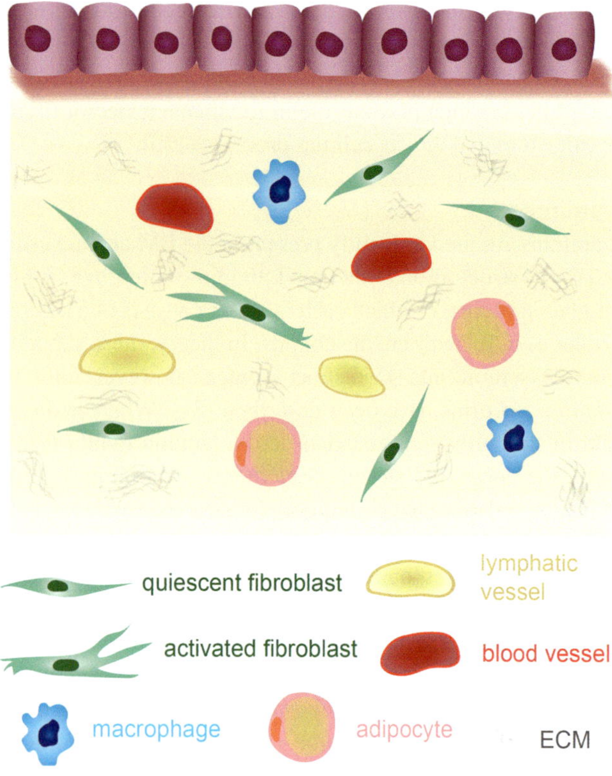

Fig. 6.2 Schematic of the epithelial tissue microenvironment

Stromal Cells of Undifferentiated Mesenchymal Cell Origin

Of tissue-resident cells, fibroblasts are the most abundant cell type in the stroma. These cells are critical for the generation and maintenance of tissue structure as the powerhouse for the synthesis of ECM molecules, including adhesive glycoproteins, GAGs, proteoglycans, and fibrous proteins. Fibroblasts in the stroma can exist in active and quiescent states, in which they exhibit periods of active synthesis and inactivity, respectively. Active fibroblasts exhibit stellate morphologies and have an enlarged nucleus and cytoplasm compared to their inactive counterparts, which are morphologically distinct and maintain an elongated spindle shape (Fig. 6.2). Fibroblasts also secrete GFs, which direct the growth and differentiation of nearby cells. In contrast, adipocytes, or fat cells, serve as an energy reservoir by storing lipids that may be used for the production of heat. Additionally, adipocytes mediate the regeneration and remodeling of stem cell-rich epithelial tissues such as the skin and mammary gland [33]. While the epithelium itself is essentially avascular, an elaborate network of endothelial and lymphatic vessels is contained within the adjacent stroma.

Endothelial cells are a specialized subtype of simple squamous epithelium that line blood and lymphatic vessels. The endothelium is a semipermeable barrier that regulates the exchange of fluid between blood plasma and interstitial fluid. In particular, blood vessels provide a source of nutrients for the connective tissue and overlying epithelium, while lymph vessels serve as a means to drain fluid, or lymph, from the tissue. Blood vessels are also supported by surrounding pericytes and smooth muscle cells, which are abundant in larger-sized vessels and mostly absent in capillaries. The capillaries are the smallest blood vessels in the body and mediate the exchange of oxygen, carbon dioxide, nutrients, and waste products within tissues. The vasculature also provides a route for circulating cells to transport throughout the body, in which the endothelium regulates the entrance of these cells into tissues as necessary to perform critical functions.

Stromal Cells of Hematopoietic Stem Cell Origin

Circulating white blood cells, or leukocytes, can enter the connective tissue and serve as resident cells or temporary surveyors and modulators of tissue activity. Of these, macrophages are phagocytic cells found in connective tissue, from which they remove material such as apoptotic cells and debris, and regulate the turnover of fibrous proteins. Tissue macrophages are derived from circulating monocytes, which cross the endothelium to exit the circulation, enter the connective tissue, and subsequently differentiate and mature to become macrophages. In addition, macrophages secrete GFs and direct interactions with other immune cell types that may be recruited to the stroma. Macrophages in the connective tissue are long-lived (months to years) and thus are referred to as resident cells. Similarly, mast cells are tissue-resident cells that mainly function to store and release chemical modulators of the immune response, and they are thus important for host tissue defense, repair, and immunity. On the other hand, other leukocyte cell types may enter the stroma and serve a short-lived residence.

Cells may be recruited to the tissue microenvironment in order to execute their functions over a short period of time. This is particularly true for a number of leukocyte cell types. For instance, plasma cells produce antibodies in response to immune reactions and live ~10–20 days, but few are found in the stroma at any given time. Other leukocytes are found in connective tissue for extremely transient periods of time (hours to days) and are known as tissue surveyors. The presence of such cells, including lymphocytes and phagocytic antigen-presenting cells, increases during periods of active inflammation and decreases once inflammation has ceased via controlled apoptosis of these cells.

The Evolving Landscape of the Aberrant Stroma in Tumor Progression

The Hallmarks of Cancer

Cancer is a complex set of diverse diseases; however, key similarities exist across these diseases, which define cancer itself. These are known as the chief hallmarks of cancer, which encompass unique capacities that enable tumor cells to grow uncontrollably, invade the adjacent stroma, and spread throughout the body. Cancer cells must overcome several barriers in order to successfully colonize distant organs. The stromal microenvironment plays a critical role in the survival and growth of disseminated tumor cells, including the priming of a pre-metastatic niche. Specifically, these hallmarks include the acquisition of capabilities to evade apoptosis, maintain self-sufficiency in growth signals, disregard anti-growth signals, replicate indefinitely, induce and sustain angiogenesis, and undergo tissue invasion and metastasis. These biological capabilities are recognized to be essential for malignant progression and are thought to be common for all human tumors; however, the mechanisms by which cancer cells adopt these phenotypes are vast [4]. With continued research and understanding of the mechanisms of cancer progression, additional "emerging hallmarks" and "enabling characteristics" of cancer have been defined to provide a more comprehensive scope of cancer evolution. The emerging hallmarks of cancer include the deregulation of cellular metabolism and the evasion of immune destruction, while the enabling characteristics include genomic instability/mutability and the promotion of tumor-supporting inflammation. Notably, the hallmarks and enabling characteristics of cancer are all intricately intertwined with the TME, in which the tumor stroma can play roles in inhibiting, initiating, and promoting cancer progression, which is discussed in detail below.

Conceiving Cancer as "A Wound That Does Not Heal"

The dysregulation of ECM composition through altered deposition and remodeling plays an important role in controlled settings such as wound healing, as well as in aberrant settings such as cancer progression. The idea that cancer involves an inflammatory and wound healing-like process dates back to 1858 when Rudolph Virchow established his irritation theory of cancer [34]. Virchow observed that abnormal tissue masses, or neoplastic lesions, frequently arose in regions of tissue associated with chronic irritation that were mechanical, chemical, or thermal in nature. Further, following the keen observation of infiltrating inflammatory cells at neoplastic sites, Virchow expanded his theory to conclude that inflammation and cancer are causally related. Since Virchow's time, scientists have continued to build upon this theory to understand the role of the ECM and development of tumor stroma in the context of wound healing gone awry in malignant progression. Notably, in his 1924 article, "First Intention," Montrose Burrows recognized that while growth ceases in tissues undergoing wound healing, growth is sustained in cancer through a variety of mechanisms linked to interactions of cancer cells with stromal cells in the surrounding microenvironment. Specifically, Burrows noted that "a change in the arrangement of cells and blood vessels" may cause cancer [35]. In the early 1970s, Alexander Haddow reinforced these themes and the link between aging, wound healing, and cancer, stating that cancer may be a process of "overhealing" [36, 37]. Later, Harold Dvorak wrote an essay in 1986 entitled, "Tumors: Wounds That Do Not Heal," which sparked great interest in the field and presented a notion that is still studied today, wherein cancer mimics an aberrant wound-healing process to sustain the necessary tumor stroma for malignant progression [38, 39]. In order for the tumor stroma to develop and evolve to promote malignant progression, a variety of cellular transitions must take place. In the next sections, we describe the processes associated with wound healing in healthy tissues and aberrant wound healing in cancer.

The Mimicry of Wound Healing in Cancer Progression

Wound healing can be simply broken down into four main phases: hemostasis, inflammatory, proliferative, and maturation phases. During hemostasis, injured blood vessels release clotting factors that induce the arrest of activated platelets and the release of fibrin at the clot site, which together with fibronectin and vitronectin form a precursor matrix. Next, neutrophils are recruited to the wound site, where they release cytokines to initiate the inflammatory phase. This leads to the recruitment and activation of fibroblasts, which deposit additional ECM proteins, notably collagens, at the wound site. Further, macrophages are recruited to clear dead cells and debris from the wound. Next, the proliferative phase begins, in which epithelial cells migrate and proliferate toward the wound gap, while simultaneously depositing BM components. Neovascularization also progresses to build new blood vessels across the wounded tissue. Lastly, during the maturation or remodeling phase, activated fibroblasts, or myofibroblasts, secrete transforming growth factor-β (TGF-β) and mediate wound contraction, which is critical for the closure of large wounds. Further, collagen III that was initially deposited during the proliferative phase is replaced by aligned collagen I through ECM remodeling to form scar tissue [40]. Analogous processes occur during tumor progression; however, in this case, the wound-healing process is chronic and unresolved. Thus, instead of scar tissue, the deposition of ECM components and extensive remodeling lead to desmoplasia, or dense fibrosis, around the primary tumor site. Together, fibroblast activation and the infiltration of immune cells play key roles in orchestrating the wound-healing process, and both contribute to the development of the tumor stroma.

The Complexity of the Stroma in Cancer: Tumor-Suppressing and Tumor-Promoting Roles

Direct and indirect interactions between malignant cells, non-malignant cells, and the ECM play pivotal roles in cancer suppression, initiation, and progression. These cell subpopulations and their surrounding microenvironment make up a complex "ecosystem" that evolves during tumor evolution and malignant progression. For instance, the stroma may initially suppress tumor initiation and progression; however, over time the suppressive factors may become diminished and outweighed by tumor-promoting factors, which tips the balance toward a pro-tumorigenic stroma. As such, the stroma initially acts to maintain tissue architecture and function, in part by inhibiting the hallmarks of cancer. Once malignant cells have been generated and a primary tumor has formed, the stroma can continue to suppress tumor progression, particularly when the stroma remains in an "inactive" state. However, as tumor growth proceeds, the local microenvironment can become hypoxic, acidic, and deficient in critical nutrients, which may activate cells in the stroma to support tumor progression [41]. For instance, many secreted factors that were once tumor-suppressive can have dual actions as tumor-promoting over time. As an example, the secretion of TGF-β by fibroblasts can suppress or promote tumor progression in a context-dependent manner. Further, the expression of tissue inhibitors of matrix metalloproteinases (TIMPs), MMPs, and a disintegrin and metalloproteinases (ADAMs) by fibroblasts can have a dramatic effect on tumor progression, in which TIMPs are typically tumor-suppressive and MMPs and ADAMs tumor-promoting, but the expression of these proteins is often dysregulated in cancer [42] and leads to alterations in the ECM. Specifically, MMPs and ADAMs are proteolytic enzymes that drive ECM degradation, whereas TIMPs inhibit these activities [43]. Separately, cellular transitions that lead to a varied state of activity or switch in phenotype can have pro-tumorigenic effects, as does the infiltration of supporting stromal cell types (immune cells, endothelial cells, etc.).

From Fibroblast to Cancer-Associated Fibroblast

Fibroblasts share mesenchymal lineage with many other cell types and, as such, they lack distinctive biomarkers that help to distinguish them from other stromal cell types. Accordingly, fibroblasts must be identified by a combination of metrics, including cell morphology and the presence and absence of biomarkers. Specifically, fibroblasts express vimentin, platelet-derived growth factor (PDGF), fibroblast activation protein (FAP), and α-smooth muscle actin, adopt an elongated shape, and lack biomarkers associated with epithelial cells and leukocytes. However, ambiguity remains in defining or identifying fibroblasts, particularly in the TME, where carcinoma cells may undergo a transition to a fibroblast-like state through the epithelial-mesenchymal transition (EMT), which is discussed below. To distinguish fibroblasts from other stromal cell types or carcinoma cells, the definition of a cancer-associated fibroblast (CAF) includes those fibroblasts that are found within the TME that are distinguishable from other resident cells based on shape, biomarkers, and the absence of mutations present in the carcinoma cells. As in wound healing, fibroblasts adjacent to cancer cells become activated to form CAFs, a process that may occur through a variety of mechanisms, including secreted factors (inflammatory cytokines, GFs), ECM changes (composition and stiffness), and more. One functional difference that distinguishes normal fibroblasts from CAFs is that tissue-resident fibroblasts rarely divide, while CAFs undergo expansion known as stromagenesis. Further, studies suggest that normal fibroblasts may be tumor-suppressive, while fibroblasts generated during stromagenesis are tumor-promoting via ECM remodeling and the secretion of GFs, cytokines, and ECM (Fig. 6.3a). Importantly, the tumor-promoting functions of CAFs are vast and make CAFs an attractive target for cancer therapy [44].

CAFs are major regulators of ECM deposition, remodeling, and cross-linking and, thus, can dramatically change the local tissue properties at the primary tumor site. For instance, in combination with force-mediated tissue remodeling, these CAF-induced ECM changes can dramatically increase tissue stiffness, which can have reciprocal effects on carcinoma cells and other stromal cells in the TME. In particular, increased tissue stiffness can trigger growth and survival pathways in the cancer cell population. Further, CAF-mediated collagen deposition, cross-linking, and alignment can lead to increased interstitial fluid pressure, reducing the efficacy of drug delivery [45]. The altered mechanical microenvironment may also lead to blood vessel collapse, generating a hypoxic and hostile TME, leading to a more aggressive cancer phenotype. CAFs also promote local proteolysis, which has been demonstrated to aid in cancer invasion. Further, the presence of CAFs has been shown to alter the infiltration of immune cells and even to promote metastasis [44]. Disseminated cancer cells can help prime local fibroblasts to generate a new CAF reservoir at secondary sites. In addition, CAFs have been found in circulation with higher frequency for patients with metastatic disease as compared to those with early-stage cancers and, as such, it is hypothesized that CAFs may play a role in priming the pre-metastatic niche and in aiding the metastatic process [42]. Overall, CAFs can dramatically alter the local TME and drive cancer progression through a variety of mechanisms that enable growth, invasion, and metastasis.

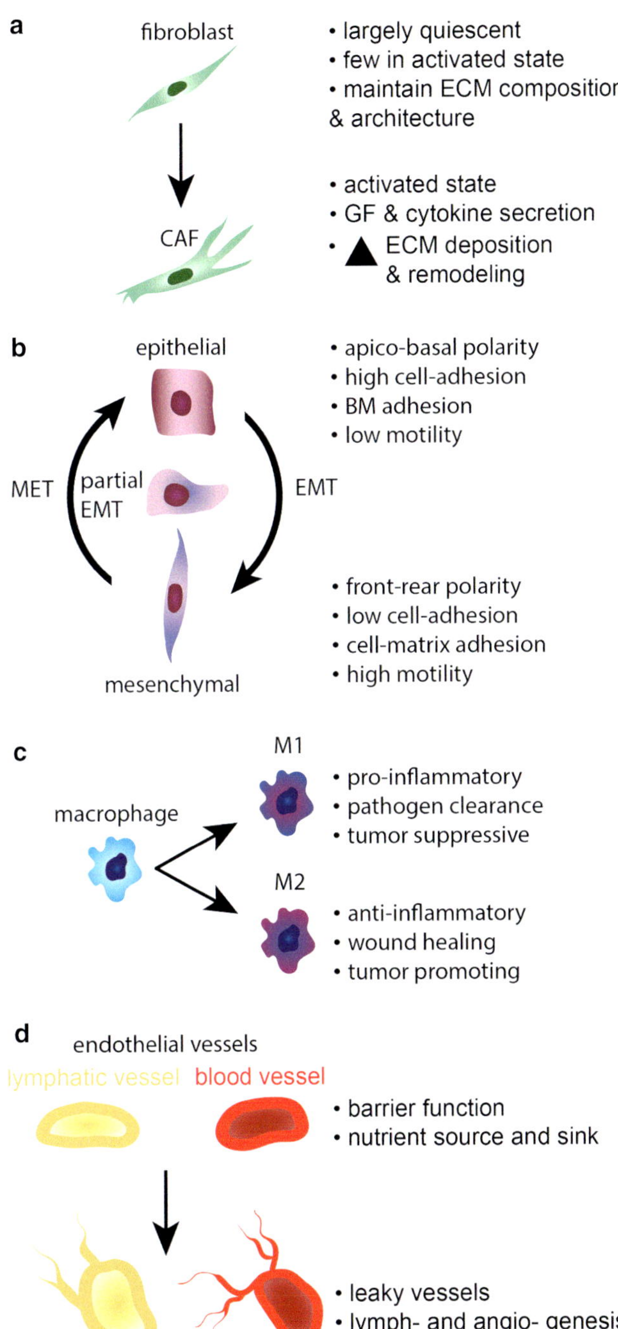

Fig. 6.3 Cellular state transitions in cancer progression. (**a**) Fibroblast to CAF transition. (**b**) The epithelial to mesenchymal transition. (**c**) Activation of immune cells. (**d**) Endothelial vessels: lymphangio- and angiogenesis

The Epithelial-Mesenchymal Transition and Epithelial-Mesenchymal Plasticity

Epithelial cells exhibit remarkable plasticity in their ability to interconvert between epithelial and mesenchymal cell phenotypes. Epithelial plasticity is critical during embryonic development, in which embryonic epithelial cells undergo EMT to migrate within the embryo and subsequently revert their phenotype via the mesenchymal-epithelial transition (MET) and differentiate into multiple cell lineages (Fig. 6.3b). Epithelial plasticity is retained after development and may be initiated in response to various stressors, such as those observed in wound healing, tissue regeneration, organ fibrosis, and cancer progression. The acquisition of a motile phenotype via EMT is critical in all of these cases. However, while many similarities exist between these EMT processes, the stability of EMT states and consequences of EMT differ substantially across these settings. As such, these context-dependent EMTs have been deemed type I, II, and III processes for phenotypic transitions that occur during development, wound healing/tissue regeneration/organ fibrosis, and cancer, respectively. Notably, during type I developmental EMTs, there is an absence of an inflammatory response, which is prevalent in type II and type III EMTs. Further, whereas type I EMT is a necessary process that occurs during the development of healthy organisms, type II and type III EMTs can be dysregulated and considered pathological, contributing to diseased states such as fibrosis, organ failure, and cancer progression [46]. Here, we focus on defining the general EMT process and the role that epithelial-mesenchymal plasticity plays in cancer progression.

In healthy, unperturbed tissue, epithelial cells are anchored to each other and to the BM, which allows for the maintenance of apical-basal polarity and restricts cell motility. EMT may be triggered by several microenvironmental stimuli including hypoxia, tissue stiffness, ECM proteins (collagen I), inflammatory stimuli, and GFs. In response to these stressors, master regulators of EMT, or transcription factors such as SLUG, SNAIL, TWIST, ZEB1/2, and E12/E47, or transcriptional co-activators YAP/TAZ, are expressed and activate EMT programs [47]. During the EMT process, cell-cell and cell-ECM contacts are disrupted, which results from the dissolution of cell-cell junctions through the transcriptional repression and downregulation of cell adhesion proteins (notably E-cadherin) and altered expression of matrix receptors (e.g., integrins and DDR) to enable a switch from BM adhesion (collagen IV and laminin) to interstitial ECM proteins such as collagen I [48]. Epithelial cell junctions are intricately linked to the cytoskeleton through association with a cortical F-actin belt and keratin intermediate filament proteins. As such, during EMT cells must undergo a dramatic reorganization of their cytoskeletons to switch from apical-basal polarity to front-rear polarity. The rearrangement and polymerization of actin to form actin-rich protrusions and stress fibers leads to an apparent change in cell shape from cuboidal to elongated, or spindle shaped. In addition, cells gain the expression of classical EMT biomarkers, including the intermediate filament protein vimentin, α-smooth muscle actin, and N-cadherin. As a consequence of EMT, cells retain minimal cell-cell adhesions and display enhanced cell-ECM interactions, which promote cell motility. EMT is also accompanied by increased MMP expression and activity, which enables cells to invade through the stroma. MMP expression is particularly critical for enabling the invasion of cancer cells through limiting pore sizes, in which cells cannot squeeze through the ECM without matrix degradation (e.g., amoeboid migration), or for the migration of wide collective invasions. Cells may also adopt "partial" EMT states, in which they retain some cell-cell contacts and co-express epithelial and mesenchymal biomarkers. Such partial EMTs are important for collective migration and may contribute to cancer progression by coordinating the migration of groups of cancer cells through the stroma [47]. Moreover, the generation of varied states along the EMT spectrum can contribute to increased functional heterogeneity within tumors, which can provide overall resilience to stressors, enhanced adaptability to new microenvironments, and increased drug resistance [49].

Infiltration of Stromal Cells in Cancer Progression

In the early stages of tumor formation, the stroma is largely tumor-suppressive; however, as tumor growth proceeds, a hostile microenvironment develops and leads to the infiltration and activation of stromal cells to promote tumor progression. These stromal cell changes aid in the adaptation to these harsh microenvironmental conditions (hypoxia, nutrient deprivation, etc.) and generate a hospitable tumor microenvironment that is able to sustain tumor growth and progression. Bone marrow-derived stromal cells have been observed to exit circulation into primary tumor sites, where they exhibit pro-tumorigenic behaviors. Similar to wound-healing processes, immune cell infiltration is also common in cancer, in which recruited immune cells become hijacked to promote tumorigenesis. For instance, infiltrating macrophages in the TME, or tumor-associated macrophages (TAMs), play important roles in cancer initiation, progression, angiogenesis, immunoregulation, and metastasis. To perform these functions, TAMs adopt the alternatively activated state, known as M2, which enables immune-suppressive and pro-tumorigenic activities. The M2 state is a stark contrast to the classically activated state of macrophages, M1, which promotes inflammation for defense against pathogens and tumor cells. Thus, macrophages can play dual roles in tumor suppression and tumor promotion, depending on their activation state (Fig. 6.3c). Of note, TAMs exert these functions by secreting cytokines to modulate inflammation via the interleukin (IL) family, various GFs to modulate cell behavior, and proteolytic enzymes to influence ECM remodeling. For instance, many of these secreted factors (TGF-β, TNF-α, MMPs, IL-1β, IL-8) can induce EMT in the carcinoma cell population, which further

exacerbates malignant progression, as discussed previously. The interaction between TAMs and tumor cells can enhance both intravasation and extravasation and, thus, augments metastasic events. In addition, TAMs can induce angiogenesis and lymphangiogenesis, both of which have dramatic effects on tumor progression [50].

The growth of new vasculature, or angiogenesis, is a hallmark of cancer and aids as a source of nutrients and waste disposal for the TME (Fig. 6.3d). The point at which tumor growth exceeds nutrient and oxygen supply and angiogenesis is initiated is known as the "angiogenic switch," which is mediated in part by TAMs, via the secretion of vascular endothelial growth factor (VEGF) and MMP-9. TAMs additionally aid in vascular remodeling, which leads to leaky, tortuous vessels associated with cancer cell dissemination and poor drug delivery. Hypoxia itself can stimulate angiogenesis through the induction of VEGF expression by tumor cells. This leads to the activation of local endothelial cells, which secrete MMPs to permit endothelial cell migration, subsequent proliferation, and reorganization into a network of nascent blood vessels that mature by angiotensin-1/2 binding to its receptor Tie-2. Neovascularization has important consequences for drug delivery to the primary tumor. For instance, leaky vessels lead to increased interstitial fluid pressure, resulting in vessel compression and central necrosis when functional lymphatics are lacking, which impedes effective drug delivery [51]. The growth of new lymphatic vessels, or lymphangiogenesis (Fig. 6.3d), is also triggered by inflammation during tumor progression and may direct metastasis to the lymph nodes. Similar to the role of VEGF in angiogenesis, lymphangiogenesis is initiated by VEGF family members, particularly VEGF-C and VEGF-D. Peritumoral lymphatics are enlarged during cancer progression, while new lymphatic vessels may be generated through lymphangiogenesis to promote lymphatic spread and metastasis [52]. As such, approaches aimed at targeting lymphangiogenesis may have a therapeutic benefit. Overall, the infiltration of immune cells and neovascularization events have pro-tumorigenic effects, which enhance tumor growth, invasion, and metastasis.

The Role of the ECM in Malignant Progression

ECM Alterations in the Tumor Stroma

The regulation of ECM composition and arrangement is critical for the maintenance of tissue homeostasis to promote normal cell- and tissue-level physiological functions. The generation of aberrant ECM through altered secretion, synthesis, and remodeling can contribute to cancer initiation and progression. The altered ECM is largely generated by CAFs and by the tumor cells themselves. ECM changes vary from cancer to cancer; however, alterations in collagen deposition,

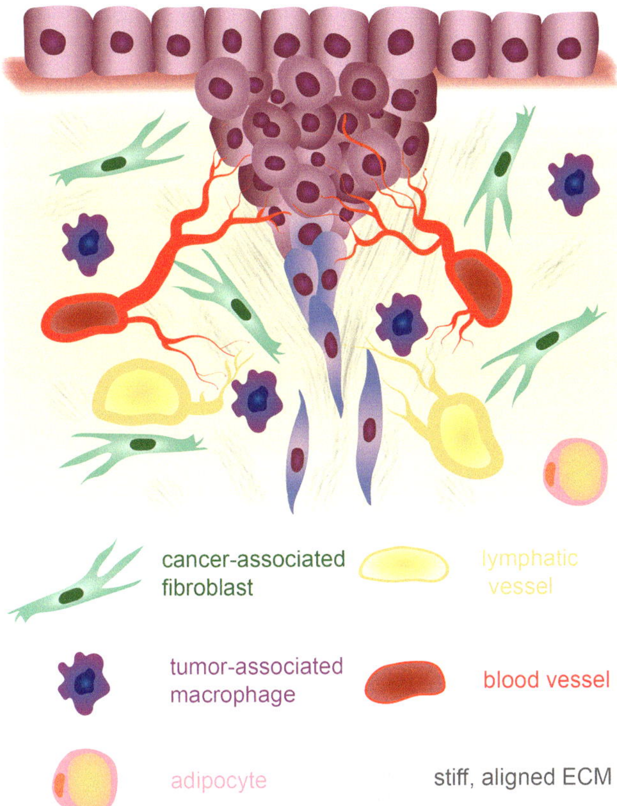

Fig. 6.4 Schematic of the tumor microenvironment

cross-linking, and organization are common features of cancer (Fig. 6.4). In general, cancer is associated with reduced levels of collagen IV and increased deposition of highly aligned collagen I fibers. Further, collagen-associated enzymes, such as lysyl hydroxylases (e.g., LOX) and prolyl hydrolases, are expressed at increased levels in the TME, which contribute to increased cross-linking of collagens and elastins, thus stiffening the ECM. Increased levels of FN, proteoglycans, and GAGs, such as hyaluronic acid (HLA), are also observed in the stroma of many epithelial tumors and are correlated with poor prognosis. Further, the organization and localization of the characteristic BM protein, laminin, is dysregulated in many cancers. For instance, laminin that was once exclusively present at the BM becomes more ubiquitously expressed in the tumor stroma. This aberrant laminin phenotype is associated with increased cancer invasion and poor prognosis in patients. Overall, these ECM changes lead to a denser and stiffer ECM, which alters cell phenotype and increases resistance to chemo-, radio-, and immuno- therapies [53].

The Intricate Interplay Between the ECM and Cell Behavior in Cancer

ECM deposition in cancer alters various cell behaviors such as polarization, adhesion, and migration. Further, ECM

remodeling leads to the release of ECM-tethered GFs, which can stimulate proliferation and cellular state transitions. ECM remodeling is particularly prevalent at the periphery of tumors, which may direct the local invasion and subsequent dissemination of tumor cells. For instance, LOX activity is often increased at the invasive front of tumors, which drives collagen cross-linking and alignment perpendicular to the tumor boundary. The locally stiffened and aligned microenvironment alters corresponding cell activities such as actin polymerization, contractility, and motility. Specifically, tumor cells have been observed to migrate along such highly aligned collagen "tracks," which may facilitate their migration and escape to nearby endothelial vessels in the TME [54]. The altered ECM phenotype is associated with increased metastasis in patients. However, in order to invade the stroma and disseminate, cancer cells must first breach the BM. Breaching the BM can occur due to local tumor growth, which leads to mechanical stress and BM rupture, the action of invadopodia that puncture through the BM, the secretion of MMPs that locally degrade and soften the BM and underlying stroma, or a combination of these activities [55].

Cell behavior is influenced by the mechanical microenvironment. That is, cells are capable of sensing the mechanical properties of their surrounding microenvironment, which activates cellular processes via mechanotransduction pathways. Specifically, the actin cytoskeleton plays a critical role in the ability of cells to sense the mechanics of the microenvironment and to generate responses to this mechanical microenvironment. As such, upstream regulators of actin bundling and associated cell contractility, such as Rho-associated protein kinase (ROCK), are important for rigidity sensing and response. YAP/TAZ transcriptional co-activators are also crucial mechanotransducers that relay biomechanical signals from the microenvironment into cellular responses. For instance, matrix elasticity, cytoskeletal tension, and cell spreading affect the subcellular localization of YAP/TAZ. Nuclear translocation of YAP/TAZ is indicative of inactive signaling for the Hippo pathway, while cytoplasmic localization of YAP/TAZ represents an active state [55]. Hippo signaling controls organ growth and development in normal settings; however, aberrant signaling of Hippo pathway components can contribute to uncontrolled tumor growth and the induction of EMT and, thus, plays dual roles in promoting tumor progression [56]. Similarly, stiff microenvironments can also induce EMT through TGF-β [57, 58] and MMP-3 via Rac1b [59]. Further, gene expression and genome integrity are affected by cytoskeletal and nuclear changes, which can be driven by the mechanical microenvironment. For instance, applied stress or local stiffness can lead to nuclear distortion and deformation, respectively, which alter gene expression and cell behavior [60]. To adapt to confinement, tumor cells themselves can soften. The capacity of cancer cells to deform may promote tumor progression by enabling invasion and metastasis [61]. Tumor growth, cancer progression, and ECM remodeling lead to a stiffened TME, altered intratumoral-generated mechanical forces at the cell and tissue level, and fluid and solid stress in the TME. Overall, the mechanical properties of the TME can induce changes in cell phenotype and behavior that promote tumor progression, thus illuminating the critical role of the ECM in cancer.

The Aberrant Stroma as a Diagnostic Tool: Early Detection and Prognostic Value

Given the prominent role that the tumor stroma and ECM play in malignant progression, it may be clinically useful to characterize these components for improved cancer staging and to inform clinical decision-making. The presence of cancer cells with EMT signatures in the primary tumor or in the circulation of patients is associated with poor prognosis and metastasis; however, EMT biomarkers have not yet translated to inform clinical outcomes [62, 63]. Although their identification is complex, CAF biomarkers may serve as clinically relevant prognostic markers. The activation state and number of CAFs present in the TME of patients are associated with patient outcomes. For instance, FAP expression is associated with decreased survival times for patients across a variety of cancers. Due to CAF-induced ECM remodeling, collagen formation and degradation products can be detected in the serum and have both diagnostic (e.g., cancer staging) and prognostic value [45]. MMPs and ADAMs produced by cells that have undergone EMT or by CAFs are particularly attractive biomarkers for patients due to their extensive roles in ECM degradation and tumor progression. In addition, these proteases can be detected in primary tumor biopsies (e.g., tissue) and liquid biopsies (e.g., plasma, serum, urine), which vary from cancer to cancer. Changes in the ECM can also be indicative of early disease and poor prognosis. For instance, ECM fragments have been found in the circulation of patients with diverse cancers (breast, colorectal, lung, ovarian), which serve as a useful diagnostic tool. Further, increased ECM deposition, cross-linking, and alignment lead to tissue stiffening and increases in density, which are prevalent in breast tissue and represent major risk factors for the development of breast cancer. As such, the palpation of tissue and examination of mammographic density are used for preventative screening and early detection of breast cancer. The presence of HLA in tumors may serve as a prognostic marker, as it is associated with EMT and cell migration [64] and has been used as a biomarker for some cancer types (breast and prostate) [55]. Since Hippo pathway members are rarely observed to exhibit

mutations, the detection of elevated levels or nuclear localization of YAP/TAZ may serve as valuable biomarkers of cancer [56]. The observation of the interaction of cancer and stromal cell types may also have predictive potential for cancer patients. The arrangement of tumor cells, TAMs, and endothelial cells has been deemed as "the tumor microenvironment of metastasis," based on clinical observations that this characteristic tripartite cell grouping is associated with increased hematogenous metastasis and poor prognosis in breast cancer patients (Fig. 6.4) [50]. Thus, the infiltration of TAMs and increased numbers of stromal cells in the TME may have predictive potential. Overall, components of the tumor stroma themselves may serve as clinically relevant biomarkers in the future, which warrants further investigation to improve patient outcomes.

Normalizing the Tumor Microenvironment: The Aberrant Stroma as a Therapeutic Target

Given the potential for components of the tumor stroma to serve as clinically relevant biomarkers for directing clinical decision-making, once identified in patients, the natural next step is to target these components for therapeutic benefit. Targeting components of the TME presents a unique opportunity for the treatment of cancer, which has historically focused on targeting and killing the cancer cells themselves. However, these classical chemotherapies have had limited success due to the high degree of resilience of cancer cells, such as their capacity to adapt to microenvironmental stress via phenotypic transitions and genomic instability that drives rapid tumor cell evolution. Several studies have demonstrated that cell phenotype can be dominant over genotype [65]. For instance, altering the microenvironment or microenvironmental signaling can have profound effects on cancer cell behavior and can even revert a malignant cell to a non-malignant phenotype [66, 67]. As such, targeting the non-malignant cells in the tumor stroma to modulate the TME, or even indirect targeting of the ECM, may provide an attractive alternative route for treatment to improve cancer patient outcomes.

Many drugs are currently in clinical trials to target CAFs using differing mechanisms, including the interference of CAF activation, the interference of CAF action, and the interference of both [44]. Specifically, therapies are aimed at targeting CAFs via blocking signaling pathways (e.g., Hedgehog; PDGF; IL-6) to revert CAFs back to a normal fibroblast phenotype, induce directed apoptosis of CAFs via FAP antibodies and PDGF mimetics as carriers of proapoptotic molecules [68], and via modulation of TGF-β signaling to block signals coming from CAFs. Attempts to inhibit angiogenesis have had little therapeutic effect to reduce mortality and metastasis and have been met with severe side effects in patients. As such, strategies to combine anti-angiogenic therapy with chemotherapy or to normalize, rather than deplete, the tumor vasculature are underway [69]. While anti-angiogenic therapies have been widely explored in the clinic, anti-lymphangiogenic therapies have shown promise in experimental systems, but have not yet made an appearance in clinical trials. Lymph node metastases have prognostic value and can guide clinical decision-making for cancer therapeutics. As such, it will be necessary to establish the clinical benefit of anti-lymphangiogenic therapies to determine if these block lymphogenous spread and lymph node metastasis in patients [70]. Another potential approach for altering the TME is to target MMPs. Next-generation antibody-based MMP inhibitors have been developed that are selective and will need to be carefully evaluated for efficacy in cancer therapy [71]. Rather than target stromal components of the TME directly, another approach is to target the mechanisms by which cancer cells transduce cues from their surroundings. Given the ability of the Hippo pathway to translate mechanical signals from the TME into cellular responses, Hippo pathway components are appealing targets for cancer therapy. As such, several Hippo pathway targets are being investigated, including inhibitors of activating kinases (MST and LATS), YAP/TAZ regulators, and the YAP/TAZ-TEAD interaction [72]. Overall, targeting the tumor stroma or its effectors represents a promising approach for the future of cancer medicine.

Concluding Remarks/Summary

Cell behavior is largely influenced by the surrounding microenvironment, which relays signals to cells in the form of physical, chemical, and mechanical cues. In the context of the epithelium, the immediate microenvironment includes the neighboring cells that are adherent to one another, the BM that the epithelial cells are anchored to, and the underlying stroma comprised of acellular ECM and stromal cells. A bidirectional relationship, or "dynamic reciprocity," exists between cells and their microenvironment, in which cells respond to their surroundings, especially the ECM. This generates a mechanism by which the microenvironment can modulate cell genotype and phenotype, resulting in cellular changes that can then lead to alterations in the cell surroundings, and the cycle continues [73]. As such, ECM architecture and composition critically affect the physiology of tissues and alterations in the ECM lead to pathological states. Dynamic reciprocity is clearly evident in cancer, which involves extensive remodeling of the ECM and stromal changes that influence cancer cell behavior. Cancer is a highly complex set of diverse diseases,

and cancers of the epithelium are known as carcinomas. Despite the heterogeneity observed across cancers, a set of unifying characteristics exist between them, which make up the hallmarks of cancer. These hallmarks enable sustained tumor growth, invasion, and spread to distant organs. The development of a pro-tumorigenic TME occurs concomitant with cancer progression, which displays striking resemblance to an aberrant wound healing response. This includes a stiffened and aligned ECM, cellular state transitions that promote ECM remodeling, and the infiltration and genesis of stromal cells. As such, the detection of these ECM and stromal cell changes may serve as valuable biomarkers to inform patient diagnosis and prognosis in a clinical setting. With the design of therapeutic agents targeted at modulating the ECM and stromal cells, the once provocative idea of targeting the tumor stroma for cancer therapy is now being realized. With careful evaluation of patient-specific biomarkers and the application of targeted therapeutics in patients, targeting the tumor stroma may lie at the forefront of personalized medicine to improve patient outcomes.

References

1. The global challenge of cancer. Nat Can. 2020; 1:1–2.
2. Faguet GB. A brief history of cancer: age-old milestones underlying our current knowledge database. Int J Cancer. 2015;136:2022–36.
3. Cagan R, Meyer P. Rethinking cancer: current challenges and opportunities in cancer research. Dis Model Mech. 2017;10:349–52.
4. Hanahan D, Weinberg RA. The Hallmarks of Cancer. Cell. 2000;100:57–70.
5. Hanahan D, Weinberg A. Robert, hallmarks of cancer: the next generation. Cell. 2011;144:646–74.
6. Farquhar MG, Palade GE. Junctional complexes in various epithelia. J Cell Biol. 1963;17:375–412.
7. Balda MS, Matter K. Tight junctions at a glance. J Cell Sci. 2008;121:3677–82.
8. Harris TJC, Tepass U. Adherens junctions: from molecules to morphogenesis. Nat Rev Mol Cell Biol. 2010;11:502–14.
9. Hatzfeld M, Keil R, Magin TM. Desmosomes and intermediate filaments: their consequences for tissue mechanics. Cold Spring Harb Perspect Biol. 2017;9:a029157.
10. Angulo-Urarte A, Van Der Wal T, Huveneers S. Cell-cell junctions as sensors and transducers of mechanical forces. Biochim Biophys Acta Biomembr. 2020;1862:183316.
11. Kumar NM, Gilula NB. The gap junction communication channel. Cell. 1996;84:381–8.
12. Guillot C, Lecuit T. Mechanics of epithelial tissue homeostasis and morphogenesis. Science. 2013;340:1185–9.
13. Frantz C, Stewart KM, Weaver VM. The extracellular matrix at a glance. J Cell Sci. 2010;123:4195–200.
14. Özbek S, Balasubramanian PG, Chiquet-Ehrismann R, Tucker RP, Adams JC. The evolution of extracellular matrix. Mol Biol Cell. 2010;21:4300–5.
15. Iozzo RV, Schaefer L. Proteoglycan form and function: a comprehensive nomenclature of proteoglycans. Matrix Biol. 2015;42:11–55.

16. Yurchenco PD, Schittny JC. Molecular architecture of basement membranes. FASEB J. 1990;4:1577–90.
17. LeBleu VS, Macdonald B, Kalluri R. Structure and function of basement membranes. Exp Biol Med (Maywood). 2007;232:1121–9.
18. Jayadev R, Sherwood DR. Basement membranes. Curr Biol. 2017;27:R207–11.
19. Rozario T, Desimone DW. The extracellular matrix in development and morphogenesis: a dynamic view. Dev Biol. 2010;341:126–40.
20. Schnaper HW, Kleinman HK. Regulation of cell function by extracellular matrix. Pediatr Nephrol. 1993;7:96–104.
21. Ricard-Blum S. The collagen family. Cold Spring Harb Perspect Biol. 2011;3:a004978.
22. Kadler KE, Holmes DF, Trotter JA, Chapman JA. Collagen fibril formation. Biochem J. 1996;316:1–11.
23. Debelle L, Tamburro AM. Elastin: molecular description and function. Int J Biochem Cell Biol. 1999;31:261–72.
24. Mithieux SM, Weiss AS. Fibrous proteins: coiled-coils, collagen and elastomers. San Diego: Elsevier; 2005. p. 437–61.
25. Brassart B, et al. Conformational dependence of collagenase (matrix metalloproteinase-1) up-regulation by elastin peptides in cultured fibroblasts. J Biol Chem. 2001;276:5222–7.
26. Rodgers UR, Weiss AS. Integrin αvβ3 binds a unique non-RGD site near the C-terminus of human tropoelastin. Biochimie. 2004;86:173–8.
27. Almine JF, Wise SG, Weiss AS. Elastin signaling in wound repair. Birth Defects Research Part C: Embryo Today: Reviews. 2012;96:248–57.
28. Potts JR, Campbell ID. Fibronectin structure and assembly. Curr Opin Cell Biol. 1994;6:648–55.
29. Singh P, Carraher C, Schwarzbauer JE. Assembly of fibronectin extracellular matrix. Annu Rev Cell Dev Biol. 2010;26:397–419.
30. To WS, Midwood KS. Plasma and cellular fibronectin: distinct and independent functions during tissue repair. Fibrogenesis Tissue Repair. 2011;4:21.
31. Durbeej M. Laminins. Cell Tissue Res. 2010;339:259–68.
32. Hamill KJ, Kligys K, Hopkinson SB, Jones JCR. Laminin deposition in the extracellular matrix: a complex picture emerges. J Cell Sci. 2009;122:4409–17.
33. Zwick RK, Guerrero-Juarez CF, Horsley V, Plikus MV. Anatomical, physiological, and functional diversity of adipose tissue. Cell Metab. 2018;27:68–83.
34. Virchow R. Die cellularpathologie in ihrer begründung auf physiologische und pathologische gewebelehre. Berlin: A. Hirschwald; 1858.
35. Burrows MT. Studies on wound healing: I. "first intention" healing of open wounds and the nature of the growth stimulus in the wound and cancer. J Med Res. 1924;44:615-644.611.
36. Haddow A. Advances in cancer research. Amsterdam: Elsevier; 1973. p. 181–234.
37. Haddow A. Advances in cancer research. Amsterdam: Elsevier; 1974. p. 343–66.
38. Flier JS, Underhill LH, Dvorak HF. Tumors: wounds that do not heal. N Engl J Med. 1986;315:1650–9.
39. Dvorak HF. Tumors: wounds that do not heal—redux. Cancer Immunol Res. 2015;3:1–11.
40. Foster DS, Jones RE, Ransom RC, Longaker MT, Norton JA. The evolving relationship of wound healing and tumor stroma. JCI Insight. 2018;3:99911.
41. Amend SR, Pienta KJ. Ecology meets cancer biology: the cancer swamp promotes the lethal cancer phenotype. Oncotarget. 2015;6:9669–78.
42. Valkenburg KC, De Groot AE, Pienta KJ. Targeting the tumour stroma to improve cancer therapy. Nat Rev Clin Oncol. 2018;15:366–81.
43. Santi A, Kugeratski FG, Zanivan S. Cancer associated fibroblasts: the architects of stroma remodeling. Proteomics. 2018;18:1700167.
44. Sahai E, et al. A framework for advancing our understanding of cancer-associated fibroblasts. Nat Rev Cancer. 2020;20:174–86.
45. Nissen NI, Karsdal M, Willumsen N. Collagens and cancer associated fibroblasts in the reactive stroma and its relation to Cancer biology. J Exp Clin Cancer Res. 2019;38(1):115.
46. Nieto MA. Epithelial plasticity: a common theme in embryonic and cancer cells. Science. 2013;342:1234850.
47. Leggett SE, Hruska AM, Guo M, Wong IY. The epithelial-mesenchymal transition and the cytoskeleton in bioengineered systems. Cell Commun Signal. 2021;19:32.
48. Leggett SE, Khoo AS, Wong IY. Multicellular tumor invasion and plasticity in biomimetic materials. Biomater Sci. 2017;5:1460–79.
49. Yang J, et al. Guidelines and definitions for research on epithelial–mesenchymal transition. Nat Rev Mol Cell Biol. 2020;21:341–52.
50. Lin Y, Xu J, Lan H. Tumor-associated macrophages in tumor metastasis: biological roles and clinical therapeutic applications. J Hematol Oncol. 2019;12:76.
51. Carmeliet P, Jain RK. Angiogenesis in cancer and other diseases. Nature. 2000;407:249–57.
52. Stacker SA, Achen MG, Jussila L, Baldwin ME, Alitalo K. Lymphangiogenesis and cancer metastasis. Nat Rev Cancer. 2002;2:573–83.
53. Henke E, Nandigama R, Ergün S. Extracellular matrix in the tumor microenvironment and its impact on cancer therapy. Front Mol Biosci. 2020;6:160.
54. Friedl P, Alexander S. Cancer invasion and the microenvironment: plasticity and reciprocity. Cell. 2011;147:992–1009.
55. Walker C, Mojares E, A. Del Río Hernández, role of extracellular matrix in development and cancer progression. Int J Mol Sci. 2018;19:3028.
56. Harvey KF, Zhang X, Thomas DM. The Hippo pathway and human cancer. Nat Rev Cancer. 2013;13:246–57.
57. Leight JL, Wozniak MA, Chen S, Lynch ML, Chen CS. Matrix rigidity regulates a switch between TGF-β1–induced apoptosis and epithelial–mesenchymal transition. Mol Biol Cell. 2012;23:781–91.
58. Kilinc AN, Han S, Barrett LA, Anandasivam N, Nelson CM. Integrin-linked kinase tunes cell–cell and cell-matrix adhesions to regulate the switch between apoptosis and EMT downstream of TGFβ1. Mol Biol Cell. 2021;32:402–12.
59. Lee K, et al. Matrix compliance regulates Rac1b localization, NADPH oxidase assembly, and epithelial–mesenchymal transition. Mol Biol Cell. 2012;23:4097–108.
60. Simi AK, Pang M-F, Nelson CM. Advances in Experimental Medicine and Biology. (Springer International Publishing; 2018. p. 57–67.
61. Rianna C, Radmacher M, Kumar S. Direct evidence that tumor cells soften when navigating confined spaces. Mol Biol Cell. 2020;31:1726–34.
62. Aktas B, et al. Stem cell and epithelial-mesenchymal transition markers are frequently overexpressed in circulating tumor cells of metastatic breast cancer patients. Breast Cancer Res. 2009;11:R46.
63. Pasquier J, Abu-Kaoud N, Al Thani H, Rafii A. Epithelial to mesenchymal transition in a clinical perspective. J Oncol. 2015;2015:1–10.
64. Mcatee CO, Barycki JJ, Simpson MA. Advances in cancer research. Amsterdam: Elsevier; 2014. p. 1–34.
65. Nelson CM, Bissell MJ. Of extracellular matrix, scaffolds, and signaling: tissue architecture regulates development, homeostasis, and cancer. Annu Rev Cell Dev Biol. 2006;22:287–309.
66. Weaver VM, et al. Reversion of the Malignant Phenotype of Human Breast Cells in Three-Dimensional Culture and In Vivo by Integrin Blocking Antibodies. J Cell Biol. 1997;137:231–45.

67. Mintz B, Illmensee K. Normal genetically mosaic mice produced from malignant teratocarcinoma cells. Proc Natl Acad Sci. 1975;72:3585–9.
68. Gascard P, Tlsty TD. Carcinoma-associated fibroblasts: orchestrating the composition of malignancy. Genes Dev. 2016;30:1002–19.
69. Teleanu RI, Chircov C, Grumezescu AM, Teleanu DM. Tumor angiogenesis and anti-angiogenic strategies for cancer treatment. J Clin Med. 2019;9:84.
70. Yamakawa M, et al. Potential lymphangiogenesis therapies: Learning from current antiangiogenesis therapies-A review. Med Res Rev. 2018;38:1769–98.
71. Fields GB. The rebirth of matrix metalloproteinase inhibitors: moving beyond the dogma. Cell. 2019;8:984.
72. Wu L, Yang X. Targeting the hippo pathway for breast cancer therapy. Cancer. 2018;10:422.
73. Bissell MJ, Aggeler J. Dynamic reciprocity: how do extracellular matrix and hormones direct gene expression? Prog Clin Biol Res. 1987;249:251–62.

Tumor-Fibroblast Interactions in Carcinomas

7

Harsh Dongre and Daniela Elena Costea

Abstract

As carcinomas evolve, mutations in cancer cells are accompanied by changes in the stroma leading to a 'reactive' or a 'desmoplastic' stroma. A reactive stroma is comparable to the activated stroma at the site of wound healing. The crosstalk between malignant cells and the surrounding stromal fibroblasts, an essential part of the reactive stroma, is a continuous, reciprocal force that modulates cancer progression. This communication unfolds at several levels and involves bidirectional growth factor and cytokine stimulations, joint extracellular matrix remodeling, and metabolic coupling. Recent findings have added even more layers of complexity by revealing the heterogeneity and plasticity of cancer-associated fibroblasts. This sheds new light on the role of cancer-associated fibroblasts in tumor progression and opens new avenues for therapeutical targeting.

H. Dongre · D. E. Costea (✉)
Centre for Cancer Biomarkers CCBIO, Department of Clinical Medicine, University of Bergen, Bergen, Norway

Department of Pathology, Haukeland University Hospital, Bergen, Norway
e-mail: Daniela.costea@uib.no

© The Author(s), under exclusive license to Springer Nature Switzerland AG 2022
L. A. Akslen, R. S. Watnick (eds.), *Biomarkers of the Tumor Microenvironment*, https://doi.org/10.1007/978-3-030-98950-7_7

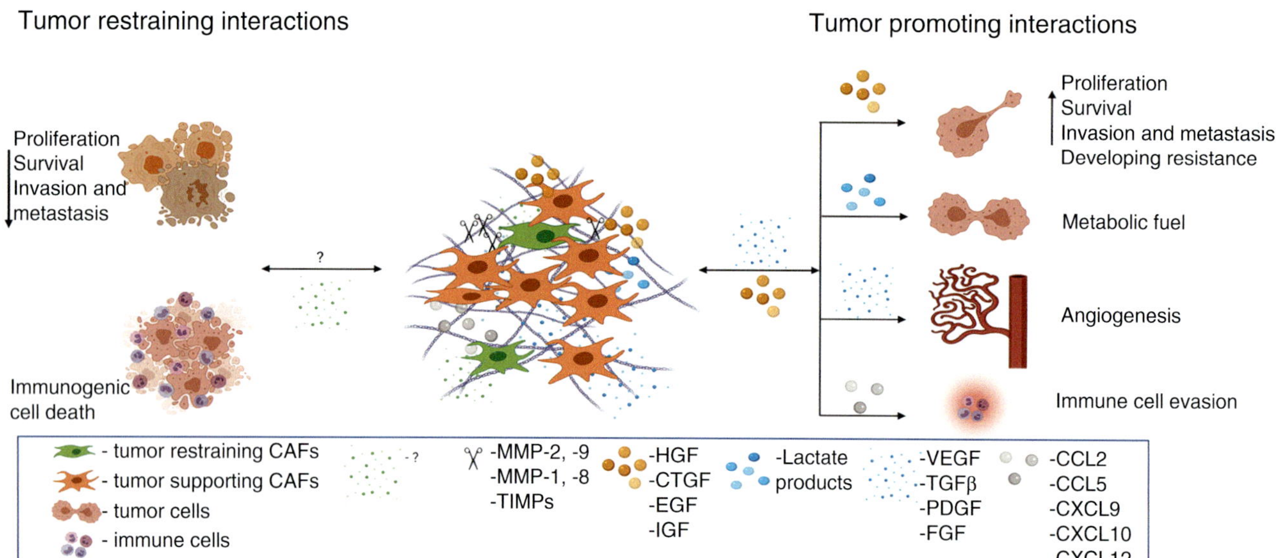

Tumour-CAF interactions in a nutshell. CAF shape the tumour microenvironment to be either tumour restraining or tumour promoting. Yet not fully characterized, tumour restraining CAF interactions have been recently demonstrated. On the other hand, CAF drives well known tumour promoting interactions such as increase in survival, invasion and metastasis, resistance to therapy and immunosuppression. The figure was created in BioRender

---

Take-Home Lessons
- Epithelial-mesenchymal interactions are deregulated early during cancer development, allegedly from premalignant stages.
- Tumor-fibroblast (the major component of tumor stroma) interactions are multifaceted, with key roles in tumor progression and drug resistance.
- In addition to growth factors, chemokines, enzymes, and extracellular matrix proteins, these interactions are mediated by metabolites.
- Cancer-associated fibroblasts display marked heterogeneity, reflected at both molecular and functional levels.
- Future anticancer therapies should target both cancer cells and stroma to improve patient outcomes.

Introduction

In mammals, all tissues and organs are heterocellular entities, and mesenchymally derived cells are a major component in most of them. These cells have important, complex, and diversified functions. The 'biological conversation' or 'crosstalk' between different cell populations in tissues and organs is essential for cell growth, differentiation, death, and replacement. One of the most studied examples of a determinative cellular crosstalk is the formation of the epithelial tissue, which is controlled by complex interactions between epithelium and the fibroblasts of the underlying mesenchyme. There is mounting evidence that these interactions are drastically modified in pathological processes, such as carcinogenesis. A plethora of studies have demonstrated that activated tumor stroma is a prerequisite for carcinoma invasion, and hence, the mesenchymal part of epithelial tumors has attracted substantial interest in recent years [1–4]. Tumor-stroma interactions can only be understood starting with the interactions between normal epithelial and stromal cells [5, 6]. Therefore, these fundamental regulatory mechanisms have also become a central area of the tumor-stromal research field, which has as a long-term goal to identify and characterize tumor-specific epithelial-mesenchymal alterations as new targets for therapy.

Fibroblasts: Definitions and Heterogeneity

Fibroblasts are the major mesenchymal cell type in the connective tissue and are often defined by a combination of morphology, spatial location, and lack of lineage markers (for epithelial cells, endothelial cells, and leukocytes), owing to a lack of markers that are specific to fibroblasts only [7]. Morphologically, fibroblasts are elongated (spindle-shaped) cells with an oval nucleus and cellular processes extending out from the cellular body (Fig. 7.1). Although lacking specific markers, pioneering work to study fibroblast functions was done by using vimentin and platelet-derived growth factor receptor-α (PDGFRα) as markers, together with other criteria such as cell shape and location.

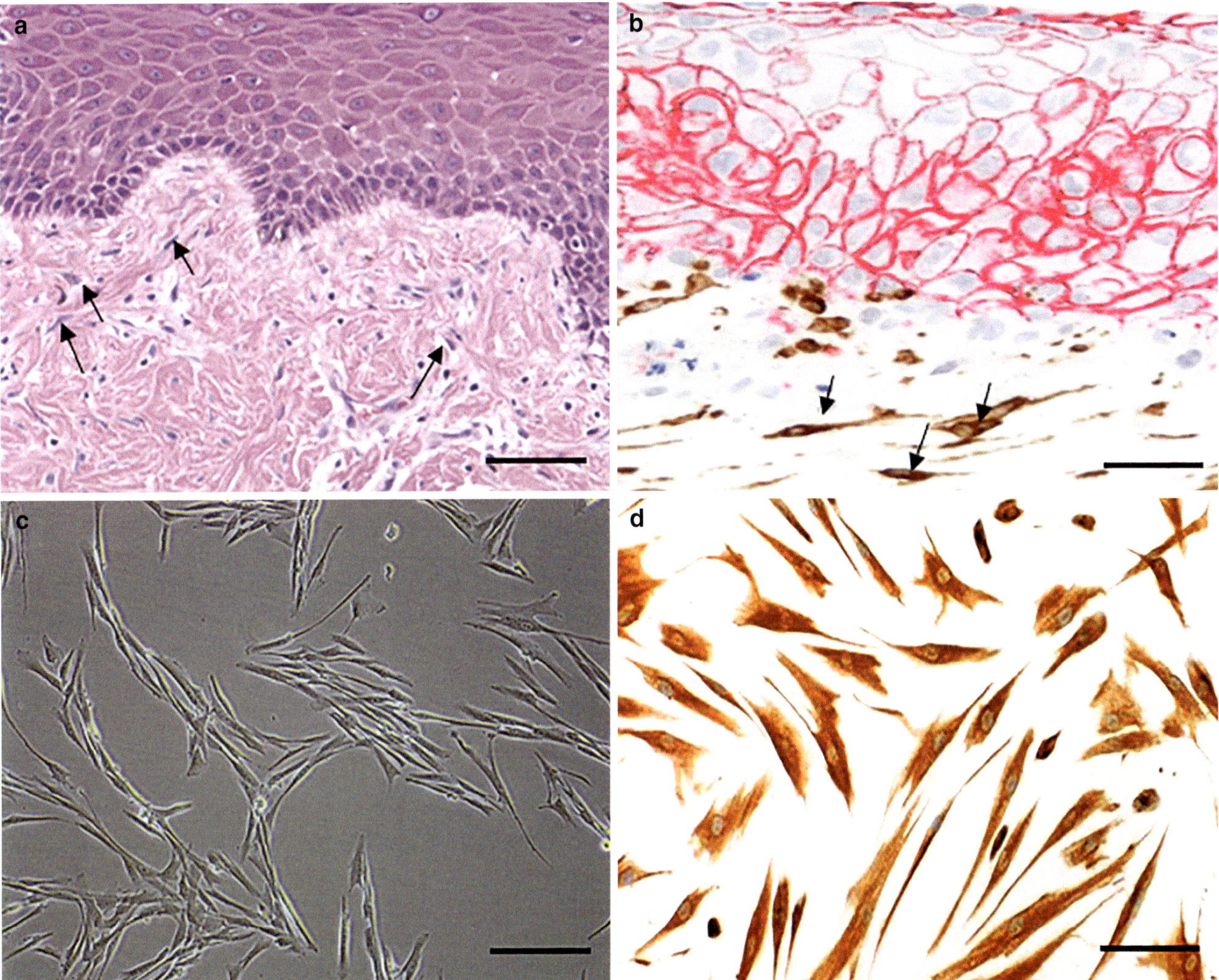

Fig. 7.1 (**a**). Hematoxylin and eosin-stained human oral mucosal tissue. Cells with elongated nuclei and cytoplasm, indicative of fibroblast morphology, are shown with black arrows. (**b**). Double immunostained (E-cadherin in red and vimentin in brown) human oral mucosal tissue. Brown cells with an elongated, fusiform shape indicative of fibroblast morphology are showed with black arrows. (**c**). Phase contrast image showing a culture of fibroblasts isolated from human vulvar mucosa. (**d**). Immunostained (vimentin–brown) cultured human fibroblasts isolated from oral mucosa. Note the marked variation in the morphology of stromal cells in **a** and **b** and of isolated fibroblasts in **c** and **d**. Scale bar of 100 μm in **a**, **b**, and **c** and of 50 μm in **d**

Fibroblasts have a variety of functions. Under homeostasis, they are responsible for maintaining the integrity and composition of the extracellular matrix (ECM) by synthesizing and degrading various matrix components. They produce tropocollagen (the precursor of collagen), the ground substance (an amorphous gel-like matrix that fills the spaces between cells and fibers in the connective tissue and is composed of water and large organic molecules, such as glycosaminoglycans (GAGs), proteoglycans, and glycoproteins), and a wide array of cytokines and growth factors [8]. Studies using three-dimensional (3D) co-cultures of fibroblasts with normal keratinocytes have demonstrated that the fibroblasts are responsible for the formation of basal lamina-anchoring zone [9]. Of interest, collagen is generally the main product of fibroblasts, and dysregulation of collagen production in cancer has attracted a lot of attention in the recent years [8]. However, in addition to collagen, fibroblasts synthesize significant amounts of GAGs and proteoglycans, and early studies of cultured fibroblasts by H. Green indicated that fibroblasts may even secrete 12 times more GAGs than collagen [10].

Fibroblasts are a heterogeneous population of cells, mainly due to their different origin, but also due to their different localization and functions of the organ/area they reside in. Their phenotype varies according to their location, age of individual, and activation state. The microscopically observed differences were recently backed up by differences between the transcriptome of the fibroblasts residing in

Table 7.1 Fibroblast cell types analyzed on the basis of biological and biochemical parameters

Parameter	MF I	MF II	MF III	PMF	Reference
Cell division potential	High	Moderate	Low	Negative	[15]
Sa-β-Gal expression	Negative	Very low	Low	High	[16]
Total collagen synthesis	Very low	Low	Low	High	[15]
KGF production	Very low	Low	Moderate	High	[15]
TGFβ1-production	Low	Low	High	High	[17]

different organs/parts of the body [11–13]. Even within a single tissue, fibroblasts exhibit remarkable functional diversity. For example, lineage tracking from the earliest stage of mesenchyme development through the adult stage identified two distinct subsets of dermal fibroblasts [14]. One subset was found responsible for the formation of the upper dermis, including the dermal papilla that regulates hair growth. The other subset formed the lower dermis, containing the reticular fibroblasts that synthesize the majority of the fibrillar ECM.

Other studies on fibroblast populations from different organs and species have classified the fibroblasts into two different populations as mitotically active fibroblasts (MF) and irreversible postmitotic fibrocytes (PMF). The MF-progenitor fibroblasts have been further classified into MF I, MF II, and MF III, subsequently differentiating into PMF. The key differences between these types of fibroblasts are described in Table 7.1.

Fibroblasts express a wide range of genes [11] and secrete several soluble growth factors like interleukin 6 (IL-6), interleukin 8 (IL-8), hepatocyte growth factor (HGF), keratinocyte growth factor (KGF), and transforming growth factor-beta (TGF-β). These different growth factors act in both autocrine and paracrine manner to maintain tissue homeostasis [18, 19].

Differences in the production level of growth factors have also been described between fibroblast from different sites. For example, HGF and KGF are produced at higher levels by oral fibroblasts when compared to skin fibroblasts [20]. One study reported increased capacity of oral mucosal fibroblasts over skin fibroblasts to organize collagen lattices, owing to an increased matrix metalloproteinase-2 (MMP-2) production [21]. Moreover, oral mucosal fibroblasts have received particular attention as they exhibit a preferential scarless wound healing [22]. Previous studies have shown that hyaluronan (an important GAG) is involved in the regulation of a distinct phenotype of oral fibroblasts which is resistant to TGF-β1-driven myofibroblast differentiation in contrast to skin fibroblasts which are readily activated into myofibroblasts upon TGF-β1 treatment [23]. Later studies of Costea et al., have shown, however, that there is a subset of normal oral fibroblasts that responds to TGF-β1 treatment and is able to differentiate into myofibroblasts with increased motility [24].

Fibroblasts play an essential role in wound healing. Following tissue injury, the resident fibroblasts of the tissue become activated mainly due to the TGF-β1 released at the site of injury by thrombocytes and are called myofibroblasts [8]. These activated fibroblasts migrate to the site of damage, where they deposit new collagen and ground substance, contract the wound, and send signals to replace the wounded tissue [12]. The cytoskeletal proteins of fibroblasts, in association with cell surface integrins and their coordination with the ECM, facilitate fibroblasts' motility. Most common markers for activated fibroblasts are α-smooth muscle actin (α-SMA; also known as ACTA2) and fibroblast activation protein (FAP) [8]. In wounded adult skin, the initial wave of dermal repair is mediated by the lower lineage, while upper dermal fibroblasts are recruited only during re-epithelialization [14].

Epithelial-Fibroblast Interactions in Normal Tissues

As early as four decades ago, experimental work clearly demonstrated that the interactions between epithelium and mesenchymal tissue play an important role not only for epithelial morphogenesis during embryonic development, but also for the differentiation and maintenance of adult epithelium [25]. To explain the influence that the connective tissue exerts on epithelial cells, two hypotheses have been proposed; (1) the connective tissue provides a physical substrate for attachment and orientation of basal keratinocytes and (2) the connective tissue cells synthesize diffusible proteins that influence both growth and differentiation of epithelial cells. Studies supporting the first hypothesis showed that the growth of a fully differentiated epithelium can be achieved in the absence of fibroblasts if the underlying physical substrate is made up of collagen type I, collagen IV, and laminin [26]. In contrast, some studies have shown that there is no need for a direct contact between skin keratinocytes and the connective tissue for a full epithelial differentiation [27]. Studies from in vitro organotypic skin cultures later confirmed that the effect of the connective tissue on epithelial morphogenesis was solely due to the diffusible factors synthesized by fibroblasts [28]. Results from Costea et al. and Dabija-Wolter et al. on 3D organotypic culture confirmed also that the fibroblasts control proliferation, differentiation, and terminal differentiation (a specific form of programmed cell death) of adjacent epithelium [29, 30].

Co-evolution of Epithelial and Stromal Fibroblasts During Malignant Transformation

As carcinoma evolves, mutations in the epithelial cells are accompanied by changes in the underlying/surrounding fibroblasts. Colon, oral, and vulvar mucosa are particularly useful for illustration of the stepwise carcinogenesis [8]. Precancerous (dysplastic) changes are classically attributed only to epithelium and are described to occur first as an epithelial 'patch'. By definition, this is an area with less than 200 mutated epithelial cells (cells with ~10 μm in diameter). This can be visualized, for example, by immunohistochemical (IHC) staining for mutated p53 (Fig. 7.2a right side). The 'patch' will develop further into a 'field', which is a larger epithelial area with mutated cells (Fig. 7.2a left side). Overtime, with the accumulation of more mutations, this patch can transform into an invasive carcinoma. However, apart from accumulation of inflammatory infiltrate under the dysplastic epithelium (Fig. 7.2a), changes in the underlying stroma are not obvious on routine hematoxylin-eosin slides before the invasive stage. Yet, some IHC studies on premalignant lesions could show early myofibroblastic changes in the stroma underlying dysplastic epithelial lesions. For example, fibroblasts from dysplastic ear lesions were shown to display increased α-SMA expression and enhanced tumor growth and angiogenesis [31]. Similar phenotypical changes have been described for oral and pancreatic carcinogenesis as well, where stromal fibroblasts with increased α-SMA expression were described as the first stromal change in the evolution toward malignancy. Initially, this might occur as a consequence of the bulging of the epithelial rete pegs (the epithelial extensions that project into the underlying connective tissue in both skin and mucous membranes) or of the epithelial buds in the glandular tissues, due to increased epithelial cell proliferation occurring at the pre-neoplastic stages. This notion is supported by the fact that cellular expression of α-SMA increases with increase in stiffness or stretching [32].

Expression of α-SMA and palladin in the stroma was found to gradually increase with progression of pancreatic tumorigenesis [33]. Fibroblasts from high-risk oral dysplastic lesions were also found to display higher α-SMA expression when compared to low-risk oral dysplastic lesions and normal mucosa [34]. A recent study on a cohort of dysplastic oral lesions showed that indeed the increased α-SMA expression occurred in the immediate subepithelial fibroblasts, juxtaposed to the bulging epithelial rete pegs in oral mucosa (Fig. 7.2b) [35]. Nevertheless, a careful review of the literature indicates that the myofibroblastic changes are not prognosticator of further development of oral premalignant lesions to carcinoma [36].

Transcriptomic analysis of 3D cultured normal fibroblasts (NF), dysplasia-associated fibroblasts (DAF), and carcinoma-associated fibroblasts (CAF) followed by unsupervised spectral clustering (Fig. 7.2c) showed a distinct grouping of DAF. This indicates global early changes in the fibroblasts located under dysplastic lesions, many of them related to TGF-β1 pathway (Fig. 7.2d) [24]. Furthermore, findings from 3D organotypic cultures showed that fibroblasts isolated from dysplastic lesions (DAF) have an intermediate phenotype between NF and CAF when it comes to supporting the invasion of carcinoma cells [24], as shown in Fig. 7.2e–g.

Carcinoma-Associated Stroma and Fibroblast Activation

Considered at first as contaminants, solid evidence has made it gradually clear that the non-neoplastic cells, and particularly the stromal fibroblasts present in carcinomas, are active and essential collaborators of tumorigenesis [37–39]. This has contributed to a paradigm shift from the traditional approach of studying cancer cells alone to studying cancer as a result of the interactions between the cancer cells and the stromal cells [37, 39]. Now we know that development of carcinoma is accompanied by a host response and complex heterotypic interactions of cancer cells with host cells and neighboring structures. This creates a complex tumor microenvironment (TME) that surrounds cancer cells and contains fibroblasts, immune cells, endothelial cells, pericytes, smooth muscle cells, adipocytes, ECM, and soluble diffusible factors [40]. However, there is a great disparity in the ratio of tumor cells to the non-tumor cells of stroma across the spectrum of human tumors. On one end are Hodgkin's lymphomas in which more than 95% of the cells are non-neoplastic cells, whereas hemangiomas (a vascular tumor derived from endothelial cells) contain almost exclusively of neoplastic cells. The ratio of stromal component between different types of carcinoma varies as well; for example, based on evaluation of the expression of α-SMA as a classical marker for activated CAF and of collagen 1 as a classical marker for fibrillar ECM, carcinomas of liver and cervix have little stroma as compared to those of colorectal or head and neck (majority of head and neck cancers being oral squamous cell carcinomas, OSCC) (Fig. 7.3a). Even within the same type of tumors, like OSCC, for example, there are significant variations between the amount of stroma present in

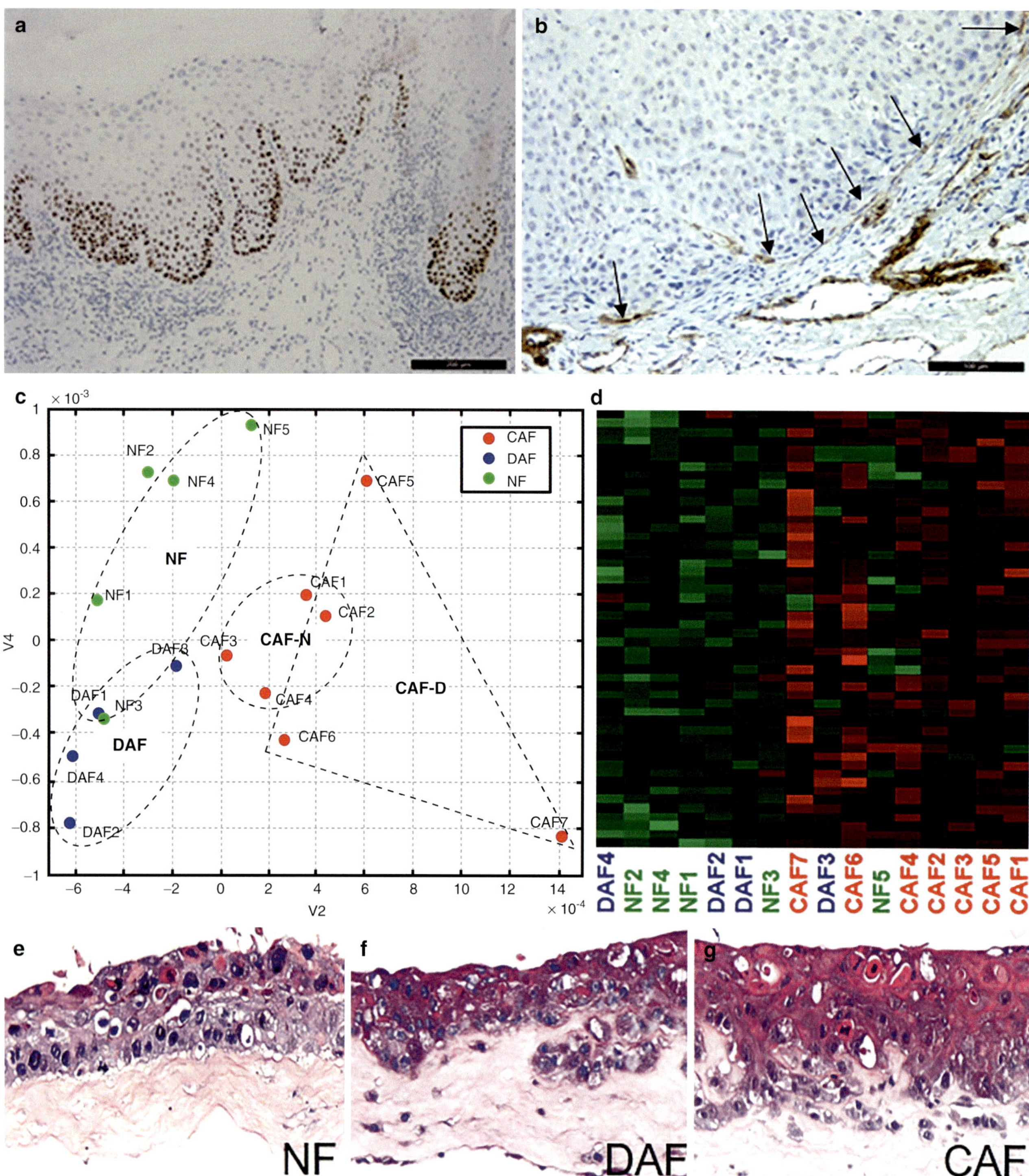

Fig. 7.2 (**a**) Immunohistochemistry for mutated p53 (brown color) showing a patch (right side) and a nearby field (left side) of transformed epithelial cells in a dysplastic oral tissue. (**b**) Immunohistochemistry for α-SMA (brown color) showing positive single cells with fibroblast morphology underneath a hyperplastic epithelial rete peg in a dysplastic oral tissue (marked with arrows). (**c**) Unsupervised spectral clustering showing distinct grouping of NF, DAF, and CAF. CAF clustered into two subgroups: one with a transcriptome closer to NF (CAF 1-4, termed CAF-N), the other with a more divergent expression profile (CAF 5-7, termed CAF-D). (**d**) Heatmap showing the top 50 differentially expressed transcripts of TGF-β target genes between NF, DAF, and CAF. Expression values are log2, mean centered (red, higher expression; green, lower expression). (**e–g**) 3D organotypic cultures showing no invasion, partial invasion, and marked invasion in the collagen gels populated with NF, DAF, and CAF, respectively

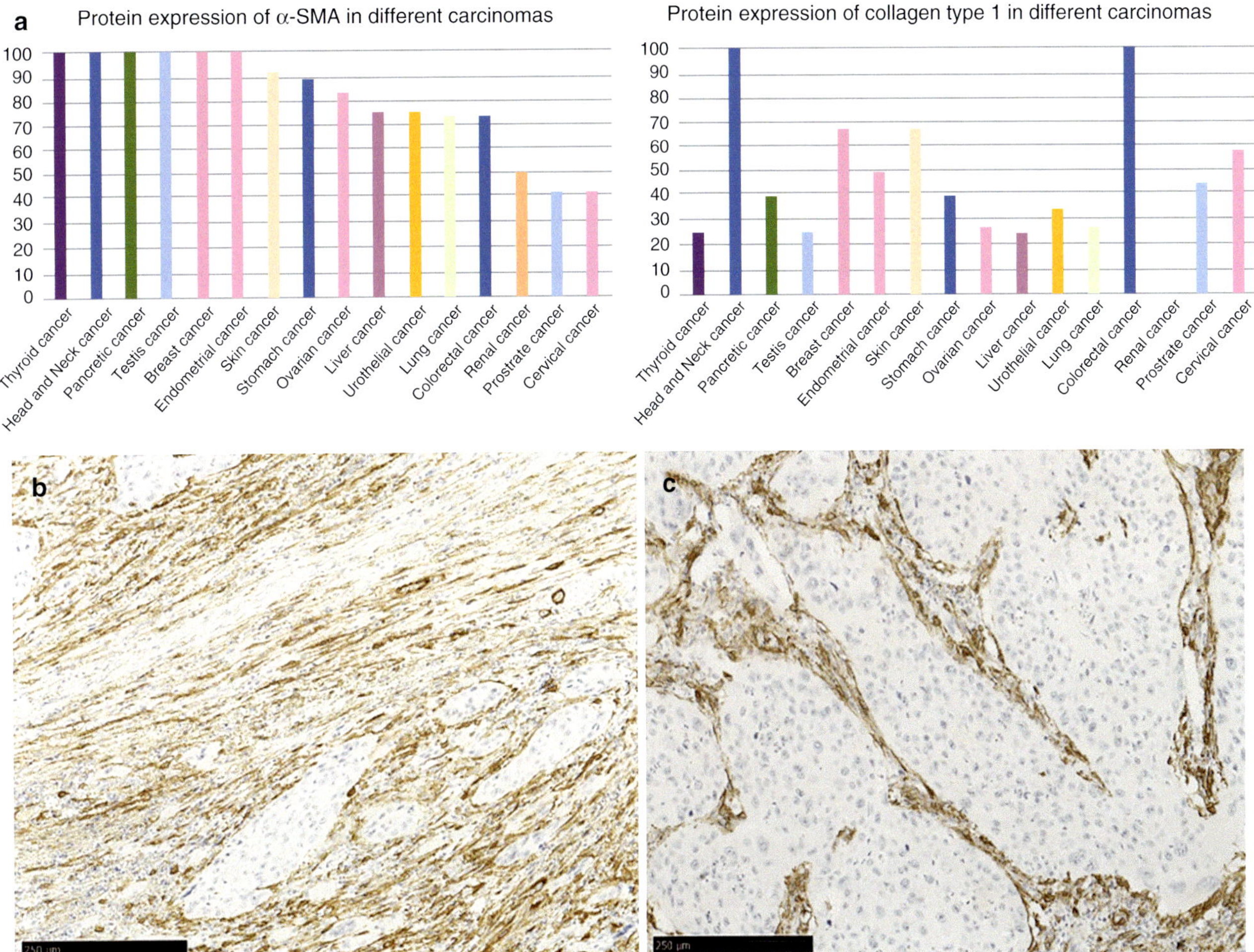

Fig. 7.3 (**a**) Graph showing the percentage of the cases containing myofibroblasts (expressing α-SMA) or fibrillar ECM (collagen 1) among different human carcinomas (based on data extracted from the Human Protein Atlas). (**b–c**) Micrographs showing various amounts of tumor stroma as evaluated by the presence of myofibroblasts (immunohistochemistry for α-SMA—brown color) in two different OSCC lesions

the OSCC lesions of different patients (Fig. 7.3b, c). Of note, in OSCC, for example, the amount of tumor stroma has been shown to predict survival [41]. As previously explained, homeostasis is maintained through heterotypic signaling between normal epithelium and underlying stroma. This signaling is mostly mediated by various mitogenic, cell-survival, and growth inhibitory signals. In contrast, the cancer cells of many carcinomas including breast, colon, prostrate, lung, and head and neck [24, 37, 39, 40, 42] continuously release higher levels of mitogenic and cell-survival signals but not growth inhibitory signals. Particularly in breast carcinomas, a potent mitogenic signal in the form of platelet-derived growth factor (PDGF) has been implicated in initiation of changes in the underlying stroma [43–45]. These changes are often referred to as 'reactive' or 'desmoplastic' stroma. Most of mesenchymal lineage cells like fibroblasts and macrophages in the stroma express the receptor for PDGF (PDGFR) which stimulates their proliferation.

The stroma induced by cancer cells differs substantially in appearance from the stroma in normal epithelial tissues due to increased deposition of ECM (Fig. 7.4). This 'reactive' or 'desmoplastic' stroma has been classically described for pancreas and breast tissues and quite widely understood as the intense stromal host reaction in the form of dense fibrosis [8, 46]. However, the desmoplastic stroma contains in addition to significant amounts of collagen types I and III, fibronectin, proteoglycans, and GAGs, as shown in Fig. 7.4 [40]. This deposition occurs progressively over months and years and gradually matures to a dense, collagenous, and acellular stroma, which is a hallmark of carcinoma-associated stroma [47, 48].

The myofibroblast phenotype is the most studied change in fibroblasts with respect to tumor progression. This is mainly due to the similarities observed between the desmoplastic stroma of tumors and the granulation tissue seen in wound healing. In wounds, normal fibroblasts tend to

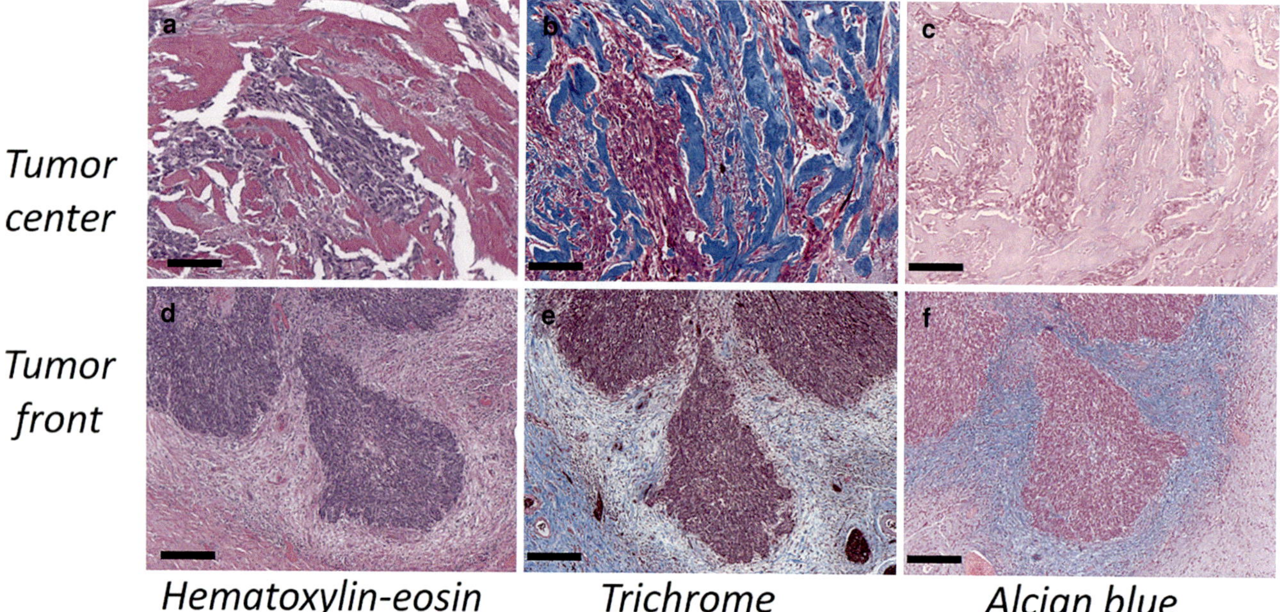

Fig. 7.4 Micrographs showing desmoplastic stroma in the same tumor (vulvar squamous cell carcinoma) with variation in content of collagen and GAGs as visualized by Trichrome (Masson's) staining and Alcian blue staining, respectively. (**a–c**) Mature, collagenous-rich stroma in the center of the tumor, which is depicted by the intense blue staining of the collagen by Trichrome staining in **b**. (**d–e**) A collagen-poor, GAGs-rich desmoplastic stroma at the tumor front of the same tumor as depicted by the intense blue staining of the GAGs by Alcian blue staining in **f**

change their phenotype to myofibroblasts, which are more contractile in nature [49]. The myofibroblast subpopulation, due to their expression of α-SMA, are proficient at using their actin-myosin machinery to generate mechanical forces required for wound closure. They are central for wound contraction in the granulation tissue during wound healing [50] as well as for synthesis of the new ECM. In wound healing, fibroblasts secrete multiple components of the ECM, including collagen types I, III, and V and fibronectin [51]. Apart from this, they are also responsible for maintaining ECM turnover by means of matrix-degrading metalloproteinases [51, 52]. In contrast to wound healing, in carcinomas, due to continuous influx of mitogenic signals and other epigenetic changes, the fibroblasts are constantly activated, and this results in an extensive deposition of ECM.

The mixed population of fibroblast and myofibroblasts that are present in the stroma of epithelial tumors is known under the common term 'carcinoma-associated fibroblasts' (CAF) [40]. Significantly altered gene pathways in CAF include regulation of substrate adhesion, tissue remodeling, cell migration, secretion, growth regulation, and angiogenesis [24]. One-third of the over-expressed genes in CAF versus NF were identified to be TGF-β1 targets [24]. In addition to a TGF-β1 response signature of CAF, an upregulation of integrin α11 expression in CAF as compared to the fibroblasts has also been reported [24].

CAF Heterogeneity

Inter- and intra-tumor heterogeneity has been recognized for long for human cancers, but it has mainly focused on the heterogeneity of the tumor parenchyma, such as the co-existence of genetically divergent clones, differences in the transcriptome, stemness, motility, or other phenotypic features [53]. Heterogeneity of the tumor stroma, although a relatively new topic, is slowly getting recognized [24, 54]. The heterogeneity of fibroblasts in normal homeostatic conditions is not something new. As discussed earlier, the fibroblasts display a different phenotype due to their differential functional specialization according to their organ of origin, body site, and spatial location [55]. It is therefore not unexpected that the CAF (which are derived, at least in part, from normal fibroblasts) are heterogenous in the tumor stroma as well.

De novo expression of α-SMA is the main and most used marker to characterize the activated fibroblasts in the tumor stroma [50, 56]. Trans-differentiation of NF toward a myofibroblastic phenotype has been described to be the key step in the activation of the stroma of carcinomas, and it was shown to be driven by IL-1, TNF-α, PDGF, FGF, and TGF-β1 [57]. Among these, TGF-β1 has been listed as the most important factor involved in the development of myofibroblasts [58, 59]. In the presence of mechanical stress and TGF-β1, proto-myofibroblasts differentiate into myofibroblasts [60]. The origin of myofibroblasts is still debated, but evidence shows that not only fibroblasts, but also other precursor cells present in TME such as endothelial cells, hematopoietic cells, and pericytes can transdifferentiate and assume a myofibroblast phenotype [61, 62].

A higher number of myofibroblasts at the invasive front of tumor stroma has been shown to be associated with poor prognosis in colorectal cancer [63], breast cancer [64], and oral cancer [65, 66]. Contrasting to this, some studies have shown that depletion of α-SMA from the myofibroblasts in an in vivo animal model increased the aggressiveness of tumors in pancreatic cancer [67, 68]. This indicates that some myofibroblasts might also have tumor-restraining effects and that other fibroblast subpopulations might also be of importance for cancer progression, especially in tumors with less myofibroblast activation. The finding that CAF strains with only 40-60% α-SMA-positive cells supported deeper invasion of malignant keratinocytes than those with a higher or lower percentage [24] points also to the suggestion that the ability of CAF to support cancer cell invasion is not dependent on their α-SMA myofibroblast phenotype. Taken together, a multitude of studies have addressed the heterogeneity of CAF in detail and some of these are summarized in Table 7.2 [69].

Table 7.2 Different subtypes of cancer-associated fibroblasts and their markers (adapted after [69])

Carcinoma type	CAF subsets	Markers		Functions	Reference
		IHC/flow cytometry	Single-cell RNA-seq		
Breast	CAF-S1	FAP^{High} $CD29^{Med-High}$ αSMA^{High} $PDPN^{High}$ $PDGFR\beta^{High}$		Proliferation, migration, metastasis, immunosuppression	[54, 70–72]
	CAF-S2	FAP^{Neg} $CD29^{Low}$ $\alpha SMA^{Neg-Low}$ $PDPN^{Low}$ $PDGFR\beta^{Low}$			
	CAF-S3	$FAP^{Neg-Low}$ $CD29^{Med}$ $\alpha SMA^{Neg-Low}$ $PDPN^{Low}$ $PDGFR\beta^{Low-Med}$			
	CAF-S4	$FAP^{Low-Med}$ $CD29^{High}$ αSMA^{High} $PDPN^{Low}$ $PDGFR\beta^{Med}$		Proliferation, migration, invasion, metastasis	
	CD10+GPR77	CD10, GRP77		Proliferation, migration, chemoresistance	[73]
Breast and PDAC	CAF-1	FSP1, VEGF, TNC		Angiogenesis, metastasis	[74–77]
	CAF-2	αSMA, NG2, PDGFRβ		Physical barrier, immunosuppression	
PDAC	rCAF	PDPN, meflin		Anti-tumorigenic	[78]
	myCAF	PDPN, αSMA	αSMA, TAGLN, TPM1, TPM2, POSTN	Proliferation, migration, invasion, metastasis	[79–81]
	iCAF	PDPN, IL-6, LIF, IL-11	IL-6, IL-8, CXCL1 [82], CXCL12, CFD, LMN, DPT	Metastasis, angiogenesis, immunosuppression	[79, 80]
	apCAF	PDPN, COL1A2	H2-Aa, H2-Ab1, CD74	Antigen presentation, immunosuppression	[80, 83]
Colorectal	CAF-A		MMP2, αFAP, COL1A2	Matrix remodeling	[84]
	CAF-B		αSMA, PDGFA, TAGLN	Proliferation, migration, invasion	
Lung cancer	Cluster 1		TGF-B	EMT, matrix remodeling	[85]
	Cluster 2		ACTA2	Proliferation, migration, invasion	
	Cluster 5		mTOR	Proliferation, immunosuppression (high mTOR signature expression, enriched in the tumor core)	
	Cluster 7		mTOR	Proliferation, immunosuppression (high mTOR signature expression, enriched in the tumor front)	
HNSCC	CAF-N	HA, MMP		Invasion, immunosuppression	[24, 86]
	CAF-D	TGF-B		Migration	
	Myofibroblasts		ACTA2, MYLK, YL9	Proliferation, migration, invasion	[87]
	CAF1		FAP, PDPN, COL1A1, VIM, THY1, MMP11, CAV1	Migration, matrix remodeling	
	CAF2		DAP, PDPN, JUN, FGF7, FOS, TGFBR	Proliferation, early response genes	
	Resting fibroblasts		–	Lacking expression of all other subsets	

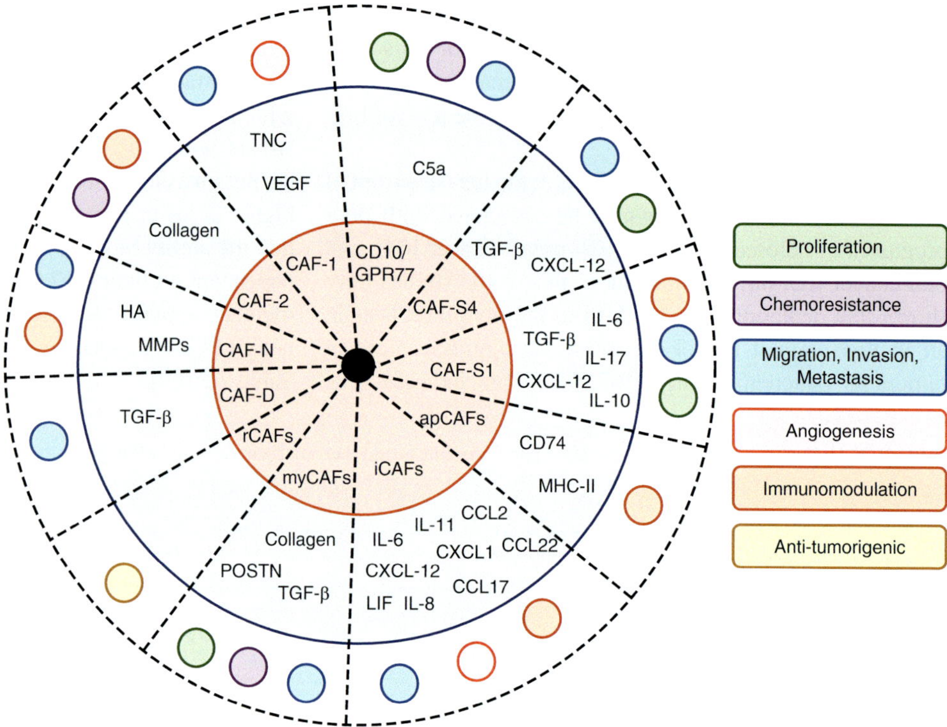

Fig. 7.5 Heterogenous function and phenotype of CAF. In the inner circle are subtypes of CAF reported by various researchers. The middle circle indicates markers and proteins secreted by each subtype, and in the outer circle, the functions attributed for each subtype are indicated by the colored circles representing one among the six CAF functions listed in the right-side margin (adapted from [69])

Evidence for different subpopulations of CAF has been shown at both transcriptional and functional levels (Fig. 7.5). Both the transcriptomics and the functional analysis identified, for example, two subgroups of CAF in oral carcinomas: one with a gene expression profile closer to NF (CAF-N) that supported the deepest invasion of malignant keratinocytes, secreted high levels of KGF, HGF, MMP3, and MMP9, and showed increased migration in response to TGF-β1 and one more divergent to NF (CAF-D) that supported a more limited invasion, secreted high levels of TGF-β1 into the tumor milieu, but did not show increased migration in response to TGF-β1.

Identification of CAF-N and CAF-D demonstrated that a mix of TGF-β-responsive and non-responsive CAF is an important driver of invasion as well as tumor initiation [24]. The relevance of a mix of TGF-β-responsive and non-responsive CAF in promoting carcinogenesis has been previously demonstrated in experimental systems by blocking TGF-β1 signaling with dominant-negative TGFBR2 [88]. This observation is also supported by tissue reconstitution experiments wherein varying the ratio of TGF-β-responsive and non-responsive cells promoted tumor induction [89]. Interestingly, some CAF subpopulations have been described to have a myeloid/monocytic phenotype and to have an impact on the clinical outcomes for tongue SCC [90].

The Multifaceted Aspects of Tumor-Fibroblast Interactions

Multiple experiments have provided direct evidence of CAF as active contributors of tumorigenesis [2, 3, 24, 91, 92]. Early experiments in prostate carcinoma demonstrated that CAF promoted tumorigenicity of non-tumorigenic, immortalized human prostate epithelial cells when implanted in immunocompromised mice [2]. The tumors formed were 500 times larger when CAF were co-injected than those formed by implanting together normal fibroblasts and immortalized human prostate epithelial cells. On the other hand, in the same experiment CAF alone did not form tumors when injected alone [2]. Such observations have been documented for many types of carcinomas, including breast [3], prostate [93], lung [94], vulva [91], and head and neck squamous cell carcinomas [24]. Though not completely understood, many aspects of the tumor-CAF crosstalk are now deciphered.

Epithelial-to-Mesenchymal Transition (EMT)

It has been documented that the transformation of NF into CAF is accompanied by ample changes in their secretome [24]. The importance of the increased secretion of TGF-β,

KGF, and HGF by CAF for supporting cancer cell invasion is well established [95, 96]. TGF-β1 is a well-known inducer of EMT, and it has been shown that CAF are able to induce EMT in head and neck and breast cancer cells due to increased secretion of TGF-β1 [24, 97]. Other growth factors and cytokines have been involved in CAF-mediated EMT induction of carcinoma cells, such as IL-8 [98], IL-6 [99], and CXCL12 [100].

Fibroblast Migration

Another major phenotypic change of CAF is toward a more motile phenotype. One of the essential roles of CAF in carcinoma progression is to stimulate the invasion of adjacent cancer cells by providing tracks into which the malignant keratinocytes can follow and migrate at distance from the primary tumor. Gaggioli et al. were the first to demonstrate that CAF are essential for cohesive invasion as they provide tracks that are used by the carcinoma cells to invade [101]. This force-mediated matrix remodeling required integrins (ITGA3 or 5), Rho and ROCK. Similar results were observed in adenoid cystic carcinoma cells (ACC) and CAF interactions albeit through CXCL12/CXCR4 pathway [102].

Complementary to generating 'tracks', some studies have showed that CAF can generate 'tunnels' by reorganizing the fibronectin and collagen fibers [103–105]. Cav1 overexpressing mouse embryonic fibroblasts (MEFs) have been shown to organize the matrix, especially fibronectin fibers into parallel fibers that favor directional cell migration with increased velocity [106]. The remodeling of matrix by Cav1-expressing fibroblasts was through actin-myosin contractility and Rho-dependent pathways [106]. In addition to this, FAP over-expressing CAF also participate in matrix reorganization [107]. Mechanistically, FAP+ CAF display altered levels of transcriptional regulators such as Twist1 and Snail1 [108, 109]. This induces increased collagen alignment and contraction leading to stiffer matrix as compared to normal matrix. Increased matrix stiffness can activate integrin-mediated receptors that can lead to activation of FAK and Src family kinases in the carcinoma cells [110]. This can in turn promote activity of YAP and TAZ transcriptional regulators that are associated with increased stem-cell properties and metastasis [110].

CAF were shown to have a higher track speed and longer track displacement than NF [24]. Increased expression of ITGA6, ITGA10, and ITGA11 that are laminin and collagen receptors, respectively, by CAF may facilitate rapid migration. Previous reports identified increased expression of ITGA3 and ITGA5 as being essential for the development of CAF-mediated tracks to support invasion of malignant kera-

tinocytes [101], but in another study, the levels of these integrins were higher in NF suggesting that the role of integrins may be context dependent [24].

The more rapid migration of CAF may also reflect the changes in the ECM components of tumors compared to normal connective tissues. Particularly at the invasive front, higher amounts of hyaluronan (HA) (as visualized in Fig. 7.4 by the Alican blue staining), syndecans, and a shift to secretion of proinvasive 14/16 tenascin isoforms were reported [111]. Using sophisticated 3D models, a significant role of HA secretion by CAF was demonstrated. In these models, reduced invasion of malignant keratinocytes was observed when they were seeded onto gels populated with CAF having downregulated the expression of hyaluronan synthetase 2 (HAS2) or onto gels populated with CAF that have had the elongation of HA chains blocked with 4-methylumbelliferone (4-MU) [24].

The CAF-induced matrix remodeling, carried by a series of matrix-metalloproteinases (MMPs), releases also a huge amount of other growth factors sequestered in the ECM. Some of these, like the families of vascular endothelial growth factors (VEGFs) and fibroblast growth factor (FGFs), are potent inducers of angiogenesis, making CAF a key regulator of tumor growth [112, 113]. Such angiogenic factors not only help in formation of new blood and lymph vessels, but they also have an autocrine effect on CAF, stimulating their own proliferation and thereby stimulating even more stromal production.

Metabolism

Another interesting aspect of the crosstalk between cancer cells and fibroblasts is their recently discovered metabolic coupling. When analyzing the metabolism of cancer cells, Warburg observed in 1920s that even in the presence of adequate oxygen, tumor cells utilized more glucose and produced more lactate than surrounding normal cells. He named this process 'aerobic glycolysis', which later was coined as the 'Warburg effect' [118]. Warburg hypothesized that cancer cells harbor dysfunctional mitochondria that are irreversibly damaged. However, the Warburg effect only partially explains tumor metabolism. Studies have shown that there is metabolic heterogeneity within tumors, with some cells maintaining a glycolytic phenotype, while others predominantly utilizing oxidative phosphorylation [119]. By investigating the metabolism of cancer cells in co-cultures with CAF, Lisanti's group revealed that it is the glycolysis in the cancer-associated stroma that metabolically supports the adjacent cancer cells [120]. His group showed a lactic acid transfer from CAF to cancer cells that allowed cancer cells to generate ATP, increase proliferation, and reduce cell death. The catabolites identified to be implicated in metabolic coupling included the monocarboxylates lactate, pyruvate, and ketone bodies [121]. Zhang et al. showed later on that carcinoma cells were able to induce a metabolic reprogramming of NF. After co-culture with cancer cells, NF were rapidly activated and acquired a CAF metabolic phenotype by undergoing aerobic glycolysis, secreting high L-lactate, and overexpressing lactate exporter MCT-4 [122]. In addition to catabolite transfer from fibroblasts to carcinoma cells, Zhang et al. also showed a unidirectional mitochondrial transfer from CAF to carcinoma cells. In addition, they demonstrated that NF were under hypoxia-like condition when co-cultured with carcinoma cells, underwent mitophagy through mitochondrial permeability transition pore (mPTP) opening via a decrease in activation of AMPK-PGC-1α axis [122]. This study corroborated well with Lisanti's studies, pointing that the energy-producing compartment in carcinomas is the fibroblasts in the tumor stroma.

Of importance, it was observed that the metabolic reprogramming with catabolite, mitochondrial transfer, and mitophagy in NF co-cultured with carcinoma cells occurred as early as 48 hours after co-culture, while the expression of α-SMA and FAP increased after NF were co-cultured with carcinoma cells for 6 and 10 days, respectively. These data point to a certain sequence of tumor-fibroblast interaction events, in which the metabolic changes and reprogramming occur earliest, before fibroblasts transition into a CAF phenotype and without concomitant cellular senescence [122]. Unrevealing this kinetic of changes from NF to CAF might have major implication on our understanding of CAF activation and on how targeting specific metabolic pathways could be employed in the treatment of carcinoma. Taken together, these findings indicate that metabolic reprogramming may act as the driver of fibroblast activation [123, 124]. These alterations can be further exploited for metabolically addressed therapy targeted at both epithelial and stromal tumor compartments.

Angiogenesis

As described above, the paracrine factors secreted by CAF involve VEGFs, PDGFs, HGF, IGFs, and other chemokines and cytokines. Of these, several are responsible for tumor vascularization. Most prominent are the family of growth factors belonging to VEGFs (VEGF-A, VEGF-B, VEGF-C, and VEGF-D) [125, 126]. Various biochemical studies have identified that the stromal CAF-derived VEGFs induce angiogenesis in breast [3, 75], pancreatic [127, 128], lung [129, 130], and hepatocellular [131] cancers. In highly angiogenic types of tumors, such as esophageal carcinoma, the essential role of CAF has been highlighted [132]. Mechanistically, the neo-angiogenic VEGF-A and VEGF-B bind to their related receptor tyrosine kinases (RTKs), VEGFR-1 and VEGFR-2 on the endothelial cells (ECs) and drive their proliferation [125]. On the other hand, the lymphangiogenic VEGF-C and VEGF-D GFs bind to VEGFR-3 and VEGFR-4 on lymph endothelial cells (LECs) and induce lymphangiogenesis [126]. This RTK activation through dimerization further drives proliferation, migration, and survival of ECs and LECs through downstream pathways like PI3K/AKT/mTor, JAK/STAT, or RAS/MEK/ERK [125]. In addition to their cognate receptors, VEGFs can bind to neuropilins (NRP1 and NRP2) on the vessels to enhance the effectiveness of signal transduction [133, 134]. Several other paracrine factors FGFs, PDGFs, HGFs, and IGFs independent of VEGFs have been shown to induce similar signal transduction to enhance ECs and LECs proliferation and vessel formation.

However, the proliferating ECs and LECs need mechanical support to form functional vessels. This support is provided by pericytes. Pericytes are cells of mesenchymal origin (and source of CAF) that promote survival of ECs but restrain their proliferation [113]. Pericytes also stabilize EC junctions to limit vascular permeability [113]. Contrary to this, the capillaries in TME display loose and uneven pericyte coverage that enables a defective and leaky vasculature [135, 136]. This further allows tumor-infiltrating cells of hematopoietic origin to accumulate in the TME and exert their pro-tumorigenic effects [113]. This knowledge has led to a plethora of studies looking at the paracrine factors secreted by CAF for clinical implications.

Apart from the paracrine effect, CAF are known to support vascular growth via mechanical force and regulation of oxygen tension [125, 130]. Recently, in a study using CAF derived from human breast cancer, the authors demonstrated that inhibition of mechano-transductive pathways involving YAP, Rock, and Snail1 in CAF attenuated vascular growth [130]. Supplementary to this, they also showed that upregulating the mechanical activity of normal breast fibroblasts induces ECM deformation and stimulates vascular growth. Further, studies have shown that as an effect of matrix remodeling, YAP is upregulated in CAF which then drives a feedforward loop into TGF-β signaling and angiogenesis that cooperates with further activation of nearby stromal fibroblasts and endothelial cells [110, 137, 138]. Moreover, oxygen tension also plays a prominent role in regulating angiogenesis. It is well established now that most solid tumors have regions of hypoxia owing to aberrant vascularization. Cancer cells then rely on HIFs to promote adaptation to such strenuous environment [139]. This in turn influences CAF to secrete cytokines and chemokines to promote metabolic reprogramming of both cancer cells and CAF [140,

141]. In breast and pancreatic carcinomas, HIF signaling is shown to induce further paracrine signaling of CAF in terms of TGF-β, FGF, and PDGF production [139, 142].

Metastasis

The role of fibroblasts for metastasis has become apparent from experiments on transgenic mice models. In a transgenic mouse lacking FSP-1 gene (*mts1*), the cancer cells did not metastasize when engrafted with highly metastatic murine mammary carcinoma cells [114]. Similarly, O'Connell et al. have showed that depletion of FSP-1(+) stromal cells reduces lung metastasis of breast cancer cells without affecting the primary tumor growth [75]. In the same study, they propose that FSP-1+ CAF-derived VEGF-A and tenascin-C plays a crucial role in establishment of pro-angiogenic microenvironment and protection from apoptosis, respectively, at the metastatic site [75]. In colorectal cancers, PDGF-stimulated CAF increase cancer cell intravasation and distant metastasis in a stanniocalcin 1 (STC1, a secreted glycoprotein)-dependent manner [115]. More recently, different CAF subsets have been shown to accumulate in metastatic lymph nodes in breast carcinoma. Although complementary in mechanisms, both subsets induced cancer cell migration and distant metastasis in either paracrine (CXCL12/TGFβ-dependent) or physically dependent (NOTCH-mediated ECM remodeling) manner [116]. The mechanisms involved in the activation or recruitment of the resident stromal cells at metastatic sites are still unknown. They may arise from primary tumor sites or be recruited from the bone marrow or yet be simply activated at the metastatic sites to remodel the metastatic soil. In addition, their multiple origin and anatomic variation can add to their functional heterogeneity. Some studies, particularly those related to hepatic metastasis, suggest that activated CAF (now termed as metastasis-associated fibroblasts, MAFs) at metastatic site support proliferation of cancer cells there and are conducive to secondary tumor growth [117]. Though not yet fully known, certain specific stimuli provided by MAFs create a metastatic niche in the secondary organ that facilitates seeding and further growth of tumors.

Concluding Remarks/Summary

Tumor-fibroblast interactions are complex and multifaceted. These interactions are mediated by chemokines, enzymes, growth factors, extracellular vesicles (e.g., exosomes), etc., and regulate enzymes activity, expression of genes and proteins, and metabolic pathways involved in tumor growth, metastasis, survival, and drug resistance. The study of the role of CAF for tumor progression has benefited enormously from their in vitro isolation in cell culture and experimenta-

tion on cultured cells. In this context, it is worth mentioning that the development of 3D matrix-cell culture models has been essential to decipher functional and biomechanical features of cell-matrix interactions in normal tissues as well as in carcinomas. Building on the knowledge derived from these experimental models on which CAF subpopulations exert a pro- versus antitumor effect will likely be beneficial for advancing cancer treatment [7, 143, 144]. Such studies could offer insights into novel combination therapies including reprogramming the CAF to control carcinoma progression and enable more efficient therapeutic responses [145].

References

1. Atula S, Grenman R, Syrjanen S. Fibroblasts can modulate the phenotype of malignant epithelial cells in vitro. Exp Cell Res. 1997;235(1):180–7.
2. Olumi AF, et al. Carcinoma-associated fibroblasts direct tumor progression of initiated human prostatic epithelium. Cancer Res. 1999;59(19):5002–11.
3. Orimo A, et al. Stromal fibroblasts present in invasive human breast carcinomas promote tumor growth and angiogenesis through elevated SDF-1/CXCL12 secretion. Cell. 2005;121(3):335–48.
4. De Wever O, et al. Tenascin-C and SF/HGF produced by myofibroblasts in vitro provide convergent pro-invasive signals to human colon cancer cells through RhoA and Rac. FASEB J. 2004;18(9):1016–8.
5. Fusenig NE, et al. Modulation of the differentiated phenotype of keratinocytes of the hair follicle and from epidermis. J Dermatol Sci. 1994;7(Suppl):S142–51.
6. Tlsty TD, Hein PW. Know thy neighbor: stromal cells can contribute oncogenic signals. Curr Opin Genet Dev. 2001;11(1):54–9.
7. Sahai E, et al. A framework for advancing our understanding of cancer-associated fibroblasts. Nat Rev Cancer. 2020;20(3):174–86.
8. Kumar V, Abbas A, Aster J. Basic pathology. Amsterdam: Elsevier; 2017. p. 952.
9. Contard P, et al. Culturing keratinocytes and fibroblasts in a three-dimensional mesh results in epidermal differentiation and formation of a basal lamina-anchoring zone. J Invest Dermatol. 1993;100(1):35–9.
10. Green H, Hemerman D. Production of hyaluronate and collagen by fibroblast clones in culture. Nature. 1964;201:710.
11. Chang HY, et al. Diversity, topographic differentiation, and positional memory in human fibroblasts. Proc Natl Acad Sci U S A. 2002;99(20):12877–82.
12. Rinn JL, et al. Anatomic demarcation by positional variation in fibroblast gene expression programs. PLoS Genet. 2006;2(7):e119.
13. Rinn JL, et al. A systems biology approach to anatomic diversity of skin. J Invest Dermatol. 2008;128(4):776–82.
14. Driskell RR, et al. Distinct fibroblast lineages determine dermal architecture in skin development and repair. Nature. 2013;504(7479):277–81.
15. Rodemann HP, et al. Selective enrichment and biochemical characterization of seven human skin fibroblasts cell types in vitro. Exp Cell Res. 1989;180(1):84–93.
16. Hakenjos L, Bamberg M, Rodemann HP. TGF-beta1-mediated alterations of rat lung fibroblast differentiation resulting in the radiation-induced fibrotic phenotype. Int J Radiat Biol. 2000;76(4):503–9.

17. Rodemann HP, Rennekampff H-O. Functional diversity of fibroblasts. In: Mueller MM, Fusenig NE, editors. Tumor-associated fibroblasts and their matrix. Dordrecht: Springer; 2011. p. 23–36.

18. Yamaguchi Y, et al. Mesenchymal-epithelial interactions in the skin: aiming for site-specific tissue regeneration. J Dermatol Sci. 2005;40(1):1–9.

19. Rodemann HP. Differential degradation of intracellular proteins in human skin fibroblasts of mitotic and mitomycin-C (MMC)-induced postmitotic differentiation states in vitro. Differentiation. 1989;42(1):37–43.

20. Gron B, et al. Oral fibroblasts produce more HGF and KGF than skin fibroblasts in response to co-culture with keratinocytes. APMIS. 2002;110(12):892–8.

21. Stephens P, et al. Skin and oral fibroblasts exhibit phenotypic differences in extracellular matrix reorganization and matrix metalloproteinase activity. Br J Dermatol. 2001;144(2):229–37.

22. Enoch S, et al. 'Young' oral fibroblasts are geno/phenotypically distinct. J Dent Res. 2010;89(12):1407–13.

23. Meran S, et al. Involvement of hyaluronan in regulation of fibroblast phenotype. J Biol Chem. 2007;282(35):25687–97.

24. Costea DE, et al. Identification of two distinct carcinoma-associated fibroblast subtypes with differential tumor-promoting abilities in oral squamous cell carcinoma. Cancer Res. 2013;73(13):3888–901.

25. Mackenzie I. Epithelial-mesencymal interactions in the development and maintenance of epithelial tissues. In: The keratinocyte handbook. Cambridge: Cambridge University Press; 1994. p. 243–57.

26. Kim SW, et al. Effects of collagen IV and laminin on the reconstruction of human oral mucosa. J Biomed Mater Res. 2001;58(1):108–12.

27. Boukamp P, et al. Mesenchyme-mediated and endogenous regulation of growth and differentiation of human skin keratinocytes derived from different body sites. Differentiation. 1990;44(2):150–61.

28. El Ghalbzouri A, Ponec M. Diffusible factors released by fibroblasts support epidermal morphogenesis and deposition of basement membrane components. Wound Repair Regen. 2004;12(3):359–67.

29. Costea DE, et al. Crucial effects of fibroblasts and keratinocyte growth factor on morphogenesis of reconstituted human oral epithelium. J Invest Dermatol. 2003;121(6):1479–86.

30. Dabija-Wolter G, et al. In vitro reconstruction of human junctional and sulcular epithelium. J Oral Pathol Med. 2013;42(5):396–404.

31. Erez N, et al. Cancer-associated fibroblasts are activated in incipient neoplasia to orchestrate tumor-promoting inflammation in an NF-kappaB-dependent manner. Cancer Cell. 2010;17(2):135–47.

32. Rothdiener M, et al. Stretching human mesenchymal stromal cells on stiffness-customized collagen type I generates a smooth muscle marker profile without growth factor addition. Sci Rep. 2016;6:35840.

33. Brentnall TA. Arousal of cancer-associated stromal fibroblasts: palladin-activated fibroblasts promote tumor invasion. Cell Adh Migr. 2012;6(6):488–94.

34. Chaudhary M, et al. Comparison of myofibroblasts expression in oral squamous cell carcinoma, verrucous carcinoma, high risk epithelial dysplasia, low risk epithelial dysplasia and normal oral mucosa. Head Neck Pathol. 2012;6(3):305–13.

35. Nguyen TH, Boe IK. Prognostic biomarkers in oral dysplasia. Bergen: University of Bergen; 2018.

36. Coletta RD, Salo T. Myofibroblasts in oral potentially malignant disorders: Is it related to malignant transformation? Oral Dis. 2018;24(1-2):84–8.

37. Giraldo NA, et al. The clinical role of the TME in solid cancer. British Journal of Cancer. 2019;120(1):45–53.

38. Hanahan D, Weinberg RA. Hallmarks of cancer: the next generation. Cell. 2011;144(5):646–74.

39. LeBleu VS, Kalluri R. A peek into cancer-associated fibroblasts: origins, functions and translational impact. Dis Model Mech. 2018;11(4):dmm029447.

40. Weinberg RA. The biology of cancer. New York: Garland Science; 2013.

41. Haave H, et al. Tumor stromal desmoplasia and inflammatory response uniquely predict survival with and without stratification for HPV tumor infection in OPSCC patients. Acta Otolaryngol. 2018;138(11):1035–42.

42. Kalluri R, Zeisberg M. Fibroblasts in cancer. Nature Reviews Cancer. 2006;6(5):392–401.

43. Östman A. PDGF receptors in tumor stroma: biological effects and associations with prognosis and response to treatment. Adv Drug Deliv Rev. 2017;121:117–23.

44. Frings O, et al. Prognostic significance in breast cancer of a gene signature capturing stromal PDGF signaling. Am J Pathol. 2013;182(6):2037–47.

45. Tsioumpekou M, et al. Specific targeting of PDGFRβ in the stroma inhibits growth and angiogenesis in tumors with high PDGF-BB expression. Theranostics. 2020;10(3):1122–35.

46. Huet E, et al. Stroma in normal and cancer wound healing. FEBS J. 2019;286(15):2909–20.

47. Valkenburg KC, de Groot AE, Pienta KJ. Targeting the tumor stroma to improve cancer therapy. Nature reviews. Clinical oncology. 2018;15(6):366–81.

48. Yamauchi M, et al. The fibrotic tumor stroma. The Journal of clinical investigation. 2018;128(1):16–25.

49. Gabbiani G. Some historical and philosophical reflections on the myofibroblast concept. Curr Top Pathol. 1999;93:1–5.

50. Gabbiani G, Ryan GB, Majno G. Presence of modified fibroblasts in granulation tissue and their possible role in wound contraction. Experientia. 1971;27(5):549–50.

51. Kalluri R. The biology and function of fibroblasts in cancer. Nat Rev Cancer. 2016;16(9):582–98.

52. Marsh T, Pietras K, McAllister SS. Fibroblasts as architects of cancer pathogenesis. Biochimica et biophysica acta. 2013;1832(7):1070–8.

53. Marusyk A, Polyak K. Tumor heterogeneity: causes and consequences. Biochim Biophys Acta. 2010;1805(1):105–17.

54. Costa A, et al. Fibroblast heterogeneity and immunosuppressive environment in human breast cancer. Cancer Cell. 2018;33(3):463–79. e10

55. Lynch MD, Watt FM. Fibroblast heterogeneity: implications for human disease. J Clin Invest. 2018;128(1):26–35.

56. Hinz B, et al. Alpha-smooth muscle actin expression upregulates fibroblast contractile activity. Molecular Biology of the Cell. 2001;12(9):2730–41.

57. Kovacs EJ, DiPietro LA. Fibrogenic cytokines and connective tissue production. The FASEB Journal. 1994;8(11):854–61.

58. Masur SK, et al. Myofibroblasts differentiate from fibroblasts when plated at low density. Proceedings of the National Academy of Sciences of the United States of America. 1996;93(9):4219–23.

59. Hautmann MB, Madsen CS, Owens GK. A Transforming Growth Factor β (TGFβ) control element drives TGFβ-induced stimulation of smooth muscle α-actin gene expression in concert with two CArG elements. Journal of Biological Chemistry. 1997;272(16):10948–56.

60. Hinz B, et al. Mechanical tension controls granulation tissue contractile activity and myofibroblast differentiation. The American Journal of Pathology. 2001;159(3):1009–20.

61. Davis J, Molkentin JD. Myofibroblasts: trust your heart and let fate decide. J Mol Cell Cardiol. 2014;70:9–18.

62. Hinz B, et al. The myofibroblast: one function, multiple origins. The American Journal of Pathology. 2007;170(6):1807–16.

63. Tsujino T, et al. Stromal myofibroblasts predict disease recurrence for colorectal cancer. Clin Cancer Res. 2007;13(7):2082–90.

64. Yazhou C, et al. Clinicopathological significance of stromal myofibroblasts in invasive ductal carcinoma of the breast. Tumor Biol. 2004;25(5-6):290–5.

65. Kellermann MG, et al. Myofibroblasts in the stroma of oral squamous cell carcinoma are associated with poor prognosis. Histopathology. 2007;51(6):849–53.

66. Bello IO, et al. Cancer-associated fibroblasts, a parameter of the tumor microenvironment, overcomes carcinoma-associated parameters in the prognosis of patients with mobile tongue cancer. Oral Oncology. 2011;47(1):33–8.

67. Özdemir BC, et al. Depletion of carcinoma-associated fibroblasts and fibrosis induces immunosuppression and accelerates pancreas cancer with diminished survival. Cancer cell. 2014;25(6):719–34.

68. [cited 2016 Jan 31]; Available from: http://www.consultant360.com/story/depleting-carcinoma-associated-myofibroblasts-may-worsen-pancreatic-cancer-outcomes.

69. Louault K, Li RR, DeClerck YA. Cancer-associated fibroblasts: understanding their heterogeneity. Cancers (Basel). 2020;12(11):3108.

70. Pelon F, et al. Cancer-associated fibroblast heterogeneity in axillary lymph nodes drives metastases in breast cancer through complementary mechanisms. Nat Commun. 2020;11(1):404.

71. Givel AM, et al. miR200-regulated CXCL12beta promotes fibroblast heterogeneity and immunosuppression in ovarian cancers. Nat Commun. 2018;9(1):1056.

72. Kieffer Y, et al. Single-cell analysis reveals fibroblast clusters linked to immunotherapy resistance in cancer. Cancer Discov. 2020;10(9):1330–51.

73. Su S, et al. CD10(+)GPR77(+) cancer-associated fibroblasts promote cancer formation and chemoresistance by sustaining cancer stemness. Cell. 2018;172(4):841–56. e16

74. Sugimoto H, et al. Identification of fibroblast heterogeneity in the tumor microenvironment. Cancer Biol Ther. 2006;5(12):1640–6.

75. O'Connell JT, et al. VEGF-A and Tenascin-C produced by S100A4+ stromal cells are important for metastatic colonization. Proc Natl Acad Sci U S A. 2011;108(38):16002–7.

76. Jiao J, et al. Depletion of S100A4(+) stromal cells does not prevent HCC development but reduces the stem cell-like phenotype of the tumors. Exp Mol Med. 2018;50(1):e422.

77. Carstens JL, et al. Spatial computation of intratumoral T cells correlates with survival of patients with pancreatic cancer. Nat Commun. 2017;8:15095.

78. Mizutani Y, et al. Meflin-positive cancer-associated fibroblasts inhibit pancreatic carcinogenesis. Cancer Res. 2019;79(20):5367–81.

79. Ohlund D, et al. Distinct populations of inflammatory fibroblasts and myofibroblasts in pancreatic cancer. J Exp Med. 2017;214(3):579–96.

80. Elyada E, et al. Cross-species single-cell analysis of pancreatic ductal adenocarcinoma reveals antigen-presenting cancer-associated fibroblasts. Cancer Discov. 2019;9(8):1102–23.

81. Hosein AN, et al. Cellular heterogeneity during mouse pancreatic ductal adenocarcinoma progression at single-cell resolution. JCI Insight. 2019;5:e129212.

82. Drapkin BJ, Farago AF. Unexpected synergy reveals new therapeutic strategy in SCLC. Trends Pharmacol Sci. 2019;40(5):295–7.

83. Lakins MA, et al. Cancer-associated fibroblasts induce antigen-specific deletion of CD8 (+) T Cells to protect tumor cells. Nat Commun. 2018;9(1):948.

84. Li H, et al. Reference component analysis of single-cell transcriptomes elucidates cellular heterogeneity in human colorectal tumors. Nat Genet. 2017;49(5):708–18.

85. Lambrechts D, et al. Phenotype molding of stromal cells in the lung tumor microenvironment. Nat Med. 2018;24(8):1277–89.

86. Hassona Y, et al. Senescent cancer-associated fibroblasts secrete active MMP-2 that promotes keratinocyte dis-cohesion and invasion. Br J Cancer. 2014;111(6):1230–7.

87. Puram SV, et al. Single-cell transcriptomic analysis of primary and metastatic tumor ecosystems in head and neck cancer. Cell. 2017;171(7):1611–24. e24

88. Franco OE, et al. Altered TGF-beta signaling in a subpopulation of human stromal cells promotes prostatic carcinogenesis. Cancer Res. 2011;71(4):1272–81.

89. Kiskowski MA, et al. Role for stromal heterogeneity in prostate tumorigenesis. Cancer Res. 2011;71(10):3459–70.

90. Vered M, et al. Cancer-associated fibroblasts in the tumor microenvironment of tongue carcinoma is a heterogeneous cell population. Acta Histochem. 2019;121(8):151446.

91. Dongre H, et al. Establishment of a novel cancer cell line derived from vulvar carcinoma associated with lichen sclerosus exhibiting a fibroblast-dependent tumorigenic potential. Experimental Cell Research. 2020;386(1):111684.

92. Costea DE, Johannessen AC, Vintermyr OK. Fibroblast control on epithelial differentiation is gradually lost during in vitro tumor progression. Differentiation. 2005;73(4):134–41.

93. Giannoni E, et al. Reciprocal activation of prostate cancer cells and cancer-associated fibroblasts stimulates epithelial-mesenchymal transition and cancer stemness. Cancer Research. 2010;70(17):6945–56.

94. Chen WJ, et al. Cancer-associated fibroblasts regulate the plasticity of lung cancer stemness via paracrine signalling. Nat Commun. 2014;5:3472.

95. Wang X, et al. Cancer-associated fibroblasts induce epithelial-mesenchymal transition through secreted cytokines in endometrial cancer cells. Oncol Lett. 2018;15(4):5694–702.

96. Lewis MP, et al. Tumor-derived TGF-beta1 modulates myofibroblast differentiation and promotes HGF/SF-dependent invasion of squamous carcinoma cells. Br J Cancer. 2004;90(4):822–32.

97. Yu Y, et al. Cancer-associated fibroblasts induce epithelial-mesenchymal transition of breast cancer cells through paracrine TGF-beta signalling. Br J Cancer. 2014;110(3):724–32.

98. Lim H, et al. Cancer-associated fibroblasts induce an aggressive phenotypic shift in non-malignant breast epithelial cells via interleukin-8 and S100A8. J Cell Physiol. 2021;236(10):7014–32.

99. Jia C, et al. Cancer-associated Fibroblasts induce epithelial-mesenchymal transition via the Transglutaminase 2-dependent IL-6/IL6R/STAT3 axis in Hepatocellular Carcinoma. Int J Biol Sci. 2020;16(14):2542–58.

100. Zhang F, et al. Cancer-associated fibroblasts induce epithelial-mesenchymal transition and cisplatin resistance in ovarian cancer via CXCL12/CXCR4 axis. Future Oncol. 2020;16(32):2619–33.

101. Gaggioli C, et al. Fibroblast-led collective invasion of carcinoma cells with differing roles for RhoGTPases in leading and following cells. Nat Cell Biol. 2007;9(12):1392–400.

102. Li J, et al. Carcinoma-associated fibroblasts lead the invasion of salivary gland adenoid cystic carcinoma cells by creating an invasive track. PLoS one. 2016;11(3):e0150247.

103. Goicoechea SM, et al. Palladin promotes invasion of pancreatic cancer cells by enhancing invadopodia formation in cancer-associated fibroblasts. Oncogene. 2014;33(10):1265–73.

104. Lugo-Cintrón KM, et al. Breast fibroblasts and ECM components modulate breast cancer cell migration through the secretion of mmps in a 3D microfluidic Co-culture model. Cancers. 2020;12(5):1173.

105. Fisher KE, et al. MT1-MMP- and Cdc42-dependent signaling co-regulate cell invasion and tunnel formation in 3D collagen matrices. J Cell Sci. 2009;122(Pt 24):4558–69.

106. Goetz JG, et al. Biomechanical remodeling of the microenvironment by stromal caveolin-1 favors tumor invasion and metastasis. Cell. 2011;146(1):148–63.

107. Lee H-O, et al. FAP-overexpressing fibroblasts produce an extracellular matrix that enhances invasive velocity and directionality of pancreatic cancer cells. BMC Cancer. 2011;11(1):245.

108. Stanisavljevic J, et al. Snail1-expressing fibroblasts in the tumor microenvironment display mechanical properties that support metastasis. Cancer Research. 2015;75(2):284–95.

109. García-Palmero I, et al. Twist1-induced activation of human fibroblasts promotes matrix stiffness by upregulating palladin and collagen α1(VI). Oncogene. 2016;35(40):5224–36.

110. Calvo F, et al. Mechanotransduction and YAP-dependent matrix remodelling is required for the generation and maintenance of cancer-associated fibroblasts. Nature Cell Biology. 2013;15(6):637–46.

111. Hancox RA, et al. Tumor-associated tenascin-C isoforms promote breast cancer cell invasion and growth by matrix metalloproteinase-dependent and independent mechanisms. Breast Cancer Res. 2009;11(2):R24.

112. Watnick RS. The role of the tumor microenvironment in regulating angiogenesis. Cold Spring Harb Perspect Med. 2012;2(12):a006676.

113. De Palma M, Biziato D, Petrova TV. Microenvironmental regulation of tumor angiogenesis. Nature Reviews Cancer. 2017;17(8):457–74.

114. Grum-Schwensen B, et al. Suppression of tumor development and metastasis formation in mice lacking the S100A4(mts1) gene. Cancer Research. 2005;65(9):3772–80.

115. Peña C, et al. STC1 expression by cancer-associated fibroblasts drives metastasis of colorectal cancer. Cancer Res. 2013;73(4):1287–97.

116. Pelon F, et al. Cancer-associated fibroblast heterogeneity in axillary lymph nodes drives metastases in breast cancer through complementary mechanisms. Nature Communications. 2020;11(1):404.

117. Pausch TM, et al. Metastasis-associated fibroblasts promote angiogenesis in metastasized pancreatic cancer via the CXCL8 and the CCL2 axes. Scientific Reports. 2020;10(1):5420.

118. Warburg O. On respiratory impairment in cancer cells. Science. 1956;124(3215):269–70.

119. Wallace DC. Mitochondria and cancer. Nat Rev Cancer. 2012;12(10):685–98.

120. Pavlides S, et al. Transcriptional evidence for the "Reverse Warburg Effect" in human breast cancer tumor stroma and metastasis: similarities with oxidative stress, inflammation, Alzheimer's disease, and "Neuron-Glia Metabolic Coupling". Aging (Albany NY). 2010;2(4):185–99.

121. Wilde L, et al. Metabolic coupling and the reverse warburg effect in cancer: implications for novel biomarker and anticancer agent development. Semin Oncol. 2017;44(3):198–203.

122. Zhang Z, et al. Metabolic reprogramming of normal oral fibroblasts correlated with increased glycolytic metabolism of oral squamous cell carcinoma and precedes their activation into carcinoma associated fibroblasts. Cell Mol Life Sci. 2020;77(6):1115–33.

123. Berridge MV, Crasso C, Neuzil J. Mitochondrial genome transfer to tumor cells breaks the rules and establishes a new precedent in cancer biology. Molecular & Cellular Oncology. 2015;5(5):e1023929.

124. Zhang Z, et al. Fibroblasts rescue oral squamous cancer cell from metformin-induced apoptosis via alleviating metabolic disbalance and inhibiting AMPK pathway. Cell Cycle. 2019;18(9):949–62.

125. Ferrara N, Gerber H-P, LeCouter J. The biology of VEGF and its receptors. Nature Medicine. 2003;9(6):669–76.

126. Rauniyar K, Jha SK, Jeltsch M. Biology of vascular endothelial growth factor c in the morphogenesis of lymphatic vessels. Frontiers in bioengineering and biotechnology. 2018;6:7–7.

127. Xu Z, et al. Role of pancreatic stellate cells in pancreatic cancer metastasis. The American Journal of Pathology. 2010;177(5):2585–96.

128. Masamune A, et al. Hypoxia stimulates pancreatic stellate cells to induce fibrosis and angiogenesis in pancreatic cancer. Am J Physiol Gastrointest Liver Physiol. 2008;295(4):G709–17.

129. Wang L, et al. Cancer-associated fibroblasts enhance metastatic potential of lung cancer cells through IL-6/STAT3 signaling pathway. Oncotarget. 2017;8:76116–28. https://doi.org/10.18632/oncotarget.18814.

130. Sewell-Loftin MK, et al. Cancer-associated fibroblasts support vascular growth through mechanical force. Scientific Reports. 2017;7(1):12574.

131. Huang B, Huang M, Li Q. Cancer-associated fibroblasts promote angiogenesis of hepatocellular carcinoma by VEGF-mediated EZH2/VASH1 pathway. Technol Cancer Res Treat. 2019;18:1533033819879905.

132. Noma K, et al. The essential role of fibroblasts in esophageal squamous cell carcinoma–induced angiogenesis. Gastroenterology. 2008;134(7):1981–93.

133. Soker S, et al. Neuropilin-1 is expressed by endothelial and tumor cells as an isoform-specific receptor for vascular endothelial growth factor. Cell. 1998;92(6):735–45.

134. Migliozzi MT, Mucka P, Bielenberg DR. Lymphangiogenesis and metastasis—A closer look at the neuropilin/semaphorin3 axis. Microvascular Research. 2014;96:68–76.

135. Armulik A, Genové G, Betsholtz C. Pericytes: developmental, physiological, and pathological perspectives, problems, and promises. Dev Cell. 2011;21(2):193–215.

136. Eberhard A, et al. Heterogeneity of angiogenesis and blood vessel maturation in human tumors: implications for antiangiogenic tumor therapies. Cancer Research. 2000;60(5):1388–93.

137. Wang X, et al. YAP/TAZ orchestrate VEGF signaling during developmental angiogenesis. Dev Cell. 2017;42(5):462–478.e7.

138. Lolo FN, et al. Tumor-stroma biomechanical crosstalk: a perspective on the role of caveolin-1 in tumor progression. Cancer and Metastasis Reviews. 2020;39(2):485–503.

139. Petrova V, et al. The hypoxic tumor microenvironment. Oncogenesis. 2018;7(1):10.

140. Ammirante M, et al. Tissue injury and hypoxia promote malignant progression of prostate cancer by inducing CXCL13 expression in tumor myofibroblasts. Proceedings of the National Academy of Sciences. 2014;111(41):14776–81.

141. Schioppa T, et al. Regulation of the chemokine receptor CXCR4 by hypoxia. Journal of Experimental Medicine. 2003;198(9):1391–402.

142. Schito L, et al. Hypoxia-inducible factor 1-dependent expression of platelet-derived growth factor B promotes lymphatic metastasis of hypoxic breast cancer cells. Proceedings of the National Academy of Sciences. 2012;109(40):E2707–16.

143. Huelsken J, Hanahan D. A subset of cancer-associated fibroblasts determines therapy resistance. Cell. 2018;172(4):643–4.

144. Kanzaki R, Pietras K. Heterogeneity of cancer-associated fibroblasts: Opportunities for precision medicine. Cancer Sci. 2020;111(8):2708–17.

145. Liu T, et al. Cancer-associated fibroblasts: an emerging target of anti-cancer immunotherapy. J Hematol Oncol. 2019;12(1):86.

Stromal PDGF Receptors; Impact on Prognosis and Response to Treatment

Carina Strell and Arne Östman

Abstract

Fibroblasts, vascular smooth muscle cells and pericytes are regulated by members of the PDGF family of growth factors. Through activation of the tyrosine kinase PDGF alpha- and beta-receptors, these growth factors stimulate proliferation and migration of target cells and regulate their contractile capacity. PDGF receptors play major roles during development as regulators of mesenchymal cells involved in paracrine instructive interactions with epithelial or endothelial cells. This chapter is focused on experimental and correlative studies which have explored the biological mechanisms and clinical significance of PDGF receptors in mesenchymal cells of the tumor microenvironment. Collectively these studies support the overall concept that the PDGF system are critical regulators of tumor growth, metastasis and drug efficacy. Furthermore, the independent expression of the two receptors, the inter-case variability and emerging explorative studies indicate potential for development of PDGFRs as biomarkers of clinical utility. Furthermore, PDGFR-beta-specific targeting remains a valid topic for future therapeutic studies that should be performed in selected patient populations.

C. Strell
Department of Immunology, Genetics and Pathology, Uppsala University, Uppsala, Sweden
e-mail: Carina.Strell@igp.uu.se

A. Östman (✉)
Department of Oncology-Pathology, Karolinska Institutet, Stockholm, Sweden
e-mail: Arne.Ostman@ki.se

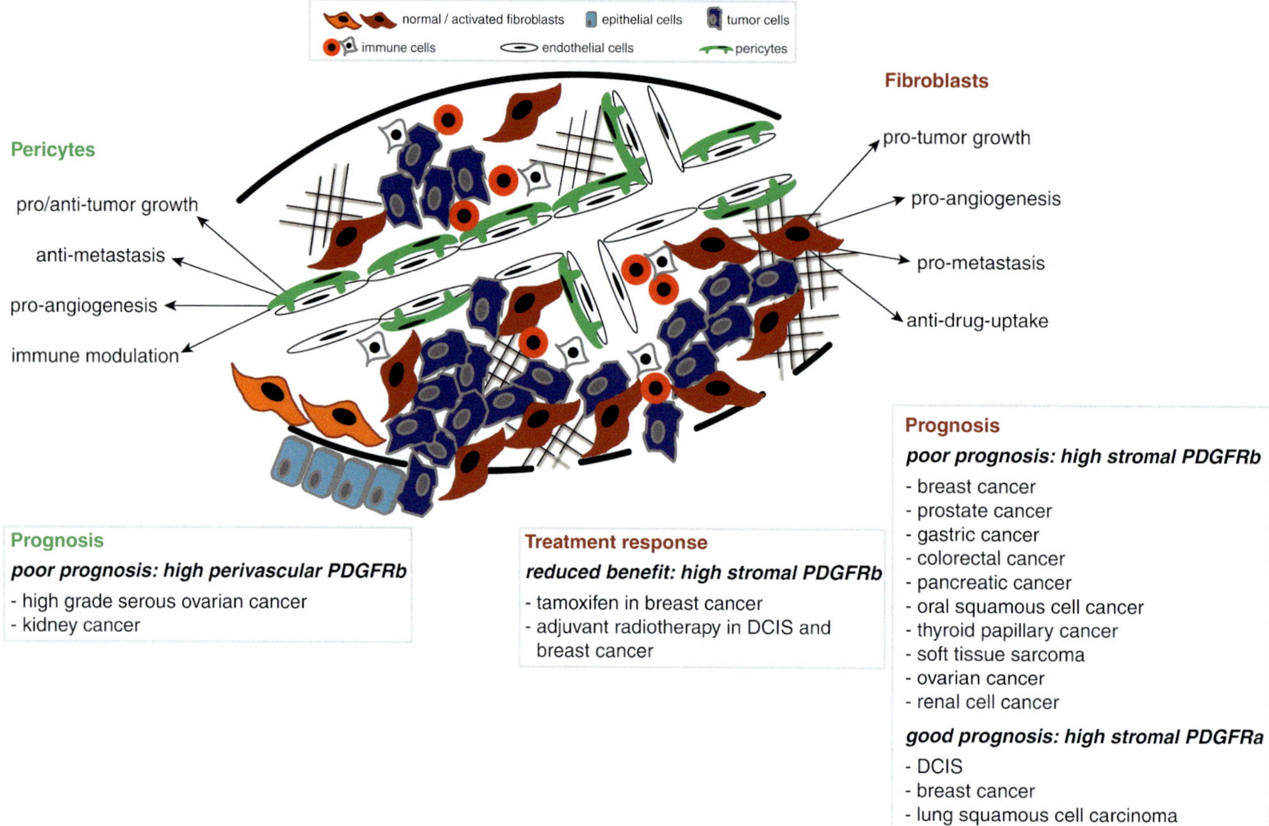

Regulatory roles and prognosis associations of stromal PDGFRb. Figure summarizes functional roles of stromal PDGFRb suggested by experimental studies (upper part) and indicates outcome associations as determined from analyses of clinical samples (lower part). Left part focuses on PDGFRb expressed on pericytes, and right part focuses on PDGFRb expressed on fibroblasts

Take-Home Lessons
- PDGF ligands and cognate tyrosine kinase receptors PDGFR-alpha and PDGFR-beta are important regulators of fibroblasts and pericytes
- PDGFR stimulation of fibroblasts affect multiple aspects of tumor biology including tumor growth, metastasis and tumor drug uptake
- PDGFR-alpha and -beta are independently expressed and their expression is associated with prognosis in many common solid tumor types, including breast and prostate cancer
- Emerging evidence suggest consistent poor prognosis associations of stromal PDGFR-beta expression, whereas PDGFR-alpha expression is possibly associated with good prognosis
- Analyses of randomized-trial-derived tissue collections imply high stromal PDGFR-beta as a biomarker for poor response to radiotherapy in breast DCIS and to tamoxifen in early-stage breast cancer

Introduction

Platelet-derived growth factor (PDGF) is a growth factor family exerting important regulatory functions on glial cells and mesenchymal cells such as fibroblasts, vascular smooth muscle cells and pericytes. First-generation cancer-related studies on PDGF family members focused on the role of oncogenic autocrine PDGF receptor signaling, based on the discovery that one of the classical retroviral oncogenes, v-sis, encoded a variant of the PDGF-B chain [1]. Rare malignancies where PDGF receptors indeed act as oncogenic drivers were identified, some of which are now also treated with PDGF receptor-blocking tyrosine kinase inhibitors such as imatinib (reviewed in [2, 3]). During the last 10–15 years, these studies have shifted focus to analyses focusing on the impact of PDGF receptor signaling in mesenchymal cells of the tumor microenvironment, such as fibroblasts and pericytes.

This chapter aims at giving an updated summary of these studies. The chapter is organized in a manner where findings from experimental studies are discussed in section "Tumor Phenotypes Controlled by PDGF Signaling", whereas analyses of clinical samples exploring biomarker potential of PDGF receptors are discussed in sections "PDGF Receptor Status and Prognosis" and "Stromal PDGF Receptors and Response to Treatment". These core parts of the text are preceded by brief introductions to the molecular biology (section "Receptor Activation and Molecular Signaling Induced by PDGF Ligands") and the developmental and physiological roles (section "Developmental and Physiological Roles of PDGF") of the PDGF system. More detailed discussions of these subtopics of PDGF biology has also been summarized in other reviews [4–9].

Molecular Cell Biology of the PDGF System

PDGF Ligands and Their Receptors

The PDGF-A and -B chains, often referred to as classical PDGFs, were initially identified upon purification from platelets; about 15 years later, the PDGF-C and -D chains were described and are referred to as novel PDGFs [5, 10–15]. The PDGF chains are encoded by four different genes located on different chromosomes in human and mice [7, 10, 16]. Two C-terminal distinct splice variants are described for the PDGF-A chain [12]. The PDGF ligand family is composed of five different PDGF dimers (PDGF-AA, -AB, -BB, -CC and -DD) linked via two inter-chain disulfide bridges in an anti-parallel manner with the conserved receptor-binding cores in each end of the dimer [5, 10, 17].

The bioavailability of PDGF ligands is not only controlled on gene expression level, but also through proteolytical post-translational activation. While PDGF-AA and PDGF-BB are activated in the *trans*-Golgi network by cleavage through proprotein convertases [18, 19], PDGF-CC and PDGF-DD are both secreted as full-length, latent dimers and activated through removal of their autoinhibitory N-terminal CUB domains by extracellular proteases [10, 13, 14, 20–23]. PDGF-A chains derived from the longer splice variant as well as PDGF-B chains hold a C-terminal retention motif, formed by a stretch of basic amino acid residues, which mediate ligand capture to proteoglycans on the cell surface and connected extracellular matrix, thereby specifically restricting ligand exposure to neighboring cells [24, 25].

PDGF ligands exert their biological effects through two structurally related type III receptor tyrosine kinases, the PDGF alpha receptor (PDGFRα) and beta receptor (PDGFRβ) [7, 26]. The receptors can form either homo- or heterodimers [27]. Both receptors are composed of an extracellular region with five Ig-like domains, a single trans-

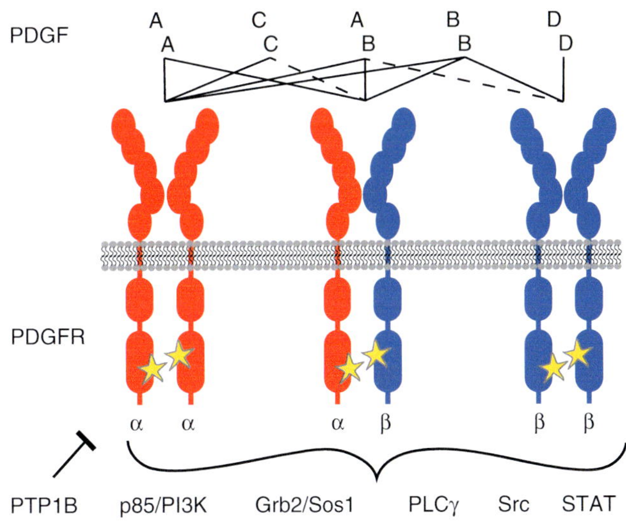

Fig. 8.1 PDGF signaling. The scheme illustrates the interaction between PDGF ligands and receptors as well as downstream signaling pathways

membrane helix region and an intracellular region with a split tyrosine kinase domain [26]. Whereas the intracellular region of the two receptors shows a high degree of conservation, larger differences are observed in the extracellular region involved in ligand binding [10]. PDGF ligands bind to the second and third extracellular Ig-like PDGFR domains causing receptor dimerization [8, 28]. Thereby the different ligands vary in their receptor specificity (Fig. 8.1). Biochemical analyses, including cell culture experiments, as well as phenotype studies in genetically modified mice indicate that PDGF-AA, -AB, -BB and -CC induce PDGFRα homodimers and that PDGF-BB and -DD are high-affinity ligands inducing PDGFRβ homodimers [4, 5, 20]. The physiological presence and role of PDGFRα/β heterodimers are still less characterized.

In cell culture, PDGF stimulation induces cell proliferation, chemotaxis and contraction of collagen matrices. These endpoints have been used in extensive experimental studies to decipher the molecular signal transduction of the PDGF growth factor family.

Receptor Activation and Molecular Signaling Induced by PDGF Ligands

Upon ligand-induced receptor dimerization, interactions via the fourth Ig-domain result in conformational changes that trigger the enzymatic activity of the kinase domain resulting in *trans* phosphorylation of tyrosine residues within the intracellular regions [29–31]. In consequence, as first step of the signal transduction cascade, the intracellular PDGFR regions become docking sites for downstream signaling proteins containing Src homology (SH2) domains [8, 32] (Fig. 8.1). These include adaptor proteins such as the p85 subunit of PI3K, the ras-activating Grb2/Sos1 and Nck, as well as proteins with intrinsic enzymatic activity like c-Src and PLC-gamma [8, 33]. The STAT transcription factor family represents a third class of SH2-domain-containing proteins activated by PDGF receptors [34]. Mechanisms for negative feedback regulation or termination of PDGFR signaling include ligand/receptor internalization and ubiquitin-dependent degradation in lysosomes as well as de-phosphorylation by tyrosine phosphatases including PTP1B, PTP-2C or SHP2 [3, 35–37].

Developmental and Physiological Roles of PDGF

Even though a certain functional redundancy in PDGFR activation and downstream signaling is recognized, developmental in vivo studies point toward crucial differences with regard to their signaling activity. Observed distinct phenotypes in mice lacking either one of the PDGF ligands or receptors might in part be explained by the characteristic, spatiotemporal expression pattern of both ligands and receptors during development and tissue homeostasis. Collectively, the theme emerging from these studies is a niche-specific paracrine signaling with PDGF ligands produced by the epithelial/endothelial cells that stimulate recruitment and proliferation of juxtaposed PDGFR-expressing mesenchymal cells.

Developmental Roles of PDGFRα, PDGF-AA and PDGF-CC/Epithelial–Mesenchymal Interactions

PDGF-A and PDGF-C are expressed by epithelial cells as well as certain muscular and neuronal cells (reviewed in [6, 38]). A particular paracrine PDGFRα signaling dependency during organ development was found in the lung, gastrointestinal tract, testis, skin and central nervous system (CNS) [5, 38]. A global knock-out of PDGF-A in mice is generally lethal, though a few mice survive postnatally with severe developmental defects. The lungs of these mice showed morphologic abnormal, enlarged alveoli with an emphysema-like phenotype, caused by the absence of PDGFRα-positive myofibroblasts in the walls of alveolar saccules [39, 40]. Conversely, lung-specific over-expression of PDGF-A resulted in a thickened mesenchymal layer through hyper-

proliferation of alveolar smooth muscle cell progenitors [41]. Overall, PDGFRα-positive fibroblasts in the murine lung were found to represent a heterogenous cell population including airway smooth muscle cells, interstitial myo- as well as matrix fibroblasts, which, depending on their spatial and temporal niche context, differ in their functionality regarding lung epithelial regulation [42, 43]. *Pdgfa* knock-out mice displayed further reduced formation and misshapen of intestinal villi together with a loss of pericryptal mesenchyme [44].

Later studies identified Wnt ligands and R-spondins derived from pericryptal PDGFRα-positive myofibroblasts as crucial regulators of crypt cell proliferation [45, 46]. A thinner dermis with defect hair follicles due to disruption of the dermal mesenchyme was also noted in *Pdgfa* knock-out mice [47]. Together these phenotypes suggest a critical role of paracrine PDGFRα signaling for the recruitment and maintenance of mesenchymal cells lining the basement membrane and their role in epithelial-instructive functions during organ development and tissue homeostasis. Outside the context of mesenchymal/epithelial interactions, PDGFRα/PDGF-A has also been shown to participate in CNS development by regulation of oligodendrocytes progenitor migration [48, 49] as well as the postnatal development of white adipose tissue [50] and the regeneration of skeletal muscle [51]. Interestingly, global *Pdgfc* knock-out mice also displayed severe developmental defects in different organs, but the phenotypes differed from PDGF-A knock-out and affected organs were mostly the skeleton, palate, CNS and skin [52–54]. As expected, observed phenotypes in *Pdgfra* knock-out mice were more severe than those observed in knock-out mice of either one of the ligands alone [54, 55].

Developmental Roles of PDGFRβ and PDGF-B and PDGF-D/Blood Vessel–Mural Cell Interactions

PDGF-B is expressed by endothelial cells in particular during angiogenic sprouting, while PDGFRβ is expressed on adjacent mural cells, namely, vascular smooth muscle cells and pericytes, but also fibroblasts (reviewed in [6, 38]). The expression pattern of PDGF-D is less well characterized, but evidence was provided for a distinct expression in arterioles, both on endothelial cells and on certain mural cell subsets, suggesting a paracrine as well as autocrine signaling network [56]. Of note, the human immunoreceptor NKp44, encoded by the *NCR2* gene, was described to recognize PDGF-DD inducing the secretion of interferon gamma and tumor necrosis factor alpha from natural killer cells [57].

In line with the described expression pattern, the observed phenotypes of *Pdgfrb* and *Pdgfb* knock-out mice support the PDGFRβ axis as a key-player in the recruitment and function of vascular mural cells [5, 38]. Both knock-out models are lethal at late embryonic stages due to widespread microvascular bleedings associated with reduced pericyte coverage, endothelial hyperplasia and abnormal capillary morphogenesis [58–62]. Interestingly, deletion of the C-terminal retention motif impacted the short-range action of PDGF-B and was sufficient to cause pericytes to detach from endothelial cells [63]. Disturbance in the PDGF-BB ligand presentation were also observed during adipose tissue expansion in a diet-induced obesity mouse model, where infiltrating M1macrophages into the obese adipose tissue were identified as a major source of PDGF-BB causing pericytes to detach from vessels [64]. These studies indicate that ligand source and presentation must act in concert to preserve pericyte recruitment. However, it was noted that mural cells within different organ sites were differently affected by the depletion of *pdgfb* or *pdgfrb* [38, 65]. This intriguing observation is the basis for ongoing efforts to better define and functionally characterize endothelial and mural cell subpopulations. The importance of the PDGF-B/PDGFRβ axis for vascular function has also been supported by human genetics data upon the identification of loss-of-function mutations of PDGF-B and PDGFRβ in familial idiopathic ganglia calcification and the concomitant demonstration of vascular defects in the etiology of the disease (reviewed in [66]).

Physiological and Pathophysiological Roles of PDGFs

The regulation of epithelial/endothelial folding and differentiation in specific niches during development and tissue homeostasis may be considered as a common trait across the PDGF growth factor family. The PDGF-A/PDGFRα epithelial–mesenchymal interaction axis is a crucial actor at folding sites of large specialized epithelial surfaces. It was suggested that this view could be extended to the PDGF-B/PDGFRβ endothelium–mural cell axis, namely, at sites of formation of large specialized vascular surfaces [38]. Ongoing research efforts employing single-cell sequencing techniques, advanced spatial mapping approaches and cell-type-specific knock-out mice models aim to decipher common as well as organ-specific traits of PDGF ligand or receptor expressing cells and to identify novel, regulatory cellular subsets in their corresponding niches.

Given the essential functions of PDGF ligands and receptors in normal physiology, dysregulation of PDGFRs was linked to several pathological conditions. Deregulation of the PDGFRα axis often is associated with not only fibrotic pro-

cesses such as pulmonary or dermal fibrosis [67–70] as well as obesity-induced white adipose tissue fibrosis [71] but also inflammatory processes such as inflammatory bowel disease, where an activation of the pericryptal, PDGFRα-positive mesenchymal niche was found to impair epithelial proliferation and maturation likely through secretion of IL6 and IL33 [46]. Deregulation of the PDGFRβ axis is commonly linked to numerous cardiovascular diseases such as atherosclerosis [72, 73], restenosis [74], stroke [75], as well as aortic aneurysm [76, 77] or pulmonary hypertension [78, 79]. The prominent role of the PDGF signaling network during development and tissue homeostasis has further encouraged numerous experimental studies and tissue-based analyses in order to investigate its role in cancer development and progression.

Tumor Phenotypes Controlled by PDGF Signaling

The following paragraphs summarize findings from experimental studies, which in concert indicate that paracrine PDGF signaling not only impacts primary tumor growth, metastasis and immune surveillance but also negatively regulates the uptake and efficacy of systemically delivered drugs (Fig. 8.2).

PDGF Signaling in Tumor Biology

First evidence for a supportive effect of paracrine PDGF signaling on tumor formation and growth was provided through in vivo models with PDGF-BB over-expressing melanoma cells, negative for PDGF receptors [80]. Although the detailed molecular mechanisms were not revealed in these initial studies, histologic analyses suggested that the growth advantage was related to increased angiogenesis and recruitment of tumor-supportive fibroblasts.

Follow-up studies using similar experimental approaches relying on over-expression of PDGF ligands in receptor-negative cells, also demonstrated tumor growth stimulatory effects for different PDGF ligands in models of e.g. skin, breast and lung cancer, in a manner associated with fibroblast recruitment [81–85]. Recruited fibroblasts secrete various growth factors, which support tumor growth, including FGF2 [86], CXCL12 [87] or HGF [88]. In line with those findings, pharmacological inhibitors of PDGFR signaling showed therapeutic effects in a genetic mouse model of cervical cancer [86].

Furthermore, pro-metastatic effects of PDGF-activated fibroblasts have been observed in different mouse models. The receptor tyrosine kinase inhibitor imatinib mesylate,

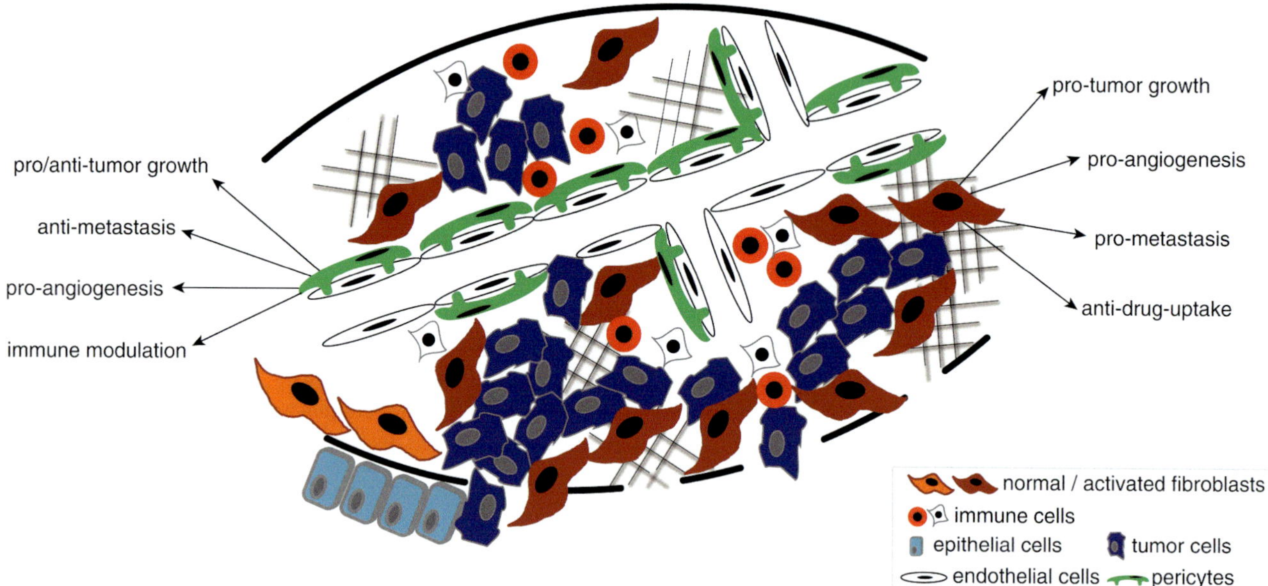

Fig. 8.2 Impact of stromal PDGF signaling on different aspects of tumor biology. The scheme summarizes findings from experimental in vitro and in vivo studies, on how paracrine PDGF signaling in peri-cytes and fibroblasts not only impacts tumor growth, metastasis, angiogenesis and immune surveillance but also negatively regulates the uptake and efficacy of systemically delivered drugs

which blocks both PDGFRs among others, significantly reduced metastasis formation in an orthotopic colorectal cancer model notably without major effects on primary tumor growth [89]. Mechanistic details were demonstrated in experimental tissue culture studies showing that PDGF-BB-stimulated fibroblasts enhance the migratory and invasive capacities of colorectal cancer cells and identifying PDGF-induced Stanniocalcin-1 (STC1) secretion as one critical component of this paracrine pathway [90]. Subsequent mouse model studies provided independent evidence for paracrine, pro-metastatic effects of fibroblast-derived STC1. It was further demonstrated that PDGF-BB-stimulated fibroblasts exhibit pro-metastatic capacities already at early stages of different tumor types using a co-implantation zebrafish model for cancer metastasis [91].

Important roles for stromal PDGF signaling in determining drug efficacy have also been postulated based on findings from mouse model studies. Initial observations in edema models noted that PDGFRβ signaling in fibroblasts increased the interstitial fluid pressure (IFP) and thereby reduced edema (reviewed in [92]). This finding initiated a series of cancer model studies, testing the hypothesis that increased tumor IFP is associated with reduced tumor drug uptake and could be overcome by targeting of stromal PDGFRs. Consistent with a role of PDGF signaling for tumoral IFP, these studies using different combination of tumor models and PDGFR inhibitors demonstrated that PDGFR inhibition indeed increased tumor drug uptake and the therapeutic efficacy of systemically delivered drugs [93–96]. Notably, the efficacy-enhancing effect of PDGF inhibitors was observed in approaches using standard chemotherapy agents including 5-FU and taxol, as well as macromolecules such as radio-labeled tumor-targeted antibodies. However, the exact molecular mechanistic relationships between PDGFR inhibition and reduced IFP as well as tumor response to chemotherapy treatment remain uncertain. One limiting factor is that inhibitors applied in experimental studies are not completely specific and often target both PDGFRα and -β. Additional studies in this area appear therefore motivated. Such studies should also aim to decipher the differential roles of PDGFRα and PDGFRβ signaling in tumor biology.

PDGFRα on Fibroblasts

The specific impact of PDGFRα-positive fibroblasts on cancer progression was analyzed in a series of breast cancer studies. Interestingly, those studies commonly identified a decrease of stromal PDGFRα expression or, respectively, a decrease in abundance of PDGFRα-positive fibroblasts with the progression from early stage to invasive cancer [97–99]. Analyses of breast ductal carcinoma in situ (DCIS) lesions implied an activation of peri-glandular fibroblasts at sites of basement membrane disruptions, a critical step in the conversion from DCIS to invasive cancer [97]. Notably, fibroblast-activation mediated DCIS-induced re-programming of mesenchymal cells via Notch signaling causing a downregulation of PDGFRα and an up-regulation of PDGFRβ and TGF-beta ligands in the affected fibroblasts. Another study reported the accumulation of PDGFRα-negative bone marrow-derived fibroblasts at the primary tumor as well as the metastatic sites of the MMTV-PyMT transgenic mouse breast cancer model, leading to a percentual decrease of resident, PDGFRα-positive fibroblasts [99]. The PDGFRα-negative fibroblasts enhanced tumor growth and angiogenesis. Single-cell sequencing of fibroblasts from this model confirmed the presence of a PDGFRα-negative fibroblast population with an angiogenic gene expression signature, as well as the presence of PDGFRα-positive fibroblasts with a matrix-remodeling-associated expression profile, resembling resident fibroblasts [98].

However, evidence is also provided that stromal PDGFRα expression can vary between different breast cancer subtypes. A paracrine cross-talk between PDGF-CC-expressing breast cancer cells and PDGFRα-positive cancer-associated fibroblasts was identified in human basal-like mammary carcinomas. PDGF-CC-activated fibroblasts expressed and secreted HGF, IGFBP3 and STC-1, of which, in particular, HGF had been previously associated to the induction of a basal-like epithelial/tumor cell fate [100]. Pharmacological intervention of this cross-talk converted the basal-like histological subtype toward a hormone receptor-positive state, sensitive to endocrine therapy, thereby highlighting a potential role of PDGF signaling in the regulation of tumor phenotypes. It will be interesting to follow upcoming studies, transferring and testing these findings in different tumor types.

PDGFRβ on Perivascular Cells

The developmental biology-based evidence linking PDGFRβ to pericyte recruitment and function, together with the recognition of the importance of angiogenesis in tumor progression, motivated studies on the role of perivascular PDGFRβ signaling as regulator of tumor angiogenesis. This concept was firstly tested using the hypomorphic PDGFB-ret/ret mouse model, which expresses a truncated form of PDGF-B, lacking the C-terminal retention motif, resulting in reduced pericyte coverage. Tumor transplants in these mice showed pericyte detachment from the vessel walls, larger tumor vessel diameter and hemorrhaging, which suggested PDGF-BB/PDGFRβ as promising, potential therapeutical target [101]. In accordance, over-expression of PDGFRβ ligands in mouse melanoma cells enhanced tumor growth in vivo, with a vascular phenotype showing increased pericyte coverage, but unchanged vessel density [102]. Later, genetic mouse model studies combining VEGFR- and PDGFRβ-inhibitors promoted forward a concept of pro-tumoral effects of PDGFRβ-positive perivascular cells mediated through tumor vessel stabilization [103]. The efficacy of VEGFR inhibitors though was found to be either un-affected or increased upon disturbance of PDGFRβ signaling in pericytes [103, 104]. However, the general significance of these findings have been challenged in more recent studies in other cancer models, where a high perivascular PDGFRβ status was instead associated with reduced tumor growth, thus implying stage- and tumor type-specific effects [105, 106].

The impact of perivascular PDGFRβ status on tumor metastasis has been experimentally explored in studies, which have used suicide-gene-mediated depletion of PDGFRβ-positive pericytes [107, 108]. In both studies, loss of PDGFRβ-positive perivascular cells induced a prometastatic tumor phenotype, including increased hypoxia, c-Met-dependent tumor cell stimulation and increased Angiopoietin-2-dependent angiogenesis.

It should also be mentioned that associations between vessel coverage and tumor immune surveillance have been noted. Flow cytometric analyses of tumors formed in the PDGFB-ret/ret mouse model displayed an increased tumoral infiltration of immune-inhibitory MDSCs together with a reduced T-cell infiltration and an immune-signature besides the histologically described angiogenic defects [109], a finding that implies reduced anti-tumoral immune activity. It is intriguing to suggest follow-up studies to analyze the impact and association of the perivascular status and the response to immune therapy.

PDGF Receptor Status and Prognosis

Experimental studies, detailed above, have implicated PDGF receptors as important stimulatory molecules for fibroblasts and perivascular cells. In parallel, tumor microenvironment studies have demonstrated that stromal cells contribute to tumor progression by interactions with both epithelial cells and immune cells. Together, these research areas have prompted a series of studies which have analyzed potential associations between stromal PDGFR status and survival in different tumor types. Differential expression of the two PDGF receptors has indeed been identified in tumor stroma of clinical samples. An important finding that is merging from these studies is that the two PDGFRs are independently expressed and that different cell populations exist expressing either only PDGFRα, only PDGFRβ or both receptors (Fig. 8.3).

Most of these studies have used conventional immunohistochemistry with antibodies recognizing PDGFRα or -β, together with manual semi-quantitative scoring of stromal expression. However, a small number of studies have also been performed in which these antibodies have been used together with digital-image-analyses-based scoring [110–112]. These novel methods, in addition to giving quantitative data, have also allowed differential analyses of PDGF

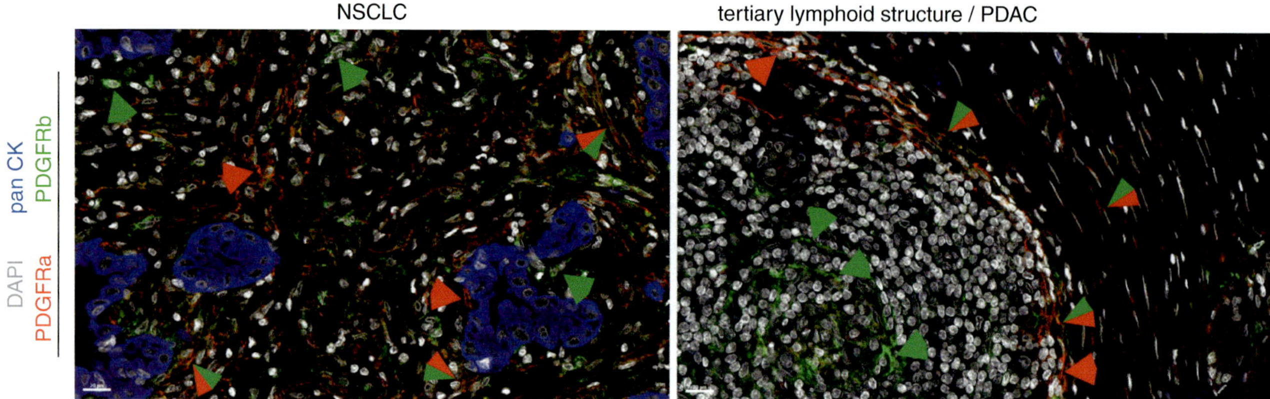

Fig. 8.3 PDGFR expression in tumor stroma. Multiplex immunofluorescence for PDGFRα (red) and PDGFRβ (green) of FFPE sections from non-small-cell lung cancer (NSCLC) and pancreatic ductal adenocarcinoma (PDAC). Tumor cells were stained with pan cytokeratin (blue), and DAPI-stained nuclei are pictured in white. Arrowheads indicate the presence of stroma cells single positive for either PDGFRα or -β (single color arrowheads) as well as double positive (red/green arrowheads). Scale bar represents 20 μm

receptor expression in perivascular areas and in fibroblast-dominated tumor regions.

Some studies have employed phosphoPDGFR antibodies to monitor expression of activated receptors [113], although concerns have been raised regarding the specificity of these reagents. A proximity ligation assay for detection of phosphorylated PDGFRs has also been described [114–116] but not yet used to report on stromal PDGFR status. A shared problem for these two approaches is the sensitivity to artifacts caused by tissue handling affecting protein phosphorylation.

PDGFRβ status in clinical samples has also, in addition to these protein-based assays, been determined by bioinformatics-based approaches. In these analyses, a "PDGFRβ-signature", derived from PDGF-BB-activated cultured fibroblasts, was used to analyze a number of different breast cancer gene-expression data sets [117]. The following paragraphs discuss results from these analyses with subsections focusing on, first, fibroblast expression of PDGFRs and, second, perivascular PDGFR expression.

PDGF-R Expression in Stromal Fibroblasts

Prognostic relevance of stromal PDGFRβ expression in breast cancer was initially described through analyses of a population-based cohort of more than 500 cases and uncovered significant associations between high stromal expression and shorter recurrence-free and breast cancer-specific survival based on univariate analyses [118]. The study also identified strong correlations between stromal PDGFRβ and poor prognosis markers such as high grade, high proliferation and HER2 amplification. Additional subsequent studies have provided overall support for these findings, by detecting shorter survival associations or links to other poor prognosis factors, through IHC studies in various cohorts, including tumor collections derived from randomized clinical trials [119–121].

Strong and robust signals linking stromal PDGFRβ signaling to poor prognosis in breast cancer were also obtained in a gene-signature study, in which a tissue-culture-derived PDGFRβ signature was used [117]. Four different breast cancer cohorts were used to dichotomize cases into "high-signature-score" and "low-signature-score" groups. Consistent associations were detected between high signature score and poor prognosis using recurrence-free survival or disease-specific survival/overall survival as endpoints. Importantly, significant prognostic association was also detected in multivariate analyses using standard clinicopathological characteristics (HR 1.2–1.3) or other stroma-related signatures (HR 1.3–1.6).

Two independent studies have also identified poor prognosis associations of stromal PDGFRβ in prostate cancer [122, 123]. Both studies, consisting of ~250 and 500 cases, respectively, identified significant associations between PDGFRβ and outcome endpoints such as biochemical relapse or cancer-specific survival. Interestingly, one of the studies also noted similar associations when PDGFRβ was scored in histologically normal prostate tissue from these cases [123].

Other conventional IHC studies have also demonstrated associations between high PDGFRβ and poor prognosis in gastric, colorectal, pancreatic, oral squamous cell and thyroid papillary cancers [124–128]. Analyses of rhabdomyosarcoma indicate that stromal PDGFRβ is also relevant for prognosis in soft tissue sarcomas through findings of significant associations between stromal PDGFRβ and development of distant metastasis [129].

In addition to these conventional IHC studies, analyses have been performed where stromal PDGFRβ status has been determined following IHC analyses and digital-image-analyses-supported automated scoring. These studies have provided novel data from ovarian and renal cell cancer showing that, also in these tumor types, high stromal/fibroblast PDGFRβ expression is associated with poor prognosis ([110]; Frödin et al., pers. comm.). In the case of ovarian cancer, the signal from univariate analyses was maintained in multivariate analyses. High PDGFRβ expression thus appears to be consistently associated with poor prognosis.

With regard to PDGFRα, less information is available [130]. Some tissue culture studies have shown that PDGFRα is down-regulated upon activation of fibroblasts by TGF-beta [131]. It is therefore possible that PDGFRα expression marks a resting, and possibly growth restraining, fibroblast population. Some studies are indeed suggesting that PDGFRα, in contrast to PDGFRβ, is associated with good prognosis. Analyses of two large DCIS cohorts demonstrated good prognosis trends for PDGFRα and could identify a poor-prognosis-associated phenotype with high PDGFRβ expression combined with low PDGFRα expression [97]. In general agreement with these findings, good prognosis associations have also been independently described for PDGFRα in invasive breast cancer [99]. Finally, analyses of the squamous cell carcinoma (SCC) subgroups of two population-based non-small-cell lung cancer cohorts have also identified association between high PDGFRα and good prognosis [132].

Perivascular PDGFRβ Expression

Perivascular cells exert important regulatory functions affecting vascular biology which in turn impact on normal physiology and the pathophysiology of tumors [133]. Based on the established role of PDGFRβ as a key regulator of pericytes (see above), studies have been initiated exploring potential inter- and intra-case heterogeneity of perivascular PDGFRβ status and associations with other vascular features, clinicopathological characteristics and survival.

Significant associations between poor prognosis and high perivascular PDGFRβ expression have been documented in high-grade serous ovarian cancer and kidney cancer [110, 112]. Both these studies used automated quantitative scoring, and the significant associations between high perivascular PDGFRβ and shorter survival were maintained in multivariate analyses.

Stromal PDGF Receptors and Response to Treatment

Preclinical evidence, as outlined above, has suggested multiple mechanisms whereby either fibroblast or perivascular PDGFRβ signaling could affect efficacy of chemotherapy and VEGF-directed anti-angiogenic therapy. Analyses of stromal PDGFRs in well-annotated tumor collections thus have the potential to uncover clinically meaningful predictive markers. Promising results from such efforts have recently been obtained in the setting of adjuvant tamoxifen treatment of early breast cancer [120]. This study relied on analyses of tumor tissue collected from women participating in two positive adjuvant tamoxifen studies recruiting pre- and post-menopausal women [134, 135]. For the biomarker study, cases were dichotomized based on stromal PDGFRβ expression. In the pre-menopausal cohort, the low-stromal PDGFRβ group displayed a significant benefit of tamoxifen with regard to recurrence-free survival. In contrast, no significant effects were detected in the high-stromal PDGFRβ group. Analysis of the postmenopausal cohort yielded results with similar trends. When analyses were restricted to cases with >75% ER-positivity, stromal PDGFRβ status divided the cohort into one "PDGFRβ-low" group that showed significant benefit and a second nonresponsive "PDGFRβ-high" group.

Additional evidence implying potential of PDGFRβ as a clinically relevant predictive biomarker has been obtained from analyses of tissue collections of a randomized trial exploring efficacy of post-surgery radiotherapy (RT) in breast DCIS [136]. Strong RT effects were detected in the low-stromal PDGFRβ group (HR 0.23 for ipsilateral recurrences), whereas RT did not show any significant effect in the high-stromal PDGFRβ group (HR 0.83). Furthermore, significant interactions were detected between marker and treatment in adjusted formal interaction tests.

Future Perspectives

Findings from the experimental interaction and correlative studies on the roles of PDGF receptor signaling in tumor stroma set the stage for continued analyses and exploration of this growth factor system. A series of questions are suggested by recent findings concerning biological mechanisms. Improved methods for monitoring of PDGF receptor status in clinical samples should facilitate development toward use of these molecules as clinical biomarkers. Finally, therapeutic targeting of stromal PDGF receptors in selected patient populations still appears as a viable research goal.

Concerning tumor biology, a series of questions are raised by the accumulating evidence for clinically relevant inter-case variability in the expression of perivascular and fibroblast expression of PDGFRα and -β. As of the writing of this chapter, the underlying basis for this variability remain unknown. Interesting possibilities to follow-up are the implications that cells with different PDGFR profile have differential cell-of-origin as suggested by some mouse studies [99]. Furthermore, paracrine pathways governing PDGFR expression, as the Jagged1/Notch2 pathway identified in breast DCIS [97], should be better defined. A key task for future studies is thus to, first, identify the molecular regulatory systems controlling PDGF receptor expression and, second, to address the fundamental question about relative contribution of host and cancer genetics in the inter-patient heterogeneity. The relationships between receptor-positive fibroblasts/CAFs and perivascular cells should also be better resolved. Emerging evidence for strong intra-case correlations between PDGFR status in fibroblasts and perivascular cells suggests that these cells might share a common cell-of-origin, which should be further explored. This notion is also supported by emerging studies identifying subpopulations of pericyte-like cells with non-perivascular locations [137]. Further studies addressing biological and prognostic differences between the two PDGF receptors are warranted and will possibly be guided by refined analyses of differential instructive roles of PDGFRα and -β during development. Notably, detailed analyses of stem-cell niches are identifying fibroblast subsets with distinct and different abilities to support stem cells or induce epithelial differentiation [138].

Future analyses of clinical cohorts are likely to benefit from improvements in methodology for analyses of PDGF receptor status. Signals linking PDGF receptor status to prognosis or response to treatment might be enhanced in analyses which integrate further spatial information in scoring algorithms such as the relative position of positive cells to epithelial or immune cells. In this context, applications of novel methodologies allowing highly multiplexed spatial tissue profiling are valuable novel resources [139, 140]. Advances allowing scoring of activated versus nonactivated receptors also appear as an important task which can possibly be achieved by assays specifically detecting activated dimeric receptors or multi-probe in situ profiling with PDGFR-activation-associated genes. Improved possibilities for PDGFR profiling of metastatic lesions might depend on noninvasive modalities. Eventually, this can be achieved with PET imaging combined with radiotracers such as derivatives of the preclinically validated PDGFRβ "affibody" [141].

The appearance of studies, relying on well-annotated tumor collections from randomized trials, implying response-predictive significance of stromal PDGFR status is very encouraging [119, 120, 136]. Continued efforts on other tumor collections, including those derived from immune-therapy trials, are expected to occur in upcoming years. Possibly, these studies will also exploit the novel multiplex methodologies to quantitate subsets of PDGF-Ra- or PDGFRβ-positive cells defined also by expression of other markers. Another important topic where progress is also expected and highly needed is PDGFR status in the tumor microenvironment of metastasis from analyses of primary tumors.

In addition to the biomarker potential, stromal PDGF receptors also remain interesting candidates for therapeutic targeting. Recent findings implying PDGFRα and -β in distinct biological processes provide a rational for development of isoform-specific antagonists, possibly including monoclonal antibodies. The inter-case variability in PDGFR status, now well established as outlined above, strongly suggests that potential upcoming PDGFR antagonists should be used in settings where patient populations have been well selected. Hopefully, results from such efforts will be reported during the upcoming 5-year period.

References

1. Doolittle RF, Hunkapiller MW, Hood LE, Devare SG, Robbins KC, Aaronson SA, et al. Simian sarcoma virus onc gene, v-sis, is derived from the gene (or genes) encoding a platelet-derived growth factor. Science. 1983;221:275–7.
2. Ehnman M, Östman A. Therapeutic targeting of platelet-derived growth factor receptors in solid tumors. Expert Opin Investig Drugs. 2014;23:211–26.
3. Heldin C-H. Targeting the PDGF signaling pathway in tumor treatment. Cell Commun Signal. 2013;11:97.
4. Heldin CH, Ostman A, Rönnstrand L. Signal transduction via platelet-derived growth factor receptors. Biochim Biophys Acta. 1998;1378:F79–113.
5. Andrae J, Gallini R, Betsholtz C. Role of platelet-derived growth factors in physiology and medicine. Genes Dev. 2008;22:1276–312.
6. Hoch RV, Soriano P. Roles of PDGF in animal development. Development. 2003;130:4769–84.
7. Kazlauskas A. PDGFs and their receptors. Gene. 2017;614:1–7.
8. Heldin C-H, Lennartsson J. Structural and functional properties of platelet-derived growth factor and stem cell factor receptors. Cold Spring Harb Perspect Biol. 2013;5:a009100.
9. Östman A. PDGF receptors in tumor stroma: biological effects and associations with prognosis and response to treatment. Adv Drug Deliv Rev. 2017;121:117–23.
10. Fredriksson L, Li H, Eriksson U. The PDGF family: four gene products form five dimeric isoforms. Cytokine Growth Factor Rev. 2004;15:197–204.
11. Johnsson A, Heldin CH, Westermark B, Wasteson A. Platelet-derived growth factor: identification of constituent polypeptide chains. Biochem Biophys Res Commun. 1982;104:66–74.
12. Betsholtz C, Johnsson A, Heldin CH, Westermark B, Lind P, Urdea MS, et al. cDNA sequence and chromosomal localization of human platelet-derived growth factor A-chain and its expression in tumour cell lines. Nature. 1986;320:695–9.
13. Li X, Pontén A, Aase K, Karlsson L, Abramsson A, Uutela M, et al. PDGF-C is a new protease-activated ligand for the PDGF α-receptor. Nat Cell Biol. 2000;2:302–9. Nature
14. Bergsten E, Uutela M, Li X, Pietras K, Östman A, Heldin C-H, et al. PDGF-D is a specific, protease-activated ligand for the PDGF β-receptor. Nat Cell Biol. 2001;3:512–6. Nature
15. LaRochelle WJ, Jeffers M, McDonald WF, Chillakuru RA, Giese NA, Lokker NA, et al. PDGF-D, a new protease-activated growth factor. Nat Cell Biol. 2001;3:517–21.
16. Bonner JC. Platelet-derived growth factor. In: Laurent GJ, Shapiro SD, editors. Encyclopedia of respiratory medicine [Internet]. Oxford: Academic; 2006. p. 343–7 [cited 18 May 2021]. Available from: https://www.sciencedirect.com/science/article/pii/B0123708796002970

17. Ostman A, Andersson M, Bäckström G, Heldin CH. Assignment of intrachain disulfide bonds in platelet-derived growth factor B-chain. J Biol Chem. 1993;268:13372–7.
18. Siegfried G, Basak A, Prichett-Pejic W, Scamuffa N, Ma L, Benjannet S, et al. Regulation of the stepwise proteolytic cleavage and secretion of PDGF-B by the proprotein convertases. Oncogene. 2005;24:6925–35.
19. Siegfried G, Khatib A-M, Benjannet S, Chrétien M, Seidah NG. The proteolytic processing of pro-platelet-derived growth factor-A at RRKR(86) by members of the proprotein convertase family is functionally correlated to platelet-derived growth factor-A-induced functions and tumorigenicity. Cancer Res. 2003;63:1458–63.
20. Fredriksson L, Ehnman M, Fieber C, Eriksson U. Structural requirements for activation of latent platelet-derived growth factor CC by tissue plasminogen activator. J Biol Chem. 2005;280:26856–62.
21. Ehnman M, Li H, Fredriksson L, Pietras K, Eriksson U. The uPA/uPAR system regulates the bioavailability of PDGF-DD: implications for tumour growth. Oncogene. 2009;28:534–44.
22. Ustach CV, Kim H-RC. Platelet-derived growth factor D is activated by urokinase plasminogen activator in prostate carcinoma cells. Mol Cell Biol. 2005;25:6279–88.
23. Ustach CV, Huang W, Conley-LaComb MK, Lin C-Y, Che M, Abrams J, et al. A novel signaling axis of matriptase/PDGF-D/ß--PDGFR in human prostate cancer. Cancer Res. 2010;70:9631–40.
24. Ostman A, Andersson M, Betsholtz C, Westermark B, Heldin CH. Identification of a cell retention signal in the B-chain of platelet-derived growth factor and in the long splice version of the A-chain. Cell Regul. 1991;2:503–12.
25. Betsholtz C, Rorsman F, Westermark B, Ostman A, Heldin CH. Analogous alternative splicing. Nature. 1990;344:299.
26. Claesson-Welsh L, Eriksson A, Westermark B, Heldin CH. cDNA cloning and expression of the human A-type platelet-derived growth factor (PDGF) receptor establishes structural similarity to the B-type PDGF receptor. Proc Natl Acad Sci U S A. 1989;86:4917–21.
27. Heldin CH, Westermark B. Mechanism of action and in vivo role of platelet-derived growth factor. Physiol Rev. 1999;79:1283–316.
28. Miyazawa K, Bäckström G, Leppänen O, Persson C, Wernstedt C, Hellman U, et al. Role of immunoglobulin-like domains 2-4 of the platelet-derived growth factor alpha-receptor in ligand-receptor complex assembly. J Biol Chem. 1998;273:25495–502.
29. Omura T, Heldin CH, Ostman A. Immunoglobulin-like domain 4-mediated receptor-receptor interactions contribute to platelet-derived growth factor-induced receptor dimerization. J Biol Chem. 1997;272:12676–82.
30. Baxter RM, Secrist JP, Vaillancourt RR, Kazlauskas A. Full activation of the platelet-derived growth factor beta-receptor kinase involves multiple events. J Biol Chem. 1998;273:17050–5.
31. Kazlauskas A, Cooper JA. Autophosphorylation of the PDGF receptor in the kinase insert region regulates interactions with cell proteins. Cell. 1989;58:1121–33.
32. Kazlauskas A, Durden DL, Cooper JA. Functions of the major tyrosine phosphorylation site of the PDGF receptor beta subunit. Cell Regul. 1991;2:413–25.
33. Basciani S, Mariani S, Spera G, Gnessi L. Role of platelet-derived growth factors in the testis. Endocr Rev. 2010;31:916–39.
34. Vignais ML, Sadowski HB, Watling D, Rogers NC, Gilman M. Platelet-derived growth factor induces phosphorylation of multiple JAK family kinases and STAT proteins. Mol Cell Biol. 1996;16:1759–69.
35. Heldin C-H, Lennartsson J, Westermark B. Involvement of platelet-derived growth factor ligands and receptors in tumorigenesis. J Intern Med. 2018;283:16–44.
36. Goh LK, Sorkin A. Endocytosis of receptor tyrosine kinases. Cold Spring Harb Perspect Biol [Internet]. 2013;5 [cited 18 May 2021]. Available from: https://www.ncbi.nlm.nih.gov/pmc/articles/PMC3632065/
37. Levkowitz G, Waterman H, Ettenberg SA, Katz M, Tsygankov AY, Alroy I, et al. Ubiquitin ligase activity and tyrosine phosphorylation underlie suppression of growth factor signaling by c-Cbl/Sli-1. Mol Cell. 1999;4:1029–40.
38. Betsholtz C. Insight into the physiological functions of PDGF through genetic studies in mice. Cytokine Growth Factor Rev. 2004;15:215–28.
39. Lindahl P, Karlsson L, Hellström M, Gebre-Medhin S, Willetts K, Heath JK, et al. Alveogenesis failure in PDGF-A-deficient mice is coupled to lack of distal spreading of alveolar smooth muscle cell progenitors during lung development. Development. 1997;124:3943–53.
40. Boström H, Willetts K, Pekny M, Levéen P, Lindahl P, Hedstrand H, et al. PDGF-A signaling is a critical event in lung alveolar myofibroblast development and alveogenesis. Cell. 1996;85:863–73.
41. Li J, Hoyle GW. Overexpression of PDGF-A in the lung epithelium of transgenic mice produces a lethal phenotype associated with hyperplasia of mesenchymal cells. Dev Biol. 2001;239:338–49.
42. Endale M, Ahlfeld S, Bao E, Chen X, Green J, Bess Z, et al. Temporal, spatial, and phenotypical changes of PDGFRα expressing fibroblasts during late lung development. Dev Biol. 2017;425:161–75.
43. Zepp JA, Zacharias WJ, Frank DB, Cavanaugh CA, Zhou S, Morley MP, et al. Distinct mesenchymal lineages and niches promote epithelial self-renewal and myofibrogenesis in the lung. Cell. 2017;170:1134–1148.e10.
44. Karlsson L, Lindahl P, Heath JK, Betsholtz C. Abnormal gastrointestinal development in PDGF-A and PDGFR-(alpha) deficient mice implicates a novel mesenchymal structure with putative instructive properties in villus morphogenesis. Development. 2000;127:3457–66.
45. Greicius G, Kabiri Z, Sigmundsson K, Liang C, Bunte R, Singh MK, et al. PDGFRα + pericryptal stromal cells are the critical source of Wnts and RSPO3 for murine intestinal stem cells in vivo. Proc Natl Acad Sci U S A. 2018;115:E3173–81.
46. Kinchen J, Chen HH, Parikh K, Antanaviciute A, Jagielowicz M, Fawkner-Corbett D, et al. Structural remodeling of the human colonic mesenchyme in inflammatory bowel disease. Cell. 2018;175:372–386.e17.
47. Karlsson L, Bondjers C, Betsholtz C. Roles for PDGF-A and sonic hedgehog in development of mesenchymal components of the hair follicle. Development. 1999;126:2611–21.
48. Calver AR, Hall AC, Yu WP, Walsh FS, Heath JK, Betsholtz C, et al. Oligodendrocyte population dynamics and the role of PDGF in vivo. Neuron. 1998;20:869–82.
49. Fruttiger M, Karlsson L, Hall AC, Abramsson A, Calver AR, Boström H, et al. Defective oligodendrocyte development and severe hypomyelination in PDGF-A knockout mice. Development. 1999;126:457–67.
50. Shin S, Pang Y, Park J, Liu L, Lukas BE, Kim SH, et al. Dynamic control of adipose tissue development and adult tissue homeostasis by platelet-derived growth factor receptor alpha. eLife. 2020;9:e56189. Horsley V, Cheah KSE, Farmer S, Sanchez-Gurmaches J, editors. eLife Sciences.
51. Wosczyna MN, Konishi CT, Perez Carbajal EE, Wang TT, Walsh RA, Gan Q, et al. Mesenchymal stromal cells are required for regeneration and homeostatic maintenance of skeletal muscle. Cell Rep. 2019;27:2029–2035.e5.
52. Fredriksson L, Nilsson I, Su EJ, Andrae J, Ding H, Betsholtz C, et al. Platelet-derived growth factor C deficiency in C57BL/6 mice leads to abnormal cerebral vascularization, loss of

neuroependymal integrity, and ventricular abnormalities. Am J Pathol. 2012;180:1136–44.

53. Andrae J, Gouveia L, Gallini R, He L, Fredriksson L, Nilsson I, et al. A role for PDGF-C/PDGFRα signaling in the formation of the meningeal basement membranes surrounding the cerebral cortex. Biol Open. 2016;5:461–74.

54. Ding H, Wu X, Boström H, Kim I, Wong N, Tsoi B, et al. A specific requirement for PDGF-C in palate formation and PDGFR-alpha signaling. Nat Genet. 2004;36:1111–6.

55. Soriano P. The PDGF alpha receptor is required for neural crest cell development and for normal patterning of the somites. Development. 1997;124:2691–700.

56. Gladh H, Folestad EB, Muhl L, Ehnman M, Tannenberg P, Lawrence A-L, et al. Mice lacking platelet-derived growth factor d display a mild vascular phenotype. PLoS One. 2016;11:e0152276.

57. Barrow AD, Edeling MA, Trifonov V, Luo J, Goyal P, Bohl B, et al. Natural killer cells control tumor growth by sensing a growth factor. Cell. 2018;172:534–548.e19.

58. Lindahl P, Johansson BR, Levéen P, Betsholtz C. Pericyte loss and microaneurysm formation in PDGF-B-deficient mice. Science. 1997;277:242–5.

59. Hellström M, Gerhardt H, Kalén M, Li X, Eriksson U, Wolburg H, et al. Lack of pericytes leads to endothelial hyperplasia and abnormal vascular morphogenesis. J Cell Biol. 2001;153:543–54.

60. Bjarnegård M, Enge M, Norlin J, Gustafsdottir S, Fredriksson S, Abramsson A, et al. Endothelium-specific ablation of PDGFB leads to pericyte loss and glomerular, cardiac and placental abnormalities. Development. 2004;131:1847–57.

61. Soriano P. Abnormal kidney development and hematological disorders in PDGF beta-receptor mutant mice. Genes Dev. 1994;8:1888–96.

62. Levéen P, Pekny M, Gebre-Medhin S, Swolin B, Larsson E, Betsholtz C. Mice deficient for PDGF B show renal, cardiovascular, and hematological abnormalities. Genes Dev. 1994;8:1875–87.

63. Lindblom P, Gerhardt H, Liebner S, Abramsson A, Enge M, Hellstrom M, et al. Endothelial PDGF-B retention is required for proper investment of pericytes in the microvessel wall. Genes Dev. 2003;17:1835–40.

64. Onogi Y, Wada T, Kamiya C, Inata K, Matsuzawa T, Inaba Y, et al. PDGFRβ regulates adipose tissue expansion and glucose metabolism via vascular remodeling in diet-induced obesity. Diabetes. 2017;66:1008–21.

65. Hellström M, Kalén M, Lindahl P, Abramsson A, Betsholtz C. Role of PDGF-B and PDGFR-beta in recruitment of vascular smooth muscle cells and pericytes during embryonic blood vessel formation in the mouse. Development. 1999;126:3047–55.

66. Betsholtz C, Keller A. PDGF, pericytes and the pathogenesis of idiopathic basal ganglia calcification (IBGC). Brain Pathol. 2014;24:387–95.

67. Bonner JC, Osornio-Vargas AR, Badgett A, Brody AR. Differential proliferation of rat lung fibroblasts induced by the platelet-derived growth factor-AA, -AB, and -BB isoforms secreted by rat alveolar macrophages. Am J Respir Cell Mol Biol. 1991;5:539–47.

68. Abdollahi A, Li M, Ping G, Plathow C, Domhan S, Kiessling F, et al. Inhibition of platelet-derived growth factor signaling attenuates pulmonary fibrosis. J Exp Med. 2005;201:925–35.

69. Takemura H, Suzuki H, Fujisawa H, Yuhara T, Akama T, Yamane K, et al. Enhanced interleukin 6 production by cultured fibroblasts from patients with systemic sclerosis in response to platelet derived growth factor. J Rheumatol. 1998;25:1534–9.

70. Iwayama T, Steele C, Yao L, Dozmorov MG, Karamichos D, Wren JD, et al. PDGFRα signaling drives adipose tissue fibrosis by targeting progenitor cell plasticity. Genes Dev. 2015;29:1106–19.

71. Marcelin G, Ferreira A, Liu Y, Atlan M, Aron-Wisnewsky J, Pelloux V, et al. A PDGFRα-mediated switch toward CD9high

adipocyte progenitors controls obesity-induced adipose tissue fibrosis. Cell Metab. 2017;25:673–85.

72. He C, Medley SC, Hu T, Hinsdale ME, Lupu F, Virmani R, et al. PDGFRβ signalling regulates local inflammation and synergizes with hypercholesterolaemia to promote atherosclerosis. Nat Commun. 2015;6:7770. Nature.

73. Kozaki K, Kaminski WE, Tang J, Hollenbach S, Lindahl P, Sullivan C, et al. Blockade of platelet-derived growth factor or its receptors transiently delays but does not prevent fibrous cap formation in ApoE null mice. Am J Pathol. 2002;161:1395–407.

74. Bilder G, Wentz T, Leadley R, Amin D, Byan L, O'Conner B, et al. Restenosis following angioplasty in the swine coronary artery is inhibited by an orally active PDGF-receptor tyrosine kinase inhibitor, RPR101511A. Circulation. 1999;99:3292–9.

75. Nakamura K, Arimura K, Nishimura A, Tachibana M, Yoshikawa Y, Makihara N, et al. Possible involvement of basic FGF in the upregulation of PDGFRβ in pericytes after ischemic stroke. Brain Res. 2016;1630:98–108.

76. Kanazawa S, Miyake T, Kakinuma T, Tanemoto K, Tsunoda T, Kikuchi K. The expression of platelet-derived growth factor and connective tissue growth factor in different types of abdominal aortic aneurysms. J Cardiovasc Surg (Torino). 2005;46:271–8.

77. Vorkapic E, Dugic E, Vikingsson S, Roy J, Mäyränpää MI, Eriksson P, et al. Imatinib treatment attenuates growth and inflammation of angiotensin II induced abdominal aortic aneurysm. Atherosclerosis. 2016;249:101–9.

78. Tannenberg P, Chang Y-T, Muhl L, Laviña B, Gladh H, Genové G, et al. Extracellular retention of PDGF-B directs vascular remodeling in mouse hypoxia-induced pulmonary hypertension. Am J Physiol Lung Cell Mol Physiol. 2018;314:L593–605.

79. Schermuly RT, Dony E, Ghofrani HA, Pullamsetti S, Savai R, Roth M, et al. Reversal of experimental pulmonary hypertension by PDGF inhibition. J Clin Invest. 2005;115:2811–21. American Society for Clinical Investigation

80. Forsberg K, Valyi-Nagy I, Heldin CH, Herlyn M, Westermark B. Platelet-derived growth factor (PDGF) in oncogenesis: development of a vascular connective tissue stroma in xenotransplanted human melanoma producing PDGF-BB. Proc Natl Acad Sci U S A. 1993;90:393–7.

81. Skobe M, Fusenig NE. Tumorigenic conversion of immortal human keratinocytes through stromal cell activation. Proc Natl Acad Sci U S A. 1998;95:1050–5.

82. Tejada ML, Yu L, Dong J, Jung K, Meng G, Peale FV, et al. Tumor-driven paracrine platelet-derived growth factor receptor alpha signaling is a key determinant of stromal cell recruitment in a model of human lung carcinoma. Clin Cancer Res. 2006;12:2676–88.

83. Campbell JS, Hughes SD, Gilbertson DG, Palmer TE, Holdren MS, Haran AC, et al. Platelet-derived growth factor C induces liver fibrosis, steatosis, and hepatocellular carcinoma. Proc Natl Acad Sci U S A. 2005;102:3389–94.

84. Anderberg C, Li H, Fredriksson L, Andrae J, Betsholtz C, Li X, et al. Paracrine signaling by platelet-derived growth factor-CC promotes tumor growth by recruitment of cancer-associated fibroblasts. Cancer Res. 2009;69:369–78.

85. Shao ZM, Nguyen M, Barsky SH. Human breast carcinoma desmoplasia is PDGF initiated. Oncogene. 2000;19:4337–45.

86. Pietras K, Pahler J, Bergers G, Hanahan D. Functions of paracrine PDGF signaling in the proangiogenic tumor stroma revealed by pharmacological targeting. PLoS Med [Internet]. 2008;5 [cited 2021 May 17]. Available from: https://www.ncbi.nlm.nih.gov/pmc/articles/PMC2214790/

87. Orimo A, Gupta PB, Sgroi DC, Arenzana-Seisdedos F, Delaunay T, Naeem R, et al. Stromal fibroblasts present in invasive human breast carcinomas promote tumor growth and angiogenesis through elevated SDF-1/CXCL12 secretion. Cell. 2005;121:335–48.

88. Lederle W, Stark H-J, Skobe M, Fusenig NE, Mueller MM. Platelet-derived growth factor-BB controls epithelial tumor phenotype by differential growth factor regulation in stromal cells. Am J Pathol. 2006;169:1767–83.

89. Shinagawa K, Kitadai Y, Tanaka M, Sumida T, Onoyama M, Ohnishi M, et al. Stroma-directed imatinib therapy impairs the tumor-promoting effect of bone marrow-derived mesenchymal stem cells in an orthotopic transplantation model of colon cancer. Int J Cancer. 2013;132:813–23.

90. Peña C, Céspedes MV, Lindh MB, Kiflemariam S, Mezheyeuski A, Edqvist P-H, et al. STC1 expression by cancer-associated fibroblasts drives metastasis of colorectal cancer. Cancer Res. 2013;73:1287–97.

91. Liu C, Zhang Y, Lim S, Hosaka K, Yang Y, Pavlova T, et al. A zebrafish model discovers a novel mechanism of stromal fibroblast-mediated cancer metastasis. Clin Cancer Res. 2017;23:4769–79. American Association for Cancer Research

92. Reed RK, Rubin K. Transcapillary exchange: role and importance of the interstitial fluid pressure and the extracellular matrix. Cardiovasc Res. 2010;87:211–7.

93. Baranowska-Kortylewicz J, Abe M, Pietras K, Kortylewicz ZP, Kurizaki T, Nearman J, et al. Effect of platelet-derived growth factor receptor-beta inhibition with STI571 on radioimmunotherapy. Cancer Res. 2005;65:7824–31.

94. Pietras K, Stumm M, Hubert M, Buchdunger E, Rubin K, Heldin C-H, et al. STI571 enhances the therapeutic index of epothilone B by a tumor-selective increase of drug uptake. Clin Cancer Res. 2003;9:3779–87.

95. Pietras K, Rubin K, Sjöblom T, Buchdunger E, Sjöquist M, Heldin C-H, et al. Inhibition of PDGF receptor signaling in tumor stroma enhances antitumor effect of chemotherapy. Cancer Res. 2002;62:5476–84.

96. Pietras K, Ostman A, Sjöquist M, Buchdunger E, Reed RK, Heldin CH, et al. Inhibition of platelet-derived growth factor receptors reduces interstitial hypertension and increases transcapillary transport in tumors. Cancer Res. 2001;61:2929–34.

97. Strell C, Paulsson J, Jin S-B, Tobin NP, Mezheyeuski A, Roswall P, et al. Impact of epithelial-stromal interactions on peritumoral fibroblasts in ductal carcinoma in situ. J Natl Cancer Inst. 2019;111:983–95.

98. Bartoschek M, Oskolkov N, Bocci M, Lövrot J, Larsson C, Sommarin M, et al. Spatially and functionally distinct subclasses of breast cancer-associated fibroblasts revealed by single cell RNA sequencing. Nat Commun. 2018;9:5150.

99. Raz Y, Cohen N, Shani O, Bell RE, Novitskiy SV, Abramovitz L, et al. Bone marrow-derived fibroblasts are a functionally distinct stromal cell population in breast cancer. J Exp Med. 2018;215:3075–93.

100. Roswall P, Bocci M, Bartoschek M, Li H, Kristiansen G, Jansson S, et al. Microenvironmental control of breast cancer subtype elicited by paracrine platelet derived growth factor-CC signaling. Nat Med. 2018;24:463–73.

101. Abramsson A, Lindblom P, Betsholtz C. Endothelial and nonendothelial sources of PDGF-B regulate pericyte recruitment and influence vascular pattern formation in tumors. J Clin Invest. 2003;112:1142–51.

102. Furuhashi M, Sjöblom T, Abramsson A, Ellingsen J, Micke P, Li H, et al. Platelet-derived growth factor production by B16 melanoma cells leads to increased pericyte abundance in tumors and an associated increase in tumor growth rate. Cancer Res. 2004;64:2725–33.

103. Pietras K, Hanahan D. A multitargeted, metronomic, and maximum-tolerated dose "chemo-switch" regimen is antiangiogenic, producing objective responses and survival benefit in a mouse model of cancer. J Clin Oncol. 2005;23:939–52.

104. Nisancioglu MH, Betsholtz C, Genové G. The absence of pericytes does not increase the sensitivity of tumor vasculature to vascular endothelial growth factor-A blockade. Cancer Res. 2010;70:5109–15.

105. McCarty MF, Somcio RJ, Stoeltzing O, Wey J, Fan F, Liu W, et al. Overexpression of PDGF-BB decreases colorectal and pancreatic cancer growth by increasing tumor pericyte content. J Clin Invest. 2007;117:2114–22.

106. Hosaka K, Yang Y, Seki T, Nakamura M, Andersson P, Rouhi P, et al. Tumour PDGF-BB expression levels determine dual effects of anti-PDGF drugs on vascular remodelling and metastasis. Nat Commun. 2013;4:2129.

107. Cooke VG, LeBleu VS, Keskin D, Khan Z, O'Connell JT, Teng Y, et al. Pericyte depletion results in hypoxia-associated epithelial-to-mesenchymal transition and metastasis mediated by met signaling pathway. Cancer Cell. 2012;21:66–81.

108. Keskin D, Kim J, Cooke VG, Wu C-C, Sugimoto H, Gu C, et al. Targeting vascular pericytes in hypoxic tumors increases lung metastasis via angiopoietin-2. Cell Rep. 2015;10:1066–81.

109. Hong J, Tobin NP, Rundqvist H, Li T, Lavergne M, García-Ibáñez Y, et al. Role of tumor pericytes in the recruitment of myeloid-derived suppressor cells. J Natl Cancer Inst. 2015;107

110. Corvigno S, Wisman GBA, Mezheyeuski A, van der Zee AGJ, Nijman HW, Åvall-Lundqvist E, et al. Markers of fibroblast-rich tumor stroma and perivascular cells in serous ovarian cancer: inter- and intra-patient heterogeneity and impact on survival. Oncotarget. 2016;7:18573–84.

111. Mezheyeuski A, Bradic Lindh M, Guren TK, Dragomir A, Pfeiffer P, Kure EH, et al. Survival-associated heterogeneity of marker-defined perivascular cells in colorectal cancer. Oncotarget. 2016;7:41948–58.

112. Frödin M, Mezheyeuski A, Corvigno S, Harmenberg U, Sandström P, Egevad L, et al. Perivascular PDGFR-β is an independent marker for prognosis in renal cell carcinoma. Br J Cancer. 2017;116:195–201. Nature

113. Suzuki S, Dobashi Y, Hatakeyama Y, Tajiri R, Fujimura T, Heldin CH, et al. Clinicopathological significance of platelet-derived growth factor (PDGF)-B and vascular endothelial growth factor-A expression, PDGF receptor-β phosphorylation, and microvessel density in gastric cancer. BMC Cancer. 2010;10:659.

114. Paulsson J, Lindh MB, Jarvius M, Puputti M, Nistér M, Nupponen NN, et al. Prognostic but not predictive role of platelet-derived growth factor receptors in patients with recurrent glioblastoma. Int J Cancer. 2011;128:1981–8.

115. Koos B, Paulsson J, Jarvius M, Sanchez BC, Wrede B, Mertsch S, et al. Platelet-derived growth factor receptor expression and activation in choroid plexus tumors. Am J Pathol. 2009;175:1631–7.

116. Jarvius M, Paulsson J, Weibrecht I, Leuchowius K-J, Andersson A-C, Wählby C, et al. In situ detection of phosphorylated platelet-derived growth factor receptor beta using a generalized proximity ligation method. Mol Cell Proteomics. 2007;6:1500–9.

117. Frings O, Augsten M, Tobin NP, Carlson J, Paulsson J, Pena C, et al. Prognostic significance in breast cancer of a gene signature capturing stromal PDGF signaling. Am J Pathol. 2013;182:2037–47.

118. Paulsson J, Sjöblom T, Micke P, Pontén F, Landberg G, Heldin C-H, et al. Prognostic significance of stromal platelet-derived growth factor β-receptor expression in human breast cancer. Am J Pathol. 2009;175:334–41.

119. Strell C, Stenmark Tullberg A, Jetne Edelmann R, Akslen LA, Malmström P, Fernö M, et al. Prognostic and predictive impact of stroma cells defined by PDGFRb expression in early breast cancer: results from the randomized SweBCG91RT trial. Breast Cancer Res Treat. 2021;187:45–55.

120. Paulsson J, Rydén L, Strell C, Frings O, Tobin NP, Fornander T, et al. High expression of stromal PDGFRβ is associated with

reduced benefit of tamoxifen in breast cancer. J Pathol Clin Res. 2016;3:38–43.

121. Jansson S, Aaltonen K, Bendahl P-O, Falck A-K, Karlsson M, Pietras K, et al. The PDGF pathway in breast cancer is linked to tumour aggressiveness, triple-negative subtype and early recurrence. Breast Cancer Res Treat. 2018;169:231–41.

122. Nordby Y, Richardsen E, Rakaee M, Ness N, Donnem T, Patel HRH, et al. High expression of PDGFR-β in prostate cancer stroma is independently associated with clinical and biochemical prostate cancer recurrence. Sci Rep [Internet]. 2017;7 [cited 18 May 2021]. Available from: https://www.ncbi.nlm.nih.gov/pmc/articles/PMC5324133/

123. Hägglöf C, Hammarsten P, Josefsson A, Stattin P, Paulsson J, Bergh A, et al. Stromal PDGFRβ expression in prostate tumors and non-malignant prostate tissue predicts prostate cancer survival. PLoS One [Internet]. 2010;5 [cited 18 May 2021]. Available from: https://www.ncbi.nlm.nih.gov/pmc/articles/PMC2873980/

124. Kodama M, Kitadai Y, Sumida T, Ohnishi M, Ohara E, Tanaka M, et al. Expression of platelet-derived growth factor (PDGF)-B and PDGF-receptor β is associated with lymphatic metastasis in human gastric carcinoma. Cancer Sci. 2010;101:1984–9.

125. Kurahara H, Maemura K, Mataki Y, Sakoda M, Shinchi H, Natsugoe S. Impact of p53 and PDGFR-β expression on metastasis and prognosis of patients with pancreatic cancer. World J Surg. 2016;40:1977–84.

126. Kitadai Y, Sasaki T, Kuwai T, Nakamura T, Bucana CD, Hamilton SR, et al. Expression of activated platelet-derived growth factor receptor in stromal cells of human colon carcinomas is associated with metastatic potential. Int J Cancer. 2006;119:2567–74.

127. Yuzawa S, Kano MR, Einama T, Nishihara H. PDGFRβ expression in tumor stroma of pancreatic adenocarcinoma as a reliable prognostic marker. Med Oncol. 2012;29:2824–30.

128. Sun W-Y, Jung W-H, Koo JS. Expression of cancer-associated fibroblast-related proteins in thyroid papillary carcinoma. Tumour Biol. 2016;37:8197–207.

129. Ehnman M, Missiaglia E, Folestad E, Selfe J, Strell C, Thway K, et al. Distinct effects of ligand-induced PDGFRα and PDGFRβ signaling in the human rhabdomyosarcoma tumor cell and stroma cell compartments. Cancer Res. 2013;73:2139–49.

130. Paulsson J, Ehnman M, Östman A. PDGF receptors in tumor biology: prognostic and predictive potential. Future Oncol. 2014;10:1695–708.

131. Crowley MR, Bowtell D, Serra R. TGF-beta, c-Cbl, and PDGFR-alpha the in mammary stroma. Dev Biol. 2005;279:58–72.

132. Kilvaer TK, Rakaee M, Hellevik T, Vik J, Petris LD, Donnem T, et al. Differential prognostic impact of platelet-derived growth factor receptor expression in NSCLC. Sci Rep. 2019;9:10163. Nature.

133. Östman A, Corvigno S. Microvascular mural cells in cancer. Trends Cancer. 2018;4:838–48.

134. Rydén L, Jönsson P-E, Chebil G, Dufmats M, Fernö M, Jirström K, et al. Two years of adjuvant tamoxifen in premenopausal patients with breast cancer: a randomised, controlled trial with long-term follow-up. Eur J Cancer. 2005;41:256–64.

135. Rutqvist LE, Johansson H. Stockholm Breast Cancer Study Group. Long-term follow-up of the randomized Stockholm trial on adjuvant tamoxifen among postmenopausal patients with early stage breast cancer. Acta Oncol. 2007;46:133–45.

136. Strell C, Folkvaljon D, Holmberg E, Schiza A, Thurfjell V, Karlsson P, et al. High PDGFRb expression predicts resistance to radiotherapy in DCIS within the SweDCIS randomized trial. Clin Cancer Res. 2021;27(12):3469–77.

137. Wu SZ, Roden DL, Wang C, Holliday H, Harvey K, Cazet AS, et al. Stromal cell diversity associated with immune evasion in human triple-negative breast cancer. EMBO J. 2020;39:e104063.

138. McCarthy N, Kraiczy J, Shivdasani RA. Cellular and molecular architecture of the intestinal stem cell niche. Nat Cell Biol. 2020;22:1033–41.

139. Jackson HW, Fischer JR, Zanotelli VRT, Ali HR, Mechera R, Soysal SD, et al. The single-cell pathology landscape of breast cancer. Nature. 2020;578:615–20.

140. Schürch CM, Bhate SS, Barlow GL, Phillips DJ, Noti L, Zlobec I, et al. Coordinated cellular neighborhoods orchestrate antitumoral immunity at the colorectal cancer invasive front. Cell. 2020;182:1341–1359.e19.

141. Lindborg M, Cortez E, Höidén-Guthenberg I, Gunneriusson E, von Hage E, Syud F, et al. Engineered high-affinity affibody molecules targeting platelet-derived growth factor receptor β in vivo. J Mol Biol. 2011;407:298–315.

Inflammation and Cancer: Lipid Autacoid and Cytokine Biomarkers of the Tumor Microenvironment

9

Molly M. Gilligan, Bruce R. Zetter, and Dipak Panigrahy

Abstract

The role of inflammation in cancer has a long and controversial history. Currently, there are two lenses through which inflammation in cancer can be viewed. Substantial evidence suggests that inflammation can not only propagate, but even initiate cancer pathogenesis, and an inflammatory microenvironment is widely acknowledged as a prerequisite for carcinogenesis. However, emerging studies indicate that inflammation may alternatively enhance host containment and destruction of tumorigenic cells. Herein, we explore how our understanding of inflammation in cancer has evolved, from the first identification of excessive inflammation in tumors two millennia ago to the complex association between inflammation and cancer pathogenesis with the recent emergence of immune-harnessing cancer therapies. Moreover, the emergence of the field of the resolution of inflammation and the discovery of specialized pro-resolving lipid autacoid mediators (SPMs) presents new opportunities for targeting cancer. Here we discuss the dynamic roles and potential clinical applications of various immune cells, cytokines, and specific lipid autacoid signaling in cancer, focusing on fatty acid-derived lipid mediators such as prostaglandins, leukotrienes, and the newly characterized specialized pro-resolving mediators.

Take-Home Lessons

- Inflammation can both propagate and initiate cancer, while also enhancing host containment and innate anti-tumor mechanisms.
- Immune cells including macrophages, dendritic cells, natural killer cells, T lymphocytes, and B lymphocytes play both pro- and anti-carcinogenic roles within the context of cancer.
- While initially understood to be pro-tumorigenic, growing evidence suggests inflammatory cytokines serve dual anti- and pro-carcinogenic roles in the tumor microenvironment complicating the paradigm use of targeted cytokine therapy.
- The resolution of inflammation is a highly bioactive pathway that has emerged as a critical inhibitor of carcinogenesis and a potential new anti-cancer therapy without the toxicity of standard cancer therapies.

Inflammation, Immunity, and Cancer

The association between inflammation and cancer dates back as early as two millennia ago, when Claudius Galen expanded on Hippocrates' theory of cancer as an excess of black bile (melancholia) by suggesting that cancer resulted from excessive inflammation [1–4]. In 1861, the German pathologist Dr. Rudolph Virchow delivered a twenty-part lecture series at the Pathological Institute of Berlin in which he was the first to describe immune cell infiltrates in tumors. Specifically, he noted the presence of white blood cells, or leukocytes, in tumor tissue and suggested that leukocytes may release factors that stimulate tumor cell proliferation [5]. By contrast, Drs. Wilhelm Busch and Friedrich Fehleisen were the first to identify a link between cancer status and immunity, noting the spontaneous regression of tumors in patients who developed the bacterial skin infection erysipelas. Thirty years later, Dr. William B. Coley alternatively linked immune stimulation to

M. M. Gilligan (✉) · D. Panigrahy
Center for Vascular Biology Research, Beth Israel Deaconess Medical Center, Harvard Medical School, Boston, MA, USA

Department of Pathology, Beth Israel Deaconess Medical Center, Harvard Medical School, Boston, MA, USA
e-mail: gilli204@umn.edu; dpanigra@bidmc.harvard.edu

B. R. Zetter
Vascular Biology Program, Boston Children's Hospital, Harvard Medical School, Boston, MA, USA
e-mail: bruce.zetter@childrens.harvard.edu

L. A. Akslen, R. S. Watnick (eds.), *Biomarkers of the Tumor Microenvironment*, https://doi.org/10.1007/978-3-030-98950-7_9

cancer regression. At the New York's Academy of Medicine, he reported three cases in which inoculating sarcoma patients with a strain of *Streptococcus* bacterium resulted in tumor regression [6]. Later coined "Coley's toxin," inoculation with this bacterium is now known to have elicited tumor regression through tumor necrosis factor-α (TNFα)-mediated activation of cytotoxic immune cells, and Dr. Coley is considered widely as the "father of modern immunotherapy." These historic discoveries set the stage for our present-day understanding of the complex role and doubled edge-sword of inflammation in cancer: while inflammation can promote carcinogenesis, stimulating the inflammatory response can also be employed as an effective anti-cancer therapeutic approach.

Inflammation in Carcinogenesis

Within the last 50 years, seminal advancements have been made in our understanding of inflammation and cancer [3]. In 1986, the eminent Harvard Medical School pathologist Dr. Harold Dvorak elegantly characterized tumors as "wounds that do not heal," noting that while tumors elicited an immune response, they also characteristically exhibited persistent, non-healing chronic inflammation [7]. Drs. Lisa Coussens, Douglas Hanahan, and Zena Werb later demonstrated that pre-malignant tissue became malignant with the assistance, or "co-conspiracy," of inflammatory cells, including mast cells, macrophages, and T lymphocytes [8, 9]. It is now recognized that inflammation plays a critical role in every stage of tumor development, and that an inflammatory microenvironment is essentially a prerequisite for tumor growth [4]. Several immune cell types, including macrophages, neutrophils, mast cells, and T lymphocytes, secrete pro-tumorigenic mediators termed cytokines, including chemokines, as well as pro-angiogenic factors and metastasis-promoting extracellular proteases [4, 10–14]. By 2011, Drs. Douglas Hanahan and Robert Weinberg added inflammation as a defining hallmark of cancer in their landmark review *Hallmarks of Cancer: The Next Generation* [15].

Chronic inflammation and inflammatory diseases are in fact known risk factors for many cancer types. For instance, chronic *Helicobacter pylori* predisposes to stomach cancer, inflammatory bowel diseases predispose to colon cancer, and hepatitis predisposes to hepatocellular carcinoma [13, 16]. Moreover, over nineteen cancers have been associated with prior bacterial, viral, or parasitic infections [16]. Chronic inflammation may even be necessary for cancer pathogenesis, as one study found that mice engineered to develop hepatitis failed to develop hepatocellular carcinoma when TNFα was neutralized [17]. NF$\kappa\beta$, a key pro-inflammatory transcription factor critical in innate and adaptive immune activation, was also suppressed in these mice [17]. Another hallmark study supporting the role of inflammation initiating cancer found that chronic pancreatitis is essential for induction of pancreatic ductal adenocarcinoma by K-Ras onco-

genes in mice [18]. Interestingly, chronic inflammatory diseases do not universally correlate with carcinogenesis or increased cancer risk. Studies have found that allergic conditions, which trigger bouts of recurrent inflammation, inversely correlate with cancer progression [19, 20].

Importantly, modern-day cytotoxic cancer therapies such as chemotherapy and radiation have been found to promote tumorigenesis through an inflammation-dependent mechanism [21–24]. Revesz was the first to demonstrate a link between radiation-generated tumor cell debris and tumor growth in the 1950s, demonstrating a paradoxical increase in tumor growth in mice treated with radiation, a therapy now known to trigger an endogenous pro-inflammatory response via pro-inflammatory mediators [22, 25]. Since then, multiple studies have found a link between cytotoxic cancer therapies and cancer progression or the occurrence of secondary malignancies such as lymphoma [21, 26, 27]. Cytotoxic therapies, while reducing tumor burden by direct killing of cancer cells, result in the rapid accumulation of cellular debris that in turn promotes pro-inflammatory eicosanoid (e.g., PGE$_2$) and cytokine (e.g., TNFα and INFγ) release by macrophages and other immune cells within the tumor microenvironment [21, 23, 24, 28]. Our growing appreciation for cytotoxic therapy-induced tumor progression not only illustrates the critical role inflammation plays in carcinogenesis, but also highlights an urgent need for novel non-inflammation-provoking cancer therapies as well as pro-resolution therapies which stimulate the clearance of cellular debris such as pro-resolving lipid mediators.

Inflammation in the Inhibition of Carcinogenesis

Despite inflammation being commonly viewed as "the other half of the tumor" [29], a growing body of evidence suggests immune cells and their mediators play more complex roles in preventing cancer progression. In 1977, Dr. Alberto Mantovani demonstrated that antibody-dependent cellular cytotoxicity (ADCC) inhibited tumor cell growth via both cytostatic (inhibiting cell growth and division) and cytolytic (cell lysis-inducing) mechanisms [30]. Cancer cells express antigens that can be identified as "non-self" by surveillance immune cells, such as natural killer cells and cytotoxic T cells, which can elicit an anti-tumor immune response. Mantovani's later seminal studies characterizing the ability of tumor-associated macrophages (TAMs) to both stimulate and inhibit tumor growth further highlighted the contrasting pro- and anti-tumorigenic functions of the immune system [31]. Expanding on Coley's observations linking immune stimulation with cancer regression, in 1987, Dr. Frances Balkwill and her colleagues discovered that treatment with inflammatory modulating cytokines such as TNFα and interferon γ (INFγ) prolonged survival of ovarian tumor-bearing mice [32]. Similar to Coley's clinical studies, the Balkwill laboratory findings suggested inflammatory signals at the tumor site may alternatively elicit endogenous anti-tumorigenic activity. Balkwill went on to characterize novel mechanisms through which TNFα can be simultaneously pro- and anti-tumorigenic depending on the context of the specific tumor microenvironment [33].

Modern-day cancer therapy targeting the immune system, known as immunotherapy, relies on inflammation to promote the detection and subsequent destruction of cancer cells. The origins of immunotherapy can be traced back to Wilhelm, Fehleisen, and Coley's early studies demonstrating a link between immune challenge and tumor regression. This concept reemerged in the twentieth century, with Dr. Paul Ehrlich hypothesizing that the immune system constantly surveys the body for cancer cells and eradicates them. Sir Frank Macfarlane Burnet, who was later awarded the 1960 Nobel Prize in Medicine for his co-discovery of acquired immunological tolerance, independently came up with the hypothesis of tumor "immunosurveillance," in which tumor antigens (neoantigens) are recognized and targeted by the immune system to prevent carcinogenesis [34]. Subsequent studies identified T cells as the key immune cells in the body's war against cancer, laying the foundation for present-day efforts to develop T cell-based immunotherapies for various cancers [35]. The first clinically implemented immunotherapy was immune checkpoint therapy, in which antibodies against conserved negative regulators of T cell activation (e.g., PD1, CTLA4) inhibited T cell recognition of cancer cells as "self," thereby preventing tumor cell evasion and promoting T cell activation against neoantigen-expressing tumor cells and initiation of their destruction [34]. Other immunotherapies, including adoptive T cell transfer therapy (e.g., chimeric antigen receptor (CAR)-T cell therapy) and cancer vaccines, have also recently emerged as promising new therapeutic avenues in which immune activation inhibits carcinogenesis [36]. Interestingly, the use of immunotherapy has been somewhat clinically limited by cytokine release syndrome (CRS), an infrequent but deadly adverse effect in which the robust, rapid release of pro-inflammatory cytokines ("cytokine storm") results in systemic organ failure and in some cases death [37]. Stimulation of resolution of inflammation via pro-resolving lipid mediators can prevent the cytokine storm in hyperinflammatory diseases such as COVID-19 and cancer via regulation of eicosanoid-driven cytokines [38, 39].

As we strive to untangle the complex, multi-faceted relationship between inflammation and cancer, our understanding of the disease has shifted radically. Cancer is increasingly illuminated as a war of self, the outcome hinging on whether our immune systems keep our mutated cells in check or assist in their progression and eventual escape. Our growing appreciation of the resolution of inflammation provides another lens through which to view cancer, and a new array of mediators and mechanisms for developing novel diagnostic, prognostic, and therapeutic approaches to cancer [13, 40, 41]. Here we will explore the immune cells, cytokines, and lipid mediators that define the tumor microenvironment and their complex roles in carcinogenesis and clinical cancer care.

Tumor Microenvironment

The tumor microenvironment has become a focus in cancer research as its constituents are the major contributors of tumor-promoting inflammation [3, 42–46]. Here, we focus specifically on the diverse roles of immune cells, cytokines, lipid mediators, and inflammatory biomarkers that actively mediate inflammation in the tumor microenvironment. While inflammation has traditionally been associated with cancer progression, current studies continue to identify both pro- and anti-tumorigenic mechanisms enacted by the immune system [3]. We explore the pro-tumorigenic mechanisms of infiltrating immune cells, pro-inflammatory cytokines, and pro-inflammatory biomarkers, while examining how these immune cells and their mediators may paradoxically play an anti-tumorigenic role in the context of cancer.

Immune Cell Biomarkers

Both the innate and adaptive immune systems contribute to cancer-associated inflammation. Immune cells such as macrophages, dendritic cells, natural killer cells, T lymphocytes, and B lymphocytes play critical pro-tumorigenic and anti-tumorigenic roles in inflammation-associated cancer pathogenesis [3, 4, 13].

Macrophages

Macrophages are traditionally viewed as scavengers of the immune system [47]. As monocytes, their immature predecessors, they circulate in the blood until they receive a signal to migrate into tissues, where they mature into macrophages. Macrophages are dual-functional: while they participate in the innate immune response by surveying tissues and destroying antigens via phagolysosomes, they also function as antigen-presenting cells within the adaptive immune system to mount specific T and B cell responses against foreign particles, microbes, or even cancer cells [48].

The view of the predominantly anti-tumorigenic role of macrophages in cancer has evolved since the 1980s to encompass their more recently characterized pro-tumorigenic actions. In the 1980s and 1990s, resident liver macrophages known as Kupffer macrophages were reported to possess anti-tumorigenic activity [48, 49]. Specifically, Kupffer macrophages were shown to phagocytose tumor cells, and their systemic depletion led to increased metastases [50]. Tumor-bearing mice lacking macrophages, a result of exogenous depletion, were shown to exhibit increased tumor differentiation and decreased survival due to aggressive tumor growth [51]. Similarly, the depletion of monocytes and macrophages in tumor models in animals demonstrated reduced tumor incidence, as well as inhibition of tumor growth and angiogenesis [52, 53]. The anti-tumorigenic nature of macrophages is further exemplified by the evolution of tumor cells to evade macrophage detection. Leukemia cell expression of CD47, an anti-apoptotic and autophagic marker, was demonstrated to inhibit macrophage phagocytosis, enabling tumor immune evasion and cancer progression [54].

Macrophages have been characterized in various tumorigenic and metastatic disease settings. For instance, glioblastoma has been associated with increased numbers of circulating monocytes [55]. Further, phagocytosis of circulating breast cancer exosomes by distant macrophages has been shown to increase macrophage secretion of pro-inflammatory cytokines via NFκβ activation [56]. Importantly, this implicates macrophages as potential mediators of metastasis, as breast cancer commonly metastasizes to the lung and brain. Indeed, pioneering studies have characterized the pro-metastatic role of macrophages in mediating the angiogenic switch via pro-inflammatory cytokines such as WNT7b and CCL2 in genetically engineered murine breast cancer models such as MMTV-PymT mouse model of mammary carcinoma [49, 57].

It is now appreciated that functionally distinct subsets of macrophages exist, and their polarization is influenced by their surroundings. Two of these polarizations are referred to as "M1" and "M2" phenotypes. However, the traditional M1/M2 categorization of macrophages appears to be an oversimplification [58, 59], as recent studies have expanded the role of M2-phenotypic macrophages to include mediating the resolution of inflammation [60]. During the resolution of inflammation, an active process, lipid autacoids stimulate M2 macrophages to efferocytose apoptotic cellular debris [47, 61–63]. Glioblastoma-associated myeloid cells are characterized as having an "M0," non-polarized phenotype. However, these non-polarized macrophages have been found to express some characteristic M2 markers, namely TGF-β and IL-10 [55]. M2-polarized macrophages in a non-cancer setting are characterized as anti-inflammatory, participating in wound healing and tissue repair; however, in a cancer setting, they are characteristically viewed as "pro-tumorigenic." Specifically, M2 macrophages have been shown to promote disease progression in numerous cancers, including lung, breast, and ovarian [64–66]. In genetically engineered murine models of lung adenocarcinoma, depletion of M2-polarized alveolar macrophages inhibited tumor growth [64]. Additionally, the polarization of macrophages to their M2 phenotype has been shown to accelerate breast cancer growth [65]. Similarly, M2-phenotype macrophages have been shown to be present in ascites fluid taken from ovarian cancer patients [66]. Interestingly, when these macrophages were cultured with lipopolysaccharide (LPS), an inflammatory stimulus, they adopted an M1 phenotype, exhibiting toll-like receptor activation and up-regulating the cytotoxic activity of natural killer (NK) cells [66]. Thus, the reprogramming of M2-macrophages to an M1-phenotype can promote their anti-tumor activity.

In contrast to M2-polarized macrophages, M1 macrophages have been characterized as anti-tumorigenic. In non-cancer settings, these macrophages mount an inflammatory response via their phagocytic and antigen-presenting activity [61, 62]. Current cancer immune-based therapies include polarizing macrophages to their M1 phenotype. Blocking TGFβ signaling in combination with stimulation of toll-like receptor 7 (characteristic of innate immune activation) results in the polarization of macrophages towards an M1 phenotype with specific anti-tumor activity [67].

In addition to M1 macrophages, studies have identified CD169+ macrophages, non-phagocytic mediators of immune tolerance, as important anti-tumorigenic cells in various cancer settings. While CD169+ macrophages are unable to phagocytose cells and debris, they are of particular importance in immune tolerance [58]. Interestingly in an inflammatory setting, these macrophages have been shown to activate cytotoxic CD8+ T cells with a greater range of targets than dendritic cells [68]. As cancers have a wide variety of constantly mutating antigenic targets, this is a potential mechanism to correlate CD169+ macrophages with documented anti-tumor activity in a variety of cancers, including endometrial carcinoma and melanoma [69–71]. CD169+ macrophages inhibit melanoma growth in orthotopic murine models via their ability to bind tumor-derived extracellular vesicles in draining lymph nodes and subsequently present them to B cells [71]. These various host macrophage-mediated mechanisms induce an adaptive immune response against the tumor, thus highlighting enhancement of the immune system as a potential cancer therapy.

Dendritic Cells

Similar to macrophages, dendritic cells exhibit both pro- and anti-tumorigenic activity in cancer. In inflammatory reactions, dendritic cells are the primary antigen-presenting cell. After binding an antigen at the site of inflammation, dendritic cells migrate to lymph nodes and activate antigen-specific immune responses from B and T lymphocytes. Dendritic cells are present in a variety of tumor types [72, 73]. Breast cancer is one tumor type characterized as having increased infiltration of dendritic cells. In a genetically engineered murine model of breast cancer (MMTV-PyMT), dendritic cells were demonstrated to be one of the most prevalent immune cells in the tumor tissue [74]. Subsequent depletion of dendritic cells ultimately inhibited tumor growth and lung metastasis [75]. While dendritic cells are pro-tumorigenic, they can also possess anti-tumor activity. The difference in their role as a double-edged sword in inflammation in cancer may be related to tumor progression. During the initial states of tumor progression, dendritic cells demonstrate anti-tumor activity. However, with tumor progression, dendritic cells lose their anti-tumor activity, unable to perform antigen presentation to T cells and can even become immunosuppressive against T cells [76]. This highlights the malleability of dendritic cell function within the tumor microenvironment and provides a potential mechanism for future immunotherapeutic approaches. In fact, dendritic cells are currently being utilized in cancer vaccination clinical trials [77–79]. Tumor-associated dendritic cells exposed to tumor antigens ex vivo are then re-introduced to glioblastoma patients. These results have demonstrated harnessing dendritic cells antigen-presenting activity increases overall and progression-free survival in glioblastoma patients [80].

Natural Killer Cells

Natural killer (NK) cells also play a key role in inflammation and cancer. NK cells mediate antibody-dependent cellular cytotoxicity within the innate immune system. Recent studies have also implicated NK cells in adaptive and memory immunity [81]. NK cells cannot only promote non-alcoholic steatohepatitis (inflammation and fat accumulation of the liver) but play a pivotal role in its progression to hepatocellular carcinoma (HCC) [82]. Here, NK cells interact with CD8+ T cells to release pro-inflammatory cytokines, contributing to tumor progression [82]. This provides implications for the role of NK cells in tumor progression within a chronic inflammatory setting and their role in adaptive immunity [81, 82]. Further, specific subsets of NK cells have been implicated in halting natural host immune responses in breast cancer patients via the expression of TGFβ and IL-10 [83].

Conversely, studies have identified various anti-tumor activities of NK cells. Prostate cancer patients with increased peripheral natural killer cells achieved improved overall survival [84]. Specifically, NK cells in these patients express NKp46, DNAm-1, and NKG2D, which contributed to the lysis of prostate tumor cells [84]. Activation of NK cells in the presence of IL-12 and IL-15 allows for the mounting of a cytotoxic response against breast cancer stem cells [85]. Importantly, IL-12 and IL-15 activate NK cells and enhance the cytotoxic activity of NK cells.

T Cells

The adaptive immune system, comprised of T and B cells, also plays a critical role in inflammation and cancer. T cells, including CD4+ T helper cells and CD8+ T cytotoxic cells, are antigen-specific cells that have a range of known phenotypes [86]. CD4+ T cells assist in B cell antibody class switching and activation of CD8+ T cells and can have both pro- and anti-tumorigenic activity. Infiltration of CD4+ T cells is increased in skin dysplasia, as well as in squamous cell carcinoma. Their role in tumor pathogenesis is evident as

demonstrated in a CD4+ T cell knockout murine model, in which tumor growth is suppressed [87]. However, it appears the tumorigenic role of CD4+ T cells varies in different malignant tissues. Specifically, the loss of CD4+ T cells in the liver accelerates tumor growth both in murine models and human patient samples of hepatocarcinogenesis. This mechanism may be due to an increase in hepatocytes' lipid concentration, resulting in CD4+ T cell death and subsequent disease progression from non-alcoholic fatty liver disease to cancer [88]. Cytotoxic CD8+ T cells also exhibit anti-tumor functions. T cells with cytotoxic phenotypes are anti-tumorigenic, specifically in genetically engineered murine breast cancer models. Their cytotoxicity against tumor cells is dependent on IL-15 and knocking out IL-15 facilitates a marked increase in tumor growth [89]. Similarly, in genetically engineered murine non-small cell lung cancer models, knocking out CD8+ T cells resulted in stimulation of tumor growth and reduced survival [90]. In recent clinical studies, CD8+ T cells appear to play a key role in anti-tumor immunity in both pancreatic and colorectal cancer. An increase in both CD8+ T cells and CD4+ T cells resulted in increased overall and disease-free survival in patients with pancreatic ductal carcinoma [91]. Reduced metastasis has been correlated with increased numbers of cytotoxic cells in colorectal cancer patient samples [92]. Similarly, depletion of CD8+ T cells in murine colorectal cancer models results in accelerated tumor growth. Thus, T cells represent the flexibility of the adaptive immune system in hindering and promoting tumor growth.

B Cells

B lymphocytic cells, another essential arm of the adaptive immune system, are best known for their role in humoral immunity, providing immune responses from a distance. B cells secrete antigen-specific antibodies, which can have a range of activity including marking cells for destruction (opsonization), providing a physical barrier on an antigen, or facilitating the creation of immune memory. Consistent with immune cells explored previously, B cells also appear to have variable roles in tumor pathogenesis [3]. Most notably, B cells have been implicated in pancreatic cancer progression. The depletion of B cells in mice inhibited orthotopic pancreatic adenocarcinoma tumor progression. The underlying mechanism is believed to be associated with B cells' role in macrophage polarization, specifically polarizing macrophages to an M2 phenotype [93]. Similarly, pancreatic tumors injected into mice lacking functional B cells exhibit decreased tumor growth as compared to wild-type mice. Alternatively, transplanting B cell-deficient mice with wild-type B cells promotes tumor growth, further highlighting the pro-tumorigenic role of B cells [94]. The presence of mature B cells has also been correlated with higher epithelial ovarian tumor grade. Additionally, increased level of plasma cells, terminally differentiated B cells, correlates with decreased overall and ovarian cancer-specific survival [95]. While largely pro-tumorigenic, B cells have also been shown to exhibit anti-tumorigenic characteristics. Gene expression studies have revealed that the presence of B cells in the microenvironment of basal-like breast tumors correlated with increased progression-free survival [96]. While the specific mechanisms in which B cells exert anti-tumorigenic action require further study, it is evident that B cells can be both anti- and pro-tumorigenic depending on the specific tumor environment.

Cytokine and Chemokine Biomarkers

We next explore the role of cytokines and chemokines in cancer-associated inflammation. Cytokines and chemokines are small protein signaling molecules that enable crosstalk between immune cells and immune cell trafficking, respectively [3]. Cytokines and chemokines in non-cancer settings may be considered pro- or anti-inflammatory, similar to immune cells, their role in tumor progression is context dependent. Although a large number of cytokines and chemokines have been implicated in inflammation in cancer, we focus here on TNFα, TGFβ, IL-1, IL-6, IL-10, and CCL2.

Tumor Necrosis Factor α

Tumor necrosis factor α (TNFα) is perhaps the most iconic cytokine in cancer-associated inflammation, however as noted by Balkwill, "tumor necrosis factor" is likely a misnomer [97]. While the name "tumor necrosis factor" would lead one to believe it has anti-tumor activity, recent research has supported a dual role in tumorigenesis for TNFα. TNFα is traditionally implicated in septic shock and is characterized as a pro-inflammatory cytokine. TNFα has also been demonstrated to have both pro- and anti-tumorigenic roles. Its contribution to cancer pathogenesis is believed to be via activation of immune cells, including B cells, which recent studies have shown is likely responsible for skin carcinogenesis. Selectively knocking out TNFα in B cells resulted in a reduction of papillomas in tumor-bearing mice [98]. Similar observations have been made in orthotopic glioblastoma tumor models, in which knocking out TNFα has led to significant increases in survival rates [99]. TNFα has been shown to be increased in non-small cell lung and pancreatic cancers, and its expression in ovarian carcinoma patient tissue correlates with high-grade serous carcinomas and endometrioid carcinomas [100–102]. While it would appear that TNFα could be an appealing target for cancer therapy, anti-TNFα therapies have been unsuccessful in cancer patients to date [103]. Insight into its therapeutic failure may be due to

TNFα's role as an anti-tumorigenic cytokine. If TNFα is expressed directly by tumor cells, it could then exert an autocrine anti-tumor activity. Mice injected with tumor cells genetically modified to secrete high levels of TNFα have little to no tumor growth as compared to control. This model has been recapitulated in breast, melanoma, and lung carcinoma models [104]. This in turn could possibly be utilized for future gene therapy, to stimulate ones' own immunity to exert autologous anti-tumor activity.

Transforming Growth Factor-β

Transforming growth factor-β (TGF-β) is widely studied for its activation of regulatory T cells and Th17 cells. TGF-β activation of regulatory T cells has been shown to dampen inflammation and activate self-tolerant immune mechanisms. Elevated levels of TGF-β secreted from natural killer cells, along with IL-10, have been reported in breast cancer patients [83]. TGF-β has also been implicated in the progression of cervical squamous cell carcinoma. TGF-β activation has been demonstrated to be the result of thrombospondin-1, an acute-phase inflammatory protein, secretion due to the interaction between cancer cells and cancer-associated fibroblasts [105]. TGF-β receptor 1 and 2 knockout mice exhibit marked decrease in pancreatic tumor growth. When the TGF-β receptor is selectively knocked out in epithelial cells, pancreatic tumor growth significantly increases [106]. This highlights the role of the tumor microenvironment in mediating pro- and anti-tumorigenic inflammation signals. Anti-TGF-β therapy in a recent clinical trial proved to have preliminary tumor reduction in advanced melanoma and renal cell carcinoma, with no apparent toxicity [107]. This establishes TGF-β as a putative viable cytokine target for future cancer therapeutic approaches alone and in combination.

However, it has been demonstrated in murine pancreatic cancer models that TGF-β may also have anti-tumor activity. In orthotopic murine and genetically engineered murine models, pharmacological inhibition of TGF-β signaling in the pancreas, using a TGF-β receptor antagonist, contributed to pancreatic ductal adenocarcinoma progression [108]. Similar to other inflammatory mediators in the tumor microenvironment, TGF-β exhibits both pro- and anti-tumorigenic activity and understanding its precise actions in cancer requires further studies.

Interleukin-1

Other cytokines and chemokines have less well-characterized roles in inflammation associated with tumor pathogenesis. Within the IL-1 family, IL-1α, IL-1β, and IL-1 receptor antagonist (IL-1Ra) tend to be a focus of many inflammatory studies. IL-1 is known to enhance CD4+ T cell proliferation and differentiation of B cells in standard inflammatory settings. It is most often associated with induction of fever in the early phase of the acute inflammatory reaction. However, it has been shown that inhibition of IL-1α and IL-1β in murine myeloma models decreases survival rates. In this model, IL-1α and IL-1β increase Th1 cells' secretion of pro-inflammatory cytokines, which in turn activate cytotoxic macrophage responses towards tumor cells [109]. IL-1α is the dominant family member in acute inflammation. However, as acute inflammation progresses to become chronic, IL-1β becomes the predominant mediator [110]. As recent studies have demonstrated, IL-1β appears to play an integral role in inflammation and cancer [3]. Decreased IL-1β secretion by tumor cells or stroma correlates with a decrease in progression-free survival in prostate cancer patients, thus highlighting the potential anti-tumor mechanisms associated with IL-1β in the tumor microenvironment [111]. However, other studies have suggested IL-1β exhibits pro-tumor effects. Specifically, infiltrating neutrophils in a colitis model will secrete IL-1β that in turn contributes to colitis-associated tumorigenesis via up-regulating the secretion of IL-6 [112]. IL-1Ra is a competitive antagonist to IL-1α and IL-1β and has been shown to inhibit their pro-inflammatory mechanisms [113]. While IL-1Ra may appear to be an alluring target for cancer therapy, recent data suggests its role in cancer progression is more complex than previously viewed. An increase in IL-1Ra has been correlated with decreased event-free and overall survival in T cell lymphoma patients [114]. Similarly, IL-Ra levels are increased in women with newly diagnosed breast cancers, as compared to breast cancer negative controls [115]. Taken together, the IL-1 cytokine family activity appears to be rather situational in its pro- and anti-tumorigenic activity.

Interleukin-6

Similar to IL-1, IL-6 is another cytokine implicated in acute inflammation, and more specifically fever. IL-6 is synthesized and secreted predominantly by macrophages and enhances macrophages' ability to present to T cells via up-regulation of B7 expression following recognition of pathogen-associated molecular patterns. Unlike the IL-1 family mediators, IL-6 has been shown to be predominantly pro-tumorigenic. In 2014, Karin and Taniguchi described IL-6 as one of the "critical lynchpins" associating inflammation and cancer [116]. They implicated IL-6's downstream signaling as contributing to tumor cell survival and proliferation, as well as to inflammation in the tumor microenvironment. Similarly, they highlighted that IL-6 is not only associated with acute inflammation but also participates in T cell activation throughout chronic inflammation. IL-6 has

also been associated with at least twelve cancer types in humans, including but not limited to stomach, pancreatic, liver, intestinal, uterine, breast, lung, esophageal, prostate, bladder, and kidney cancers [116]. In a murine model of pancreatitis (a chronic inflammatory condition), knocking out IL-6 has led to the recovery of normal pancreatic tissue as compared to wild-type mice, which ultimately develop pancreatic tumors [117]. IL-6 secretion from fibroblasts has even been implicated as a mechanism for angiogenesis, again highlighting the pro-tumorigenic role of IL-6 [118]. IL-6 has been implicated in the progression of both triple-negative breast cancer and pancreatic cancer [102, 117, 119]. Blocking the IL-6 receptor on breast cancer cells has been shown to render the tumor cells unable to adhere to endothelium, which is a key step in metastasis [119]. Thus, IL-6 not only possesses the potential to promote primary tumor growth, but also to stimulate tumor angiogenesis and metastasis.

Interleukin-10

In non-cancer settings, IL-10 is traditionally characterized as an anti-inflammatory cytokine, namely for its' inhibition of NFκβ, a transcription factor implicated in both cancer and inflammation. Recent studies, however, have shown that IL-10 may contribute to tumor growth and even cancer therapy resistance. IL-10 is increased in breast tumor tissue, with a corresponding increase in macrophage infiltration [120]. Further, increased secretion of IL-10 by macrophages in the tumor stroma has been associated with drug resistance in breast cancer [120]. This again presents an interesting paradigm, in which a characteristically anti-inflammatory cytokine contributing to tumor growth.

Chemokine Ligand 2

Chemokine ligand 2 (CCL2), also known as monocyte chemoattractant protein 1 (MCP1), is involved in macrophage chemotaxis, signaling macrophages to traffic to a specific tissue site. CCL2 plays a critical role in inflammation and cancer, particularly for its role in breast cancer metastasis. CCL2 secreted by tumor cells and macrophages increases metastatic seeding of breast cancer cells via stimulating the secretion of CCL3 [121]. Interestingly, CCL3, also known as macrophage inflammatory protein 1-α (MIP1-α), is known to play a role in acute inflammation, again demonstrating the intertwined role of inflammation and cancer. Further, a recent clinical trial implicated antagonizing CCL2 activity in pancreatic tumor inhibition. Pharmacologically inhibiting CCR2, the receptor for CCL2, in combination with chemotherapy, significantly inhibited tumor growth [122]. In this study, inhibition of CCR2 significantly decreased tumor-associated macrophages and regulatory T cells, while increasing CD8+ and CD4+ T cells.

Eicosanoids: Lipid Autacoid Biomarkers in Cancer

Another lens to view inflammation and cancer is through inflammatory lipid autacoid mediators and proteins. Lipids biosynthesized from arachidonic acid such as prostaglandins, leukotrienes, and thromboxane are collectively termed eicosanoids, and are potent locally acting mediators which initiate inflammation [13, 14, 47, 123] (Fig. 9.1). Here we will discuss the critical role of eicosanoids in cancer, including prostaglandin E_2 (PGE$_2$), epoxyeicosatrienoic acids (EETs), omega-3 fatty acids, and leukotrienes.

Prostaglandin E$_2$

Prostaglandin E_2 is a characteristically pro-inflammatory bioactive lipid synthesized from arachidonic acid initially by cyclooxygenase 1 (COX-1) and cyclooxygenase 2 (COX-2), and then by PGE synthase. Both PGE$_2$ and COX-2 expression have been implicated in inflammation and cancer [14]. PGE$_2$ has been most notably characterized in colon cancer, where knocking out PGE synthase and thus inhibiting PGE$_2$ synthesis decreases colon tumor formation in genetically engineered murine models of colon cancer [124]. Further, levels of PGE$_2$ positively correlate with cancer stem cell markers in colorectal cancer patient tumor samples [125]. PGE$_2$ exhibits pro-metastatic activity, as administration of PGE$_2$ results in increased tumor and liver metastasis in a genetically engineered model of colorectal cancer [125]. Mechanistically PGE$_2$ promotes tumor growth through stimulation of angiogenesis and immune suppression in several cancers, including colon cancer [126, 127]. PGE$_2$ generated by tumor cells additionally stimulates myeloid-derived suppressor cells to inhibit natural killer cells, contributing to immune suppression [128]. In addition to PGE$_2$'s well-characterized activity in colon cancer, deleting COX or PGE synthase in melanoma cells results in tumor rejection in immunocompetent mice [129]. However, in Rag1 knockout (KO) mice, melanoma tumor cells lacking PGE synthase

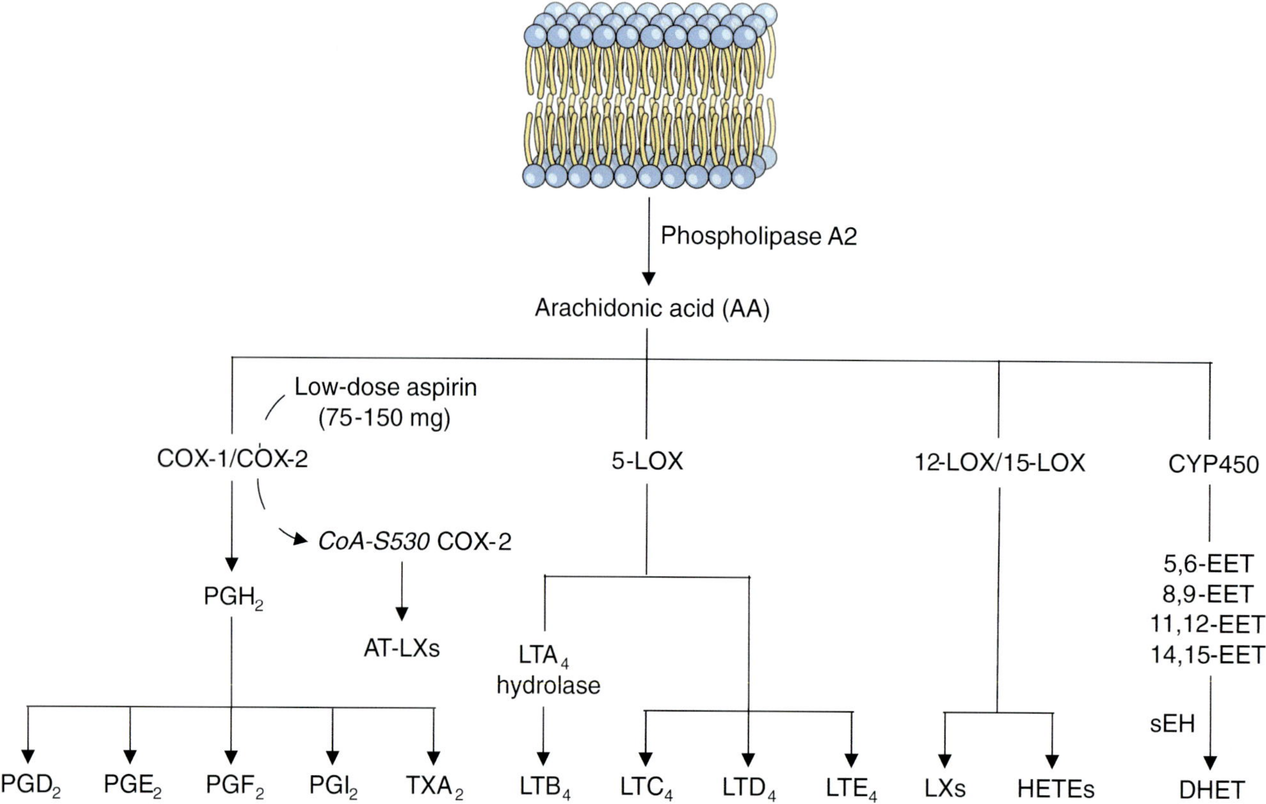

Fig. 9.1 Arachidonic acid metabolism via cyclooxygenase (COX), lipoxygenase (LOX) and cytochrome P450 (CYP450). AA metabolism via COX-1/2 generates prostaglandins (PGs), thromboxanes (TXs), and aspirin-triggered lipoxins (AT-LXs). *CoA-S530,* acetylated serine 530 residue on COX-2. AA metabolism via 5-LOX generates leukotrienes (LTs), and metabolism via 12-LOX/15-LOX generates lipoxins (LXs) and HETEs. AA metabolism by CYP450 generates epoxide intermediates (5,6-EET, 8,9-EET, 11,12-EET, 14,15-EET) that are hydrolyzed to DHET by soluble epoxide hydrolase (sEH)

form growing tumors [129]. As Rag1 KO mice are unable to generate mature T and B lymphocytes, this result highlights the relationship between PGE_2, immune cells and tumor progression [127]. We analyze the characterization of PGE_2 within this paradigm in regard to its relationship with omega-3 fatty acids and aspirin in the sections below, entitled "Omega-3 Fatty Acids and Derivatives" and "Inflammation, Resolution, and Cancer: Clinical Applications," respectively.

Epoxyeicosatrienoic Acids

Epoxyeicosatrienoic acids (EETs) are locally acting lipid signaling molecules with a short-half life and both autocrine and paracrine activity [130]. EETs are the products of arachidonic acid metabolism by cytochrome P450 enzymes. EETs are then further metabolized by soluble epoxide hydrolase (sEH) into dihydroxyeicosatrienoic acid (DHET) [123]. EETs have been extensively studied in various inflammatory diseases. While EETs are known to mediate proliferation, migration, and inflammation in human tissues, their molecular mechanisms in doing so remain poorly characterized [43]. EETs are known to play a role in coronary arteriole dilation [131], stimulate tissue and organ regeneration [132], promote wound healing [133], delay seizure onset [134], and participate in many other disease processes with an inflammatory component [135]. Interestingly, their role in specific inflammatory diseases appears to be somewhat complex. EETs have been shown to be cardioprotective, inhibit pathogenesis of diabetes, exert renal and neuronal protection [123]. EETs also promote tumor cell proliferation and regulate host anti-tumor immunity [43, 45, 136]. Thus, the role of EETs in cancer has been neglected and continues to be an active area of study [42]. It has been demonstrated that both exogenous systemic and endogenous endothelium-derived EETs not only can promote tumor growth and angiogenesis in murine models but also metastasis and tumor dormancy escape [45]. The underlying mechanism in these models revealed to be mediated in part by increasing VEGF secretion from endothelium in the tumor microenvironment [45]. In fact, the pro-tumorigenic role of EETs has also been demonstrated in human breast tumor tissue. Increased levels of 14,15-EET correlate with greater malignancy potential in breast cancer patients [137]. While the role of EETs in cancer still requires further elucidation, modulation of EET levels via soluble epoxide hydrolase (sEH) has been proposed as a possible new direction in cancer therapy [43, 138]. Specifically, the promotion of EET metabolism by the endogenous over-expression of sEH in transgenic mice has been shown to reduce tumor burden [45]. Moreover, the dual inhibitors of sEH and COX2 inhibit primary tumor growth and metastasis via resolution of an eicosanoid and cytokine

storm [23, 28, 139]. Taken together, the role of EETs in cancer remains an interesting vantage point in which to target inflammation and cancer, while also providing insight into possible new therapeutic approaches.

Leukotrienes

Analogous to EETs, leukotrienes are another class of eicosanoids generated by the metabolism of arachidonic acid, namely by members of the lipoxygenase enzyme family. Leukotrienes are traditionally viewed as pro-inflammatory molecules and have been intensely studied in inflammatory lung diseases. Similar to the other lipid mediators, their role in inflammation is being actively elucidated. Leukotrienes are mainly synthesized by leukocytes, contributing to both innate and adaptive immunity responses [140]. In acute inflammatory settings, leukotriene B_4 (LTB_4) increases leukocyte trafficking, as well as pro-inflammatory cytokines such as IL-6 and TNFα. In fact, cellular secretion of LTB_4 is a crucial first step in potentiating inflammation-induced tumorigenesis in a lung cancer model [141]. The mechanism of LTB_4 pro-tumorigenic activity was demonstrated to be mediated by signaling through binding of its receptor BLT1, characteristically expressed on peripheral blood leukocytes [141]. LC-MS-MS-based profiling revealed an increase in leukotrienes LTC_4 and LTE_4, which correlates with tumor progression in aggressive murine lung cancer models [142]. Interestingly in these models, resident alveolar macrophages demonstrated high expression of 5-lipoxygenase (5-LOX), and subsequent increases in LTB_4, LTC_4, and LTD_4 secretion, as compared to infiltrating macrophages which did not produce leukotrienes [142]. This study provides insight into leukotrienes' locally acting inflammatory mechanisms in the tumor microenvironment. Similarly, the deletion of 5-LOX in a murine lung cancer model stimulates primary tumor growth and liver metastasis [143].

Recent evidence implicating 5-LOX as an inhibitor of tumor growth suggests that leukotrienes produced by this enzyme potentially enact anti-tumorigenic programs in addition to their well-characterized pro-tumorigenic activities. Inhibition of 5-LOX in murine model has been demonstrated to reduce polyp burden in intestinal mucosa, a known mechanistic step in the APC-driven adenoma-carcinoma sequence of colon cancer [144]. In this model, the inhibition of 5-LOX was further accompanied by a reduction in inflammatory infiltrate, including cytokines and immune cells [144]. Further, the inhibition of 5-LOX has been shown to selectively induce apoptosis in prostate cancer cells via decreased expression of c-Myc mRNA [145]. C-Myc is a commonly mutated gene in various cancers, allowing for unregulated cell proliferation. However, in pancreatic cancer models, the opposite was found to be true; 5-LOX knockout mice were shown to have increased pancreatic lesions, precursors to pancreatic ductal adenocarcinoma [146]. Thus, the integral role of leukotrienes in inflammation and cancer requires further studies, although it is apparent their modulation could provide important insight into cancer pathogenesis and potentially open new therapeutic avenues.

The Resolution of Inflammation in Cancer

Acute inflammation in response to physiologic stress (e.g., infection, injury, allergens, or cell death) serves as the body's defense against the outside world and has long been understood to be a complex process dictated by chemical signaling [147, 148]. In fact, Sune Bergström, Bengt Samuelsson, and Sir John Vane shared the 1982 Nobel Prize for their independent discoveries on cyclooxygenase (COX-2)-mediated prostaglandin synthesis and the COX-2 inhibitory mechanisms of aspirin's anti-inflammatory activity. While previously thought to be a passively self-limited process, recent evidence from Prof. Charles Serhan and colleagues demonstrate the bioactive cessation, or "resolution," of inflammation is an active process [47]. The notion of resolution can be traced back to ancient times with "resolvent mollificants" being referenced in the eleventh-century medical text *Canon of Medicine* [149]. While the 1970s saw the recognition of resolution as a distinct process from inflammation [150], it wasn't until the 1980s that studies led

by Savill and colleagues shed light on the characteristic cellular mechanisms of resolution [151, 152]. Specifically, these studies identified the consumption of apoptotic polymorphonuclear neutrophils (PMN) such as neutrophils, the first responders in acute inflammation, and inflammatory exudates (cell debris) by macrophages as key events in inflammation resolution [151, 152].

Parallel studies led to the discovery of the first class of resolution-mediating lipid autacoids now known as specialized pro-resolving mediators (SPMs), termed lipoxins (LXs) [153]. The subsequent discovery that LXs exert differential activities on neutrophils and macrophages, namely inhibiting neutrophil infiltration while recruiting macrophages for non-phlogistic (non-inflammation provoking) consumption of inflammation-induced cellular debris, shifted the field from studying LXs' anti-inflammatory activities towards uncovering their remarkable tissue-restorative mechanisms [154–159]. Since the discovery of LXs, the field of resolution and our understanding of pro-resolving lipid mediators and mechanisms has grown exponentially. The past two decades have seen the discovery of several classes of SPMs, derived from the omega-3 fatty acids docosahexaenoic acid (DHA) and eicosapentaenoic acid (EPA), including the resolvins (RvDs, RvEs, RvTs, respectively), the maresins (MaRs), the protectins (PD1, AT-PD1), and the maresin, resolvin, and protectin conjugates in tissue regeneration (MCTRs, RCTRs, and PCTRs, respectively) [47, 160, 161] (Fig. 9.2). Moreover, the G protein-coupled receptors (GPCRs) for many SPMs

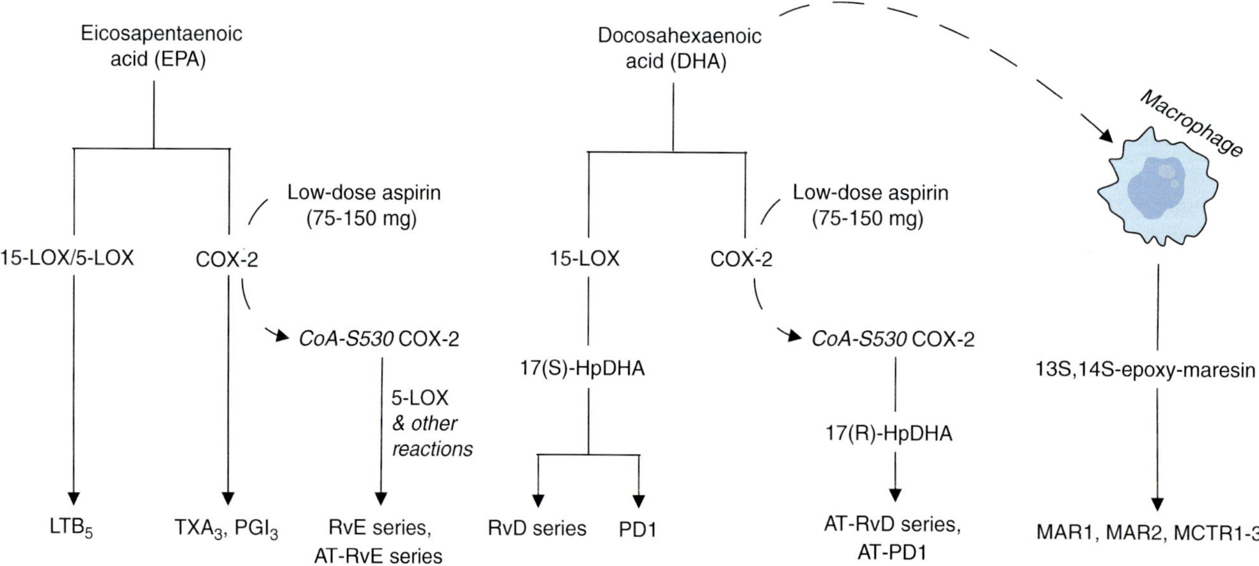

Fig. 9.2 Eicosapentaenoic acid (EPA) and docosahexaenoic acid (DHA) metabolism via 15-LOX, 5-LOX, COX-2, and 15-LOX, COX-2, respectively. Metabolism of EPA via 15-LOX/5-LOX generates leukotriene B5 (LTB5), metabolism via COX-2 generates TXA3 and PGI3, and metabolism via acetylated COX-2 (*CoA-S530* COX-2) generates E series resolinvs (RvEs) and their aspirin-triggered epimers (AT-RvEs). DHA metabolism via 15-LOX generates D series resolvins (RvDs) and protectin D1 (PD1), and metabolism via *CoA-S530* COX-2 generates aspirin-triggered RvDs (AT-RvDs) and aspirin-triggered PD1 (AT-PD1). DHA metabolism by macrophages generates Maresins (MaRs) and their epoxy-intermediates

have been discovered to date [161], facilitating robust efforts to characterize SPM mechanisms and potential therapeutic applications in a broad array of acute and chronic inflammatory diseases, including cancer [21, 40].

Specialized Pro-resolving Mediators and Their Precursors: Lipid Biomarkers in Cancer

A growing body of evidence suggests SPMs may be potential cancer biomarkers, prognostic markers, and novel therapeutic targets for the development of novel anti-cancer pharmaceuticals [13]. While many eicosanoids promote carcinogenesis, SPMs have thus far been found to exert broad potent anti-tumor activity across many animal cancer models [13]. Moreover, low endogenous levels of SPMs and/or dysfunctional resolution circuits are emerging as a contributor to the chronic inflammatory state that underlies most cancers. Here we will discuss the present and potential future roles of SPMs and their precursors in cancer, including omega-3 fatty acids, lipoxins, resolvins, and aspirin-triggered SPMs.

Omega-3 Fatty Acids and Derivatives

Omega-3 fatty acids are essential dietary polyunsaturated fatty acids that are metabolized in the human body to other essential lipid metabolites, including prostaglandins, thromboxane, and leukotrienes. Omega-3 fatty acids and their derivatives have recently gained widespread public attention for their potential wide-ranging health benefits. Eicosapentaenoic acid (EPA) and docosahexaenoic acid (DHA) are omega-3 fatty acids that are frequently marketed as dietary supplements to promote heart health. The possible role of these fatty acids in cancer pathogenesis is also of interest, as diets rich in omega-3 fatty acids correlate with a reduction in cancer-related deaths [162]. The anti-inflammatory mechanism of omega-3 fatty acids has been significantly attributed to their metabolites, EPA and DHA. These molecules saturate enzymes that classically metabolize arachidonic acid into pro-inflammatory molecules, and instead produce metabolites with more anti-inflammatory characteristics [163]. EPA and DHA can also activate peroxisome proliferator-activated receptors (PPARs), transcription factors with known anti-inflammatory effects [163] and, interestingly, anti-tumor activity [164, 165]. Dietary supplementation of omega-3 fatty acids has been associated with decreased risk of colorectal cancer mortality [166]. Of note, chronic inflammation, such as ulcerative colitis, is a risk factor for colorectal cancer pathogenesis [167].

Omega-3 fatty acid supplementation has also been demonstrated to suppress prostate cancer progression in murine models via a macrophage-mediated mechanism [168]. Dietary DHA in these models reduced tumor-associated macrophage viability, as well as pro-inflammatory cytokines and NF$\kappa\beta$-mediated gene expression. Induction of tumor cell apoptosis may mediate, at least in part, the anti-tumor activity of omega-3 fatty acids [169]. Studies have further indicated omega-3 fatty acids are capable of inducing apoptosis in a range of solid cancers in vitro, ranging from gastrointestinal origin to neural tissue, and even hematological cancers [169]. While the underlying mechanism remains to be fully elucidated, it appears that omega-3 fatty acids play a role in inducing both the intrinsic and extrinsic apoptosis pathways [169]. In addition to inducing apoptotic programs, omega-3 fatty acids play an anti-tumorigenic role also through increasing tumor cell susceptibility to cytotoxic therapies and are being investigated as adjuvant cancer therapies [170]. Omega-3 fatty acid supplementation was also found to enrich tumor cell membranes in unsaturated fatty acids, in turn making the cells more susceptible to destruction by free radicals [170].

An important process in tumor malignancy is epithelial-mesenchymal transition, an example of tumor plasticity. This transformation is critical for tumor cell invasion into neighboring tissues and sets the foundation for tumor metastasis. DHA has proven to be efficacious in inhibiting epithelial-mesenchymal transition in colorectal cancer models [171]. The mechanism of DHA's direct action in halting this process remains relatively unknown. As previously described, the actions of PGE_2 and COX-2 characteristically are pro-tumorigenic molecules. Recent studies in endometrial cancer suggest omega-3 fatty acid supplementation exerts its anti-tumor activity through downregulating COX-2 expression, and thus subsequently decreasing endogenous PGE_2 levels [172]. This mechanism has also been demonstrated in a colon cancer model, in which researchers further found that EPA and DHA supplementation increased LXA_4, an anti-inflammatory and pro-resolving endogenous lipid mediator [173, 174]. While the intricate workings of omega-3 fatty acids still required further research, their potential in cancer therapeutics appears promising.

Lipoxins

The 12-lipoxygenase (12-LOX)/15-lipoxygenase (15-LOX) metabolism of arachidonic acid (AA) produces lipoxins, the first pro-resolving mediators to be discovered [153] (Fig. 9.2). Lipoxins levels have been found to correlate with cancer, however evidence is limited. For instance, one study found that Kaposi Sarcoma cell cultures had decreased lipoxin A_4 levels (LXA_4) compared to non-neoplastic control cultures [175]. When treated with LXA₄, neoplastic cell cultures exhibited decreased pro-inflammatory cytokine production (e.g., NF-κB) as well as reduced inflammatory enzyme expression (e.g., COX-2, 5-LOX). Platelet production of LXA₄ and lipoxin B₄ (LXB) was also found to be decreased in blood samples from patients with chronic myelogenous leukemia, suggesting the failure of resolution via the loss of pro-resolving lipid mediator production may result in carcinogenesis [176]. Colorectal cancer is associated with a loss of LXA₄ and RvD1 [177]. Compared with healthy volunteers, the levels of serum inflammatory cytokines in colon cancer patients increase significantly while the level of RvD1 decreases significantly. Both inflammatory cytokines and RvD1 are associated with higher TNM stages of colon cancer [178]. The inflammatory response associated with hepatobiliary surgery is associated with low circulating concentrations of lipoxin A4 and resolvin D that mirror, in an opposite manner, the kinetics of interleukin 6 and cortisol [179]. The regulation of lipoxin and other SPM production will require further studies in murine cancer models or clinical cancer specimens to better understand the failure of resolution in cancer [13].

Despite limited evidence for their altered production in cancers, lipoxins have been shown to have anti-cancer activity in both animal and human pre-clinical cancer studies. Specifically, LXA₄ and the synthetic LXA₄ analog BML-111 as well as other SPMs such as resolvins reduce disease severity and prolong survival in murine models of hepatocellular carcinoma [180], liver metastasis [181], and pancreatic cancer [182]. Pre-clinical human studies have also identified therapeutic benefits of LXA₄, lipoxin B₄ (LXB₄), BML-111, and Resolvin D1 in gastric cancer [183], hepatocellular carcinoma [184, 185], and leukemia [186]. Importantly, lipoxins have also been found to be beneficial in decreasing bone cancer pain [187] and radiation-induced skin inflammation [188] in murine cancer models. BML-111 has also been shown to inhibit angiogenesis in cultured human tumor cells as well as tumor angiogenesis [189–191]. Lipoxins may be novel therapeutic targets and promising adjuvant therapy in cancer treatment, however additional pre-clinical and clinical studies are required to further evaluate their potential clinical applications in cancer.

Resolvins

As found with lipoxins, recent studies have identified decreased levels of SPMs such as resolvins in various cancers. One study found that resolvin D1 (RvD1) is decreased and inflammatory cytokines (IL-6, IL-10, IL-1β, TNFα) are increased in sera of patients with more advanced colorectal carcinoma by tumor-node-metastasis (TNM) staging as compared to those with less advanced disease [178]. RvD1

was also shown to be increased in association with tumor blood flow in hysterectomy specimens from patients with endometrial cancer [192].

In 2017, studies led by Sulciner, Serhan, Gilligan, and colleagues characterized the broad anti-tumorigenic, anti-metastatic, and anti-angiogenic activity of resolvins in murine lung, prostate, breast, and lymphoma tumor models [21]. As discussed above, cytotoxic cancer therapies create an inflammatory response within the tumor microenvironment, involving the accumulation of inflammatory tumor cell debris and the release of pro-inflammatory cytokines. As reported by Sulciner et al., resolvins potently stimulated macrophage clearance of cellular debris and counter-regulated pro-inflammatory cytokine production in multiple tumor cell lines and murine models [21]. Resolvins were also demonstrated to decrease CD31+ staining, a marker for angiogenesis, in murine tumor specimens, illuminating their anti-angiogenic activity [21]. Other studies have further identified resolvins' potent anti-cancer activity in pre-clinical animal and human models of a huge range of primary and metastatic cancers, including lung [40, 44, 193], liver [180], hematological (e.g., lymphoma) [21], nasopharyngeal [194], head and neck/oral [195], pancreatic [21, 196], prostatic [21, 197], colorectal [21, 198], and gastric cancers [183]. Like lipoxins, resolvins also exhibit beneficial therapeutic effects in bone cancer pain [199] and radiation-induced skin inflammation [200], as well as chemotherapy-induced cardiotoxicity and peripheral neuropathy [201, 202]. Thus, resolvins may hold enormous therapeutic potential in a broad range of cancers for both their anti-cancer activity as well as their benefit in treating the adverse effects of cytotoxic therapies. Similar to lipoxins and other SPMs, additional studies are required for the clinical translation of resolvins to treat cancer. Moreover, their rapid endogenous degradation (within minutes) highlights the need for alternative synthetic SPMs with longer half-lives for use in clinical settings.

Aspirin and Aspirin-Triggered SPMs

Low-dose aspirin (81–100 mg), which is known to stimulate cyclooxygenase-2 (COX-2) production of aspirin-triggered SPMs (AT-SPMs) [47] (Figs. 9.1 and 9.2), has also been linked to cancer prevention in multiple clinical trials [203]. Initial efforts to harness aspirin's anti-cancer activity focused on coxib development, a class of COX-2-inhibiting pharmaceutical agents. However, prolonged COX-2 inhibition via coxibs resulted in significant clinical toxicity and thus indicated an important role for COX-2 in endogenous inflammation-resolving processes [204]. Aspirin acetylation of COX-1/2 inhibits prostaglandin synthesis, thus decreasing the pro-inflammatory and pro-tumorigenic activities of PGE₂, as well as decreasing platelet activation. It has been hypothesized that aspirin also inhibits immune cell activation [205].

Importantly, it is now appreciated that aspirin acetylation of COX-2 also jumpstarts the enzyme's production of aspirin-triggered SPMs (AT-SPMs), which are epimers of their non-AT SPM counterparts [47]. Aspirin regiments have been associated with decreased risks of epithelial ovarian cancer and gastric cancer [206–208]. Aspirin has also been associated with decreased risk of breast cancer related-death following breast cancer diagnosis [209]. However, retrospective studies assessing aspirin's anti-cancer benefits remain controversial. One review concluded that there was no statistically significant correlation between low-dose aspirin use and reduction in overall cancer risk, and that aspirin's chemo-preventative activity was limited to colorectal cancer risk [210]. Similarly, other non-steroidal anti-inflammatory drugs have proved to decrease risk of colorectal and prostate cancer [211–213].

While aspirin's anti-cancer activity was initially attributed solely to prostaglandin E_2 (PGE$_2$) inhibition, aspirin-triggered SPMs (e.g., AT-LXA$_4$, AT-resolvin D1 (AT-RvD1), AT-resolvin D3 (AT-RvD3)) may contribute to aspirin inhibition of cancer. Studies from Gilligan et al. demonstrated the tumor- and metastases-inhibitory activity of AT-SPMs that may in part account for aspirin's clinical efficacy in cancer prevention, specifically in murine lung carcinoma and breast cancer models [40]. These lipid mediators are especially promising new therapeutic targets as they lack the toxicity of aspirin and other COX-2 inhibitors. However, more studies are required to determine whether they have significant diagnostic and prognostic value in cancer.

Inflammation, Resolution, and Cancer: Clinical Applications

Chronic inflammation is a known risk factor for various cancers. For example, pancreatitis is known risk factor for pancreatic cancer, ulcerative colitis and Crohn's disease are known risk factors for colon cancer, and *Helicobacter pylori* infections are known to increase the risk of stomach cancer [13]. Other associations include cystitis and bladder cancer, Barrett's esophagus and esophageal carcinoma, and bronchitis and lung cancer [12, 16]. However, the extent to which underlying inflammation contributes to tumor growth remains elusive. Inflammatory reactions appear to have a threshold for which they can either play a pro-tumorigenic role or anti-tumorigenic role. Thus, characterizing the point at which inflammation transitions from facilitating tumor inhibition to promoting disease progression has been the aim of many recent clinical studies. These studies evaluate the "overall inflammatory score" in relation to specific cancers and highlight a potential threshold between acute and chronic inflammation that, when surpassed, could contribute to cancer pathogenesis.

In a recent study, in which the inflammatory score reflected the neutrophil to lymphocyte ratio, an increased neutrophil to leukocyte ratio was associated with head and neck squamous cell carcinoma patients. This increased ratio was also associated with a decreased in overall survival and recurrence-free survival [214]. Another study found men who demonstrated either acute or chronic inflammation in prostate tissue with a negative prostate biopsy have a decreased risk in prostate cancer pathogenesis 2 years post-biopsy. However, 4 years post-biopsy, decreased risk in prostate cancer was found to be positively associated with acute inflammation [215]. In a similar study on prostate cancer, chronic inflammation, defined by the presence of lymphocytes, plasma cells and macrophages, was associated with lower prostate tumor volume [216]. In a large-scale study evaluating the overall risk of cancer, a combination of CRP levels and leukocyte count was used as an inflammatory score. An increase in the inflammatory score correlated with an increase in prostate, lung, and colorectal cancer risk [217]. A correlation between decreased inflammation and increased cancer survival has also been shown in cervical cancer, in which a decreased platelet to lymphocyte ratio correlates with an increase in overall and disease-free survival in patients [218]. Recent studies further highlight the importance of lymphocyte to monocyte ratio in several cancers. Interestingly, a decrease in lymphocyte to monocyte ratio was found to be consistent with decrease in overall survival in colorectal cancer, lung cancer, pancreatic cancer, and Hodgkin's lymphoma [219]. An additional large-scale, retrospective study demonstrated that a greater ratio of lymphocytes to monocytes resulted in increased overall and disease-free survival in non-small cell lung cancer patients [220].

As discussed above, lipoxins, resolvins, and other SPMs may hold great therapeutic benefit in cancer. Evidence pointing towards dysregulated SPM production in cancer suggests they may serve as important diagnostic or prognostic markers in cancers. Additionally, abundant studies demonstrating their anti-cancer activity and ability to counter cancer-promoting inflammation suggests they may be novel therapeutic targets in many cancers. This is especially important given the toxicity and adverse effects of current cancer therapies (e.g., chemotherapy, radiation) discussed above, as well as aspirin and synthetic COX-2 inhibitors. SPMs moreover may be a more precise and effective way to harness the observed anti-cancer activity of omega-3 dietary supplementation and low-dose aspirin. Despite their promise, additional studies are needed to better understand the role of SPMs in cancer pathogenesis and to facilitate the development of their various clinical applications in the realm of cancer.

Concluding Remarks/Summary

The pleiotropic role of inflammation and cancer has been well documented, from the first observation of inflammation in tumors hundreds of years ago to current studies that have characterized the malleable and complex roles inflammatory cells and their mediators play in cancer progression. Experimental and clinical studies provide mechanisms that can be harnessed as targets for future cancer therapy, with the aim to halt pro-tumorigenic inflammatory signaling or harness the anti-tumorigenic pathways embedded in the human immune system. Many of the lipid mediators discussed in this chapter have potential as cancer biomarkers and exhibit a dual role in tumorigenesis, highlighting the diverse biological activity in various tumor microenvironments. The frame to view inflammation and cancer is not one of strictly "protumor" or "anti-tumor;" rather there exists a multitude of environmental influences that ultimately direct the role inflammation plays within the context of cancer. Future studies will be required to elucidate both the pro- and anti-tumorigenic roles inflammation plays as well as to provide novel therapies to harness the immune system to inhibit or prevent cancer.

References

1. Trinchieri G. Cancer and inflammation: an old intuition with rapidly evolving new concepts. Annu Rev Immunol. 2012;30:677–706. https://doi.org/10.1146/annurev-immunol-020711-075008.
2. Reedy J. Galen on cancer and related diseases. Clio Med. 1975;10:227–38.
3. Greten FR, Grivennikov SI. Inflammation and cancer: triggers, mechanisms, and consequences. Immunity. 2019;51:27–41. https://doi.org/10.1016/j.immuni.2019.06.025.
4. Grivennikov SI, Greten FR, Karin M. Immunity, inflammation, and cancer. Cell. 2010;140:883–99. https://doi.org/10.1016/j.cell.2010.01.025. S0092-8674(10)00060-7 [pii]
5. Virchow R. Cellular pathology as based upon physiological and pathological histology: twenty lectures delivered in the pathological institute of berlin during the months of February, March, and April. New York: Robert M. De Witt; 1860. Print 1858.
6. Coley WB II. Contribution to the knowledge of sarcoma. Ann Surg. 1891;14:199–220.
7. Dvorak HF. Tumors: wounds that do not heal. Similarities between tumor stroma generation and wound healing. N Engl J Med. 1986;315:1650–9. https://doi.org/10.1056/NEJM198612253152606.
8. Coussens LM, et al. Inflammatory mast cells up-regulate angiogenesis during squamous epithelial carcinogenesis. Genes Dev. 1999;13:1382–97.
9. Coussens LM, Tinkle CL, Hanahan D, Werb Z. MMP-9 supplied by bone marrow-derived cells contributes to skin carcinogenesis. Cell. 2000;103:481–90. S0092-8674(00)00139-2 [pii].
10. Di Carlo E, et al. The intriguing role of polymorphonuclear neutrophils in antitumor reactions. Blood. 2001;97:339–45.
11. Kitamura T, Qian BZ, Pollard JW. Immune cell promotion of metastasis. Nat Rev Immunol. 2015;15:73–86. https://doi.org/10.1038/nri3789.
12. Greene ER, Huang S, Serhan CN, Panigrahy D. Regulation of inflammation in cancer by eicosanoids. Prostaglandins Other Lipid Mediat. 2011;96:27–36. https://doi.org/10.1016/j.prostaglandins.2011.08.004.
13. Fishbein A, Hammock BD, Serhan CN, Panigrahy D. Carcinogenesis: failure of resolution of inflammation? Pharmacol Ther. 2020;107670. https://doi.org/10.1016/j.pharmthera.2020.107670.
14. Wang D, Dubois RN. Eicosanoids and cancer. Nat Rev Cancer. 2010;10:181–93. https://doi.org/10.1038/nrc2809. nrc2809 [pii]
15. Hanahan D, Weinberg RA. Hallmarks of cancer: the next generation. Cell. 2011;144:646–74. https://doi.org/10.1016/j.cell.2011.02.013. S0092-8674(11)00127-9 [pii]
16. Coussens LM, Werb Z. Inflammation and cancer. Nature. 2002;420:860–7.
17. Pikarsky E, et al. NF-kappaB functions as a tumour promoter in inflammation-associated cancer. Nature. 2004;431:461–6.
18. Guerra C, et al. Chronic pancreatitis is essential for induction of pancreatic ductal adenocarcinoma by K-Ras oncogenes in adult mice. Cancer Cell. 2007;11:291–302. https://doi.org/10.1016/j.ccr.2007.01.012.
19. Turner MC, Chen Y, Krewski D, Ghadirian P. An overview of the association between allergy and cancer. Int J Cancer. 2006;118:3124–32. https://doi.org/10.1002/ijc.21752.
20. Ritter B, Greten FR. Modulating inflammation for cancer therapy. J Exp Med. 2019;216:1234–43. https://doi.org/10.1084/jem.20181739.
21. Sulciner ML, et al. Resolvins suppress tumor growth and enhance cancer therapy. J Exp Med. 2018;215:115–40. https://doi.org/10.1084/jem.20170681.
22. Revesz L. Effect of tumour cells killed by x-rays upon the growth of admixed viable cells. Nature. 1956;178:1391–2.
23. Gartung A, et al. Suppression of chemotherapy-induced cytokine/lipid mediator surge and ovarian cancer by a dual COX-2/sEH inhibitor. Proc Natl Acad Sci U S A. 2019;116:1698–703. https://doi.org/10.1073/pnas.1803999116.
24. Chang J, et al. Chemotherapy-generated cell debris stimulates colon carcinoma tumor growth via osteopontin. FASEB J. 2019;33:114–25. https://doi.org/10.1096/fj.201800019RR.
25. Revesz L. Effect of lethally damaged tumor cells upon the development of admixed viable cells. J Natl Cancer Inst. 1958;20:1157–86.
26. Krishnan B, Morgan GJ. Non-Hodgkin lymphoma secondary to cancer chemotherapy. Cancer Epidemiol Biomarkers Prev. 2007;16:377–80. https://doi.org/10.1158/1055-9965.EPI-06-1069.
27. Faguet GB. A brief history of cancer: age-old milestones underlying our current knowledge database. Int J Cancer. 2015;136:2022–36. https://doi.org/10.1002/ijc.29134.
28. Fishbein A, et al. Resolution of eicosanoid/cytokine storm prevents carcinogen and inflammation-initiated hepatocellular cancer progression. Proc Natl Acad Sci U S A. 2020;117:21576–87. https://doi.org/10.1073/pnas.2007412117.
29. Mantovani A, Allavena P, Sica A, Balkwill F. Cancer-related inflammation. Nature. 2008;454:436–44. https://doi.org/10.1038/nature07205.
30. Mantovani A, Caprioli V, Gritti P, Spreafico F. Human mature macrophages mediate antibody-dependent cellular cytotoxicity on tumour cells. Transplantation. 1977;24:291–3.
31. Mantovani A, Bottazzi B, Colotta F, Sozzani S, Ruco L. The origin and function of tumor-associated macrophages. Immunol Today. 1992;13:265–70. https://doi.org/10.1016/0167-5699(92)90008-U.
32. Balkwill FR, Ward BG, Moodie E, Fiers W. Therapeutic potential of tumor necrosis factor-alpha and gamma-interferon in experimental human ovarian cancer. Cancer Res. 1987;47:4755–8.

33. Balkwill F, Mantovani A. Inflammation and cancer: back to Virchow? Lancet. 2001;357:539–45. https://doi.org/10.1016/S0140-6736(00)04046-0. S0140-6736(00)04046-0 [pii]

34. Waldman AD, Fritz JM, Lenardo MJ. A guide to cancer immunotherapy: from T cell basic science to clinical practice. Nat Rev Immunol. 2020;20:651–68. https://doi.org/10.1038/s41577-020-0306-5.

35. Halliday GM, Patel A, Hunt MJ, Tefany FJ, Barnetson RS. Spontaneous regression of human melanoma/nonmelanoma skin cancer: association with infiltrating CD4+ T cells. World J Surg. 1995;19:352–8. https://doi.org/10.1007/BF00299157.

36. Sharma P, Allison JP. The future of immune checkpoint therapy. Science. 2015;348:56–61. https://doi.org/10.1126/science.aaa8172.

37. Shimabukuro-Vornhagen A, et al. Cytokine release syndrome. J Immunother Cancer. 2018;6:56. https://doi.org/10.1186/s40425-018-0343-9.

38. Panigrahy D, et al. Inflammation resolution: a dual-pronged approach to averting cytokine storms in COVID-19? Cancer Metastasis Rev. 2020;39:337–40. https://doi.org/10.1007/s10555-020-09889-4.

39. Hammock BD, Wang W, Gilligan MM, Panigrahy D. Eicosanoids: the overlooked storm in coronavirus disease 2019 (COVID-19)? Am J Pathol. 2020;190:1782–8. https://doi.org/10.1016/j.ajpath.2020.06.010.

40. Gilligan MM, et al. Aspirin-triggered proresolving mediators stimulate resolution in cancer. Proc Natl Acad Sci U S A. 2019;116:6292–7. https://doi.org/10.1073/pnas.1804000116.

41. Sulciner ML, Gartung A, Gilligan MM, Serhan CN, Panigrahy D. Targeting lipid mediators in cancer biology. Cancer Metastasis Rev. 2018;37:557–72. https://doi.org/10.1007/s10555-018-9754-9.

42. Panigrahy D, Kaipainen A, Greene ER, Huang S. Cytochrome P450-derived eicosanoids: the neglected pathway in cancer. Cancer Metastasis Rev. 2010;29:723–35. https://doi.org/10.1007/s10555-010-9264-x.

43. Panigrahy D, Greene ER, Pozzi A, Wang DW, Zeldin DC. EET signaling in cancer. Cancer Metastasis Rev. 2011;30:525–40. https://doi.org/10.1007/s10555-011-9315-y.

44. Panigrahy D, et al. Preoperative stimulation of resolution and inflammation blockade eradicates micrometastases. J Clin Invest. 2019;129:2964–79. https://doi.org/10.1172/JCI127282.

45. Panigrahy D, et al. Epoxyeicosanoids stimulate multiorgan metastasis and tumor dormancy escape in mice. J Clin Invest. 2012;122:178–91. https://doi.org/10.1172/JCI58128. 58128 [pii]

46. Panigrahy D, et al. PPARgamma ligands inhibit primary tumor growth and metastasis by inhibiting angiogenesis. J Clin Invest. 2002;110:923–32. https://doi.org/10.1172/JCI15634.

47. Serhan CN. Pro-resolving lipid mediators are leads for resolution physiology. Nature. 2014;510:92–101. https://doi.org/10.1038/nature13479.

48. Qian BZ, Pollard JW. Macrophage diversity enhances tumor progression and metastasis. Cell. 2010;141:39–51. https://doi.org/10.1016/j.cell.2010.03.014. S0092-8674(10)00287-4 [pii]

49. Qian BZ, et al. CCL2 recruits inflammatory monocytes to facilitate breast-tumour metastasis. Nature. 2011;475:222–5. https://doi.org/10.1038/nature10138.

50. Heuff G, et al. Enhanced tumour growth in the rat liver after selective elimination of Kupffer cells. Cancer Immunol Immunother. 1993;37:125–30.

51. Oosterling SJ, et al. Macrophages direct tumour histology and clinical outcome in a colon cancer model. J Pathol. 2005;207:147–55. https://doi.org/10.1002/path.1830.

52. Weber C, et al. Macrophage infiltration and alternative activation during wound healing promote MEK1-induced skin carcinogenesis. Cancer Res. 2016;76:805–17. https://doi.org/10.1158/0008-5472.CAN-14-3676.

53. Zeisberger SM, et al. Clodronate-liposome-mediated depletion of tumour-associated macrophages: a new and highly effective antiangiogenic therapy approach. Br J Cancer. 2006;95:272–81. https://doi.org/10.1038/sj.bjc.6603240. 6603240 [pii]

54. Jaiswal S, et al. CD47 is upregulated on circulating hematopoietic stem cells and leukemia cells to avoid phagocytosis. Cell. 2009;138:271–85. https://doi.org/10.1016/j.cell.2009.05.046.

55. Gabrusiewicz K, et al. Glioblastoma-infiltrated innate immune cells resemble M0 macrophage phenotype. JCI Insight. 2016;1. https://doi.org/10.1172/jci.insight.85841.

56. Chow A, et al. Macrophage immunomodulation by breast cancer-derived exosomes requires Toll-like receptor 2-mediated activation of NF-kappaB. Sci Rep. 2014;4:5750. https://doi.org/10.1038/srep05750.

57. Yeo EJ, et al. Myeloid WNT7b mediates the angiogenic switch and metastasis in breast cancer. Cancer Res. 2014;74:2962–73. https://doi.org/10.1158/0008-5472.CAN-13-2421.

58. Chavez-Galan L, Olleros ML, Vesin D, Garcia I. Much more than M1 and M2 macrophages, there are also CD169(+) and TCR(+) macrophages. Front Immunol. 2015;6:263. https://doi.org/10.3389/fimmu.2015.00263.

59. Van Overmeire E, Laoui D, Keirsse J, Van Ginderachter JA, Sarukhan A. Mechanisms driving macrophage diversity and specialization in distinct tumor microenvironments and parallelisms with other tissues. Front Immunol. 2014;5:127. https://doi.org/10.3389/fimmu.2014.00127.

60. Dalli J, Serhan CN. Pro-resolving mediators in regulating and conferring macrophage function. Front Immunol. 2017;8:1400. https://doi.org/10.3389/fimmu.2017.01400.

61. Dey A, Allen J, Hankey-Giblin PA. Ontogeny and polarization of macrophages in inflammation: blood monocytes versus tissue macrophages. Front Immunol. 2014;5:683. https://doi.org/10.3389/fimmu.2014.00683.

62. Noy R, Pollard JW. Tumor-associated macrophages: from mechanisms to therapy. Immunity. 2014;41:49–61. https://doi.org/10.1016/j.immuni.2014.06.010.

63. Fullerton JN, Gilroy DW. Resolution of inflammation: a new therapeutic frontier. Nat Rev Drug Discov. 2016;15:551–67. https://doi.org/10.1038/nrd.2016.39.

64. Zaynagetdinov R, et al. Chronic NF-kappaB activation links COPD and lung cancer through generation of an immunosuppressive microenvironment in the lungs. Oncotarget. 2016;7:5470–82. https://doi.org/10.18632/oncotarget.6562.

65. Zonari E, et al. A role for miR-155 in enabling tumor-infiltrating innate immune cells to mount effective antitumor responses in mice. Blood. 2013;122:243–52. https://doi.org/10.1182/blood-2012-08-449306.

66. Bellora F, et al. TLR activation of tumor-associated macrophages from ovarian cancer patients triggers cytolytic activity of NK cells. Eur J Immunol. 2014;44:1814–22. https://doi.org/10.1002/eji.201344130.

67. Peng J, et al. Inhibition of TGF-beta signaling in combination with TLR7 ligation re-programs a tumoricidal phenotype in tumor-associated macrophages. Cancer Lett. 2013;331:239–49. https://doi.org/10.1016/j.canlet.2013.01.001.

68. Bernhard CA, Ried C, Kochanek S, Brocker T. CD169+ macrophages are sufficient for priming of CTLs with specificities left out by cross-priming dendritic cells. Proc Natl Acad Sci U S A. 2015;112:5461–6. https://doi.org/10.1073/pnas.1423356112.

69. Ohnishi K, et al. Prognostic significance of CD169-positive lymph node sinus macrophages in patients with endometrial carcinoma. Cancer Sci. 2016;107:846–52. https://doi.org/10.1111/cas.12929.

70. Saito Y, et al. Prognostic significance of CD169+ lymph node sinus macrophages in patients with malignant melanoma. Cancer

Immunol Res. 2015;3:1356–63. https://doi.org/10.1158/2326-6066.CIR-14-0180.

71. Pucci F, et al. SCS macrophages suppress melanoma by restricting tumor-derived vesicle-B cell interactions. Science. 2016;352:242–6. https://doi.org/10.1126/science.aaf1328.

72. Palucka K, Coussens LM, O'Shaughnessy J. Dendritic cells, inflammation, and breast cancer. Cancer J. 2013;19:511–6. https://doi.org/10.1097/PPO.0000000000000007.

73. Tran Janco JM, Lamichhane P, Karyampudi L, Knutson KL. Tumor-infiltrating dendritic cells in cancer pathogenesis. J Immunol. 2015;194:2985–91. https://doi.org/10.4049/jimmunol.1403134.

74. Martelli C, et al. In vivo imaging of lymph node migration of MNP- and (111)In-labeled dendritic cells in a transgenic mouse model of breast cancer (MMTV-Ras). Mol Imaging Biol. 2012;14:183–96. https://doi.org/10.1007/s11307-011-0496-0.

75. Lohela M, et al. Intravital imaging reveals distinct responses of depleting dynamic tumor-associated macrophage and dendritic cell subpopulations. Proc Natl Acad Sci U S A. 2014;111:E5086–95. https://doi.org/10.1073/pnas.1419899111.

76. Scarlett UK, et al. Ovarian cancer progression is controlled by phenotypic changes in dendritic cells. J Exp Med. 2012;209:495–506. https://doi.org/10.1084/jem.20111413.

77. Prue RL, et al. A phase I clinical trial of CD1c (BDCA-1)+ dendritic cells pulsed with HLA-A*0201 peptides for immunotherapy of metastatic hormone refractory prostate cancer. J Immunother. 2015;38:71–6. https://doi.org/10.1097/CJI.0000000000000063.

78. Kranz LM, et al. Systemic RNA delivery to dendritic cells exploits antiviral defence for cancer immunotherapy. Nature. 2016;534:396–401. https://doi.org/10.1038/nature18300.

79. Cornelissen R, et al. Extended tumor control after dendritic cell vaccination with low-dose cyclophosphamide as adjuvant treatment in patients with malignant pleural mesothelioma. Am J Respir Crit Care Med. 2016;193:1023–31. https://doi.org/10.1164/rccm.201508-1573OC.

80. Phuphanich S, et al. Phase I trial of a multi-epitope-pulsed dendritic cell vaccine for patients with newly diagnosed glioblastoma. Cancer Immunol Immunother. 2013;62:125–35. https://doi.org/10.1007/s00262-012-1319-0.

81. Geiger TL, Sun JC. Development and maturation of natural killer cells. Curr Opin Immunol. 2016;39:82–9. https://doi.org/10.1016/j.coi.2016.01.007.

82. Wolf MJ, et al. Metabolic activation of intrahepatic CD8+ T cells and NKT cells causes nonalcoholic steatohepatitis and liver cancer via cross-talk with hepatocytes. Cancer Cell. 2014;26:549–64. https://doi.org/10.1016/j.ccell.2014.09.003.

83. Ostapchuk YO, et al. Peripheral blood NK cells expressing HLA-G, IL-10 and TGF-beta in healthy donors and breast cancer patients. Cell Immunol. 2015;298:37–46. https://doi.org/10.1016/j.cellimm.2015.09.002.

84. Pasero C, et al. Highly effective NK cells are associated with good prognosis in patients with metastatic prostate cancer. Oncotarget. 2015;6:14360–73. https://doi.org/10.18632/oncotarget.3965.

85. Yin T, et al. Human cancer cells with stem cell-like phenotype exhibit enhanced sensitivity to the cytotoxicity of IL-2 and IL-15 activated natural killer cells. Cell Immunol. 2016;300:41–5. https://doi.org/10.1016/j.cellimm.2015.11.009.

86. Masopust D, Schenkel JM. The integration of T cell migration, differentiation and function. Nat Rev Immunol. 2013;13:309–20. https://doi.org/10.1038/nri3442.

87. Daniel D, et al. Immune enhancement of skin carcinogenesis by CD4+ T cells. J Exp Med. 2003;197:1017–28. https://doi.org/10.1084/jem.20021047.

88. Ma C, et al. NAFLD causes selective CD4(+) T lymphocyte loss and promotes hepatocarcinogenesis. Nature. 2016;531:253–7. https://doi.org/10.1038/nature16969.

89. Dadi S, et al. Cancer immunosurveillance by tissue-resident innate lymphoid cells and innate-like T cells. Cell. 2016;164:365–77. https://doi.org/10.1016/j.cell.2016.01.002.

90. Ganesan AP, et al. Tumor-infiltrating regulatory T cells inhibit endogenous cytotoxic T cell responses to lung adenocarcinoma. J Immunol. 2013;191:2009–17. https://doi.org/10.4049/jimmunol.1301317.

91. Ino Y, et al. Immune cell infiltration as an indicator of the immune microenvironment of pancreatic cancer. Br J Cancer. 2013;108:914–23. https://doi.org/10.1038/bjc.2013.32.

92. Mlecnik B, et al. The tumor microenvironment and Immunoscore are critical determinants of dissemination to distant metastasis. Sci Transl Med. 2016;8:327ra326. https://doi.org/10.1126/scitranslmed.aad6352.

93. Gunderson AJ, et al. Bruton tyrosine kinase-dependent immune cell cross-talk drives pancreas cancer. Cancer Discov. 2016;6:270–85. https://doi.org/10.1158/2159-8290.CD-15-0827.

94. Pylayeva-Gupta Y, et al. IL35-producing B cells promote the development of pancreatic neoplasia. Cancer Discov. 2016;6:247–55. https://doi.org/10.1158/2159-8290.CD-15-0843.

95. Lundgren S, Berntsson J, Nodin B, Micke P, Jirstrom K. Prognostic impact of tumour-associated B cells and plasma cells in epithelial ovarian cancer. J Ovarian Res. 2016;9:21. https://doi.org/10.1186/s13048-016-0232-0.

96. Iglesia MD, et al. Prognostic B-cell signatures using mRNA-seq in patients with subtype-specific breast and ovarian cancer. Clin Cancer Res. 2014;20:3818–29. https://doi.org/10.1158/1078-0432.CCR-13-3368.

97. Balkwill F. Tumor necrosis factor or tumor promoting factor? Cytokine Growth Factor Rev. 2002;13:135–41.

98. Schioppa T, et al. B regulatory cells and the tumor-promoting actions of TNF-alpha during squamous carcinogenesis. Proc Natl Acad Sci U S A. 2011;108:10662–7. https://doi.org/10.1073/pnas.1100994108.

99. Kusne Y, et al. Targeting aPKC disables oncogenic signaling by both the EGFR and the proinflammatory cytokine TNFalpha in glioblastoma. Sci Signal. 2014;7:ra75. https://doi.org/10.1126/scisignal.2005196.

100. Gupta M, Babic A, Beck AH, Terry K. TNF-alpha expression, risk factors, and inflammatory exposures in ovarian cancer: evidence for an inflammatory pathway of ovarian carcinogenesis? Hum Pathol. 2016;54:82–91. https://doi.org/10.1016/j.humpath.2016.03.006.

101. Liao C, et al. Association between Th17-related cytokines and risk of non-small cell lung cancer among patients with or without chronic obstructive pulmonary disease. Cancer. 2015;121(Suppl 17):3122–9. https://doi.org/10.1002/cncr.29369.

102. Blogowski W, et al. Selected cytokines in patients with pancreatic cancer: a preliminary report. PLoS One. 2014;9:e97613. https://doi.org/10.1371/journal.pone.0097613.

103. Roberts NJ, Zhou S, Diaz LA Jr, Holdhoff M. Systemic use of tumor necrosis factor alpha as an anticancer agent. Oncotarget. 2011;2:739–51. https://doi.org/10.18632/oncotarget.344.

104. Dondossola E, et al. Self-targeting of TNF-releasing cancer cells in preclinical models of primary and metastatic tumors. Proc Natl Acad Sci U S A. 2016;113:2223–8. https://doi.org/10.1073/pnas.1525697113.

105. Nagura M, et al. Invasion of uterine cervical squamous cell carcinoma cells is facilitated by locoregional interaction with cancer-associated fibroblasts via activating transforming growth factor-beta. Gynecol Oncol. 2015;136:104–11. https://doi.org/10.1016/j.ygyno.2014.11.075.

106. Principe DR, et al. TGFbeta signaling in the pancreatic tumor microenvironment promotes fibrosis and immune evasion to facilitate tumorigenesis. Cancer Res. 2016;76:2525–39. https://doi.org/10.1158/0008-5472.CAN-15-1293.

107. Morris JC, et al. Phase I study of GC1008 (fresolimumab): a human anti-transforming growth factor-beta (TGFbeta) monoclonal antibody in patients with advanced malignant melanoma or renal cell carcinoma. PLoS One. 2014;9:e90353. https://doi.org/10.1371/journal.pone.0090353.

108. Zhao Z, Xi H, Xu D, Li C. Transforming growth factor beta receptor signaling restrains growth of pancreatic carcinoma cells. Tumour Biol. 2015;36:7711–6. https://doi.org/10.1007/s13277-015-3466-3.

109. Haabeth OA, Lorvik KB, Yagita H, Bogen B, Corthay A. Interleukin-1 is required for cancer eradication mediated by tumor-specific Th1 cells. Oncoimmunology. 2016;5:e1039763. https://doi.org/10.1080/2162402X.2015.1039763.

110. Dinarello CA, van der Meer JW. Treating inflammation by blocking interleukin-1 in humans. Semin Immunol. 2013;25:469–84. https://doi.org/10.1016/j.smim.2013.10.008.

111. Rodriguez-Berriguete G, et al. Clinical significance of both tumor and stromal expression of components of the IL-1 and TNF-alpha signaling pathways in prostate cancer. Cytokine. 2013;64:555–63. https://doi.org/10.1016/j.cyto.2013.09.003.

112. Wang Y, et al. Neutrophil infiltration favors colitis-associated tumorigenesis by activating the interleukin-1 (IL-1)/IL-6 axis. Mucosal Immunol. 2014;7:1106–15. https://doi.org/10.1038/mi.2013.126.

113. Palomo J, Dietrich D, Martin P, Palmer G, Gabay C. The interleukin (IL)-1 cytokine family—balance between agonists and antagonists in inflammatory diseases. Cytokine. 2015;76:25–37. https://doi.org/10.1016/j.cyto.2015.06.017.

114. Gupta M, et al. Comprehensive serum cytokine analysis identifies IL-1RA and soluble IL-2Ralpha as predictors of event-free survival in T-cell lymphoma. Ann Oncol. 2016;27:165–72. https://doi.org/10.1093/annonc/mdv486.

115. Patel SK, et al. Inflammatory biomarkers, comorbidity, and neurocognition in women with newly diagnosed breast cancer. J Natl Cancer Inst. 2015;107. https://doi.org/10.1093/jnci/djv131.

116. Taniguchi K, Karin M. IL-6 and related cytokines as the critical lynchpins between inflammation and cancer. Semin Immunol. 2014;26:54–74. https://doi.org/10.1016/j.smim.2014.01.001.

117. Zhang Y, et al. Interleukin-6 is required for pancreatic cancer progression by promoting MAPK signaling activation and oxidative stress resistance. Cancer Res. 2013;73:6359–74. https://doi.org/10.1158/0008-5472.CAN-13-1558-T.

118. Nagasaki T, et al. Interleukin-6 released by colon cancer-associated fibroblasts is critical for tumour angiogenesis: anti-interleukin-6 receptor antibody suppressed angiogenesis and inhibited tumour-stroma interaction. Br J Cancer. 2014;110:469–78. https://doi.org/10.1038/bjc.2013.748.

119. Geng Y, et al. Phenotypic switch in blood: effects of pro-inflammatory cytokines on breast cancer cell aggregation and adhesion. PLoS One. 2013;8:e54959. https://doi.org/10.1371/journal.pone.0054959.

120. Yang C, et al. Increased drug resistance in breast cancer by tumor-associated macrophages through IL-10/STAT3/bcl-2 signaling pathway. Med Oncol. 2015;32:352. https://doi.org/10.1007/s12032-014-0352-6.

121. Kitamura T, et al. CCL2-induced chemokine cascade promotes breast cancer metastasis by enhancing retention of metastasis-associated macrophages. J Exp Med. 2015;212:1043–59. https://doi.org/10.1084/jem.20141836.

122. Nywening TM, et al. Targeting tumour-associated macrophages with CCR2 inhibition in combination with FOLFIRINOX in patients with borderline resectable and locally advanced pancreatic cancer: a single-centre, open-label, dose-finding, non-randomised, phase 1b trial. Lancet Oncol. 2016;17:651–62. https://doi.org/10.1016/S1470-2045(16)00078-4.

123. Imig JD, Hammock BD. Soluble epoxide hydrolase as a therapeutic target for cardiovascular diseases. Nat Rev Drug Discov. 2009;8:794–805. https://doi.org/10.1038/nrd2875. nrd2875 [pii].

124. Montrose DC, et al. The role of PGE2 in intestinal inflammation and tumorigenesis. Prostaglandins Other Lipid Mediat. 2015;116–117:26–36. https://doi.org/10.1016/j.prostaglandins.2014.10.002.

125. Wang D, Fu L, Sun H, Guo L, DuBois RN. Prostaglandin E2 promotes colorectal cancer stem cell expansion and metastasis in mice. Gastroenterology. 2015;149:1884–1895 e1884. https://doi.org/10.1053/j.gastro.2015.07.064.

126. Xu L, et al. COX-2 inhibition potentiates antiangiogenic cancer therapy and prevents metastasis in preclinical models. Sci Transl Med. 2014;6:242ra284. https://doi.org/10.1126/scitranslmed.3008455.

127. Wang D, DuBois RN. Role of prostanoids in gastrointestinal cancer. J Clin Invest. 2018;128:2732–42. https://doi.org/10.1172/JCI97953.

128. Mao Y, et al. Inhibition of tumor-derived prostaglandin-e2 blocks the induction of myeloid-derived suppressor cells and recovers natural killer cell activity. Clin Cancer Res. 2014;20:4096–106. https://doi.org/10.1158/1078-0432.CCR-14-0635.

129. Zelenay S, et al. Cyclooxygenase-dependent tumor growth through evasion of immunity. Cell. 2015;162:1257–70. https://doi.org/10.1016/j.cell.2015.08.015.

130. Zhang X, Zhu Z, Zhong S, Xu T, Shen Z. Ureteral tumours showing a worse prognosis than renal pelvis tumours may be attributed to ureteral tumours more likely to have hydronephrosis and less likely to have haematuria. World J Urol. 2013;31:155–60. https://doi.org/10.1007/s00345-012-0885-2.

131. Larsen BT, et al. Epoxyeicosatrienoic and dihydroxyeicosatrienoic acids dilate human coronary arterioles via BK(Ca) channels: implications for soluble epoxide hydrolase inhibition. Am J Physiol Heart Circ Physiol. 2006;290:H491–9. https://doi.org/10.1152/ajpheart.00927.2005. 00927.2005 [pii]

132. Panigrahy D, et al. Epoxyeicosanoids promote organ and tissue regeneration. Proc Natl Acad Sci U S A. 2013; https://doi.org/10.1073/pnas.1311565110.

133. Sander AL, et al. Cytochrome P450-derived epoxyeicosatrienoic acids accelerate wound epithelialization and neovascularization in the hairless mouse ear wound model. Langenbecks Arch Surg. 2011;396:1245–53. https://doi.org/10.1007/s00423-011-0838-z.

134. Inceoglu B, et al. Epoxy fatty acids and inhibition of the soluble epoxide hydrolase selectively modulate GABA mediated neurotransmission to delay onset of seizures. PLoS One. 2013;8:e80922. https://doi.org/10.1371/journal.pone.0080922.

135. Zhang G, Kodani S, Hammock BD. Stabilized epoxygenated fatty acids regulate inflammation, pain, angiogenesis and cancer. Prog Lipid Res. 2014;53:108–23. https://doi.org/10.1016/j.plipres.2013.11.003.

136. Wang D, Dubois RN. Epoxyeicosatrienoic acids: a double-edged sword in cardiovascular diseases and cancer. J Clin Invest. 2012;122:19–22. https://doi.org/10.1172/JCI61453.

137. Wei X, et al. Elevated 14,15-epoxyeicosatrienoic acid by increasing of cytochrome P450 2C8, 2C9 and 2J2 and decreasing of soluble epoxide hydrolase associated with aggressiveness of human breast cancer. BMC Cancer. 2014;14:841. https://doi.org/10.1186/1471-2407-14-841.

138. Morisseau C, Hammock BD. Impact of soluble epoxide hydrolase and epoxyeicosanoids on human health. Annu Rev Pharmacol Toxicol. 2013;53:37–58. https://doi.org/10.1146/annurev-pharmtox-011112-140244.

139. Zhang G, et al. Dual inhibition of cyclooxygenase-2 and soluble epoxide hydrolase synergistically suppresses primary tumor growth and metastasis. Proc Natl Acad Sci U S A. 2014;111:11127–32. https://doi.org/10.1073/pnas.1410432111.

140. Di Gennaro A, Haeggstrom JZ. The leukotrienes: immune-modulating lipid mediators of disease. Adv Immunol. 2012;116:51–92. https://doi.org/10.1016/B978-0-12-394300-2.00002-8.

141. Satpathy SR, et al. Crystalline silica-induced leukotriene B4-dependent inflammation promotes lung tumour growth. Nat Commun. 2015;6:7064. https://doi.org/10.1038/ncomms8064.

142. Poczobutt JM, et al. Eicosanoid profiling in an orthotopic model of lung cancer progression by mass spectrometry demonstrates selective production of leukotrienes by inflammatory cells of the microenvironment. PLoS One. 2013;8:e79633. https://doi.org/10.1371/journal.pone.0079633.

143. Poczobutt JM, et al. Deletion of 5-lipoxygenase in the tumor microenvironment promotes lung cancer progression and metastasis through regulating T cell recruitment. J Immunol. 2016;196:891–901. https://doi.org/10.4049/jimmunol.1501648.

144. Gounaris E, et al. Zileuton, 5-lipoxygenase inhibitor, acts as a chemopreventive agent in intestinal polyposis, by modulating polyp and systemic inflammation. PLoS One. 2015;10:e0121402. https://doi.org/10.1371/journal.pone.0121402.

145. Sarveswaran S, Chakraborty D, Chitale D, Sears R, Ghosh J. Inhibition of 5-lipoxygenase selectively triggers disruption of c-Myc signaling in prostate cancer cells. J Biol Chem. 2015;290:4994–5006. https://doi.org/10.1074/jbc.M114.599035.

146. Knab LM, et al. Ablation of 5-lipoxygenase mitigates pancreatic lesion development. J Surg Res. 2015;194:481–7. https://doi.org/10.1016/j.jss.2014.10.021.

147. Weissmann G, Smolen JE, Korchak HM. Release of inflammatory mediators from stimulated neutrophils. N Engl J Med. 1980;303:27–34. https://doi.org/10.1056/NEJM198007033030109.

148. Houck JC. Chemical messengers of the inflammatory process. Amsterdam: Elsevier/North-Holland Biomedical Press; 1979.

149. Sina AAA. The canon of medicine (al-Qanun fi'l-tibb) (adapted by Bahktiar L). Great Books of the Islamic World; 1999.

150. Robbins SL, Cotran R. Pathologic basis of disease. 2nd ed. Philadelphia: W.B. Saunders; 1979.

151. Savill JS, Henson PM, Haslett C. Phagocytosis of aged human neutrophils by macrophages is mediated by a novel "charge-sensitive" recognition mechanism. J Clin Invest. 1989;84:1518–27. https://doi.org/10.1172/JCI114328.

152. Savill JS, et al. Macrophage phagocytosis of aging neutrophils in inflammation. Programmed cell death in the neutrophil leads to its recognition by macrophages. J Clin Invest. 1989;83:865–75. https://doi.org/10.1172/JCI113970.

153. Serhan CN, Hamberg M, Samuelsson B. Lipoxins: novel series of biologically active compounds formed from arachidonic acid in human leukocytes. Proc Natl Acad Sci U S A. 1984;81:5335–9.

154. Maddox JF, Serhan CN. Lipoxin A4 and B4 are potent stimuli for human monocyte migration and adhesion: selective inactivation by dehydrogenation and reduction. J Exp Med. 1996;183:137–46. https://doi.org/10.1084/jem.183.1.137.

155. Bandeira-Melo C, et al. Cyclooxygenase-2-derived prostaglandin E2 and lipoxin A4 accelerate resolution of allergic edema in Angiostrongylus costaricensis-infected rats: relationship with concurrent eosinophilia. J Immunol. 2000;164:1029–36. https://doi.org/10.4049/jimmunol.164.2.1029.

156. Godson C, et al. Cutting edge: lipoxins rapidly stimulate nonphlogistic phagocytosis of apoptotic neutrophils by monocyte-derived macrophages. J Immunol. 2000;164:1663–7., ji_v164n4p1663 [pii].

157. Serhan CN. A search for endogenous mechanisms of anti-inflammation uncovers novel chemical mediators: missing links to resolution. Histochem Cell Biol. 2004;122:305–21. https://doi.org/10.1007/s00418-004-0695-8.

158. Takano T, Clish CB, Gronert K, Petasis N, Serhan CN. Neutrophil-mediated changes in vascular permeability are inhibited by topical application of aspirin-triggered 15-epi-lipoxin A4 and novel lipoxin B4 stable analogues. J Clin Invest. 1998;101:819–26. https://doi.org/10.1172/JCI1578.

159. Takano T, et al. Aspirin-triggered 15-epi-lipoxin A4 (LXA4) and LXA4 stable analogues are potent inhibitors of acute inflammation: evidence for anti-inflammatory receptors. J Exp Med. 1997;185:1693–704. https://doi.org/10.1084/jem.185.9.1693.

160. Serhan CN. The resolution of inflammation: the devil in the flask and in the details. FASEB J. 2011;25:1441–8. https://doi.org/10.1096/fj.11-0502ufm. 25/5/1441 [pii].

161. Chiang N, Serhan CN. Specialized pro-resolving mediator network: an update on production and actions. Essays Biochem. 2020;64:443–62. https://doi.org/10.1042/EBC20200018.

162. Bell GA, et al. Intake of long-chain omega-3 fatty acids from diet and supplements in relation to mortality. Am J Epidemiol. 2014;179:710–20. https://doi.org/10.1093/aje/kwt326.

163. Yates CM, Calder PC, Ed Rainger G. Pharmacology and therapeutics of omega-3 polyunsaturated fatty acids in chronic inflammatory disease. Pharmacol Ther. 2014;141:272–82. https://doi.org/10.1016/j.pharmthera.2013.10.010.

164. Panigrahy D, et al. PPARalpha agonist fenofibrate suppresses tumor growth through direct and indirect angiogenesis inhibition. Proc Natl Acad Sci U S A. 2008;105:985–90. https://doi.org/10.1073/pnas.0711281105.

165. Kaipainen A, et al. PPARalpha deficiency in inflammatory cells suppresses tumor growth. PLoS One. 2007;2:e260. https://doi.org/10.1371/journal.pone.0000260.

166. Song M, et al. Marine omega-3 polyunsaturated fatty acid intake and survival after colorectal cancer diagnosis. Gut. 2016; https://doi.org/10.1136/gutjnl-2016-311990.

167. Wang D, DuBois RN. The role of anti-inflammatory drugs in colorectal cancer. Annu Rev Med. 2013;64:131–44. https://doi.org/10.1146/annurev-med-112211-154330.

168. Liang P, et al. Effect of dietary omega-3 fatty acids on tumor-associated macrophages and prostate cancer progression. Prostate. 2016;76:1293–302. https://doi.org/10.1002/pros.23218.

169. D'Eliseo D, Velotti F. Omega-3 fatty acids and cancer cell cytotoxicity: implications for multi-targeted cancer therapy. J Clin Med. 2016;5. https://doi.org/10.3390/jcm5020015.

170. Nabavi SF, et al. Omega-3 polyunsaturated fatty acids and cancer: lessons learned from clinical trials. Cancer Metastasis Rev. 2015;34:359–80. https://doi.org/10.1007/s10555-015-9572-2.

171. D'Eliseo D, et al. Epitelial-to-mesenchymal transition and invasion are upmodulated by tumor-expressed granzyme B and inhibited by docosahexaenoic acid in human colorectal cancer cells. J Exp Clin Cancer Res. 2016;35:24. https://doi.org/10.1186/s13046-016-0302-6.

172. Pan J, et al. Elevation of omega-3 polyunsaturated fatty acids attenuates PTEN-deficiency induced endometrial cancer development through regulation of COX-2 and PGE2 production. Sci Rep. 2015;5:14958. https://doi.org/10.1038/srep14958.

173. Zhang C, Yu H, Ni X, Shen S, Das UN. Growth inhibitory effect of polyunsaturated fatty acids (PUFAs) on colon cancer cells via their growth inhibitory metabolites and fatty acid composition changes. PLoS One. 2015;10:e0123256. https://doi.org/10.1371/journal.pone.0123256.

174. Serhan CN, Levy BD. Resolvins in inflammation: emergence of the pro-resolving superfamily of mediators. J Clin Invest. 2018;128:2657–69. https://doi.org/10.1172/JCI97943.

175. Chandrasekharan JA, Huang XM, Hwang AC, Sharma-Walia N. Altering the anti-inflammatory lipoxin microenvironment: a new insight into Kaposi's sarcoma-associated herpesvirus patho-

genesis. J Virol. 2016;90:11020–31. https://doi.org/10.1128/JVI.01491-16.

176. Stenke L, Edenius C, Samuelsson J, Lindgren JA. Deficient lipoxin synthesis: a novel platelet dysfunction in myeloproliferative disorders with special reference to blastic crisis of chronic myelogenous leukemia. Blood. 1991;78:2989–95.

177. Liu H, et al. Colorectal cancer is associated with a deficiency of lipoxin A4, an endogenous anti-inflammatory mediator. J Cancer. 2019;10:4719–30. https://doi.org/10.7150/jca.32456.

178. Zhuang Q, Meng Q, Xi Q, Wu G. [Association of serum inflammatory cytokines and Resolvin D1 concentration with pathological stage of colon cancer]. Zhonghua Wei Chang Wai Ke Za Zhi. 2018;21:1285–90.

179. Cata JP, et al. Inflammation and pro-resolution inflammation after hepatobiliary surgery. World J Surg Oncol. 2017;15:152. https://doi.org/10.1186/s12957-017-1220-6.

180. Kuang H, Hua X, Zhou J, Yang R. Resolvin D1 and E1 alleviate the progress of hepatitis toward liver cancer in long-term concanavalin A-induced mice through inhibition of NF-kappaB activity. Oncol Rep. 2016;35:307–17. https://doi.org/10.3892/or.2015.4389.

181. Zong L, et al. Lipoxin A4 reverses mesenchymal phenotypes to attenuate invasion and metastasis via the inhibition of autocrine TGF-beta1 signaling in pancreatic cancer. J Exp Clin Cancer Res. 2017;36:181. https://doi.org/10.1186/s13046-017-0655-5.

182. Schnittert J, Heinrich MA, Kuninty PR, Storm G, Prakash J. Reprogramming tumor stroma using an endogenous lipid lipoxin A4 to treat pancreatic cancer. Cancer Lett. 2018;420:247–58. https://doi.org/10.1016/j.canlet.2018.01.072.

183. Prevete N, et al. Formyl peptide receptor 1 suppresses gastric cancer angiogenesis and growth by exploiting inflammation resolution pathways. Oncoimmunology. 2017;6:e1293213. https://doi.org/10.1080/2162402X.2017.1293213.

184. Lu Y, Xu Q, Yin G, Xu W, Jiang H. Resolvin D1 inhibits the proliferation of lipopolysaccharide-treated HepG2 hepatoblastoma and PLC/PRF/5 hepatocellular carcinoma cells by targeting the MAPK pathway. Exp Ther Med. 2018;16:3603–10. https://doi.org/10.3892/etm.2018.6651.

185. Zhang B, et al. Depletion of regulatory T cells facilitates growth of established tumors: a mechanism involving the regulation of myeloid-derived suppressor cells by lipoxin A4. J Immunol. 2010;185:7199–206. https://doi.org/10.4049/jimmunol.1001876. jimmunol.1001876 [pii]

186. Tsai WH, et al. Role of lipoxin A4 in the cell-to-cell interaction between all-trans retinoic acid-treated acute promyelocytic leukemic cells and alveolar macrophages. J Cell Physiol. 2012;227:1123–9. https://doi.org/10.1002/jcp.22832.

187. Hu S, et al. Lipoxins and aspirin-triggered lipoxin alleviate bone cancer pain in association with suppressing expression of spinal proinflammatory cytokines. J Neuroinflammation. 2012;9:278. https://doi.org/10.1186/1742-2094-9-278.

188. Martinez RM, et al. The lipoxin receptor/FPR2 agonist BML-111 protects mouse skin against ultraviolet B radiation. Molecules. 2020;25. https://doi.org/10.3390/molecules25122953.

189. Lin L, et al. BML-111, the lipoxin A4 agonist, modulates VEGF or CoCl2-induced migration, angiogenesis and permeability in tumor-derived endothelial cells. Immunol Lett. 2020;230:27–35. https://doi.org/10.1016/j.imlet.2020.12.007.

190. Chen Y, et al. Lipoxin A4 and its analogue suppress the tumor growth of transplanted H22 in mice: the role of antiangiogenesis. Mol Cancer Ther. 2010;9:2164–74. https://doi.org/10.1158/1535-7163.MCT-10-0173. 1535-7163.MCT-10-0173 [pii]

191. Hao H, et al. Lipoxin A4 and its analog suppress hepatocellular carcinoma via remodeling tumor microenvironment. Cancer Lett. 2011;309:85–94. https://doi.org/10.1016/j.canlet.2011.05.020.

192. Eritja N, et al. Tumour-microenvironmental blood flow determines a metabolomic signature identifying lysophospholipids and resolvin D as biomarkers in endometrial cancer patients. Oncotarget. 2017;8:109018–26. https://doi.org/10.18632/oncotarget.22558.

193. Bai X, et al. Inhibition of lung cancer growth and metastasis by DHA and its metabolite, RvD1, through miR-138-5p/FOXC1 pathway. J Exp Clin Cancer Res. 2019;38:479. https://doi.org/10.1186/s13046-019-1478-3.

194. Yang P, et al. ResolvinD1 attenuates high-mobility group box 1-induced epithelial-to-mesenchymal transition in nasopharyngeal carcinoma cells. Exp Biol Med (Maywood). 2019;244:1608–18. https://doi.org/10.1177/1535370219885320.

195. Ye Y, et al. Anti-cancer and analgesic effects of resolvin D2 in oral squamous cell carcinoma. Neuropharmacology. 2018;139:182–93. https://doi.org/10.1016/j.neuropharm.2018.07.016.

196. Halder RC, et al. Curcuminoids and omega-3 fatty acids with antioxidants potentiate cytotoxicity of natural killer cells against pancreatic ductal adenocarcinoma cells and inhibit interferon gamma production. Front Physiol. 2015;6:129. https://doi.org/10.3389/fphys.2015.00129.

197. Shan K, et al. Resolvin D1 and D2 inhibit tumour growth and inflammation via modulating macrophage polarization. J Cell Mol Med. 2020; https://doi.org/10.1111/jcmm.15436.

198. Zhong X, Lee HN, Surh YJ. RvD1 inhibits TNFalpha-induced c-Myc expression in normal intestinal epithelial cells and destabilizes hyper-expressed c-Myc in colon cancer cells. Biochem Biophys Res Commun. 2018;496:316–23. https://doi.org/10.1016/j.bbrc.2017.12.171.

199. Khasabova IA, Golovko MY, Golovko SA, Simone DA, Khasabov SG. Intrathecal administration of Resolvin D1 and E1 decreases hyperalgesia in mice with bone cancer pain: involvement of endocannabinoid signaling. Prostaglandins Other Lipid Mediat. 2020;151:106479. https://doi.org/10.1016/j.prostaglandins.2020.106479.

200. Saito P, et al. The lipid mediator resolvin D1 reduces the skin inflammation and oxidative stress induced by UV irradiation in hairless mice. Front Pharmacol. 2018;9:1242. https://doi.org/10.3389/fphar.2018.01242.

201. Zhang J, et al. Resolvin E1 protects against doxorubicin-induced cardiotoxicity by inhibiting oxidative stress, autophagy and apoptosis by targeting AKT/mTOR signaling. Biochem Pharmacol. 2020;180:114188. https://doi.org/10.1016/j.bcp.2020.114188.

202. Luo X, Gu Y, Tao X, Serhan CN, Ji RR. Resolvin D5 inhibits neuropathic and inflammatory pain in male but not female mice: distinct actions of D-series resolvins in chemotherapy-induced peripheral neuropathy. Front Pharmacol. 2019;10:745. https://doi.org/10.3389/fphar.2019.00745.

203. Qiao Y, et al. Associations between aspirin use and the risk of cancers: a meta-analysis of observational studies. BMC Cancer. 2018;18:288. https://doi.org/10.1186/s12885-018-4156-5.

204. Gilroy DW, et al. Inducible cyclooxygenase may have anti-inflammatory properties. Nat Med. 1999;5:698–701. https://doi.org/10.1038/9550.

205. Drew DA, Cao Y, Chan AT. Aspirin and colorectal cancer: the promise of precision chemoprevention. Nat Rev Cancer. 2016;16:173–86. https://doi.org/10.1038/nrc.2016.4.

206. Baandrup L, Kjaer SK, Olsen JH, Dehlendorff C, Friis S. Low-dose aspirin use and the risk of ovarian cancer in Denmark. Ann Oncol. 2015;26:787–92. https://doi.org/10.1093/annonc/mdu578.

207. Trabert B, et al. Aspirin, nonaspirin nonsteroidal anti-inflammatory drug, and acetaminophen use and risk of invasive epithelial ovarian cancer: a pooled analysis in the Ovarian Cancer Association Consortium. J Natl Cancer Inst. 2014;106:djt431. https://doi.org/10.1093/jnci/djt431.

208. Ye X, et al. Frequency-risk and duration-risk relationships between aspirin use and gastric cancer: a systematic review and meta-analysis. PLoS One. 2013;8:e71522. https://doi.org/10.1371/journal.pone.0071522.

209. Fraser DM, Sullivan FM, Thompson AM, McCowan C. Aspirin use and survival after the diagnosis of breast cancer: a population-based cohort study. Br J Cancer. 2014;111:623–7. https://doi.org/10.1038/bjc.2014.264.

210. Chubak J, et al. Aspirin for the prevention of cancer incidence and mortality: systematic evidence reviews for the U.S. Preventive Services Task Force. Ann Intern Med. 2016;164:814–25. https://doi.org/10.7326/M15-2117.

211. Friis S, Riis AH, Erichsen R, Baron JA, Sorensen HT. Low-dose aspirin or nonsteroidal anti-inflammatory drug use and colorectal cancer risk: a population-based, case-control study. Ann Intern Med. 2015;163:347–55. https://doi.org/10.7326/M15-0039.

212. Nan H, et al. Association of aspirin and NSAID use with risk of colorectal cancer according to genetic variants. JAMA. 2015;313:1133–42. https://doi.org/10.1001/jama.2015.1815.

213. Vidal AC, et al. Aspirin, NSAIDs, and risk of prostate cancer: results from the REDUCE study. Clin Cancer Res. 2015;21:756–62. https://doi.org/10.1158/1078-0432.CCR-14-2235.

214. Charles KA, et al. Systemic inflammation is an independent predictive marker of clinical outcomes in mucosal squamous cell carcinoma of the head and neck in oropharyngeal and non-oropharyngeal patients. BMC Cancer. 2016;16:124. https://doi.org/10.1186/s12885-016-2089-4.

215. Moreira DM, et al. Baseline prostate inflammation is associated with a reduced risk of prostate cancer in men undergoing repeat prostate biopsy: results from the REDUCE study. Cancer. 2014;120:190–6. https://doi.org/10.1002/cncr.28349.

216. Moreira DM, Nickel JC, Andriole GL, Castro-Santamaria R, Freedland SJ. Chronic baseline prostate inflammation is associated with lower tumor volume in men with prostate cancer on repeat biopsy: results from the REDUCE study. Prostate. 2015;75:1492–8. https://doi.org/10.1002/pros.23041.

217. Morrison L, et al. Inflammatory biomarker score and cancer: a population-based prospective cohort study. BMC Cancer. 2016;16:80. https://doi.org/10.1186/s12885-016-2115-6.

218. Zheng RR, et al. Cervical cancer systemic inflammation score: a novel predictor of prognosis. Oncotarget. 2016;7:15230–42. https://doi.org/10.18632/oncotarget.7378.

219. Gu L, et al. Prognostic role of lymphocyte to monocyte ratio for patients with cancer: evidence from a systematic review and meta-analysis. Oncotarget. 2016;7:31926–42. https://doi.org/10.18632/oncotarget.7876.

220. Hu P, et al. Prognostic significance of systemic inflammation-based lymphocyte-monocyte ratio in patients with lung cancer: based on a large cohort study. PLoS One. 2014;9:e108062. https://doi.org/10.1371/journal.pone.0108062.

Role of Lymphocytes in Cancer Immunity and Immune Evasion Mechanisms

10

Kushi Kushekhar, Stalin Chellappa, Einar M. Aandahl, and Kjetil Taskén

Abstract

It is well established that the immune system is involved in the initiation, development, and progression of cancer. The tumor microenvironment is highly infiltrated by a complex network of immune cells, which includes innate (macrophages, mast cells, neutrophils, dendritic cells, natural killer cells, innate lymphoid cells, and myeloid-derived suppressor cells) and adaptive T and B lymphocytes. This diverse set of cells, their interactions, and secretion of anti- or pro-inflammatory immune mediators create an immunologically active tumor microenvironment. It is the composition of immune cells, their functional phenotype, and their secretions that dictate either tumor regression or tumor progression. The CD4+ T cells are instrumental in eliminating cancer cells by secreting various pro-inflammatory cytokines that act directly and indirectly by activating and recruiting other cell types such as macrophages, and granulocytes to eliminate cancer. However, CD8+ T cells with the help of CD4+ T cells represent the major effector mechanism of anti-tumor immunity. On the other hand, regulatory T cells, a subset of CD4+ T cells, are involved in promoting tumor growth by suppressing both CD4+ and CD8+ T cells. With the advancement of high-throughput and multiplex analysis techniques, immune cells are characterized in detail with advanced functional roles in relation to cancer development and progression. In this chapter, we review and discuss the current knowledge with respect to the evolving functional role and prognostic significance of individual T cell subsets in various malignancies.

Take-Home Lessons

- Anti-tumor immunity mediated by lymphocytes is predetermined as well as adapted during the course of disease.
- Adaptive CD4+Th1 and CD8+ Tc1 cells have well-defined roles in anti-tumor immunity while CD4+ Tregs have pro-tumoral role and are tumor-antigen specific.
- CD4+ Th2, Th9, Th17, Th22, Tfh, and CD8+ Tc2 subsets can be both anti-tumoral and pro-tumoral depending on the context of the tumor microenvironment and cancer type.
- Unconventional, innate-like T cells have more potent anti-tumoral effects in a non-tumor antigen-specific manner, especially in solid tumors.

K. Kushekhar · S. Chellappa
Department of Cancer Immunology, Institute for Cancer Research, Oslo University Hospital, Oslo, Norway

Nykode Therapeutics AS, Oslo, Norway

E. M. Aandahl
Department of Cancer Immunology, Institute for Cancer Research, Oslo University Hospital, Oslo, Norway

Department of Transplantation Medicine, Oslo University Hospital Rikshospitalet, Oslo, Norway

K. Taskén (✉)
Department of Cancer Immunology, Institute for Cancer Research, Oslo University Hospital, Oslo, Norway

Institute Clinical Medicine, University of Oslo, Oslo, Norway
e-mail: kjetil.tasken@medisin.uio.no

Box 10.1

- The tumor microenvironment consists of CD4 T cells, CD8 T cells, Tregs, antigen-presenting cells, unconventional T cells, stromal cells, and the tumor cells and harbors active processes of immunosurveillance and immune escape.
- CD4 T cell subtypes may, depending on the tumor immune context, act in both tumor killing and tumor promotion.

- CD8 T cell subtypes are the primary effectors of anti-tumor immunity and eliminate tumor cells by direct killing through secretion of cytokines and cytotoxic granules.
- Tregs suppress the anti-tumor immunity by expressing immune checkpoint inhibitors and secreting immunosuppressive cytokines and inflammatory mediators.
- Unconventional, innate-like T cells have broad and nonspecific anti-tumor immunity, especially in solid cancer types.
- The type of T cells, their phenotypic plasticity, location, the niche they share with other immune cells, cancer cells, and stromal cells along with their complex interactions play a crucial role in modulating tumor progression, therapeutic response, and patient outcomes.

Cancer Immunoediting and Tumor Immune Evasion Mechanisms

While the role of the immune system in controlling microbial pathogens is well appreciated, the notion that the immune system can also control tumor initiation, development, and progression has been subject to controversy for over a century. In 1909, Paul Ehrlich was the first to suggest that the immune system could protect the host from malignancies [1]. Nearly 50 years later, Thomas and Burnet predicted that adaptive immunity is responsible for preventing tumor formation and progression in an immunocompetent host and proposed the concept of cancer immunosurveillance [2, 3]. Currently, the term immunosurveillance is used to describe the processes by which cells of the immune system look for and recognize foreign pathogens, such as bacteria and viruses, or precancerous and cancerous cells in the body. However, due to inadequate experimental support, the cancer immunosurveillance concept was abandoned at that time. This was largely due to the lack of mouse models with pure genetic backgrounds available at that time. By the 1990s, with improved genetically modified mouse models available, several seminal works have validated the role of cancer immunosurveillance in both chemically induced and spontaneous tumor models [4]. Multiple components of the immune system have been identified as having central roles in cancer immunosurveillance, such as T cells, B cells, natural killer (NK) cells, and cytokines such as interferon-gamma (INF-γ) and perforins [4, 5]. Similarly, several experimental and clinical studies have confirmed the existence of cancer immunosurveillance (T cell-mediated cancer immunosur-

veillance is described in detail in the following sections) [5]. These findings suggest that cancer immunosurveillance is an active process that happens in the tumor microenvironment. However, despite the presence of an active cancer immunosurveillance process, many immunocompetent individuals still develop cancer. This paradox is explained via seminal mice studies showing that the immune system not only eliminates but also reduces the immunogenicity of the tumor, thereby promoting tumor growth [4]. This led to a significant revision of the original cancer immunosurveillance concept wherein Robert Schreiber and colleagues proposed a new concept termed "cancer immunoediting," which emphasized the dual role of the cancer-promoting and suppressing role of the immune system during tumor growth [4, 6].

Cancer immunoediting consists of three phases: elimination, equilibrium, and escape, termed "the three E's of cancer immunoediting" [6]. The elimination phase represents the original concept of cancer immunosurveillance, in which the cooperative actions of the innate and adaptive immune system eliminates the tumor before it is clinically manifest. Studies suggest that the immune component required for the elimination of tumors depends on specific tumor characteristics such as origin (spontaneous vs. carcinogen-induced), anatomical location, histology, and growth rate. During the elimination phase, rare tumor cell variants may survive and enter into an equilibrium state. Generally, the equilibrium state is the longest phase and it can extend throughout the life of the host. In this period, tumor cells undergo a process called antigenicity sculpting, where the immune cells apply a selective pressure (to deplete susceptible tumor cells) leading to the survival of the fittest/fastest-growing cells that escape elimination by the immune system. This process results in reduced immunogenicity of tumors and acquired resistance to immune effector cells. At the end of the equilibrium and the antigenicity sculpting phase, several tumor clones with immune evasive mutations and epigenetic instability will survive and start to proliferate. These cells ultimately enter into the escape phase and develop into visible tumors and successfully avoid immune destruction, which is now considered an emerging hallmark of cancers as described by Hanahan and Weinberg [7].

Tumor cells may evade the protective immunity by a number of mechanisms as presented in Table 10.1, for example, by loss of human leukocyte antigen (HLA, also called as major histocompatibility complex (MHC) in mice) display of foreign peptides thereby impairing tumor immune recognition, by inhibition of mechanisms that promote immune cell trafficking into the tumor microenvironment, by promoting immune suppression or subversion, or by inducing tumor cell resistance to apoptosis by altering the expression of anti- and pro-apoptotic molecules. The array of immunosuppressive mechanisms that may be active include secretion soluble inhibitors (adenosine, prostaglandin E2 (PGE2), IL-10,

Table 10.1 Tumor immune evasion mechanisms

Evasion strategy	Mechanisms
Impaired tumor antigen presentation to immune cells	• Downregulation of tumor antigens or antigen processing machinery (e.g., lack of LMP and TAP proteins) [9] • Downregulation of HLA genes [10]
Impaired trafficking of immune cells into tumor microenvironment	• Epigenetic silencing of chemokine expression [11] • Lack of endothelial adhesion molecules [12–14] • Physical barrier by stroma [15] • Lack of tumor antigens in lymphoid organs [16]
Immune cell dysfunction or subversion	• Immune suppression is mediated by CD4+FOXP3+ regulatory T cells (Tregs) and myeloid-derived suppressor cells (MDSCs) [17–21] • Secretion of suppressive cytokines (TGFβ, IL-10, etc.) [22–24], and other soluble immunosuppressive factors (prostaglandin E2, VEGF, RCAS1, extracellular adenosine, reactive oxygen and nitrogen species, etc.) [25–29] • Expression of IDO in tumor cells leading to secretion of immunosuppressive tryptophan metabolites [30] • Induction of T cell tolerance by expressing cognate ligands for T cell checkpoint inhibitory receptors such as CTLA-4, PD-1, LAG-3, Tim-3 [31, 32] • Apoptosis of immune cells induced by tumor cell expression of CD95L (FasL) (tumor counterattack) [33] triggering CD95 (Fas)-mediated T cell apoptosis • Immune cell deviation and plasticity [34–37]
Tumor cell resistance to apoptosis	• Abnormal expression of antiapoptotic molecules (Bcl-2 and IAPs family protein) [38] • Mutations or loss of pro-apoptotic molecules (TRAIL and CD95 receptors) [38] • Interference with granzyme/perforin pathway [39, 40]

IL-35, transforming growth factor-β1 (TGF-β1), etc.), overexpression of indoleamine 2,3-Dioxygenase, activation of inhibitory immune checkpoints or migration or formation and activation of regulatory T cells (Tregs) locally in the tumor to suppress bystander tumor-infiltrating effector T cells [8].

Targeting the immune escape mechanisms has proven to be a promising strategy for cancer treatment. The introduction of immune checkpoint inhibitors has been very successful and ICIs provide a cure or long-term remission for many patients, particularly patients with cancers with high tumor mutational burden (TMB) such as melanoma, lung, and kidney cancer [41, 42]. However, immune checkpoint inhibitors only appear to work for a subgroup (40–50%) of patients in each of these indications whereas it does not work despite high TMB in some cancers [43]. Thus, many of the other tumor immune evasion mechanisms (Table 10.1) may also be acting in parallel and have clinical importance. Therapeutic strategies for blocking these mechanisms to rescue anti-tumor immunity could add to the current repertoire of immunostimulating therapies, in a precision immune oncology approach in patients not responding to immune checkpoint inhibitors. Currently, targeting one or more of these mechanisms clinically holds the most promising approach to improving anti-tumor immunity [25].

Our group studies tumor immune evasion strategies by soluble inhibitors secreted by cancer cells (PGE2, adenosine, and cAMP), immune suppression by Tregs and interaction with immune checkpoint inhibitors [44–46]. We have studied anti-tumor immunity in colorectal cancer, pancreatic ductal adenocarcinoma, cholangiocarcinoma, ovarian cancer, and leukemias [47–53], which are discussed in detail under specific sections. In this chapter, we review and discuss the complex role of immune cells, particularly T lymphocytes and TILs in cancer immunity and tumor immune evasion mechanisms.

T Lymphocytes and Cancer Immunity

T cells are mainly classified into two lineages. CD4+ T cells and CD8+ T cells. CD4+ T cells are further subclassified into CD4+ T-helper cells (Th) that mediate tumor immunity and CD4+ forkhead protein 3+ (FOXP3) Tregs that suppress anti-tumor immunity. Naïve T cells that express a unique T cell receptor (TCR) on the surface develop through stringent positive and negative selection pathways in the thymus. T cells migrate through tissues and scan for cognate antigen peptides in the context of HLA complex on antigen-presenting cells (APCs) that activate their TCR downstream signaling, resulting in functional differentiation into a variety of T cell subsets [54]. Here we focus on conventional TCRα/β T cell subsets, unconventional T lymphocytes, and their role in tumor immunity.

CD4+ T Cells and Anti-tumor Immunity

CD4+ T cells are an important component of adaptive immune responses and are crucial in orchestrating humoral and cell-mediated immune responses [55]. However, their role in anticancer immunity is complex and reflects the diverse role of various CD4+ Th cells subsets (discussed in subsequent sections) [34]. The naïve CD4+ T cell TCR recognizes antigenic epitopes in the form of 12–20 peptide residues, presented on HLA class II expressed on professional APCs such as dendritic cells (DCs), macrophages, and B cells [56]. For a successful T cell activation, naïve CD4+ T cells require two signals [57]. Signal-1 involves TCR recognition of antigen in the context of HLA class II expressed on the surface of APCs. Signal-2 involves an interaction of co-stimulatory receptors such as CD28 on T cells with its ligands CD80/86 on APCs, which results in clonal expansion, triggered effector functions, and subsequent memory formation. In addition, a third signal from the cytokines in the microenvironment defines the "maturation" of CD4+ T cells into its Th subtypes. The fate and functional specialization of activated CD4+ T cells are dependent on the concentration, source of antigen, type of APC, the co-stimulatory receptors, and most importantly, the polarizing cytokine milieu of the microenvironment at the time of activation [54]. Together, these polarizing factors contribute to the specific expression of key subset defining transcriptional factors and the subsequent secretion of effector cytokines that defines the functional subsets of CD4+ Th cells [54]. The cytokines secreted by CD4+ Th subsets then activate and recruit a variety of other immune effector cells that together define the type of immune response [55]. Table 10.2 summarizes the CD4+ Th cell subsets in the human and murine systems, the polarizing cytokines that drive their development, their master transcription factors, and the effector cytokines they secrete.

Conventional Role of CD4+ T Cells in Tumor Immunity

One of the important roles of CD4+ Th cells in anti-tumor immunity is to induce priming, activation, and expansion of cytotoxic T lymphocyte (CTL) responses, a concept known as CD4+ T cell help [58, 59]. CD4+ T cell help is complex and involves multiple mechanisms broadly classified into indirect and direct help. During the primary immune response to the tumor, the major indirect help from activated CD4+ Th cells comes through CD40/CD40L interaction with APCs that leads to maturation of the APCs [60–62]. This process provides all three necessary signals for CD8+ T cell activation, including antigen-mediated TCR triggering, co-stimulation, and stimulatory cytokines, most notably IL-12, that are critically important for naïve antigen-specific CD8+ T cells to differentiate into CTLs. Alternatively, CD4+ Th cells can directly activate CTLs through CD40/CD40L [63]. Activated CD4+ Th cells also directly help CTLs through the secretion of IL-2, which supports the growth and expansion of T cells [64, 65]. Furthermore, secretion of INF-γ by CD4+ Th1 cells upregulates the expression of HLA molecules on the surface of tumor cells leading to a feed-forward loop of enhanced CTL responses as well as CD4+ Th responses [66]. Recent reports also suggest the presence of cytotoxic CD4+ T cells with tumor killing by direct cytotoxicity. These cytotoxic CD4+ T cells can directly recognize tumor antigens presented in the context of HLA class II and degranulate

cytotoxic compounds such as granzyme-B killing the tumor cells, for example, in melanoma and bladder cancer [67, 68].

In addition to priming the primary CTL response, CD4+ Th cells also help during the post-priming stage that takes place in the tumor microenvironment [69, 70]. Tumor-specific CD4+ T cells accelerate the recruitment of CTLs into the tumor microenvironment (TILs) by IFN-γ-dependent production of chemokines. Production of IL-2 by tumor resident CD4+ T cells enhances CD8+ T cell proliferation and upregulates the expression of granzyme-B [70]. In addition, the tumor-specific CD4+ Th cells have been shown to enhance the expansion of both low-avidity [71], and cognate [72] CTLs in the tumor microenvironment and enhance tumor killing.

Memory T cells are antigen-specific T cells that remain long-term after an infection or tumor has been eliminated. The memory T cells quickly converted into large numbers of effector T cells upon re-exposure to the specific antigen, thus providing a rapid response to past infection. In addition to their support to optimize CTL responses, CD4+ Th cells also play an essential role in the generation and maintenance of memory CD8+ T cells during active CTL responses and homeostatic proliferation [73, 74]. Hosts lacking CD4+ Th cells have been shown to have a reduced number of CD8+ memory T cells and impaired secondary CD8+ T cell responses [75]. Moreover, CTLs that develop in the absence of CD4+ T cell help are less likely to exhibit an effector-memory function and instead tend toward an exhausted phenotype [76].

Unconventional Role of CD4+ T Cells in Tumor Immunity

CD4+ Th cell-mediated anti-tumor immunity is primarily thought to be involved in activation and maintenance of CTL responses. However, recent studies have shown that CD4+ Th subsets also play independent roles in tumor immunity. Here we discuss the specific roles of different CD4+ Th cell subsets in tumor immunity.

CD4+ Th1 Cells

In 1991, *Romagnani* and colleagues discovered that human CD4+ Th clones specific for intracellular *Mycobacterium tuberculosis* were mostly Th1 type CD4+ T cells, whereas the CD4+ T clones specific for the extracellular helminth *Toxocara canis* were mainly Th2 cells [77]. The Th1 lineage is controlled by the key transcription factor T-bet and the key polarizing cytokine IL-12 [54, 78, 79]. CD4+ Th1 cells secrete a set of pro-inflammatory cytokines that includes IL-2, INF-γ, TNF-α, and the chemokines CCL2 and CCL3 that attract macrophages (Table 10.2). Th1 cells are best characterized for their role in the clearance of intracellular pathogens such as viruses and in the pathogenesis of autoim-

Table 10.2 CD4+Th cell subsets: polarizing cytokines, master transcription factors, and effector cytokines

Th subset	Polarizing cytokines	Transcription factors	Effector cytokines
Th1	IL-12, IL-18, INF-γ, IL-27	T-bet, STAT4	IL-2, IL-10, INF-γ, TNF-α, TNF-β (LT-α), CCL2, CCL3
Th2	IL-4, IL-25, IL-33, TSLP	GATA3, IRF4, STAT6	IL-4, IL-5, IL-9, IL-10, IL-13, IL-21, IL-31, TNF-α
Th9	TGF-β, IL-4	PU.1, IRF4	IL-9, IL10
Th17	TGF-β, IL-1β, IL-6, IL-21, IL-23	RORγt, RORα, IRF4 Batf, STAT3	IL-17A, IL-17F, IL-21, IL-22, IL-26 (human), CCL20
Th22	IL-6, IL-13, TNF-α	AhR, Batf, STAT3	IL-10, IL-13, IL-22, IL-21, TNF-α, IL-26 (human),
Tfh	IL-6, IL-21	Bcl6, BATF, c-MAF	IL-4, IL-10, IL-12, IL-21, INF-γ

mune conditions [80]. Th1 cells are considered to have potent anti-tumor activity due to their secretion of INF-γ, IL-2, and CD40/CD40L co-stimulation to help initiate CD8+ T cell responses as described earlier [73]. Human Th1 cells can also mediate anti-tumor immunity independently of helping CTL responses. For example, INF-γ acts directly on tumor cells and directs the immunogenic phenotype of tumors that arise in an immunocompetent host [81]. In mice, it has been demonstrated that Th1 cell-mediated INF-γ secretion in the tumor microenvironment is essential for inhibiting angiogenesis and regression of tumors that do not express HLA class II [82]. Similarly, a study of mouse B cell cancer suggests that Th1 cell-mediated INF-γ secretion in the tumor microenvironment is essential for eliminating MHC class II negative tumor cells through activation of type 1 macrophages (M1) and angiogenic inhibitors like IP-10 [83]. However, their mechanistic relevance in human cancer is yet to be determined.

A key function of Th1-derived INF-γ in tumor-bearing hosts is to substantially increase the IL-12 secretion by DCs, which serves to further polarize the naïve CD4+T cells into a Th1 phenotype thereby contributing to their own development and maintenance [84]. In addition, secretion of cytokines and chemokines by Th1 cells also leads to recruitment and activation of pro-inflammatory M1 macrophages, and NK cells at the tumor site [85–87]. The cytotoxic mediators secreted from M1 and NK cells have multiple anti-tumor properties [88, 89]. In line with this, patient studies show that the presence of Th1 cells and increased levels of their associated cytokines correlate with superior anti-tumor immunity and good clinical outcome in a majority of cancers [90]. Despite their potent anti-tumor role, Th1 cell functions are efficiently hindered by tumor cells by varying suppressive factors (Table 10.1 and described later), and imbalance or alterations in Th1/Th2 ratio in many human cancers lead to

poor clinical outcomes [91]. Th1 cells are an attractive treatment option in cancer cell therapies. Adoptive transfer of tumor antigen-specific Th1 cells in patients with metastatic melanoma [92] and metastatic cholangiocarcinoma [93] was shown to induce regression of the tumor for prolonged periods. In contrast, responses in melanoma patients that received only in vitro-expanded, autologous CD8+ TILs were found to be sub-optimal in tumor clearing [94]. These findings clearly underpin the importance of inducing tumor antigen-specific Th1 cells for successful anti-tumor immunity.

CD4+ Th2 Cells

CD4+ Th2 cells are recognized for their role in the host defense against extracellular parasites and their involvement in allergy and asthma [54]. In both mice and humans, Th2 lineage commitment is controlled by the transcription factor GATA (nucleotide sequence) binding protein 3 (GATA3) and the polarizing cytokine IL-4 in the microenvironment [54, 95]. Activated Th2 cells produce their signature cytokines such as IL-4, IL-5, IL-13, and IL-10 (Table 10.2). Initial studies from murine models and in vitro studies showed that IL-4 secreted from Th2 cells has a direct antiangiogenic and tumoricidal activity [96–98]. Both IL-4 and IL-13 bind to type-II IL-4 receptor alpha (IL-4RA) and signals through signal transducer and activator 6 (Stat6) [99]. IL-4 and IL-13 are critical for the recruitment of eosinophils, macrophages, neutrophils, and CD8+ T cells to the tumor site and result in regression of the tumor [100–104]. Conversely, Th2 cytokines also interfere with anti-tumor activity, which is largely attributed to cytokines that antagonize the development of INF-γ secreting Th1 and CTLs at the tumor site. IL-4 and IL-13 have an anti-apoptotic role [99, 105–107] and IL-13 has a pro-fibrotic role [108, 109] that may affect anti-tumor activity. Activating polymorphisms in IL-4, IL-13, and STAT6 genes have been implicated in a higher risk of developing Hodgkin lymphoma [110].

Numerous studies indicate altered Th1/Th2 ratio in a variety of cancers [90, 91]. Th2 cytokines mutually antagonize the development of Th1 cells [54, 111]. This hypothesis was demonstrated using Th2-deficient Stat6-KO mice which rejected tumors through the action of tumor-specific CD8+ CTLs [99]. Immune deviation toward Th2 suppresses Th1 development, and it has been thought that induction affecting a Th2 immune response is one of the mechanisms that downregulate effective tumor immune responses. Initial murine studies suggested that both Th1 and Th2 cells contribute to anti-tumor immunity [87, 112, 113]. However, the increased presence of Th2 cells was found to be pro-carcinogenic in many human cancers [34, 90, 114, 115]. These pro-tumorigenic roles of Th2 cells were proposed to be cancer-specific rather than constituting a global effect, as the Th1 response in these patients was not impaired [116, 117]. Multiple tumor-derived factors may favor the development of Th2 cells. Tumor cell-derived IL-10 induces skewing toward Th2 cells and inhibits the maturation of DCs, which effectively reduces the secretion of INF-γ and IL-12 from T cells resulting in impaired Th1 anti-tumor activity [118, 119]. Early reports demonstrated that human renal cell carcinoma and non-small cell lung cancer actively produced Th2 polarizing cytokines [120, 121]. Pancreatic cancer, an aggressive malignancy, is typically infiltrated by Th2 cells [122]. A clinical study from pancreatic cancer patients showed that the skewing toward Th2 was primarily due to the secretion of thymic stromal lymphopoietin from cancer-associated fibroblasts that activate DCs to produce Th2-associated cytokines and polarize T cells toward Th2 cells [123]. A similar mechanism was observed in mouse models of breast cancer [124], and chronic gastritis [125], which is the causative factor for gastric cancer. Studies in mice have shown that expression of the human tumor antigen, epithelial cell adhesion molecule (EpCAM), strongly promotes Th2 skewing despite the presence of strong Th1 polarizing conditions [126]. Moreover, Th2 cells are capable of clearing established lung and visceral metastases of a CTL-resistant melanoma [104]. Clearance of lung metastases by the Th2 cells was found to be dependent on the eosinophil chemokine, eotaxin, and Stat6, with degranulating eosinophils within the tumors inducing tumor regression. In contrast, tumor-specific CD4+ Th1 cells, that recruited macrophages into the tumors, had no effect on tumor growth. Thus, the involvement of Th2 cells in anti-tumor immunity is evolving, but still controversial, and their effect may be context-dependent.

CD4+ Th17 Cells

In 2005, the third subset of CD4+ Th cells was identified in mice as Th17 cells based on the production of the key cytokine IL-17 [127, 128]. Two years later, the existence of Th17 cells was confirmed in the human immune system [129]. The development of Th17 cells is controlled by the master transcription factor RAR-related orphan receptor gamma t (RORγt) and multiple polarizing cytokines [130–132] (Table 10.2). Th17 cells play an important inflammatory role in the host defense against extracellular bacteria and fungi, but are pathogenic in many inflammatory and autoimmune diseases [35, 130, 133–135]. Th17 cells are shown to infiltrate several cancer types in both mice and humans [35]. However, their exact role in anti-tumor immunity is controversial and still elusive. Contradictory findings with respect to their role in anti-tumor versus pro-tumoral role may be due to the existence of multiple flavors of Th17 cells that are fostered by different cancerous cell types and mediators in the tumor microenvironment. Depending on the type of cancer encountered, a number of factors could alter the effect of Th17 cells on tumor pathology, including the source of the Th17 cells (arising naturally via tumor growth or adoptively

transferred following ex vivo manipulation), the functional phenotype of the cells and/or exposure to therapeutic interventions such as chemotherapy [35].

To understand the dual role of Th17 cells in promoting and antagonizing tumors, studies were conducted using a variety of mouse tumor models. Evidence for the role of Th17 cells in anti-tumor immunity came from studies with established murine models of B16 melanoma [136], and B16/F10 lung metastatic melanoma [137], in which adoptive transfer of in vitro-expanded, tumor antigen-specific Th17 cells induced regression of cancer to a larger extent than Th1 cells transferred in a parallel experiment. The transfused Th17 cells were found to promote the infiltration of DCs and enhanced cross-antigen presentation to naïve CD8+ T cells, as well as to induce the secretion of CCL20 from cancer residing lung cells to further recruit CD8+ CTLs into the tumor site [137]. Therefore, the Th17 cells were proposed to have a synergistic function with CD8+ CTLs. In contrast, other tumor models in mice, including leukemia [138], cervical cancer [139], non-small cell lung cancer [140], lung cancer [141], and colon cancer [142], suggested that Th17 cell-secreted inflammatory cytokines in the tumor microenvironment promoted neutrophil recruitment and secretion of elastase, a pro-tumorigenic factor [143]. Th17 cells also promoted the secretion of pro-angiogenic factors and pro-inflammatory cytokines from tumor cells, which promote angiogenesis and cancer progression [143]. Studies with genetically modified mice with colon cancer [144] and pancreatic cancer [145] showed that the preinvasive epithelial layer expressed large amounts of IL-17R that facilitated the infiltration of Th17 cells further substantiating the above findings. Subsequently, IL-17A derived from Th17 cells triggered the oncogenic signal through the IL-17R-STAT3 pathway and accelerated the transformation of epithelial cells into invasive neoplasia. β-catenin signaling is also implicated in the development of Th17 cells in colon cancer [146]. Similar dichotomous findings were observed in human cancers where infiltration of Th17 cells was positively associated with CD8+ T cell count and better survival in ovarian cancer [147] and esophageal cancer [148], but associated with poor prognosis in colon or pancreatic cancer [35, 90].

Th17 cells are a major fraction of TILs in human cancers, attracted by tumor-derived CCL5 and monocyte chemoattractant protein-1 (MCP-1) [149, 150]. Human Th17 cells also undergo functional plasticity, secreting cytokines of other Th lineages [131, 134]. Interestingly, in vitro-expanded, tumor antigen-specific Th17 clones from melanoma, breast, and colon cancer produced large amounts of polyfunctional cytokines including IL-8 and TNF-α, but not IL-2, IL-4, IL-12, or IL-23 [149]. Furthermore, it is also suggested that Th17 cells can be converted into FOXP3 expressing Tregs that produce IL-10 and TGF-β1, indicating a possible regulatory function [151]. In contrast, other studies suggest that in vitro-expanded, tumor antigen-specific Th17 clones from colon cancer and ulcerative colitis mainly produce IL-2, TNF-α, INF-γ, GM-CSF, and exhibite plasticity to convert into both FOXP3- and INF-γ expressing cells with suppressive properties [143, 147, 152]. These findings were contrasted by the proposed cytokine signature of freshly isolated Th17 cells from healthy donors [153] and argue that these differences may arise from in vitro induced changes or may reflect their actual function in the tumor microenvironment.

The conversion of Th17 cells into Th1 cells is well documented in autoimmune diseases and cancer [131, 134]. Additionally, studies have also shown that ex vivo isolated Th17 cells from peripheral blood mononuclear cells of human pancreatic cancer patients can also produce Th2 and Th17 cytokines [154]. Notably, these findings demonstrate that Th17 cells from human cancers not only correlate with IL-17 secretion but can also acquire Th1- or Th2-associated features. To summarize, Th17 cell-mediated anti-tumor immunity is due to the enhancement of DC and CD8+ CTL functions. However, Th17 cells also contribute to cancer-promoting inflammation and angiogenesis. Further, their plasticity-associated complexity in the tumor microenvironment may determine their pro-tumorigenic, suppressive, or anti-tumorigenic role that may influence cancer prognosis.

CD4+ Th9 Cells

In 2008, Th9 cells, a novel subset of CD4+ Th cells characterized by the secretion of IL-9 and IL-10 were reported for the first time [155]. Although the role of the IL-9 cytokine in cancer has previously been explored [156, 157], the role of Th9-derived IL-9 in effective anti-tumor responses came from a study on melanoma that exhibited superior anti-tumor properties over Th1 and Th17 cells [158, 159]. However, recent advancements in the biology of Th9 cells have resulted in a dual role, both anti-tumor and pro-tumor effects in tumor progression.

In most solid tumors such as melanoma, lung adenocarcinoma, colon cancer, and breast cancer Th9 has anti-tumor effects. Growth of B16F10 melanomas was inhibited in RORγ-deficient mice, which presented a greater number of infiltrating CD4+ and CD8+ T cells at tumor sites and secreted a high level of IL-9. The neutralization of IL-9 successfully reversed this effect, suggesting an anti-tumor role of IL-9 against melanoma [159]. The same study also revealed that the Th9 anti-tumor effect was superior compared to Th1, Th2, or Th17. In lung and colon cancer models the anti-tumor effects of IL-9 depended on mast cells [147, 148]. Inhibiting the activity of mast cells with cromoglycate or depleting mast cells with anti-CD117 antibodies reversed the anti-tumor efficacy. DC-based immunotherapy has great promise for cancer treatment. Studies have demonstrated that dectin-1-activated DCs triggers potent anti-tumor Th9 cells in vivo [160].

In contrast to its effect in most solid tumors, Th9 has pro-tumoral effects in hematological malignancies such as non-Hodgkin's lymphoma, chronic lymphocytic leukemia, adult T cell leukemia, Hodgkin's lymphoma, cutaneous T cell lymphoma, anaplastic large-cell lymphoma, and NKT cell lymphoma. It has been reported that IL-9 promotes the immunosuppression mediated by Tregs in B cell non-Hodgkin's lymphoma [161]. Overexpression of IL-9 has shown a direct contribution to the development of chronic lymphocytic leukemia in the presence of the transcription factor STAT6 [162]. High expression of IL-9 was also detected in adult T cell leukemia, Hodgkin's lymphoma, anaplastic large-cell lymphoma, and NKT cell lymphoma suggesting that IL-9 might be a potential target for the development of novel therapeutic strategies against hematological malignancies [163–166].

Intriguingly, a tumor-promoting role for Th9 cells was also suggested in hepatocellular carcinoma through CCL20 and STAT3 pathways [167]. Frequencies of Th9 cells were higher in peri-tumor and tumor tissues compared to unaffected tissues and patients with higher Th9 infiltrates appeared to exhibit shorter disease-free survival [167]. Moreover, Th17/IL-17 and Th9/IL-9 exhibit critical, but often opposing, roles in tumor progression. A recent study shows that while IL-17 and IL-9 induced distinct but complementary molecular pathways, both cytokines also induced epithelial–mesenchymal transition (EMT) in lung cancer cells and promoted metastatic spreading [168]. Overall, important progress has recently been made in understanding the role of Th9 in both pro- and anti-tumor immunity. However, the complex differentiation process and high plasticity of the Th9 subset make it difficult to pinpoint and target the Th9 cells for cancer treatment.

CD4+ Th22 Cells

Like Th9 cells, Th22 cells have only gained recognition as a distinct CD4+ T cell lineage within the past decade. Th22 cells compose another novel T cell subset with polarizing transcription factors such as aryl hydrocarbon receptor (AhR), basic leucine zipper transcription factor (BATF), and STAT3 characterized to produce IL-22, IL-26, and IL-33 [169] (Table 10.2). Expression of IL-22 is not restricted to the Th22 subsets, as Th17 cells and NK cells are also capable of IL-22 production. However, Th22 T cells are unique in their expression of IL-22 in the absence of IL-17 and IFN-γ [169].

Early studies revealed that IL-22 promotes the growth of tumor cells in many types of cancers, including lung adenocarcinoma and hepatocellular carcinoma [170, 171]. Studies have shown that IL-22 has a direct proliferative effect on colonic epithelial cells thereby modulating the tumorigenesis in the intestine [172, 173]. Furthermore, IL-22 potentially stimulates intestinal epithelial cells to secrete IL-10, the main contributor to the formation of an immunosuppressive milieu in colorectal cancer [174]. In addition, IL-22 genetic polymorphisms have shown to be a risk factor for colon cancer and elevated serum IL-22 levels correlate with chemoresistance in patients with colorectal cancer [175, 176]. Using both murine and human breast and lung cancer models, Voigt et al. demonstrated that cancer cells directly induce IL-22 production from memory CD4+ T cells via IL-1 to promote tumor growth [177]. In addition, the authors show the existence of IL-22-producing Th1, Th17, and Th22 cells in tumor tissue of patients. Use of the clinically approved IL-1 receptor antagonist anakinra in vivo reduced IL-22 production and reduced tumor growth in a breast cancer model [177]. A recent study showed that the prevalence of Th22 cells was gradually increased in normal, para-tumor, and tumor tissues of triple-negative breast cancer, promoting migration and paclitaxel resistance through JAK-STAT3/MAPKs/AKT signaling pathways [178]. Taken together, most current data suggest a promoting effect of Th22/IL-22 on the development of various cancers making it an attractive target for anticancer therapy.

CD4+ T Follicular Helper Cells

T follicular helper (Tfh) cells are a subset of activated CD4+ Th cells characterized by expression of CXCR5, PD-1, BCL-6, and ICOS. Tfh cells are specialized in promoting germinal center reactions that support B cell proliferation and maturation, and in the development of humoral immunity [179, 180]. Evidence of Tfh in cancer came from a study of angio-immunoblastic T cell lymphoma, where the tumors phenotypically resemble the Tfh cells by the expression of CXCL13, ICOS, CD154, CD40L, and NFATC1 [181]. A mutated Rho GTPase protein (RHOA G17V) is shown to induce Tfh cell specification and promotes lymphomagenesis [182]. In follicular T cell lymphomas, TILs resemble the phenotype of Tfh cells and play a role in the regulation of Treg and Th2 cell migration into the tumor site [183]. Additionally, FOXP3+ Tfr cells are also found within tumor follicles and the number of Tfr cells is elevated during lymphomagenesis. However, in nonlymphoid tumors, Tfh cells appear to have protective roles. Higher levels of Tfh cell infiltrates and tertiary lymphoid structures within tumors have been associated with increased survival and reduced immunosuppression in breast cancer [184]. It was suggested that IL-21 and CXCL13 might play a key role in the protective functions of Tfh cells via the modulation of local leukocyte recruitment. Infiltrating Tfh cells have also been reported in chronic lymphocytic leukemia, non-small cell lung cancer, osteosarcoma, and colorectal cancer, where they positively correlated with patient survival [185–188]. To date, there is limited understanding in the functions of Tfh and Tfr subsets in lymphomagenesis further studies will be important for a better understanding of their role in cancer.

CD8+ T Cells and Cancer Immunity

CD8+ CTLs recognize their cognate antigen through binding of their TCR to antigen-HLA class I complex expressed on the surface of tumor cells. CD4+Th cells also provide help to CTL responses (section "Conventional Role of CD4+ T Cells in Tumor Immunity"). CTLs are considered as the primary effectors of anti-tumor immunity and potentially eliminate the tumor cells and are shown to correlate with a good prognosis in almost every type of human malignancy (Table 10.3). CTLs use multiple mechanisms to kill tumor cells mediated by granzyme-B, perforin, and the triggering

Table 10.3 The association of tumor-infiltrating T cell subsets and prognosis (indicated as good or poor)

Cancer types	CD8+ T cells	CD4+ Th1 cells	CD4+ Th2 cells	CD4+ Th17 cells	CD4+ Treg cells
Head and neck cancers	Good [192, 193]				Good [193]
Esophageal cancer	Good [194, 195]	Good [196]		Good [148]	
Lung cancer	Good [197]	Good [197]		Poor [198]	Poor [199]
Pancreatic cancer	Good [200, 201]		Poor [123]	Poor [202]	Poor [202, 203]
Distal bile cancer	Good [204]				Good [204]
Breast cancer	Good [205]	Good [206]	Good [207]	Poor [208]	Poor [209, 210] Good [211]
Gastric cancer	Poor [212, 213]	Good [214]	Poor [214]	Good [215] Poor [216]	Good [216] Poor [217]
Hepatocellular carcinoma	Good [218, 219] Poor [219]	Good [220]		Poor [221]	Poor [219, 222]
Colon cancer	Good [223–229]	Good [223–225]	None [224]	Poor [224, 230, 231]	Good [224, 231–233] Poor [234] None [227]
Ovarian cancer	Good [235]	Good [236, 237]	Poor [237]	Good [147]	Good [238, 239] Poor [240]
Renal cell carcinoma	Good [241]	Good [242]			Poor [242]

Table 10.3 (continued)

Cancer types	CD8+ T cells	CD4+ Th1 cells	CD4+ Th2 cells	CD4+ Th17 cells	CD4+ Treg cells
Prostate cancer	Good [243]				
Urothelial carcinoma	Good [244]				
Endometrial cancer	Good [245]				
Cervical cancer	Good [246] Poor [247]				
Melanoma	Good [248, 249]				None [250] Poor [251, 252]
Follicular and Hodgkin's lymphoma			Good [253]		Good [254, 255] Poor [253]

of the Fas signaling pathway through Fas ligand (FasL). Major CTL activities are mediated either directly, through synaptic exocytosis of cytotoxic granules containing perforin and granzymes into the target, resulting in cancer cell destruction, or indirectly, through secretion of pro-inflammatory cytokines. CTLs and target cell interactions are characterized by sustained motility of the CD8+ T cell on the target cell [189]. FasL expressed on CTLs binds to its Fas receptor on the tumor cell surface activates death domains, which, in turn, activates caspases and endonucleases, leading to the fragmentation of target cell DNA [190]. In parallel, perforin secreted by activated CTLs forms pores on the surface of tumor cells that aid in the directed delivery of granzyme-B into the tumor cell cytoplasm subsequently inducing apoptosis. Alternatively, a complex of granulysin, perforin, and granzymes are ingested by target cells through endocytosis of CTL membranes. Granulysin and perforin subsequently create pores in the endosomal membrane and release several granzymes into the cytoplasm [191].

Similar to CD4+ T cells subset differentiation (Th1, Th2, and Th17), after antigen recognition, the naïve CD8+ T cells also differentiate into different T cell cytotoxic (Tc) subsets. The CD8+ T cells differentiation is controlled by the master regulator transcription factors and cytokines, such as Tc1 (T-bet+ Eomes+ INF-γ+), Tc2 (GATA3+ IL4+), and Tc17 (RORγt+ T-bet+ IL17+) cells (Table 10.2 and Fig. 10.1). Since type 1, 2, and 17 related cytokines are primarily produced by Th subsets rather than Tc subsets in the tumor microenvironment, their functional relevance is not yet clearly known. Studies in mice suggest that T cells secrete INF-γ and IL-2 directly into the immune synapse targeting antigen-presenting tumor cells, whereas TNF-α and CCL3 were released multidirectional [256]. It is possible that INF-γ secreted by tumor-infiltrating Tc1 cells can have direct anti-tumor activity by enhancing HLA expression on cancer cells, inducing angiostatic effects, and also recruiting macrophages [85]. IFN-γ produced by CTLs supports their further differentiation to effector CTLs [257]. IFN-γ is responsible for the induction of the CD8+ T cells into being antigen-specific CTLs, which leads to the expansion of immunological memory cells for combatting tumors. The role of IL-4 secreting Tc2 cells in the tumor microenvironment is largely unknown, although a study from breast cancer [258] showed their association with cancer progression. In contrast to Tc1 cells, IL-17 secreting Tc17 cells were found to be impaired in their cytotoxic activity [259, 260]. However, adoptive transfer studies in mouse tumor models have shown that Tc17 cells inhibited tumor growth, which was primarily associated with their plasticity to convert into Tc17/Tc1 cells that produced INF-γ along with IL-17A [261]. Moreover, Tc17 cells were identified in gastric cancer [212], hepatocellular carcinoma [262], cervical cancer [247], breast cancer [258], and endometrial carcinoma [263], primarily found to be less cytotoxic and rather promoted cancer. Especially, in gastric cancer [212] and cervical cancer [247], Tc17 cells are shown to promote angiogenesis and recruit immune suppressor cells, including myeloid-derived suppressor cells (MSDCs) and Tregs. In addition, our study on CD8+ T Cells that co-express RORγt and T-bet were functionally impaired in Distal Bile Duct Cancer [51]. Therefore, emerging results suggest that the cytotoxic activity of CTL secreted cytokines is context-dependent, and under specific polarizing conditions, they may potentially lose their cytotoxic activity. Continued activation of CTLs can cause expression of co-inhibitory receptors on them restricting priming of newly recruited CD8+ T cells to the tumor stroma or their exhaustion, predominantly dampening immune-activating signals within the tumor microenvironment, all of which are in favor of tumor progression and invasiveness. Additionally, cancer cells can also develop defense mechanisms by downregulating the expression of surface HLA molecules, secreting perforin-degrading enzymes, as seen in melanoma cells [264] or by upregulation of checkpoint inhibitors (discussed below).

Regulatory T Cells and Cancer Immunity

Tregs are a highly immune-suppressive fraction of CD4+ T cells, which were originally reported as CD4+ T cells expressing the IL-2 receptor alpha chain (CD25) by Sakaguchi et al. in 1995 [265]. Tregs are a dynamic subset of CD4+ T lymphocytes that modulate physiological (peripheral tolerance) and pathological (autoimmunity) responses thereby maintaining immune homeostasis [266]. Tregs can

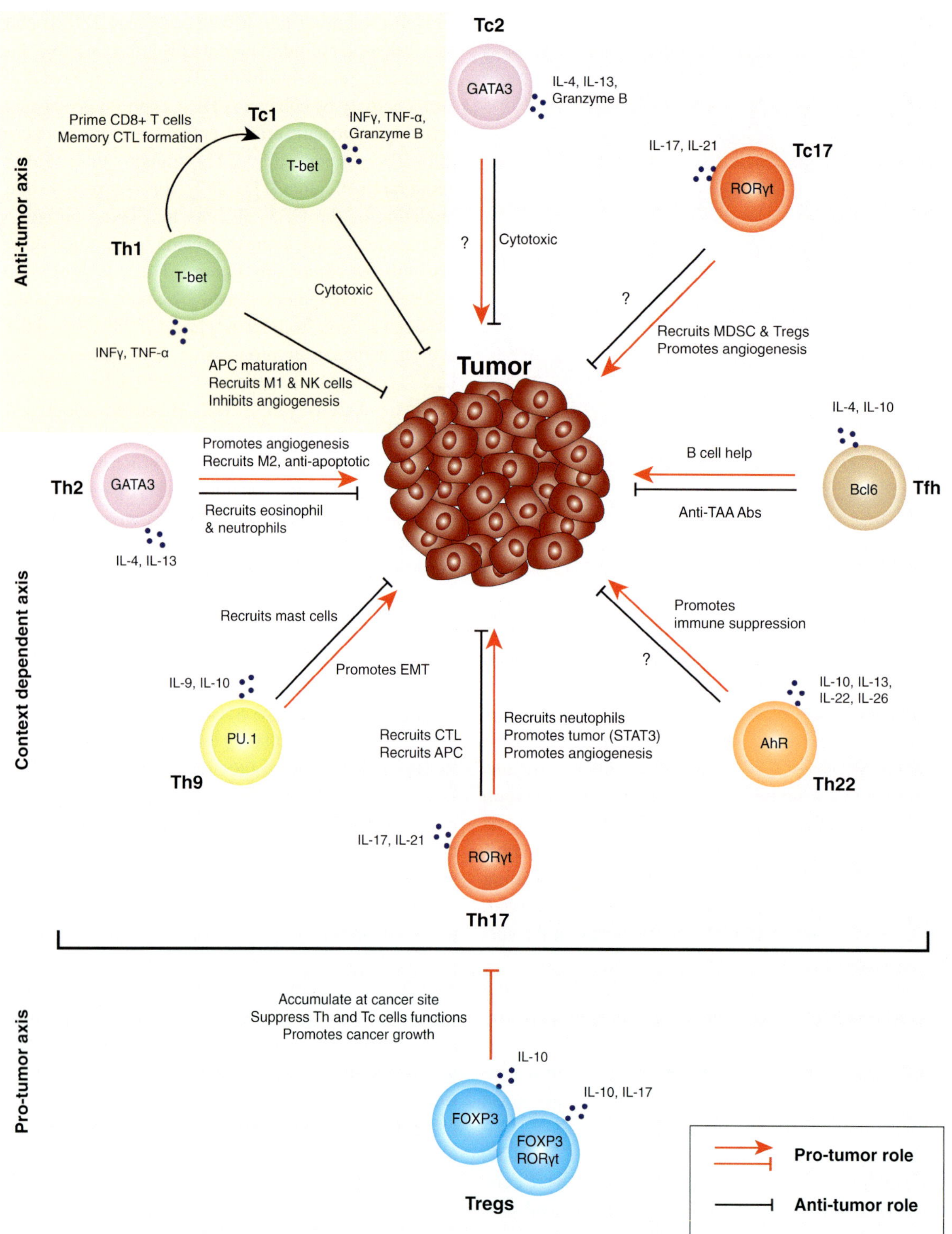

Fig. 10.1 Role of T cell subsets in anti-tumor immunity. Th1 cells express T-bet, INFγ, and IL-12. Th1 cells are superior in anti-tumor activity primarily due to their activation of APC, recruitment of M1 macrophages and NK cells, and their priming of the CTL (Tc1 cells) response. Both Th1 cells and Tc2 cells associate with good prognosis in many cancers and form a prominent anti-tumor axis in humans. Th2 cells express GATA3, IL-4, and IL-13 and contribute to cancer regression via recruiting eosinophils and neutrophils. Furthermore, cytokines produced by Th2 cells also contribute to angiogenesis, recruit M2 macrophages, and have an anti-apoptotic role. Their counterpart the Tc2 cells contribute to cancer regression through their cytotoxic activity but their possible cancer-promoting features are not clearly known. Th17 cells contribute to cancer regression via activating APC and CTL. However, they may also contribute to cancer progression by various mechanisms. Similarly, their counterpart Tc17 also primarily contributes to cancer progression by recruiting suppressor cells into cancer stroma, mainly Treg and MDSC. Both Th17 and Tc17 cells contribute to angiogenesis. Tregs contribute to cancer progression by suppressing effector functions of Th and Tc subsets. Tregs also largely accumulate at the cancer site and their phenotypic heterogeneity and plasticity also contribute to pro-carcinogenic inflammation and cancer progression. Therefore, Th2, Th17, Tc17, and Treg subsets form a context-dependent axis in anti-tumor immunity in human malignancies

be broadly divided into natural or thymus-derived (nTregs or tTregs), which are TCR reactive to self-peptides presented on HLA molecules and peripherally induced Tregs (pTregs or iTregs) in response to TCR stimulation with retinoic acid or TGF-β [267]. The master transcription factor FOXP3 is essential for the development and function of Tregs [266]. In humans, FOXP3 expression alone cannot delineate the suppressive function of Tregs, since FOXP3 is also upregulated following the activation of naive T cells. Based on expression levels of FOXP3 and the naive T cell marker CD45RA, Tregs can be functionally classified into naive Tregs (nTregs: CD45RA+ FOXP3low CD4+ cells), effector Tregs (eTregs: CD45RA-FOXP3high CD4+cells), and non-Tregs (CD45RA– FOXP3low CD4+ cells) [268]. The essential function of Tregs is to suppress the activation, clonal expansion, and effector functions of various immune cells including CD4+ T cells, CD8+ T cells, NKT cells, and APCs through a myriad of mechanisms [269, 270].

The role of Tregs in tumor immunity was first established by animal studies where Treg depletion by anti-CD25 depleting antibody or CD4 depletion in mice prevented the tumor growth [271]. In human tumor biopsies, the proportion of Tregs was significantly higher in tumor sites (i.e., TILs) than in peripheral blood (also see the section below) [272]. Accumulating evidence suggests that naturally occurring Tregs are specifically attracted to the tumor site by chemokines or their receptors expressed by tumor cells [17]. Several chemokines and their cognate receptors are involved in the recruitment of Tregs into TILs, such as CCR4 with CCL22, CCR4 with CCL17, CCR10 with CCL28, and CXCR4 with CXCL1 [209, 273–275]. Tumors may establish resistance to immunotherapy by regulating Treg recruitment via CCR4 [276]. The tumor microenvironment provides a niche to strongly expand Tregs [277] and the Tregs next contribute to the suppression of anti-tumor immunity initiated by Th cells, CTLs and other innate immune cells tumor [18]. In addition, the conversion of Th cells into Tregs also contributes to the presence of Tregs in tumor tissue [278]. Within the tumor, Tregs exhibit highly activated phenotypes, such as high expression of suppressive immune checkpoint molecules like CTLA-4, TIGIT, ICOS, and GITR [279–281]. It is critical to decipher their role in the immune response in order to fully utilize the potential of immune checkpoint inhibitors and other immune-modulating agents. Moreover, tumor-infiltrating Tregs can also be activated by a large number of self-antigens released from tumor cells, because Tregs usually harbor high-affinity TCRs against self-antigens, compared to conventional T cells [282].

Apart from their suppressive function through the surface expression of checkpoint inhibitors, cytokines such as IL-10 secreted by Tregs can also skew Th subsets in the tumor into a Th2 phenotype, which is associated with poor prognosis in many tumor types (Table 10.3). Tregs are known to produce TGF-β, which can promote differentiation of naive CD4+ T cells into Treg cells via FOXP3 expression [283]. Further, TGF-β is also known to dampen effector T cells and APCs [284]. Findings from many solid tumors such as colon cancer [285], pancreatic cancer [154], and breast cancer [286] suggest that IL17+FOXP3+ Tregs retain their suppressive function, but also contribute to Th17 associated inflammation, which is associated with poor prognosis in these tumor types (Table 10.3).

Several immune escape mechanisms involving Tregs rely on cAMP-dependent pathways to suppress Teffs [287]. Tregs may utilize a COX-2-dependent mechanism of suppression [48, 288] where PGE2 is produced by Tregs and can bind to its cognate receptors (EP1-EP4) on effector T cells, thus inhibiting their activation through the TCR [44–46]. In particular, EP2 and EP4 signal through a cAMP inhibitory pathway (cAMP-PKA-Csk-Lck) that was identified in the Taskén laboratory [45, 289–292]. A parallel mechanism that also turns on cAMP is the production of adenosine from ATP via the exoenzymes CD73 and CD39 expressed on Tregs. Adenosine signals through adenosine A2A receptors (A2AR) on Teffs and signaling converges on the inhibitory cAMP pathway [48, 288, 293–295]. Yet another mechanism involves direct transfer of cAMP from Tregs to Teffs through gap junctions [296, 297]. Monocyte-mediated PGE$_2$ production is also a significant source of cAMP in Teff [298]. Furthermore, antagonists targeting PGE$_2$ signaling through its EP4 receptor (Grapiprant, E7046, and ONO-4578/BMS-986310), adenosine A2a receptor (A2AR) antagonists (Ciforadenant), and CD73 and CD39 blocking antibodies (CPI-006, TTX-030) are in clinical use or under development reviewed in [299–301].

Our studies on Tregs reveal their complex nature in the tumor microenvironment. Tregs contribute to an immunosuppressive microenvironment in colorectal cancer and inhibit effector T cells by a COX-2-PGE2-dependent mechanism and thereby facilitating tumor growth. Thus targeting Tregs and the PGE2-cAMP pathway may enhance the anti-tumor immune activity in colorectal carcinoma patients [49, 302]. Intriguingly, in human pancreatic cancer Tregs that co-express RORγt and FOXP3 are both pro-inflammatory and immunosuppressive [50]. Due to the anti-tumor activity of Tregs through various mechanisms, anticancer drugs often fail to activate the endogenous immune cells against cancer. Currently, there are several strategies to enhance the specificity of Treg targeting, especially checkpoint inhibitors like CTLA-4, PD1, LAG3, and TIGIT either alone or in combination for cancer immunotherapy are underway [303].

Unconventional T Cells and Cancer Immunity

T cells make up a central part of the adaptive immune system. Certain T cell populations, frequently referred to as unconventional T cells, share functional profiles of both innate and adaptive immunity. The unconventional, innate-like T cell population consists 20–50% of CD3+ T cells such as mucosal-associated invariant T cells (MAIT), TCR γδ T cells, and innate lymphoid cells (ILCs) and invariant NKT (iNKT). Broadly, unconventional T cells comprise cells with invariant TCRs, different from conventional TCR αβ T cells that most commonly reside in an epithelial environment such as the skin, gastrointestinal tract, or genitourinary tract. Their role is to recognize infections and cancer cells and regulate inflammatory responses that arise in these tissues [304]. These innate-like T cells have the capacity to rapidly respond to non-cognate stimulation by releasing large amounts of cytokines. Use of unconventional T cells have certain advantages in anticancer treatment compared to conventional Th1 and Th17 cells. These cells are non-HLA restricted, meaning that they can have off-the-shelf applicability irrespective of an individual's genotype without HLA-dependent graft versus host disease [305]. While most conventional T cells are rather ineffective in solid tumors, unconventional T cells have the advantage of being tissue resident in most cases [305]. Here we summarize the role of iNKT cells, MAIT cells, and γδ T cells in cancer.

Invariant NKT Cells

Invariant NKT cells are characterized by their semi-invariant Vα24Jα18 and TCRβ chains, which recognize glycolipid antigen in the context of the nonclassical HLA molecule CD1d [306]. Several studies have demonstrated the anti-tumor potential for iNKT cells in mice [307]. Activated iNKT cells also express cytotoxic factors such as perforin, granzymes, FasL, and TNF-related apoptosis-inducing ligand (TRAIL), and are capable of directly lysing tumors [308, 309]. Activated iNKT cells in turn activate many other cells of the immune system and in particular DCs where multifactorial crosstalk involving CD40L-CD40, IFN-γ, and IL-12 production leads to increased expression of CD80, CD86, CD70, and IL-12 production by the DCs. This translates to more potent activation of conventional CD4 and CD8 T cells [310]. In addition, other bystander cells are activated in this environment that contribute to tumor rejection, including NK cells [308] and γδ T cells [311], leading to enhanced effector function at many levels. Studies have shown that low iNKT cell frequencies are associated with poor prognosis in head and neck carcinoma, acute myeloid leukemia, neuroblastoma, and chronic lymphocytic leukemia [312–314]. Overall, targeting iNKT cells appears to engage several arms of the immune system at once, reducing the potential for tumor escape from a more focused immune response.

Mucosal-Associated Invariant T Cells

MAIT cells reside, as their name implies, in the mucosa, but they are also found in the peripheral blood, lymphoid tissues, and organs such as the liver. MAIT cells can be activated by viruses in a TCR-independent manner, or through the MAIT TCR-MR1 axis and are thought to play a role in protection against bacteria [315, 316]. In addition, MAIT cells are also implicated in several autoimmune disorders including diabetes [317, 318]. MAIT cells are reminiscent of type I NKT cells, rapidly secreting cytokines including IFN-γ, TNF, and, in some situations IL-17, following TCR-mediated activation [319]. While there are no defined MR1-binding tumor antigens that activate MAIT cells, it is conceivable that MAIT cells may encounter microbial antigens in tumor types, such as mucosal cancers, where bacterial infiltrates are likely to be present. MAIT cells can be activated in the presence of virus-induced inflammatory cytokines, such as IL-12 and IL-18, without specific antigen stimulation [320]. The first report to document the role of MAIT cells in human cancers is in brain and kidney tumors [321]. More recently MAIT cells were found to be diminished in the circulation of mucosal-associated cancers (gastric, colon, and lung), but not in association with non-mucosal cancers (breast, liver, and thyroid) [322]. MAIT cells are highly abundant in the human liver. In hepatocellular carcinoma patients' liver samples, MAIT cells were found to be abundant in healthy liver tissue, but diminished in number in the tumor site correlating with poor prognosis [323]. In multiple myeloma patients, MAIT cells are also numerically and functionally diminished in blood and bone marrow [324]. These studies suggest that inhibition of MAIT cell infiltration and/or function may be important for tumor survival.

Gamma Delta T Cells

In humans, γδ T cells represent approximately 1–5% of circulating T cells, also localized in peripheral sites such as skin and large intestine. The γδ T cells are Th1-type cytokine bias with strong IFN-γ production and potent cytotoxicity that are closely correlated with tumor destruction. Many γδ T cells have unique homing properties compared to αβ T cells, typically migrating to peripheral sites, such as epithelial tissues and solid tumors. While the major focus for the function of γδ T cells has been their role in homeostasis, wound repair, and infection [325], there is also a great interest in the role that these cells play in cancer, especially as intra-tumoral γδ T cells represent the most favorable prognostic indicator across different cancers [326]. Evidence for the role of γδ T cells in cancer surveillance first came from studies using γδ T cell-deficient mice showing a significantly elevated incidence of tumors of skin and prostate adenocarcinoma [327, 328]. Human γδ T cells can also elicit strong anti-tumor responses in vitro. Activated γδ T cells recognize and kill a broad range of tumor target cells in vitro [329–331].

However, the association between γδ T cells and tumor progression and/or patient survival is still controversial. In melanoma patients, an abundance of γδ T cells in TILs was positively associated with survival [332]. In several leukemias, patients receiving allogenic bone marrow transplantation revealed a strong correlation between γδ T cell abundance and overall survival or disease-free survival [333, 334]. In contrast, γδ T cells also have been shown to be associated with poor outcomes or high tumor burden, indicative of a pro-tumorigenic role. A study in rectal cancer showed the γδ T cells among TILs to positively correlate with tumor burden [335]. Another study also found an association between IL-17-producing γδ T cells and poor survival in gall bladder patients [336]. In primary breast cancer patients, γδ T cells were associated with more severe disease and reduced overall survival, indicating a pro-tumor role [337]. Peng et al. isolated regulatory γδ T cells from breast cancer TILs that specifically recognized a tumor epitope via the γδ TCR and exhibited immune-suppressive functions [338]. Collectively these studies highlight the importance of further research to understand the key factors involved in driving pro- versus anti-tumor immunity by γδ T cells.

Tumor-Infiltrating Lymphocytes and Cancer Prognosis

The tumor microenvironment plays a crucial role in tumor progression, therapeutic response, and patient outcomes. The tumor microenvironment primarily includes TILs, blood, and lymphatic vessels [7]. There are anticancer and pro-cancer immune cells. In general, infiltration of anticancer immune cells, such as CTLs, is associated with a favorable patient prognosis. In contrast, infiltration of pro-cancer immune cells, such as Tregs, TAMs, and MDSCs is associated with a poor prognosis. These characteristics of T cell subtype distribution are incorporated for example in IMMUNOSCORE, a test used in clinics to measure the response of a patient's immune system to a tumor [339].

Despite the importance of TIL characteristics described above, phenotyping of tumor-infiltrating T cell subsets as a prognostic marker is a complicated endeavor. In addition to the complex interactions in the tumor microenvironment, CD4+ Th cells in the tumor are found in different maturation states such as activated, exhausted, or regulatory. Moreover, they may share phenotypic markers with other immune cells adding more complexity to the analyses and interpretations of individual patient TIL profiles. Conflicting conclusions with respect to TIL phenotype could also potentially be due to differences in methodologies used, such as polymerase chain reaction, immunohistochemistry, multicolor flow cytometry, and CyTOF. Nonetheless, similar conclusions drawn for a particular cancer type by several groups substantiate the need for studying the link between Th cell subsets and prognosis and/or response to therapy. Here, we summarize the prognostic value of analyzing the abundance of Th subsets, Tc subsets, and Tregs in several human malignancies (Table 10.3).

The Th1 cells and CD8+ CTLs are strongly associated with good prognosis in many human cancers including esophageal cancer [194–196], colon cancer [223–229], head and neck cancer [192, 193], lung cancer [197], pancreatic cancer [200, 201], distal bile duct cancer [204], breast cancer [205, 206], gastric cancer [214], prostate cancer [243], urothelial cancer [244], ovarian cancer [235–237], endometrial cancer [245], cervical cancer [246], hepatocellular carcinoma [218–220], melanoma [248, 249], and renal cell carcinoma [241, 242]. The CD8+ CTLs lead target cancer cells to apoptosis in a series of steps, known as the cancer-immunity cycle [340]. Neo-antigens released by tumor cells are captured and processed by DCs and presented to CTLs. The CTLs are primed and activated to cancer-specific neo-antigens. Activated CTLs are attracted by chemokines such as CCL5 and CXCL10 and infiltrated into the tumor site. Infiltrated CTLs bind to tumor cells through the TCR-HLA class I and secrete granzymes to induce apoptosis of the target cells. Dead cells release additional neo-antigens, further fueling the cancer-immunity cycle. Therefore, high infiltration of CTLs is a favorable prognostic marker in many cancers. Th1 cells produce pro-inflammatory cytokines, such as IFN-γ and IL-2, to assist CTLs. Despite this, the presence of CD8+ T cells has also been reported to associate with poor outcomes, particularly in hepatocellular carcinoma, gastric cancer, and cervical cancer (Table 10.3), which is thought primarily to be due to the conversion of CD8+ T cells into Tc17 cells [212, 247]. However, CD8+ CTLs within tumors manifest a broad spectrum of dysfunctional states, molded by multiple suppressive signals in the tumor microenvironment. The mechanisms underlying CD8+ T cell failure in the tumor microenvironment may include: (1) exclusion by stromal cells; (2) exhaustion associated with the expression of inhibitory receptors and their ligands; (3) lack of intratumoral niches which maintain CD8+ CTL functions; (4) loss of HLA class I; (5) recruitment of immunosuppressive cells; (6) direct inhibition of CD8+ CTL functions by suppressive cytokines; (7) direct suppression of CD8+ CTL functions by generated metabolites; and (8) physiological stress conditions such as hypoxia, low pH, and nutrient deprivation. One or more of these mechanisms are related to the failure of current immunotherapies. Hence, current translational research has a significant focus on how to reinvigorate the suppressed CTLs [341].

In contrast to Th1 cells and CD8+ CTL cells, Th2 and Th17 cells correlate with either good or poor prognosis (Table 10.3). Th17 cells have been associated with a good prognosis in esophageal cancer [148], ovarian cancer [147], and gastric cancer [215], but correlated with poor prognosis in colon cancer [224, 230], lung cancer [198], pancreatic cancer [202], breast cancer [208], gastric cancer [216], and hepatocellular carcinoma [221] (Table 10.3). Whereas the presence of Th2 cells is associated with a good prognosis in breast cancer [207], follicular lymphoma, and Hodgkin's lymphoma [253], their presence associates with poor prognosis in pancreatic cancer [123], gastric cancer [214], and ovarian cancer [237], but does not appear to have an impact on colon cancer prognosis [224] (Table 10.3). Interestingly, in gastric cancer accumulation of Th17 cells has been shown to associate with either good prognosis irrespective of the cancer stage [215] or poor prognosis at an early stage of cancer [216]. These disparities could originate from differences in experimental setup and markers used to define Th17 and Th2 cells. Some of the above-mentioned studies used only IL-17 as a predictor, investigating the CD4+IL17+ T cells. This may affect the results as other immune cell types including $\gamma\delta$ T cells, myeloid cells, and innate lymphoid cells can also produce IL-17 [55, 135]. In addition, as described earlier (section "Unconventional Role of CD4+ T Cells in Tumor Immunity"), Th17 cells also undergo plasticity and therefore the conflicting observation of Th17 cells and Th2 cells may also reflect the fundamental differences in the inflammatory tumor microenvironment and stress the importance of well-delineated Th lineage analysis in these patients. In addition, Fridman et al. proposed a concept termed "immune contexture" in which the location and density of CD8+ T cells and CD4+ Th cells in both the invasive margin and intra-tumoral region predicted a favorable outcome in colorectal cancer patients [223, 342]. Currently, this particular immune contexture has been demonstrated in other cancer types such as biliary cancer, pancreatic cancer, breast cancer, and gliomas [204, 343–346]. In our own study on ovarian cancer, TILs in malignant ascites were distinctly different from peripheral blood T cells [52]. This indicates that test systems predicting patient responsiveness to immunotherapy may need to explore both tumor-infiltrating immune cells and circulating cells. These findings provide a framework to further standardize the studies that involve T cell subset association with prognosis in human cancers.

Tumor-infiltrating Tregs have been extensively studied and the prognostic value of their presence varies in different tumors. Specific depletion of Tregs in vivo can effectively stimulate the anti-tumor immune response of cancer patients. The cytokines IL-10 and IL-35 expressed by Tregs in the tumor microenvironment promote intra-tumoral T cell exhaustion by regulating the expression of several inhibitory receptors and the exhaustion-associated transcriptomic signatures of CD8+ TILs [347]. Tregs have been reported to correlate with poor outcomes in colon cancer [234], lung cancer [199, 348], pancreas cancer [202, 203], breast cancer [209, 210], gastric cancer [217], ovarian cancer [240], renal

cell carcinoma [242], and hepatocellular carcinoma [219, 222] as well as melanoma, follicular lymphoma, and Hodgkin's lymphoma [253]. In contrast, the presence of Tregs was found to be associated with a good prognosis in colon cancer [224, 232, 233], head and neck cancer [193], distal bile duct cancer [204], gastric cancer [216], ovarian cancer and breast cancer [211], as well as follicular lymphoma and Hodgkin's lymphoma [254, 255]. Intriguingly, associations with both good and poor prognoses were observed within the same cancer type for colon, breast, gastric, and ovarian cancer and Hodgkin's lymphoma. Moreover, some studies have reported that the presence of Tregs has no impact on colon cancer and melanoma (Table 10.3).

These discrepancies in prognostic value may arise from the use of different markers to define Tregs. Both CD25 and FoxP3, the bona fide Treg markers, can also be expressed by activated T cells [268]. Other factors that may contribute to these discrepancies are tumor subtypes, tumor stage and the location of the characterized Tregs (within the tumor tissue, at the margin of the tumor, or in the inflamed tissue outside the tumor). Finally, the role of Tregs in cancer progression may also be dependent on whether the cancers were preceded or stimulated by inflammation. In addition, many of these studies have not reported Treg-suppressive function or their phenotypic plasticity. The positive impact of Tregs in some tumor types may reflect their anti-inflammatory role in suppressing tumor-promoting inflammation. Discrepancies within the same tumor type such as colon, breast, and gastric cancer may indicate that Tregs may predominantly share other Th lineage phenotypes, such as IL17+FOXP3+ Treg, which have been found to be the major Treg pool in colon, breast, and pancreatic cancer patients [154, 286, 349]. Remarkably, Tregs are further categorized into type 1 (Tr1), Th3 Tregs, and CD8+ Tregs based on their mechanisms of suppression and cytokine profiles which lack FOXP3 expression [350–352]. Hence, it is imperative to add phenotypic plasticity of Tregs to characterize the immune suppression in the tumor and then draw conclusions on the prognosis of cancer patients. Nonetheless, these data suggest that the original view of Tregs suppressing anti-tumor immunity is oversimplified and that Tregs may have multiple roles in influencing inflammation and shaping the tumor microenvironment as well as in suppressing anti-tumor immunity.

Concluding Remarks/Summary

Experimental and clinical studies now indicate that T cells play a pivotal, albeit sometimes paradoxical role in shaping anti-tumor immunity (Fig. 10.1). Nonetheless, the presence of Th1 and CTL cells is strongly associated with favorable outcomes in many tumor types and indicates that active cancer immunosurveillance is an integral part of many human malignancies. However, the potency of CTLs' function in several malignant tumors is generally compromised. The main factors contributing to tumor immune evasion include reduced HLA class I and class II expression by tumor cells to eliminate the direct detection by CTLs, along with reduced help from CD4+ Th tumor cells. In addition, the differentiation of CD8+ T cells into less cytotoxic and anti-inflammatory subsets under polarizing conditions in the tumor microenvironment together with Treg-mediated immunosuppression at the cancer site contribute to the functional defect in tumor-specific Th1 cells and CTLs that ultimately lead to tumor progression. In addition, Th2, Th17, and Tregs are largely associated with poor outcomes in many tumor types. The bifurcation of the pro- and anti-tumorigenic nature of T cell subsets is too complex to predict, as it largely depends on cytokines secreted in the cancer microenvironment. To add to this complexity, recent reports suggest that T cells share different lineage-specific transcription factors and exhibit heterogeneity and plasticity. This may explain the paradoxical role of Th2, Th17, and Treg subsets observed, as many earlier studies assessed the prognostic value of individual subsets but did not consider the potential of phenotypic plasticity. It is also inevitable that the location of T cells and the niche they share with other immune cells, cancer cells, and stromal cells along with their complex interactions dictate their functional status. An integrated picture of all these factors will shed more light on the role of T cells in cancer and enable us to better tailor T cell therapies in the future.

Acknowledgments We apologize to all authors whose work we were unable to cite due to space restrictions. Our work is supported by grants from the Research Council of Norway (Grants 294916 and 315538 to K. Taskén), Norwegian Cancer Society (Grants 182794 and 215850 to K. Taskén), South-Eastern Norway Regional Health Authority (grant 2018065 to E.M. Aandahl and grant 2017119 and 2020045 to K. Taskén), and Stiftelsen Kristian Gerhard Jebsen (Grants SKGJ-MED-09 and SKGJ-MED-19).

References

1. Ehrlich P. Über den jetzigen Stand der Karzinomforschung. Ned Tijdschr Genceskd. 1909;5:273–90.
2. Burnet M. Cancer: a biological approach. III. Viruses associated with neoplastic conditions. IV. Practical applications. Br Med J. 1957;1(5023):841–7.
3. Thomas L. Discussion. In: Lawrence H, editor. Cellular and humoral aspects of the hypersensitive states. New York: Hoeber-Harper; 1959.
4. Dunn GP, Bruce AT, Ikeda H, Old LJ, Schreiber RD. Cancer immunoediting: from immunosurveillance to tumor escape. Nat Immunol. 2002;3(11):991–8.
5. Kim R, Emi M, Tanabe K. Cancer immunoediting from immune surveillance to immune escape. Immunology. 2007;121(1):1–14.
6. Dunn GP, Old LJ, Schreiber RD. The three Es of cancer immunoediting. Annu Rev Immunol. 2004;22(1):329–60.
7. Hanahan D, Weinberg RA. Hallmarks of cancer: the next generation. Cell. 2011;144(5):646–74.
8. Schreiber RD, Old LJ, Smyth MJ. Cancer immunoediting: integrating immunity's roles in cancer suppression and promotion. Science. 2011;331(6024):1565.
9. Khanna R. Tumour surveillance: missing peptides and MHC molecules. Immunol Cell Biol. 1998;76(1):20–6.
10. Bubenik J. MHC class I down-regulation: tumour escape from immune surveillance? (review). Int J Oncol. 2004;25(2):487–91.
11. Peng D, Kryczek I, Nagarsheth N, Zhao L, Wei S, Wang W, et al. Epigenetic silencing of TH1-type chemokines shapes tumour immunity and immunotherapy. Nature. 2015;527(7577):249–53.
12. Onrust SV, Hartl PM, Rosen SD, Hanahan D. Modulation of L-selectin ligand expression during an immune response accompanying tumorigenesis in transgenic mice. J Clin Invest. 1996;97(1):54–64.
13. Wu T-C. The role of vascular cell adhesion molecule-1 in tumor immune evasion. Cancer Res. 2007;67(13):6003–6.
14. Piali L, Fichtel A, Terpe HJ, Imhof BA, Gisler RH. Endothelial vascular cell adhesion molecule 1 expression is suppressed by melanoma and carcinoma. J Exp Med. 1995;181(2):811–6.
15. Turley SJ, Cremasco V, Astarita JL. Immunological hallmarks of stromal cells in the tumour microenvironment. Nat Rev Immunol. 2015;15(11):669–82.
16. Ochsenbein AF. Principles of tumor immunosurveillance and implications for immunotherapy. Cancer Gene Ther. 2002;9(12):1043–55.
17. Mailloux AW, Young MR. Regulatory T-cell trafficking: from thymic development to tumor-induced immune suppression. Crit Rev Immunol. 2010;30(5):435–47.
18. Savage PA, Malchow S, Leventhal DS. Basic principles of tumor-associated regulatory T cell biology. Trends Immunol. 2013;34(1):33–40.
19. Wolf D, Sopper S, Pircher A, Gastl G, Wolf AM. Treg(s) in cancer: friends or foe? J Cell Physiol. 2015;230(11):2598–605.
20. Marvel D, Gabrilovich DI. Myeloid-derived suppressor cells in the tumor microenvironment: expect the unexpected. J Clin Invest. 2015;125(9):3356–64.
21. Töpfer K, Kempe S, Müller N, Schmitz M, Bachmann M, Cartellieri M, et al. Tumor evasion from T cell surveillance. J Biomed Biotechnol. 2011;2011:19.
22. Pickup M, Novitskiy S, Moses HL. The roles of TGF[beta] in the tumour microenvironment. Nat Rev Cancer. 2013;13(11):788–99.
23. Sato T, Terai M, Tamura Y, Alexeev V, Mastrangelo MJ, Selvan SR. Interleukin 10 in the tumor microenvironment: a target for anticancer immunotherapy. Immunol Res. 2011;51(2-3):170–82.
24. Germano G, Allavena P, Mantovani A. Cytokines as a key component of cancer-related inflammation. Cytokine. 2008;43(3):374–9.
25. Smyth MJ, Ngiow SF, Ribas A, Teng MWL. Combination cancer immunotherapies tailored to the tumour microenvironment. Nat Rev Clin Oncol. 2016;13(3):143–58.
26. Antonioli L, Blandizzi C, Pacher P, Hasko G. Immunity, inflammation and cancer: a leading role for adenosine. Nat Rev Cancer. 2013;13(12):842–57.
27. Brudvik KW, Tasken K. Modulation of T cell immune functions by the prostaglandin E(2) - cAMP pathway in chronic inflammatory states. Br J Pharmacol. 2012;166(2):411–9.
28. Sonoda K. RCAS1 is a promising therapeutic target against cancer: its multifunctional bioactivities and clinical significance. Expert Rev Obstet Gynecol. 2012;7(3):261–7.
29. Grivennikov SI, Greten FR, Karin M. Immunity, inflammation, and cancer. Cell. 2010;140(6):883–99.
30. Platten M, Wick W, Van den Eynde BJ. Tryptophan catabolism in cancer: beyond IDO and tryptophan depletion. Cancer Res. 2012;72(21):5435–40.

31. Crespo J, Sun H, Welling TH, Tian Z, Zou W. T cell anergy, exhaustion, senescence, and stemness in the tumor microenvironment. Curr Opin Immunol. 2013;25(2):214–21.

32. Pauken KE, Wherry EJ. Overcoming T cell exhaustion in infection and cancer. Trends Immunol. 2015;36(4):265–76.

33. Peter ME, Hadji A, Murmann AE, Brockway S, Putzbach W, Pattanayak A, et al. The role of CD95 and CD95 ligand in cancer. Cell Death Differ. 2015;22(4):549–59.

34. Kim HJ, Cantor H. CD4 T-cell subsets and tumor immunity: the helpful and the not-so-helpful. Cancer Immunol Res. 2014;2(2):91–8.

35. Bailey SR, Nelson MH, Himes RA, Li Z, Mehrotra S, Paulos CM. Th17 cells in cancer: the ultimate identity crisis. Front Immunol. 2014;5:276.

36. Protti MP, De Monte L. Cross-talk within the tumor microenvironment mediates Th2-type inflammation in pancreatic cancer. OncoImmunology. 2012;1(1):89–91.

37. Ostuni R, Kratochvill F, Murray PJ, Natoli G. Macrophages and cancer: from mechanisms to therapeutic implications. Trends Immunol. 2015;36(4):229–39.

38. Fulda S. Tumor resistance to apoptosis. Int J Cancer. 2009;124(3):511–5.

39. Lehmann C, Zeis M, Schmitz N, Uharek L. Impaired binding of perforin on the surface of tumor cells is a cause of target cell resistance against cytotoxic effector cells. Blood. 2000;96(2):594–600.

40. Medema JP, de Jong J, Peltenburg LTC, Verdegaal EME, Gorter A, Bres SA, et al. Blockade of the granzyme B/perforin pathway through overexpression of the serine protease inhibitor PI-9/SPI-6 constitutes a mechanism for immune escape by tumors. Proc Natl Acad Sci U S A. 2001;98(20):11515–20.

41. Larkin J, Chiarion-Sileni V, Gonzalez R, Grob JJ, Cowey CL, Lao CD, et al. Combined nivolumab and ipilimumab or monotherapy in untreated melanoma. N Engl J Med. 2015;373(1):23–34.

42. Brahmer J, Reckamp KL, Baas P, Crinò L, Eberhardt WEE, Poddubskaya E, et al. Nivolumab versus docetaxel in advanced squamous-cell non-small-cell lung cancer. N Engl J Med. 2015;373(2):123–35.

43. Sharma P, Hu-Lieskovan S, Wargo JA, Ribas A. Primary, adaptive, and acquired resistance to cancer immunotherapy. Cell. 2017;168(4):707–23.

44. Lone AM, Taskén K. Proinflammatory and immunoregulatory roles of eicosanoids in T cells. Front Immunol. 2013;4:130.

45. Wehbi VL, Taskén K. Molecular mechanisms for cAMP-mediated immunoregulation in T cells—role of anchored protein kinase A signaling units. Front Immunol. 2016;7:222.

46. Lone AM, Taskén K. Phosphoproteomics-based characterization of prostaglandin E(2) signaling in T cells. Mol Pharmacol. 2021;99(5):370–82.

47. Wang D, Floisand Y, Myklebust CV, Burgler S, Parente-Ribes A, Hofgaard PO, et al. Autologous bone marrow Th cells can support multiple myeloma cell proliferation in vitro and in xenografted mice. Leukemia. 2017;31(10):2114–21.

48. Yaqub S, Henjum K, Mahic M, Jahnsen FL, Aandahl EM, Bjornbeth BA, et al. Regulatory T cells in colorectal cancer patients suppress anti-tumor immune activity in a COX-2 dependent manner. Cancer Immunol Immunother. 2008;57(6):813–21.

49. Brudvik KW, Henjum K, Aandahl EM, Bjornbeth BA, Tasken K. Regulatory T-cell-mediated inhibition of antitumor immune responses is associated with clinical outcome in patients with liver metastasis from colorectal cancer. Cancer Immunol Immunother. 2012;61(7):1045–53.

50. Chellappa S, Hugenschmidt H, Hagness M, Line PD, Labori KJ, Wiedswang G, et al. Regulatory T cells that co-express RORgammat and FOXP3 are pro-inflammatory and immunosuppressive and expand in human pancreatic cancer. Oncoimmunology. 2016;5(4):e1102828.

51. Chellappa S, Hugenschmidt H, Hagness M, Subramani S, Melum E, Line PD, et al. CD8+ T cells that coexpress RORgammat and T-bet are functionally impaired and expand in patients with distal bile duct cancer. J Immunol. 2017;198(4):1729–39.

52. Landskron J, Helland O, Torgersen KM, Aandahl EM, Gjertsen BT, Bjorge L, et al. Activated regulatory and memory T-cells accumulate in malignant ascites from ovarian carcinoma patients. Cancer Immunol Immunother. 2015;64(3):337–47.

53. Landskron J, Kraggerud SM, Wik E, Dorum A, Bjornslett M, Melum E, et al. C77G in PTPRC (CD45) is no risk allele for ovarian cancer, but associated with less aggressive disease. PLoS One. 2017;12(7):e0182030.

54. Zhu J, Yamane H, Paul WE. Differentiation of effector CD4 T cell populations. Annu Rev Immunol. 2010;28(1):445–89.

55. Annunziato F, Romagnani C, Romagnani S. The 3 major types of innate and adaptive cell-mediated effector immunity. J Allergy Clin Immunol. 2015;135(3):626–35.

56. Rossjohn J, Gras S, Miles JJ, Turner SJ, Godfrey DI, McCluskey J. T cell antigen receptor recognition of antigen-presenting molecules. Annu Rev Immunol. 2015;33(1):169–200.

57. Neefjes J, Jongsma MLM, Paul P, Bakke O. Towards a systems understanding of MHC class I and MHC class II antigen presentation. Nat Rev Immunol. 2011;11(12):823–36.

58. Keene JA, Forman J. Helper activity is required for the in vivo generation of cytotoxic T lymphocytes. J Exp Med. 1982;155(3):768–82.

59. Ossendorp F, Mengede E, Camps M, Filius R, Melief CJ. Specific T helper cell requirement for optimal induction of cytotoxic T lymphocytes against major histocompatibility complex class II negative tumors. J Exp Med. 1998;187(5):693–702.

60. Bennett SR, Carbone FR, Karamalis F, Flavell RA, Miller JF, Heath WR. Help for cytotoxic-T-cell responses is mediated by CD40 signalling. Nature. 1998;393(6684):478–80.

61. Schoenberger SP, Toes RE, van der Voort EI, Offringa R, Melief CJ. T-cell help for cytotoxic T lymphocytes is mediated by CD40-CD40L interactions. Nature. 1998;393(6684):480–3.

62. Ridge JP, Di Rosa F, Matzinger P. A conditioned dendritic cell can be a temporal bridge between a CD4+ T-helper and a T-killer cell. Nature. 1998;393(6684):474–8.

63. Bourgeois C, Rocha B, Tanchot C. A role for CD40 expression on CD8+ T cells in the generation of CD8+ T cell memory. Science. 2002;297(5589):2060–3.

64. Williams MA, Tyznik AJ, Bevan MJ. Interleukin-2 signals during priming are required for secondary expansion of CD8+ memory T cells. Nature. 2006;441(7095):890–3.

65. Tham EL, Shrikant P, Mescher MF. Activation-induced nonresponsiveness: a Th-dependent regulatory checkpoint in the CTL response. J Immunol. 2002;168(3):1190–7.

66. Mescher MF, Curtsinger JM, Agarwal P, Casey KA, Gerner M, Hammerbeck CD, et al. Signals required for programming effector and memory development by CD8+ T cells. Immunol Rev. 2006;211:81–92.

67. Quezada SA, Simpson TR, Peggs KS, Merghoub T, Vider J, Fan X, et al. Tumor-reactive CD4(+) T cells develop cytotoxic activity and eradicate large established melanoma after transfer into lymphopenic hosts. J Exp Med. 2010;207(3):637–50.

68. Oh DY, Kwek SS, Raju SS, Li T, McCarthy E, Chow E, et al. Intratumoral CD4+ T cells mediate anti-tumor cytotoxicity in human bladder cancer. Cell. 2020;181(7):1612–25.e13.

69. Baxevanis CN, Voutsas IF, Tsitsilonis OE, Gritzapis AD, Sotiriadou R, Papamichail M. Tumor-specific CD4+ T lympho-

cytes from cancer patients are required for optimal induction of cytotoxic T cells against the autologous tumor. J Immunol. 2000;164(7):3902–12.

70. Bos R, Sherman LA. CD4+ T-cell help in the tumor milieu is required for recruitment and cytolytic function of CD8+ T lymphocytes. Cancer Res. 2010;70(21):8368–77.

71. Wong SB, Bos R, Sherman LA. Tumor-specific CD4+ T cells render the tumor environment permissive for infiltration by low-avidity CD8+ T cells. J Immunol. 2008;180(5):3122–31.

72. Hwang ML, Lukens JR, Bullock TN. Cognate memory CD4+ T cells generated with dendritic cell priming influence the expansion, trafficking, and differentiation of secondary CD8+ T cells and enhance tumor control. J Immunol. 2007;179(9):5829–38.

73. Shedlock DJ, Shen H. Requirement for CD4 T cell help in generating functional CD8 T cell memory. Science. 2003;300(5617):337–9.

74. Hamilton SE, Wolkers MC, Schoenberger SP, Jameson SC. The generation of protective memory-like CD8+ T cells during homeostatic proliferation requires CD4+ T cells. Nat Immunol. 2006;7(5):475–81.

75. Belz GT, Wodarz D, Diaz G, Nowak MA, Doherty PC. Compromised influenza virus-specific CD8(+)-T-cell memory in CD4(+)-T-cell-deficient mice. J Virol. 2002;76(23):12388–93.

76. Provine NM, Larocca RA, Aid M, Penaloza-MacMaster P, Badamchi-Zadeh A, Borducchi EN, et al. Immediate dysfunction of vaccine-elicited CD8+ T cells primed in the absence of CD4+ T cells. J Immunol. 2016;197(5):1809–22.

77. Del Prete GF, De Carli M, Mastromauro C, Biagiotti R, Macchia D, Falagiani P, et al. Purified protein derivative of Mycobacterium tuberculosis and excretory-secretory antigen(s) of Toxocara canis expand in vitro human T cells with stable and opposite (type 1 T helper or type 2 T helper) profile of cytokine production. J Clin Invest. 1991;88(1):346–50.

78. Szabo SJ, Kim ST, Costa GL, Zhang X, Fathman CG, Glimcher LH. A novel transcription factor, T-bet, directs Th1 lineage commitment. Cell. 2000;100(6):655–69.

79. Hsieh CS, Macatonia SE, Tripp CS, Wolf SF, O'Garra A, Murphy KM. Development of TH1 CD4+ T cells through IL-12 produced by Listeria-induced macrophages. Science. 1993;260(5107):547–9.

80. Raphael I, Nalawade S, Eagar TN, Forsthuber TG. T cell subsets and their signature cytokines in autoimmune and inflammatory diseases. Cytokine. 2015;74(1):5–17.

81. Zaidi MR, Merlino G. The two faces of interferon-gamma in cancer. Clin Cancer Res. 2011;17(19):6118–24.

82. Qin Z, Blankenstein T. CD4+ T cell-mediated tumor rejection involves inhibition of angiogenesis that is dependent on IFN gamma receptor expression by nonhematopoietic cells. Immunity. 2000;12(6):677–86.

83. Haabeth OA, Lorvik KB, Hammarstrom C, Donaldson IM, Haraldsen G, Bogen B, et al. Inflammation driven by tumour-specific Th1 cells protects against B-cell cancer. Nat Commun. 2011;2:240.

84. Palucka K, Banchereau J. Cancer immunotherapy via dendritic cells. Nat Rev Cancer. 2012;12(4):265–77.

85. Schroder K, Hertzog PJ, Ravasi T, Hume DA. Interferon-γ: an overview of signals, mechanisms and functions. J Leukoc Biol. 2004;75(2):163–89.

86. Murray HW, Spitalny GL, Nathan CF. Activation of mouse peritoneal macrophages in vitro and in vivo by interferon-gamma. J Immunol. 1985;134(3):1619–22.

87. Hung K, Hayashi R, Lafond-Walker A, Lowenstein C, Pardoll D, Levitsky H. The central role of CD4(+) T cells in the antitumor immune response. J Exp Med. 1998;188(12):2357–68.

88. Waldhauer I, Steinle A. NK cells and cancer immunosurveillance. Oncogene. 2008;27(45):5932–43.

89. Noy R, Pollard JW. Tumor-associated macrophages: from mechanisms to therapy. Immunity. 2014;41(1):49–61.

90. Fridman WH, Pagès F, Sautès-Fridman C, Galon J. The immune contexture in human tumours: impact on clinical outcome. Nat Rev Cancer. 2012;12(4):298–306.

91. Shurin MR, Lu L, Kalinski P, Stewart-Akers AM, Lotze MT. Th1/Th2 balance in cancer, transplantation and pregnancy. Springer Semin Immunopathol. 1999;21(3):339–59.

92. Hunder NN, Wallen H, Cao J, Hendricks DW, Reilly JZ, Rodmyre R, et al. Treatment of metastatic melanoma with autologous CD4+ T cells against NY-ESO-1. N Engl J Med. 2008;358(25):2698–703.

93. Tran E, Turcotte S, Gros A, Robbins PF, Lu YC, Dudley ME, et al. Cancer immunotherapy based on mutation-specific CD4+ T cells in a patient with epithelial cancer. Science. 2014;344(6184):641–5.

94. Chandran SS, Paria BC, Srivastava AK, Rothermel LD, Stephens DJ, Dudley ME, et al. Persistence of CTL clones targeting melanocyte differentiation antigens was insufficient to mediate significant melanoma regression in humans. Clin Cancer Res. 2015;21(3):534–43.

95. Zheng W, Flavell RA. The transcription factor GATA-3 is necessary and sufficient for Th2 cytokine gene expression in CD4 T cells. Cell. 1997;89(4):587–96.

96. Tepper RI, Pattengale PK, Leder P. Murine interleukin-4 displays potent anti-tumor activity in vivo. Cell. 1989;57(3):503–12.

97. Volpert OV, Fong T, Koch AE, Peterson JD, Waltenbaugh C, Tepper RI, et al. Inhibition of angiogenesis by interleukin 4. J Exp Med. 1998;188(6):1039–46.

98. Shen Y, Fujimoto S. A tumor-specific Th2 clone initiating tumor rejection via primed CD8+ cytotoxic T-lymphocyte activation in mice. Cancer Res. 1996;56(21):5005–11.

99. Terabe M, Park JM, Berzofsky JA. Role of IL-13 in regulation of anti-tumor immunity and tumor growth. Cancer Immunol Immunother. 2004;53(2):79–85.

100. Modesti A, D'Orazi G, Masuelli L, Modica A, Scarpa S, Bosco MC, et al. Ultrastructural evidence of the mechanisms responsible for interleukin-4-activated rejection of a spontaneous murine adenocarcinoma. Int J Cancer. 1993;53(6):988–93.

101. Musiani P, Allione A, Modica A, Lollini PL, Giovarelli M, Cavallo F, et al. Role of neutrophils and lymphocytes in inhibition of a mouse mammary adenocarcinoma engineered to release IL-2, IL-4, IL-7, IL-10, IFN-alpha, IFN-gamma, and TNF-alpha. Lab Invest. 1996;74(1):146–57.

102. Pericle F, Giovarelli M, Colombo MP, Ferrari G, Musiani P, Modesti A, et al. An efficient Th2-type memory follows CD8+ lymphocyte-driven and eosinophil-mediated rejection of a spontaneous mouse mammary adenocarcinoma engineered to release IL-4. J Immunol. 1994;153(12):5659–73.

103. Lebel-Binay S, Laguerre B, Quintin-Colonna F, Conjeaud H, Magazin M, Miloux B, et al. Experimental gene therapy of cancer using tumor cells engineered to secrete interleukin-13. Eur J Immunol. 1995;25(8):2340–8.

104. Mattes J, Hulett M, Xie W, Hogan S, Rothenberg ME, Foster P, et al. Immunotherapy of cytotoxic T cell-resistant tumors by T helper 2 cells: an eotaxin and STAT6-dependent process. J Exp Med. 2003;197(3):387–93.

105. Conticello C, Pedini F, Zeuner A, Patti M, Zerilli M, Stassi G, et al. IL-4 protects tumor cells from anti-CD95 and chemotherapeutic agents via up-regulation of antiapoptotic proteins. J Immunol. 2004;172(9):5467–77.

106. Zhang WJ, Li BH, Yang XZ, Li PD, Yuan Q, Liu XH, et al. IL-4-induced Stat6 activities affect apoptosis and gene expression in breast cancer cells. Cytokine. 2008;42(1):39–47.

107. Aspord C, Pedroza-Gonzalez A, Gallegos M, Tindle S, Burton EC, Su D, et al. Breast cancer instructs dendritic cells to prime interleukin 13-secreting CD4+ T cells that facilitate tumor development. J Exp Med. 2007;204(5):1037–47.

108. Wynn TA. Fibrotic disease and the T(H)1/T(H)2 paradigm. Nat Rev Immunol. 2004;4(8):583–94.

109. Wynn TA. IL-13 effector functions. Annu Rev Immunol. 2003;21(1):425–56.

110. Kushekhar K, van den Berg A, Nolte I, Hepkema B, Visser L, Diepstra A. Genetic associations in classical Hodgkin lymphoma: a systematic review and insights into susceptibility mechanisms. Cancer Epidemiol Biomarkers Prev. 2014;23(12):2737–47.

111. Kanno Y, Vahedi G, Hirahara K, Singleton K, O'Shea JJ. Transcriptional and epigenetic control of T helper cell specification: molecular mechanisms underlying commitment and plasticity. Annu Rev Immunol. 2012;30(1):707–31.

112. Schuler T, Qin Z, Ibe S, Noben-Trauth N, Blankenstein T. T helper cell type 1-associated and cytotoxic T lymphocyte-mediated tumor immunity is impaired in interleukin 4-deficient mice. J Exp Med. 1999;189(5):803–10.

113. Nishimura T, Iwakabe K, Sekimoto M, Ohmi Y, Yahata T, Nakui M, et al. Distinct role of antigen-specific T helper type 1 (Th1) and Th2 cells in tumor eradication in vivo. J Exp Med. 1999;190(5):617–27.

114. Wormann SM, Diakopoulos KN, Lesina M, Algul H. The immune network in pancreatic cancer development and progression. Oncogene. 2014;33(23):2956–67.

115. Kristensen VN, Vaske CJ, Ursini-Siegel J, Van Loo P, Nordgard SH, Sachidanandam R, et al. Integrated molecular profiles of invasive breast tumors and ductal carcinoma in situ (DCIS) reveal differential vascular and interleukin signaling. Proc Natl Acad Sci U S A. 2012;109(8):2802–7.

116. Tassi E, Gavazzi F, Albarello L, Senyukov V, Longhi R, Dellabona P, et al. Carcinoembryonic antigen-specific but not antiviral CD4+ T cell immunity is impaired in pancreatic carcinoma patients. J Immunol. 2008;181(9):6595–603.

117. Tatsumi T, Kierstead LS, Ranieri E, Gesualdo L, Schena FP, Finke JH, et al. Disease-associated bias in T helper type 1 (Th1)/Th2 CD4(+) T cell responses against MAGE-6 in HLA-DRB10401(+) patients with renal cell carcinoma or melanoma. J Exp Med. 2002;196(5):619–28.

118. Fiorentino DF, Zlotnik A, Vieira P, Mosmann TR, Howard M, Moore KW, et al. IL-10 acts on the antigen-presenting cell to inhibit cytokine production by Th1 cells. J Immunol. 1991;146(10):3444–51.

119. Steinbrink K, Wolfl M, Jonuleit H, Knop J, Enk AH. Induction of tolerance by IL-10-treated dendritic cells. J Immunol. 1997;159(10):4772–80.

120. Huang M, Wang J, Lee P, Sharma S, Mao JT, Meissner H, et al. Human non-small cell lung cancer cells express a type 2 cytokine pattern. Cancer Res. 1995;55(17):3847–53.

121. Maeurer MJ, Martin DM, Castelli C, Elder E, Leder G, Storkus WJ, et al. Host immune response in renal cell cancer: interleukin-4 (IL-4) and IL-10 mRNA are frequently detected in freshly collected tumor-infiltrating lymphocytes. Cancer Immunol Immunother. 1995;41(2):111–21.

122. Ochi A, Nguyen AH, Bedrosian AS, Mushlin HM, Zarbakhsh S, Barilla R, et al. MyD88 inhibition amplifies dendritic cell capacity to promote pancreatic carcinogenesis via Th2 cells. J Exp Med. 2012;209(9):1671–87.

123. De Monte L, Reni M, Tassi E, Clavenna D, Papa I, Recalde H, et al. Intratumor T helper type 2 cell infiltrate correlates with cancer-associated fibroblast thymic stromal lymphopoietin production and reduced survival in pancreatic cancer. J Exp Med. 2011;208(3):469–78.

124. Pedroza-Gonzalez A, Xu K, Wu T-C, Aspord C, Tindle S, Marches F, et al. Thymic stromal lymphopoietin fosters human breast tumor growth by promoting type 2 inflammation. J Exp Med. 2011;208(3):479–90.

125. Kido M, Tanaka J, Aoki N, Iwamoto S, Nishiura H, Chiba T, et al. Helicobacter pylori promotes the production of thymic stromal lymphopoietin by gastric epithelial cells and induces dendritic cell-mediated inflammatory Th2 responses. Infect Immun. 2010;78(1):108–14.

126. Ziegler A, Heidenreich R, Braumuller H, Wolburg H, Weidemann S, Mocikat R, et al. EpCAM, a human tumor-associated antigen promotes Th2 development and tumor immune evasion. Blood. 2009;113(15):3494–502.

127. Harrington LE, Hatton RD, Mangan PR, Turner H, Murphy TL, Murphy KM, et al. Interleukin 17-producing CD4+ effector T cells develop via a lineage distinct from the T helper type 1 and 2 lineages. Nat Immunol. 2005;6(11):1123–32.

128. Park H, Li Z, Yang XO, Chang SH, Nurieva R, Wang YH, et al. A distinct lineage of CD4 T cells regulates tissue inflammation by producing interleukin 17. Nat Immunol. 2005;6(11):1133–41.

129. Annunziato F, Cosmi L, Santarlasci V, Maggi L, Liotta F, Mazzinghi B, et al. Phenotypic and functional features of human Th17 cells. J Exp Med. 2007;204(8):1849–61.

130. Korn T, Bettelli E, Oukka M, Kuchroo VK. IL-17 and Th17 cells. Annu Rev Immunol. 2009;27:485–517.

131. Annunziato F, Cosmi L, Liotta F, Maggi E, Romagnani S. Main features of human T helper 17 cells. Ann N Y Acad Sci. 2013;1284:66–70.

132. Annunziato F, Cosmi L, Liotta F, Maggi E, Romagnani S. The phenotype of human Th17 cells and their precursors, the cytokines that mediate their differentiation and the role of Th17 cells in inflammation. Int Immunol. 2008;20(11):1361–8.

133. Kleinewietfeld M, Hafler DA. The plasticity of human Treg and Th17 cells and its role in autoimmunity. Semin Immunol. 2013;25(4):305–12.

134. Sundrud MS, Trivigno C. Identity crisis of Th17 cells: many forms, many functions, many questions. Semin Immunol. 2013;25(4):263–72.

135. Jin W, Dong C. IL-17 cytokines in immunity and inflammation. Emerg Microbes Infect. 2013;2:e60.

136. Muranski P, Boni A, Antony PA, Cassard L, Irvine KR, Kaiser A, et al. Tumor-specific Th17-polarized cells eradicate large established melanoma. Blood. 2008;112(2):362–73.

137. Martin-Orozco N, Muranski P, Chung Y, Yang XO, Yamazaki T, Lu S, et al. T helper 17 cells promote cytotoxic T cell activation in tumor immunity. Immunity. 2009;31(5):787–98.

138. Cho BS, Lim JY, Yahng SA, Lee SE, Eom KS, Kim YJ, et al. Circulating IL-17 levels during the peri-transplant period as a predictor for early leukemia relapse after myeloablative allogeneic stem cell transplantation. Ann Hematol. 2012;91(3):439–48.

139. Tartour E, Fossiez F, Joyeux I, Galinha A, Gey A, Claret E, et al. Interleukin 17, a T-cell-derived cytokine, promotes tumorigenicity of human cervical tumors in nude mice. Cancer Res. 1999;59(15):3698–704.

140. Numasaki M, Watanabe M, Suzuki T, Takahashi H, Nakamura A, McAllister F, et al. IL-17 enhances the net angiogenic activity and in vivo growth of human non-small cell lung cancer in SCID mice through promoting CXCR-2-dependent angiogenesis. J Immunol. 2005;175(9):6177–89.

141. Chang SH, Mirabolfathinejad SG, Katta H, Cumpian AM, Gong L, Caetano MS, et al. T helper 17 cells play a critical pathogenic role in lung cancer. Proc Natl Acad Sci U S A. 2014;111(15):5664–9.

142. De Simone V, Pallone F, Monteleone G, Stolfi C. Role of T(H)17 cytokines in the control of colorectal cancer. Oncoimmunology. 2013;2(12):e26617.

143. Wei S, Zhao E, Kryczek I, Zou W. Th17 cells have stem cell-like features and promote long-term immunity. OncoImmunology. 2012;1(4):516–9.

144. Wang K, Kim MK, Di Caro G, Wong J, Shalapour S, Wan J, et al. Interleukin-17 receptor a signaling in transformed enterocytes promotes early colorectal tumorigenesis. Immunity. 2014;41(6):1052–63.

145. McAllister F, Bailey JM, Alsina J, Nirschl CJ, Sharma R, Fan H, et al. Oncogenic Kras activates a hematopoietic-to-epithelial IL-17 signaling axis in preinvasive pancreatic neoplasia. Cancer Cell. 2014;25(5):621–37.

146. Keerthivasan S, Aghajani K, Dose M, Molinero L, Khan MW, Venkateswaran V, et al. beta-Catenin promotes colitis and colon cancer through imprinting of proinflammatory properties in T cells. Sci Transl Med. 2014;6(225):225ra28.

147. Kryczek I, Banerjee M, Cheng P, Vatan L, Szeliga W, Wei S, et al. Phenotype, distribution, generation, and functional and clinical relevance of Th17 cells in the human tumor environments. Blood. 2009;114(6):1141–9.

148. Lv L, Pan K, Li XD, She KL, Zhao JJ, Wang W, et al. The accumulation and prognosis value of tumor infiltrating IL-17 producing cells in esophageal squamous cell carcinoma. PLoS One. 2011;6(3):e18219.

149. Su X, Ye J, Hsueh EC, Zhang Y, Hoft DF, Peng G. Tumor microenvironments direct the recruitment and expansion of human Th17 cells. J Immunol. 2010;184(3):1630–41.

150. De Simone V, Franze E, Ronchetti G, Colantoni A, Fantini MC, Di Fusco D, et al. Th17-type cytokines, IL-6 and TNF-alpha synergistically activate STAT3 and NF-kB to promote colorectal cancer cell growth. Oncogene. 2015;34(27):3493–503.

151. Ye J, Su X, Hsueh EC, Zhang Y, Koenig JM, Hoft DF, et al. Human tumor-infiltrating Th17 cells have the capacity to differentiate into IFN-gamma+ and FOXP3+ T cells with potent suppressive function. Eur J Immunol. 2011;41(4):936–51.

152. Kryczek I, Zhao E, Liu Y, Wang Y, Vatan L, Szeliga W, et al. Human TH17 cells are long-lived effector memory cells. Sci Transl Med. 2011;3(104):104ra100.

153. Liu H, Rohowsky-Kochan C. Regulation of IL-17 in human CCR6+ effector memory T cells. J Immunol. 2008;180(12):7948–57.

154. Chellappa S, Hugenschmidt H, Hagness M, Line PD, Labori KJ, Wiedswang G, et al. Regulatory T cells that co-express RORγt and FOXP3 are pro-inflammatory and immunosuppressive and expand in human pancreatic cancer. OncoImmunology. 2015;5(4):e1102828.

155. Veldhoen M, Uyttenhove C, van Snick J, Helmby H, Westendorf A, Buer J, et al. Transforming growth factor-β 'reprograms' the differentiation of T helper 2 cells and promotes an interleukin 9-producing subset. Nat Immunol. 2008;9(12):1341–6.

156. Renauld JC, van der Lugt N, Vink A, van Roon M, Godfraind C, Warnier G, et al. Thymic lymphomas in interleukin 9 transgenic mice. Oncogene. 1994;9(5):1327–32.

157. Lee JE, Zhu Z, Bai Q, Brady TJ, Xiao H, Wakefield MR, et al. The role of interleukin-9 in cancer. Pathol Oncol Res. 2020;26(4):2017–22.

158. Lu Y, Hong S, Li H, Park J, Hong B, Wang L, et al. Th9 cells promote antitumor immune responses in vivo. J Clin Invest. 2012;122(11):4160–71.

159. Purwar R, Schlapbach C, Xiao S, Kang HS, Elyaman W, Jiang X, et al. Robust tumor immunity to melanoma mediated by interleukin-9-producing T cells. Nat Med. 2012;18(8):1248–53.

160. Chen J, Zhao Y, Chu X, Lu Y, Wang S, Yi Q. Dectin-1-activated dendritic cells: a potent Th9 cell inducer for tumor immunotherapy. Oncoimmunology. 2016;5(11):e1238558.

161. Feng LL, Gao JM, Li PP, Wang X. IL-9 contributes to immunosuppression mediated by regulatory T cells and mast cells in B-cell non-Hodgkin's lymphoma. J Clin Immunol. 2011;31(6):1084–94.

162. Chen N, Lv X, Li P, Lu K, Wang X. Role of high expression of IL-9 in prognosis of CLL. Int J Clin Exp Pathol. 2014;7(2):716–21.

163. Qiu L, Lai R, Lin Q, Lau E, Thomazy DM, Calame D, et al. Autocrine release of interleukin-9 promotes Jak3-dependent survival of ALK+ anaplastic large-cell lymphoma cells. Blood. 2006;108(7):2407–15.

164. Nagato T, Kobayashi H, Kishibe K, Takahara M, Ogino T, Ishii H, et al. Expression of interleukin-9 in nasal natural killer/T-cell lymphoma cell lines and patients. Clin Cancer Res. 2005;11(23):8250.

165. Ju W, Zhang M, Jiang J-k, Thomas CJ, Oh U, Bryant BR, et al. CP-690,550, a therapeutic agent, inhibits cytokine-mediated Jak3 activation and proliferation of T cells from patients with ATL and HAM/TSP. Blood. 2011;117(6):1938–46.

166. Abdul-Wahid A, Cydzik M, Prodeus A, Alwash M, Stanojcic M, Thompson M, et al. Induction of antigen-specific TH9 immunity accompanied by mast cell activation blocks tumor cell engraftment. Int J Cancer. 2016;139(4):841–53.

167. Tan H, Wang S, Zhao L. A tumour-promoting role of Th9 cells in hepatocellular carcinoma through CCL20 and STAT3 pathways. Clin Exp Pharmacol Physiol. 2017;44(2):213–21.

168. Salazar Y, Zheng X, Brunn D, Raifer H, Picard F, Zhang Y, et al. Microenvironmental Th9 and Th17 lymphocytes induce metastatic spreading in lung cancer. J Clin Invest. 2020;130(7):3560–75.

169. Duhen T, Geiger R, Jarrossay D, Lanzavecchia A, Sallusto F. Production of interleukin 22 but not interleukin 17 by a subset of human skin-homing memory T cells. Nat Immunol. 2009;10(8):857–63.

170. Jiang R, Tan Z, Deng L, Chen Y, Xia Y, Gao Y, et al. Interleukin-22 promotes human hepatocellular carcinoma by activation of STAT3. Hepatology. 2011;54(3):900–9.

171. Khosravi N, Caetano MS, Cumpian AM, Unver N, De la Garza Ramos C, Noble O, et al. IL22 promotes *Kras*-mutant lung cancer by induction of a protumor immune response and protection of stemness properties. Cancer Immunol Res. 2018;6(7):788.

172. Sun D, Lin Y, Hong J, Chen H, Nagarsheth N, Peng D, et al. Th22 cells control colon tumorigenesis through STAT3 and Polycomb Repression complex 2 signaling. OncoImmunology. 2016;5(8):e1082704.

173. Huber S, Gagliani N, Zenewicz LA, Huber FJ, Bosurgi L, Hu B, et al. IL-22BP is regulated by the inflammasome and modulates tumorigenesis in the intestine. Nature. 2012;491(7423):259–63.

174. Cella M, Fuchs A, Vermi W, Facchetti F, Otero K, Lennerz JKM, et al. A human natural killer cell subset provides an innate source of IL-22 for mucosal immunity. Nature. 2009;457(7230):722–5.

175. Thompson CL, Plummer SJ, Tucker TC, Casey G, Li L. Interleukin-22 genetic polymorphisms and risk of colon cancer. Cancer Causes Control. 2010;21(8):1165–70.

176. Wu T, Cui L, Liang Z, Liu C, Liu Y, Li J. Elevated serum IL-22 levels correlate with chemoresistant condition of colorectal cancer. Clin Immunol. 2013;147(1):38–9.

177. Voigt C, May P, Gottschlich A, Markota A, Wenk D, Gerlach I, et al. Cancer cells induce interleukin-22 production from memory CD4+ T cells via interleukin-1 to promote tumor growth. Proc Natl Acad Sci USA. 2017;114(49):12994.

178. Wang S, Yao Y, Yao M, Fu P, Wang W. Interleukin-22 promotes triple negative breast cancer cells migration and paclitaxel resistance through JAK-STAT3/MAPKs/AKT signaling pathways. Biochem Biophys Res Commun. 2018;503(3):1605–9.

179. Qi H. T follicular helper cells in space-time. Nat Rev Immunol. 2016;16(10):612–25.

180. Campbell DJ, Kim CH, Butcher EC. Separable effector T cell populations specialized for B cell help or tissue inflammation. Nat Immunol. 2001;2(9):876–81.

181. de Leval L, Rickman DS, Thielen C, Reynies A, Huang Y-L, Delsol G, et al. The gene expression profile of nodal peripheral T-cell lymphoma demonstrates a molecular link between angio-immunoblastic T-cell lymphoma (AITL) and follicular helper T (TFH) cells. Blood. 2007;109(11):4952–63.

182. Cortes JR, Ambesi-Impiombato A, Couronné L, Quinn SA, Kim CS, da Silva Almeida AC, et al. RHOA G17V induces T follicular helper cell specification and promotes lymphomagenesis. Cancer Cell. 2018;33(2):259–73. e7

183. Ochando J, Braza MS. T follicular helper cells: a potential therapeutic target in follicular lymphoma. Oncotarget. 2017;8(67):112116.

184. Gu-Trantien C, Loi S, Garaud S, Equeter C, Libin M, De Wind A, et al. CD4+ follicular helper T cell infiltration predicts breast cancer survival. J Clin Invest. 2013;123(7):2873–92.

185. Xiao H, Luo G, Son H, Zhou Y, Zheng W. Upregulation of peripheral CD4+ CXCR5+ T cells in osteosarcoma. Tumor Biol. 2014;35(6):5273–9.

186. Shi W, Li X, Cha Z, Sun S, Wang L, Jiao S, et al. Dysregulation of circulating follicular helper T cells in nonsmall cell lung cancer. DNA Cell Biol. 2014;33(6):355–60.

187. Cha Z, Zang Y, Guo H, Rechlic JR, Olasnova LM, Gu H, et al. Association of peripheral CD4+ CXCR5+ T cells with chronic lymphocytic leukemia. Tumor Biol. 2013;34(6):3579–85.

188. Wang Z, Wang Z, Diao Y, Qian X, Zhu N, Dong W. Circulating follicular helper T cells in Crohn's disease (CD) and CD-associated colorectal cancer. Tumor Biol. 2014;35(9):9355–9.

189. Ritter AT, Angus KL, Griffiths GM. The role of the cytoskeleton at the immunological synapse. Immunol Rev. 2013;256(1):107–17.

190. Fu Q, Fu T-M, Cruz Anthony C, Sengupta P, Thomas Stacy K, Wang S, et al. Structural basis and functional role of intramembrane trimerization of the Fas/CD95 death receptor. Mol Cell. 2016;61(4):602–13.

191. Gordy C, He YW. Endocytosis by target cells: an essential means for perforin- and granzyme-mediated killing. Cell Mol Immunol. 2012;9(1):5–6.

192. Shibuya TY, Nugyen N, McLaren CE, Li KT, Wei WZ, Kim S, et al. Clinical significance of poor CD3 response in head and neck cancer. Clin Cancer Res. 2002;8(3):745–51.

193. Badoual C, Hans S, Rodriguez J, Peyrard S, Klein C, Agueznay Nel H, et al. Prognostic value of tumor-infiltrating CD4+ T-cell subpopulations in head and neck cancers. Clin Cancer Res. 2006;12(2):465–72.

194. Cho Y, Miyamoto M, Kato K, Fukunaga A, Shichinohe T, Kawarada Y, et al. CD4+ and CD8+ T cells cooperate to improve prognosis of patients with esophageal squamous cell carcinoma. Cancer Res. 2003;63(7):1555–9.

195. Schumacher K, Haensch W, Roefzaad C, Schlag PM. Prognostic significance of activated CD8(+) T cell infiltrations within esophageal carcinomas. Cancer Res. 2001;61(10):3932–6.

196. van Sandick JW, Boermeester MA, Gisbertz SS, ten Berge IJ, Out TA, van der Pouw Kraan TC, et al. Lymphocyte subsets and T(h)1/T(h)2 immune responses in patients with adenocarcinoma of the oesophagus or oesophagogastric junction: relation to pTNM stage and clinical outcome. Cancer Immunol Immunother. 2003;52(10):617–24.

197. Dieu-Nosjean MC, Antoine M, Danel C, Heudes D, Wislez M, Poulot V, et al. Long-term survival for patients with non-small-cell lung cancer with intratumoral lymphoid structures. J Clin Oncol. 2008;26(27):4410–7.

198. Chen X, Wan J, Liu J, Xie W, Diao X, Xu J, et al. Increased IL-17-producing cells correlate with poor survival and lymphangiogenesis in NSCLC patients. Lung Cancer. 2010;69(3):348–54.

199. Tao H, Mimura Y, Aoe K, Kobayashi S, Yamamoto H, Matsuda E, et al. Prognostic potential of FOXP3 expression in non-small cell lung cancer cells combined with tumor-infiltrating regulatory T cells. Lung Cancer. 2012;75(1):95–101.

200. Fukunaga A, Miyamoto M, Cho Y, Murakami S, Kawarada Y, Oshikiri T, et al. CD8+ tumor-infiltrating lymphocytes together with CD4+ tumor-infiltrating lymphocytes and dendritic cells improve the prognosis of patients with pancreatic adenocarcinoma. Pancreas. 2004;28(1):e26–31.

201. Bazhin AV, Shevchenko I, Umansky V, Werner J, Karakhanova S. Two immune faces of pancreatic adenocarcinoma: possible implication for immunotherapy. Cancer Immunol Immunother. 2014;63(1):59–65.

202. Vizio B, Novarino A, Giacobino A, Cristiano C, Prati A, Ciuffreda L, et al. Potential plasticity of T regulatory cells in pancreatic carcinoma in relation to disease progression and outcome. Exp Ther Med. 2012;4(1):70–8.

203. Hiraoka N, Onozato K, Kosuge T, Hirohashi S. Prevalence of FOXP3+ regulatory T cells increases during the progression of pancreatic ductal adenocarcinoma and its premalignant lesions. Clin Cancer Res. 2006;12(18):5423–34.

204. Goeppert B, Frauenschuh L, Zucknick M, Stenzinger A, Andrulis M, Klauschen F, et al. Prognostic impact of tumour-infiltrating immune cells on biliary tract cancer. Br J Cancer. 2013;109(10):2665–74.

205. Mahmoud SM, Paish EC, Powe DG, Macmillan RD, Grainge MJ, Lee AH, et al. Tumor-infiltrating CD8+ lymphocytes predict clinical outcome in breast cancer. J Clin Oncol. 2011;29(15):1949–55.

206. Teschendorff AE, Gomez S, Arenas A, El-Ashry D, Schmidt M, Gehrmann M, et al. Improved prognostic classification of breast cancer defined by antagonistic activation patterns of immune response pathway modules. BMC Cancer. 2010;10:604.

207. Yoon NK, Maresh EL, Shen D, Elshimali Y, Apple S, Horvath S, et al. Higher levels of GATA3 predict better survival in women with breast cancer. Hum Pathol. 2010;41(12):1794–801.

208. Chen WC, Lai YH, Chen HY, Guo HR, Su IJ, Chen HH. Interleukin-17-producing cell infiltration in the breast cancer tumour microenvironment is a poor prognostic factor. Histopathology. 2013;63(2):225–33.

209. Gobert M, Treilleux I, Bendriss-Vermare N, Bachelot T, Goddard-Leon S, Arfi V, et al. Regulatory T cells recruited through CCL22/CCR4 are selectively activated in lymphoid infiltrates surrounding primary breast tumors and lead to an adverse clinical outcome. Cancer Res. 2009;69(5):2000–9.

210. Bates GJ, Fox SB, Han C, Leek RD, Garcia JF, Harris AL, et al. Quantification of regulatory T cells enables the identification of high-risk breast cancer patients and those at risk of late relapse. J Clin Oncol. 2006;24(34):5373–80.

211. West NR, Kost SE, Martin SD, Milne K, Deleeuw RJ, Nelson BH, et al. Tumour-infiltrating FOXP3(+) lymphocytes are associated with cytotoxic immune responses and good clinical outcome in oestrogen receptor-negative breast cancer. Br J Cancer. 2013;108(1):155–62.

212. Zhuang Y, Peng LS, Zhao YL, Shi Y, Mao XH, Chen W, et al. CD8(+) T cells that produce interleukin-17 regulate myeloid-derived suppressor cells and are associated with survival time of patients with gastric cancer. Gastroenterology. 2012;143(4):951–62.e8.

213. Saito H, Yamada Y, Takaya S, Osaki T, Ikeguchi M. Clinical relevance of the number of interleukin-17-producing CD 8+ T cells in patients with gastric cancer. Surg Today. 2015;45(11):1429–35.

214. Ubukata H, Motohashi G, Tabuchi T, Nagata H, Konishi S, Tabuchi T. Evaluations of interferon-gamma/interleukin-4 ratio and neutrophil/lymphocyte ratio as prognostic indicators in gastric cancer patients. J Surg Oncol. 2010;102(7):742–7.

215. Chen JG, Xia JC, Liang XT, Pan K, Wang W, Lv L, et al. Intratumoral expression of IL-17 and its prognostic role in gastric adenocarcinoma patients. Int J Biol Sci. 2011;7(1):53–60.

216. Maruyama T, Kono K, Mizukami Y, Kawaguchi Y, Mimura K, Watanabe M, et al. Distribution of Th17 cells and FoxP3(+) regulatory T cells in tumor-infiltrating lymphocytes, tumor-draining lymph nodes and peripheral blood lymphocytes in patients with gastric cancer. Cancer Sci. 2010;101(9):1947–54.

217. Shen Z, Zhou S, Wang Y, Li RL, Zhong C, Liang C, et al. Higher intratumoral infiltrated Foxp3+ Treg numbers and Foxp3+/CD8+ ratio are associated with adverse prognosis in resectable gastric cancer. J Cancer Res Clin Oncol. 2010;136(10):1585–95.

218. Cai XY, Gao Q, Qiu SJ, Ye SL, Wu ZQ, Fan J, et al. Dendritic cell infiltration and prognosis of human hepatocellular carcinoma. J Cancer Res Clin Oncol. 2006;132(5):293–301.

219. Gao Q, Qiu SJ, Fan J, Zhou J, Wang XY, Xiao YS, et al. Intratumoral balance of regulatory and cytotoxic T cells is associated with prognosis of hepatocellular carcinoma after resection. J Clin Oncol. 2007;25(18):2586–93.

220. Gao Q, Wang XY, Qiu SJ, Zhou J, Shi YH, Zhang BH, et al. Tumor stroma reaction-related gene signature predicts clinical outcome in human hepatocellular carcinoma. Cancer Sci. 2011;102(8):1522–31.

221. Zhang JP, Yan J, Xu J, Pang XH, Chen MS, Li L, et al. Increased intratumoral IL-17-producing cells correlate with poor survival in hepatocellular carcinoma patients. J Hepatol. 2009;50(5):980–9.

222. Kobayashi N, Hiraoka N, Yamagami W, Ojima H, Kanai Y, Kosuge T, et al. FOXP3+ regulatory T cells affect the development and progression of hepatocarcinogenesis. Clin Cancer Res. 2007;13(3):902–11.

223. Galon J, Costes A, Sanchez-Cabo F, Kirilovsky A, Mlecnik B, Lagorce-Pages C, et al. Type, density, and location of immune cells within human colorectal tumors predict clinical outcome. Science. 2006;313(5795):1960–4.

224. Tosolini M, Kirilovsky A, Mlecnik B, Fredriksen T, Mauger S, Bindea G, et al. Clinical impact of different classes of infiltrating T cytotoxic and helper cells (Th1, th2, treg, th17) in patients with colorectal cancer. Cancer Res. 2011;71(4):1263–71.

225. Camus M, Tosolini M, Mlecnik B, Pages F, Kirilovsky A, Berger A, et al. Coordination of intratumoral immune reaction and human colorectal cancer recurrence. Cancer Res. 2009;69(6):2685–93.

226. Mlecnik B, Tosolini M, Kirilovsky A, Berger A, Bindea G, Meatchi T, et al. Histopathologic-based prognostic factors of colorectal cancers are associated with the state of the local immune reaction. J Clin Oncol. 2011;29(6):610–8.

227. Sinicrope FA, Rego RL, Ansell SM, Knutson KL, Foster NR, Sargent DJ. Intraepithelial effector (CD3+)/regulatory (FoxP3+) T-cell ratio predicts a clinical outcome of human colon carcinoma. Gastroenterology. 2009;137(4):1270–9.

228. Naito Y, Saito K, Shiiba K, Ohuchi A, Saigenji K, Nagura H, et al. CD8+ T cells infiltrated within cancer cell nests as a prognostic factor in human colorectal cancer. Cancer Res. 1998;58(16):3491–4.

229. Nosho K, Baba Y, Tanaka N, Shima K, Hayashi M, Meyerhardt JA, et al. Tumour-infiltrating T-cell subsets, molecular changes in colorectal cancer, and prognosis: cohort study and literature review. J Pathol. 2010;222(4):350–66.

230. Liu J, Duan Y, Cheng X, Chen X, Xie W, Long H, et al. IL-17 is associated with poor prognosis and promotes angiogenesis via stimulating VEGF production of cancer cells in colorectal carcinoma. Biochem Biophys Res Commun. 2011;407(2):348–54.

231. Yoshida N, Kinugasa T, Miyoshi H, Sato K, Yuge K, Ohchi T, et al. A high RORgammaT/CD3 ratio is a strong prognostic factor for postoperative survival in advanced colorectal cancer: analysis of helper T cell lymphocytes (Th1, Th2, Th17 and regulatory T cells). Ann Surg Oncol. 2015;23(3):919–27.

232. Frey DM, Droeser RA, Viehl CT, Zlobec I, Lugli A, Zingg U, et al. High frequency of tumor-infiltrating FOXP3(+) regulatory T cells predicts improved survival in mismatch repair-proficient colorectal cancer patients. Int J Cancer. 2010;126(11):2635–43.

233. Salama P, Phillips M, Grieu F, Morris M, Zeps N, Joseph D, et al. Tumor-infiltrating FOXP3+ T regulatory cells show strong prognostic significance in colorectal cancer. J Clin Oncol. 2009;27(2):186–92.

234. Blatner NR, Mulcahy MF, Dennis KL, Scholtens D, Bentrem DJ, Phillips JD, et al. Expression of RORγt marks a pathogenic regulatory T cell subset in human colon cancer. Sci Transl Med. 2012;4(164):164ra59.

235. Sato E, Olson SH, Ahn J, Bundy B, Nishikawa H, Qian F, et al. Intraepithelial CD8+ tumor-infiltrating lymphocytes and a high CD8+/regulatory T cell ratio are associated with favorable prognosis in ovarian cancer. Proc Natl Acad Sci U S A. 2005;102(51):18538–43.

236. Marth C, Fiegl H, Zeimet AG, Muller-Holzner E, Deibl M, Doppler W, et al. Interferon-gamma expression is an independent prognostic factor in ovarian cancer. Am J Obstet Gynecol. 2004;191(5):1598–605.

237. Kusuda T, Shigemasa K, Arihiro K, Fujii T, Nagai N, Ohama K. Relative expression levels of Th1 and Th2 cytokine mRNA are independent prognostic factors in patients with ovarian cancer. Oncol Rep. 2005;13(6):1153–8.

238. Milne K, Kobel M, Kalloger SE, Barnes RO, Gao D, Gilks CB, et al. Systematic analysis of immune infiltrates in high-grade serous ovarian cancer reveals CD20, FoxP3 and TIA-1 as positive prognostic factors. PLoS One. 2009;4(7):e6412.

239. Leffers N, Gooden MJ, de Jong RA, Hoogeboom BN, ten Hoor KA, Hollema H, et al. Prognostic significance of tumor-infiltrating T-lymphocytes in primary and metastatic lesions of advanced stage ovarian cancer. Cancer Immunol Immunother. 2009;58(3):449–59.

240. Curiel TJ, Coukos G, Zou L, Alvarez X, Cheng P, Mottram P, et al. Specific recruitment of regulatory T cells in ovarian carcinoma fosters immune privilege and predicts reduced survival. Nat Med. 2004;10(9):942–9.

241. Nakano O, Sato M, Naito Y, Suzuki K, Orikasa S, Aizawa M, et al. Proliferative activity of intratumoral CD8(+) T-lymphocytes as a prognostic factor in human renal cell carcinoma: clinicopathologic demonstration of antitumor immunity. Cancer Res. 2001;61(13):5132–6.

242. Kondo T, Nakazawa H, Ito F, Hashimoto Y, Osaka Y, Futatsuyama K, et al. Favorable prognosis of renal cell carcinoma with increased expression of chemokines associated with a Th1-type immune response. Cancer Sci. 2006;97(8):780–6.

243. Karja V, Aaltomaa S, Lipponen P, Isotalo T, Talja M, Mokka R. Tumour-infiltrating lymphocytes: a prognostic factor of PSA-free survival in patients with local prostate carcinoma treated by radical prostatectomy. Anticancer Res. 2005;25(6C):4435–8.

244. Sharma P, Shen Y, Wen S, Yamada S, Jungbluth AA, Gnjatic S, et al. CD8 tumor-infiltrating lymphocytes are predictive of survival in muscle-invasive urothelial carcinoma. Proc Natl Acad Sci U S A. 2007;104(10):3967–72.

245. de Jong RA, Leffers N, Boezen HM, ten Hoor KA, van der Zee AG, Hollema H, et al. Presence of tumor-infiltrating lymphocytes is an independent prognostic factor in type I and II endometrial cancer. Gynecol Oncol. 2009;114(1):105–10.

246. Piersma SJ, Jordanova ES, van Poelgeest MI, Kwappenberg KM, van der Hulst JM, Drijfhout JW, et al. High number of intraepithelial CD8+ tumor-infiltrating lymphocytes is associated with the absence of lymph node metastases in patients with large early-stage cervical cancer. Cancer Res. 2007;67(1):354–61.

247. Zhang Y, Hou F, Liu X, Ma D, Zhang Y, Kong B, et al. Tc17 cells in patients with uterine cervical cancer. PLoS One. 2014;9(2):e86812.

248. Taylor RC, Patel A, Panageas KS, Busam KJ, Brady MS. Tumor-infiltrating lymphocytes predict sentinel lymph node positivity in patients with cutaneous melanoma. J Clin Oncol. 2007;25(7):869–75.

249. Clemente CG, Mihm MC Jr, Bufalino R, Zurrida S, Collini P, Cascinelli N. Prognostic value of tumor infiltrating lymphocytes in the vertical growth phase of primary cutaneous melanoma. Cancer. 1996;77(7):1303–10.

250. Ladanyi A, Mohos A, Somlai B, Liszkay G, Gilde K, Fejos Z, et al. FOXP3+ cell density in primary tumor has no prognostic

impact in patients with cutaneous malignant melanoma. Pathol Oncol Res. 2010;16(3):303–9.

251. Mougiakakos D, Johansson CC, Trocme E, All-Ericsson C, Economou MA, Larsson O, et al. Intratumoral forkhead box P3-positive regulatory T cells predict poor survival in cyclooxygenase-2-positive uveal melanoma. Cancer. 2010;116(9):2224–33.

252. Miracco C, Mourmouras V, Biagioli M, Rubegni P, Mannucci S, Monciatti I, et al. Utility of tumour-infiltrating CD25+FOXP3+ regulatory T cell evaluation in predicting local recurrence in vertical growth phase cutaneous melanoma. Oncol Rep. 2007;18(5):1115–22.

253. Schreck S, Friebel D, Buettner M, Distel L, Grabenbauer G, Young LS, et al. Prognostic impact of tumour-infiltrating Th2 and regulatory T cells in classical Hodgkin lymphoma. Hematol Oncol. 2009;27(1):31–9.

254. Tzankov A, Meier C, Hirschmann P, Went P, Pileri SA, Dirnhofer S. Correlation of high numbers of intratumoral FOXP3+ regulatory T cells with improved survival in germinal center-like diffuse large B-cell lymphoma, follicular lymphoma and classical Hodgkin's lymphoma. Haematologica. 2008;93(2):193–200.

255. Carreras J, Lopez-Guillermo A, Fox BC, Colomo L, Martinez A, Roncador G, et al. High numbers of tumor-infiltrating FOXP3-positive regulatory T cells are associated with improved overall survival in follicular lymphoma. Blood. 2006;108(9):2957–64.

256. Huse M, Lillemeier BF, Kuhns MS, Chen DS, Davis MM. T cells use two directionally distinct pathways for cytokine secretion. Nat Immunol. 2006;7(3):247–55.

257. Borst J, Ahrends T, Bąbała N, Melief CJ, Kastenmüller W. CD4+ T cell help in cancer immunology and immunotherapy. Nat Rev Immunol. 2018;18(10):635–47.

258. Faghih Z, Rezaeifard S, Safaei A, Ghaderi A, Erfani N. IL-17 and IL-4 producing CD8+ T cells in tumor draining lymph nodes of breast cancer patients: positive association with tumor progression. Iran J Immunol IJI. 2013;10(4):193–204.

259. Tsai JP, Lee MH, Hsu SC, Chen MY, Liu SJ, Chang JT, et al. CD4+ T cells disarm or delete cytotoxic T lymphocytes under IL-17-polarizing conditions. J Immunol. 2012;189(4):1671–9.

260. Huber M, Heink S, Grothe H, Guralnik A, Reinhard K, Elflein K, et al. A Th17-like developmental process leads to CD8(+) Tc17 cells with reduced cytotoxic activity. Eur J Immunol. 2009;39(7):1716–25.

261. Tajima M, Wakita D, Satoh T, Kitamura H, Nishimura T. IL-17/IFN-gamma double producing CD8+ T (Tc17/IFN-gamma) cells: a novel cytotoxic T-cell subset converted from Tc17 cells by IL-12. Int Immunol. 2011;23(12):751–9.

262. Kuang DM, Peng C, Zhao Q, Wu Y, Zhu LY, Wang J, et al. Tumor-activated monocytes promote expansion of IL-17-producing CD8+ T cells in hepatocellular carcinoma patients. J Immunol. 2010;185(3):1544–9.

263. Zhang W, Hou F, Zhang Y, Tian Y, Jiao J, Ma D, et al. Changes of Th17/Tc17 and Th17/Treg cells in endometrial carcinoma. Gynecol Oncol. 2014;132(3):599–605.

264. Khazen R, Müller S, Gaudenzio N, Espinosa E, Puissegur MP, Valitutti S. Melanoma cell lysosome secretory burst neutralizes the CTL-mediated cytotoxicity at the lytic synapse. Nat Commun. 2016;7:10823.

265. Sakaguchi S, Sakaguchi N, Asano M, Itoh M, Toda M. Immunologic self-tolerance maintained by activated T cells expressing IL-2 receptor alpha-chains (CD25). Breakdown of a single mechanism of self-tolerance causes various autoimmune diseases. J Immunol. 1995;155(3):1151–64.

266. Sakaguchi S, Yamaguchi T, Nomura T, Ono M. Regulatory T cells and immune tolerance. Cell. 2008;133(5):775–87.

267. Pohar J, Simon Q, Fillatreau S. Antigen-specificity in the thymic development and peripheral activity of CD4(+)FOXP3(+) T regulatory cells. Front Immunol. 2018;9:1701.

268. Miyara M, Yoshioka Y, Kitoh A, Shima T, Wing K, Niwa A, et al. Functional delineation and differentiation dynamics of human CD4+ T cells expressing the FoxP3 transcription factor. Immunity. 2009;30(6):899–911.

269. Sakaguchi S, Miyara M, Costantino CM, Hafler DA. FOXP3+ regulatory T cells in the human immune system. Nat Rev Immunol. 2010;10(7):490–500.

270. Shevach EM. Mechanisms of Foxp3+ T regulatory cell-mediated suppression. Immunity. 2009;30(5):636–45.

271. Shimizu J, Yamazaki S, Sakaguchi S. Induction of tumor immunity by removing CD25+CD4+ T cells: a common basis between tumor immunity and autoimmunity. J Immunol. 1999;163(10):5211–8.

272. Nishikawa H, Sakaguchi S. Regulatory T cells in cancer immunotherapy. Curr Opin Immunol. 2014;27:1–7.

273. Ishida T, Ishii T, Inagaki A, Yano H, Komatsu H, Iida S, et al. Specific recruitment of CC chemokine receptor 4-positive regulatory T cells in Hodgkin lymphoma fosters immune privilege. Cancer Res. 2006;66(11):5716–22.

274. Facciabene A, Peng X, Hagemann IS, Balint K, Barchetti A, Wang LP, et al. Tumour hypoxia promotes tolerance and angiogenesis via CCL28 and T(reg) cells. Nature. 2011;475(7355):226–30.

275. Tan MC, Goedegebuure PS, Belt BA, Flaherty B, Sankpal N, Gillanders WE, et al. Disruption of CCR5-dependent homing of regulatory T cells inhibits tumor growth in a murine model of pancreatic cancer. J Immunol. 2009;182(3):1746–55.

276. Marshall LA, Marubayashi S, Jorapur A, Jacobson S, Zibinsky M, Robles O, et al. Tumors establish resistance to immunotherapy by regulating T(reg) recruitment via CCR4. J Immunother Cancer. 2020;8(2)

277. Banerjee A, Vasanthakumar A, Grigoriadis G. Modulating T regulatory cells in cancer: how close are we? Immunol Cell Biol. 2013;91(5):340–9.

278. Waight JD, Takai S, Marelli B, Qin G, Hance KW, Zhang D, et al. Cutting edge: epigenetic regulation of Foxp3 defines a stable population of CD4+ regulatory T cells in tumors from mice and humans. J Immunol. 2015;194(3):878–82.

279. Sugiyama D, Nishikawa H, Maeda Y, Nishioka M, Tanemura A, Katayama I, et al. Anti-CCR4 mAb selectively depletes effector-type FoxP3+CD4+ regulatory T cells, evoking antitumor immune responses in humans. Proc Natl Acad Sci U S A. 2013;110(44):17945–50.

280. Li DY, Xiong XZ. ICOS(+) Tregs: a functional subset of tregs in immune diseases. Front Immunol. 2020;11:2104.

281. Buzzatti G, Dellepiane C, Del Mastro L. New emerging targets in cancer immunotherapy: the role of GITR. ESMO Open. 2020;4(Suppl 3).

282. Nishikawa H, Kato T, Tawara I, Saito K, Ikeda H, Kuribayashi K, et al. Definition of target antigens for naturally occurring CD4(+) CD25(+) regulatory T cells. J Exp Med. 2005;201(5):681–6.

283. Tone Y, Furuuchi K, Kojima Y, Tykocinski ML, Greene MI, Tone M. Smad3 and NFAT cooperate to induce Foxp3 expression through its enhancer. Nat Immunol. 2008;9(2):194–202.

284. Sanjabi S, Oh SA, Li MO. Regulation of the immune response by TGF-β: from conception to autoimmunity and infection. Cold Spring Harb Perspect Biol. 2017;9(6)

285. Yang S, Wang B, Guan C, Wu B, Cai C, Wang M, et al. Foxp3+IL-17+ T cells promote development of cancer-initiating cells in colorectal cancer. J Leukoc Biol. 2011;89(1):85–91.

286. Thibaudin M, Chaix M, Boidot R, Végran F, Derangère V, Limagne E, et al. Human ectonucleotidase-expressing CD25high

Th17 cells accumulate in breast cancer tumors and exert immunosuppressive functions. OncoImmunology. 2015;5(1):e1055444.

287. Scott JD, Dessauer CW, Tasken K. Creating order from chaos: cellular regulation by kinase anchoring. Annu Rev Pharmacol Toxicol. 2013;53:187–210.

288. Mahic M, Yaqub S, Johansson CC, Tasken K, Aandahl EM. FOXP3+CD4+CD25+ adaptive regulatory T cells express cyclooxygenase-2 and suppress effector T cells by a prostaglandin E2-dependent mechanism. J Immunol. 2006;177(1):246–54.

289. Vang T, Torgersen KM, Sundvold V, Saxena M, Levy FO, Skalhegg BS, et al. Activation of the COOH-terminal Src kinase (Csk) by cAMP-dependent protein kinase inhibits signaling through the T cell receptor. J Exp Med. 2001;193(4):497–507.

290. Torgersen KM, Vang T, Abrahamsen H, Yaqub S, Horejsi V, Schraven B, et al. Release from tonic inhibition of T cell activation through transient displacement of C-terminal Src kinase (Csk) from lipid rafts. J Biol Chem. 2001;276(31):29313–8.

291. Ruppelt A, Mosenden R, Gronholm M, Aandahl EM, Tobin D, Carlson CR, et al. Inhibition of T cell activation by cyclic adenosine 5′-monophosphate requires lipid raft targeting of protein kinase A type I by the A-kinase anchoring protein ezrin. J Immunol. 2007;179(8):5159–68.

292. Mosenden R, Singh P, Cornez I, Heglind M, Ruppelt A, Moutschen M, et al. Mice with disrupted type I protein kinase A anchoring in T cells resist retrovirus-induced immunodeficiency. J Immunol. 2011;186(9):5119–30.

293. Deaglio S, Dwyer KM, Gao W, Friedman D, Usheva A, Erat A, et al. Adenosine generation catalyzed by CD39 and CD73 expressed on regulatory T cells mediates immune suppression. J Exp Med. 2007;204(6):1257–65.

294. Whiteside TL, Jackson EK. Adenosine and prostaglandin e2 production by human inducible regulatory T cells in health and disease. Front Immunol. 2013;4:212.

295. Ohta A, Sitkovsky M. Role of G-protein-coupled adenosine receptors in downregulation of inflammation and protection from tissue damage. Nature. 2001;414(6866):916–20.

296. Bopp T, Becker C, Klein M, Klein-Hessling S, Palmetshofer A, Serfling E, et al. Cyclic adenosine monophosphate is a key component of regulatory T cell-mediated suppression. J Exp Med. 2007;204(6):1303–10.

297. Tasken K. Waking up regulatory T cells. Blood. 2009;114(6):1136–7.

298. Bryn T, Yaqub S, Mahic M, Henjum K, Aandahl EM, Tasken K. LPS-activated monocytes suppress T-cell immune responses and induce FOXP3+ T cells through a COX-2-PGE2-dependent mechanism. Int Immunol. 2008;20(2):235–45.

299. Take Y, Koizumi S, Nagahisa A. Prostaglandin E receptor 4 antagonist in cancer immunotherapy: mechanisms of action. Front Immunol. 2020;11:324.

300. Congreve M, Brown GA, Borodovsky A, Lamb ML. Targeting adenosine A2A receptor antagonism for treatment of cancer. Expert Opin Drug Discov. 2018;13(11):997–1003.

301. Willingham SB, Ho PY, Hotson A, Hill C, Piccione EC, Hsieh J, et al. A2AR antagonism with CPI-444 induces antitumor responses and augments efficacy to anti-PD-(L)1 and anti-CTLA-4 in preclinical models. Cancer Immunol Res. 2018;6(10):1136–49.

302. Yaqub S, Henjum K, Mahic M, Jahnsen FL, Aandahl EM, Bjørnbeth BA, et al. Regulatory T cells in colorectal cancer patients suppress anti-tumor immune activity in a COX-2 dependent manner. Cancer Immunol Immunother. 2008;57(6):813–21.

303. Dees S, Ganesan R, Singh S, Grewal IS. Regulatory T cell targeting in cancer: emerging strategies in immunotherapy. Eur J Immunol. 2021;51(2):280–91.

304. Roberts S, Girardi M. Conventional and unconventional T cells. In: Gaspari AA, Tyring SK, editors. Clinical and basic immunodermatology. London: Springer; 2008. p. 85–104.

305. Godfrey DI, Le Nours J, Andrews DM, Uldrich AP, Rossjohn J. Unconventional T cell targets for cancer immunotherapy. Immunity. 2018;48(3):453–73.

306. Lantz O, Bendelac A. An invariant T cell receptor alpha chain is used by a unique subset of major histocompatibility complex class I-specific CD4+ and CD4-8- T cells in mice and humans. J Exp Med. 1994;180(3):1097–106.

307. McEwen-Smith RM, Salio M, Cerundolo V. The regulatory role of invariant NKT cells in tumor immunity. Cancer Immunol Res. 2015;3(5):425–35.

308. Smyth MJ, Crowe NY, Pellicci DG, Kyparissoudis K, Kelly JM, Takeda K, et al. Sequential production of interferon-γ by NK1. 1+ T cells and natural killer cells is essential for the antimetastatic effect of α-galactosylceramide. Blood. 2002;99(4):1259–66.

309. Metelitsa LS, Naidenko OV, Kant A, Wu H-W, Loza MJ, Perussia B, et al. Human NKT cells mediate antitumor cytotoxicity directly by recognizing target cell CD1d with bound ligand or indirectly by producing IL-2 to activate NK cells. J Immunol. 2001;167(6):3114–22.

310. Fujii S-i, Shimizu K, Smith C, Bonifaz L, Steinman RM. Activation of natural killer T cells by α-galactosylceramide rapidly induces the full maturation of dendritic cells in vivo and thereby acts as an adjuvant for combined CD4 and CD8 T cell immunity to a coadministered protein. J Exp Med. 2003;198(2):267–79.

311. Paget C, Chow MT, Duret H, Mattarollo SR, Smyth MJ. Role of γδ T cells in α-galactosylceramide-mediated immunity. J Immunol. 2012;188(8):3928–39.

312. Molling JW, Langius JA, Langendijk JA, Leemans CR, Bontkes HJ, van der Vliet HJ, et al. Low levels of circulating invariant natural killer T cells predict poor clinical outcome in patients with head and neck squamous cell carcinoma. J Clin Oncol. 2007;25(7):862–8.

313. Chuc AEN, Cervantes LAM, Retiguin FP, Ojeda JV, Maldonado ER. Low number of invariant NKT cells is associated with poor survival in acute myeloid leukemia. J Cancer Res Clin Oncol. 2012;138(8):1427–32.

314. Hishiki T, Mise N, Harada K, Ihara F, Takami M, Saito T, et al. Invariant natural killer T infiltration in neuroblastoma with favorable outcome. Pediatr Surg Int. 2018;34(2):195–201.

315. Loh L, Wang Z, Sant S, Koutsakos M, Jegaskanda S, Corbett AJ, et al. Human mucosal-associated invariant T cells contribute to antiviral influenza immunity via IL-18-dependent activation. Proc Natl Acad Sci USA. 2016;113(36):10133–8.

316. Meierovics A, Yankelevich W-JC, Cowley SC. MAIT cells are critical for optimal mucosal immune responses during in vivo pulmonary bacterial infection. Proc Natl Acad Sci USA. 2013;110(33):E3119–E28.

317. Rouxel O, Beaudoin L, Nel I, Tard C, Cagninacci L, Kiaf B, et al. Cytotoxic and regulatory roles of mucosal-associated invariant T cells in type 1 diabetes. Nat Immunol. 2017;18(12):1321–31.

318. Godfrey DI, Uldrich AP, McCluskey J, Rossjohn J, Moody DB. The burgeoning family of unconventional T cells. Nat Immunol. 2015;16(11):1114.

319. Salio M, Silk JD, Yvonne Jones E, Cerundolo V. Biology of CD1- and MR1-restricted T cells. Annu Rev Immunol. 2014;32:323–66.

320. Ussher JE, Willberg CB, Klenerman P. MAIT cells and viruses. Immunol Cell Biol. 2018;96(6):630–41.

321. Peterfalvi A, Gomori E, Magyarlaki T, Pal J, Banati M, Javorhazy A, et al. Invariant Vα7. 2-Jα33 TCR is expressed in human kidney and brain tumors indicating infiltration by mucosal-associated invariant T (MAIT) cells. Int Immunol. 2008;20(12): 1517–25.

322. Won EJ, Ju JK, Cho Y-N, Jin H-M, Park K-J, Kim T-J, et al. Clinical relevance of circulating mucosal-associated invariant T cell levels and their anti-cancer activity in patients with mucosal-associated cancer. Oncotarget. 2016;7(46):76274.

323. Zheng C, Zheng L, Yoo J-K, Guo H, Zhang Y, Guo X, et al. Landscape of infiltrating T cells in liver cancer revealed by single-cell sequencing. Cell. 2017;169(7):1342–56. e16

324. Gherardin NA, Loh L, Admojo L, Davenport AJ, Richardson K, Rogers A, et al. Enumeration, functional responses and cytotoxic capacity of MAIT cells in newly diagnosed and relapsed multiple myeloma. Sci Rep. 2018;8(1):1–14.

325. Nielsen MM, Witherden DA, Havran WL. γδ T cells in homeostasis and host defence of epithelial barrier tissues. Nat Rev Immunol. 2017;17(12):733–45.

326. Gentles AJ, Newman AM, Liu CL, Bratman SV, Feng W, Kim D, et al. The prognostic landscape of genes and infiltrating immune cells across human cancers. Nat Med. 2015;21(8):938–45.

327. Girardi M, Oppenheim DE, Steele CR, Lewis JM, Glusac E, Filler R, et al. Regulation of cutaneous malignancy by γδ T cells. Science. 2001;294(5542):605–9.

328. Liu Z, Eltoum I-EA, Guo B, Beck BH, Cloud GA, Lopez RD. Protective immunosurveillance and therapeutic antitumor activity of γδ T cells demonstrated in a mouse model of prostate cancer. J Immunol. 2008;180(9):6044–53.

329. Bouet-Toussaint F, Cabillic F, Toutirais O, Le Gallo M, de la Pintière CT, Daniel P, et al. Vγ9Vδ2 T cell-mediated recognition of human solid tumors. Potential for immunotherapy of hepatocellular and colorectal carcinomas. Cancer Immunol Immunother. 2008;57(4):531–9.

330. Kunzmann V, Bauer E, Feurle J, Weissinger F, Tony HP, Wilhelm M. Stimulation of γδ T cells by aminobisphosphonates and induction of antiplasma cell activity in multiple myeloma. Blood. 2000;96(2):384–92.

331. Lanca T, Correia DV, Moita CF, Raquel H, Neves-Costa A, Ferreira C, et al. The MHC class Ib protein ULBP1 is a nonredundant determinant of leukemia/lymphoma susceptibility to γδ T-cell cytotoxicity. Blood. 2010;115(12):2407–11.

332. Wu R, Forget M-A, Chacon J, Bernatchez C, Haymaker C, Chen JQ, et al. Adoptive T-cell therapy using autologous tumor-infiltrating lymphocytes for metastatic melanoma: current status and future outlook. Cancer J (Sudbury, Mass). 2012;18(2):160.

333. Godder K, Henslee-Downey P, Mehta J, Park B, Chiang K, Abhyankar S, et al. Long term disease-free survival in acute leukemia patients recovering with increased γδ T cells after partially mismatched related donor bone marrow transplantation. Bone Marrow Transplant. 2007;39(12):751–7.

334. Lamb L Jr, Henslee-Downey P, Parrish R, Godder K, Thompson J, Lee C, et al. Increased frequency of TCR gamma delta+ T cells in disease-free survivors following T cell-depleted, partially mismatched, related donor bone marrow transplantation for leukemia. J Hematother. 1996;5(5):503–9.

335. Rong L, Li K, Li R, Liu H-M, Sun R, Liu X-Y. Analysis of tumor-infiltrating gamma delta T cells in rectal cancer. World J Gastroenterol. 2016;22(13):3573.

336. Patil RS, Shah SU, Shrikhande SV, Goel M, Dikshit RP, Chiplunkar SV. IL17 producing γδT cells induce angiogenesis and are associated with poor survival in gallbladder cancer patients. Int J Cancer. 2016;139(4):869–81.

337. Ma C, Zhang Q, Ye J, Wang F, Zhang Y, Wevers E, et al. Tumor-infiltrating γδ T lymphocytes predict clinical outcome in human breast cancer. J Immunol. 2012;189(10):5029–36.

338. Peng G, Wang HY, Peng W, Kiniwa Y, Seo KH, Wang R-F. Tumor-infiltrating γδ T cells suppress T and dendritic cell function via mechanisms controlled by a unique toll-like receptor signaling pathway. Immunity. 2007;27(2):334–48.

339. Galon J, Lanzi A. Immunoscore and its introduction in clinical practice. Q J Nucl Med Mol Imaging. 2020;64(2):152–61.

340. Chen DS, Mellman I. Oncology meets immunology: the cancer-immunity cycle. Immunity. 2013;39(1):1–10.

341. Hossain MA, Liu G, Dai B, Si Y, Yang Q, Wazir J, et al. Reinvigorating exhausted CD8+ cytotoxic T lymphocytes in the tumor microenvironment and current strategies in cancer immunotherapy. Med Res Rev. 2021;41(1):156–201.

342. Bindea G, Mlecnik B, Tosolini M, Kirilovsky A, Waldner M, Obenauf Anna C, et al. Spatiotemporal dynamics of intratumoral immune cells reveal the immune landscape in human cancer. Immunity. 2013;39(4):782–95.

343. Xu YF, Lu Y, Cheng H, Shi S, Xu J, Long J, et al. Abnormal distribution of peripheral lymphocyte subsets induced by PDAC modulates overall survival. Pancreatology. 2014;14(4):295–301.

344. Jochems C, Schlom J. Tumor-infiltrating immune cells and prognosis: the potential link between conventional cancer therapy and immunity. Exp Biol Med. 2011;236(5):567–79.

345. Zanker DJ, Owen KL, Baschuk N, Spurling AJ, Parker BS. Loss of type I IFN responsiveness impairs natural killer cell antitumor activity in breast cancer. Cancer Immunol Immunother. 2021;70(8):2125–38.

346. Zhou Q, Yan X, Liu W, Yin W, Xu H, Cheng D, et al. Three immune-associated subtypes of diffuse glioma differ in immune infiltration, immune checkpoint molecules, and prognosis. Front Oncol. 2020;10:586019.

347. Sawant DV, Yano H, Chikina M, Zhang Q, Liao M, Liu C, et al. Adaptive plasticity of IL-10(+) and IL-35(+) T(reg) cells cooperatively promotes tumor T cell exhaustion. Nat Immunol. 2019;20(6):724–35.

348. O'Callaghan DS, Rexhepaj E, Gately K, Coate L, Delaney D, O'Donnell DM, et al. Tumour islet Foxp3+ T-cell infiltration predicts poor outcome in nonsmall cell lung cancer. Eur Respir J. 2015;46(6):1762–72.

349. Rizzo A, Di Giovangiulio M, Stolfi C, Franzè E, Fehling HJ, Carsetti R, et al. RORγt-expressing tregs drive the growth of colitis-associated colorectal cancer by controlling IL6 in dendritic cells. Cancer Immunol Res. 2018;6(9):1082–92.

350. Groux H, O'Garra A, Bigler M, Rouleau M, Antonenko S, De Vries JE, et al. A CD4+ T-cell subset inhibits antigen-specific T-cell responses and prevents colitis. Nature. 1997;389(6652):737–42.

351. Chen Y, Kuchroo VK, Inobe J-i, Hafler DA, Weiner HL. Regulatory T cell clones induced by oral tolerance: suppression of autoimmune encephalomyelitis. Science. 1994;265(5176):1237–40.

352. Kiniwa Y, Miyahara Y, Wang HY, Peng W, Peng G, Wheeler TM, et al. CD8+ Foxp3+ regulatory T cells mediate immunosuppression in prostate cancer. Clin Cancer Res. 2007;13(23):6947–58.

Drivers of EMT and Immune Evasion

Rolf A. Brekken and Katarzyna Wnuk-Lipinska

11

Abstract

The heterogeneity of tumor cells and the complexity of the surrounding microenvironment make the process of predicting patient outcomes and selection of the most suitable treatment regimen very difficult. Many biomarkers have been evaluated for prognostic value with success more consistently seen with targeted therapy. The advent of immune therapy as a frontline treatment for some cancers has moved immune phenotyping into the forefront of biomarker and predictive marker research. Here, we review some of the regulatory mechanisms of the host immune response and epithelial plasticity and highlight their potential as biomarkers of the hallmark of immune evasion.

Take-Home Lessons
- TAM receptors downregulate inflammatory pathways in sentinel cells and contribute to tumor immune suppression.
- PrdSer, an immune suppressive lipid, is exposed in the tumor microenvironment and contributes to the evasion of immune surveillance.
- Epithelial-to-mesenchymal transition (EMT) is associated with reduced immune activation in tumors and tumor progression.
- VEGF-induced angiogenesis is a driver of a vascular immune barrier in tumors and VEGF signaling in myeloid cells can induce an immune suppressive phenotype.

R. A. Brekken (✉)
UT Southwestern Medical Center, Dallas, TX, USA
e-mail: rolf.brekken@utsouthwestern.edu

K. Wnuk-Lipinska
Novartis Pharma, Basel, Switzerland
e-mail: katarzyna.wnuk-lipinska@novartis.com

Introduction

Tumors are a complex network of transformed cells, immune cells, stromal cells, vascular and lymphatic vessels, and extracellular matrix (ECM). Tumor progression is dependent on the interaction between tumor cells and the normal, non-cancerous cells and ECM of the surrounding microenvironment. The immune component of the tumor microenvironment is of particular interest as it controls or promotes tumor progression, underscored by the fact that tumor-associated inflammation and immune evasion have been recognized as hallmarks of cancer [1]. Indeed, every type of immune cell can be found within a tumor, including dendritic cells (DCs), macrophages, myeloid-derived suppressor cells (MDSCs), natural killer (NK) cells, lymphocytes, mast cells, and B cells.

It is clear that location, density, and the level of interaction between different immune cell populations impact clinical outcomes [2]. For instance, high infiltration of tumors by CD3$^+$CD8$^+$ cytotoxic T cells (CTLs) and T helper 1 cells (T$_H$1) is generally associated with good clinical outcome [2]. In contrast, elevated levels of CD4$^+$ regulatory T cells (T$_{reg}$) in tumors are typically linked with poor prognosis [3, 4]. It is not just the presence of immune cells but also the activity of those cells that affects tumor progression. For example, in many tumors, NK cells are present at a high level but are anergic, as evidenced by the downregulation of such markers as NKp30, NKp80, DNAX, or CD16 in lung, cervical and ovarian carcinomas [5, 6]. This anergic state is maintained by tumor-derived suppressive factors, such as TGFβ, IDO, or PGE2, which downregulate NK cell effector functions and allow tumors to escape from NK-mediated recognition [2]. In addition, B cells have been observed to enhance the progression of spontaneous murine tumors due to the release of anti-inflammatory IL-10, which stimulates polarization of macrophages into a pro-tumorigenic phenotype [7, 8] and enhances immune suppression. However, B cells are not always associated with poor prognosis, as in some subtypes of breast and ovarian carcinomas the presence of B cells was found to be beneficial, because they can

L. A. Akslen, R. S. Watnick (eds.), *Biomarkers of the Tumor Microenvironment*, https://doi.org/10.1007/978-3-030-98950-7_11

function as antigen-presenting cells and participate in the induction of memory T cells [9].

The cytokine/chemokine pathways that control immune cell infiltration and activity in tumors are complex, yet there is a strong impetus to determine if quantification of the factors that drive these pathways have predictive value for the outcome of therapy. Here we discuss some of those mechanisms. In particular, we focus on molecules that can drive the immunosuppressive state in the tumor microenvironment and can potentially serve as biomarkers for poor prognosis. These markers include the TAM (Tyro3, Axl, Mer) family of receptors, externalized phosphatidylserine (PtdSer), and vascular endothelial growth factor (VEGF). We will also highlight the link between epithelial plasticity (e.g., EMT programs) and immune escape in tumors.

TAM Receptors in Inflammation

The TAM receptor family of tyrosine kinases (RTKs) is comprised of Tyro3, Axl, and Mer. TAM receptors are involved in the clearance of apoptotic cells in healthy adult tissues [10], the regulation of the innate immune response [11, 12], viral infection [13], as well as cancer progression and metastatic dissemination [14–16]. TAM receptors are particularly important for the processes driven by sentinel cells, (DCs and macrophages), such as innate inflammatory responses and the clearance of apoptotic cells through efferocytosis [12]. TAM receptor signaling is pivotal in the inflammatory cycle and constitutes an "off switch" for dynamic innate immunity. This regulation prevents prolonged inflammation from occurring and restores homeostasis to adult tissues [12].

An innate immune response in sentinel cells often initiates with the activation of toll-like receptors (TLRs) by danger-associated molecular patterns (DAMPs) or pathogen-associated molecular patterns (PAMPs) resulting in the secretion of pro-inflammatory cytokines, including tumor necrosis factor-α (TNFα), interleukin-6 (IL-6), IL-12 and type I interferons (IFNs) [17], which form a positive feed-forward loop with their receptors, resulting in amplification of the pro-inflammatory cascade [18] (Fig. 11.1a). Constitutive secretion of TNF-α, and other pro-inflammatory molecules, can lead to chronic inflammation and subsequent endotoxic shock [19]. Hence, the levels of these cytokines are tightly controlled. Simultaneous with TLR activation, as proposed by Rothlin et al., [12], IFN α/β receptor (IFNAR) and STAT1 form a complex with ligand-activated TAM receptors. This results in activation of STAT1, which translocates to the nucleus and triggers expression of the cytoplasmic suppressors of cytokine signaling 1 and 3 (SOCS1 and SOCS3). SOCS1 mediates polyubiquitylation and subsequent degradation of the TLR connecting molecule myelin and lymphocyte protein MAL, preventing MAL-dependent p65 phosphorylation and transactivation of NF-κB leading to inhibition of inflammatory responses [20]

(Fig. 11.1b). SOCS3 prevents ubiquitination of TLR downstream effector TNF receptor-associated factor 6 (TRAF6), thereby inhibiting the TLR signal transduction pathway [21] (Fig. 11.1c). As described above TAM-regulated signal transduction pathway is pivotal for the suppression of inflammatory responses [11, 12, 22].

Furthermore, SOCS1 and SOCS3 can inhibit JAK/STAT1 signaling and subsequently impair the synthesis of pro-inflammatory cytokines, such as IL-1, IL-6, IL-12, CCL9, CCL10, and TNFα [23]. Additionally, activation of Axl and/or Mer stimulates Twist activation, which transcriptionally suppresses TNFα expression [24, 25]. Thus, as a consequence of the interaction with SOCS proteins, TAM receptors govern repression of the pro-inflammatory cascade by blocking TLR signaling and hindering cytokine-receptor feed-forward signaling loops.

TAM signaling is also essential for efferocytosis, the phagocytic clearance of apoptotic cells [26]. Efferocytosis initiates an immunosuppressive signal in phagocytic cells, which is a critical defense against auto-immunity and is required for the maintenance of tissue homeostasis [27]. However, tumors are able to co-opt this biologic process to evade immune surveillance [28].

As described above, TAM signaling profoundly influences the function of sentinel cells. Specifically, TAM activation has an inhibitory effect on the innate immune response, and downregulation of TAM signaling promotes autoimmunity. TAM receptors, despite their similarity, are likely to perform distinct functions. Axl and Mer were identified as central in the control of the innate immune system, yet they exhibit divergent expression and activity depending on the condition of surrounding tissue. While both are immunosuppressive phagocytic receptors, Mer appears to be a principal RTK in the tolerogenic environment, whereas Axl operates during inflammation [29]. Furthermore, Axl and Mer are differentially dependent on their ligands. AXL is activated by dimerization through binding to Gas6 in a 2:2 stoichiometry [30]. Gas6 is a ligand for each TAM receptor, whereas Tyro3 and Mer are also activated by Protein S [31]. Gas6 is required for activation of Axl, whereas Axl maintains Gas6 expression in vivo [29]. This co-dependence and continuous presence of Gas6-Axl complex suggests that there may be another trigger of full Axl activation. Indeed, it was shown that basal Gas6-Axl activity was greatly enhanced upon exposure to apoptotic cells with membranes rich in externalized PtdSer and PtdSer has been shown to be a critical stimulus driving Axl activation [29]. Gas6 binds to PtdSer via a gamma carboxyglutamic acid-rich (GLA) domain [32]. The immunoglobulin-like (Ig) domains of Axl function as a docking site for the laminin G-like (LG) domains of Gas6, which drives Axl dimerization [30]. PtdSer bound to the GLA domain of Gas6 appears to stabilize Axl dimerization and induce optimal Axl signaling [33]. Furthermore, Axl can be activated through ligand-independent dimerization with other TAM receptors or members of other RTK families, such as ErBb [34, 35]. In contrast, Mer has only one docking site for Gas6 and exhibits a much lower affinity for its ligands.

TAM signaling is also important for the maturation and differentiation of NK cells [36]. NK cells are an essential component of the innate immune system that recognizes infected or malignant cells in the absence of "education" or priming [37]. In the presence of Gas6 or Protein S, TAM receptors expressed by immature NK cells are activated. TAM signaling stimulates the acquisition of inhibitory, e.g., members of Ly49 and CD94 families, or activating receptors (CD69) required for target-cell recognition [38, 39]. Thus,

TAM-deficient NK cells lack inhibitory and activating receptors and fail to secrete certain cytokines, such as macrophage-inducing IFNγ even though they produce normal levels of perforins and granzymes [36]. The lack of TAM signaling results in NK cells that have a tenfold lower activity against target cells [36].

Signaling of principal TAM receptors, Axl and Mer, is particularly important in sentinel cells of the immune system [12]. Signaling of either receptor drives an intrinsic negative feedback for immune activation. Importantly, activation of Axl and Mer is specific for different environments, where Axl is specialized to function in inflammatory, and Mer in

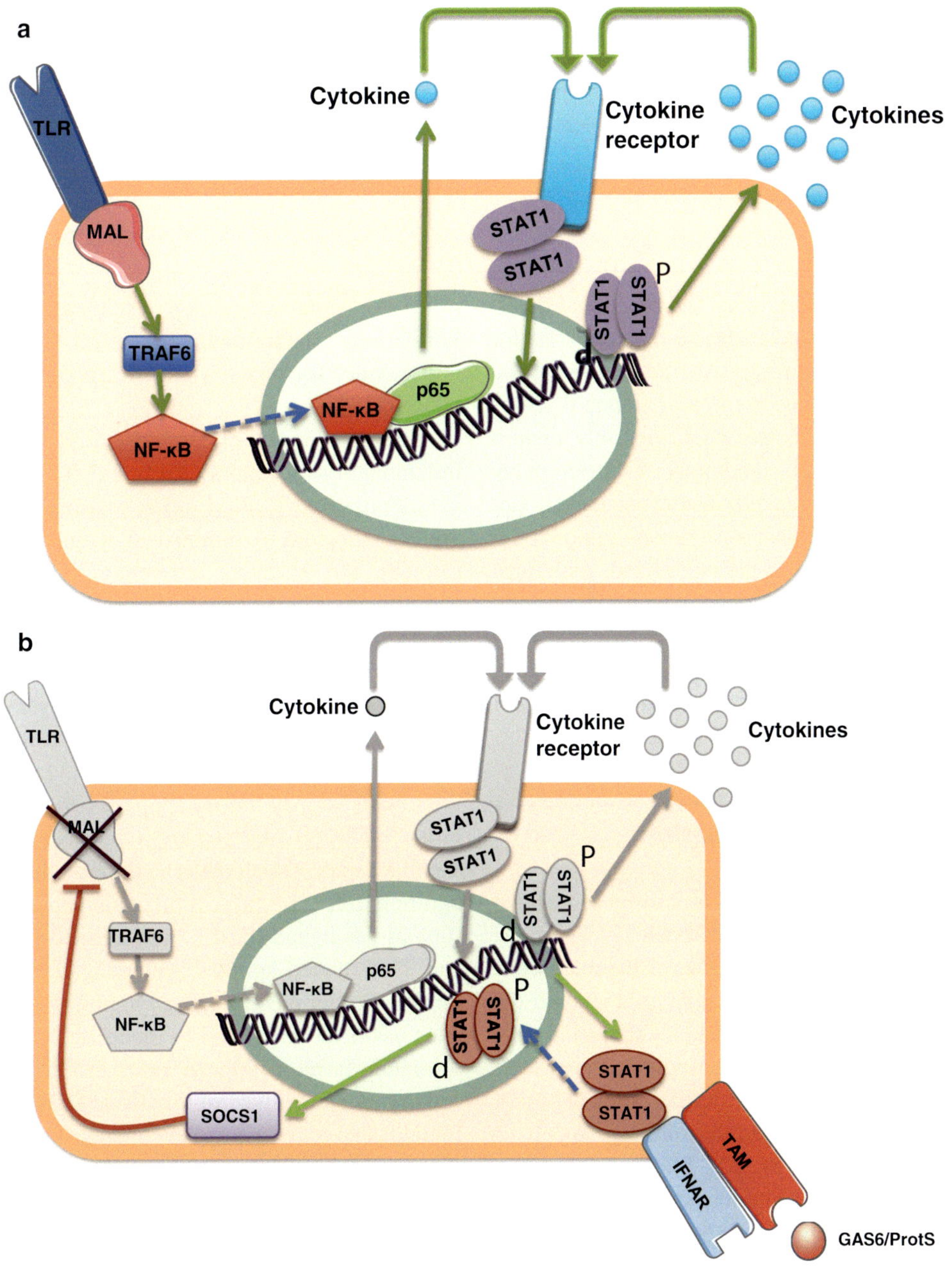

Fig. 11.1 TAM-regulated suppression of inflammatory response in sentinel cells of the innate immune system. Activation of TLR results in secretion of pro-inflammatory cytokines, which are in positive feed-forward loop with their receptors (**a**) TAM mediated activation of SOCS1 (**b**) and SOCS3 (**c**) inhibits signaling of MAL and TRAF6, subsequently resulting in immunosuppressive environment

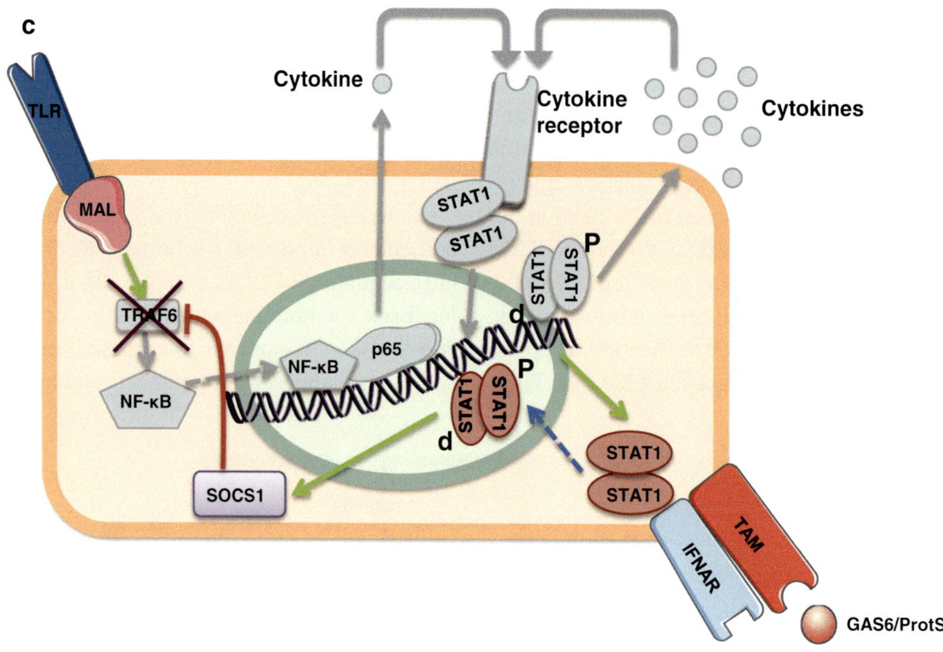

Fig. 11.1 (continued)

tolerogenic settings [29]. Accordingly, the functional divergence of these receptors can have adverse repercussions for the development of new therapies. TAM activation can be beneficial for patients suffering from autoimmune diseases [40]. Long-term inhibition of Mer could possibly disturb homeostasis of healthy tissues and may result in many adverse side effects. An example of potential expected toxicity of Mer inhibition is loss of photoreceptor cells upon long-term Mer inhibition [41, 42]. On the other hand, prolonged Axl inhibition may be less harmful and potentially advantageous for cancer patients. Hence, antibody-based [43] or highly selective targeted treatments [44] are promising approaches to treating human disease through modulation of TAM signaling [45–47].

Phosphatidylserine in Inflammation

PtdSer is an anionic phospholipid that is actively segregated to the inner leaflet of the plasma membrane. In apoptotic cells, PtdSer is flipped to the outer leaflet of the membrane where it functions as a signal for macrophages to engulf the cell [48]. PtdSer is externalized on vascular endothelial cells in tumors [49] and is constitutively present in the outer leaflet of some tumor cells [50]. PtdSer externalization on tumor cells is significantly increased when they undergo apoptosis upon chemo- or radiotherapy [51, 52]. PtdSer is an evolutionarily conserved driver of immunosuppression in the tumor microenvironment [53], a topic that has recently been reviewed [54]. As mentioned above, PtdSer is required for full activation of TAM receptors [29, 33], whose signaling has an inhibitory effect on the innate immune response [12]. Specifically, low basal activity of Axl-Gas6 complex is sig-

nificantly reinforced upon bridging with PtdSer [29]. Furthermore, the formation of the Axl-Gas6-PtdSer complex is necessary for phagocytosis of apoptotic cells by macrophages [10].

PtdSer-dependent efferocytosis triggers secretion of anti-inflammatory mediators TGFβ and IL-10 by macrophages [55]. Furthermore, tumor microenvironments rich in PtdSer are characterized by diminished adaptive immune response [56–58]. For instance, intratumoral dendritic cells, upon engulfment of PtdSer-opsonized cells, maintain an immature phenotype, resulting in failed antigen presentation [59]. Also, PtdSer has been linked to the suppression of cytotoxic T-cell responses [60]. PtdSer-rich microvesicles, released by lymphocytes upon TCR activation, also transmit cell-death signals to activated T cells [61, 62]. Lymphocyte-derived microvesicles may induce apoptosis and nonreversible inhibition of T-cell function by suppression of CD3-ζ chain T-cell receptor, which plays an important role in antigen recognition [62] or by expression of apoptosis-inducing ligands, such as Fas ligand (FasL), programmed-death ligand (PDL) and TNF-related apoptosis-inducing ligand (TRAIL) [63]. Further, PtdSer present on the lymphocyte-derived microvesicles has been postulated to modulate T-cell activation in a reversible fashion [60]. As such, PtdSer seems to enhance activity of diacylglycerol kinase-α (DGK-α) [60], which is found in excessive amounts in anergic T cells [64]. Although primarily reversible, suppression of T-cell function through contact with PtdSer may become non-reversible, as a consequence of chronic exposure to PtdSer-rich membranes, resulting in T-cell exhaustion [60, 65].

PtdSer also activates a second class of receptors, T-cell immunoglobulin and mucin receptors (TIMs) [66]. There are three subtypes of TIM receptors (TIM-1, TIM-3, and TIM-

4). All TIM family members have been shown to recognize PtdSer through a conserved N-terminal IgV extracellular domain [67–69]; however, their expression varies between different immune cells [66]. TIM-1 is highly expressed on T-helper 2 (T_H2) cells and functions as a co-stimulatory receptor important for T-cell activation [66]. TIM-3 is preferentially expressed on T_C1 (a subset of CD8+ lymphocytes producing IFNγ) and T_H1 cells and mediates apoptosis of those cells [66]. TIM-3 expressed by dendritic cells and macrophages enhances phagocytosis of apoptotic cells and antigen presentation [66]. TIM-4 is important for the maintenance of a tolerogenic state and phagocytosis of apoptotic cells and is solely expressed by antigen-presenting cells [66, 69].

TIM-3 is known to be immunosuppressive when activated and is thought to be a biomarker for T-cell exhaustion [70]. Hence, its function in cancer has been studied extensively. Recent studies on TIM-3 signaling revealed that TIM-3 abrogates Lck function and prevents TCR signal transduction [71]. Lck-mediated phosphorylation can be however rescued by HLA-B-associated transcript 3 (Bat3), which was postulated to positively regulate the catalytic activity of Lck and as result prevent induction of T-cell exhaustion [72]. Consequently, the shortage of Bat3 expression in T cells causes the accumulation of inactive Lck [72], which reduces the efficacy of the T-cell receptor (TCR) complex.

In summary, PtdSer, by impinging upon multiple innate and adaptive pathways, functions as a negative regulator of immune responses in the tumor microenvironment. It has been shown that PtdSer can serve as a versatile biomarker of tumor cells [73] and tumor vasculature [49], as well as a novel target for therapeutic approaches [53].

Epithelial-Mesenchymal Transition

Epithelial-mesenchymal transition (EMT) is a biological process in which epithelial cells adopt a mesenchymal phenotype [74]. EMT endows epithelial cells, that normally are polarized and interact with a basement membrane, with motile and invasive properties and increased production of extracellular matrix components (ECM) [74].

EMT is critical for morphogenesis in the developing embryo [75]. In adult tissue, EMT is restricted and occurs primarily during wound healing or organ regeneration and fibrosis [76, 77]. EMT has been linked to cancer progression [78] where it is associated with the acquisition of a metastatic phenotype, chemoresistance, and immune suppression in epithelial tumors [79–83].

Physiologically, regulatory networks exist that function to support the homeostasis of every cell; however, when these networks are disturbed, dedifferentiation may be triggered [84]. It was proposed that during primary tumor formation tumor cells become receptive to EMT inducers whose source is often the tumor-associated stroma [74, 80]. Thus, changing microenvironmental conditions regulate the epithelial-mesenchymal plasticity of tumor cells. There are several major players involved in EMT induction, such as HGF, EGF, PDGF, and TGF-β [85–88]. These in turn act on a range of transcription factors that directly or indirectly orchestrate EMT machinery [79]. EMT and its reverse process mesenchymal to epithelial transition (MET) are regulated by at least four different regulatory networks: transcriptional control, non-coding RNA regulation, differential splicing, and post-translational control, where EMT-inducing transcription factors are central in this network, as they are interconnected with remaining regulatory layers [84, 89–91].

To undergo EMT, an epithelial cell must be in a permissive state, allowing it to circumvent normalizing cues from the microenvironment [84, 90]. In the case of tumors, inflammation and hypoxia are common environmental factors that disturb the equilibrium between these regulatory networks [78] and promote cellular transition [90]. Response to oxygen levels is mainly regulated by hypoxia-inducible factor 1α (HIF1α), expression of which correlates with metastasis) in many cancers [92–94]. HIF1α upregulates the expression of zinc transcript protein 1 (SNAI1), which in turn functions as negative regulator of transcription of the cell-cell adhesion molecule E-cadherin [95]. Due to the disturbed formation of adherens junctions within the epithelium, cells become motile and able to avoid anoikis [96–98].

There are several other transcription factors involved in EMT, such as zinc finger protein 2 (SNAI2), zinc finger E-box-binding homeobox 1 (ZEB1), zinc finger E-box-binding homeobox 2 (ZEB2) and Twist family BHLH transcription factor 1 (TWIST1) [99–101], that also repress the expression of several junctional proteins such as E-cadherin, claudins or desmosomes and promote EMT [96–98]. EMT-transcription factors also have exceptionally high potency in causing genome-wide changes in gene expression by their interaction with epigenetic modulators [102]. Among the epigenetic mechanisms, DNA methylation, histone modifications, and microRNA expression changes have been observed in cells undergoing EMT [103]. As an example, SNAI1 expression is associated with methylation of regulatory regions of *CDH1* [104], where methylation represses *CDH1* expression and promotes EMT [105, 106]. SNAI1 was also found to stimulate histone deacetylase activity, which in turn silences the *CDH1* promoter [107]. High SNAI1 expression also correlates with immunosuppression in melanoma, which is demonstrated by impaired DC recruitment and poor infiltration of cytotoxic T cells [108]. Further, the mesenchymal phenotype and high expression of SNAI1 in murine preclinical models are associated with higher expression of PD-L1 and lower of MHC-I. In these tumors, the presence of cytotoxic T cells diminishes, with simultaneous enrichment for immunosuppressive components, including M2 macrophages and T_{regs} cells [109].

Among microRNAs (miRNAs) that are implicated in EMT are members of the miR-200 and miR-34 families. These miRNAs are in a reciprocal feedback loop with ZEB1/ZEB2 [110, 111] and SNAI1 [112], respectively, and are known to be drivers of an epithelial phenotype [113]. Therefore, miR-200 and miR-34 family members are considered to be tumor suppressors [114]. Recent work by Chen et al. [115] suggests that the miR-200/ZEB1 axis regulates EMT and PD-L1 expression on tumor cells and it is therefore an indirect cause of immunosuppression. Hence, miR-200 and ZEB1 are in a negative feedback loop and while tied to EMT regulation, they mediate CD8+ T-cell impairment via increased PD-L1 expression, which promotes tumor growth and metastasis.

Overexpression of EMT-related transcription factors, such as SNAI1, SNAI2, ZEB1 and ZEB2, TWIST1 also leads to increased expression of Axl [14]. Moreover, high levels of Axl expression support the maintenance of a mesenchymal phenotype by stimulating SNAI1, SNAI2, and TWIST expression [14, 44]. Bearing in mind that Axl is involved in sustaining mesenchymal traits, such as motility and invasiveness, the contribution of Axl in tumor initiation and metastasis takes on additional clarity [44, 116]. Elevated Axl expression is linked with unfavorable overall prognosis in breast cancer [14], non-small cell lung carcinoma [117], pancreatic cancer [118], glioblastoma multiforme [119], esophageal adenocarcinoma [120], acute myeloid leukemia [121], and ovarian cancer [122]. Significantly, abundant expression of Axl is predominantly related to metastatic dissemination and survival, rather than primary tumor growth [14, 44, 116, 123].

Many recent studies have revealed elevated expression of Axl in tumors resistant to chemotherapies [35, 85, 124–127]. More importantly, these studies suggest that chemoresistance is a repercussion of EMT [128], while inducing MET restores sensitivity. Axl expression is associated with an aggressive mesenchymal phenotype and with immunosuppression. Thus, inhibition of Axl signaling has the potential to reduce tumor invasion and immunosuppression. However, while high Axl levels have been correlated with poor clinical outcome, the predictive value of Axl expression for immune phenotype has not been yet evaluated.

Normal and neoplastic epithelial cells that undergo EMT have also been shown to acquire stem cell-like properties [129, 130]. Interestingly, EMT seems to serve as a universal mechanism for acquisition of stem-like traits and therefore epithelial cells within tumors appear to undergo the same program as normal antecedent cells [129, 131]. The mesenchymal phenotype is associated with increased motility, invasiveness, and resistance to apoptosis, all traits that predispose to metastatic dissemination [132, 133]. Furthermore, cancer stem cells (CSCs) are thought to have the ability to initiate tumors at distant sites upon MET [134] and form macro-metastases through self-renewal [131]. The invasive phenotype of these cancer stem cells is a reflection of their plasticity and ability to reversibly change phenotype across the epithelial-mesenchymal axis [135]. The increasing awareness of the importance of tumor cell plasticity in tumor progression resulted in drafting a Consensus Statement by "the EMT International Association" (TEMTIA). As such, the changes along an EMT axis should be referred to as Epithelial-Mesenchymal Plasticity (EMP) [136]. EMP has been closely associated with the acquisition of stem cell-like traits in tumors. The intermediate states between epithelial and mesenchymal phenotypes are common and seem to have the highest metastatic potential [137, 138]. Congruently, EMP warrants stemness and contributes to a multidrug resistance phenotype [134, 139–145]. As a result, CSCs are thought to be a major cause of treatment failure, and development of targeted therapeutics directed against them is an attractive concept [134]. However, while CSCs can give rise to a new tumor that includes non-stem-like tumor cells, the reverse is also true, implying that CSCs may be regenerated from non-cancer stem cells within a treated carcinoma [146]. Therefore, propitious therapy should include agents targeting CSC and normal cancer cells, eliminating CSCs and their descendants [147].

Immunoregulation

EMT, genotypic and phenotypic heterogeneity, and dynamic epigenetic interactions have been linked to tumor relapse and resistance to systemic therapy [148]. Also, reciprocal interactions between tumor cells and components of the surrounding microenvironment, such as soluble inflammatory mediators, can confer resistance to therapy [149]. Additionally, therapy-induced injury, which occurs in response to systemic treatment disrupting established tumor structure, causes secretion of pro-inflammatory cytokines, which can mediate tumor cell plasticity. For instance, chemotherapy, in parallel to killing cancer cells, stimulates macrophages to produce TNF-α and IL-6. TNF-α in turn promotes chemoresistance by activating its downstream effector nuclear factor-κB (NF-κB) and then CXCL1 and CXCL2 [150]. Interestingly, TNF-α also has a protective effect toward BRAF-mutant melanoma cells, in which case TNF-α and NF-κB signaling enable cancer cells to bypass apoptosis induced by BRAF inhibitors [151]. Furthermore, TNF-α and IL-6 were found to elicit transition of tumor cells to a mesenchymal phenotype by modulating the expression of EMT-transcription factors, such as Twist, Snail, or Slug [152–156]. Accordingly, plasma TNF-α was proposed to be suitable as a biomarker, when combined with TNM classification of malignant tumors, for predicting survival of head and neck squamous cell carcinoma and may be useful for designing treatment strategies [157].

T cells also constitute an important part of the reciprocal interactions between immune and tumor cells. Melanoma-specific cytotoxic T leukocytes (CTLs) secrete IFNγ, which in turn induces expression of PD-L1 by tumor cells. PD-L1 inhibits the function of 0.effector T cells by binding to its receptor PD1 [158, 159]. It is, however, possible to block the formation of the PD1:PD-L1 axis by treatment with immune checkpoint inhibitors and thereby restore a pro-inflammatory environment with tumor-specific CTLs [158, 160]. The recent advances in the field of immuno-oncology have brought to light T-cell immunoreceptor with immunoglobulin and ITIM domain (TIGIT) as a novel immune checkpoint receptor target [161]. TIGIT is upregulated by various immune cells, including T cells, NK cells, and T_{regs} cells [162]. TIGIT interacts with CD155 expressed on antigen-presenting cells or tumor cells to downregulate T cell and natural killer (NK) cell functions [163]. Particularly dual PD-1/TIGIT blockade seems to be a rational therapeutic approach, as it potently increases tumor antigen-specific CD8+ T-cell expansion in vitro and promotes tumor rejection in murine tumor models [162]. The possibility of reactivation of CTLs in the tumor microenvironment is one of the indications of the functional plasticity of the tumor immune component.

Additionally, alterations in metabolic pathways contribute to the interplay between tumor and immune cells. For instance, hypoxia-induced tumor subclones with pronounced mesenchymal phenotypes exhibited an increased propensity to resist cytotoxic T lymphocytes (CTL) and natural killer (NK) cell-mediated lysis. This resistance was driven by a defective immune synapse signaling [164]. Hypoxia was also proposed to stimulate expression of CCL28, followed by recruitment of regulatory T cells (T_{reg}) stimulating tumor tolerance [165]. Hypoxia-induced release of VEGF by tumor cells also contributes to the recruitment of T_{reg} cells [166], indicating that immune tolerance and angiogenesis are closely related mechanisms mediating immune evasion [167].

VEGF and Inflammation

To maintain the dynamic interactions between tumor and immune cells there is an extensive vascular network. The complex organization of blood vessels within the tumor may allow mesenchymal tumor cells to escape and encourage metastatic spread. On the other hand, dense vasculature favors the recruitment of immune cells to the tumor environment. VEGF is a key inducer of tumor neovascularization and is abundantly produced by tumor cells [168]. VEGF release is regulated by VEGF receptor 2 (VEGFR2)-dependent activation of mTOR. The VEGF-mTOR autocrine feed-forward loop intensifies the primary angiogenic signal and leads to the formation of new blood vessels in cancer [169], which is essential for tumor growth, further expansion and metastatic dissemination [1, 170]. Moreover, it was suggested that CXCL1/CXCR2 stimulates VEGF release through activation of its downstream JAK/STAT3 signaling cascade [171]. The CXCL1/CXCR2 axis amplifies VEGF signaling, and possibly rescues the proangiogenic phenotype upon VEGF inhibition. It was also revealed that activation of Src homology 2 domain-containing protein tyrosine phosphatase 2 (SHP-2) by Axl inhibits vascular endothelial growth factor receptor 2 (VEGFR2) during morphogenesis of endothelial cells [172]. Interestingly VEGFR2 is expressed not only on the surface of endothelial cells but also on macrophages, neutrophils, myeloid-derived suppressor cells (MDSCs), DCs, and T cells [173–177]. Hence, it is not surprising that anti-angiogenic therapy affects immune function in the tumor microenvironment. Further, anti-VEGF therapy can reduce macrophage and MDSCs infiltration and increase mature DCs in the tumor suggesting that anti-VEGF therapy can function to restore a pro-inflammatory tumor microenvironment [178–180].

Concluding Remarks/Summary

Tumors are a complex network of dependencies between tumor cells, immune cells, and the microenvironment. The immune contexture varies between tumors and may be associated with different overall prognoses, depending on the histological and molecular type of the tumor, stage and organ-specific microenvironment. There are different approaches to modulating immune response. Certain approaches, for instance immune checkpoint blockade or adaptive cell transfer, can result in long-term durable efficacy. However, multiple evolutionarily conserved programs active in the tumor microenvironment promote immune suppression. For example, the processes of efferocytosis and EMT function to promote local immune suppression, and these programs are co-opted by the tumor to evade immune surveillance. These pathways exploit signaling modules including those driven by the TAM receptors, PtdSer, and EMT inducing growth factors and as result these molecules or pathways are attractive as targets for prognostic exploration.

References

1. Hanahan D, Weinberg RA. Hallmarks of cancer: the next generation. Cell. 2011;144(5):646–74.
2. Fridman WH, Pages F, Sautes-Fridman C, Galon J. The immune contexture in human tumours: impact on clinical outcome. Nat Rev Cancer. 2012;12(4):298–306.
3. Jacobs JF, Idema AJ, Bol KF, Grotenhuis JA, de Vries IJ, Wesseling P, et al. Prognostic significance and mechanism of Treg infiltration in human brain tumors. J Neuroimmunol. 2010;225(1–2):195–9.
4. Fu J, Xu D, Liu Z, Shi M, Zhao P, Fu B, et al. Increased regulatory T cells correlate with CD8 T-cell impairment and poor survival in hepatocellular carcinoma patients. Gastroenterology. 2007;132(7):2328–39.
5. Katou F, Ohtani H, Watanabe Y, Nakayama T, Yoshie O, Hashimoto K. Differing phenotypes between intraepithelial and stromal lymphocytes in early-stage tongue cancer. Cancer Res. 2007;67(23):11195–201.

6. Schleypen JS, Von Geldern M, Weiss EH, Kotzias N, Rohrmann K, Schendel DJ, et al. Renal cell carcinoma-infiltrating natural killer cells express differential repertoires of activating and inhibitory receptors and are inhibited by specific HLA class I allotypes. Int J Cancer. 2003;106(6):905–12.

7. Wong SC, Puaux AL, Chittezhath M, Shalova I, Kajiji TS, Wang X, et al. Macrophage polarization to a unique phenotype driven by B cells. Eur J Immunol. 2010;40(8):2296–307.

8. Mantovani A. B cells and macrophages in cancer: yin and yang. Nat Med. 2011;17(3):285–6.

9. Iglesia MD, Vincent BG, Parker JS, Hoadley KA, Carey LA, Perou CM, et al. Prognostic B-cell signatures using mRNA-seq in patients with subtype-specific breast and ovarian cancer. Clin Cancer Res. 2014;20(14):3818–29.

10. Lemke G, Burstyn-Cohen T. TAM receptors and the clearance of apoptotic cells. Ann N Y Acad Sci. 2010;1209:23–9.

11. Lemke G, Rothlin CV. Immunobiology of the TAM receptors. Nat Rev Immunol. 2008;8(5):327–36.

12. Rothlin CV, Ghosh S, Zuniga EI, Oldstone MB, Lemke G. TAM receptors are pleiotropic inhibitors of the innate immune response. Cell. 2007;131(6):1124–36.

13. Bhattacharyya S, Zagorska A, Lew ED, Shrestha B, Rothlin CV, Naughton J, et al. Enveloped viruses disable innate immune responses in dendritic cells by direct activation of TAM receptors. Cell Host Microbe. 2013;14(2):136–47.

14. Gjerdrum C, Tiron C, Hoiby T, Stefansson I, Haugen H, Sandal T, et al. Axl is an essential epithelial-to-mesenchymal transition-induced regulator of breast cancer metastasis and patient survival. Proc Natl Acad Sci U S A. 2010;107(3):1124–9.

15. Schlegel J, Sambade MJ, Sather S, Moschos SJ, Tan AC, Winges A, et al. MERTK receptor tyrosine kinase is a therapeutic target in melanoma. J Clin Invest. 2013;123(5):2257–67.

16. Meyer AS, Miller MA, Gertler FB, Lauffenburger DA. The receptor AXL diversifies EGFR signaling and limits the response to EGFR-targeted inhibitors in triple-negative breast cancer cells. Sci Signal. 2013;6(287):ra66.

17. Beutler B, Jiang Z, Georgel P, Crozat K, Croker B, Rutschmann S, et al. Genetic analysis of host resistance: Toll-like receptor signaling and immunity at large. Annu Rev Immunol. 2006;24:353–89.

18. Honda K, Takaoka A, Taniguchi T. Type I interferon [corrected] gene induction by the interferon regulatory factor family of transcription factors. Immunity. 2006;25(3):349–60.

19. Camenisch TD, Koller BH, Earp HS, Matsushima GK. A novel receptor tyrosine kinase, Mer, inhibits TNF-alpha production and lipopolysaccharide-induced endotoxic shock. J Immunol. 1999;162(6):3498–503.

20. Mansell A, Smith R, Doyle SL, Gray P, Fenner JE, Crack PJ, et al. Suppressor of cytokine signaling 1 negatively regulates Toll-like receptor signaling by mediating Mal degradation. Nat Immunol. 2006;7(2):148–55.

21. Frobose H, Ronn SG, Heding PE, Mendoza H, Cohen P, Mandrup-Poulsen T, et al. Suppressor of cytokine Signaling-3 inhibits interleukin-1 signaling by targeting the TRAF-6/TAK1 complex. Mol Endocrinol. 2006;20(7):1587–96.

22. Zong C, Yan R, August A, Darnell JE Jr, Hanafusa H. Unique signal transduction of Eyk: constitutive stimulation of the JAK-STAT pathway by an oncogenic receptor-type tyrosine kinase. EMBO J. 1996;15(17):4515–25.

23. Li HS, Watowich SS. Innate immune regulation by STAT-mediated transcriptional mechanisms. Immunol Rev. 2014;261(1):84–101.

24. Sharif MN, Sosic D, Rothlin CV, Kelly E, Lemke G, Olson EN, et al. Twist mediates suppression of inflammation by type I IFNs and Axl. J Exp Med. 2006;203(8):1891–901.

25. Sosic D, Richardson JA, Yu K, Ornitz DM, Olson EN. Twist regulates cytokine gene expression through a negative feedback loop that represses NF-kappaB activity. Cell. 2003;112(2):169–80.

26. Seitz HM, Camenisch TD, Lemke G, Earp HS, Matsushima GK. Macrophages and dendritic cells use different Axl/Mertk/Tyro3 receptors in clearance of apoptotic cells. J Immunol. 2007;178(9):5635–42.

27. Arandjelovic S, Ravichandran KS. Phagocytosis of apoptotic cells in homeostasis. Nat Immunol. 2015;16(9):907–17.

28. Schreiber RD, Old LJ, Smyth MJ. Cancer immunoediting: integrating immunity's roles in cancer suppression and promotion. Science. 2011;331(6024):1565–70.

29. Zagorska A, Traves PG, Lew ED, Dransfield I, Lemke G. Diversification of TAM receptor tyrosine kinase function. Nat Immunol. 2014;15(10):920–8.

30. Sasaki T, Knyazev PG, Clout NJ, Cheburkin Y, Gohring W, Ullrich A, et al. Structural basis for Gas6-Axl signalling. EMBO J. 2006;25(1):80–7.

31. Prasad D, Rothlin CV, Burrola P, Burstyn-Cohen T, Lu Q, Garcia de Frutos P, et al. TAM receptor function in the retinal pigment epithelium. Mol Cell Neurosci. 2006;33(1):96–108.

32. Geng K, Kumar S, Kimani SG, Kholodovych V, Kasikara C, Mizuno K, et al. Requirement of gamma-carboxyglutamic acid modification and phosphatidylserine binding for the activation of Tyro3, Axl, and Mertk receptors by growth arrest-specific 6. Front Immunol. 2017;8:1521.

33. Lew ED, Oh J, Burrola PG, Lax I, Zagorska A, Traves PG, et al. Differential TAM receptor-ligand-phospholipid interactions delimit differential TAM bioactivities. Elife. 2014;3.

34. Burchert A, Attar EC, McCloskey P, Fridell YW, Liu ET. Determinants for transformation induced by the Axl receptor tyrosine kinase. Oncogene. 1998;16(24):3177–87.

35. Linger RM, Keating AK, Earp HS, Graham DK. TAM receptor tyrosine kinases: biologic functions, signaling, and potential therapeutic targeting in human cancer. Adv Cancer Res. 2008;100:35–83.

36. Caraux A, Lu Q, Fernandez N, Riou S, Di Santo JP, Raulet DH, et al. Natural killer cell differentiation driven by Tyro3 receptor tyrosine kinases. Nat Immunol. 2006;7(7):747–54.

37. Papazahariadou M, Athanasiadis GI, Papadopoulos E, Symeonidou I, Hatzistilianou M, Castellani ML, et al. Involvement of NK cells against tumors and parasites. Int J Biol Markers. 2007;22(2):144–53.

38. Vivier E, Nunes JA, Vely F. Natural killer cell signaling pathways. Science. 2004;306(5701):1517–9.

39. Roth C, Rothlin C, Riou S, Raulet DH, Lemke G. Stromal-cell regulation of natural killer cell differentiation. J Mol Med (Berl). 2007;85(10):1047–56.

40. Rothlin CV, Lemke G. TAM receptor signaling and autoimmune disease. Curr Opin Immunol. 2010;22(6):740–6.

41. Sayama A, Okado K, Nakamura K, Kawaguchi T, Iguchi T, Makino T, et al. UNC569-induced morphological changes in pigment epithelia and photoreceptor cells in the retina through MerTK inhibition in mice. Toxicol Pathol. 2018;46(2):193–201.

42. Sayama A, Okado K, Yamaguchi M, Samata N, Imaoka M, Kai K, et al. The impact of the timing of dosing on the severity of UNC569-induced ultrastructural changes in the mouse retina. Toxicol Pathol. 2020;48(5):669–76.

43. Ye X, Li Y, Stawicki S, Couto S, Eastham-Anderson J, Kallop D, et al. An anti-Axl monoclonal antibody attenuates xenograft tumor growth and enhances the effect of multiple anticancer therapies. Oncogene. 2010;29(38):5254–64.

44. Holland SJ, Pan A, Franci C, Hu Y, Chang B, Li W, et al. R428, a selective small molecule inhibitor of Axl kinase, blocks tumor spread and prolongs survival in models of metastatic breast cancer. Cancer Res. 2010;70(4):1544–54.

45. Aehnlich P, Powell RM, Peeters MJW, Rahbech A, Thor Straten P. TAM receptor inhibition-implications for cancer and the immune system. Cancers (Basel). 2021;13(6).

46. Burstyn-Cohen T, Maimon A. TAM receptors, phosphatidylserine, inflammation, and cancer. Cell Commun Signal. 2019;17(1):156.

47. Peeters MJW, Rahbech A, Thor Straten P. TAM-ing T cells in the tumor microenvironment: implications for TAM receptor targeting. Cancer Immunol Immunother. 2020;69(2):237–44.

48. Verhoven B, Schlegel RA, Williamson P. Mechanisms of phosphatidylserine exposure, a phagocyte recognition signal, on apoptotic T lymphocytes. J Exp Med. 1995;182(5):1597–601.

49. Ran S, Thorpe PE. Phosphatidylserine is a marker of tumor vasculature and a potential target for cancer imaging and therapy. Int J Radiat Oncol Biol Phys. 2002;54(5):1479–84.

50. Utsugi T, Schroit AJ, Connor J, Bucana CD, Fidler IJ. Elevated expression of phosphatidylserine in the outer membrane leaflet of human tumor cells and recognition by activated human blood monocytes. Cancer Res. 1991;51(11):3062–6.

51. He J, Luster TA, Thorpe PE. Radiation-enhanced vascular targeting of human lung cancers in mice with a monoclonal antibody that binds anionic phospholipids. Clin Cancer Res. 2007;13(17):5211–8.

52. Huang X, Bennett M, Thorpe PE. A monoclonal antibody that binds anionic phospholipids on tumor blood vessels enhances the antitumor effect of docetaxel on human breast tumors in mice. Cancer Res. 2005;65(10):4408–16.

53. Yin Y, Huang X, Lynn KD, Thorpe PE. Phosphatidylserine-targeting antibody induces M1 macrophage polarization and promotes myeloid-derived suppressor cell differentiation. Cancer Immunol Res. 2013;1(4):256–68.

54. Birge RB, Boeltz S, Kumar S, Carlson J, Wanderley J, Calianese D, et al. Phosphatidylserine (PS) is a global immunosuppressive signal in efferocytosis, infectious disease, and cancer. Cell Death Discov. 2016;23(6):962–78.

55. Fadok VA, Bratton DL, Konowal A, Freed PW, Westcott JY, Henson PM. Macrophages that have ingested apoptotic cells in vitro inhibit proinflammatory cytokine production through autocrine/paracrine mechanisms involving TGF-beta, PGE2, and PAF. J Clin Invest. 1998;101(4):890–8.

56. Kumar S, Calianese D, Birge RB. Efferocytosis of dying cells differentially modulate immunological outcomes in tumor microenvironment. Immunol Rev. 2017;280(1):149–64.

57. Park M, Kang KW. Phosphatidylserine receptor-targeting therapies for the treatment of cancer. Arch Pharm Res. 2019;42(7):617–28.

58. Zhou Y, Yao Y, Deng Y, Shao A. Regulation of efferocytosis as a novel cancer therapy. Cell Commun Signal. 2020;18(1):71.

59. He J, Yin Y, Luster TA, Watkins L, Thorpe PE. Antiphosphatidylserine antibody combined with irradiation damages tumor blood vessels and induces tumor immunity in a rat model of glioblastoma. Clin Cancer Res. 2009;15(22):6871–80.

60. Kelleher RJ Jr, Balu-Iyer S, Loyall J, Sacca AJ, Shenoy GN, Peng P, et al. Extracellular vesicles present in human ovarian tumor microenvironments induce a phosphatidylserine-dependent arrest in the T-cell signaling cascade. Cancer Immunol Res. 2015;3(11):1269–78.

61. Perone MJ, Larregina AT, Shufesky WJ, Papworth GD, Sullivan ML, Zahorchak AF, et al. Transgenic galectin-1 induces maturation of dendritic cells that elicit contrasting responses in naive and activated T cells. J Immunol. 2006;176(12):7207–20.

62. Blanchard N, Lankar D, Faure F, Regnault A, Dumont C, Raposo G, et al. TCR activation of human T cells induces the production of exosomes bearing the TCR/CD3/zeta complex. J Immunol. 2002;168(7):3235–41.

63. Kim JW, Wieckowski E, Taylor DD, Reichert TE, Watkins S, Whiteside TL. Fas ligand-positive membranous vesicles isolated from sera of patients with oral cancer induce apoptosis of activated T lymphocytes. Clin Cancer Res. 2005;11(3):1010–20.

64. Mueller DL. Linking diacylglycerol kinase to T cell anergy. Nat Immunol. 2006;7(11):1132–4.

65. Wherry EJ. T cell exhaustion. Nat Immunol. 2011;12(6):492–9.

66. Freeman GJ, Casasnovas JM, Umetsu DT, DeKruyff RH. TIM genes: a family of cell surface phosphatidylserine receptors that regulate innate and adaptive immunity. Immunol Rev. 2010;235(1):172–89.

67. Santiago C, Ballesteros A, Tami C, Martinez-Munoz L, Kaplan GG, Casasnovas JM. Structures of T cell immunoglobulin mucin receptors 1 and 2 reveal mechanisms for regulation of immune responses by the TIM receptor family. Immunity. 2007;26(3):299–310.

68. DeKruyff RH, Bu X, Ballesteros A, Santiago C, Chim YL, Lee HH, et al. T cell/transmembrane, Ig, and mucin-3 allelic variants differentially recognize phosphatidylserine and mediate phagocytosis of apoptotic cells. J Immunol. 2010;184(4):1918–30.

69. Albacker LA, Karisola P, Chang YJ, Umetsu SE, Zhou M, Akbari O, et al. TIM-4, a receptor for phosphatidylserine, controls adaptive immunity by regulating the removal of antigen-specific T cells. J Immunol. 2010;185(11):6839–49.

70. Ferris RL, Lu B, Kane LP. Too much of a good thing? Tim-3 and TCR signaling in T cell exhaustion. J Immunol. 2014;193(4):1525–30.

71. Lee J, Su EW, Zhu C, Hainline S, Phuah J, Moroco JA, et al. Phosphotyrosine-dependent coupling of Tim-3 to T-cell receptor signaling pathways. Mol Cell Biol. 2011;31(19):3963–74.

72. Rangachari M, Zhu C, Sakuishi K, Xiao S, Karman J, Chen A, et al. Bat3 promotes T cell responses and autoimmunity by repressing Tim-3-mediated cell death and exhaustion. Nat Med. 2012;18(9):1394–400.

73. Riedl S, Rinner B, Asslaber M, Schaider H, Walzer S, Novak A, et al. In search of a novel target - phosphatidylserine exposed by non-apoptotic tumor cells and metastases of malignancies with poor treatment efficacy. Biochim Biophys Acta. 2011;1808(11):2638–45.

74. Kalluri R, Weinberg RA. The basics of epithelial-mesenchymal transition. J Clin Invest. 2009;119(6):1420–8.

75. Acloque H, Adams MS, Fishwick K, Bronner-Fraser M, Nieto MA. Epithelial-mesenchymal transitions: the importance of changing cell state in development and disease. J Clin Invest. 2009;119(6):1438–49.

76. Zeisberg M, Yang C, Martino M, Duncan MB, Rieder F, Tanjore H, et al. Fibroblasts derive from hepatocytes in liver fibrosis via epithelial to mesenchymal transition. J Biol Chem. 2007;282(32):23337–47.

77. Kim KK, Kugler MC, Wolters PJ, Robillard L, Galvez MG, Brumwell AN, et al. Alveolar epithelial cell mesenchymal transition develops in vivo during pulmonary fibrosis and is regulated by the extracellular matrix. Proc Natl Acad Sci U S A. 2006;103(35):13180–5.

78. Thiery JP, Acloque H, Huang RY, Nieto MA. Epithelial-mesenchymal transitions in development and disease. Cell. 2009;139(5):871–90.

79. Thiery JP. Epithelial-mesenchymal transitions in tumour progression. Nat Rev Cancer. 2002;2(6):442–54.

80. Bissell MJ, Radisky DC, Rizki A, Weaver VM, Petersen OW. The organizing principle: microenvironmental influences in the normal and malignant breast. Differentiation. 2002;70(9–10):537–46.

81. Aggarwal V, Montoya CA, Donnenberg VS, Sant S. Interplay between tumor microenvironment and partial EMT as the driver of tumor progression. iScience. 2021;24(2):102113.

82. Lambert AW, Weinberg RA. Linking EMT programmes to normal and neoplastic epithelial stem cells. Nat Rev Cancer. 2021;21(5):325–38.

83. Taki M, Abiko K, Ukita M, Murakami R, Yamanoi K, Yamaguchi K, et al. Tumor immune microenvironment during epithelial-mesenchymal transition. Clin Cancer Res. 2021;27(17):4669–79.

84. De Craene B, Berx G. Regulatory networks defining EMT during cancer initiation and progression. Nat Rev Cancer. 2013;13(2):97–110.

85. Zhang Z, Lee JC, Lin L, Olivas V, Au V, LaFramboise T, et al. Activation of the AXL kinase causes resistance to EGFR-targeted therapy in lung cancer. Nat Genet. 2012;44(8):852–60.

86. Niessen K, Fu Y, Chang L, Hoodless PA, McFadden D, Karsan A. Slug is a direct Notch target required for initiation of cardiac cushion cellularization. J Cell Biol. 2008;182(2):315–25.

87. Medici D, Hay ED, Olsen BR. Snail and Slug promote epithelial-mesenchymal transition through beta-catenin-T-cell factor-4-dependent expression of transforming growth factor-beta3. Mol Biol Cell. 2008;19(11):4875–87.

88. Kokudo T, Suzuki Y, Yoshimatsu Y, Yamazaki T, Watabe T, Miyazono K. Snail is required for TGFbeta-induced endothelial-mesenchymal transition of embryonic stem cell-derived endothelial cells. J Cell Sci. 2008;121(Pt 20):3317–24.

89. Morel AP, Hinkal GW, Thomas C, Fauvet F, Courtois-Cox S, Wierinckx A, et al. EMT inducers catalyze malignant transformation of mammary epithelial cells and drive tumorigenesis towards claudin-low tumors in transgenic mice. PLoS Genet. 2012;8(5):e1002723.

90. Rhim AD, Mirek ET, Aiello NM, Maitra A, Bailey JM, McAllister F, et al. EMT and dissemination precede pancreatic tumor formation. Cell. 2012;148(1-2):349–61.

91. Boutet A, De Frutos CA, Maxwell PH, Mayol MJ, Romero J, Nieto MA. Snail activation disrupts tissue homeostasis and induces fibrosis in the adult kidney. EMBO J. 2006;25(23):5603–13.

92. Miyake K, Yoshizumi T, Imura S, Sugimoto K, Batmunkh E, Kanemura H, et al. Expression of hypoxia-inducible factor-1alpha, histone deacetylase 1, and metastasis-associated protein 1 in pancreatic carcinoma: correlation with poor prognosis with possible regulation. Pancreas. 2008;36(3):e1–9.

93. Liao D, Corle C, Seagroves TN, Johnson RS. Hypoxia-inducible factor-1alpha is a key regulator of metastasis in a transgenic model of cancer initiation and progression. Cancer Res. 2007;67(2):563–72.

94. Chen HH, Su WC, Lin PW, Guo HR, Lee WY. Hypoxia-inducible factor-1alpha correlates with MET and metastasis in node-negative breast cancer. Breast Cancer Res Treat. 2007;103(2):167–75.

95. Evans AJ, Russell RC, Roche O, Burry TN, Fish JE, Chow VW, et al. VHL promotes E2 box-dependent E-cadherin transcription by HIF-mediated regulation of SIP1 and snail. Mol Cell Biol. 2007;27(1):157–69.

96. Batlle E, Sancho E, Franci C, Dominguez D, Monfar M, Baulida J, et al. The transcription factor snail is a repressor of E-cadherin gene expression in epithelial tumour cells. Nat Cell Biol. 2000;2(2):84–9.

97. Cano A, Perez-Moreno MA, Rodrigo I, Locascio A, Blanco MJ, del Barrio MG, et al. The transcription factor snail controls epithelial-mesenchymal transitions by repressing E-cadherin expression. Nat Cell Biol. 2000;2(2):76–83.

98. Hajra KM, Chen DY, Fearon ER. The SLUG zinc-finger protein represses E-cadherin in breast cancer. Cancer Res. 2002;62(6):1613–8.

99. De Craene B, Gilbert B, Stove C, Bruyneel E, van Roy F, Berx G. The transcription factor snail induces tumor cell invasion through modulation of the epithelial cell differentiation program. Cancer Res. 2005;65(14):6237–44.

100. Moreno-Bueno G, Cubillo E, Sarrio D, Peinado H, Rodriguez-Pinilla SM, Villa S, et al. Genetic profiling of epithelial cells expressing E-cadherin repressors reveals a distinct role for Snail, Slug, and E47 factors in epithelial-mesenchymal transition. Cancer Res. 2006;66(19):9543–56.

101. Yang J, Mani SA, Donaher JL, Ramaswamy S, Itzykson RA, Come C, et al. Twist, a master regulator of morphogenesis, plays an essential role in tumor metastasis. Cell. 2004;117(7):927–39.

102. Wang Y, Shang Y. Epigenetic control of epithelial-to-mesenchymal transition and cancer metastasis. Exp Cell Res. 2013;319(2):160–9.

103. McDonald OG, Wu H, Timp W, Doi A, Feinberg AP. Genome-scale epigenetic reprogramming during epithelial-to-mesenchymal transition. Nat Struct Mol Biol. 2011;18(8):867–74.

104. Espada J, Peinado H, Lopez-Serra L, Setien F, Lopez-Serra P, Portela A, et al. Regulation of SNAIL1 and E-cadherin function by DNMT1 in a DNA methylation-independent context. Nucleic Acids Res. 2011;39(21):9194–205.

105. Graff JR, Gabrielson E, Fujii H, Baylin SB, Herman JG. Methylation patterns of the E-cadherin 5′ CpG island are unstable and reflect the dynamic, heterogeneous loss of E-cadherin expression during metastatic progression. J Biol Chem. 2000;275(4):2727–32.

106. Lombaerts M, van Wezel T, Philippo K, Dierssen JW, Zimmerman RM, Oosting J, et al. E-cadherin transcriptional downregulation by promoter methylation but not mutation is related to epithelial-to-mesenchymal transition in breast cancer cell lines. Br J Cancer. 2006;94(5):661–71.

107. Peinado H, Ballestar E, Esteller M, Cano A. Snail mediates E-cadherin repression by the recruitment of the Sin3A/histone deacetylase 1 (HDAC1)/HDAC2 complex. Mol Cell Biol. 2004;24(1):306–19.

108. Kudo-Saito C, Shirako H, Takeuchi T, Kawakami Y. Cancer metastasis is accelerated through immunosuppression during Snail-induced EMT of cancer cells. Cancer Cell. 2009;15(3):195–206.

109. Dongre A, Rashidian M, Reinhardt F, Bagnato A, Keckesova Z, Ploegh HL, Weinberg RA. Epithelial-to-mesenchymal transition contributes to immunosuppression in breast carcinomas. Cancer Res. 2017;77(15):3982–9.

110. Park SM, Gaur AB, Lengyel E, Peter ME. The miR-200 family determines the epithelial phenotype of cancer cells by targeting the E-cadherin repressors ZEB1 and ZEB2. Genes Dev. 2008;22(7):894–907.

111. Gregory PA, Bert AG, Paterson EL, Barry SC, Tsykin A, Farshid G, et al. The miR-200 family and miR-205 regulate epithelial to mesenchymal transition by targeting ZEB1 and SIP1. Nat Cell Biol. 2008;10(5):593–601.

112. Kim NH, Kim HS, Li XY, Lee I, Choi HS, Kang SE, et al. A p53/miRNA-34 axis regulates Snail1-dependent cancer cell epithelial-mesenchymal transition. J Cell Biol. 2011;195(3):417–33.

113. Korpal M, Lee ES, Hu G, Kang Y. The miR-200 family inhibits epithelial-mesenchymal transition and cancer cell migration by direct targeting of E-cadherin transcriptional repressors ZEB1 and ZEB2. J Biol Chem. 2008;283(22):14910–4.

114. Burk U, Schubert J, Wellner U, Schmalhofer O, Vincan E, Spaderna S, et al. A reciprocal repression between ZEB1 and members of the miR-200 family promotes EMT and invasion in cancer cells. EMBO Rep. 2008;9(6):582–9.

115. Chen L, Gibbons DL, Goswami S, Cortez MA, Ahn YH, Byers LA, et al. Metastasis is regulated via microRNA-200/ZEB1 axis control of tumour cell PD-L1 expression and intratumoral immunosuppression. Nat Commun. 2014;5:5241.

116. Li Y, Ye X, Tan C, Hongo JA, Zha J, Liu J, et al. Axl as a potential therapeutic target in cancer: role of Axl in tumor growth, metastasis and angiogenesis. Oncogene. 2009;28(39):3442–55.

117. Shieh YS, Lai CY, Kao YR, Shiah SG, Chu YW, Lee HS, et al. Expression of axl in lung adenocarcinoma and correlation with tumor progression. Neoplasia. 2005;7(12):1058–64.

118. Koorstra JB, Karikari CA, Feldmann G, Bisht S, Rojas PL, Offerhaus GJ, et al. The Axl receptor tyrosine kinase confers an

adverse prognostic influence in pancreatic cancer and represents a new therapeutic target. Cancer Biol Ther. 2009;8(7):618–26.

119. Hutterer M, Knyazev P, Abate A, Reschke M, Maier H, Stefanova N, et al. Axl and growth arrest-specific gene 6 are frequently overexpressed in human gliomas and predict poor prognosis in patients with glioblastoma multiforme. Clin Cancer Res. 2008;14(1):130–8.

120. Hector A, Montgomery EA, Karikari C, Canto M, Dunbar KB, Wang JS, et al. The Axl receptor tyrosine kinase is an adverse prognostic factor and a therapeutic target in esophageal adenocarcinoma. Cancer Biol Ther. 2010;10(10):1009–18.

121. Rochlitz C, Lohri A, Bacchi M, Schmidt M, Nagel S, Fopp M, et al. Axl expression is associated with adverse prognosis and with expression of Bcl-2 and CD34 in de novo acute myeloid leukemia (AML): results from a multicenter trial of the Swiss Group for Clinical Cancer Research (SAKK). Leukemia. 1999;13(9):1352–8.

122. Rankin EB, Fuh KC, Taylor TE, Krieg AJ, Musser M, Yuan J, et al. AXL is an essential factor and therapeutic target for metastatic ovarian cancer. Cancer Res. 2010;70(19):7570–9.

123. Song X, Wang H, Logsdon CD, Rashid A, Fleming JB, Abbruzzese JL, et al. Overexpression of receptor tyrosine kinase Axl promotes tumor cell invasion and survival in pancreatic ductal adenocarcinoma. Cancer. 2011;117(4):734–43.

124. Liu L, Greger J, Shi H, Liu Y, Greshock J, Annan R, et al. Novel mechanism of lapatinib resistance in HER2-positive breast tumor cells: activation of AXL. Cancer Res. 2009;69(17):6871–8.

125. Dufies M, Jacquel A, Belhacene N, Robert G, Cluzeau T, Luciano F, et al. Mechanisms of AXL overexpression and function in Imatinib-resistant chronic myeloid leukemia cells. Oncotarget. 2011;2(11):874–85.

126. Hong CC, Lay JD, Huang JS, Cheng AL, Tang JL, Lin MT, et al. Receptor tyrosine kinase AXL is induced by chemotherapy drugs and overexpression of AXL confers drug resistance in acute myeloid leukemia. Cancer Lett. 2008;268(2):314–24.

127. Hong J, Peng D, Chen Z, Sehdev V, Belkhiri A. ABL regulation by AXL promotes cisplatin resistance in esophageal cancer. Cancer Res. 2013;73(1):331–40.

128. Byers LA, Diao L, Wang J, Saintigny P, Girard L, Peyton M, et al. An epithelial-mesenchymal transition gene signature predicts resistance to EGFR and PI3K inhibitors and identifies Axl as a therapeutic target for overcoming EGFR inhibitor resistance. Clin Cancer Res. 2013;19(1):279–90.

129. Mani SA, Guo W, Liao MJ, Eaton EN, Ayyanan A, Zhou AY, et al. The epithelial-mesenchymal transition generates cells with properties of stem cells. Cell. 2008;133(4):704–15.

130. Morel AP, Lievre M, Thomas C, Hinkal G, Ansieau S, Puisieux A. Generation of breast cancer stem cells through epithelial-mesenchymal transition. PLoS One. 2008;3(8):e2888.

131. Scheel C, Weinberg RA. Cancer stem cells and epithelial-mesenchymal transition: concepts and molecular links. Semin Cancer Biol. 2012;22(5-6):396–403.

132. Thomson S, Petti F, Sujka-Kwok I, Mercado P, Bean J, Monaghan M, et al. A systems view of epithelial-mesenchymal transition signaling states. Clin Exp Metastasis. 2011;28(2):137–55.

133. Wang Y, Zhou BP. Epithelial-mesenchymal transition—a hallmark of breast cancer metastasis. Cancer Hallmarks. 2013;1(1):38–49.

134. Gupta PB, Onder TT, Jiang G, Tao K, Kuperwasser C, Weinberg RA, et al. Identification of selective inhibitors of cancer stem cells by high-throughput screening. Cell. 2009;138(4):645–59.

135. Nieto MA. Epithelial plasticity: a common theme in embryonic and cancer cells. Science. 2013;342(6159):1234850.

136. Yang J, Antin P, Berx G, Blanpain C, Brabletz T, Bronner M, et al. Guidelines and definitions for research on epithelial–mesenchymal transition. Nat Rev Mol Cell Biol. 2020;341–52.

137. Pastushenko I, Brisebarre A, Sifrim A, Fioramonti M, Revenco T, Boumahdi S, Van Keymeulen A, Brown D, Moers V, Lemaire S, De Clercq S, Minguijón E, Balsat C, Sokolow Y, Dubois C, De Cock F, Scozzaro S, Sopena F, Lanas A, D'Haene N, Salmon I, Marine JC, Voet T, Sotiropoulou PA, Blanpain C. Identification of the tumour transition states occurring during EMT. Nature. 2018;463–8.

138. Gupta PB, Pastushenko I, Skibinski A, Blanpain C, Kuperwasser C. Phenotypic plasticity: driver of cancer initiation, progression, and therapy resistance. Cell Stem Cell. 2019;24(1):65–78.

139. Shibue T, Weinberg RA. EMT, CSCs, and drug resistance: the mechanistic link and clinical implications. Nat Rev Clin Oncol. 2017;611–29.

140. Arumugam T, Ramachandran V, Fournier KF, Wang H, Marquis L, Abbruzzese JL, et al. Epithelial to mesenchymal transition contributes to drug resistance in pancreatic cancer. Cancer Res. 2009;69(14):5820–8.

141. Thomson S, Buck E, Petti F, Griffin G, Brown E, Ramnarine N, et al. Epithelial to mesenchymal transition is a determinant of sensitivity of non-small-cell lung carcinoma cell lines and xenografts to epidermal growth factor receptor inhibition. Cancer Res. 2005;65(20):9455–62.

142. Yang Q, Huang J, Wu Q, Cai Y, Zhu L, Lu X, et al. Acquisition of epithelial-mesenchymal transition is associated with Skp2 expression in paclitaxel-resistant breast cancer cells. Br J Cancer. 2014;110(8):1958–67.

143. Lee CG, McCarthy S, Gruidl M, Timme C, Yeatman TJ. MicroRNA-147 induces a mesenchymal-to-epithelial transition (MET) and reverses EGFR inhibitor resistance. PLoS One. 2014;9(1):e84597.

144. Wang H, Zhang G, Zhang H, Zhang F, Zhou B, Ning F, et al. Acquisition of epithelial-mesenchymal transition phenotype and cancer stem cell-like properties in cisplatin-resistant lung cancer cells through AKT/beta-catenin/Snail signaling pathway. Eur J Pharmacol. 2014;723:156–66.

145. Tan J, You Y, Xu T, Yu P, Wu D, Deng H, et al. Par-4 downregulation confers cisplatin resistance in pancreatic cancer cells via PI3K/Akt pathway-dependent EMT. Toxicol Lett. 2014;224(1):7–15.

146. Chaffer CL, Brueckmann I, Scheel C, Kaestli AJ, Wiggins PA, Rodrigues LO, et al. Normal and neoplastic nonstem cells can spontaneously convert to a stem-like state. Proc Natl Acad Sci U S A. 2011;108(19):7950–5.

147. Shackleton M. Moving targets that drive cancer progression. N Engl J Med. 2010;363(9):885–6.

148. Marusyk A, Almendro V, Polyak K. Intra-tumour heterogeneity: a looking glass for cancer? Nat Rev Cancer. 2012;12(5):323–34.

149. Correia AL, Bissell MJ. The tumor microenvironment is a dominant force in multidrug resistance. Drug Resist Updat. 2012;15(1-2):39–49.

150. Acharyya S, Oskarsson T, Vanharanta S, Malladi S, Kim J, Morris PG, et al. A CXCL1 paracrine network links cancer chemoresistance and metastasis. Cell. 2012;150(1):165–78.

151. Gray-Schopfer VC, Karasarides M, Hayward R, Marais R. Tumor necrosis factor-alpha blocks apoptosis in melanoma cells when BRAF signaling is inhibited. Cancer Res. 2007;67(1):122–9.

152. Sullivan NJ, Sasser AK, Axel AE, Vesuna F, Raman V, Ramirez N, et al. Interleukin-6 induces an epithelial-mesenchymal transition phenotype in human breast cancer cells. Oncogene. 2009;28(33):2940–7.

153. Yadav A, Kumar B, Datta J, Teknos TN, Kumar P. IL-6 promotes head and neck tumor metastasis by inducing epithelial-mesenchymal transition via the JAK-STAT3-SNAIL signaling pathway. Mol Cancer Res. 2011;9(12):1658–67.

154. Rokavec M, Oner MG, Li H, Jackstadt R, Jiang L, Lodygin D, et al. IL-6R/STAT3/miR-34a feedback loop promotes

EMT-mediated colorectal cancer invasion and metastasis. J Clin Invest. 2014;124(4):1853–67.

155. Li CW, Xia W, Huo L, Lim SO, Wu Y, Hsu JL, et al. Epithelial-mesenchymal transition induced by TNF-alpha requires NF-kappaB-mediated transcriptional upregulation of Twist1. Cancer Res. 2012;72(5):1290–300.

156. Wang H, Wang HS, Zhou BH, Li CL, Zhang F, Wang XF, et al. Epithelial-mesenchymal transition (EMT) induced by TNF-alpha requires AKT/GSK-3beta-mediated stabilization of snail in colorectal cancer. PLoS One. 2013;8(2):e56664.

157. Andersson BA, Lewin F, Lundgren J, Nilsson M, Rutqvist LE, Lofgren S, et al. Plasma tumor necrosis factor-alpha and C-reactive protein as biomarker for survival in head and neck squamous cell carcinoma. J Cancer Res Clin Oncol. 2014;140(3):515–9.

158. Seton-Rogers S. Melanoma: dual effects of PD1 blockade. Nat Rev Cancer. 2015;15(11):637.

159. Landsberg J, Kohlmeyer J, Renn M, Bald T, Rogava M, Cron M, et al. Melanomas resist T-cell therapy through inflammation-induced reversible dedifferentiation. Nature. 2012;490(7420):412–6.

160. Peng W, Liu C, Xu C, Lou Y, Chen J, Yang Y, et al. PD-1 blockade enhances T-cell migration to tumors by elevating IFN-gamma inducible chemokines. Cancer Res. 2012;72(20):5209–18.

161. Dougall WC, Kurtulus S, Smyth MJ, Anderson AC. TIGIT and CD96: new checkpoint receptor targets for cancer immunotherapy. Immunol Rev. 2017;276(1):112–20.

162. Chauvin JM, Zarour HM. TIGIT in cancer immunotherapy. J Immunother Cancer. 2020;8(2):e000957.

163. Harjunpää H, Guillerey C. TIGIT as an emerging immune checkpoint. Clin Exp Immunol. 2020;200(2):108–19.

164. Terry S, Buart S, Tan TZ, Gros G, Noman MZ, Lorens JB, Mami-Chouaib F, Thiery JP, Chouaib S. Acquisition of tumor cell phenotypic diversity along the EMT spectrum under hypoxic pressure: consequences on susceptibility to cell-mediated cytotoxicity. Oncoimmunology. 2017;6(2):e1271858.

165. Facciabene A, Peng X, Hagemann IS, Balint K, Barchetti A, Wang LP, et al. Tumour hypoxia promotes tolerance and angiogenesis via CCL28 and T(reg) cells. Nature. 2011;475(7355):226–30.

166. Hansen W, Hutzler M, Abel S, Alter C, Stockmann C, Kliche S, et al. Neuropilin 1 deficiency on CD4+Foxp3+ regulatory T cells impairs mouse melanoma growth. J Exp Med. 2012;209(11):2001–16.

167. Stockmann C, Schadendorf D, Klose R, Helfrich I. The impact of the immune system on tumor: angiogenesis and vascular remodeling. Front Oncol. 2014;4:69.

168. Holmes K, Roberts OL, Thomas AM, Cross MJ. Vascular endothelial growth factor receptor-2: structure, function, intra-cellular signalling and therapeutic inhibition. Cell Signal. 2007;19(10):2003–12.

169. Chatterjee S, Heukamp LC, Siobal M, Schottle J, Wieczorek C, Peifer M, et al. Tumor VEGF:VEGFR2 autocrine feed-forward loop triggers angiogenesis in lung cancer. J Clin Invest. 2013;123(4):1732–40.

170. Bergers G, Benjamin LE. Tumorigenesis and the angiogenic switch. Nat Rev Cancer. 2003;3(6):401–10.

171. Wei ZW, Xia GK, Wu Y, Chen W, Xiang Z, Schwarz RE, et al. CXCL1 promotes tumor growth through VEGF pathway activation and is associated with inferior survival in gastric cancer. Cancer Lett. 2015;359(2):335–43.

172. Goruppi S, Ruaro E, Varnum B, Schneider C. Requirement of phosphatidylinositol 3-kinase-dependent pathway and Src for Gas6-Axl mitogenic and survival activities in NIH 3T3 fibroblasts. Mol Cell Biol. 1997;17(8):4442–53.

173. Murdoch C, Muthana M, Coffelt SB, Lewis CE. The role of myeloid cells in the promotion of tumour angiogenesis. Nat Rev Cancer. 2008;8(8):618–31.

174. Dikov MM, Ohm JE, Ray N, Tchekneva EE, Burlison J, Moghanaki D, et al. Differential roles of vascular endothelial growth factor receptors 1 and 2 in dendritic cell differentiation. J Immunol (Baltimore, MD: 1950). 2005;174(1):215–22.

175. Folkman J. Angiogenesis: an organizing principle for drug discovery? Nat Rev Drug Discov. 2007;6(4):273–86.

176. Iwami D, Brinkman CC, Bromberg JS. Vascular endothelial growth factor c/vascular endothelial growth factor receptor 3 signaling regulates chemokine gradients and lymphocyte migration from tissues to lymphatics. Transplantation. 2015;99(4):668–77.

177. Voron T, Colussi O, Marcheteau E, Pernot S, Nizard M, Pointet AL, et al. VEGF-A modulates expression of inhibitory checkpoints on CD8+ T cells in tumors. J Exp Med. 2015;212(2):139–48.

178. Roland CL, Lynn KD, Toombs JE, Dineen SP, Udugamasooriya DG, Brekken RA. Cytokine levels correlate with immune cell infiltration after anti-VEGF therapy in preclinical mouse models of breast cancer. PLoS One. 2009;4(11):e7669.

179. Dineen SP, Lynn KD, Holloway SE, Miller AF, Sullivan JP, Shames DS, et al. Vascular endothelial growth factor receptor 2 mediates macrophage infiltration into orthotopic pancreatic tumors in mice. Cancer Res. 2008;68(11):4340–6.

180. Roland CL, Dineen SP, Lynn KD, Sullivan LA, Dellinger MT, Sadegh L, et al. Inhibition of vascular endothelial growth factor reduces angiogenesis and modulates immune cell infiltration of orthotopic breast cancer xenografts. Mol Cancer Ther. 2009;8(7):1761–71.

Inflammatory Biomarkers for Cancer

12

Alexandre Corthay and Guttorm Haraldsen

Abstract

Cancer is associated with various degrees of inflammation locally and systemically, due to an immunological response towards the malignant lesions. Here, we review several inflammatory parameters as biomarkers and prognostic tools for cancer. Colorectal cancer (CRC) represents the paradigm of a causative relationship between chronic inflammatory disease and cancer development. However, close examination of the data reveals that the risk of CRC in patients with inflammatory bowel disease (IBD) has been largely overestimated. In fact, IBD patients only have a slightly increased risk of developing CRC (standardized incidence ratio ~1.7), which only weakly supports the link between chronic inflammation and cancer. However, long-term immunosuppressive treatment of IBD patients is associated with an increased risk of cancer in general, particularly hematologic and skin cancers. In contrast, there is a strong association between infection with the bacterium *Helicobacter pylori*, gastritis, and gastric cancer. Therefore, *H. pylori* seropositivity or the associated gastritis should be considered risk factors for gastric cancer, and treatment to eradicate *H. pylori* in infected individuals is recommended. We also review several cytokines of the interleukin-1 family and cytokines that converge on STAT3 signalling because they are suitable to illustrate the multitude of cytokine actions that makes interpretation of one single cytokine as a cancer biomarker very complex.

Take-Home Lessons
- Patients with inflammatory bowel disease have only a slightly increased risk of developing colorectal cancer.
- Infection with the bacterium *Helicobacter pylori* is a risk factor for gastric cancer, and treatment to eradicate *H. pylori* is recommended.
- Proinflammatory cytokines of several subfamilies are found to affect tumour development, often because they are secreted from tumour cells and recruit immune cells to influence tumour progression.
- The interleukin-1-family member IL-33 can play both pro- and anti-tumourigenic roles in tumour growth and progression.

Introduction

Cancer elicits an inflammatory immune response within and around tumours as well as systemically. The role of the immune system in cancer is complex as both tumour-promoting and tumour-suppressive effects have been observed [1]. Some chronic inflammatory diseases are associated with increased cancer risk, suggesting a causative relationship between chronic inflammation and cancer development [2]. Therefore, one may consider using a diagnosis of inflammatory disease as a predictive biomarker for cancer. In the first two sections of this chapter, we present current knowledge about two inflammatory conditions that are reported to predispose to cancer, namely inflammatory bowel disease and gastritis. The usefulness of these diseases as risk biomarkers of cancer is critically discussed. In the following sections, we critically review several cytokines as biomarkers of inflammation and cancer prognosis.

A. Corthay
Tumor Immunology Lab, Department of Pathology, Oslo University Hospital and University of Oslo, Oslo, Norway
e-mail: alexandre.corthay@medisin.uio.no

G. Haraldsen (✉)
Vascular Biology Lab, Department of Pathology, Oslo University Hospital and University of Oslo, Oslo, Norway
e-mail: guttorm.haraldsen@medisin.uio.no

© The Author(s), under exclusive license to Springer Nature Switzerland AG 2022
L. A. Akslen, R. S. Watnick (eds.), *Biomarkers of the Tumor Microenvironment*, https://doi.org/10.1007/978-3-030-98950-7_12

Inflammatory Bowel Disease and Colorectal Cancer Risk

Crohn's disease (CD) and ulcerative colitis (UC) are the two main types of inflammatory bowel diseases (IBD). People with CD have 40 % greater mortality than the general population, whereas those who suffer from UC do not show increased mortality [3]. An increased risk of developing colorectal cancer (CRC) has been reported for patients with IBD. In fact, colon cancer represents a paradigm of the causative relationship between chronic inflammatory disease and cancer development [2]. In the official guidelines from the American Gastroenterological Association concerning CRC risk, surveillance colonoscopy is recommended every 1–3 years for patients with IBD [4]. A fundament for these guidelines is a landmark meta-analysis published in 2001 by Eaden et al., that reported the cumulative probabilities of patients with UC to develop CRC of 2% by 10 years, 8% by 20 years, and as high as 18% by 30 years [5]. These numbers have been much referred to and represent a pillar for the paradigm of chronic inflammation causing cancer. However, the validity of these high estimates has been questioned since their publication.

Herrinton and colleagues (see Table 12.1) reported that the incidence of CRC in Northern California from 1998 to 2010, among 16,500 individuals with IBD, was only 60% higher than in the general population and was stable over time [6]. The standardized CRC mortality ratios were 2.3 and 2.0 for individuals with CD and UC, respectively [6]. In a prospective study of >19,000 patients with IBD in France, the standardized incidence ratio (SIR) of CRC was 2.2 for all patients [7]. Patients with IBD and long-standing extensive colitis were found to have an increased risk for CRC with a SIR of 7.0 [7]. In contrast, CRC risk was lower among IBD patients receiving thiopurine therapy [7]. Thus, these two studies are consistent with a 1.6–2.2 times increased risk of developing CRC in patients with IBD. These numbers are in accordance with a meta-analysis of population-based cohort

studies that was published in 2013 and found a SIR for CRC of 1.7 for patients with IBD [8]. Close examination of population-based cohort studies from several countries reveals a consistent but modest increased risk for CRC in the range of 0.7–2.7 both for patients with UC (Table 12.1) and CD (Table 12.2).

There is strong evidence that the risk of CRC for IBD patients may have decreased considerably over the past 30 years [14, 15]. A large cohort study in Denmark with >47,000 patients with IBD over a 30-year period (1979–2008) showed that the overall risk of CRC among patients with IBD was comparable with that of the general population [15]. However, increased CRC risk was observed for subgroups of patients with UC such as patients diagnosed in childhood or adolescence, those with long duration of disease, and those with concomitant primary sclerosing cholangitis [15]. For patients with UC, the overall relative risk for CRC had decreased from 1.34 in 1979–1988 to 0.57 in 1999–2008. For CD patients, the relative CRC risk was 0.85 and did not change over time. Therefore, the authors of this large Danish cohort study concluded that a diagnosis of UC or CD no longer appears to increase the patients' risk of CRC, presumably due to improved therapies for patients with IBD [15]. Similarly, a nationwide study in the Netherlands including 78 general hospitals concluded that the risk of developing CRC in IBD patients was very low [20]. Interestingly, reduced CRC incidence was observed in IBD patients treated with immunosuppressive therapy or by tumour necrosis factor α (TNF-α) blockade [20].

Thus, one can conclude that the CRC risk in IBD has been overestimated in the past, presumably due to bias in patient inclusion and flaws in statistical analysis. A major pitfall appears to be the use of referral centre-based rather than population-based cohorts which tend to overestimate the risks by including patients with more severe diseases [8]. An approximately twofold increased risk of developing CRC in patients with IBD is a more reliable estimate, which only weakly supports the proposed link between chronic inflam-

Table 12.1 Reported risk of colorectal cancer in patients with ulcerative colitis (UC)

First author	Publication year	Country	No. of UC patients	SIR[a]	Reference
Stewenius	1995	Sweden	471	2.1	[9]
Wandall	2000	Denmark	801	1.7	[10]
Palli	2000	Italy	689	1.8	[11]
Jess	2006	USA	378	1.1	[12]
Jess	2007	Denmark	1575	1.1	[13]
Söderlund	2009	Sweden	4125	2.7	[14]
Herrinton	2012	USA	10,895	1.6	[6]
Jess	2012	Denmark	32,911	1.1[b]	[15]
Manninen	2013	Finland	1253	1.99	[16]
van den Heuvel	2016	The Netherlands	1644	0.7	[17]
Cheddani	2016	France	474	0.9	[18]

[a]Standardized Incidence Ratio, i.e. the ratio of the observed number of cancer cases to the expected number of cases
[b]This study reported Relative Risk (RR) instead of SIR

Table 12.2 Reported risk of colorectal cancer in patients with Crohn's disease (CD)

First author	Publication year	Country	No. of CD patients	SIR[a]	Reference
Palli	2000	Italy	231	1.4	[11]
Jess	2004	Denmark	374	1.6	[19]
Jess	2006	USA	314	1.9	[12]
Jess	2007	Denmark	641	1.4	[13]
Söderlund	2009	Sweden	3482	2.1	[14]
Herrinton	2012	USA	5603	1.6	[6]
Jess	2012	Denmark	14,463	0.9[b]	[15]
Manninen	2013	Finland	551	1.92	[16]
Beaugerie	2013	France	11,759	2.4	[7]
van den Heuvel	2016	The Netherlands	1157	2.0	[17]
Cheddani	2016	France	370	2.5	[18]

[a]Standardized Incidence Ratio
[b]This study reported Relative Risk (RR) instead of SIR

mation and cancer. In contrast, long-term immunosuppressive treatment of IBD patients is associated with an increased risk for overall cancer including hematologic and skin cancers [17], which is consistent with a key role of the immune system in preventing cancer [21]. Thus, a diagnosis of IBD may be considered a risk factor for immunosuppression-associated cancers rather than CRC only.

Helicobacter pylori **Infection and the Risk of Gastritis**

Helicobacter pylori is a Gram-negative bacterium which colonizes the stomachs of about half of the world population. The prevalence of *H. pylori* infection varies widely in different geographic areas [22]. Sequencing data from a worldwide collection of *H. pylori* strains suggest that anatomically modern humans were already infected with the bacterium before their migrations out of Africa [23]. A complete *H. pylori* genome was recovered from the stomach of a 5300-year-old mummy of an early European farmer (*the Iceman*), formally demonstrating that *H. pylori* has been a human pathogen for >5000 years [24]. Although the vast majority (>90%) of *H. pylori* infected people remain asymptomatic, *H. pylori* is considered the main causative agent behind gastritis and peptic ulcer. *H. pylori* (originally named *Campylobacter*) was first isolated from stomach biopsies by the Australian scientists J. Robin Warren and Barry Marshall [25]. *H. pylori* was reported to grow in close contact with the epithelium of the stomach, presumably near the neutral end of the pH gradient and protected by the overlying mucus [25]. Importantly, *H. pylori* was almost always detected in patients with active chronic gastritis, suggesting a causal relationship between *H. pylori* infection and inflammation. This hypothesis was strengthened by the analysis of biopsy specimens from 100 consecutive patients, revealing that the bacterium was present in almost all patients with active

chronic gastritis, duodenal ulcers, or gastric ulcers [26]. Several studies have confirmed this association [27, 28].

Helicobacter pylori **Infection and Gastric Cancer Risk**

Several studies have revealed that infection with *H. pylori* is associated with an increased risk of developing gastric cancer. For example, in a cohort of American men of Japanese ancestry living in Hawaii, 94% of patients with gastric carcinoma, but only 76% of the matched controls, had a positive test for *H. pylori* antibodies, implying an odds ratio of 6.0 [29]. Increased levels of antibody to *H. pylori* were associated with an increased risk of gastric carcinoma [29]. Another American study in California with 109 patients with gastric adenocarcinoma reported an 84% infection rate among patients and 61% for the matched controls [30]. Similar findings were made with patient cohorts in Japan and Norway [31–33]. Thus, although most *H. pylori*-infected individuals remain healthy, there is a strong association between *H. pylori* infection and gastric cancer. Essentially, all patients with gastric cancer are colonized by *H. pylori*. Infection by *H. pylori* is now established as a risk factor for developing gastric cancer, and *H. pylori* was classified as a carcinogen by the World Health Organization (WHO) in 1994 [34]. Therefore, gastric carcinoma is considered a paradigm of infection-associated cancer.

Can *H. pylori* **Infection or Gastritis Be Used as Risk Biomarkers for Gastric Cancer?**

Although it is well known that most people infected with *H. pylori* never develop gastric cancer, several investigators have attempted to use *H. pylori* infection and/or gastritis as predictors of gastric cancer development. For example, in a prospective study, 1526 Japanese patients with various gastrointestinal diseases (duodenal ulcers, gastric ulcers, gastric hyperplasia, or non-ulcer dyspepsia) at the time of enrolment were followed. Gastric cancer developed in 36 of 1246 *H. pylori*-infected patients (2.9%) but in none of the 280 uninfected patients ($p < 0.001$) [35]. Interestingly, gastric cancer did not develop in any of the 253 patients with *H. pylori* infection who had received eradication therapy [35]. Thus, *H. pylori* sero-positivity or the associated gastritis may be used as biomarkers to predict the development of gastric cancer. This may be particularly useful in populations with a high incidence of gastric cancer such as in Japan [36]. Importantly, the Kyoto global consensus report concluded in 2015 that *H. pylori* gastritis should be considered as an infectious disease. As such, treatment was recommended for *H. pylori* gastritis, whether or not it is associated with symptoms, because it represents a condition that may evolve towards serious complications, including peptic ulcer and gastric neoplasia [37].

Cytokines as Biomarkers of Inflammation and Cancer Prognosis

Central to the consideration of inflammation-associated biomarkers is the important role of soluble cytokines and other signalling factors that serve to initiate and maintain inflammation. Some of these are released from the liver, whereas others originate either from leukocytes or tissue resident cells of inflammatory lesions. In the following section, we will focus on some selected cytokines. We give a detailed account of their sources, targets and the signalling pathways they activate, as this information is critical to understanding inflammatory biomarkers in cancer.

MyD88 and Interleukin-1 (IL-1) Family Members

IL-1 is elevated in various types of cancers, and it is known that patients with IL-1-producing tumours have a poor prognosis [38]. This knowledge has called for strategies to target IL-1 which will be detailed below. However, before we explain the possible functions of IL-1 and put them into the context of other IL-1-like cytokines (IL-18 and IL-33), we shall first describe the mechanisms by which these cytokines affect the immune system and may act to affect tumour development. Signalling induced by most members of the IL-1 family of cytokines and also the Toll-like receptor (TLR) family, converge on MyD88 (myeloid differentiation primary response gene 88), a central adapter of the IL-1 receptor/TLR superfamily [39]. This central position of MyD88 (Fig. 12.1) in inflammation has boosted a strong interest in assessing tumour development when MyD88 is

inactivated, and starting this account of the IL-1 family can be better explained by first examining the signalling events downstream from MyD88 activation.

MyD88

The majority of studies imply that MyD88 signalling promotes carcinogenesis in many cancer models. In chemical carcinogenesis models of skin and liver, tumour induction was inhibited in response to a genetic lack of *MyD88* [40, 41]. Reduced intestinal tumour growth was also observed in *Myd88*$^{-/-}$ mice subjected to multiple injections of the carcinogen azoxymethane (AOM) in comparison with WT controls [42]. Furthermore, MyD88 signalling was shown to be required for AOM-enhanced colon carcinogenesis in *Il10*$^{-/-}$ mice [43], and, in the *Apc*$^{Min/+}$ mouse model of spontaneous intestinal tumourigenesis, MyD88 signalling contributed to adenoma growth and progression [42].

On the other hand, when combining AOM with the chemical irritant dextran sodium sulphate (DSS), MyD88 was found to protect against the development of colitis-induced cancer [44], contrasting the findings obtained in response to AOM alone [42]. Moreover, MyD88 activation protects against the development of myeloproliferative neoplasia (MPN) [45]. A protective role of MyD88 against cancer may be explained by the fact that the immune system naturally protects against cancer and that certain types of inflammation prevent malignancies, whereas other types promote cancer [1, 46, 47].

These observations have nevertheless raised the following question: what are the signals that act upstream of MyD88? Central to the activation of IL-1 and IL-18 are their cleavage by caspase-1, generated by the inflammasome, a composite protein complex strongly involved in the regulation of inflammation and autoimmunity [48]. Indeed, inflammasome defects have been shown to increase tumour growth in several colitis-derived murine cancer models [49–53]. However, the biological effects of IL-1 and IL-18 differ in many respects. Despite the fact that both cytokines signal via MyD88, IL-1 is a strong driver of NF-kB signalling and the MAPK p38 pathway, whereas IL-18 signal transduction mainly involves the latter [54].

Interleukin-1

In carcinogenesis-driven experimental skin cancer, lack of IL-1β led to slower tumour growth, and conversely, when IL-1 receptor antagonist was lacking, tumour growth was accelerated [55]. In the same vein, IL-1 contributes to the development of preneoplastic gastric lesions in the *Helicobacter*-driven model of intestinal neoplasia [56]. On the other hand, genetic lack of IL-1R does not alter the outcome of the AOM/DSS-driven colitis model [44]. Several studies in mice have also documented protective functions of IL-1α and IL-1β against cancer [46, 57].

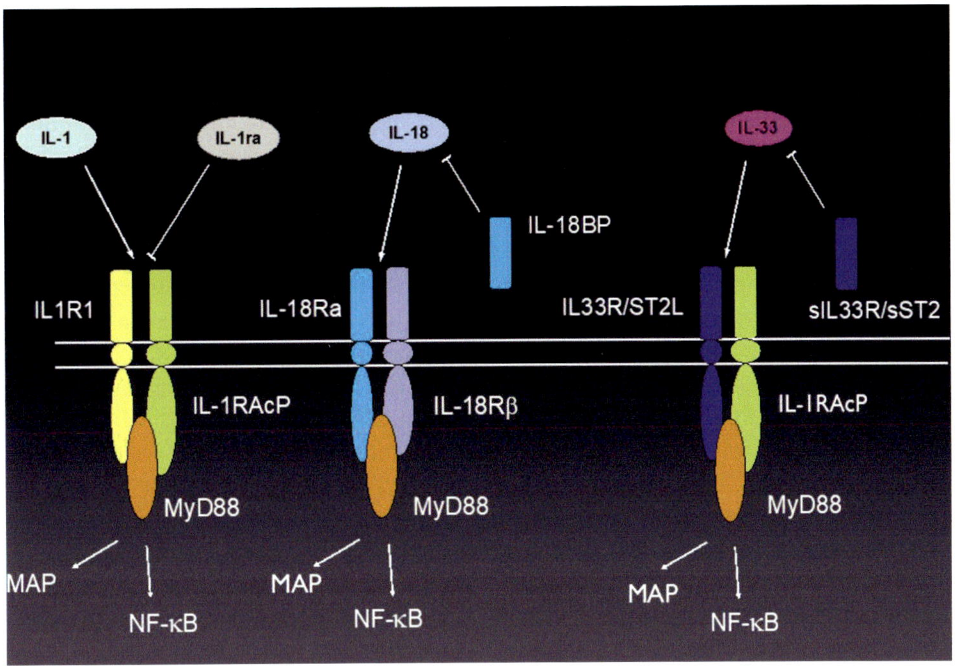

Fig. 12.1 Schematic representation of receptors for IL-1, IL-18 and IL-33. IL-1 receptor (IL1R1) forms a heterodimer with the IL-1 receptor accessory protein (IL-RAcP, aka IL1R3) upon binding of IL-1α or IL-1β, leading to intracellular recruitment of MyD88 and downstream signalling to NFkB and p38MAP. Interleukin-1 receptor antagonist (IL1Ra, aka IL1F3) competes with IL-1 for binding to IL1R1. IL-18 receptor (IL-18Rα, aka IL1R5) forms heterodimer with IL-18Rβ (aka IL1R7) to mediate signalling after binding IL18. IL18 binding protein (IL18BP) acts as a decoy to intercept IL-18. IL-33 receptor (IL-33Ra, aka ST2 or IL1R4) forms heterodimer with IL-RAcP upon binding of IL-33. Soluble IL33R/ST2 acts as decoy to intercept IL-33

The effect of targeting IL-1 signalling in cancer treatment has been assessed in some clinical trials. A phase 2 clinical trial with patients with smouldering or indolent multiple myeloma indicated that blocking of IL-1 activity by recombinant IL-1 receptor antagonist (Anakinra) may result in prolongation of progression-free disease [58]. Moreover, a human antibody to IL-1α was tested in a phase I trial of patients that were refractory to anti-tumour therapies and losing weight and found to induce a significant increase in lean body mass [59]. In a phase 3 study of advanced CRC, treatment with anti-IL-1α antibody was reported to reduce the disease-associated symptoms and improve the global quality of life [60].

Interleukin-18

IL-18 is a member of the IL-1 family of cytokines best known for its role in promoting IFN-γ production and Th1 polarization of T cells [61] and a cytokine that has also attracted interest in the field of immuno-oncology. In the Helicobacter-driven model of intestinal neoplasia, IL-18, in contrast to IL-1, appears to prevent the onset of gastric cancer [56], perhaps by mediating conversion of T cells to a regulatory phenotype [62]. Likewise, mice lacking either IL-18 or IL-18R were highly susceptible to tumour formation in a colitis-driven model of CRC [44]. Indeed, several studies have implicated IL-18 production as the main mediator that confers protection against colorectal tumour formation downstream of the Nlrp3 inflammasome [49]. In fact, in a model lacking caspase-1, substitution with bioactive IL-18 could reverse epithelial dysplasia [51]. IL-18 administration also mediated regression of melanoma and sarcoma [63], apparently mediated by IFN-γ [64] and perhaps involving the antiangiogenic effect of IFN-γ-responsive chemokines CXCL9 and CXCL10 [65]. It deserves mention that IL18-primed human NK cells develop a distinct helper phenotype that shows the reduced cytotoxic function and instead, via production of IFN-γ, promotes tumour-specific Th1 and CTL responses [66].

The experimental evidence of an antineoplastic role of IL-18 is in apparent contradiction to the elevated levels of IL-18 seen for example in human ovarian cancer [67]. However, it appears that while tumour cells have the capacity to synthesize high levels of IL-18, it is the full-length pro-IL-18 that has not been processed by capase-1, and accordingly, it has no biological activity [67]. Likewise, elevated levels of soluble IL-18 binding protein have the capacity to neutralize the effect of IL-18 [68, 69]. The preclinical efficacy of IL-18 has initiated clinical trials of IL-18 alone or in combination, showing that IL-18 has low toxicity in man but a limited therapeutic effect as a single agent [61].

Interleukin-33

Interleukin-33 (IL-33, also known as IL1F11) is the most recently identified member of the IL-1 family of cytokines [70]. IL-33 has a complex biology based on the observation that it acts as a nuclear factor in many cell types, yet when released by damaged cells, it binds to a more conventional surface membrane receptor (IL-33R, also known as ST2 or IL-1R4) that resembles other members of the IL-1/Toll-like receptor (TIR) superfamily. It is important to understand this dual function when interpreting results in cancer biology studies that modulate the function of IL-33 and its receptor.

The identification of IL-33 was initiated by the discovery that serum-stimulated fibroblasts expressed a molecule that partly resembled the IL-1 receptor [71]. This putative IL-1 family receptor member was designated ST2 and widely characterized as an orphan receptor until scientists working at Genentech identified IL-33 as its ligand [70]. In a genome-wide search and modelling for novel members of the IL-1 family, Schmitz et al. [70] selected a transcript that had been characterized in vasospastic vessels of subarachnoid haemorrhage previously [72]. We also identified this transcript in high endothelial venules of human tonsils [73] and later found it to be abundantly expressed in the nuclei of endothelial cells in most healthy human tissues, yet strikingly absent in angiogenic tumour vessels [74]. Later, its expression was also reported in some epithelia and in the fibroblastic reticular cells of lymphoid tissues [74, 75]. In lesions of inflammation, it is also expressed by activated myofibroblasts [76], and the repertoire of epithelial cells that express IL-33 is expanded [77]. There are also important species differences [77] but as a general principle, IL-33 is expressed in intact cells as a nuclear protein thought to affect transcriptional behaviour.

The other aspect of IL-33 biology occurs when IL-33 is released by necrotic or otherwise damaged cells and acts as an active cytokine that binds to the IL-33 receptor (IL-33, previously designed ST2) and initiates a signalling cascade that also involves signalling via MyD88, p38MAPK, and NF-kB (Fig. 12.1) [70]. Very interestingly, the signalling pathways activated by IL-33 show very strong similarities to those well-characterized in response to IL-1. Indeed, despite numerous papers that analysed IL-33 signalling, only one publication reported a side-by-side comparison of the transcriptional response, concluding a virtually identical profile and instead describing mechanisms of regulation related to the expression of IL-33R in relation to cell cycle [78]. Further complicating the biology of ST2 is the fact that alternative splicing of mRNA results in transcripts that also encode a shorter, soluble form of ST2 (sST2) that lacks the transmembrane region and is thought to act as a decoy receptor.

Since the first edition of this book, several new studies have expanded our understanding of IL-33 in tumour biology and publications mentioned in the previous edition that were largely describing associations between IL-33 and tumour behaviour are not given further attention here. Several subsequent studies now indicate that IL-33 can play both pro- and anti-tumourigenic roles in tumour growth and progression. In some cancer types, IL-33 appears to promote tumourigenesis by directly affecting tumour cells [79, 80] while in other cases IL-33 regulates immune cells in the tumour microenvironment [81, 82].

The first functional evidence for a role of IL-33 in cancer development came from a study that, based on the known association of inflammation and myeloproliferative neoplasia (MPN), used a model of MPN-like disease in which *styx*, a mutant of the inositol phosphatase SHIP, leads to increased numbers of granulocyte-macrophage progenitors and myeloid cell proliferation in multiple organs [45]. First, demonstrating that deletion of MyD88 abrogated fatal MPN-like disease, a systematic search for involved upstream receptors identified IL-33/ST2 signalling as a non-redundant requirement in this process, because deletion of ST2 prevented the aberrant haematopoiesis in *styx* mice [45]. Moreover, IL-33 was shown to originate from tissue-resident, non-haematopoietic cells, as lethally irradiated IL-33–/– mice reconstituted with *styx* bone marrow failed to develop MPN-like disease [45].

Several studies report data to indicate that IL-33 is secreted from tumour cells and affects the behaviour of tumour-associated immune cells. For example, pro-tumoural type 2 innate lymphoid cells (ILC2) appear to be driven by IL-33-secreting cancer cells [83]. IL-33 also appears to reduce experimental CRC growth via the recruitment and activation of eosinophils [84]. IL-33-induced activation of lung-resident group 2 innate lymphoid cells (ILC2s) orchestrated suppression of natural killer (NK) cell-mediated innate antitumour immunity, leading to increased lung metastases and mortality [85]. A recent study of murine carcinoma development revealed that tumour-initiating cells release IL-33 in an antioxidant response, inducing differentiation of macrophages that in turn release of TGF-β, feeding back to further upregulation of IL-33 and promoting malignant progression [86].

Recent attention to *nuclear* IL-33 found it to drive phosphorylation of SMAD2/3 and SMAD1/5 in epithelial cells by repressing the expression of inhibitory Smad6. Blocking TGF-β/SMAD signalling attenuated the IL-33-induced cell proliferation in vitro and inhibited IL-33-dependent epidermal hyperplasia and skin cancer development in vivo [87]. Nuclear IL-33 was also found to mediate release of inflammatory cytokines in glioblastoma and accelerate tumour progression [88].

Cytokines That Converge on STAT3 Signalling

STAT3 (Signal transducer and activator of transcription 3) is a transcription factor that has received much attention in cancer biology because of its function as an oncogene [89]. While much focus has been given to IL-6 and its signalling from the IL-6 receptor towards the activation of STAT3, several other cytokine pathways converge on this central transcription factor and we shall give examples of how this should be considered in different settings of cancer development.

Interleukin-6 Family

The interleukin-6 family of cytokines is defined by the shared use of the gp130 receptor beta-subunit. IL-6 family members, with the exception of IL-31, can activate the STAT3 pathway, as well as the Erk and PI3K pathways. Included in this family is IL-6, recognized for its role as a systemic acute phase mediator, and IL-11, a cytokine that stimulates platelet production. IL-6 is one of the best characterized tumourigenic cytokines [90]. Elevated IL-6 levels in patients with CRC are associated with advanced-stage cancer and an independent prognostic marker of reduced survival [91]. A common feature of IL-6 family signalling is the downstream activation of STAT3, and it is clear that manipulation of STAT3 signalling indeed affects tumourigenesis and that its activation can be driven by other upstream mediators that signal via STAT3.

First, evidence suggests that IL-11 is more strongly correlated to elevated STAT3 activation than IL-6 in gastrointestinal cancers [92]. This became evident from the observation that TGF-β (see below) can drive the stromal production of IL-11 in this context [93]. Additionally, STAT3 signalling can induce microsatellite instability in CRC by activation of the human mismatch repair mediator MSH3 (mutS homologue 3) [94]. Moreover, excessive STAT3 activation is a prominent feature of the majority of solid cancers and indeed, some carcinomas also show activating somatic mutations in *STAT3* and *gp130*, as well as epigenetic silencing of SOCS3 that encodes a critical negative regulator of STAT3 signalling [95, 96].

IL-22

Several cytokines not related to the IL-6 family of cytokines also signal via STAT3. IL-22 is a member of the IL-10 family produced by T helper 17 (Th17) cells, Th22 cells and innate lymphoid cells. IL-22 is involved in the resolution of tissue damage [97] and, in fact, IL-22-deficiency delays wound healing [98]. A possible involvement of IL-22 in cancer development and progress comes from the following studies: Elevated levels of IL-22 are associated with non-small cell lung cancer [99], and in human CRC, elevated IL-22 is associated with resistance to chemotherapy [100, 101]. At a functional level, exogenous IL-22 promoted the growth of non-melanoma ectopic skin cancers in nude mice [102] and conversely, in a model of CRC. In fact, neutralization of IL-22 blocked several target genes of the IL-22/STAT3 axis and led to a reduction in dysplasia and invasiveness [103]. Moreover, transgenic IL-22 expression driven by the albumin promoter increased susceptibility to carcinogen-induced liver cancer [104] and in addition, IL-22 stimulates the synthesis of VEGF-A – itself a STAT3 activator.

TGF-β

TGF-β is a pleiotropic cytokine that has complex roles in cancer, wound healing and tissue homeostasis. In breast and prostate cancer, TGF-β appears to induce a variety of pro-metastatic programs [105], whereas in the development of CRC, TGF-β is generally thought of as having a tumour-suppressive function [106]. Whereas normal cells may produce small amounts of TGF-β, cancer cells often secrete large quantities [107]. TGF-β also affects the functions of the non-transformed cells that are present in the tumour mass, in particular by inhibiting immune cells, presumably as a mechanism to dampen the antitumour immune response. For various cancer types, an association has been reported between elevated serum levels of TGF-β and poor prognosis [107]. Amazingly, TGF-β has the ability to function both as a tumour suppressor and a tumour promoter, this duality being known as the TGF-β paradox [108].

In the early stages of tumourigenicity, TGF-β potently induces growth arrest of cancer cells. Downstream mediators of TGF-β signalling are SMAD2/3, which interact with SMAD4 to regulate gene expression. In a model of CRC induced by *Helicobacter bilis*, Smad3-deficient mice showed more rapid disease development, and intriguingly, Smad4-deficiency is associated with poor prognosis in human CRC and leads to elevated levels of CCL15, thought to recruit CCR1+ myeloid cells to liver metastases [109].

In contrast, in later stages of cancer development, TGF-β signalling pathways are severely deregulated, and TGF-β promotes tumour growth instead [108]. Perhaps accordingly, high levels of TGF-β are associated with a poor prognosis for patients with established CRC. This paradox may rest on the recent demonstration that TGF-β drives the synthesis of IL-11 in cancer-associated fibroblasts that feeds back on tumour cells to promote STAT3 signalling and metastasis, perhaps by suppressing apoptotic stimuli encountered during colonization [106].

Concluding Remarks/Summary

Previous estimates of risk for colorectal cancer in IBD have been overestimated but immunosuppressive treatment of IBD is nevertheless associated with an increased risk for overall cancer. On the other hand, there is a strong association of *H. pylori* infection and gastric cancer, and treatment of infection is recommended. Cytokines of several subfamilies are found to affect tumour development, often because they are secreted from tumour cells and recruit immune cells to modulate tumour progression.

Acknowledgements This work was supported by the Norwegian Cancer Society (grant no. 198040), the Research Council of Norway (Grants 2009-2014) under project contract NFI/R/2014/051 and the South-Eastern Norway Regional Health Authority (2016116, 2019080).

References

1. Haabeth OA, Bogen B, Corthay A. A model for cancer-suppressive inflammation. Oncoimmunology. 2012;1:1146–55.
2. Danese S, Mantovani A. Inflammatory bowel disease and intestinal cancer: a paradigm of the Yin-Yang interplay between inflammation and cancer. Oncogene. 2010;29:3313–23.
3. Zhao M, Gonczi L, Lakatos PL, Burisch J. The burden of inflammatory bowel disease in Europe in 2020. J Crohns Colitis. 2021;15(9):1573–87.
4. Farraye FA, Odze RD, Eaden J, Itzkowitz SH, McCabe RP, Dassopoulos T, Lewis JD, Ullman TA, James T 3rd, McLeod R, Burgart LJ, Allen J, Brill JV, AGA Institute Medical Position Panel on Diagnosis and Management of Colorectal Neoplasia in Inflammatory Bowel Disease. AGA medical position statement on the diagnosis and management of colorectal neoplasia in inflammatory bowel disease. Gastroenterology. 2010;138:738–45.
5. Eaden JA, Abrams KR, Mayberry JF. The risk of colorectal cancer in ulcerative colitis: a meta-analysis. Gut. 2001;48:526–35.
6. Herrinton LJ, Liu L, Levin TR, Allison JE, Lewis JD, Velayos F. Incidence and mortality of colorectal adenocarcinoma in persons with inflammatory bowel disease from 1998 to 2010. Gastroenterology. 2012;143:382–9.
7. Beaugerie L, Svrcek M, Seksik P, Bouvier AM, Simon T, Allez M, Brixi H, Gornet JM, Altwegg R, Beau P, Duclos B, Bourreille A, Faivre J, Peyrin-Biroulet L, Flejou JF, Carrat F, CESAME Study Group. Risk of colorectal high-grade dysplasia and cancer in a prospective observational cohort of patients with inflammatory bowel disease. Gastroenterology. 2013;145:166–75 e8.
8. Lutgens MW, van Oijen MG, van der Heijden GJ, Vleggaar FP, Siersema PD, Oldenburg B. Declining risk of colorectal cancer in inflammatory bowel disease: an updated meta-analysis of population-based cohort studies. Inflamm Bowel Dis. 2013;19:789–99.
9. Stewenius J, Adnerhill I, Anderson H, Ekelund GR, Floren CH, Fork FT, Janzon L, Lindstrom C, Ogren M. Incidence of colorectal cancer and all cause mortality in non-selected patients with ulcerative colitis and indeterminate colitis in Malmo, Sweden. Int J Colorectal Dis. 1995;10:117–22.
10. Wandall EP, Damkier P, Moller Pedersen F, Wilson B, Schaffalitzky de Muckadell OB. Survival and incidence of colorectal cancer in patients with ulcerative colitis in Funen county diagnosed between 1973 and 1993. Scand J Gastroenterol. 2000;35:312–7.
11. Palli D, Trallori G, Bagnoli S, Saieva C, Tarantino O, Ceroti M, d'Albasio G, Pacini F, Amorosi A, Masala G. Hodgkin's disease risk is increased in patients with ulcerative colitis. Gastroenterology. 2000;119:647–53.
12. Jess T, Loftus EV Jr, Velayos FS, Harmsen WS, Zinsmeister AR, Smyrk TC, Schleck CD, Tremaine WJ, Melton LJ 3rd, Munkholm P, Sandborn WJ. Risk of intestinal cancer in inflammatory bowel disease: a population-based study from Olmsted County, Minnesota. Gastroenterology. 2006;130:1039–46.
13. Jess T, Riis L, Vind I, Winther KV, Borg S, Binder V, Langholz E, Thomsen OO, Munkholm P. Changes in clinical characteristics, course, and prognosis of inflammatory bowel disease during the last 5 decades: a population-based study from Copenhagen, Denmark. Inflamm Bowel Dis. 2007;13:481–9.
14. Soderlund S, Brandt L, Lapidus A, Karlen P, Brostrom O, Lofberg R, Ekbom A, Askling J. Decreasing time-trends of colorectal cancer in a large cohort of patients with inflammatory bowel disease. Gastroenterology. 2009;136:1561–7. Quiz 818–9
15. Jess T, Simonsen J, Jorgensen KT, Pedersen BV, Nielsen NM, Frisch M. Decreasing risk of colorectal cancer in patients with inflammatory bowel disease over 30 years. Gastroenterology. 2012;143:375–81 e1; quiz e13–4.
16. Manninen P, Karvonen AL, Huhtala H, Aitola P, Hyoty M, Nieminen I, Hemminki H, Collin P. The risk of colorectal cancer in patients with inflammatory bowel diseases in Finland: a follow-up of 20 years. J Crohns Colitis. 2013;7:e551–7.
17. van den Heuvel TR, Wintjens DS, Jeuring SF, Wassink MH, Romberg-Camps MJ, Oostenbrug LE, Sanduleanu S, Hameeteman WH, Zeegers MP, Masclee AA, Jonkers DM, Pierik MJ. Inflammatory bowel disease, cancer and medication: cancer risk in the Dutch population-based IBDSL cohort. Int J Cancer. 2016;139:1270–80.
18. Cheddani H, Dauchet L, Fumery M, Charpentier C, Marie Bouvier A, Dupas JL, Pariente B, Peyrin-Biroulet L, Savoye G, Gower-Rousseau C. Cancer in elderly onset inflammatory bowel disease: a population-based study. Am J Gastroenterol. 2016;111:1428–36.
19. Jess T, Winther KV, Munkholm P, Langholz E, Binder V. Intestinal and extra-intestinal cancer in Crohn's disease: follow-up of a population-based cohort in Copenhagen County, Denmark. Aliment Pharmacol Ther. 2004;19:287–93.
20. Baars JE, Looman CW, Steyerberg EW, Beukers R, Tan AC, Weusten BL, Kuipers EJ, van der Woude CJ. The risk of inflammatory bowel disease-related colorectal carcinoma is limited: results from a nationwide nested case-control study. Am J Gastroenterol. 2011;106:319–28.
21. Corthay A. Does the immune system naturally protect against cancer? Front Immunol. 2014;5:197.
22. Hooi JKY, Lai WY, Ng WK, Suen MMY, Underwood FE, Tanyingoh D, Malfertheiner P, Graham DY, Wong VWS, Wu JCY, Chan FKL, Sung JJY, Kaplan GG, Ng SC. Global prevalence of helicobacter pylori infection: systematic review and meta-analysis. Gastroenterology. 2017;153:420–9.
23. Linz B, Balloux F, Moodley Y, Manica A, Liu H, Roumagnac P, Falush D, Stamer C, Prugnolle F, van der Merwe SW, Yamaoka Y, Graham DY, Perez-Trallero E, Wadstrom T, Suerbaum S, Achtman M. An African origin for the intimate association between humans and Helicobacter pylori. Nature. 2007;445:915–8.
24. Maixner F, Krause-Kyora B, Turaev D, Herbig A, Hoopmann MR, Hallows JL, Kusebauch U, Vigl EE, Malfertheiner P, Megraud F, O'Sullivan N, Cipollini G, Coia V, Samadelli M, Engstrand L, Linz B, Moritz RL, Grimm R, Krause J, Nebel A, Moodley Y, Rattei T, Zink A. The 5300-year-old Helicobacter pylori genome of the Iceman. Science. 2016;351:162–5.
25. Warren JR, Marshall B. Unidentified curved bacilli on gastric epithelium in active chronic gastritis. Lancet. 1983;1:1273–5.

26. Marshall BJ, Warren JR. Unidentified curved bacilli in the stomach of patients with gastritis and peptic ulceration. Lancet. 1984;1:1311–5.

27. Fiocca R, Villani L, Turpini F, Turpini R, Solcia E. High incidence of Campylobacter-like organisms in endoscopic biopsies from patients with gastritis, with or without peptic ulcer. Digestion. 1987;38:234–44.

28. Niemela S, Karttunen T, Lehtola J. Campylobacter-like organisms in patients with gastric ulcer. Scand J Gastroenterol. 1987;22:487–90.

29. Nomura A, Stemmermann GN, Chyou PH, Kato I, Perez-Perez GI, Blaser MJ. Helicobacter pylori infection and gastric carcinoma among Japanese Americans in Hawaii. N Engl J Med. 1991;325:1132–6.

30. Parsonnet J, Friedman GD, Vandersteen DP, Chang Y, Vogelman JH, Orentreich N, Sibley RK. Helicobacter pylori infection and the risk of gastric carcinoma. N Engl J Med. 1991;325:1127–31.

31. Enomoto H, Watanabe H, Nishikura K, Umezawa H, Asakura H. Topographic distribution of Helicobacter pylori in the resected stomach. Eur J Gastroenterol Hepatol. 1998;10:473–8.

32. Hansen S, Melby KK, Aase S, Jellum E, Vollset SE. Helicobacter pylori infection and risk of cardia cancer and non-cardia gastric cancer. A nested case-control study. Scand J Gastroenterol. 1999;34:353–60.

33. Sasazuki S, Inoue M, Iwasaki M, Otani T, Yamamoto S, Ikeda S, Hanaoka T, Tsugane S, Japan Public Health Center Study Group. Effect of Helicobacter pylori infection combined with CagA and pepsinogen status on gastric cancer development among Japanese men and women: a nested case-control study. Cancer Epidemiol Biomarkers Prev. 2006;15:1341–7.

34. Infection with Helicobacter pylori. IARC Monogr Eval Carcinog Risks Hum. 1994;61:177–240.

35. Uemura N, Okamoto S, Yamamoto S, Matsumura N, Yamaguchi S, Yamakido M, Taniyama K, Sasaki N, Schlemper RJ. Helicobacter pylori infection and the development of gastric cancer. N Engl J Med. 2001;345:784–9.

36. Ford AC, Forman D, Hunt RH, Yuan Y, Moayyedi P. Helicobacter pylori eradication therapy to prevent gastric cancer in healthy asymptomatic infected individuals: systematic review and meta-analysis of randomised controlled trials. BMJ. 2014;348:g3174.

37. Sugano K, Tack J, Kuipers EJ, Graham DY, El-Omar EM, Miura S, Haruma K, Asaka M, Uemura N, Malfertheiner P, faculty members of Kyoto Global Consensus. Kyoto global consensus report on Helicobacter pylori gastritis. Gut. 2015;64:1353–67.

38. Dinarello CA. Why not treat human cancer with interleukin-1 blockade? Cancer Metastasis Rev. 2010;29:317–29.

39. O'Neill LA. The interleukin-1 receptor/Toll-like receptor superfamily: 10 years of progress. Immunol Rev. 2008;226:10–8.

40. Naugler WE, Sakurai T, Kim S, Maeda S, Kim K, Elsharkawy AM, Karin M. Gender disparity in liver cancer due to sex differences in MyD88-dependent IL-6 production. Science. 2007;317:121–4.

41. Swann JB, Vesely MD, Silva A, Sharkey J, Akira S, Schreiber RD, Smyth MJ. Demonstration of inflammation-induced cancer and cancer immunoediting during primary tumorigenesis. Proc Natl Acad Sci U S A. 2008;105:652–6.

42. Rakoff-Nahoum S, Medzhitov R. Regulation of spontaneous intestinal tumorigenesis through the adaptor protein MyD88. Science. 2007;317:124–7.

43. Uronis JM, Muhlbauer M, Herfarth HH, Rubinas TC, Jones GS, Jobin C. Modulation of the intestinal microbiota alters colitis-associated colorectal cancer susceptibility. PLoS One. 2009;4:e6026.

44. Salcedo R, Worschech A, Cardone M, Jones Y, Gyulai Z, Dai RM, Wang E, Ma W, Haines D, O'HUigin C, Marincola FM, Trinchieri G. MyD88-mediated signaling prevents development of adenocarcinomas of the colon: role of interleukin 18. J Exp Med. 2010;207:1625–36.

45. Mager LF, Riether C, Schurch CM, Banz Y, Wasmer MH, Stuber R, Theocharides AP, Li X, Xia Y, Saito H, Nakae S, Baerlocher GM, Manz MG, McCoy KD, Macpherson AJ, Ochsenbein AF, Beutler B, Krebs P. IL-33 signaling contributes to the pathogenesis of myeloproliferative neoplasms. J Clin Invest. 2015;125:2579–91.

46. Haabeth OA, Lorvik KB, Hammarstrom C, Donaldson IM, Haraldsen G, Bogen B, Corthay A. Inflammation driven by tumour-specific Th1 cells protects against B-cell cancer. Nat Commun. 2011;2:240.

47. Lorvik KB, Hammarstrom C, Fauskanger M, Haabeth OA, Zangani M, Haraldsen G, Bogen B, Corthay A. Adoptive transfer of tumor-specific Th2 cells eradicates tumors by triggering an in situ inflammatory immune response. Cancer Res. 2016;76:6864–76.

48. Guo H, Callaway JB, Ting JP. Inflammasomes: mechanism of action, role in disease, and therapeutics. Nat Med. 2015;21:677–87.

49. Dupaul-Chicoine J, Yeretssian G, Doiron K, Bergstrom KS, McIntire CR, LeBlanc PM, Meunier C, Turbide C, Gros P, Beauchemin N, Vallance BA, Saleh M. Control of intestinal homeostasis, colitis, and colitis-associated colorectal cancer by the inflammatory caspases. Immunity. 2010;32:367–78.

50. Allen IC, TeKippe EM, Woodford RM, Uronis JM, Holl EK, Rogers AB, Herfarth HH, Jobin C, Ting JP. The NLRP3 inflammasome functions as a negative regulator of tumorigenesis during colitis-associated cancer. J Exp Med. 2010;207:1045–56.

51. Zaki MH, Vogel P, Body-Malapel M, Lamkanfi M, Kanneganti TD. IL-18 production downstream of the Nlrp3 inflammasome confers protection against colorectal tumor formation. J Immunol. 2010;185:4912–20.

52. Allen IC, Wilson JE, Schneider M, Lich JD, Roberts RA, Arthur JC, Woodford RM, Davis BK, Uronis JM, Herfarth HH, Jobin C, Rogers AB, Ting JP. NLRP12 suppresses colon inflammation and tumorigenesis through the negative regulation of noncanonical NF-kappaB signaling. Immunity. 2012;36:742–54.

53. Karki R, Kanneganti TD. Diverging inflammasome signals in tumorigenesis and potential targeting. Nat Rev Cancer. 2019;19:197–214.

54. Lee JK, Kim SH, Lewis EC, Azam T, Reznikov LL, Dinarello CA. Differences in signaling pathways by IL-1beta and IL-18. Proc Natl Acad Sci U S A. 2004;101:8815–20.

55. Krelin Y, Voronov E, Dotan S, Elkabets M, Reich E, Fogel M, Huszar M, Iwakura Y, Segal S, Dinarello CA, Apte RN. Interleukin-1beta-driven inflammation promotes the development and invasiveness of chemical carcinogen-induced tumors. Cancer Res. 2007;67:1062–71.

56. Hitzler I, Sayi A, Kohler E, Engler DB, Koch KN, Hardt WD, Muller A. Caspase-1 has both proinflammatory and regulatory properties in Helicobacter infections, which are differentially mediated by its substrates IL-1beta and IL-18. J Immunol. 2012;188:3594–602.

57. Haabeth OA, Lorvik KB, Yagita H, Bogen B, Corthay A. Interleukin-1 is required for cancer eradication mediated by tumor-specific Th1 cells. Oncoimmunology. 2016;5:e1039763.

58. Lust JA, Lacy MQ, Zeldenrust SR, Dispenzieri A, Gertz MA, Witzig TE, Kumar S, Hayman SR, Russell SJ, Buadi FK, Geyer SM, Campbell ME, Kyle RA, Rajkumar SV, Greipp PR, Kline MP, Xiong Y, Moon-Tasson LL, Donovan KA. Induction of a chronic disease state in patients with smoldering or indolent multiple myeloma by targeting interleukin 1{beta}-induced interleukin 6 production and the myeloma proliferative component. Mayo Clin Proc. 2009;84:114–22.

59. Hong DS, Hui D, Bruera E, Janku F, Naing A, Falchook GS, Piha-Paul S, Wheler JJ, Fu S, Tsimberidou AM, Stecher M, Mohanty

P, Simard J, Kurzrock R. MABp1, a first-in-class true human antibody targeting interleukin-1alpha in refractory cancers: an open-label, phase 1 dose-escalation and expansion study. Lancet Oncol. 2014;15:656–66.

60. Hickish T, Andre T, Wyrwicz L, Saunders M, Sarosiek T, Kocsis J, Nemecek R, Rogowski W, Lesniewski-Kmak K, Petruzelka L, Apte RN, Mohanty P, Stecher M, Simard J, de Gramont A. MABp1 as a novel antibody treatment for advanced colorectal cancer: a randomised, double-blind, placebo-controlled, phase 3 study. Lancet Oncol. 2017;18:192–201.

61. Fabbi M, Carbotti G, Ferrini S. Context-dependent role of IL-18 in cancer biology and counter-regulation by IL-18BP. J Leukoc Biol. 2015;97:665–75.

62. Oertli M, Sundquist M, Hitzler I, Engler DB, Arnold IC, Reuter S, Maxeiner J, Hansson M, Taube C, Quiding-Jarbrink M, Muller A. DC-derived IL-18 drives Treg differentiation, murine Helicobacter pylori-specific immune tolerance, and asthma protection. J Clin Invest. 2012;122:1082–96.

63. Nishio S, Yamada N, Ohyama H, Yamanegi K, Nakasho K, Hata M, Nakamura Y, Fukunaga S, Futani H, Yoshiya S, Ueda H, Taniguchi M, Okamura H, Terada N. Enhanced suppression of pulmonary metastasis of malignant melanoma cells by combined administration of alpha-galactosylceramide and interleukin-18. Cancer Sci. 2008;99:113–20.

64. Osaki T, Peron JM, Cai Q, Okamura H, Robbins PD, Kurimoto M, Lotze MT, Tahara H. IFN-gamma-inducing factor/IL-18 administration mediates IFN-gamma- and IL-12-independent antitumor effects. J Immunol. 1998;160:1742–9.

65. Coughlin CM, Salhany KE, Gee MS, LaTemple DC, Kotenko S, Ma X, Gri G, Wysocka M, Kim JE, Liu L, Liao F, Farber JM, Pestka S, Trinchieri G, Lee WM. Tumor cell responses to IFNgamma affect tumorigenicity and response to IL-12 therapy and antiangiogenesis. Immunity. 1998;9:25–34.

66. Wong JL, Mailliard RB, Moschos SJ, Edington H, Lotze MT, Kirkwood JM, Kalinski P. Helper activity of natural killer cells during the dendritic cell-mediated induction of melanoma-specific cytotoxic T cells. J Immunother. 2011;34:270–8.

67. Orengo AM, Fabbi M, Miglietta L, Andreani C, Bruzzone M, Puppo A, Cristoforoni P, Centurioni MG, Gualco M, Salvi S, Boccardo S, Truini M, Piazza T, Canevari S, Mezzanzanica D, Ferrini S. Interleukin (IL)-18, a biomarker of human ovarian carcinoma, is predominantly released as biologically inactive precursor. Int J Cancer. 2011;129:1116–25.

68. Fujita K, Ewing CM, Isaacs WB, Pavlovich CP. Immunomodulatory IL-18 binding protein is produced by prostate cancer cells and its levels in urine and serum correlate with tumor status. Int J Cancer. 2011;129:424–32.

69. Carbotti G, Barisione G, Orengo AM, Brizzolara A, Airoldi I, Bagnoli M, Pinciroli P, Mezzanzanica D, Centurioni MG, Fabbi M, Ferrini S. The IL-18 antagonist IL-18-binding protein is produced in the human ovarian cancer microenvironment. Clin Cancer Res. 2013;19:4611–20.

70. Schmitz J, Owyang A, Oldham E, Song Y, Murphy E, McClanahan TK, Zurawski G, Moshrefi M, Qin J, Li X, Gorman DM, Bazan JF, Kastelein RA. IL-33, an interleukin-1-like cytokine that signals via the IL-1 receptor-related protein ST2 and induces T helper type 2-associated cytokines. Immunity. 2005;23:479–90.

71. Tominaga S. A putative protein of a growth specific cDNA from BALB/c-3T3 cells is highly similar to the extracellular portion of mouse interleukin 1 receptor. FEBS Lett. 1989;258:301–4.

72. Onda H, Kasuya H, Takakura K, Hori T, Imaizumi T, Takeuchi T, Inoue I, Takeda J. Identification of genes differentially expressed in canine vasospastic cerebral arteries after subarachnoid hemorrhage. J Cereb Blood Flow Metab. 1999;19:1279–88.

73. Baekkevold ES, Roussigne M, Yamanaka T, Johansen FE, Jahnsen FL, Amalric F, Brandtzaeg P, Erard M, Haraldsen G, Girard JP. Molecular characterization of NF-HEV, a nuclear factor preferentially expressed in human high endothelial venules. Am J Pathol. 2003;163:69–79.

74. Kuchler AM, Pollheimer J, Balogh J, Sponheim J, Manley L, Sorensen DR, De Angelis PM, Scott H, Haraldsen G. Nuclear interleukin-33 is generally expressed in resting endothelium but rapidly lost upon angiogenic or proinflammatory activation. Am J Pathol. 2008;173:1229–42.

75. Moussion C, Ortega N, Girard JP. The IL-1-like cytokine IL-33 is constitutively expressed in the nucleus of endothelial cells and epithelial cells in vivo: a novel 'alarmin'? PLoS One. 2008;3:e3331.

76. Sponheim J, Pollheimer J, Olsen T, Balogh J, Hammarstrom C, Loos T, Kasprzycka M, Sorensen DR, Nilsen HR, Kuchler AM, Vatn MH, Haraldsen G. Inflammatory bowel disease-associated interleukin-33 is preferentially expressed in ulceration-associated myofibroblasts. Am J Pathol. 2010;177:2804–15.

77. Sundnes O, Pietka W, Loos T, Sponheim J, Rankin AL, Pflanz S, Bertelsen V, Sitek JC, Hol J, Haraldsen G, Khnykin D. Epidermal expression and regulation of interleukin-33 during homeostasis and inflammation: strong species differences. J Invest Dermatol. 2015;135:1771–80.

78. Pollheimer J, Bodin J, Sundnes O, Edelmann RJ, Skanland SS, Sponheim J, Brox MJ, Sundlisaeter E, Loos T, Vatn M, Kasprzycka M, Wang J, Kuchler AM, Tasken K, Haraldsen G, Hol J. Interleukin-33 drives a proinflammatory endothelial activation that selectively targets nonquiescent cells. Arterioscler Thromb Vasc Biol. 2013;33:e47–55.

79. Fang M, Li Y, Huang K, Qi S, Zhang J, Zgodzinski W, Majewski M, Wallner G, Gozdz S, Macek P, Kowalik A, Pasiarski M, Grywalska E, Vatan L, Nagarsheth N, Li W, Zhao L, Kryczek I, Wang G, Wang Z, Zou W, Wang L. IL33 promotes colon cancer cell stemness via JNK activation and macrophage recruitment. Cancer Res. 2017;77:2735–45.

80. Zhang JF, Wang P, Yan YJ, Li Y, Guan MW, Yu JJ, Wang XD. IL33 enhances glioma cell migration and invasion by upregulation of MMP2 and MMP9 via the ST2-NF-kappaB pathway. Oncol Rep. 2017;38:2033–42.

81. Wasmer MH, Krebs P. The role of IL-33-dependent inflammation in the tumor microenvironment. Front Immunol. 2016;7:682.

82. Fournie JJ, Poupot M. The pro-tumorigenic IL-33 involved in antitumor immunity: a Yin and Yang cytokine. Front Immunol. 2018;9:2506.

83. Ercolano G, Gomez-Cadena A, Dumauthioz N, Vanoni G, Kreutzfeldt M, Wyss T, Michalik L, Loyon R, Ianaro A, Ho PC, Borg C, Kopf M, Merkler D, Krebs P, Romero P, Trabanelli S, Jandus C. PPAR drives IL-33-dependent ILC2 pro-tumoral functions. Nat Commun. 2021;12:2538.

84. Kienzl M, Hasenoehrl C, Valadez-Cosmes P, Maitz K, Sarsembayeva A, Sturm E, Heinemann A, Kargl J, Schicho R. IL-33 reduces tumor growth in models of colorectal cancer with the help of eosinophils. Oncoimmunology. 2020;9:1776059.

85. Schuijs MJ, Png S, Richard AC, Tsyben A, Hamm G, Stockis J, Garcia C, Pinaud S, Nicholls A, Ros XR, Su J, Eldridge MD, Riedel A, Serrao EM, Rodewald HR, Mack M, Shields JD, Cohen ES, McKenzie ANJ, Goodwin RJA, Brindle KM, Marioni JC, Halim TYF. ILC2-driven innate immune checkpoint mechanism antagonizes NK cell antimetastatic function in the lung. Nat Immunol. 2020;21:998–1009.

86. Taniguchi S, Elhance A, Van Duzer A, Kumar S, Leitenberger JJ, Oshimori N. Tumor-initiating cells establish an IL-33-TGF-beta niche signaling loop to promote cancer progression. Science. 2020;369

87. Park JH, Ameri AH, Dempsey KE, Conrad DN, Kem M, Mino-Kenudson M, Demehri S. Nuclear IL-33/SMAD signaling axis promotes cancer development in chronic inflammation. EMBO J. 2021;40:e106151.

88. De Boeck A, Ahn BY, D'Mello C, Lun X, Menon SV, Alshehri MM, Szulzewsky F, Shen Y, Khan L, Dang NH, Reichardt E, Goring KA, King J, Grisdale CJ, Grinshtein N, Hambardzumyan D, Reilly KM, Blough MD, Cairncross JG, Yong VW, Marra MA, Jones SJM, Kaplan DR, McCoy KD, Holland EC, Bose P, Chan JA, Robbins SM, Senger DL. Glioma-derived IL-33 orchestrates an inflammatory brain tumor microenvironment that accelerates glioma progression. Nat Commun. 2020;11:4997.

89. Bromberg JF, Wrzeszczynska MH, Devgan G, Zhao Y, Pestell RG, Albanese C, Darnell JE Jr. Stat3 as an oncogene. Cell. 1999;98:295–303.

90. Taniguchi K, Karin M. IL-6 and related cytokines as the critical lynchpins between inflammation and cancer. Semin Immunol. 2014;26:54–74.

91. Belluco C, Nitti D, Frantz M, Toppan P, Basso D, Plebani M, Lise M, Jessup JM. Interleukin-6 blood level is associated with circulating carcinoembryonic antigen and prognosis in patients with colorectal cancer. Ann Surg Oncol. 2000;7:133–8.

92. Putoczki TL, Thiem S, Loving A, Busuttil RA, Wilson NJ, Ziegler PK, Nguyen PM, Preaudet A, Farid R, Edwards KM, Boglev Y, Luwor RB, Jarnicki A, Horst D, Boussioutas A, Heath JK, Sieber OM, Pleines I, Kile BT, Nash A, Greten FR, McKenzie BS, Ernst M. Interleukin-11 is the dominant IL-6 family cytokine during gastrointestinal tumorigenesis and can be targeted therapeutically. Cancer Cell. 2013;24:257–71.

93. Musolino C, Allegra A, Profita M, Alonci A, Saitta S, Russo S, Bonanno A, Innao V, Gangemi S. Reduced IL-33 plasma levels in multiple myeloma patients are associated with more advanced stage of disease. Br J Haematol. 2013;160:709–10.

94. Tseng-Rogenski SS, Hamaya Y, Choi DY, Carethers JM. Interleukin 6 alters localization of hMSH3, leading to DNA mismatch repair defects in colorectal cancer cells. Gastroenterology. 2015;148:579–89.

95. He B, You L, Uematsu K, Zang K, Xu Z, Lee AY, Costello JF, McCormick F, Jablons DM. SOCS-3 is frequently silenced by hypermethylation and suppresses cell growth in human lung cancer. Proc Natl Acad Sci U S A. 2003;100:14133–8.

96. Rebouissou S, Amessou M, Couchy G, Poussin K, Imbeaud S, Pilati C, Izard T, Balabaud C, Bioulac-Sage P, Zucman-Rossi J. Frequent in-frame somatic deletions activate gp130 in inflammatory hepatocellular tumours. Nature. 2009;457:200–4.

97. Rutz S, Wang X, Ouyang W. The IL-20 subfamily of cytokines—from host defence to tissue homeostasis. Nat Rev Immunol. 2014;14:783–95.

98. McGee HM, Schmidt BA, Booth CJ, Yancopoulos GD, Valenzuela DM, Murphy AJ, Stevens S, Flavell RA, Horsley V. IL-22 promotes fibroblast-mediated wound repair in the skin. J Invest Dermatol. 2013;133:1321–9.

99. Liao C, Yu ZB, Meng G, Wang L, Liu QY, Chen LT, Feng SS, Tu HB, Li YF, Bai L. Association between Th17-related cytokines and risk of non-small cell lung cancer among patients with or without chronic obstructive pulmonary disease. Cancer. 2015;121(Suppl 17):3122–9.

100. Wu T, Cui L, Liang Z, Liu C, Liu Y, Li J. Elevated serum IL-22 levels correlate with chemoresistant condition of colorectal cancer. Clin Immunol. 2013;147:38–9.

101. Wu T, Wang Z, Liu Y, Mei Z, Wang G, Liang Z, Cui A, Hu X, Cui L, Yang Y, Liu CY. Interleukin 22 protects colorectal cancer cells from chemotherapy by activating the STAT3 pathway and inducing autocrine expression of interleukin 8. Clin Immunol. 2014;154:116–26.

102. Nardinocchi L, Sonego G, Passarelli F, Avitabile S, Scarponi C, Failla CM, Simoni S, Albanesi C, Cavani A. Interleukin-17 and interleukin-22 promote tumor progression in human nonmelanoma skin cancer. Eur J Immunol. 2015;45:922–31.

103. Kirchberger S, Royston DJ, Boulard O, Thornton E, Franchini F, Szabady RL, Harrison O, Powrie F. Innate lymphoid cells sustain colon cancer through production of interleukin-22 in a mouse model. J Exp Med. 2013;210:917–31.

104. Park O, Wang H, Weng H, Feigenbaum L, Li H, Yin S, Ki SH, Yoo SH, Dooley S, Wang FS, Young HA, Gao B. In vivo consequences of liver-specific interleukin-22 expression in mice: implications for human liver disease progression. Hepatology. 2011;54:252–61.

105. Massague J. TGFbeta in cancer. Cell. 2008;134:215–30.

106. Calon A, Espinet E, Palomo-Ponce S, Tauriello DV, Iglesias M, Cespedes MV, Sevillano M, Nadal C, Jung P, Zhang XH, Byrom D, Riera A, Rossell D, Mangues R, Massague J, Sancho E, Batlle E. Dependency of colorectal cancer on a TGF-beta-driven program in stromal cells for metastasis initiation. Cancer Cell. 2012;22:571–84.

107. Lippitz BE. Cytokine patterns in patients with cancer: a systematic review. Lancet Oncol. 2013;14:e218–28.

108. Principe DR, Doll JA, Bauer J, Jung B, Munshi HG, Bartholin L, Pasche B, Lee C, Grippo PJ. TGF-beta: duality of function between tumor prevention and carcinogenesis. J Natl Cancer Inst. 2014;106:djt369.

109. Itatani Y, Kawada K, Fujishita T, Kakizaki F, Hirai H, Matsumoto T, Iwamoto M, Inamoto S, Hatano E, Hasegawa S, Maekawa T, Uemoto S, Sakai Y, Taketo MM. Loss of SMAD4 from colorectal cancer cells promotes CCL15 expression to recruit CCR1+ myeloid cells and facilitate liver metastasis. Gastroenterology. 2013;145:1064–75 e11.

Tumor Infiltrating Lymphocytes in Breast Cancer: Implementation of a New Histopathological Biomarker

13

Giuseppe Floris, Glenn Broeckx, Asier Antoranz,
Maxim De Schepper, Roberto Salgado,
Christine Desmedt, Dieter J. E. Peeters,
and Gert G. G. M. Van den Eynden

Abstract

In this chapter we describe a promising new histopatho-logical biomarker in immuno-pathology/oncology: tumor infiltrating lymphocytes (TILs). The semiquantitative assessment of TILs in breast cancer (and other tumors) is a well-defined histopathological parameter of which the assessment can easily be integrated in the standard examination of biopsies and resection specimens by the (surgical) pathologist. Focusing on breast cancer, we first summarize available evidence on the prognostic and predictive value of TILs in DCIS, ER+/HER2-, triple-negative, and Her2-positive breast cancer. We also describe the correlation between TILs and other biomarkers, the most notorious among pathologists being programmed death-ligand 1 (PD-L1).

Secondly, we describe the efforts of the International Immuno-Oncology Biomarkers Working Group (www.tilsinbreastcancer.org) to standardize TIL assessment (leading to standardized international guidelines), create awareness, and educate pathologists and oncologists. Finally, we briefly introduce new concepts and techniques that will in the coming years be introduced to further characterize the immune microenvironment in tumors and the interaction between tumor cells and inflammatory cells, such as the use of spatial single cell technologies and artificial intelligence. We believe these techniques should be integrated with the use of TILs and other biomarkers in clinical practice, for the benefit of our patients.

G. Floris
Department of Imaging and Pathology, KU Leuven, Translational Cell and Tissue Research Unit, Leuven, Belgium

Department of Pathology, University Hospitals Leuven, Leuven, Belgium
e-mail: giuseppe.floris@uzleuven.be

G. Broeckx
Department of Histopathology, Antwerp University Hospital, Edegem, Belgium
e-mail: glenn.broeckx@uza.be

A. Antoranz
Department of Imaging and Pathology, KU Leuven, Translational Cell and Tissue Research Unit, Leuven, Belgium
e-mail: asier.antoranzmartinez@kuleuven.be

M. De Schepper
Department of Pathology, University Hospitals Leuven, Leuven, Belgium

Department of Oncology, Laboratory for Translational Breast Cancer Research, KU Leuven, Leuven, Belgium
e-mail: maxim.deschepper@uzleuven.be

R. Salgado · G. G. G. M. Van den Eynden (✉)
Laboratory of Pathology and Cytology PA2, GZA/ZNA Hospitals, Antwerp, Belgium
e-mail: roberto@salgado.be

C. Desmedt
Department of Oncology, Laboratory for Translational Breast Cancer Research, KU Leuven, Leuven, Belgium
e-mail: christine.desmedt@uzleuven.be

D. J. E. Peeters
Histopathology, Imaging and Quantification Unit, CellCarta, Antwerp, Belgium

Laboratory of Pathology, AZ Sint-Maarten, Mechelen, Belgium

Human Molecular Genetics, University of Antwerp, Edegem, Belgium

L. A. Akslen, R. S. Watnick (eds.), *Biomarkers of the Tumor Microenvironment*, https://doi.org/10.1007/978-3-030-98950-7_13

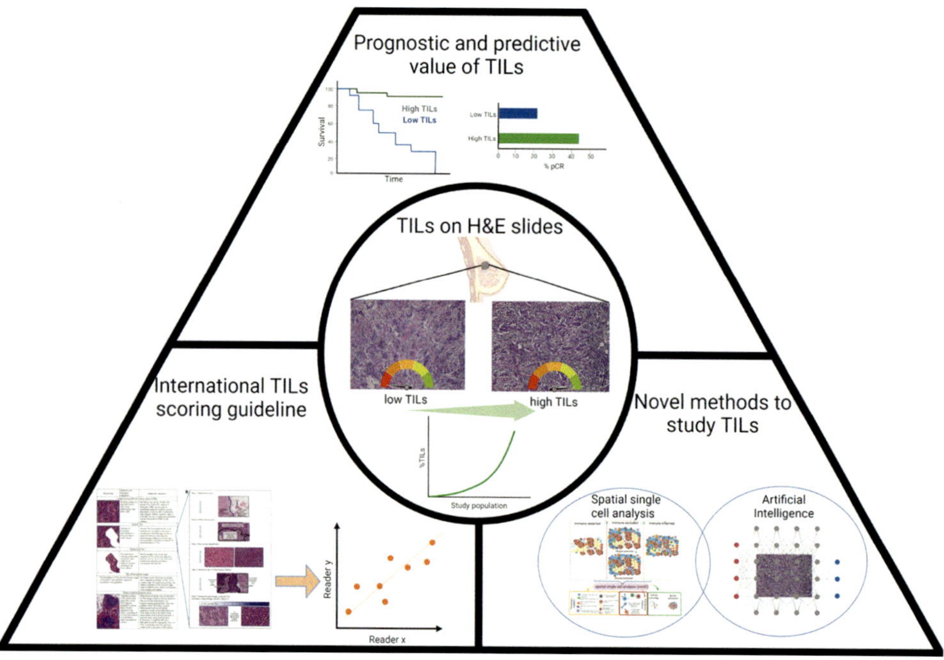

Key Content Graphic. Figure created with BioRender.com

Take Home Lessons

- Tumor infiltrating lymphocytes (TILs) is a continuous marker showing strong positive correlation with survival outcomes especially in breast cancer patients with TNBC and HER2+ phenotypes, reaching level Ib of evidence for these groups of patients. The value of TILs in ER+/HER2- is currently discussed and poorly understood.
- The predictive value of TILs has been extensively investigated, being predictive for pathologic complete response in breast cancer patients treated with neoadjuvant chemotherapy. More recently, the introduction of immune checkpoint blocking therapy has shown promising positive interactions between TILs levels, PD-L1 expression, and response to therapy, strongly suggesting TILs as a potential predictive marker also in this context.
- Standardized international guidelines for the assessment of TILs on routine H&E stained slides are available, showing high grade of concordance among pathologists.
- A learning tool is freely available at www.tilsinbreastcancer.org to teach and assist in the scoring activities in the scientific community.
- The use of spatial single cell technologies and artificial intelligence will be the next step to understand the underpinning mechanisms of immune editing and unravel the interactions between tumor cells and the tumor immune microenvironment.

Part 1: Introduction

Over the last decade, our understanding of the interactions between cancer cells and the different components of the immune system has increased exponentially. Furthermore, we are developing strategies and medications to exploit this complex interplay for treating patients with cancer. The rapidly increasing number of possible targets and therapeutic options also makes it necessary to develop biomarkers that enable selection of the right therapy for the right patients. One of the reasons being that these innovative agents are extremely expensive.

The purpose of this chapter is to describe a very promising histopathological biomarker that can easily be incorporated in the standard assessment by (surgical) pathologists, namely tumor infiltrating lymphocytes (TILs). As further described, TILs can be assessed on a standard hematoxylin and eosin (H&E) stained slide, no special staining or additional test is needed. Although the same assessment method can be used for TILs in almost every tumor type and data show that its usefulness is not limited to breast cancer (BC) at all, the prognostic and predictive value has been most extensively demonstrated in BC. Therefore, this chapter will mainly focus on the use of TILs in the latter.

First, we will give an overview on the available evidence of the prognostic and predictive value of TILs in BC. We will furthermore give an overview of the guidelines as developed by the International Immuno-Oncology Biomarker Working Group on Breast Cancer and on the efforts and initiatives to standardize, teach, and distribute TILs assessment among pathologists. The purpose of these international, academic efforts is to harmonize and streamline TILs assessment and to avoid the origination of an unworkable chaos as we have seen happening, for instance, in the field of PD-L1 assessment, with many different assays and assessment methodologies. In the last section we will shortly elaborate on future evolutions in TILs assessment.

Part 2: Evidence on Prognostic and Predictive Value of TILs

Evidence of the Prognostic and Predictive Use of TILs in Breast Cancer

Depending on the expression at the protein level of estrogen receptor (ER), progesterone receptor (PgR), human epidermal growth factor receptor 2 (HER-2), and Ki-67, BC patients are subdivided into clinically and biologically meaningful surrogate intrinsic molecular categories. Treatment decisions are largely dependent on the combinations of these biomarkers, which show strong predictive value concerning anti-hormonal therapy in ER-positive tumors and anti-HER2 therapy in HER-2 positive tumors. A subset of tumors lacking expression ER, PgR, and HER2 (i.e., triple-negative breast cancers, TNBC) are associated with a poor prognosis and are mostly treated with standard chemotherapy [1, 2]. Interestingly, a growing body of evidence suggests that also in BC the amount of TILs relate to a better prognosis and are potentially predictive for response to chemotherapy [3]. The association with higher TILs and better prognosis in breast pathology was first proposed long time ago in a series investigating pathological features linked to improved prognosis after radical mastectomy [4]. Also, the paradox of the so-called medullary carcinoma of the breast which is a poorly differentiated BC (usually TNBC) associated with high level of peritumoral inflammation and indolent clinical course provided further evidence for this observation [5]. This is in line with the concept that a tumor mass is composed not only by tumor cells but also by non-neoplastic cells forming the so-called tumor microenvironment (TME). Stromal cells in the tumor microenvironment establish intimate interactions with the cancer cells, functioning as an external layer of modulation in cancer progression [6, 7]. Inflammatory cells play a major role in this process, as postulated by the theory of the cancer immunoediting [8]. Three phases, namely elimination, equilibrium, and escape seem to modulate the interactions between cancer cells and immune system. Although not yet fully understood, this process seems to be strongly regulated by the underlying genetic alterations in cancer cells and their capacity to escape or stimulate the immune system [8–10]. Overall, in cancer, high levels of immune infiltrates are a pre-requisite for response to novel therapeu-

tic strategies like immune checkpoint blocking immunotherapy (ICB) and are considered to be a surrogate for high level of antigenicity (i.e., the presence of "foreign" epitopes in the cancer cells to be recognized by the immune system) [11, 12]. However, only a small number of cancers actually display a positive relation between tumor mutational burden (TMB), neoantigens, and CD8+ TILs (melanoma, endometrial cancer, non-small cell lung cancer, colorectal cancer). Breast cancer generally exhibits relatively lower TMB and neoantigens, with no clear correlation with CD8+ T-cell infiltration [13]. This apparent paradox will be further discussed in the section about novel methods to assess TILs.

The International Immuno-Oncology Biomarkers Working Group (see further; also referred to as TILs-WG) has recently issued guidelines to help pathologists in scoring the mononuclear immune infiltrate with a standardized scoring method, based on regular H&E staining [14–16]. The strength of this method resides in its prompt implementation, which can be easily translated into daily clinical practice. Like BC tumor grading which arguably constitutes the most important prognostic tool in breast pathology, the TILs scoring method is based on evaluation of H&E stained slides, making this tool accessible to all pathology laboratories around the world, and it is promising to become a novel standard of practice in breast pathology [17, 18].

TILs are not normally distributed across the BC molecular subtypes and in addition the clinical context may add a further layer of heterogeneity. In older series, about 17% of BC showed dense TILs infiltration within the tumor border irrespective of age, and high TILs were independently positively associated with a better survival only in patients younger than 40, implying strong differences in the interaction between BC and immune system according to tumor biology [19]. Specific associations with mutations or copy number alterations may also influence their prognostic impact [20–23]. A systematic review of 15 studies including almost 14.000 patients provided a global picture of the heterogeneous distribution of TILs across BC molecular subtypes. The median percentage of BC patient showing no evidence of TILs is 16%, while 11% show high level of TILs. The comparison between the specific molecular BC subtypes indicated that a higher level of TILs infiltration is generally observed in TNBC and HER2+ tumors which show a median value of high TILs level in 20% and 16% of the patients, respectively. On the contrary, patients with ER+ tumors showed about three times less frequently high TILs level as compared to TNBC and HER2+. These results were also reflected by the amount of CD8+ T-cells, suggesting a different activation of the adaptive immune system depending on the molecular BC subtype [24]. A pooled analysis of six randomized clinical trials in the neoadjuvant setting performed by the German Breast Cancer Group confirmed in over 3000 patients that TNBC and HER2+ tumors have the highest incidence of TILs as compared to ER+ BC [25]. High TILs levels were defined according to the definition of lymphocytic predominant breast cancer (LPBC), which is a terminology adapted from the hematopathological literature. LPBC refers from a pragmatic point of view to BC for which the relative percentage of mononuclear inflammatory infiltrate in tumor nests or stroma "outnumbers" the tumor cells, the cut-off values most frequently used are 50% or 60% of TILs [26, 27]. Currently no cut-offs are recommended by the TILs-WG, and the TILs scoring should be considered rather as a continuous variable [28]. Nevertheless, efforts made by the TILs group around specific cut-points show excellent level of concordance among pathologists (intraclass correlation coefficient [ICC] ≥0.7), being higher than those reported for established methods like the Nottingham grading system [16, 29].

Prognostic Significance of TILs in Ductal Carcinoma In Situ (DCIS)

Ductal carcinoma in situ (DCIS) is a segmental disease of the terminal duct-lobular units and represents a non-obligate precursor of invasive BC which is historically related to higher risk of developing invasive carcinoma as compared to normal population. DCIS is extremely heterogeneous and treatment options involve usually either breast conserving surgery with or without radiotherapy or radical mastectomy. However, the natural history of DCIS remains poorly understood, posing the question of patient overtreatment and better selection for treatment [30]. For this reason, the search for reliable prognostic markers of recurrence in patients with DCIS has enormously flourished in the past years, including research on TILs. A scoring method to assess the density of immune infiltrates in the periductal stroma has been proposed as well by the TILs-WG [28]. Cases of pure DCIS tend to have less dense immune infiltrate as compared to DCIS associated with micro-invasive focus or compared to invasive BC [31]. Higher nuclear grades, solid growth pattern, and comedo-necrosis are generally associated with higher TILs levels [32]. Comparably to invasive BC, the quantity and the quality of the immune infiltrate in DCIS seems to be related to the protein expression of ER, PR, and HER2. Agahozo et al. described high TILs levels in over 60% of HER2+ and TN DCIS, while ER+ DCIS showed remarkably lower levels of TILs with ER+/HER2+ DCIS showing intermediate levels [33]. Analysis of the qualitative composition of the TILs (e.g., higher levels of FOXP3+ cells, increased number of PD-L1+ cells, and lower levels of granzyme B) suggests that mechanisms of immune editing implicated in immune escape may be involved in the development of invasive BC, occurring as recurrence after DCIS or in invasive BC associated with DCIS [33–35]. However, the DCIS phenotype does not sig-

nificantly influence the composition of the immune infiltrate [33]. DCIS carrying *TP53* mutations and higher levels of aneuploidy seems also to be related to higher TILs levels [34, 36]. Interestingly the proportion of DCIS cases with high TILs varies depending on the scoring method used [33, 37]. This discrepancy might be explained by the location and the density of immune infiltrates which may be extremely variable around ducts affected by DCIS. Therefore, the identification of the portion of periductal stroma that need to be considered for the scoring might be particularly challenging and have a strong impact on the results and their interpretation. Benchmarking of seven different scoring methods for TILs in DCIS has identified that the count of TILs touching the basement membrane of the ducts is the most reproducible and reliable method of all (so-called touching TILs) [38]. However, efforts made by different groups have revealed that scoring histopathological features in DCIS, including TILs, results in fair to moderate interobserver agreement requiring further refinement in the definition and education of pathologists [39–41]. These observations may explain the discrepancy in results reported by diverse independent groups in recent years, when the prognostic value of periductal TILs density was interrogated as prognostic marker for (ipsilateral) breast recurrence. Indeed, at present it remains unclear whether the density of DCIS-associated periductal TILs can predict recurrence [34, 38, 42–45] or not [36, 37, 40, 46] calling for a profound revision and harmonization of scoring methods to be used. Unraveling the interactions existing between DCIS and its periductal inflammatory microenvironment will be important to understand mechanisms of BC immune escape that may contribute to the selection of patients for ICB therapies [35].

Prognostic Significance of TILs in ER+/HER2- Breast Cancer in the Adjuvant Setting

ER+/HER2- BC largely corresponds to the IHC surrogate of the luminal molecular BC intrinsic subtype, as defined by transcriptome analysis. Depending on the proliferation markers, ER+/HER2- BC is subdivided into low proliferative (also referred to as luminal A-like) or high proliferative BC (also referred to as luminal B-like) [47]. Tumor grade, tumor size, and lymph-node status are traditionally used in the adjuvant setting to guide systemic therapy decisions in BC patients with luminal disease [48]. The recent clinical validation of the use of multigene signatures (MGS) has further refined this decision-making process, especially for post-menopausal patients [49–51]. Interestingly, high levels of TILs are supposed to influence MGS results when they are associated with BC that would be allocated to the luminal A-like category by standard histopathology [52]. This observation is perhaps the result of a bias introduced by the higher proliferation level of the TILs, which may influence MGS results in these cases [53]. Data describing how TILs values influences MGS results in patients with luminal disease are limited and conflicting. In one study studying TILs densities in a retrospective monocentric cohort including 344 early BC patients (of which 187 ER+) treated with surgery and adjuvant systemic treatment, TILs level was not prognostic for overall survival and disease-free survival in ER+ tumors despite a negative correlation between TILs value and recurrence scores measured by the MGS Oncotype Dx [54]. On the contrary, another small retrospective monocentric study focusing on luminal tumors in the adjuvant setting showed a weak but statistically significant correlation between continuous TILs values and continuous recurrence scores values measured by Oncotype Dx [55]. However multivariable analysis demonstrated that Oncotype Dx scores was not an independent factor able to predict high TILs in this study, suggesting that tumor immune microenvironment may contribute to prognosis as well in luminal tumors [55]. Similarly, the retrospective-prospective translational analysis of the West German Study PlanB trial found a strong and significant correlation between TILs levels and recurrence scores as measured by Oncotype Dx. A model based on hormone receptor status, Ki67 and TILs levels was found to be predictive of Oncotype Dx results with an area under the curve of 0.80. The authors concluded that the impact of the TILs on prognosis might not necessarily be dependent on the association with proliferation [56]. Interestingly, previous in silico analysis performed on 15 publicly available databases illustrated that the interaction between inflammatory metagenes and prognosis in ER+ tumors may have a dual effect depending on the molecular subtype and proliferation status. In their study, Nagalla et al. found that 23% of highly proliferative ER+ tumors displayed high expression levels of inflammatory metagenes and were associated with excellent distant metastasis-free survival while an inverse relationship was observed in luminal B tumors with low proliferative activity [57]. Indeed, mitotic stress is considered a strong regulator of the immune surveillance in cancer cells [58, 59].

In this regard the integration of BC transcriptome and genome analysis seems to provide a novel twist to this complex background in ER+ tumors. Smid and collaborators found that the upregulation of TIL signatures and better prognosis may be triggered only by specific patterns of somatic mutations (also referred to as mutational signatures) independently from the cell cycle [60]. In their study the mutational signatures 3 and 13 were particularly associated to higher TILs signatures and better prognosis. A recent study performed on TNBC patients with or without germline *BRCA* mutations (which possibly correspond to signature 3) seems to confirm this observation. Indeed, the number of patients with TILs >10% was significantly higher in the patients carrying the mutation as opposed to the wild-type

group, although the TILs infiltrates were globally similar between the two groups [61]. Conversely, a high number of non-synonymous mutations are generally linked to high proliferation, high tumor grade, and poor prognosis [60, 62]. However, specific mutational signatures or other genetic mutations that may trigger TILs (e.g., microsatellite instability) may be rarely encountered in BC with luminal biology (e.g., 86% of ER+ BC did not show the mutational signature 3 in the report from Smid et al.) [60, 63]. Importantly, TILs scores measured on tumor tissue are strongly correlated to the expression level of immune signatures in transcriptome analyses and represent a reliable surrogate of the immune response within a tumor [64, 65]. It remains to be ascertained whether the presence of high level of TILs on histology is a reliable predictor for a specific mutational signature in ER+ tumors and if the LPBC category is a clinically meaningful category in these tumors, despite its inconsistent definition.

Considering the previous observations, it is not surprising that the literature reports conflicting results when it comes to study the prognostic value of TILs in ER+ tumors in the adjuvant setting. Indeed, in a recent systematic review, the percentage of non-LPBC ER+ BC cases was estimated to be almost 95% [24]. Many authors failed in finding significant associations between TILs densities evaluated on H&E stained slides and prognosis in different clinical trials, however no particular distinction was made between luminal subtypes [26, 66, 67]. Others confirmed the lack of prognostic information of TILs in the global population of ER+ BC patients, but in subgroup analysis found a positive prognostic association in the high proliferative tumors (although in [68] this was only borderline) and an inverse prognostic correlation in the low proliferative tumors [68, 69]. In addition, a recent meta-analysis has revealed that LPBC category in ER+ tumors displays worse overall survival but has no effect on disease-free survival in the 4 high quality studies included. However, the authors acknowledge that results should be taken with caution considering the limited number of studies available [70]. Interestingly, special BC types that are usually associated to a luminal phenotype like invasive lobular and micropapillary carcinomas show generally low TILs densities and inverse prognostic correlation [23, 71–73]. On the contrary, male BC, which is characterized by ER expression in about 99% of the cases and displays lower incidences of BC with special histology, shows a positive correlation with prognosis in cases with high TILs levels [74, 75]. The reduced presence of CD8+ T-cells in the epithelial compartment of luminal invasive BC has been advocated as possible cause for the adverse prognosis observed in some studies [76, 77].

Given the highly heterogeneous outcomes observed in the ER-positive disease, it is conceivable that subgrouping breast carcinomas by ER expression alone can be insufficient to describe clinically meaningful associations between outcomes and immune response. So far clinical utility and validity of TILs assessment in ER+/HER2- tumors has been inconsistent and warrants further studies before standard application in the clinic [78].

Prognostic Significance of TILs in HER2+ Breast Cancer in the Adjuvant Setting

HER2+ BC is classically defined by its peculiar strong membranous HER2 expression which is readily visible by IHC on low magnification under the microscope [79]. The strong HER2 protein expression is generally the consequence of the *HER2* gene amplification, which renders HER2+ BC cells addicted to the activation of its metabolic cascade [80]. The major evidence for this oncogenic addition is provided by the dramatic improvement of survival outcomes that have been achieved thanks to the introduction of the targeted anti-HER2 therapy in combination with cytotoxic chemotherapy as standard of care [81, 82]. Nevertheless, HER2+ BC remains very heterogeneous disease that can be driven by different underlying molecular mechanisms depending in first instance on the ER+ or ER- status [83]. Additionally, as illustrated by transcriptomic analysis with the PAM50 MGS classifier, both ER+/HER2+ and ER-/HER2+ IHC BC subgroups can be further divided into four major molecular BC subtypes, although with different proportions. This observation has led to the introduction of a new classification within HER2+ tumors, resulting in the category of the HER2-enriched tumors, which also may benefit from anti-HER2 therapy despite lacking strong HER2 protein expression, for which a different distribution of TILs has been observed depending on HER2 IHC score levels [84, 85]. Based on these observations, one may argue that mechanisms of immune editing may have a different impact on prognostic and predictive outcomes in HER+ BC. For instance, ER+/HER2+ BC generally displays less TILs as compared to ER-/HER2+ BC [66, 86]. Moreover, the ER status seems also to influence survival outcomes and response to treatment in HER2+ BC. However, transcriptomic analysis suggests that when dealing with HER2-enriched tumors, the ER status may lose its relationship with clinical outcomes [83]. In this regard, the study of the expression of T-cell metagenes in BC molecular subtypes indicated a strong positive prognostic correlation between high expression level of the lymphocyte-specific kinase (LCK) metagene and HER2-enriched tumors, irrespective of the ER status [87].

The BIG 02-98 trial as well as the FinHER trial failed to find a positive prognostic association between high TILs level and disease-free or overall survival [26, 66]. On the contrary, Dieci and collaborators found that both intratumoral TILs (iTILs) and stromal TILs (sTILs) were associated with improved OS in two multicentric phase III trials in the adjuvant setting. For each 10% sTILs increase, an 18% reduction in death risk was observed for HER2+ patients (adjusted HR 0.82, 85% CI 0.69–0.96, p = 0.02) [67]. In a selection of 945 out of 3505 HER2+ BC patients enrolled in the phase III N9831 adjuvant study (<50% of the entire cohort), sTILs infiltrates were investigated to study recurrence-free survival in relation to type of systemic treatment (i.e., chemotherapy alone *vs* chemotherapy + trastuzumab). The predefined cut-point at 60% was used to define LPBC on whole slide sections. Of the 945 cases analyzed 94 (± 10%) were LPBC, the majority of the LPBC showed ER+/HER2+ phenotype and displayed less recurrence events as compared to non-LPBC (*n* = 8 vs 154, respectively) [88]. Similarly to what was observed in the BIG 02-98, patients with high TILs level in the N9831 study had improved recurrence-free survival in the chemotherapy arm [26, 88]. However, as opposed to the FinHER study in the N9831, the benefit of adding trastuzumab to the backbone of systemic chemotherapy was not observed; the statistical power to exclude or confirm ER influence was too limited [66, 88]. A retrospective analysis of the NRG/NSABP-B31, a large phase III trial assessing the benefit of trastuzumab in combination with chemotherapy in BC patients with HER2+ disease in the adjuvant setting, revealed that higher TILs values measured on H&E (both semicontinuous and categorical, LPBC = 50%) were significantly associated with improved disease-free survival but were not predictive of trastuzumab benefit. Of note, whole slide sections of about 82% of the patient population enrolled in the trial (*n* = 1581/1931) were analyzed, 100 of which were additionally reviewed by 6 pathologists of the TILs-WG achieving 90.8% concordance between the main reviewer and the 6 additional observers (mean value). Interestingly, high TILs scores showed also strong correlation with groups of patients showing high benefit from anti-HER2 targeted therapy as defined by an 8-gene prediction signature on transcriptome analysis [89]. Intriguingly, the same predictive signature has been recently validated in the B-31 and N9831 study by an independent validation, suggesting that specific immune markers may capture different biological outcomes as opposed to global TILs assessment by H&E [89, 90] Biomarker analysis performed in about 70% (*n* = 866/1253) of the samples collected in the negative non-inferiority phase III ShortHER trial (i.e., 9 weeks vs 52 weeks adjuvant Trastuzumab) showed an improved five-year rate distant disease-free survival for patients with ≥20% sTILs as compared to patients with <20% sTILs (95.7% vs 91.1%; p = 0.025), and it was found that the distant disease-free survival rate was excellent for both treatment arms in patients with higher TILs value suggesting TILs guided de-escalation options for HER2+ BC patients [91]. *PIK3CA* mutations were associated with higher sTILs and provided a favorable five-year disease-free survival in the HER2-enriched tumors as established by PAM50 MGS [20]. More recently TILs have been included in a multivariable prognostic tool that has the potential to inform treatment choices in BC patients with HER2+ disease [92].

Altogether the evidence collected in the adjuvant setting suggests a strong positive prognostic value for high level of TILs in HER2+ BC. Two recent meta-analyses confirmed these results [70, 93]. HER2-enriched tumors are supposed to retain higher TILs level as compared to luminal molecular subtypes assessed by PAM50.

Somatic activating mutations in the *HER2* are rare events encountered in not more than 1–3% of BC causing HER2 activation in an alternative way as compared to BC with *HER2* gene amplification. BC carrying *HER2* mutations are not mutually exclusive with *HER2* gene amplification, correlate more frequently with lobular histology, and are supposed to be a mechanism of endocrine resistance and for anti-HER2 therapy as well [84, 94]. Recent clinic-pathologic review of primary tumors of metastatic BC patients carrying *HER2* mutations revealed low sTILs in nine out of 13 patients and LPBC in one out of 13 patients (median sTILs = 5%; mean sTILs = 15%; LPBC defined as ≥50% sTILs); the distribution across the surrogate molecular subtypes was overall comparable to that observed in the general BC population [95].

Prognostic Significance of TILs in TNBC in the Adjuvant Setting

Almost one fifth of all BC lacks ER, PR, and HER2 expression and is referred to as TNBC. This group of BC is generally characterized by aggressive biological behavior, poor prognosis, earlier age at presentation, and higher risk of metastasis. Although the TNBC definition is clinically meaningful and reflects the lack of specific therapeutic options, this terminology is from the biological point of view highly inaccurate [96]. Therefore, it was not surprising that at the transcriptomic level TNBC could be subdivided into at least four different intrinsic molecular subtypes, including the immunomodulatory or the basal-like immune activated which display a favorable prognosis [97, 98]. Bridging the TNBC gene expression profiles to the clinic represents the main challenge in the coming years (e.g., tumors showing high AR expression by IHC may be considered a surrogate for Luminal Androgen Receptor (LAR) subtype) [99]. Interestingly, as already suggested by Lehmann and colleagues, the immunomodulatory subtype shared transcriptomic features with those described in medullary carcinomas of the breast, which are classically characterized by TNBC status, high inflammatory infiltrates, and good prognosis despite their high grade on histology [5, 100]. TILs assessment on H&E is thus potentially the best surrogate marker available to date to recapitulate the immune-related molecular subtype within the TNBC group, which may be not necessarily seen as distinct entity [25, 101]. What is thus the evidence accumulated so far in TNBC using the TILs scoring method proposed by the TILs-WG?

In the retrospective analysis of the BIG 02-98 about 70% (2009/2887 patients enrolled in the study) of the tumor tissue was retrieved to measure iTILs, sTILs as continuous variable and LPBC as categorical variable with cut-point at 50%; outcomes were overall survival and disease-free survival. Receptor status was unknown in a bit more than 400 patients, leaving 256 patients in the TNBC category. In this subgroup of patients 10% increment of TILs as continuous variable in the stromal compartment was associated with a statistically significant improved disease-free and overall survival with 15% and 17% reduction in risk, respectively. Categorical TILs for TNBC with the LPBC phenotype showed 92% five-year disease-free and overall survival rates, which were comparable to that observed in the luminal subgroup where the TILs had no prognostic significance. Of note, interactions with the type of systemic chemotherapy (anthracycline only *vs* anthracycline-docetaxel) were observed only in the group of BC patients with HER2+ disease [26]. In the FinHER study (*n* = 134 TNBC patients) no association with overall survival was observed probably due to the low number of events [66]. In another retrospective analysis of two large phase III trials in the adjuvant setting including 199 TNBC patients, similar results were observed. The ten-year overall survival rate was 89% and 68% for high TILs and low TILs, respectively (HR 0.44, 95% CI 0.18–1.10, *p* = 0.07), no interaction with anthracycline-based chemotherapy was found [67]. Two independent groups at both sides of the Atlantic Ocean validated further the strong prognostic value of TILs in TNBC. Adams and colleagues measured TILs on whole tissue slides stained by H&E in a selection of 481 out of 506 tumor blocks of TNBC patients enrolled in two phase III studies sponsored by the Eastern Cooperative Group (ECOG E2197 and E1199) [102]. Pruneri and coworkers analyzed TILs scores in whole slide H&E-stained sections from 647 tumors collected in the context of the adjuvant phase III trial from the International Breast Cancer Study Group Trial 22-00 [103]. Both studies showed in multivariable analysis a remarkable similarity in hazard ratio values when sTILs were considered as continuous variable to assess the risk reduction in disease-free survival (HR = 0.90 [95% CI 0.82–0.97;*p* = 0.01] in Pruneri et al., HR = 0.86 [95% CI 0.76–0.98; *p* = 0.02] in Adams et al., respectively), distant recurrence-free interval (HR = 0.83 [95% CI 0.74–0.94; *p* = 0.004] in Pruneri et al., HR = 0.81 [95% CI 0.69–0.95; *p* = 0.01] in Adams et al., respectively), and overall survival (HR = 0.83 [95% CI 0.74–0.93; *p* = 0.001] in Pruneri et al., HR = 0.82 [95% CI, 0.68–0.99; *p* = 0.04] in Adams et al., respectively), confirming the strong prognostic value of TILs in TNBC patients. The LPBC category showed similar results as well [102, 103]. In 2019 a pooled analysis of prospective-retrospective data collected from over 2100 TNBC patients enrolled in 9 large studies performed in the adjuvant setting was published and confirmed the strong prognostic value of the TILs scoring method on H&E, finally reaching level Ib evidence [104]. In this study the average sTILs value was 23% (mean 15%, quartile range 10–30%), lower TILs quantities were significantly associated with older age, larger tumors, more lymph-node involvement, and tumors with lower grade. This pooled analysis confirmed a very strong, statistically significant linear correlation between increment in sTILs quantity and better invasive disease-free, distant disease-free, and overall survival with hazard ratio in the range of 0.83 and 0.86, being very similar to what was observed in the original studies. A test for heterogeneity indicated no or minimal heterogeneity among the studies; iTILs showed similar results. Interactions with the type of adjuvant systemic chemotherapy (anthracycline alone *versus* anthracycline-taxane) were found to be not statistically significant. Further analysis was performed to test the performance of a predefined cut-point in predicting prognosis. To this extent the higher quartile of the sTILs values across the entire cohort was chosen (30%) and tested for the three endpoints. The cut point at 30% remained statistically significant for all outcomes and it contributed significant improved prognostic value in all nodal categories. Further statistical analysis was performed to demonstrate the additional independent prognostic value of TILs quantities as compared to standard clinic-pathological parameters; however, this was true only for the stromal component of the TILs. Based on these results a clinicopathological prognostic model combining classical clinic-pathological features with sTILs values has been made freely available on the website of the TILs-WG: www.tilsinbreastcancer.org [104].

The Role of TILs in the Neoadjuvant Setting, in the Metastatic Setting and in Immune Checkpoint Blocking Immunotherapy

Neoadjuvant Setting

The achievement of pCR provides improved overall survival and better event-free survival but is not validated as surrogate endpoint yet [105]. For BC patients not achieving pCR, the measurement of residual disease remaining in the tumor bed after neoadjuvant treatment entails as well important prognostic information which is better captured by standardized scoring methods [106–108]. Therefore, the identification of reliable biomarkers able to predict pCR may have important implications for the prognosis of BC, especially for those carrying luminal B-like, HER2+, and TNBC tumors and may inform further treatment approaches in postneoadjuvant phase [105, 109, 110]. The current TILs scoring method has been applied for the first time by Denkert et al. as a predictive tool to predict pathologic complete response

(pCR) in patients enrolled in two neoadjuvant anthracycline/taxane-based studies (GeparDuo, $n = 218$, training cohort; and GeparTrio, $n = 840$, validation cohort) in a total of 1058 diagnostic core needle biopsies [27]. In this seminal paper the investigators demonstrated that the percentage of sTILs and iTILs was significantly and independently associated with increased pCR values. When exploring the so-called LPBC phenotype (defined as 60% TILs), the authors observed a significant improvement with pCR rates of 41.7% and 40% in the GeparDuo and GeparTrio, respectively. They concluded that TILs scores were able to identify a subpopulation of patients showing improved response to neoadjuvant chemotherapy and observed that LPBC displayed different histomorphological features as compared to the criteria of medullary carcinoma [27]. Perhaps also for this reason the medullary carcinoma is no longer considered a special subtype of BC in the latest edition of the World Health Organization Classification of breast tumors [18]. The addition of carboplatin to the anthracycline/taxane backbone in the neoadjuvant scheme showed an increase in pCR rates up to 59.9% in LPBC suggesting for the first time a strong interaction between TILs and the type of treatment when carboplatin was added (the odds of pCR increased 3.71-fold in LPBC tumors compared with a 1.01-fold increase in non-LPBCs) [64]. This finding, however, was not further validated in another trial from the same group performed at a later point in time [111]. TILs were found to be a strong and independent predictor of pCR especially in TNBC and HER2+ tumors [27, 64, 111, 112]. Independent confirmation of the predictive value of TILs on the diagnostic pretherapeutic core biopsy is also available from the literature.

In the NeoALTTO study 455 women with HER2+ early breast cancer were randomly assigned to 1 of 3 neoadjuvant treatment arms: trastuzumab, lapatinib, or the combination for 6 weeks followed by the addition of weekly paclitaxel for 12 weeks, followed by 3 cycles of fluorouracil, epirubicin, and cyclophosphamide after surgery. Retrospective review on H&E of 85% ($n = 387/455$) of the diagnostic biopsies collected in this study revealed a non-linear correlation between TILs level and pCR rates, with an odds ratio of 2.6 [(95%CI, 1.26–5.39; $p = 0.01$] when TILs levels were greater than 5%. Importantly, patients with sTILs levels greater than 40% achieved excellent 3-year event-free survival rates regardless of pCR status, being equal to those observed in patients achieving pCR, confirming the strong prognostic value of the TILs [86]. The positive correlation between TILs quantity and pCR was also observed in a multi-institutional study. In this study experienced breast pathologists across Europe tested the reproducibility of the TILs scoring method on pretreatment biopsies of TNBC patients treated with neoadjuvant chemotherapy (anthracycline- taxane+/− carboplatin). TILs scores done on the same set of slides in two consecutive circulations (initially by 16 and then subsequently by 19 participants) demonstrated on multivariable analysis that increasing TILs levels (both as continuous variable and with 10% increment) were predictive for higher pCR rates [113]. Moreover, albeit modestly, the interobserver concordance was improved in the second circulation possibly pointing to a beneficial effect of the training, as suggested by the TILs-WG [113, 114]. Asano and colleagues reviewed retrospectively 177 cases of early BC patients treated in their institution with neoadjuvant chemotherapy and found positive association with increased pCR and improved survival endpoints in TNBC and HER2+ tumors but not in the luminal ones [115]. In the LAR-like subtype TILs values as categorical variable measured on the pre-treatment core biopsy ($\geq 30\%$) were predictive for pCR but association with AR expression levels on IHC lacked statistical significance. Interestingly, the multiple correspondence analysis described in one of the clusters a possible association of high AR expression with low TILs, older age, obesity, and residual disease after therapy, possibly indicating a different response to therapy in relation to AR status, body weight, and TILs [116]. Recently, a large retrospective analysis performed by Hamy et al. described the association between sTILs quantity on pretherapeutic core needle biopsies and pCR by reviewing over 700 institutional cases encompassing all surrogate molecular subtypes. The authors found that pCR was positively associated with higher levels of TILs only in patients with TNBC disease and described a non-linear association. Similarly, the levels of TILs in the pretherapeutic biopsy showed a non-linear improvement of disease-free survival only in the whole population and in the TNBC patients. This effect was additionally related to the type of therapy used, since a statistically significant positive interaction was observed only in patients who received other treatment than anthracyclines $+/-$ taxane or taxane alone (HR = 0.968; 95% CI, 0.944–0.994; $p = 0.014$). No significant associations were observed in the luminal-like and HER2+ subtypes concerning TILs scores in the pre-treatment biopsy [117]. On the contrary, the pooled analysis performed by the German Breast Cancer Group in 3771 pre-treatment biopsies collected from patients treated in six neoadjuvant clinical trials showed a significant association between improved pCR rates and increased TILs quantities, regardless of surrogate molecular subtype. In the whole population the pCR rates were indeed significantly higher in the tumors with high TILs level as compared to those observed in the intermediate or low TILs groups (High$^{\geq 60\%TILs}$ = 44% vs Intermediate$^{11-59\%TILs}$ = 27% vs Low$^{\leq 10\%TILs}$ = 22%; $p < 0.0001$). The magnitude of pCR rates was the highest in the TNBC category, nevertheless the effect of TILs in diverse clinicopathological categories seemed to be the same in all molecular subtype according to a post-hoc univariate logistic regression analysis. When prognostic outcomes were investigated in the 2570 patients of which complete follow-up data were available, the scientists found that disease-free and overall survival were differentially affected by molecular subtype. In univariate analysis high TILs predicted a longer disease-free survival in TNBC and HER2+ tumors, a longer overall survival only in the TNBC subgroup, and a reverse association with overall survival in the luminal category. In the multivariate analysis, the inclusion of baseline features and pCR rates showed that high TILs were no longer associated with better outcomes in TNBC and HER2+ tumor, while the inverse association with overall survival was retained in the luminal tumors. Kaplan-Meier analysis showed similar results. Interestingly, a post-hoc analysis of the survival performed on the surrogate molecular subtypes showed for both endpoints a mixed effect in the luminal category. For instance, high TILs were associated with a shorter disease-free survival in the grade 1–2 tumors (HR = 1.132; 95% CI = 1.04–1.233; $p = 0.004$) as opposed to grade 3 tumors, where high TILs predicted longer recurrence outcome (HR = 0.879; 95%CI = 0.787–0.981; $p = 0.021$) possibly suggesting once again a dual effect of TILs based on proliferation [25, 57, 69]. Specific analysis on ER status in the HER2+ tumors showed no statistically significant difference on both outcomes in the study of Denkert and colleagues [25]. A recent meta-analysis confirms the results from Denkert et al. concerning pCR rates but suggested a publication bias for the results observed in the luminal tumors [70]. While another meta-analysis specifically focused on TNBC studies confirmed, after review of 37 studies, the predictive value of high TILs for achieving higher pCR rates and improved survival endpoints [118].

In the past years, the variation in quantities of sTILs in response to chemotherapy has gained interest, because of the reported retained prognostic value of the TILs in relation to the partial response after neoadjuvant chemotherapy. In particular, the combination of the residual cancer burden (RCB) score and class with TILs may provide additional prognostic information that might be useful to inform clinicians for further therapies [109, 119]. The interest in this type of approach stemmed from initial reports based on small series, in which increasing densities of TILs were observed in relation to increasing level of response to neoadjuvant paclitaxel therapy in core biopsy-resection specimen matched samples and correlated with the level of apoptotic activity [120]. The evidence so far collected is greater for TNBC as compared to the other molecular subtype/surrogate. Dieci et al. performed a retrospective multi-institutional study, where sTILs and iTILs were assessed on a representative H&E slide from the resection specimen post-neoadjuvant chemotherapy ($n = 278$). Chemotherapy regimens were based on anthracycline $+/-$ taxane schemes, and further adjuvant chemotherapy was given to 32% of the patients. High TILs levels were associated with tumor size smaller than 20 mm and negative lymph node status. In multivariate analysis, 10% increment in sTILs were associated with a statistically significant reduction in risk of metastasis (HR = 0.86; 95% CI = 0.77–0.96; $p = 0.01$) and reduction in risk of death (HR = 0.86;

95% CI = 0.77–0.97; p = 0.01). High TILs in residual disease predicted a longer metastasis-free and overall survival 5-year rates as compared to low TILs levels (81.5% vs 46% and 91% vs 55%, respectively). This difference remained significant only in the category of patients with positive lymph nodes +/− ypT2 tumors for the metastasis-free survival endpoint (p = 0.005) [121]. However, no correlations with RCB scores or classes were made. Patients with high TILs in residual disease showed an increase of TILs in the post-neoadjuvant resection specimen as compared to diagnostic biopsy (n = 19) [121]. This contrasted with what is reported by Loi and colleagues in which the matched pre- and post-neoadjuvant specimens showed a reduction in TILs levels associated with residual disease (n = 39/111; p = 0.07). No meaningful associations with survival endpoints were observed based on the TILs changes occurred during neoadjuvant treatment. Nevertheless, TILs in the residual disease post-neoadjuvant treatment did show a linear and statistically significant association with improved relapse free and overall survival also after correction for confounders in the multivariate analysis [122]. In another retrospective analysis Luen et al. matched sTILs pre-treatment on core biopsy with sTILs values post-treatment in 375 BC patients with TNBC disease. pCR cases were excluded from analysis. About 50% of the patients showed either increase or decrease in sTILs after neoadjuvant treatment, globally resulting on average in a non-statistically significant reduction of −3% in the post-treatment specimen. sTILs were statistically significantly inversely correlated with the ypTN and with the stage, however no correlation was observed with RCB class. Survival analysis showed that high sTILs in the residual disease were significantly associated with longer relapse free and overall survival only in patients with RCB class II, but not in the RCB class III. These results indicate that TILs can provide independent and additional prognostic information in patients with RCB class II [123]. Hamy and colleagues provided description of the pre- and post-neoadjuvant dynamics in a more comprehensive cohort of patients involving over 700 cases encompassing all molecular subtypes. TILs level in the residual disease indicated a dismal prognosis only in the HER2+ tumors, while it had no impact on prognosis in TNBC or luminal tumors. Additionally, they also demonstrated a reduction in TILs level following neoadjuvant chemotherapy across the whole study population (mean pre-treatment TILs = 24.1% vs mean post-treatment TILs = 13%; p = <0.001); this difference remained significant also in all molecular subtypes, but the magnitude was higher in HER2+ and TNBC samples. In addition, they found an inverse correlation between TILs level variations and TILs level pre-therapy, while a decrease in TILs was strongly associated with pCR [117]. Similar results have been reported on studies based on computational pathology in a series of over 500 cases, in which the increase of TILs density post-neoadjuvant therapy was negatively associated with the likelihood of pCR [124, 125].

The value of TILs scores as a predictive marker of response in chemotherapy-free schemes of neoadjuvant treatment is less established in the literature and to some extent controversial. Dieci et al. reported on the added value of baseline high TILs scores and high Ki-67 labeling index in predicting response, in a hypothesis generating study in which 77 patients treated with neoadjuvant aromatase inhibitors were enrolled. In this study non-ductal histology was found to be predictor of poor response [126]. A subsequent analysis done on the same cohort of patients showed that high TILs were significantly associated with non-luminal subtypes (26%) with basal-like showing the highest levels when tumors were classified according to the PAM50 MGS classifier. CIBERSORT analysis provided evidence for a more pro-inflammatory background in these tumors, suggesting that these tumors may be better candidate for other treatment strategies [127]. Reduced PR expression in the post-therapy specimens has been found to be related to lack of inflammatory infiltrate post-neoadjuvant endocrine treatment according to a retrospective monocentric study of 132 patients [128]. The dynamics of TILs and relationship with neoadjuvant endocrine therapy was studied in 119 patients treated with neoadjuvant letrozole for 4 months prior to curative intended surgery as part of a clinical phase II study conducted by the Danish Breast Cancer Group (DBCG). Diverse histopathological methods for response were applied and correlated with pre- and post-therapy TILs shifts. The investigators recorded globally a 6% increase in TILs values after neoadjuvant letrozole. Nevertheless, ductal histology and reduction of TILs after therapy were predictive for pCR (regardless of type of evaluation method used) [129]. The increase in TILs was thus associated with poor response being consistent with results coming from transcriptomic analysis indicating resistance to letrozole in ER+ tumors with higher lymphocytic inflammation [130] However, in the CARMINA study the response to aromatase inhibitors was observed following an increase of TILs post-treatment [131]. The increase in CD8+ T-cells and in the ratio CD8+/Treg has been proposed as marker for response in patients treated with endocrine treatment in the neoadjuvant setting [132]. In the HER2+ tumors, novel chemo-free neoadjuvant approaches have been recently tested in BC patients with HER2+ tumors. In these clinical trials, the molecular HER2-enriched subtype as defined by the PAM50 MGS classifier was a strong predictor of response [133]. In addition, TILs have been also studied in this context providing further knowledge about the interaction of the tumor-associated immune environment in response to anti-HER2 therapies in HER2+ tumors. In the neoadjuvant PAMELA trial, 151 HER2 + BC patients have been treated with trastuzumab and lapatinib (+/− hormone treatment depending on ER status) for 18 weeks [133]. This trial provides valuable insights in the dynamic changes of TILs during treatment with targeted anti HER2 therapy, because it provides the comparison between the core biopsy collected at baseline *versus* the one collected at day 15 despite evaluations at the moment of surgery are missing. As already observed in other studies, TILs levels were statistically significantly differently distributed across molecular subtypes as defined by the PAM50 classifier. sTILs at baseline were found to be significantly associated with pCR only in univariable analysis. Combined anti-HER2 therapy induced a significant increase in TILs in most patients at day 15. These induced sTILs were found independently associated with pCR in multivariate analysis. Tumor cellularity was also evaluated at the two points in time and found to be positively associated with pCR in multivariate analysis. A combined score called CelTIL was then derived from both variables and was found to be a good predictor (both categorical and continuous) at day 15 for pCR [134]. The CelTIL score have been recently validated as categorical variable in the NeoALTTO trial, showing better 5-year event-free and overall survival rates in the high CelTIL tumors as compared to the low CelTIL tumors (EFS = 76.4%$^{CelTIL\text{-}HIGH}$ vs 59.7%$^{CelTIL\text{-}LOW}$; OS = 86.4% $^{CelTIL\text{-}HIGH}$ vs 73.5% $^{CelTIL\text{-}LOW}$) [135].

Finally, important patient related conditions may also influence the interactions between tumor cells and its surrounding microenvironment. Obesity is becoming a novel pandemic in the western countries, which is strongly associated with cardio-vascular conditions and cancer resulting in poor survival outcomes. Recently, Desmedt et al. have demonstrated that lipophilic cytotoxic drugs may result in reduced disease-free and overall survival in relation to increasing value of body mass index (BMI), which is probably related to the high distribution volume of these drugs in patients with obesity [136]. Based on these observations, a recent study reviewed 445 diagnostic biopsies collected from TNBC patients treated with neoadjuvant chemotherapy in two large tertiary centers, to study the relations between TILs and BMI [137]. High TILs were statistically significantly associated with pCR in lean patients but not in overweighted patients. The association between TILs and BMI was linear after formal statistical testing and showed a statistically significant interaction between TILs and BMI. A model showing the odds ratio of having pCR was built in function of TILs and BMI. This model clearly showed that the likelihood of having pCR in lean patients with high TILs was higher than that of overweighted patients with high TILs. Survival analysis showed better event-free and overall survival rates only in lean patients but not in overweighted BC patients (HR = 0.22[95% CI = 0.08 to 0.62; *p* = 0.004] vs 0.53 [95% CI = 0.26 to 1.08; *p* = 0.08] and HR = 0.22 [95% CI = 0.07 to 0.70; *p* = 0.01] vs HR = 0.65, 95% CI = 0.31 to 1.35; *p* = 0.25), although in multivariate analysis the interaction term was not statistically significant [137]. These results indicate qualitative differences in the composition of the inflammatory tumor microenvironment according to BMI which considering recent findings may be potentially informative for hypothesis generating trials using ICB therapy specifically in overweighted BC patients [138].

Metastatic Setting

The knowledge about immune and tumor interactions is quite limited and fragmented in the BC metastatic setting. One of the major hurdles in this field of research is tissue procurement, which prevents researchers in most of the cases from comparing matched samples. Indeed, metastasis can be anatomically difficult to reach, sample processing may impair the quality of the material or the tissue available is very limited. Nevertheless, testing metastasis for receptor status is now regarded a mainstay because it may better inform clinicians about therapeutic options and unravel molecular mechanisms of resistance and progression [139]. Given the strong prognostic information showed by the TILs in the early setting it is anticipated that also in the metastatic setting will be retained, providing useful insights in the understanding of the process of immune escape [140].

In general, the tumor microenvironment in metastasis shows lower densities of lymphocytic aggregates as compared to primary tumors, suggesting upregulation of mechanisms of immune evasion by the tumor cells [141–145]. BC metastasis in the lung displays higher TILs level as compared to other metastatic sites, while brain, skin, and liver show reduced TILs quantities [146]. Interestingly, liver metastases show different histologic growth patterns within the liver, each associated with prognosis in BC patients with oligo-metastatic disease [147, 148]. It remains to be ascertained how TILs relate to these histologic patterns and whether TILs can provide further prognostic information. BC patients with brain metastasis, for instance, show improved overall survival in the presence of immune infiltrate, gliosis, or hemorrhages, while necrosis is associated with shorter overall survival [149]. Additionally, transcriptomic analysis performed on matched samples demonstrated a significant downregulation of molecules that are associated with immune activation and upregulation of immune suppressive molecules in metastatic specimens in comparison to primary tumors, supporting the hypothesis of immune evasion in BC metastatic sites [150]. Survival analysis performed in a retrospective study in which metastatic lesions collected from 94 TNBC and HER2+ BC patients were evaluated to study TILs revealed a significant association between TILs and prognosis in both TNBC and HER2+ tumors [151]. Higher TILs in TNBC metastatic patients showed longer overall survival rates, while in HER2+ BC patients an inverse relation was observed [151]. In the Cleopatra study, on the contrary, after review of over 670 samples collected from HER2+ BC patients with metastatic disease, a significant positive association between high TILs and prolonged overall survival was observed. Of note, in this study only a minority of samples were collected from metastatic sites ($n = 58$), and in less than 30 cases, it was possible to make a matched comparison with the primary tumors [152]. Two important considerations can be made based on these findings. First the survival analysis of the Cleopatra study most likely informs more about the interactions existing between the primary tumor and TILs rather than about those observed between metastatic site and TILs. Secondly, the biomarker analysis of this large clinical trials reflects the difficulties encountered in the tissue procurement in the metastatic setting. A possible solution to this problem may come from the establishment of post-mortem tissue donation programs that may provide useful information and unravel the underlying mechanisms of resistance, progression, and immune escape in metastatic BC patients [153, 154]. Several programs of this kind are currently running in no more than 15 locations around the world, including one recently initiated at our institution (University Hospitals Leuven; clinical trial number NCT04531696).

Immune Checkpoint Blocking Immunotherapy

High immune infiltrates together with high antigenicity are considered a pre-requisite for response to ICB therapies. Nevertheless, there seems to be a dissociation between TILs and formation of neoantigens in BC [13]. To date, the assessment of the program death-ligand receptor 1 (PD-L1) by IHC constitutes the only reliable predictive marker of response to ICB therapies. Two companion diagnostic antibodies have been validated and approved in the context of randomized clinical trial to select patients who may potentially respond to ICB therapies. The Ventana PD-L1 SP142 (Medical System Inc., Tucson, AZ, USA) and the PDL1 22C3 pharmDx (Dako North America, Inc., Carpinteria, CA, USA) are currently indicated as the companion diagnostics for selecting advanced TNBC patients for atezolizumab (anti PD-L1 antibody) and pembrolizumab (anti PD-1 antibody), respectively. Additionally, two different scoring methods should be applied to assess expression in BC specimens [155]. Table 13.1 provides a summary of the different scoring methods to be applied according to ICB therapy.

Figure 13.1 illustrates the PD1-PD-L1 interaction and mechanism of action of anti PD1/PD-L1 ICB therapy.

For the SP142 PD-L1 assay (Ventana, AZ, USA), the immune cell (IC) area score with cut-off at 1% has been validated in the context of the phase III randomized controlled trial for unresectable locally advanced or metastatic TNBC (IMpassion130: atezolizumab/placebo + first-line chemotherapy with nab-paclitaxel). A statistically significant longer progression free survival was observed in the intended to treat population as well as in the PD-L1+ population. The overall survival was not improved in the intended to treat population. Despite not formally tested due to the design of the study, an improved overall survival was observed in the PD-L1+ population treated with atezolizumab [157, 158]. The use of the PD-L1 IHC 22C3 pharmDx assay (Agilent, CA, USA) has been validated in the KEYNOTE-355 trial comparing physician's best choice systemic treatment (i.e., diverse cytotoxic agents) in combination with either placebo or pembrolizumab for the first-line treatment of inoperable locally recurrent or metastatic TNBC. The combined positive score (CPS) was used to identify patient populations that may respond to pembrolizumab. The CPS measures PD-L1 expression not only in immune cells (lymphocytes and macrophages) but also on tumor cells. The trial showed a significantly longer progression free survival for patients treated with the combination of chemotherapy+ pembrolizumab as compared to chemotherapy alone and CPS $\geq$ 10 [159]. However, the use of PD-L1 IHC as predictive marker remains controversial given the results obtained in another phase III trial, IMpassion131, which compared first-line paclitaxel with either placebo or atezolizumab in a similar population of patients with unresectable locally advanced or metastatic TNBC. In this trial, which showed negative results, the PD-L1+ status as measured by the SP142 assay did not show effect on outcomes end points [160]. Several factors may be responsible for these results, including treatment choice or the fact that PD-L1 assessment may be a poor predictive

Table 13.1 General overview of PD-L1 assays used in clinical trials and (for validated indications) in clinical practice, their companion staining platforms, associated scoring methods applied in clinical trials and companion anti-PD1/anti-PD-L1 monoclonal antibody drugs across tumor indications. In bold are indicated the drugs and respective companion diagnostic assays and scoring algorithms validated in clinical trials for patients with TNBC

Clone	Manufacturer/Platform	Scoring method	Companion drug
22c3	Agilent Dako/Dako Autostainer Link	TPS (%) = (#TC^{+ve} /total #TC) × 100	**Pembrolizumab**
28-8	48	**CPS = (#TC^{+ve} + #IC$_{Ly/M\varphi}$$^{+ve}$ /total #TC) × 100**	Nivolumab
73-10		TPS (%) = (#TC^{+ve} /total #TC) × 100	Avelumab
SP263	Ventana/Benchmark Ultra	IC$_{proportion}$ (%) = (#IC$_{mononuclear}$$^{+ve}$ /total #IC) × 100	Durvalumab
		IC$_{area}$ (%) = (area occupied by IC$_{anytype}$$^{+ve}$/total tumor area) × 100	Avelumab
SP142		**IC$_{area}$ (%) = (area occupied by IC$_{anytype}$$^{+ve}$/total tumor area) × 100**	**Atezolizumab**
		TPS (%) = (#TC^{+ve} /total #TC) × 100	

TPS tumor proportion score, *CPS* combined positive score, *IC* immune cells, *TC* tumor cells, *Ly* lymphocyte, *Mφ* macrophage, *#* number/cell count

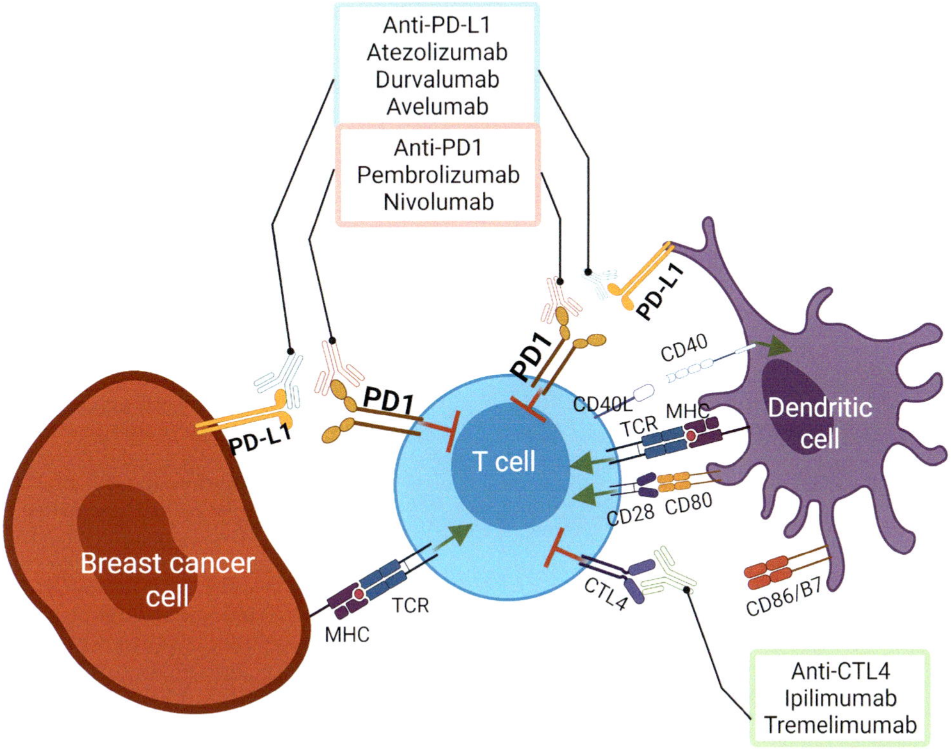

Fig. 13.1 Immune checkpoint localization in tumor cells, T cells, and antigen presenting cells. The figure illustrates the interactions between T cells, dendritic cells, and breast cancer cells. The interaction between check-point molecules results either in stimulatory signals (green arrow) or inhibitory signals (red). In the text boxes are shown the sites of action of the major monoclonal antibodies directed against immune checkpoint molecules, tested in different types of cancer. Treatment with one of the monoclonal immune checkpoint antibody blockers is supposed to block the inhibitory signals preventing activation of T cells and cytotoxic elimination of cancer cells. Figure created with BioRender.com. Adapted from [156]

marker of response [161]. Remarkably, also in the neoadjuvant setting of the phase III KEYNOTE-522 trial, where the addition of pembrolizumab to neoadjuvant anthracycline–taxane–carboplatin-based chemotherapy was studied, pCR rates were significantly improved in the combination treatment arm regardless of PD-L1 status as determined with the 22C3 pharmDx assay assessed with CPS at a cut-off of 1 or greater [162]. Similar results were observed in the phase III Impassion031 trial investigating the addition of atezolizumab to nab-paclitaxel and anthracycline-based chemotherapy in the neoadjuvant treatment of patients with early stage TNBC, suggesting a potentially different role for PD-L1 assessment in TNBC in the primary as opposed to the metastatic disease setting [163]. Additionally, the use of different antibodies may result in the identification of diverse cohort of patients when applied to the same study population. In a retrospective exploratory analysis of Impassion130 trial data comparing three commercially available PD-L1 assays (Ventana SP142, Ventana SP263 and Agilent 22C3 pharmDx) scored with two different scoring algorithms (ICarea and CPS), PD-L1 assays and scoring algorithms were shown to be overlapping but not entirely interchangeable in selecting patients with metastatic TNBC who are most likely to benefit from atezolizumab plus nab-paclitaxel [164]. Further studies are warranted to identify better predictive markers of response in the context of ICB-therapies [165]. Table 13.2 provides a summary of the available evidence on PD-L1 status in phase 3 clinical trials testing ICB therapy in triple-negative breast cancer (TNBC). Table 13.3 shows ongoing phase 3 trials, registered at clinicaltrials.gov.

Different types of therapies, different regimens of chemotherapy, different assays, and diverse types of tissue tested may have been responsible for the heterogeneity and inconsistency of these results. Moreover, in some trials the cut point selection has been directly dictated by the sponsor itself or even changed during the conduct of the trial following a "bottom-up" strategy which recently has received severe criticism [189, 190]. There is an urgent need to better understand the TME and help health care professionals in the search of reliable biomarkers of response to cancer treatment, such as ICB therapies, to improve patient selection as proposed by a joint action of major groups of pathologists coordinated by the TILs working group [191]. However, the evidence accumulated in these trials suggests also that there is a strong relation between PD-L1 expression and TILs in general. When looking at the patterns of PD-L1 expression,

Table 13.2 Overview of relevant phase 3 trials testing ICB therapy in breast cancer with available evidence on PD-L1 status

Acronym/ID *NCT number*	Phase *Enrollment*	BC type	Stage	Study design	Results concerning PD-L1
Triple-negative breast cancer					
IMpassion-130 *NCT02425891* [166]	Phase 3 *N = 902*	TNBC	Locally advanced Metastatic	Arm 1: First-line **Atezolizumab** + Nab-paclitaxel Arm 2: First-line *Placebo* + Nab-paclitaxel	*PD-L1 SP142 IC score cut-off 1%* Improved PFS in PD-L1+ group: hazard ratio 0.62 (95% CI 0.49–0.78, *p* < 0.001) [158] Trend to improved OS in PD-L1+ group: hazard ratio 0.71 (95% CI 0.54–0.94; exploratory, not tested) [167] *Post-hoc analysis PD-L1 SP142 IC 1%, SP263 IC 1% and 22C3 CPS > 1* [168]: Similar predictive value for PFS observed with all assays based on hazard rates for atezolizumab vs placebo with highest median survival benefits observed in SP142 IC >1% patients. **Conclusion on PD-L1:** • **PD-L1 SP142 validated for Atezolizumab + Nab-Paclitaxel in metastatic TNBC.** • **SP142, SP263 and 22C3 PD-L1 assays not analytically equivalent.**
IMpassion-131 *NCT03125902* [169]	Phase 3 *N = 651*	TNBC	Locally advanced Metastatic	Arm 1: First-line **Atezolizumab** + Paclitaxel Arm 2: First-line *Placebo* + Paclitaxel	*PD-L1 SP142 IC score cut-off 1%* [170] No improved PFS: hazard ratio 0.82 (95% CI 0.60–1.12, *p* = 0.20) Negative impact on OS: hazard ratio 1.55 (95% CI 0.86–2.80, trial not powered for OS) **Conclusion on PD-L1: no role of PD-L1 SP142 for Atezolizumab + Paclitaxel in metastatic TNBC**
IMpassion-031 *NCT03197935* [171]	Phase 3 *N = 324*	TNBC	Early BC	Arm 1: Neoadjuvant **Atezolizumab** + chemotherapy Arm 2: Neoadjuvant *Placebo* + chemotherapy	*PD-L1 SP142 IC score cut-off 1%* [163] Improved pCR rate for Atezolizumab arm (58% vs 41%, *p* = 0.0044) No difference in pCR rate for PD-L1 positive vs negative • PD-L1+: 69% vs 49%, diff. 20% (95% CI 6–27%, *p* = 0.021, not significant). • PD-L1-: 48% vs 34%, diff. 13% (95% CI 4–35%). Trial not powered for EFS, DFS, or OS and results are immature **Conclusion on PD-L1: Role of PD-L1 SP142 for Atezolizumab in early TNBC not demonstrated (similar to KEYNOTE-522)**
KEYNOTE-119 *NCT02555657* [172]	Phase 3 *N = 622*	TNBC	Locally advanced Metastatic	Arm 1: Pembrolizumab Arm 2: chemotherapy	*PD-L1 22C3 CPS cut-off 10* [173] No significant improvement of OS: hazard ratio 0·78 (95% CI 0·57–1·06, *p* = 0·057) PFS is not a primary endpoint *PD-L1 22C3 CPS cut-off 1* [173] No significant improvement of OS: hazard ratio: 0·86 (95% CI 0·69–1·06, *p* = 0·073) PFS is not a primary endpoint **Conclusion on PD-L1: Role of PD-L1 22C3 not demonstrated for Pembrolizumab monotherapy in metastatic TNBC**

Table 13.2 (continued)

Acronym/ID NCT number	Phase Enrollment	BC type	Stage	Study design	Results concerning PD-L1
KEYNOTE-355 NCT02819518 [174]	Phase 3 N = 882	TNBC	Locally advanced Metastatic	Arm 1: First-line **Pembrolizumab** + chemotherapy Arm 2: First-line *Placebo* + chemotherapy	*PD-L1 22C3 CPS cut-off 10* [159] Improved PFS in PD-L1+ group: hazard ratio 0.65 (95% CI 0.49–0.86, p = 0.0012) OS assessment ongoing *PD-L1 22C3 CPS cut-off 1* [159] Improved PFS in PD-L1+ group: hazard ratio 0.74 (95% CI 0.61–0.90, p = 0.0014, not significant) OS assessment ongoing **Conclusion on PD-L1:** • **Role of PD-L1 22C3 demonstrated for Pembrolizumab in metastatic TNBC** • **Significant improvement of PFS from cut-off CPS 10.**
KEYNOTE-522 NCT03036488 [175]	Phase 3 N = 1174	TNBC	Neoadjuvant	Arm 1: Neoadjuvant **Pembrolizumab** + Chemotherapy and adjuvant **Pembrolizumab** Arm 2: Neoadjuvant *Placebo* + Chemotherapy and adjuvant *Placebo*	*PD-L1 22C3 CPS cut-off 1/10* [162] Improved pCR rate for Pembrolizumab arm (64.8% vs 51.2%, p < 0.001) No difference in pCR rate for PD-L1 positive vs negative • PD-L1+: 68.9% vs 54.9%, diff. 14.2% (95% CI 5.3–23.1%) • PD-L1−: 45.3% vs 30.3%, diff. 18.3% (95% CI 3.3–36.8%) **Conclusion on PD-L1: Role of PD-L1 22C3 for Pembrolizumab in early TNBC not demonstrated (similar to IMpassion-030)**

it has been observed that PD-L1 expression in BC is predominant in immune cells rather than in tumor cells [165, 192]. In addition, evidence coming from mouse experiments suggests that a sufficient T cell infiltration is essential for response to PD-L1 blockade [193]. In general, high levels of TILs are strongly related to high PD-L1 expression, suggesting that TILs may be a useful surrogate for activated cytotoxic T cells. Early biomarkers of response to ICB have been investigated in the the phase 0, window of opportunity trial, Biokey. In this study, a single dose of 200 mg Pembrolizumab was administered to 54 patients in the window between time of diagnosis and surgery, either in the adjuvant or in the neoadjuvant setting. All molecular subtypes were allowed. Fresh tumor tissue and blood were collected from these patients before and 6–14 days after pembrolizumab administration. In the post-treatment samples after one single administration of pembrolizumab, significant clonotype changes in the T-cells and rearrangement of the T-cell receptor were observed, suggesting activity of the drug even after one single dose [194]. Importantly, these changes were also associated with a large shift in TILs abundancy. Notably, these results were in line with the results described in the KEYNOTE-173, in which after one dose of single-agent pembrolizumab, TILs count increased significantly as compared to baseline values, predicting pCR. In this study, high levels of PD-L1 expression and TILs were generally related to higher rates of pCR. However, because of the lack of a control arm without pembrolizumab the predictive role of TILs remains uncertain in this study [11]. In the KEYNOTE-086 patients defined as responders based on the overall response rate under pembrolizumab showed greater levels of sTILs as compared to non-responders [143, 195]. The KEYNOTE-119 trial suggested a potential role of sTILs in predicting response to pembrolizumab in a cohort of heavily pre-treated advanced TNBC patients. In this study, sTILs, both continuous and categorical with a cutoff at 5%, were significantly associated with all clinical outcomes only in the immunotherapy arm [173]. In the biomarker analysis of the IMPASSION-130 study, tumors considered as TILs+ (i.e., with a predefined cut point ≥10% sTILs; n = 284/892) were also PD-L1+ (i.e., IC score ≥ 1%) in almost 67% of the cases (n = 190/284) showing a statistically significant correlation. In the comparator arm without Atezolizumab, sTILs+ tumors did not influence the survival outcomes. Only patients exhibiting TILs+ and PD-L1 expression showed the longest improvement in progression free survival, leading to the conclusion that sTILs do not provide additional predictive value beyond that observed with PD-L1+ in patients under ICB therapy [196]. Conversely based on the analysis of the hazard ratios of benefit to atezolizumab one can speculate that in the absence of access to a PD-L1 assay, stromal TILs values of >10% assessed on H&E are able to identify a (smaller) subgroup of patients deriving benefit from ICB therapy with Atezolizumab. In a phase I/II trial testing the efficacy of the

Table 13.3 Overview of ongoing phase 3 trials testing ICB therapy in breast cancer with available evidence on PD-L1 status

Acronym/ID *NCT number*	Phase *Enrollment*	BC type	Stage	Study design	Results concerning PD-L1
Triple-negative breast cancer					
EL1SSAR *NCT04148911* [176]	Phase 3 *N = 180*	TNBC	Locally advanced Metastatic	Arm 1: **Atezolizumab** + Nab-Paclitaxel Arm 2: *Placebo* + Nab-Paclitaxel	*No results available yet (October 2024)*
GeparDouze *NCT03281954* [177]	Phase 3 *N = 1520*	TNBC	Early BC	Arm 1: Neoadjuvant chemotherapy + **Atezolizumab** followed by adjuvant **Atezolizumab** Arm 2: Neoadjuvant chemotherapy + *Placebo* followed by adjuvant *Placebo*	*No results available yet (December 2023)*
KEYLYNK-009 *NCT04191135* [178]	Phase 3 *N = 932*	TNBC	Early BC	Arm 1: Induction **Pembrolizumab** + chemotherapy followed by Olaparib + **Pembrolizumab** Arm 2: Induction **Pembrolizumab** + chemotherapy followed by chemotherapy + **Pembrolizumab**	*No results available yet (January 2026)*
IMpassion-132 *NCT03371017* [179]	Phase 3 *N = 572*	TNBC	Locally advanced Metastatic	Arm 1: **Atezolizumab** + chemotherapy Arm 2: *Placebo* + chemotherapy	*No results available yet (January 2023)*
IMpassion-030 *NCT03498716* [180]	Phase 3 *N = 2300*	TNBC	Early BC	Arm 1: Adjuvant **Atezolizumab** + Anthracycline/Taxane-Based Chemotherapy Arm 2: Adjuvant *Placebo* + Anthracycline/Taxane-Based Chemotherapy	*No results available yet (January 2022)*
NeoTRIPaPDL1 *NCT02620280* [181]	Phase 3 278	TNBC	Early BC	Arm 1: **Atezolizumab** + Carboplatin + Nab-Paclitaxel Arm 2: *Placebo* + Carboplatin + Nab-Paclitaxel	*Failed/No results available yet?*
SHR-1210-III-318 *NCT04335006* [182]	Phase 3 *N = 780*	TNBC	Locally advanced Metastatic	Arm 1: **Camrelizumab** + Nab-paclitaxel + Apatinib Arm 2: **Camrelizumab** + Nab-paclitaxel Arm 3: *Placebo* + Nab-paclitaxel	*No results available yet (January 2025)*
SHR1210-III-322 *NCT04613674* [183]	Phase 3 *N = 581*	TNBC	Early BC	Arm 1: Neoadjuvant **Camrelizumab** + chemotherapy Arm 2: Neoadjuvant *Placebo* + chemotherapy	*No results available yet (July 2023)*
TORCHLIGHT *NCT04085276* [184]	Phase 3 *N = 660*	TNBC	Locally advanced Metastatic	Arm 1: All lines Toripalimab + Nab-Paclitaxel Arm 2: All lines Placebo + Nab-Paclitaxel	*No results available yet (February 2022)*
HER2-amplified breast cancer					
IMpassion-050 *NCT03726879* [185]	Phase 3 *N = 454*	HER2 + BC	Early BC	Arm 1: Neoadjuvant Doxorubicin + cyclophosphamide + **Atezolizumab** followed by paclitaxel + Trastuzumab + Pertuzumab Arm 2: Neoadjuvant Doxorubicin + cyclophosphamide + *Placebo* followed by paclitaxel + Trastuzumab + Pertuzumab	*No results available yet (February 2021?)*
KATE3 *NCT04740918* [186]	Phase 3 *N = 350*	HER2+ BC	Locally advanced Metastatic	Arm 1: Trastuzumab Emtansine + **Atezolizumab** Arm 2: Trastuzumab Emtansine + *Placebo*	*No results available yet (May 2024)*
ER-positive HER2-negative breast cancer					
AMBITION *NCT04732598* [187]	Phase 3 *N = 280*	ER+/HER2- BC	Locally advanced Metastatic	Arm 1: Bevacizumab + Paclitaxel + **Atezolizumab** Arm 2: Bevacizumab + Paclitaxel + *Placebo*	*No results available yet (June 2025)*
KEYNOTE-756 *NCT03725059* [188]	Phase 3 *N = 1140*	ER+/HER2- BC	Early BC	Arm 1: Pembrolizumab + neoadjuvant chemotherapy + adjuvant endocrine therapy Arm 2: Placebo + neoadjuvant chemotherapy + adjuvant endocrine therapy	*No results available yet (January 2031)*

anti PD-1 antibody durvalumab in the neoadjuvant setting of TNBC patients, higher levels of PD-L1 expression by IHC (Ventana SP263 assay) were numerically associated with higher pCR rates as compared to PD-L1 negative tumors under ICB therapy. However, this difference was statistically not significant. On the opposite high stromal TILs by H&E were statistically significantly associated with higher pCR rates under ICB therapy. Higher TILs were also associated with higher PD-L1 expression levels [197]. Table 13.4 provides a summary of the current evidence of the potential clinical utility of TILs in BC patients treated with ICB therapies.

Table 13.4 Overview of clinical trials concerning ICB therapy in which sTILs are investigated

Acronym/ID NCT number	Phase Enrollment	BC type	Stage	Study design	Nature testing	sTIL cut-off	Results concerning sTIL
IMpassion-130 NCT02425891	Phase 3 N = 900	TNBC	Locally advanced Metastatic	*Arm 1*: First-line **Atezolizumab** + Nab-paclitaxel *Arm 2*: First-line *Placebo* + Nab-paclitaxel	*Retrospective*	10%	*sTIL in post-hoc biomarker analysis* [198] sTIL positive samples are associated with PD-L1 expression (Fisher's exact test, $p < 0.001$) Combo of sTIL positive and PD-L1 expression showed best improvement of PFS sTIL $\geq$10% alone (regardless of PD-L1 status) still predictive for PFS benefit of atezolizumab **Conclusion on sTIL: sTIL $\geq$ 10% predictive for benefit of atezolizumab as single marker or combined with PD-L1 testing.**
KEYNOTE-119 NCT02555657	Phase 3 N = 622	TNBC	Locally advanced Metastatic	*Arm 1*: Pembrolizumab *Arm 2*: chemotherapy	*Retrospective*	5% (median)	*TIL continuous percentage* [199] TIL levels are higher in responders than in non-responders (significant) TIL associated with all clinical outcomes ($p < 0.05$) Improved overall survival: hazard ratio 0.75 (95% CI0.59–0.96, $p = 0.0001$) TIL vs CPS: moderate correlation (0.45); multivariate analysis showed independent predictive value **Conclusion on sTIL: high sTIL levels are associated with better clinical outcome in case of Pembrolizumab therapy**
KEYNOTE-173 NCT02819518	Phase 1b N = 882	TNBC	Early BC	6 cohorts of neoadjuvant regimes with • Pembrolizumab. • (Nab-)Paclitaxel. • Carboplatin. • Doxorubicin. • Cyclophosphamide.	Prospective	/	*sTIL continuous percentage* [11] Trend toward Increase in sTIL after first administration of pembrolizumab High sTIL pre-treatment predicts pCR: 40% (95%CI 10–75%) vs 10% (95%CI 5–38%), $p = 0.0091$ Increase in sTIL on-treatment predicts pCR: 65% (95%CI 5–86%) vs 25% (95%CI 3–60%), $p = 0.0097$ sTIL and PD-L1 22C3 expression are significantly correlated: pre-treatment ρ 0.622 ($p < 0.0001$), on-treatment ρ 0.626 ($p < 0.0001$) **Conclusion on sTIL:** **• sTIL and on-treatment sTIL increase help identify responders,** **• sTILs are correlated with PD-L1 expression,** **• Unclear if sTIL and PD-L1 expression are independent predictive or prognostic biomarkers.**
KEYNOTE-086 NCT03036488	Phase 2 N = 170	TNBC	Locally advanced Metastatic	*Cohort A*: **Pembrolizumab** monotherapy, any PD-L1 expression, previously treated *Cohort B*: **Pembrolizumab** monotherapy, PD-L1 positive, previously treated	Retrospective	Median Cohort A: 17.5% Cohort B: 5%	*sTIL dichotomized by median* [200] Responders have higher levels of sTIL compared to non-responders: 10% (95%CI 7.5–25%) vs 5% (95%CI 1–10%) Improved ORR for TIL more than median: odds ratio 1.26 (95% CI 1.03–1.55, $p = 0.01$) Improved DCR: odds ratio 1.22 (95% CI 1.02–1.46, $p = 0.01$) PD-L1 22C3 is significantly correlated with sTIL% ($\rho = 0.4962$, $p < 0.001$) **Conclusion on sTIL: sTIL can help identify metastatic TNBC amenable for pembrolizumab monotherapy**

(continued)

Table 13.4 (continued)

Acronym/ID NCT number	Phase Enrollment	BC type	Stage	Study design	Nature testing	sTIL cut-off	Results concerning sTIL
Panacea NCT02129556	Phase 1b-2	HER2	Locally advanced Metastatic	Trastuzumab + **Pembrolizumab**	Retrospective	Continuous	*sTIL continuous percentage* [142] Correlation with ORR ($p = 0.006$) Correlation with DCR ($p = 0.0006$) **Conclusion on sTIL: sTIL levels are associated with ORR and DCR**
KATE-2 NCT02924883	Phase 2	HER2	Locally advanced Metastatic	*Arm 1:* **Atezolizumab** + TDM1 *Arm 2: Placebo* + TDM1	Retrospective	5%	*sTIL dichotomized by cut-off* [201] High sTIL associated with improved PFS: hazard ratio 1.43 (95% CI 0.51–4.01) vs 0.55 (95% CI 0.26–1.12) **Conclusion on sTIL: high sTIL levels are associated with better clinical outcome in case of Atezolizumab + T-DM1 therapy**
GeparNuevo NCT02685059	Phase 2	TNBC	Neoadjuvant	*Arm 1:* **Durvalumab** followed by **Durvalumab** + Nab-Paclitaxel, followed by **Durvalumab** + Epirubicin + Cyclophosphamide *Arm 2: Placebo* followed by *Placebo* + Nab-Paclitaxel, followed by *Placebo* + Epirubicin + Cyclophosphamide	Retrospective	10% 60%	*sTIL dichotomized by cut-offs* [202] High sTIL associated with improved pCR rate: OR 1.23 (95% CI 1.04–1.6, $p = 0.019$) vs OR = 1.39 (95% CI 1.12–1.74, $p = 0.003$) Pre-treatment sTIL not predictive for Durvalumab benefit Increase in sTIL on-treatment associated with Durvalumab benefit **Conclusion on sTIL:** **• high sTIL levels are associated with improved pCR rate regardless of Durvalumab benefit,** **• Increase in on-treatment sTIL associated with Durvalumab benefit.**
NeoTRIPaPDL1 NCT02620280	Phase 3	TNBC	Neoadjuvant	*Arm 1:* **Atezolizumab** + Carboplatinum + Nab-paclitaxel *Arm 2: Placebo* + Carboplatinum + Nab-paclitaxel	Retrospective	40%	*sTIL dichotomized by cut-off* [203] High sTIL associated with improved pCR rate: • Atezolizumab arm: pCR rate 71.43% vs. 28.07% ($p = 0.001$). • Placebo arm: pCR rate 63.16% vs. 33.90% ($p = 0.009$). **Conclusion on sTIL: high sTIL levels are associated with higher pCR rates**
GIADA NCT04659551	Phase 2	Luminal B	Neoadjuvant	Epirubicin + Cyclophosphamide followed by endocrine therapy + **Nivolumab**	Retrospective	Continuous	*sTIL continuous percentage* [204] sTIL levels associated with pCR rates ($p = 0.001$) **Conclusion on sTIL: sTIL levels are associated with pCR rates**

More recently ICB therapy has been tested also in HER2+ and luminal BC. In the PANACEA study which included advanced HER2+ BC patients a correlation between PD-L1+ and higher level of TILs has been observed in patients showing objective response as well as in those with stable disease. The lack of a control arm prevents from drawing final conclusions about the role of TILs as predictive marker of response [142]. In the KATE2 trial, the combination of either TDM1 + placebo or TDM1 + atezolizumab showed only borderline significant association between higher TILs and benefit from the combination therapy [201]. In the GIADA trial 43 luminal-B-like early BC patients were randomized to receive, in the neoadjuvant setting, anthracycline-based induction chemotherapy followed by the combination of nivolumab plus endocrine therapy. Higher level of sTILs was associated with pCR, while cytotoxic chemotherapy induced increase in TILs value, increase in cytotoxic T cells, and decrease in regulatory T cell in the post-treatment samples as compared to baseline [204].

Part 3: Implementation of International TIL Scoring Guidelines

Summary of the Scoring Guidelines

As mentioned above, the most widely spread methodology to assess TILs has been developed and harmonized by the founders of the TILs-WG. This international group of academic pathologists in collaboration with expert clinical oncologists, scientists, computational pathology experts, and statisticians has set up an appropriate framework for adoption of well-validated immuno-oncology biomarkers in daily and clinical trial practice, focusing mostly on TILs. It currently has over 600 members, most of them anatomic pathologists, from 43 different countries, across 6 continents. The TILs-WGs website—www.tilsinbreastcancer.org—has had nearly 30,000 visitors so far. The wide global reach of the TILs-WG enables it to understand all different viewpoints on immuno-oncology biomarkers across the world. All authors that contributed to this chapter are member of this working group.

On behalf of the TILs-WG, Salgado et al. published in 2014 in Annals of Oncology this methodology and how it has been developed [14]. Table 13.5 lists these guidelines.

The TILs in these guidelines refer to stromal tumor infiltrating lymphocytes (sTILs). sTILs are located in the tumor stroma between carcinoma cells and are not in direct contact with these carcinoma cells. This is in contrast to intratumoral TILs (iTILs), which are located within the tumor nests and interact directly with the carcinoma cells. Irrespective of the biological significance of both types of TILs, sTILs seem to be more relevant for histological diagnostic purposes at the moment. sTILs are more numerously present in tumors, less

Table 13.5 Guidelines for assessment of tumor infiltrating lymphocytes (TILs) in breast, according to the International Immuno-Oncology Biomarker Working Group on Breast Cancer (14, By permission of Oxford University Press on behalf of the European Society for Medical Oncology)

1   TILs should be reported for the stromal compartment (= % sTILs). The denominator used to determine the % sTILs is the area of stromal tissue (i.e., area occupied by mononuclear inflammatory cells over total intratumoral stromal area), not the number of stromal cells (i.e., fraction of total stromal nuclei that represent mononuclear inflammatory cell nuclei).

2   TILs should be evaluated within the borders of the invasive tumor.

3   Exclude TILs outside of the tumor border and around DCIS and normal lobules.

4   Exclude TILs in tumor zones with crush artifacts, necrosis, regressive hyalinization as well as in the previous core biopsy site.

5   All mononuclear cells (including lymphocytes and plasma cells) should be scored, but polymorphonuclear leukocytes are excluded.

6   One section (4–5 μm, magnification ×200–400) per patient is currently considered to be sufficient.

7   Full sections are preferred over biopsies whenever possible. Cores can be used in the pretherapeutic neoadjuvant setting; currently no validated methodology has been developed to score TILs after neoadjuvant treatment.

8   A full assessment of average TILs in the tumor area by the pathologist should be used. Do not focus on hotspots.

9   The working group's consensus is that TILs may provide more biological relevant information when scored as a continuous variable, since this will allow more accurate statistical analyses, which can later be categorized around different thresholds. However, in daily practice, most pathologists will rarely report for example 13.5% and will round up to the nearest 5%–10%, in this example thus 15%. Pathologist should report their scores in as much detail as the pathologist feels comfortable with.

10   TILs should be assessed as a continuous parameter. The percentage of sTILs is a semiquantitative parameter for this assessment, for example, 80% sTILs means that 80% of the stromal area shows a dense mononuclear infiltrate. For assessment of percentage values, the dissociated growth pattern of lymphocytes needs to be considered. Lymphocytes typically do not form solid cellular aggregates; therefore, the designation "100% sTILs" would still allow some empty tissue space between the individual lymphocytes.

11   No formal recommendation for a clinically relevant TIL threshold(s) can be given at this stage. The consensus was that a valid methodology is currently more important than issues of thresholds for clinical use, which will be determined once a solid methodology is in place. Lymphocyte predominant breast cancer can be used as a descriptive term for tumors that contain "more lymphocytes than tumor cells." However, the thresholds vary between 50% and 60% stromal lymphocytes.

variably dispersed and more easily to appreciate on H&E-stained slides, without the use of additional techniques, such as immunohistochemistry or immunofluorescence. These are important advantages for its use as an easy-to-assess and reproducible histopathological tumor parameter. Figure 13.2, adapted from Salgado et al. [14], illustrates the difference between sTILs, iTILs, and other types of lymphoid infiltrates

a

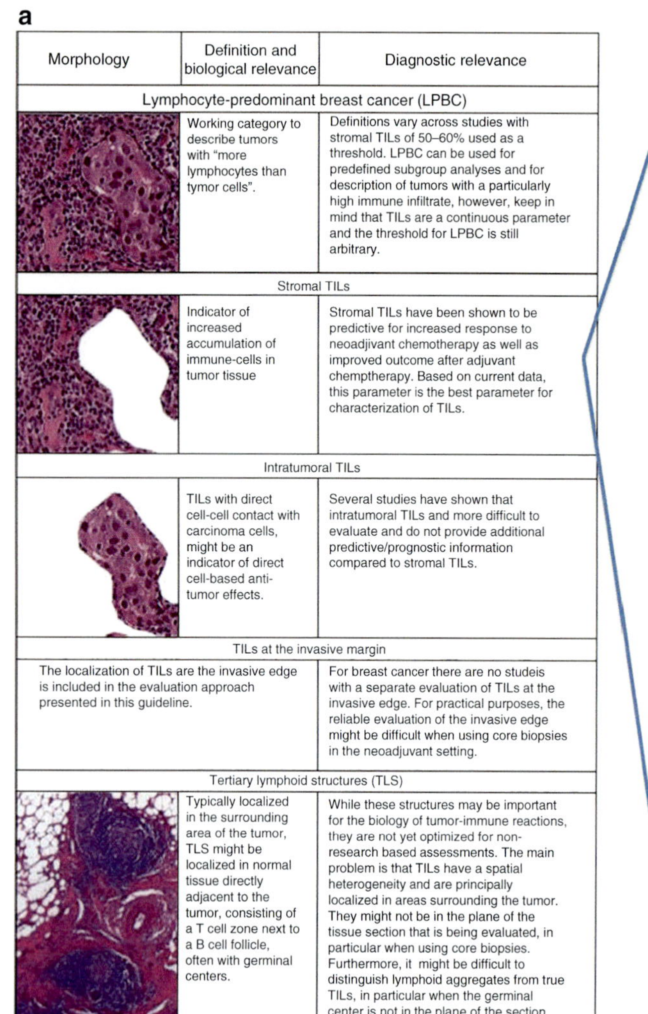

b

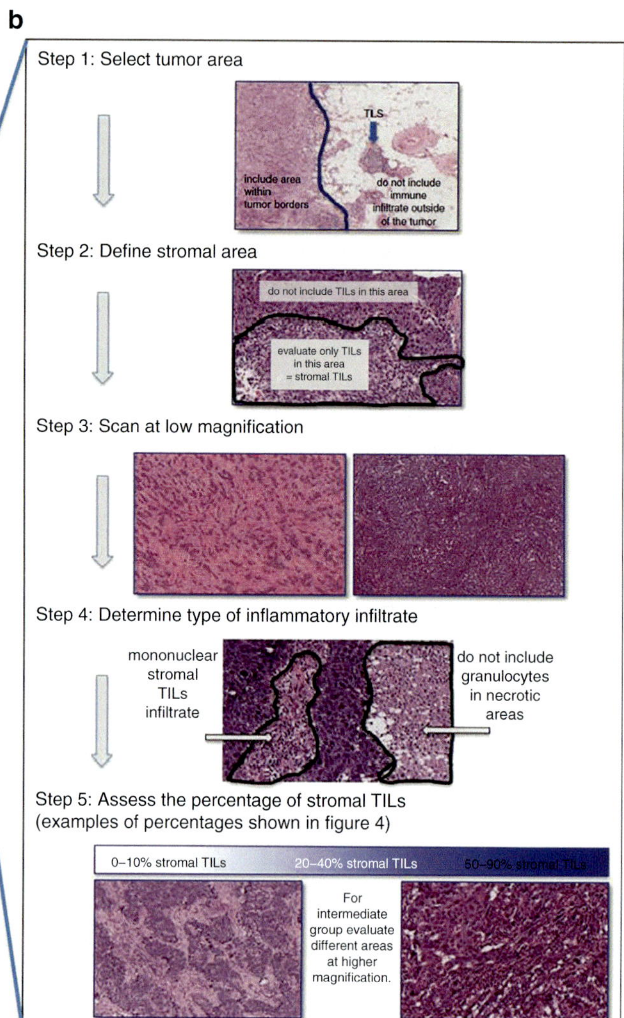

Fig. 13.2 (**a**) Morphology, definitions, biological and diagnostic relevance of the different immune infiltrates found in breast cancer. (**b**) Standardized approach for sTILs evaluation in breast cancer (14, By permission of Oxford University Press on behalf of the European Society for Medical Oncology)

and gives an overview on the scoring method for sTILs. For a more detailed discussion, we refer to the original publication.

Guidelines Include TIL Scoring

International expert committees like those of the St. Gallen Breast Cancer Conference and European Society of Medical Oncology recognize in their latest published recommendations the prognostic importance of TILs in TNBC, encouraging reporting in daily practice, while cautioning that TILs should not be used solely to determine treatment options, as treatments are governed by stage. It needs to be emphasized that the level IB evidence of the TILs as a prognostic factor in TNBC does not mean that TILs should be used as a binary variable for treatment selection, either for de-escalation of chemotherapy or for immunotherapeutic approaches. Binary use of any biomarker, to decide to treat or not to treat the patient based on the result of the biomarker, depends on prospective randomized controlled trials designed to address the utility of the biomarker at predefined cut-offs, thus on level IA-evidence. This level IA-evidence is not yet present for the TILs, suggesting that TILs should be used in conjunction with other prognostic variables such as tumor size and lymph node status to inform the clinician on the outcome of the patient. The clinician then informs the patient, to take in mutual agreement with the patient, the most optimal treatment. Clinical trials where TILs are used as an inclusive biomarker to decide on treatment are in development. In daily practice, some clinicians are still reluctant to include the TILs in their daily practice because there is no level IA evidence, however most other prognostic factors used in breast cancer practice do not have that level of evidence either. Treatments were escalated based on the worse outcome with the prognostic factors and were not designed to assess prospective in a binary value the value of that biomarker. For predictive purposes, two phase 3 clinical trials, namely KEYNOTE-119 [173] and IMpassion130 [196], showed that TILs predict benefit to immunotherapy, so conceptually level of evidence IB, yet because the TILs are used as a predictive biomarker, a binary approach is needed, hence level of evidence IA. So, TILs should not be used for immunotherapeutic treatment decisions, and in this context, TILs can be used to support PD-L1-assessment, as if there are no TILs, any PD-L1 assay is likely to be negative, while if many TILs are present, any PD-L1-assay is likely to be positive.

This interpretation is important, as some clinicians in daily practice do not consider the TILs as a binary variable, since it has no level IA-evidence so they do not ask for it, while others recognize that TILs can be used together with other prognostic variables, and hence they ask for it. This difference is also informative for discussion at international expert committees, as it all depends on how the question about the use of TILs counts is posed. We believe that experts should answer to the question whether there is enough evidence to use TILs quantities in combination with other features, instead of answering to questions about the use of TILs for treatment decisions. Formal endorsement of the use of TILs by pathology societies is also variable and fragmented depending on the country.

Practical Aspects of the Implementation of TILs in Breast Cancer

Section "Summary of the Scoring Guidelines" illustrates in detail the scoring guidelines for sTILs as proposed by the TILs-WG. In this section, we provide a practical guide for sTILs scoring and interpretation in clinical practice, challenges and pitfalls pathologists may encounter and we give an overview of training resources that are freely available.

Pitfalls When Scoring sTILs and Their Remediation

In 2015, the TIL-WG published the first practical guideline to evaluate sTILs in H&E stained tissue section of breast cancer specimens [14]. Subsequently, several reproducibility studies evaluating the robustness of this method among pathologists were conducted, both by the TIL-WG and other research groups [89, 113, 114, 205–207]. While these studies showed on average acceptable to—in some studies—excellent interobserver reproducibility of this method, these pivotal reproducibility studies also identified sources of variability and difficulties pathologists may face when applying sTILs evaluation in their daily practices. A systematic analysis of such sources of variability and recommendations on how to handle these was published by Kos et al. in 2020

[16]. For this study, data were analyzed from three different RING trials conducted by the TIL-WG. For each of these RING studies sTILs were evaluated by 6–32 dedicated pathologists on H&E stained slides (core needle biopsies or whole tumor sections) of 60–100 invasive breast carcinomas [89, 114]. Based on the highest variation between individual pathologist's sTILs scores, 4 categories of pitfalls in sTILs assessment were identified. Here, we briefly discuss each of these categories and provide some tips and tricks on how to cope with them when evaluating sTILs. Extensive description can be found in the original paper by Kos et al. [16].

1. *Heterogeneity in sTILs distribution:* Heterogeneity in sTILs distribution was identified as the most important factor contributing to variability in pathologist's sTILs scores. When assessing sTILs, all peri- and intratumoral stroma associated with invasive carcinoma is to be included in the denominator. When sTILs are heterogeneously distributed within this stroma, the pathologist has to average the different density levels of sTILs relative to the area they occupy into a single score.

   Frequent patterns of heterogenous distribution of the immune infiltrate in a tumor that can render sTILs evaluation challenging, consist of increased density of sTILs at the invasive front as opposed to the center of the tumor, when a tumor is composed of variably spaced tumoral cell nests associated with sTILs, or abundant stroma that is sparse in lymphocytic infiltrate in between. In such situations, it is advised to evaluate sTILs in multiple (at least three) fields of view that are representative of the overall pattern of sTILs observed at low magnification and average the results into one global sTILs score rather than trying to eye-ball a single global sTILs score all at once.

2. *Technical factors:* A lot of different technical factors such as fixation (mainly underfixation), microtomy, and crush artifacts, fading of H&E stainings over time and—as more and more labs are adopting digital pathology—scanning focus errors can all contribute to poor reproducibility of sTILs evaluation. Keeping such variables as much as possible under control is a primary focus of every pathology lab. When artifacts are only focally present, sTILs should be scored in unaffected areas and in general pathologists should have a low threshold not to evaluate prognostic or predictive biomarkers when reliable assessment is hampered by technical factors.

3. *Problems with identifying area or cells of interest:* As outlined above, for the tumor area all peri- and intratumoral tumor-associated stroma should be taken into account and included in the denominator when evaluating sTILs. An exception to this rule is the presence of a central hyalinized scar or fibrotic focus, which is excluded from sTILs scoring. Challenging cases can be encountered

when DCIS or pre-existent benign structures are present with the boundaries of an invasive carcinoma. Lymphocytic infiltrate clearly associated with DCIS or benign structures should not be included in the sTILs score. In cases with a very heterogenous composition of invasive carcinoma, DCIS and pre-existent normal structures, a similar representative field-of-view scoring approach as described above focusing on invasive carcinoma can be helpful.

With respect to the cells of interest, by definition sTILs evaluation is restricted to loosely organized infiltrate of lymphocytes and plasma cells in a tumor. Cases of invasive carcinoma with abundant infiltrate of histiocytes, neutrophils, or abundant presence of apoptotic cells—which can at low magnification mimic lymphocytes—can be challenging to score. These cases often require more detailed evaluation of the immune infiltrate at high magnification in different areas of the tumor before assessing the sTILs score. In addition, confined dense lymphoid aggregates and organized lymphoid structures such as tertiary lymphoid structures (TLS) are also excluded from the sTILs score.

4. *Cases with little evaluable stroma:* A final category of cases in which sTILs evaluation can be challenging are those with only limited stroma present within the tumor. This can be encountered in highly cellular tumors with a high tumor-stroma ratio, micropapillary carcinomas, mucinous tumors with only slender fibrovascular cores in between the mucus lakes or tumors with abundant necrosis obscuring fibrous stroma. In such cases, even an apparently paucicellular stromal immune infiltrate in absolute numbers can result in paradoxically high sTILs scores. There is currently no formal guideline defined on minimal sample requirements for scoring sTILs, neither in terms of minimal number of tumor cells nor in terms of minimal amount of evaluable tumor-associated stroma to be present. As a general rule of thumb, pathologists should use judgment. Also, important to keep in mind when scoring sTILs in samples with little stroma is that iTILs, i.e. immune cells that are present with the epithelial cell nests, should not be included in the sTILs score.

Similarly O'Loughlin and colleagues found that factors contributing to discrepancies between pathologist were intratumoral heterogeneity of TILs, necrosis, biopsy fragmentation, tumor cellularity, and difficulties in the identification of the tumor border [113]. Figure 13.3 illustrates some of the most frequently encountered pitfalls.

Available Resources for Pathologists

To aid pathologists and researchers in getting familiar with how sTILs were scored in clinical trials that have shown clinical validity and potential clinical utility of this biomarker, the TIL-WG has developed a wealth of educational tools and resources that are freely available via their website www.tilsinbreastcancer.org. On this website, an extensive training section can be found where literature references, video tutorials, tutorial slide decks with step-by-step explanations on how to score TILs in different cancer types (invasive breast cancer, DCIS, and breast cancer after neoadjuvant chemotherapy, but also melanoma, NSCLC adenocarcinoma, endometrial carcinoma, urothelial carcinoma, and colorectal carcinoma) and sheets of reference images that can be used as a visual guide when scoring sTILs are centralized. Specific guidance on how to handle challenging cases can be found in a separate section on the website at www.tilsinbreastcancer.org/pitfalls.

The use of a well-calibrated set of reference images together with a structured representative sampling approach for heterogeneous cases has been shown to be the most effective way to improve reproducibility and to reduce scaling differences among pathologists. This was clearly illustrated in one of the RING trials conducted by the TILs-WG in which ICC values amongst an identical group of 28 pathologists improved considerably from 0.71 (95% CI 0.63–0.79) to 0.89 (95% CI 0.85–0.92) after the implementation of a software tool that guided pathologists to select different areas for sTILs evaluation and provided direct visual feedback for provided sTILs values [114].

In addition, the website hosts an interactive scoring platform (available through the link "Teach yourself to score TILs") with two functionalities. First, a large collection of training images that have been assigned a consensus sTILs score by expert members of the TIL-WG is available. Here, pathologists can run training sessions in which these images are randomly presented, sTILs can be scored with or without the use of reference images and a progress report of training status summarizing the concordance c.q. deviation of assigned scores compared to the reference scores can be generated. A second functionality of this interactive tool provides the users with the possibility to upload snapshot images (ideally .jpeg or .png images of 20× fields-of-view) from own clinical cases and compare these images to a reference set of images of invasive breast cancer with verified sTILs. Multiple images per case can be uploaded and can then be assigned a sTILs score with 10% increments after which a summary report with automatic calculation of an average sTILs score for the entire case can be generated. This tool is particularly helpful in case of heterogenous distribution of sTILs where eyeballing a single global sTILs sore is not recommended, as explained earlier.

Currently, projects on the development of imaging analysis tools for automated measurement of sTILs in invasive breast cancer images using machine learning techniques are ongoing [208].

Finally, during the first half of 2021, the TIL-WG, in collaboration with the Biomedical Quality Assurance Research

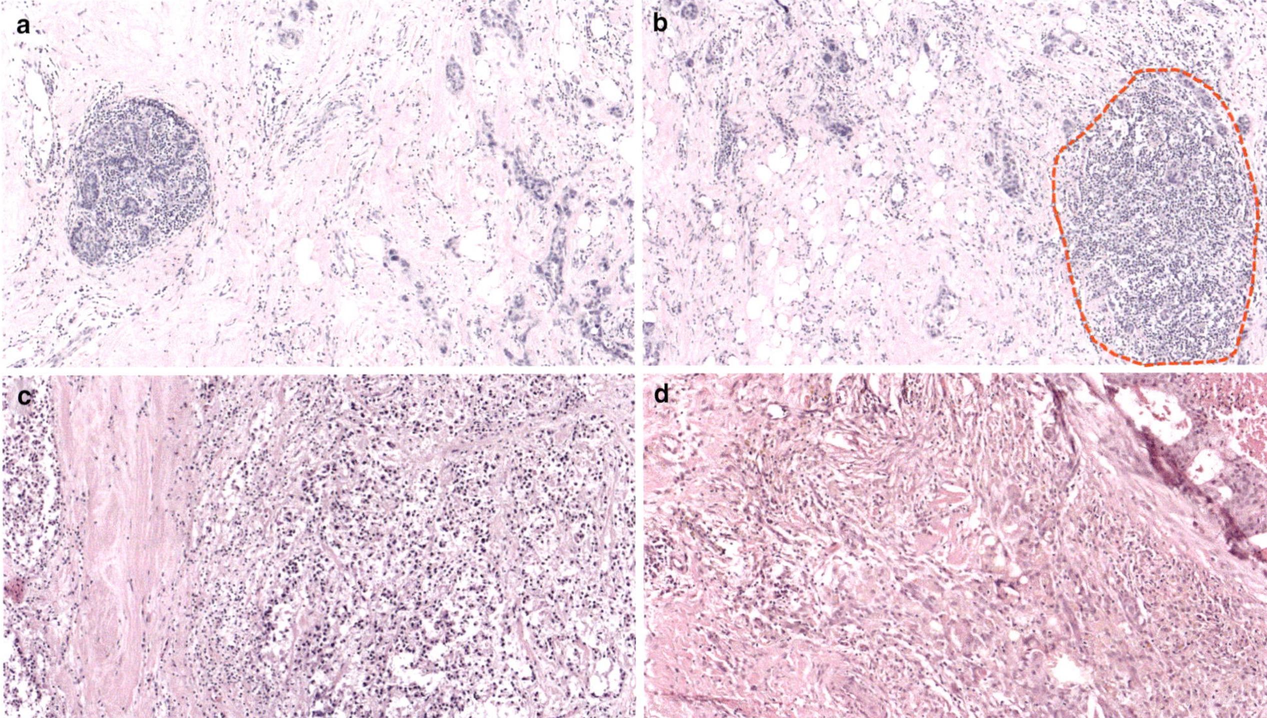

Fig. 13.3 H&E stained slides of invasive breast carcinoma specimens illustrating some frequently encountered pitfalls when scoring sTILs. All images were extracted from digitized whole slide images at 200x magnification. (**a**) sTILs are evaluated in tumor-associated stroma only. Lymphoid infiltrate clearly associated with normal lobules should be disregarded. In this field of view, consensus sTILs score within the boundaries of the invasive carcinoma was determined by two expert pathologists of the TIL-WG to be 10%. (**b**) Confined dense lymphoid aggregates and especially organized lymphoid elements such as tertiary lymphoid structures (TLS) are not included in the sTILs score. In this example, the encircled dense lymphoid aggregate should not be taken into account for the sTILs score. Consensus score for sTILs in this field of view as determined by two expert pathologists of the TIL-WG is 20%. (**c**) This case clearly illustrates the difficulties one may encounter to distinguish tumor cells from immune infiltrate when breast cancer tissue is not properly fixed. General principles of good laboratory practice for handling breast cancer specimens should be strictly adhered to (including limiting delay to fixation to less than 30 min and minimum duration of fixation for breast cancer specimens to more than 6 h as much as possible). (**d**) This image shows a confined area of inflammation with many iron macrophages consistent with a biopsy site. Apart from macrophages never to be included into the sTILs score, sTILs should always be scored outside areas of inflammation attributable to iatrogenic manipulation (biopsy sites, implantation site of radiographic markers)

Unit of the Catholic University Leuven (Leuven, Belgium) will launch an external quality assessment (EQA) scheme for sTILs in triple-negative breast cancer (TNBC) for laboratories and pathologists worldwide. In addition to the EQA scheme for sTILs, also exploratory data will be collected on the real-world implementation of PD-L1 assays and scoring algorithms in TNBC. This EQA program will be available at https://tils.agoko.be.

Choice of Sample Types, Interobserver Reproducibility, and Impact on Clinical Validity

As mentioned above, the interobserver reproducibility of the described method has been documented in multiple studies including 2 to up to 40 different pathologists evaluating biopsies or full-face sections of invasive [89, 113, 114, 205–207] carcinoma. In these studies, intraclass correlation coefficients for concordance between pathologists ranged from around 0.60 to 0.95 when evaluating sTILs as continuous variable. Measures resulting in a marked positive effect on scoring reproducibility include the use of reference images and structured representative sampling approaches for assessing cases with heterogenous sTILs distribution [114]. While these data are reassuring for the evaluation of sTILs in biomarker driven treatment decision schemes in the years to come, they also clearly highlight the need for sustained training efforts and participation in external quality assessment and reader proficiency testing programs when sTILs evaluation is introduced in clinical practice. An important question is how the observed interobserver variability affects the clinical validity and clinical utility of a biomarker, especially when discrete cut-offs are taken into consideration. In an effort to statistically defer the impact of variability in sTILs assessment on pathological complete response (pCR) prediction, the TILs-WG calculated for the neoadjuvant GeparSixto trial [209], that for any intraclass correlation coefficient for scoring concordance between pathologists (ranging from 0.6

to 0.9), comparable odds ratios for pCR prediction would be obtained [210]. Several studies specifically designed to evaluate the impact of interobserver variability in sTILs assessment on prediction of response to neoadjuvant chemotherapy in a real-life sample sets are currently underway (personal communication Dr. Van Bockstal and Dr. Callagy).

Finally, given the fact that the currently most robust data supporting clinical application of sTILs assessment are situated within the primary disease setting, a relevant question to ask is to what extent sTILs assessment in small core needle biopsies is representative for the overall immune infiltrate in the whole tumor. As previously mentioned, no minimum sample requirements for sTILs evaluation in terms of number of invasive tumor cells or amount of evaluable tumor-associated stroma that must be present in order to be able to reliable assess the sTILs have currently been defined. At least two studies have shown excellent correlation of sTILs evaluation of core needle biopsies as compared to full-face sections of the corresponding primary resection specimen, especially when multiple cores per biopsy were examined [211, 212]. In addition, in a study by Althobiti et al. no statistically significant difference could be observed in sTILs scores evaluated on slides from different tissue blocks of the same tumor [213]. Together, these data further underscore the robustness of the proposed sTILs evaluation system in heterogenous sample types.

Part 4: Novel Methods

As described above, the quantification of (s)TILs can easily be incorporated in a standard pathology examination of (breast cancer) biopsies and resection specimens. It is a good general semiquantitative histopathological measure of the immune reaction in a tumor. New developments will aim at more standard and more quantitative measurement, on the one hand, or further, more detailed, characterization of the immune response, on the other hand. The purpose of this section is to briefly describe new evolutions and technologies that are emerging in this field.

Tumor Mutational Burden

The measure of the TILs on H&E is generally regarded as a surrogate of tumor immunogenicity. However, the quantification of TILs alone may not be sufficient to capture clinically and biologically meaningful differences between the different breast cancer subtypes. From an immunological point of view, the presence of foreign antigens is crucial for the activation of the adaptive immune system and elimination of potentially harmful organisms. Several mechanisms contribute to the accumulation of mutations in cancer genes

and contribute to cancer progression. This process is supposed to generate a number of neoantigens that are capable of laying the basis of the interactions with the immune system and promote immune editing [8]. The ultimate aggregate of all mutations found in a tumor is defined as tumor mutational burden (TMB). As indicated by recent studies based on whole genome sequencing analysis, some types of cancers more than others are characterized by the accumulation of higher numbers of non-synonymous mutations across the whole DNA. Melanoma and lung carcinoma are typical examples of tumor types with high TMB, microsatellite instability also attributes to high TMB to colon, while mutations in the DNA polymerase genes may contribute to hyper mutant cancer phenotypes in endometrial carcinoma [214]. Tumors with high TMB profiles seem to respond better to ICB therapies, providing proof for the concept that higher TMB is synonymous of higher antigenicity. Based on these observations pembrolizumab has been approved in a tumor agnostic manner in all cancer types showing microsatellite instability defects [215]. However, as briefly mentioned before microsatellite instability has an incidence of <2% in BC and BC are considered as "cold tumors" with poor antigenicity because of the low TMB [63, 216]. Despite this observation, ICB has also in BC the potential to become a new mainstay of treatment for at least certain patients [157, 162]. Therefore, there is an urgent need to better understand this paradox and help health care professionals in the search of reliable biomarkers of response to ICB therapy to increase patient selection [217]. In this regard recent evidence suggests that contrary to what initially thought, TMB in general is unlikely to become a pancancer marker for predicting response to ICB therapy. McGrail and colleagues found that overall response rates to ICB therapy above 20% were present only in TMB-high tumors with a positive correlation between CD8+ T cells and neoantigen load, while in the tumors lacking this type of correlation (e.g., breast, prostate, glioma, etc.) the overall response rates were <20% and were statistically significantly lower when compared to the TMB low tumors [13]. A recent meta-analysis performed by Litchfield et al. demonstrated in a pancancer study, comprising over 1000 patients, that clonal TMB has a better predictive value for the response to therapy when comparing to total TMB or subclonal TMB, suggesting that it is the early signatures in tumor development that makes a tumor sensitive for ICB [218]. Examples are the APOBEC signature, the UV-signature in melanoma, and Tobacco signature in NSCLC. The diversity of further subclonal mutational signatures would "confuse" the immune system, resulting in an ineffective response. Nevertheless, there is quite some heterogeneity between different cancer types and histologies that renders the effect small when looking at single histology type. Therefore, a multimodal approach for assessing sensitivity to ICB is more likely to be effective in choosing the right therapy for the patient, integrating (clonal) TMB, specific TMB signatures, and immune infiltrate abundance and phenotypes [161].

CD8+ T Lymphocytes

The CD8+ T lymphocytes play a major role in the recognition of tumor-specific epitopes which are presented by antigen presenting cells. The T-cell mediated antigen recognition depends on the interaction of T cell receptor (TCR) with the antigen-major histocompatibility complex molecules. Only activated CD8+ cytotoxic T cells can efficiently kill tumor cells upon specific recognition of tumor-specific antigens [219]. A large amount of evidence accumulated in the past strongly suggest that the presence of cytotoxic CD8+ T cells is associated with longer survival rates and higher rates of pCR after neoadjuvant chemotherapy in BC patients [76, 77, 220–223]. In addition, recent evidence based on multiomics analysis suggests that estimates of CD8 + T-cells abundance may represent the most robust predictive biomarker for the response to anti PD-1/PD-L1 therapy across multiple types of cancers including breast [224]. However, the biomarker analysis of the IMpassion130 study showed that CD8+ tumors were associated with improved survival outcomes only when also PD-L1 was positive [196]. Prolonged exposure to tumor neoantigens may induce sustained expression of immune checkpoint molecules that eventually may result in a dysfunctional T-cell state or apoptotic CD8+ T cells which is not resolved even when antigens are removed (tumor immunotolerance and tumor immunosuppression) [225]. Metabolic signals coming from the tumor microenvironment or other factors that are intrinsically related to the tumor cells may contribute to the dysfunctional status of the cytotoxic T cells, explaining at least in part why ICB therapies are successful only in a minority of patients [226, 227]. In this regard, the study of specific subset of TILs may give a substantial contribution in the understanding of the involved mechanisms of immune editing. In treatment naïve TNBC important quantitative and qualitative variations in the composition of CD8+ T cells were recently observed. T cells with CD8 + CD103+ displayed a distinctive phenotype as compared to the subset of CD8 + CD103- T cells, indicating in the former group higher PD1 expression levels, ability of clonal expansion and cytotoxic activity suggesting important immune surveillance functions. Interestingly, higher levels of TILs were associated with the CD8 + CD103+ phenotype proposing a mechanistic relation between high TILs levels and good prognosis in TNBC patients [228]. In the window of opportunity trial Biokey, after one single administration of pembrolizumab, significant clonotype changes in the T-cells were observed. In particular Pembrolizumab induced expansion of the PD1+ T-cells expressing CD8 or CD4 markers.

These cells showed mainly markers which suggested activation of T cells based on the expression of immune checkpoint (LAG3, HAVCR2, PDCD1), effector (IFNG, NKG7) and cytotoxic (GZMB, PRF1) markers; only a small portion of the expanded T cells showed a CD8+ effector/memory phenotype [194]. These data strongly suggest that the identification of specific subset of TILs may be important for the identification of functional markers that can improve patient selection for ICB therapies.

Spatial Heterogeneity of Immune Infiltrate in the Breast

The spatial resolution of the lymphocytes present in the tumor microenvironment can further refine the classification of BC in meaningful prognostic categories [228, 229]. In this regard, tumors can be classified as immune-inflamed, immune-excluded, and immune deserted tumors based on the quantity and the topographical localization of the immune cells in relation to stroma and tumor cells [229] (Fig. 13.4). For instance, luminal BC and special histologic subtypes of BC have been regarded as immune-excluded tumors because of the lack of intraepithelial CD8+ T cells [23, 77]. The topographical identification on H&E of lymphocytic hot spot seems also to have important implications for the prognosis of BC, as illustrated by studies performed with the aid of computational pathology [230, 231]. In an exploratory study performed on luminal B tumors across three different age groups, it has been observed that CD20+ and FOXP3+ inflammatory cells were more abundant at the periphery and in the inner part of the tumor regardless of age, respectively [232, 233]. The spatial pattern of TILs seems to be comparable when primary tumors are matched to their metastasis, suggesting in the metastasis a kind of TILs imprinting which is derived from the primary tumor [234]. Additionally, as recently suggested, the immune-excluded BC category can be further classified as margin-restricted or stroma-restricted. On the other hand, the inflamed tumors can be distinguished in stromal-intraepithelial and stromal-restricted both potentially associated with different prognostic information [228, 235]. However, the biological meaning of these categories is not fully understood yet and, importantly, studies performed on tissue microarray or with small pieces of tissue may introduce sampling bias and prevent to fully understand spatial heterogeneity in BC [236, 237].

Spatial Single Cell Technologies

A detailed map of the interactions existing between tumor cells and its surrounding microenvironment requires the availability of highly specialized technologies that can mea-

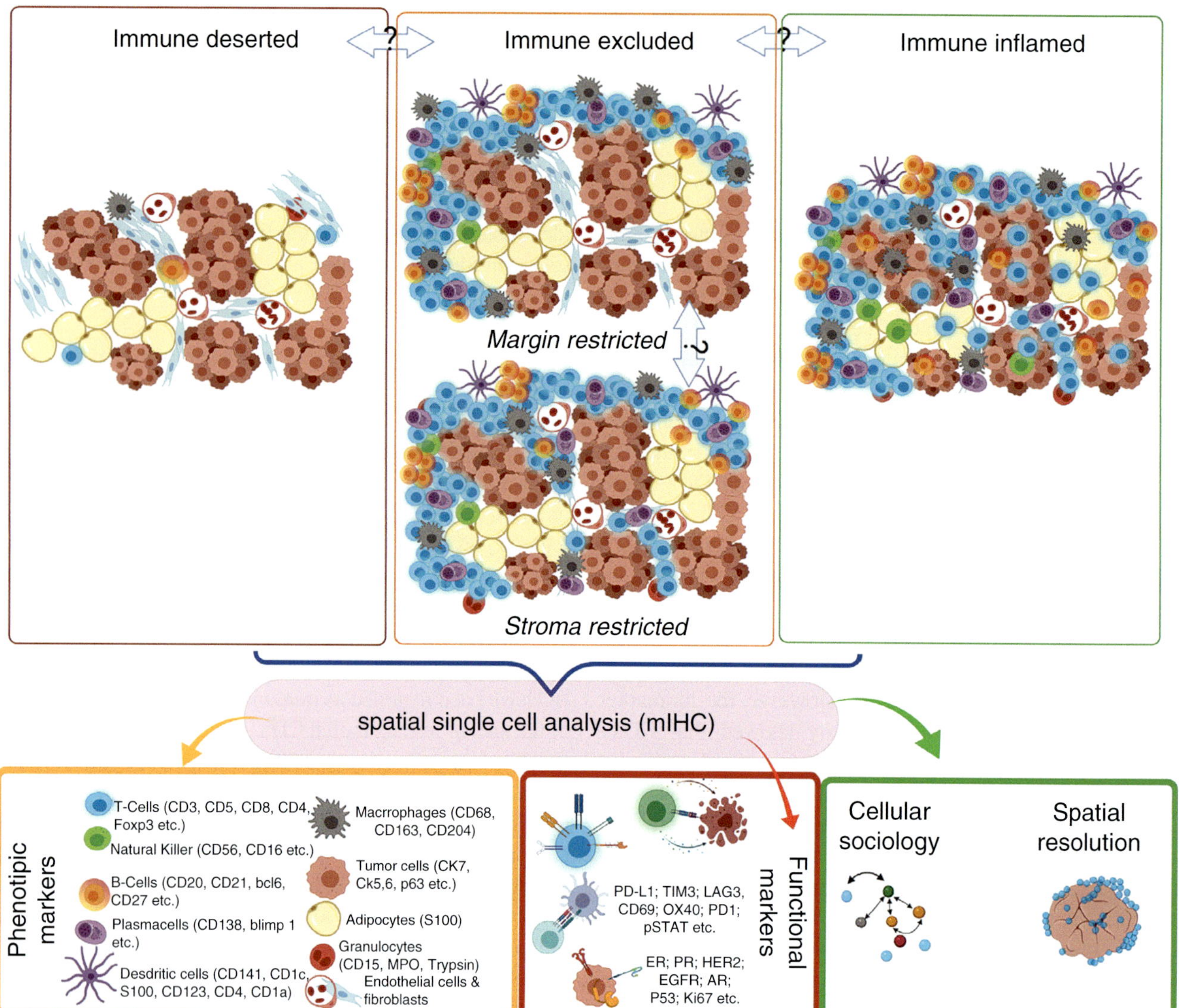

Fig. 13.4 The spatial lymphocytic phenotypes of immune infiltration in BC. BC are often divided into poorly infiltrated (immune deserted, left panel), immune excluded (central panel), and inflamed (right panel). "Immune deserted" tumors show almost total lack of lymphocytes. "Immune excluded" tumors show a lack of lymphocytes within the epithelial nests of the tumor, but lymphocytes may be present at the invasive margin (margin restricted) or spread in the whole surface but restricted only to the stroma (stroma restricted). "Inflamed tumors" show lymphocytic infiltration lymphocytic infiltration in the stroma and intratumorally. To date it is unclear whether these patterns are related to specific biological features existing between tumor cells and its microenvironment or represent different magnitude of infiltration. It is anticipated that the use of spatial single cells technologies like m-IHC will allow us to achieve four goals using one tumor section: (1) identify each single cellular component of a tumor mass (orange panel); (2) infer about the functionality of the different cells (red box); (3) understand the interactions between cells using neighborhood analysis (cellular sociology, green panel); (4) topographical mapping of all the components to resolve at the spatial level the interactions between tumor cells and its microenvironment. Figure created with BioRender.com

sure a multitude of features in single cells while maintaining their original position in a tissue. Such technologies are now becoming available, from which multiplexed immunohistochemistry (m-IHC) is the most advanced [238]. By using m-IHC, the interactions between tumor cells and its TME are preserved, overcoming the shortcomings provided by cell dissociation and cell enrichment of other single cell technologies [239].

The use of m-IHC in BC pathology is emerging as useful tool to gain better insight in the cellular composition of the tumor microenvironment, understand relationship between different cells including mechanisms of activation, and most importantly acquire spatial information. Using imaging mass cytometry, Jackson et al. recently described the complex structure of BC at single cell level. With a panel of 35 metal-labeled antibodies, used simultaneously to detect different cell populations, the researchers have been able to identify different cellular communities which were correlated to different molecular subtypes, beyond those already known. Tumors also showed some level of spatial heterogeneity in about 60% of the cases and related to spatial heterogeneity. Interestingly, survival analysis performed on spatially identified cellular communities was able to provide strong prognostic information beyond current clinical classification [240]. Using multiplexed ion beam imaging, Keren et al. were able describe the spatial organization of inflammatory infiltrates in TNBC [235, 240]. In their experiment using simultaneously over 30 different Ab in 41 samples of TNBC patients they found two main cellular compartments: epithelial and inflammatory cell compartment. Depending on the quantity and spatial interactions between epithelial and inflammatory cells tumors were subdivided into cold (low number of inflammatory cells), mixed (heterogeneous mixture of the two compartment), and compartmentalized (physical separation of either of the two compartment). Expression of PD1 was associated with either CD8+ or CD4+ T cells in mixed or compartmentalized tumors, cold tumors were rarely observed. CD4 + PD1+ were found to be more frequently associated with the compartmentalized tumors and were spatially segregated showing additional co-expression of other immune-modulatory markers like IDO or PD-L1. Conversely, mixed tumors showed higher level of CD8 + PD1+ T cells which were more frequently admixed with tumor cells expressing IDO or PD-L1 immune-modulatory molecules. Survival analysis showed improved survival outcomes in the compartmentalized tumors as compared to the mixed ones. These findings were in contrast with those reported by Gruosso et al., however in the latter no co-expression analysis or CD4 assessment was performed [228, 235]. Alternatively, the spatial identification of CD8 + CD103+ T cells with resident memory phenotype suggests that these cells are associated with nests of epithelial cancer cells being associated with improved relapse free survival as suggested by multiplex analysis using low-plex methods with multiple cycles of staining [141, 241, 242].

Pre- and post-treatment matched samples of patients with inflammatory breast carcinoma treated with neoadjuvant chemotherapy have been studied by "first-generation" m-IHC with medium-plex panel of inflammatory ad myeloid cell lineages. Low level of macrophages in the pre-treatment biopsy was associated with higher pCR rates, while spatial analysis revealed a significant association between mast cells, CD163+ cells, and CD8+ cells in patients with residual disease, suggesting a potential mechanism of resistance [243]. In BC patients with HER2+ disease low- to medium plex m-IHC studies have been conducted as well to understand spatial immune profiling in relation to anti HER2-therapy. These studies linked the activity of trastuzumab directly to extracellular domain of HER2 and co-localization of CD8+ T cells providing further evidence for the involvement of the immune system in the mechanism of action of monoclonal Ab directed against HER2 [244]. Similarly, in another study from an independent group it was observed that HER2+ BC showing immune cells spatially interacting with tumor cells had higher responses to anti-HER2 therapies [245]. Tumors characterized by high stromal CD4+, CD8+, CD20+, and high intratumoral CD20+ immune cells showed higher rates of pCR in another analysis performed on HER2+ BC [246].

Artificial Intelligence

Another technological (r)evolution that will influence the field of pathology in general and that of TILs assessment in particular in the near future will be artificial intelligence (AI). The use of AI is currently under immense investigation (the big boom of AI is expected to happen in the next 10–15 years), and there are in fact already clinically validated algorithms for quantification or categorization of well-known histopathological biomarkers [247]. Some of these algorithms are already CE-IVD (Europe) approved. Concerning TILs, there are several methods described in the literature. The most accessible method is scoring of sTILs on H&E slides. On top of the application of TILs in H&E, more and more investigators are also trying to dissect the tumor microenvironment by using multiplex immunohistochemistry as discussed above [247]. To this date, no CE-IVD labeled algorithm for AI-based sTIL assessment exists. Yet, this topic is under thorough investigation for several types of cancer, among which breast cancer, melanoma, colorectal cancer, and lung cancer [231, 248–257]. The general principles for assessing TILs are simple. The AI-based algorithm analyzes the whole slide image via convolutional neural networks (CNN) or other another artificial neural network, differentiating tumor stroma from tumoral structures. In a next step TILs are differentiated in the stroma from other (inflammatory cells) that cannot be considered when scoring TILs. To have the most accurate result, the application needs to follow the TIL scoring guidelines as closely as possible [247].

An extensive review of computational assessment of sTIL was written by Amgad et al. in 2020 on behalf of the TILs-WG. It does not only graphically describe the aforementioned general steps, but also describes all possible approaches and methods used in literature for automated sTIL evaluation. The author divides the overview into H&E based approaches and immunohistochemistry based approaches. Table 13.6 is adapted from this data to give an overview of all possible methods and approaches and their strengths and weaknesses as reported by the authors [208].

Although AI is a promising addition to pathological evaluation of whole slide images, there are some important challenges to overcome. Tizhoosh et al. mentioned three key elements: interoperability, cost, and trust [260]. For a more in-depth general discussion on these factors, we refer to the original papers [260, 261]. Specifically in the context of

Table 13.6 Overview of methods of automated sTIL assessment in tumors. Adapted with permission from Amgad et al. [208]

Method	Approach	Stain	Notes
CNN [249]	Patch classification	H&E	*Strengths*: spatial information on sTIL. Molecular correlations *Limitations*: no distinction between sTIL and iTIL. No classification of individual TILs
FCN [258]	Semantic segmentation	H&E	*Strengths*: large sample size and regions. Delineation of tumor, stroma, and necrosis regions. *Limitations*: only detects dense TIL infiltrates. No classification of individual TILs.
Seeding + FCN [259]	Semantic segmentation + object detection	H&E	*Limitations*: heavy ground truth requirement
SVM	Object detection	H&E	*Strengths*: robust analysis and correlation with molecular TIL *Limitations*: individual labeled nuclei are limited. No distinction of TILs in different histologic regions
	Object detection + inferred TIL localization	H&E	*Strengths*: spatial localization and patterns. Robust. *Limitations*: individual labeled nuclei are limited. 1:1 correspondence clustering vs regions unclear
RG + MRF [250]	Object detection	H&E	*Strengths*: explainable model and modular pipeline. *Limitations*: no distinction between sTIL and iTIL. No classification of individual TILs
Watershed + SVM	Object detection	H&E	*Strengths*: explainable model. Robust. Spatial TIL clustering. *Limitations*: no distinction between sTIL and iTIL
Complex pipeline	Object detection + manual regions	IHC	*Strengths*: assessment of manual regions, including invasive margin.

TILs assessment, there are certainly trust challenges to overcome. These challenges are usually the reason for a high discordance rate between manual and automated assessment. Differences between both assessments can explain the discordance rate for the major part. Manual assessment is usually an estimation of the amount of mononuclear inflammatory cells in the stroma, while automated assessments predict a more accurate percentage. Moreover, in some tumor types (e.g., melanoma) different systems are used for categorization of the percentage of TILs, further explaining discordance. Another challenge in automated sTIL assessment is the characterization of the cells in the stroma. Not all of these cells are lymphocytes and not all lymphocytes have the same phenotype. Other cells that might be encountered are macrophages, fibroblasts, plasma cells, granulocytes, mast cells, etc. In normal circumstances, the AI-algorithm takes the size of the cell, the size of the nucleus and the area of the cytoplasm into consideration, but it is not aware that these measurements are highly dependent on the cut level through the cell, which might lead to a wrong identification of a cell. This is also an issue in manual assessment, although the human mind can easily consider this pitfall. Nonetheless, the prognostic value of sTIL is more robust when assessed with automated algorithms.

To have the most accurate result, the automated TILS assessment needs to follow the guidelines for scoring TILs as closely as possible. Therefore the efforts of the TILs-WG to standardize TILs assessment methodology from the very beginning are important to create a stable framework that contributes to development of reproducible algorithms. A good biomarker is considered analytically valid, reproducible, affordable, accessible, and clinically useful. It is in this context that Gonzalez-Ericsson et al. applied a risk management framework for the implementation of TILS next to PD-L1 assessment as immune-oncology biomarkers in daily practice and clinical trials. This application paves the pathway for further recommendations and guidelines regarding TILS scoring, improving reproducibility. The authors also mention the use of AI-based methods, but like any other biomarker computer-aided analysis should be analytically and clinically valid [165].

The predictive use of AI-based analysis of TILs is still somewhat controversial. To this date, no clinical trials concerning computer-aided TILs assessment exist, evaluating the efficacy of immune checkpoint inhibition. This is in contrast to the growing body of evidences illustrating that AI-assisted assessment of TILs is linked to prognosis. But of course, as AI is becoming more and more prominent, it is just a matter of time before the first trials with automated analysis of TILs counts will appear.

CNN convolutional neural networks, *sTIL* stromal tumor infiltrating lymphocytes, *iTIL* intratumoral infiltrating lymphocytes, *FCN* full convolutional neural network, *SVM* support vector machine, *RG* region growing, *MRF* Markov random field, *DL* deep learning

Concluding Remarks/Summary

The semiquantitative assessment of TILs in breast cancer (and in other tumors) is a well-defined histopathological parameter of which the assessment can easily be integrated in the standard examination of biopsies and resection specimens by the (surgical) pathologist. It contributes valuable prognostic and predictive information that should be taken into account—together with other tumor characteristics—when discussing treatment options, especially in Her2-positive and TNBC. Over the past years, the International Immuno-Oncology Biomarkers Working Group (www.tilsinbreastcancer.org) has been involved in multiple studies to further characterize its value as a biomarker and it has also taken several educational initiatives and developed several tools to create awareness, to teach pathologists how to assess TILs according to a reproducible methodology and to integrate TILs assessment with other (new) biomarkers in immuno-oncology. Without any doubt, progressively TILs assessment will further enter clinical practice in the coming years. A structured, coordinated, and scientific approach—as the Immuno-Oncology Biomarkers Working Group tries to propagate and support—should aim to avoid the chaos PD-L1 testing has brought to this field.

Putting genomic/transcriptomic/proteomic information into a spatial context is considered as "the next step" in understanding cancer and establishing novel standards of personalized treatment [217]. Pathologists have been using spatial expression profiling using antibody- DNA-, RNA- and morphology-based methods for decades, but traditional IHC or in situ hybridization methods only allow the simultaneous assessment of a handful of markers in a single tissue slide, which are subsequently evaluated in a semiquantitative way [232]. Multiplex IHC represent the ideal bridge between non-spatial single cell technologies and the traditional monoplex approach of standard pathology providing useful insight about the spatial distribution of the diverse cellular components in a tumor mass. It is anticipated that using these types of approaches in well-designed early phase clinical trials will boost our knowledge about ICB therapies and improve personalized medicine [149, 154, 197, 233].

Furthermore, it is undebatable that computer-assisted TILs assessment can further characterize the tumor microenvironment beyond the capabilities of human minds. It is anticipated that AI-enabled methods will confirm more and more the prognostic and predictive value of TILs, therefore it seems logic to proceed with the implementation of these AI models in practice and in clinical trials. The robustness of these assessments will only increase when combined with the power of multiplexing immunohistochemistry for further characterization of the inflammatory infiltrate [208, 248].

As several AI models also investigate spatial information concerning sTIL, this spatial information can become part of the investigational subjects to further research the prognostic and predictive value of TILs. Not only distances between infiltrates or infiltrates and tumor cells can be considered, but also heterogeneity will also become more important [231, 248, 249].

Many current AI algorithms are based on image analysis, but in a next step additional clinical information and genomic data can be integrated in the analysis as well in order to create more robust models toward personalized and precision medicine. By integrating more and more data, these models are able to detect other prognostic or predictive patterns that are at first, invisible to human perception [208, 248].

References

1. Harbeck N, Penault-Llorca F, Cortes J, Gnant M, Houssami N, Poortmans P, et al. Breast cancer. Nat Rev Dis Primers. 2019;5:66.
2. Loibl S, Poortmans P, Morrow M, Denkert C, Curigliano G. Seminar Breast cancer. Lancet. 2021;397:1750–69. https://doi.org/10.1016/S0140-6736.
3. Savas P, Salgado R, Denkert C, Sotiriou C, Darcy PK, Smyth MJ, et al. Clinical relevance of host immunity in breast cancer: from TILs to the clinic. Nat Rev Clin Oncol. 2015;13(4):228–41.
4. Sistrunk WE, MacCarty WCMD. Life expectancy following radical amputation for carcinoma of the breast. Ann Surg. 1922;75(1):61–9.
5. Moore OS, Foote FW. The relatively favorable prognosis of medullary carcinoma of the breast. Cancer. 1949;2(4):635–42.
6. Hanahan D, Weinberg RA. Hallmarks of cancer: the next generation. Cell. 2011;144:646–74.
7. Vitale I, Shema E, Loi S, Galluzzi L. Dynamic heterogeneity of cancer cells Intratumoral heterogeneity in cancer progression and response to immunotherapy. Nat Med. 2022;14(2):280. https://doi.org/10.1038/s41591-021-01233-9.
8. Dunn GP, Bruce AT, Ikeda H, Old LJ, Schreiber RD. Cancer immunoediting: from immunosurveillance to tumor escape. Nat Immunol. 2002;3:991–8.
9. Zitvogel L, Tesniere A, Kroemer G. Cancer despite immunosurveillance: immunoselection and immunosubversion. Nat Rev Immunol. 2006;6:715–27.
10. Teng MWL, Galon J, Fridman WH, Smyth MJ. From mice to humans: developments in cancer immunoediting. J Clin Invest. 2015;125:3338–46.
11. Schmid P, Salgado R, Park YH, Muñoz-Couselo E, Kim SB, Sohn J, et al. Pembrolizumab plus chemotherapy as neoadjuvant treatment of high-risk, early-stage triple-negative breast cancer: results from the phase 1b open-label, multicohort KEYNOTE-173 study. Ann Oncol. 2020;31(5):569–81.
12. Samstein RM, Lee CH, Shoushtari AN, Hellmann MD, Shen R, Janjigian YY, et al. Tumor mutational load predicts survival after immunotherapy across multiple cancer types. Nat Genet. 2019;51:202–6.
13. McGrail DJ, Pilié PG, Rashid NU, Voorwerk L, Slagter M, Kok M, et al. High tumor mutation burden fails to predict immune checkpoint blockade response across all cancer types. Ann Oncol. 2021;32(5):661–72.
14. Salgado R, Denkert C, Demaria S, Sirtaine N, Klauschen F, Pruneri G, et al. The evaluation of tumor-infiltrating lymphocytes (TILS) in breast cancer: recommendations by an International TILS Working Group 2014. Ann Oncol. 2015;26:259–71.
15. Hendry S, Salgado R, Gevaert T, Russell PA, John T, Thapa B, et al. Assessing tumor-infiltrating lymphocytes in solid tumors: a practical review for pathologists and proposal for a standardized method from the international immunooncology biomarkers working group: part 1: assessing the host immune response, TILs in invasi breast carcinoma and ductal carcinoma in situ, metastatic

tumor deposits and areas for further research. Adv Anat Pathol. 2017;24:235–51.

16. Kos Z, Roblin E, Kim RS, Michiels S, Gallas BD, Chen W, et al. Pitfalls in assessing stromal tumor infiltrating lymphocytes (sTILs) in breast cancer. npj Breast Cancer. 2020;6(1):17.

17. Rakha EA, El-Sayed ME, Lee AHS, Elston CW, Grainge MJ, Hodi Z, et al. Prognostic significance of nottingham histologic grade in invasive breast carcinoma. J Clin Oncol. 2008;26(19):3153–8.

18. WHO Classification of Tumours Editorial Board. Breast Tumours WHO Classification of Tumours, 5th Edition, Volume 2. oard WC of tumours editorial, editor. International Agency for Research on Cancer; 2019.

19. Monard S, Gorana T, Patrizia C, Andrea B, Silvana P, Natale C, et al. Lymphoid infiltration as a prognostic variable for early-onset breast carcinomas. Clin Cancer Res. 1997;3:817–9.

20. Guarneri V, Dieci MV, Bisagni G, Brandes AA, Frassoldati A, Cavanna L, et al. PIK3CA mutation in the shortHER randomized adjuvant trial for patients with early HER2þ breast cancer: Association with prognosis and integration with PAM50 subtype. Clin Cancer Res. 2020;26(22):5843–51.

21. Sasaki R, Horimoto Y, Yanai Y, Kurisaki-Arakawa A, Arakawa A, Nakai K, et al. Molecular characteristics of lymphocyte-predominant triple-negative breast cancer. Anticancer Res. 2021;41(4):2133–40.

22. Craven KE, Gökmen-Polar Y, Badve SS. CIBERSORT analysis of TCGA and METABRIC identifies subgroups with better outcomes in triple negative breast cancer. Sci Rep. 2021;11(1):4691.

23. Desmedt C, Salgado R, Fornili M, Pruneri G, van den Eynden G, Zoppoli G, et al. Immune infiltration in invasive lobular breast cancer. J Natl Cancer Inst. 2018;110(7):768–76.

24. Stanton SE, Adams S, Disis ML. Variation in the incidence and magnitude of tumor-infiltrating lymphocytes in breast cancer subtypes. JAMA Oncol. 2016;2(10):1354.

25. Denkert C, von Minckwitz G, Darb-Esfahani S, Lederer B, Heppner BI, Weber KE, et al. Tumour-infiltrating lymphocytes and prognosis in different subtypes of breast cancer: a pooled analysis of 3771 patients treated with neoadjuvant therapy. Lancet Oncol. 2018;19(1):40–50.

26. Loi S, Sirtaine N, Piette F, Salgado R, Viale G, van Eenoo F, et al. Prognostic and predictive value of tumor-infiltrating lymphocytes in a phase III randomized adjuvant breast cancer trial in node-positive breast cancer comparing the addition of docetaxel to doxorubicin with doxorubicin-based chemotherapy: BIG 02-98. J Clin Oncol. 2013;31(7):860–7.

27. Denkert C, Loibl S, Noske A, Roller M, Müller BM, Komor M, et al. Tumor-associated lymphocytes as an independent predictor of response to neoadjuvant chemotherapy in breast cancer. J Clin Oncol. 2010;28(1):105–13.

28. Hendry S, Salgado R, Gevaert T, Russell PA, John T, Thapa B, et al. Assessing tumor-infiltrating lymphocytes in solid tumors: a practical review for pathologists and proposal for a standardized method from the international immunooncology biomarkers working group: part 1: assessing the host immune response, TILs in invasive breast carcinoma and ductal carcinoma in situ, metastatic tumor deposits and areas for further research. In: Advances in anatomic pathology, vol. 24. Lippincott Williams and Wilkins; 2017. p. 235–51.

29. Rakha EA, Bennett RL, Coleman D, Pinder SE, Ellis IO. Review of the national external quality assessment (EQA) scheme for breast pathology in the UK. J Clin Pathol. 2017;70(1):51–7.

30. Morrow M, Schnitt SJ, Norton L. Current management of lesions associated with an increased risk of breast cancer. Nat Rev Clin Oncol. 2015;12(4):227–38.

31. Kim M, Chung YR, Kim HJ, Woo JW, Ahn S, Park SY. Immune microenvironment in ductal carcinoma in situ: a comparison with invasive carcinoma of the breast. Breast Cancer Res. 2020;22(1):32.

32. Chen X-Y, Yeong J, Thike AA, Bay BH, et al. Prognostic role of immune infiltrates in breast ductal carcinoma in situ. Breast Cancer Res Treat. 2019;177:17–27. https://doi.org/10.1007/s10549-019-05272-2.

33. Agahozo MC, van Bockstal MR, Groenendijk FH, van den Bosch TPP, Westenend PJ, van Deurzen CHM. Ductal carcinoma in situ of the breast: immune cell composition according to subtype. Mod Pathol. 2020;33(2):196–205.

34. Toss MS, Abidi A, Lesche D, Joseph C, Mahale S, Saunders H, et al. The prognostic significance of immune microenvironment in breast ductal carcinoma in situ. Br J Cancer. 2020;122(10):1496–506.

35. Gil Del Alcazar CR, Huh SJ, Ekram MB, Trinh A, Liu LL, Beca F, et al. Immune escape in breast cancer during in situ to invasive carcinoma transition. Cancer Discov. 2017;7(10):1098–115.

36. Hendry S, Pang JMB, Byrne DJ, Lakhani SR, Cummings MC, Campbell IG, et al. Relationship of the breast ductal carcinoma in situ immune microenvironment with clinicopathological and genetic features. Clin Cancer Res. 2017;23(17):5210–7.

37. Pruneri G, Lazzeroni M, Bagnardi V, Tiburzio GB, Rotmensz N, DeCensi A, et al. The prevalence and clinical relevance of tumor-infiltrating lymphocytes (TILs) in ductal carcinoma in situ of the breast. Ann Oncol. 2017;28(2):321–8.

38. Toss MS, Miligy I, Al-Kawaz A, Alsleem M, Khout H, Rida PC, et al. Prognostic significance of tumor-infiltrating lymphocytes in ductal carcinoma in situ of the breast. Mod Pathol. 2018;31(8):1226–36.

39. Dano H, Altinay S, Arnould L, Bletard N, Colpaert C, Dedeurwaerdere F, et al. Interobserver variability in upfront dichotomous histopathological assessment of ductal carcinoma in situ of the breast: the DCISion study. Mod Pathol. 2020;33(3):354–66.

40. Groen EJ, Hudecek J, Mulder L, van Seijen M, Almekinders MM, Alexov S, et al. Prognostic value of histopathological DCIS features in a large-scale international interrater reliability study. Breast Cancer Res Treat. 2020;183(3):759–70.

41. Cserni G, Sejben A. Grading ductal carcinoma in situ (DCIS) of the breast – what's wrong with it? Pathol Oncol Res. 2020;26:665–71.

42. Van Bockstal M, Lambein K, Smeets A, Slembrouck L, Neven P, Nevelsteen I, et al. Stromal characteristics are adequate prognosticators for recurrence risk in ductal carcinoma in situ of the breast. Eur J Surg Oncol. 2019;45(4):550–9.

43. Darvishian F, Ozerdem U, Adams S, Chun J, Pirraglia E, Kaplowitz E, et al. Tumor-infiltrating lymphocytes in a contemporary cohort of women with ductal carcinoma in situ (DCIS). Ann Surg Oncol. 2019;26(10):3337–43.

44. Thike AA, Chen X, Koh VCY, Binte md Nasir ND, JPS Y, Bay BH, et al. Higher densities of tumour-infiltrating lymphocytes and CD4+ T cells predict recurrence and progression of ductal carcinoma in situ of the breast. Histopathology. 2020;76(6):852–64.

45. Xu FF, Zheng SF, Xu C, Cai G, Wang SB, Qi WX, et al. Prognostic and predictive significance of tumor infiltrating lymphocytes for ductal carcinoma in situ. OncoImmunology. 2021;10(1):1875637.

46. Farolfi A, Petracci E, Serra L, Ravaioli A, Bravaccini S, Ravaioli S, et al. Tumor-infiltrating lymphocytes (TILs) and risk of a second breast event after a ductal carcinoma in situ. Front Oncol. 2020;10:1486.

47. Ades F, Zardavas D, Bozovic-Spasojevic I, Pugliano L, Fumagalli D, De Azambuja E, et al. Luminal B breast cancer: molecular characterization, clinical management, and future perspectives. J Clin Oncol. 2014;32:2794–803.

48. Pondé NF, Zardavas D, Piccart M. Progress in adjuvant systemic therapy for breast cancer. Nat Rev Clin Oncol. 2019;16:27–44.

49. Sparano JA, Gray RJ, Ravdin PM, Makower DF, Pritchard KI, Albain KS, et al. Clinical and genomic risk to guide the

use of adjuvant therapy for breast cancer. N Engl J Med. 2019;380(25):2395–405.

50. Piccart M, van 't Veer LJ, Poncet C, Lopes Cardozo JMN, Delaloge S, Pierga JY, et al. 70-gene signature as an aid for treatment decisions in early breast cancer: updated results of the phase 3 randomised MINDACT trial with an exploratory analysis by age. Lancet Oncol. 2021;22(4):476–88.

51. Laws A, Garrido-Castro AC, Poorvu PD, Winer EP, Mittendorf EA, King TA. Utility of the 21-gene recurrence score in node-positive breast cancer. Oncology. 2021;35:77–84.

52. Acs G, Esposito NN, Kiluk J, Loftus L, Laronga C. A mitotically active, cellular tumor stroma and/or inflammatory cells associated with tumor cells may contribute to intermediate or high Oncotype DX Recurrence Scores in low-grade invasive breast carcinomas. Mod Pathol. 2012;25(4):556–66.

53. Desmedt C, Haibe-Kains B, Wirapati P, Buyse M, Larsimont D, Bontempi G, et al. Biological processes associated with breast cancer clinical outcome depend on the molecular subtypes. Clin Cancer Res. 2008;14(16):5158–65.

54. Krishnamurti U, Wetherilt CS, Yang J, Peng L, Li X. Tumor-infiltrating lymphocytes are significantly associated with better overall survival and disease-free survival in triple-negative but not estrogen receptor–positive breast cancers. Hum Pathol. 2017;64:7–12.

55. Ahn SG, Cha YJ, Bae SJ, Yoon C, Lee HW, Jeong J. Comparisons of tumor-infiltrating lymphocyte levels and the 21-gene recurrence score in ER-positive/HER2-negative breast cancer. BMC Cancer. 2018;18(1):320.

56. Kolberg-Liedtke C, Oleg G, Fred H, Friedrich F, Hans K, Michael C, et al. Association of TILs with clinical parameters, Recurrence Score® results, and prognosis in patients with early HER2-negative breast cancer (BC) - a translational analysis of the prospective WSG PlanB trial. Breast Cancer Res. 2020;22(1):47.

57. Nagalla S, Chou JW, Willingham MC, Ruiz J, Vaughn JP, Dubey P, et al. Interactions between immunity, proliferation and molecular subtype in breast cancer prognosis. Genome Biol. 2013;14(4):R34.

58. Seelige R, Searles S, Jack ·, Bui D. Mechanisms regulating immune surveillance of cellular stress in cancer. Cell Mol Life Sci. 2018;75:225–40.

59. López-Soto A, Gonzalez S, López-Larrea C, Kroemer G. Immunosurveillance of malignant cells with complex karyotypes. Trends Cell Biol. 2017;27:880–4.

60. Smid M, Rodríguez-González FG, Sieuwerts AM, Salgado R, Prager-Van Der Smissen WJC, van der Vlugt-Daane M, et al. Breast cancer genome and transcriptome integration implicates specific mutational signatures with immune cell infiltration. Nat Commun. 2016;7:12910.

61. Solinas C, Marcoux D, Garaud S, Vitória JR, van den Eynden G, de Wind A, et al. BRCA gene mutations do not shape the extent and organization of tumor infiltrating lymphocytes in triple negative breast cancer. Cancer Lett. 2019;450:88–97.

62. Haricharan S, Bainbridge MN, Scheet P, Brown PH. Somatic mutation load of estrogen receptor-positive breast tumors predicts overall survival: An analysis of genome sequence data. Breast Cancer Res Treat. 2014;146(1):211–20.

63. Davies H, Morganella S, Purdie CA, Jang SJ, Borgen E, Russnes H, et al. Whole-genome sequencing reveals breast cancers with mismatch repair deficiency. Cancer Res. 2017;77(18):4755–62.

64. Denkert C, Von Minckwitz G, Brase JC, Sinn BV, Gade S, Kronenwett R, et al. Tumor-infiltrating lymphocytes and response to neoadjuvant chemotherapy with or without carboplatin in human epidermal growth factor receptor 2-positive and triple-negative primary breast cancers. J Clin Oncol. 2015;33(9):983–91.

65. Heng YJ, Lester SC, Tse GMK, Factor RE, Allison KH, Collins LC, et al. The molecular basis of breast cancer pathological phenotypes. J Pathol. 2017;241(3):375–91.

66. Loi S, Michiels S, Salgado R, Sirtaine N, Jose V, Fumagalli D, et al. Tumor infiltrating lymphocytes are prognostic in triple negative breast cancer and predictive for trastuzumab benefit in early breast cancer: results from the FinHER trial. Ann Oncol. 2014;25(8):1544–50.

67. Dieci MV, Mathieu MC, Guarneri V, Conte P, Delaloge S, Andre F, et al. Prognostic and predictive value of tumor-infiltrating lymphocytes in two phase III randomized adjuvant breast cancer trials. Ann Oncol. 2015;26(8):1698–704.

68. Fujimoto Y, Watanabe T, Hida AI, Higuchi T, Miyagawa Y, Ozawa H, et al. Prognostic significance of tumor-infiltrating lymphocytes may differ depending on Ki67 expression levels in estrogen receptor-positive/HER2-negative operated breast cancers. Breast Cancer. 2019;26(6):738–47.

69. Criscitiello C, Vingiani A, Maisonneuve P, Viale G, Viale G, Curigliano G. Tumor-infiltrating lymphocytes (TILs) in ER+/HER2− breast cancer. Breast Cancer Res Treat. 2020;183(2):347–54.

70. Hua GZ, Xin LC, Liu M, Yuan JJ. Predictive and prognostic role of tumour-infiltrating lymphocytes in breast cancer patients with different molecular subtypes: a meta-analysis. BMC Cancer. 2020;20(1):1150.

71. Deman F, Punie K, Laenen A, Neven P, Oldenburger E, Smeets A, et al. Assessment of stromal tumor infiltrating lymphocytes and immunohistochemical features in invasive micropapillary breast carcinoma with long-term outcomes. Breast Cancer Res Treat. 2020;184(3):985–98.

72. Richard F, Majjaj S, Venet D, Rothé F, Pingitore J, Boeckx B, et al. Characterization of stromal tumor-infiltrating lymphocytes and genomic alterations in metastatic lobular breast cancer. Clin Cancer Res. 2020;26(23):6254–65.

73. Guo X, Chen L, Lang R, Fan Y, Zhang X, Fu L. Invasive micropapillary carcinoma of the breast: association of pathologic features with lymph node metastasis. Am J Clin Pathol. 2006;126(5):740–6.

74. Gucalp A, Traina TA, Eisner JR, Parker JS, Selitsky SR, Park BH, et al. Male breast cancer: a disease distinct from female breast cancer. Breast Cancer Res Treat. 2019;173:37–48.

75. Vermeulen MA, Slaets L, Cardoso F, Giordano SH, Tryfonidis K, van Diest PJ, et al. Pathological characterisation of male breast cancer: results of the EORTC 10085/TBCRC/BIG/NABCG International Male Breast Cancer Program. Eur J Cancer. 2017;82:219–27.

76. Ali HR, Provenzano E, Dawson S-J, Blows FM, Liu B, Shah M, et al. Association between CD8+ T-cell infiltration and breast cancer survival in 12 439 patients. Ann Oncol. 2014;25:1536–43.

77. Mahmoud SMA, Paish EC, Powe DG, Macmillan RD, Grainge MJ, Lee AHS, et al. Tumor-infiltrating CD8+ lymphocytes predict clinical outcome in breast cancer. J Clin Oncol. 2011;29(15):1949–55.

78. Dieci MV, Miglietta F, Guarneri V. Immune infiltrates in breast cancer: recent updates and clinical implications. Cells. 2021;10:223.

79. Scheel AH, Penault-Llorca F, Hanna W, Baretton G, Middel P, Burchhardt J, et al. Physical basis of the "magnification rule" for standardized Immunohistochemical scoring of HER2 in breast and gastric cancer. Diagn Pathol. 2018;13(1)

80. Wolff AC, McShane LM, Hammond MEH, Allison KH, Fitzgibbons P, Press MF, et al. Human epidermal growth factor receptor 2 testing in breast cancer: American Society of Clinical Oncology/College of American Pathologists Clinical Practice Guideline Focused Update. Arch Pathol Lab Med. 2018;142:1364–82.

81. Goutsouliak K, Veeraraghavan J, Sethunath V, Angelis C, Kent Osborne C, Rimawi MF, et al. Towards personalized treatment for early stage HER2-positive breast cancer. Nat Rev Clin Oncol. 2020;17(4):233–50.

82. Rimawi MF, Schiff R, Osborne CK. Targeting HER2 for the treatment of breast cancer. Annu Rev Med. 2015;66:111–28.

83. Brandão M, Caparica R, Malorni L, Prat A, Carey LA, Piccart M. What is the real impact of estrogen receptor status on the prognosis and treatment of HER2-positive early breast cancer? Clin Cancer Res. 2020;26:2783–8.

84. Marchiò C, Annaratone L, Marques A, Casorzo L, Berrino E, Sapino A. Evolving concepts in HER2 evaluation in breast cancer: heterogeneity, HER2-low carcinomas and beyond. Semin Cancer Biol. 2021;72:123–35.

85. Schettini F, Chic N, Brasó-Maristany F, Paré L, Pascual T, Conte B, et al. Clinical, pathological, and PAM50 gene expression features of HER2-low breast cancer. NPJ Breast Cancer. 2021;7(1):1.

86. Salgado R, Denkert C, Campbell C, Savas P, Nuciforo P, Aura C, et al. Tumor-infiltrating lymphocytes and associations with pathological complete response and event-free survival in HER2-positive early-stage breast cancer treated with lapatinib and trastuzumab: A secondary analysis of the NeoALTTO trial. JAMA Oncol. 2015;1(4):448–55.

87. Rody A, Holtrich U, Pusztai L, Liedtke C, Gaetje R, Ruckhaeberle E, et al. T-cell metagene predicts a favorable prognosis in estrogen receptor-negative and HER2-positive breast cancers. Breast Cancer Res. 2009;11(2):R15.

88. Perez EA, Ballman KV, Tenner KS, Thompson EA, Badve SS, Bailey H, et al. Association of stromal tumor-infiltrating lymphocytes with recurrence-free survival in the n9831 adjuvant trial in patients with early-stage HER2-positive breast cancer. JAMA Oncol. 2016;2(1):56–64.

89. Kim RS, Song N, Gavin PG, Salgado R, Bandos H, Kos Z, et al. Stromal tumor-infiltrating lymphocytes in NRG oncology/NSABP B-31 adjuvant trial for early-stage HER2-positive breast cancer. J Natl Cancer Inst. 2019;111(8):867–71.

90. Pogue-Geile KL, Song N, Serie DJ, Wang Y, Gavin PG, Kim RS, et al. Validation of the NSABP/NRG Oncology 8-gene trastuzumab-benefit signature in alliance/NCCTG N9831. JNCI Cancer Spectr. 2020;4(5):pkaa058.

91. Dieci MV, Conte P, Bisagni G, Brandes AA, Frassoldati A, Cavanna L, et al. Association of tumor-infiltrating lymphocytes with distant disease-free survival in the ShortHER randomized adjuvant trial for patients with early HER2+ breast cancer. Ann Oncol. 2019;30(3):418–23.

92. Prat A, Guarneri V, Paré L, Griguolo G, Pascual T, Dieci MV, et al. A multivariable prognostic score to guide systemic therapy in early-stage HER2-positive breast cancer: a retrospective study with an external evaluation. Lancet Oncol. 2020;21(11):1455–64.

93. He L, Wang Y, Wu Q, Song Y, Ma X, Zhang B, et al. Association between levels of tumor-infiltrating lymphocytes in different subtypes of primary breast tumors and prognostic outcomes: a meta-analysis. BMC Women's Health. 2020;20(1):194.

94. Desmedt C, Zoppoli G, Sotiriou C, Salgado R. Transcriptomic and genomic features of invasive lobular breast cancer. Semin Cancer Biol. 2017;44:98–105.

95. Jongen L, Floris G, Boeckx B, Smeets D, Lambrechts D, van der Borght S, et al. Identification, clinical-pathological characteristics and treatment outcomes of patients with metastatic breast cancer and somatic human epidermal growth factor receptor 2 (ERBB2) mutations. Breast Cancer Res Treat. 2019;174(1):55–63.

96. Geyer FC, Pareja F, Weigelt B, Rakha E, Ellis IO, Schnitt SJ, et al. The spectrum of triple-negative breast disease: high- and low-grade lesions. Am J Pathol. 2017;187:2139–51.

97. Lehmann BD, Bauer JA, Chen X, Sanders ME, Chakravarthy AB, Shyr Y, et al. Identification of human triple-negative breast cancer subtypes and preclinical models for selection of targeted therapies. J Clin Investig. 2011;121(7):2750–67.

98. Burstein MD, Tsimelzon A, Poage GM, Covington KR, Contreras A, Fuqua SAW, et al. Comprehensive genomic analysis identifies novel subtypes and targets of triple-negative breast cancer. Clin Cancer Res. 2015;21(7):1688–98.

99. Turner NC, Reis-Filho JS. Tackling the diversity of Triple-negative breast cancer. Clin Cancer Res. 2013;19(23):6380–8.

100. Bertucci F, Finetti P, Cervera N, Charafe-Jauffret E, Mamessier E, Adélaïdev JA, et al. Gene expression profiling shows medullary breast cancer is a subgroup of basal breast cancers. Cancer Res. 2006;66(9):4636–80.

101. Lehmann BD, Jovanović B, Chen X, Estrada MV, Johnson KN, Shyr Y, et al. Refinement of triple-negative breast cancer molecular subtypes: implications for neoadjuvant chemotherapy selection. 2016. Available from: http://cancer

102. Adams S, Gray RJ, Demaria S, Goldstein L, Perez EA, Shulman LN, et al. Prognostic value of tumor-infiltrating lymphocytes in triple-negative breast cancers from two phase III randomized adjuvant breast cancer trials: ECOG 2197 and ECOG 1199. J Clin Oncol. 2014;32:2959–66.

103. Pruneri G, Gray KP, Vingiani A, Viale G, Curigliano G, Criscitiello C, et al. Tumor-infiltrating lymphocytes (TILs) are a powerful prognostic marker in patients with triple-negative breast cancer enrolled in the IBCSG phase III randomized clinical trial 22-00. Breast Cancer Res Treat. 2016;158:323–31.

104. Loi S, Drubay D, Adams S, Pruneri G, Francis PA, Lacroix-Triki M, et al. Tumor-infiltrating lymphocytes and prognosis: a pooled individual patient analysis of early-stage triple-negative breast cancers. J Clin Oncol. 2019;37:559–69.

105. Cortazar P, Zhang L, Untch M, Mehta K, Costantino JP, Wolmark N, et al. Pathological complete response and long-term clinical benefit in breast cancer: the CTNeoBC pooled analysis. The Lancet. 2014;384(9938):164–72.

106. Provenzano E, Bossuyt V, Viale G, Cameron D, Badve S, Denkert C, et al. Standardization of pathologic evaluation and reporting of postneoadjuvant specimens in clinical trials of breast cancer: recommendations from an international working group. 2015. Available from: www.modernpathology.org

107. Symmans WF, Peintinger F, Hatzis C, Rajan R, Kuerer H, Valero V, et al. Measurement of residual breast cancer burden to predict survival after neoadjuvant chemotherapy. J Clin Oncol. 2007;25(28):4414–22.

108. Ogston KN, Miller ID, Payne S, Hutcheon AW, Sarkar TK, Smith I, et al. A new histological grading system to assess response of breast cancers to primary chemotherapy: prognostic significance and survival. Breast. 2003;12(5):320–7.

109. Wein L, Luen SJ, Savas P, Salgado R, Loi S. Checkpoint blockade in the treatment of breast cancer: current status and future directions. 2018. https://doi.org/10.1038/s41416-018-0126-6.

110. von Minckwitz G, Untch M, Blohmer JU, Costa SD, Eidtmann H, Fasching PA, et al. Definition and impact of pathologic complete response on prognosis after neoadjuvant chemotherapy in various intrinsic breast cancer subtypes. J Clin Oncol. 2012;30(15):1796–804.

111. Schneeweiss A, Möbus V, Tesch H, Hanusch C, Denkert C, Lübbe K, et al. Intense dose-dense epirubicin, paclitaxel, cyclophosphamide versus weekly paclitaxel, liposomal doxorubicin (plus carboplatin in triple-negative breast cancer) for neoadjuvant treatment of high-risk early breast cancer (GeparOcto—GBG 84): a randomised phase III trial. Eur J Cancer. 2019;106:181–92.

112. Issa-Nummer Y, Darb-Esfahani S, Loibl S, Kunz G, Nekljudova V, Schrader I, et al. Prospective validation of immunological infiltrate for prediction of response to neoadjuvant chemotherapy in HER2-negative breast cancer – a substudy of the neoadjuvant GeparQuinto trial. PLoS One. 2013;8(12):e79775. https://doi.org/10.1371/journal.pone.0079775.

113. O'Loughlin M, Andreu X, Bianchi S, Chemielik E, Cordoba A, Cserni G, et al. Reproducibility and predictive value of scoring stromal tumour infiltrating lymphocytes in triple-negative breast

cancer: a multi-institutional study. Breast Cancer Res Treat. 2021;171(1):1–9.

114. Denkert C, Wienert S, Poterie A, Loibl S, Budczies J, Badve S, et al. Standardized evaluation of tumor-infiltrating lymphocytes in breast cancer: results of the ring studies of the international immuno-oncology biomarker working group. Mod Pathol. 2016;29(10):1155–64.

115. Asano Y, Kashiwagi S, Goto W, Takada K, Takahashi K, Hatano T, et al. Prediction of treatment response to neoadjuvant chemotherapy in breast cancer by subtype using tumor-infiltrating lymphocytes. Anticancer Res. 2018;38(4):2311–21.

116. Jongen L, Floris G, Wildiers H, Claessens F, Richard F, Laenen A, et al. Tumor characteristics and outcome by androgen receptor expression in triple-negative breast cancer patients treated with neo-adjuvant chemotherapy. Br Cancer Res Treat. 2019;176:699–708. https://doi.org/10.1007/s10549-019-05252-6.

117. Hamy AS, Bonsang-Kitzis H, de Croze D, Laas E, Darrigues L, Topciu L, et al. Interaction between molecular subtypes and stromal immune infiltration before and after treatment in breast cancer patients treated with neoadjuvant chemotherapy. Clin Cancer Res. 2019;25(22):6731–41.

118. Gao G, Wang Z, Qu X, Zhang Z. Prognostic value of tumor-infiltrating lymphocytes in patients with triple-negative breast cancer: a systematic review and meta-analysis. BMC Cancer. 2020;20(1):179.

119. Luen SJ, Salgado R, Loi S. Residual disease and immune infiltration as a new surrogate endpoint for TNBC post neoadjuvant chemotherapy. Oncotarget. 2019;10:4612–4.

120. Demaria S, Volm MD, Shapiro RL, Yee HY, Oratz R, Formenti SC, et al. Development of tumor-infiltrating lymphocytes in breast cancer after neoadjuvant paclitaxel chemotherapy. Clin Cancer Res. 2001;7(10):3025–30.

121. Dieci MV, Criscitiello C, Goubar A, Viale G, Conte P, Guarneri V, et al. Prognostic value of tumor-infiltrating lymphocytes on residual disease after primary chemotherapy for triple-negative breast cancer: a retrospective multicenter study. Ann Oncol. 2014;25(3):611–8.

122. Loi S, Dushyanthen S, Beavis PA, Salgado R, Denkert C, Savas P, et al. RAS/MAPK activation is associated with reduced tumor-infiltrating lymphocytes in triple-negative breast cancer: Therapeutic cooperation between MEK and PD-1/PD-L1 immune checkpoint inhibitors. Clin Cancer Res. 2016;22(6):1499–509.

123. Luen SJ, Salgado R, Dieci MV, Vingiani A, Curigliano G, Gould RE, et al. Prognostic implications of residual disease tumor-infiltrating lymphocytes and residual cancer burden in triple-negative breast cancer patients after neoadjuvant chemotherapy. Ann Oncol. 2019;30(2):236–42.

124. Ali HR, Dariush A, Thomas J, Provenzano E, Dunn J, Hiller L, et al. Lymphocyte density determined by computational pathology validated as a predictor of response to neoadjuvant chemotherapy in breast cancer: secondary analysis of the ARTemis trial. Ann Oncol. 2017;28(8):1832–5.

125. Ali HR, Dariush A, Provenzano E, Bardwell H, Abraham JE, Iddawela M, et al. Computational pathology of pre-treatment biopsies identifies lymphocyte density as a predictor of response to neoadjuvant chemotherapy in breast cancer. Breast Cancer Res. 2016;18(1):21.

126. Dieci MV, Frassoldati A, Generali D, Bisagni G, Piacentini F, Cavanna L, et al. Tumor-infiltrating lymphocytes and molecular response after neoadjuvant therapy for HR+/HER2− breast cancer: results from two prospective trials. Br Cancer Res Treat. 2017;163(2):295–302.

127. Griguolo G, Dieci MV, Paré L, Miglietta F, Generali DG, Frassoldati A, et al. Immune microenvironment and intrinsic subtyping in hormone receptor-positive/HER2-negative breast cancer. NPJ Br Cancer. 2021;7(1):1–5. https://doi.org/10.1038/s41523-021-00223-x.

128. Badr NM, Spooner D, Steven J, Stevens A, Shaaban AM. Morphological and molecular changes following neoadjuvant endocrine therapy of ER positive breast cancer: implications for clinical practice. Histopathology. 2021;79(1):47–56.

129. Skriver SK, Jensen MB, Knoop AS, Ejlertsen B, Laenkholm AV. Tumour-infiltrating lymphocytes and response to neoadjuvant letrozole in patients with early oestrogen receptor-positive breast cancer: analysis from a nationwide phase II DBCG trial. Breast Cancer Res. 2020;22(1):46.

130. Dunbier AK, Ghazoui Z, Anderson H, Salter J, Nerurkar A, Osin P, et al. Molecular profiling of aromatase inhibitor-treated postmenopausal breast tumors identifies immune-related correlates of resistance. Clin Cancer Res. 2013;19(10):2775–86.

131. Liang X, Briaux A, Becette V, Benoist C, Boulai A, Chemlali W, et al. Molecular profiling of hormone receptor-positive, HER2-negative breast cancers from patients treated with neoadjuvant endocrine therapy in the CARMINA 02 trial (UCBG-0609). J Hematol Oncol. 2018;11(1):124.

132. Chan MSM, Wang L, Felizola SJA, Ueno T, Toi M, Loo W, et al. Changes of tumor infiltrating lymphocyte subtypes before and after neoadjuvant endocrine therapy in estrogen receptor-positive breast cancer patients - an immunohistochemical study of cd8+ and foxp3+ using double immunostaining with correlation to the pathobiological response of the patients. Int J Biol Markers. 2012;27(4):e295–304.

133. Llombart-Cussac A, Cortés J, Paré L, Galván P, Bermejo B, Martínez N, et al. HER2-enriched subtype as a predictor of pathological complete response following trastuzumab and lapatinib without chemotherapy in early-stage HER2-positive breast cancer (PAMELA): an open-label, single-group, multicentre, phase 2 trial. Lancet Oncol. 2017;18(4):545–54.

134. Nuciforo P, Pascual T, Cortés J, Llombart-Cussac A, Fasani R, Paré L, et al. A predictive model of pathologic response based on tumor cellularity and tumor-infiltrating lymphocytes (CelTIL) in HER2-positive breast cancer treated with chemo-free dual HER2 blockade. Ann Oncol. 2018;29(1):170–7.

135. Chic N, Luen SJ, Nuciforo P, Salgado R, Fumagalli D, Hilbers F, et al. Tumor cellularity and infiltrating lymphocytes (CelTIL) as a survival surrogate in HER2-positive breast cancer. J Natl Cancer Inst. 2022;114(3):467–70.

136. Desmedt C, Fornili M, Clatot F, Demicheli R, de Bortoli D, di Leo A, et al. Differential benefit of adjuvant docetaxel-based chemotherapy in patients with early breast cancer according to baseline body mass index. J Clin Oncol. 2020;38(25):2883–91.

137. Floris G, Richard F, Hamy A-S, Jongen L, Wildiers H, Ardui J, et al. Body mass index and tumor-infiltrating lymphocytes in triple-negative breast cancer. J Natl Cancer Inst. 2021;113(2):146–53.

138. Murphy WJ, Longo DL. The surprisingly positive association between obesity and cancer immunotherapy efficacy. J Am Med Assoc. 2019;321:1247–8.

139. Cardoso F, Paluch-Shimon S, Senkus E, Curigliano G, Aapro MS, André F, et al. 5th ESO-ESMO international consensus guidelines for advanced breast cancer (ABC 5). Ann Oncol. 2020;31(12):1623–49.

140. Wein L, Savas P, Luen SJ, Virassamy B, Salgado R, Loi S. Clinical validity and utility of tumor-infiltrating lymphocytes in routine clinical practice for breast cancer patients: current and future directions. Front Oncol. 2017;7:156.

141. Savas P, Virassamy B, Ye C, Salim A, Mintoff CP, Caramia F, et al. Single-cell profiling of breast cancer T cells reveals a tissue-resident memory subset associated with improved prognosis. Nat Med. 2018;24(7):986–93.

142. Loi S, Giobbie-Hurder A, Gombos A, Bachelot T, Hui R, Curigliano G, et al. Pembrolizumab plus trastuzumab in

trastuzumab-resistant, advanced, HER2-positive breast cancer (PANACEA): a single-arm, multicentre, phase 1b–2 trial. Lancet Oncol. 2019;20(3):371–82.

143. Adams S, Schmid P, Rugo HS, Winer EP, Loirat D, Awada A, et al. Pembrolizumab monotherapy for previously treated metastatic triple-negative breast cancer: cohort A of the phase II KEYNOTE-086 study. Ann Oncol. 2019;30(3):397–404.

144. Ogiya R, Niikura N, Kumaki N, Bianchini G, Kitano S, Iwamoto T, et al. Comparison of tumor-infiltrating lymphocytes between primary and metastatic tumors in breast cancer patients. Cancer Sci. 2016;107(12):1730–5.

145. Cimino-Mathews A, Ye X, Meeker A, Argani P, Emens LA. Metastatic triple-negative breast cancers at first relapse have fewer tumor-infiltrating lymphocytes than their matched primary breast tumors: a pilot study. Hum Pathol. 2013;44(10):2055–63.

146. Ogiya R, Niikura N, Kumaki N, Yasojima H, Iwasa T, Kanbayashi C, et al. Comparison of immune microenvironments between primary tumors and brain metastases in patients with breast cancer. Oncotarget. 2017;8(61):103671–81.

147. Vermeulen PB, Bohlok A, Leduc S, Richard F, Botzenhart L, Ignatiadis M, et al. Abstract P3-01-13: Association between the histopathological growth patterns (HGP) of liver metastases (LM) and survival after hepatic surgery in patients with oligometastatic breast cancer (BC). In: Cancer Research. American Association for Cancer Research (AACR); 2020. p. P3-01-13-P3-01-13. Available from: https://cancerres.aacrjournals.org/content/80/4_Supplement/P3-01-13

148. van Dam PJ, van der Stok EP, Teuwen LA, van den Eynden GG, Illemann M, Frentzas S, et al. International consensus guidelines for scoring the histopathological growth patterns of liver metastasis. Br J Cancer. 2017;117:1427–41.

149. Sambade MJ, Prince G, Deal AM, Trembath D, McKee M, Garrett A, et al. Examination and prognostic implications of the unique microenvironment of breast cancer brain metastases. Brest Cancer Res Treat. 2019;176(2):321–8.

150. Szekely B, Bossuyt V, Li X, Wali VB, Patwardhan GA, Frederick C, et al. Immunological differences between primary and metastatic breast cancer. Ann Oncol. 2018;29(11):2232–9.

151. Dieci MV, Tsvetkova V, Orvieto E, Piacentini F, Ficarra G, Griguolo G, et al. Immune characterization of breast cancer metastases: Prognostic implications. Breast Cancer Res. 2018;20(1):62.

152. Luen SJ, Salgado R, Fox S, Savas P, Eng-Wong J, Clark E, et al. Tumour-infiltrating lymphocytes in advanced HER2-positive breast cancer treated with pertuzumab or placebo in addition to trastuzumab and docetaxel: a retrospective analysis of the CLEOPATRA study. Lancet Oncol. 2017;18(1):52–62.

153. Iacobuzio-Donahue CA, Michael C, Baez P, Kappagantula R, Hooper JE, Hollman TJ. Cancer biology as revealed by the research autopsy. Nat Rev Cancer. 2019;19(12):686–97.

154. Dankner M, Issa-Chergui B, Bouganim N. Post-mortem tissue donation programs as platforms to accelerate cancer research. J Pathol Clin Res. 2020;6(3):163–70.

155. Doroshow DB, Bhalla S, Beasley MB, Sholl LM, Kerr KM, Gnjatic S, et al. PD-L1 as a biomarker of response to immune-checkpoint inhibitors. Nat Rev Clin Oncol. 2021;18(6):345–62.

156. Paver EC, Cooper WA, Colebatch AJ, Ferguson PM, Hill SK, Lum T, et al. Programmed death ligand-1 (PD-L1) as a predictive marker for immunotherapy in solid tumours: a guide to immunohistochemistry implementation and interpretation. Pathology. 2021;53:141–56.

157. Schmid P, Rugo HS, Adams S, Schneeweiss A, Barrios CH, Iwata H, et al. Atezolizumab plus nab-paclitaxel as first-line treatment for unresectable, locally advanced or metastatic triple-negative breast cancer (IMpassion130): updated efficacy results from a randomised, double-blind, placebo-controlled, phase 3 trial. Lancet Oncol. 2020;21(1):44–59.

158. Schmid P, Adams S, Rugo HS, Schneeweiss A, Barrios CH, Iwata H, et al. Atezolizumab and nab-paclitaxel in advanced triple-negative breast cancer. N Engl J Med. 2018;379(22):2108–21.

159. Cortes J, Cescon DW, Rugo HS, Nowecki Z, Im SA, Yusof MM, et al. Pembrolizumab plus chemotherapy versus placebo plus chemotherapy for previously untreated locally recurrent inoperable or metastatic triple-negative breast cancer (KEYNOTE-355): a randomised, placebo-controlled, double-blind, phase 3 clinical trial. The Lancet. 2020;396(10265):1817–28.

160. Miles DW, Gligorov J, André F, Cameron D, Schneeweiss A, Barrios CH, et al. LBA15 Primary results from IMpassion131, a double-blind placebo-controlled randomised phase III trial of first-line paclitaxel (PAC) ± atezolizumab (atezo) for unresectable locally advanced/metastatic triple-negative breast cancer (mTNBC). Ann Oncol. 2020;31:S1147–8.

161. Lu S, Stein JE, Rimm DL, Wang DW, Bell JM, Johnson DB, et al. Comparison of biomarker modalities for predicting response to PD-1/PD-L1 checkpoint blockade: a systematic review and meta-analysis. JAMA Oncol. 2019;5:1195–204.

162. Schmid P, Cortes J, Pusztai L, McArthur H, Kümmel S, Bergh J, et al. Pembrolizumab for early triple-negative breast cancer. N Engl J Med. 2020;382(9):810–21.

163. Mittendorf EA, Zhang H, Barrios CH, Saji S, Jung KH, Hegg R, et al. Neoadjuvant atezolizumab in combination with sequential nab-paclitaxel and anthracycline-based chemotherapy versus placebo and chemotherapy in patients with early-stage triple-negative breast cancer (IMpassion031): a randomised, double-blind, phase 3 trial. Lancet. 2020;396(10257):1090–100.

164. Rugo H, Loi S, Adams S, Schmid P, Schneeweiss A, Barrios CH, et al. PD1-07. Exploratory analytical harmonization of PD-L1 immunohistochemistry assays in advanced triple-negative breast cancer: a retrospective substudy of IMpassion130. 42nd Annual CTRC-AACR San Antonio Breast Cancer Symposium, San Antonio, TX, December 10–14, 2019.

165. Gonzalez-Ericsson PI, Stovgaard ES, Sua LF, Reisenbichler E, Kos Z, Carter JM, et al. The path to a better biomarker: application of a risk management framework for the implementation of PD-L1 and TILs as immuno-oncology biomarkers in breast cancer clinical trials and daily practice. J Pathol. 2020;250:667–84.

166. Roche H-L (2015) A study of atezolizumab in combination with nab-paclitaxel compared with placebo with nab-paclitaxel for participants with previously untreated metastatic triple-negative breast cancer (IMpassion130), https://ClinicalTrials.gov/show/NCT02425891

167. Schmid P, et al. Atezolizumab plus nab-paclitaxel as first-line treatment for unresectable, locally advanced or metastatic triple-negative breast cancer (IMpassion130): updated efficacy results from a randomised, double-blind, placebo-controlled, phase 3 trial. Lancet Oncol. 2020;21(1):44–59.

168. Rugo HS, Loi S, Adams S, Schmid P, Schneeweiss A, Barrios CH, et al. LBA20: performance of PD-L1 immunohistochemistry (IHC) assays in unresectable locally advanced or metastatic triple-negative breastcancer (mTNBC): post-hoc analysis of IMpassion130. Ann Oncol. 2019;30(S5):v858–9.

169. A study of atezolizumab and paclitaxel versus placebo and paclitaxel in participants with previously untreated locally advanced or metastatic triple negative breast cancer (TNBC), https://ClinicalTrials.gov/show/NCT03125902

170. Miles DW, Gligorov J, André F, Cameron D, Schneeweiss A, Barrios CH, et al. LBA15 - primary results from IMpassion131, a double-blind placebo-controlled randomised phase III trial of first-line paclitaxel (PAC) ± atezolizumab (atezo) for unresectable locally advanced/metastatic triple-negative breast cancer (mTNBC). Ann Oncol. 2020;31(suppl_4):S1142–215. https://doi.org/10.1016/annonc/annonc325.

171. A study to investigate atezolizumab and chemotherapy compared with placebo and chemotherapy in the neoadjuvant setting in participants with early stage triple negative breast cancer, https://ClinicalTrials.gov/show/NCT03197935

172. Study of single agent pembrolizumab (MK-3475) versus single agent chemotherapy for metastatic triple negative breast cancer (MK-3475-119/KEYNOTE-119), https://ClinicalTrials.gov/show/NCT02555657

173. Winer EP, Lipatov O, Im S-A, Goncalves A, Muñoz-Couselo E, Lee KS, et al. Pembrolizumab versus investigator-choice chemotherapy for metastatic triple-negative breast cancer (KEYNOTE-119): a randomised, open-label, phase 3 trial. Lancet Oncol. 2021;22(4):499–511.

174. Study of pembrolizumab (MK-3475) plus chemotherapy vs. placebo plus chemotherapy for previously untreated locally recurrent inoperable or metastatic triple negative breast cancer (MK-3475-355/KEYNOTE-355), https://ClinicalTrials.gov/show/NCT02819518

175. Study of pembrolizumab (MK-3475) plus chemotherapy vs placebo plus chemotherapy as neoadjuvant therapy and pembrolizumab vs placebo as adjuvant therapy in participants with triple negative breast cancer (TNBC) (MK-3475-522/KEYNOTE-522), https://ClinicalTrials.gov/show/NCT03036488

176. Roche H-L (2019) A study of atezolizumab plus nab-paclitaxel in the treatment of unresectable locally advanced or metastatic PD-L1-positive triple-negative breast cancer, https://ClinicalTrials.gov/show/NCT04148911.

177. Inc NF et al. (2017) Clinical trial of neoadjuvant chemotherapy with atezolizumab or placebo in patients with triple-negative breast cancer followed after surgery by atezolizumab or placebo, https://ClinicalTrials.gov/show/NCT03281954.

178. Sharp M, Corp D (2019) Study of olaparib plus pembrolizumab versus chemotherapy plus pembrolizumab after induction with first-line chemotherapy plus pembrolizumab in triple negative breast cancer (TNBC) (MK-7339-009/KEYLYNK-009), https://ClinicalTrials.gov/show/NCT04191135

179. Roche H-L (2018) A study of the efficacy and safety of atezolizumab plus chemotherapy for patients with early relapsing recurrent triple-negative breast cancer, https://ClinicalTrials.gov/show/NCT03371017

180. Roche H-L, et al (2018) A study comparing atezolizumab (anti PD-L1 antibody) in combination with adjuvant anthracycline/taxane-based chemotherapy versus chemotherapy alone in patients with operable triple-negative breast cancer, https://ClinicalTrials.gov/show/NCT03498716

181. Michelangelo F (2016) Neoadjuvant therapy in TRIPle negative breast cancer with antiPDL1, https://ClinicalTrials.gov/show/NCT02620280

182. Jiangsu HengRui Medicine Co., L. (2020) A phase 3 study comparing carelizumab plus nab-paclitaxel and apatinib, carelizumab plus nab-paclitaxel, and nab-paclitaxel in patients with advanced triple negative breast cancer, https://ClinicalTrials.gov/show/NCT04335006

183. Jiangsu HengRui Medicine Co., L. (2020) A study of camrelizumab plus chemotherapy vs placebo plus chemotherapy as neoadjuvant therapy in participants with triple negative breast cancer (TNBC), https://ClinicalTrials.gov/show/NCT04613674

184. Shanghai Junshi Bioscience Co., L. (2018). Toripalimab in combination with nab-paclitaxel for patients with metastatic or recurrent triple-negative breast cancer (TNBC) with or without systemic treatment, https://ClinicalTrials.gov/show/NCT04085276

185. Roche H-L, Chugai Pharmaceutical (2019) A study to evaluate the efficacy and safety of atezolizumab or placebo in combination with neoadjuvant doxorubicin + cyclophosphamide followed by paclitaxel + trastuzumab + pertuzumab in early her2-positive breast cancer, https://ClinicalTrials.gov/show/NCT03726879

186. Roche H-L (2021) A study of trastuzumab emtansine in combination with atezolizumab or placebo as a treatment for participants with human epidermal growth factor 2 (HER2)-positive and programmed death-ligand 1 (PD-L1)-positive locally advanced (LABC) or metastatic breast cancer (MBC), https://ClinicalTrials.gov/show/NCT04740918

187. Japanese Foundation for Cancer Research and Chugai Pharmaceutical (2021) A phase III study of bevacizumab and paclitaxel in combination with atezolizumab as a treatment for locally advanced unresectable or metastatic hormone receptor-positive HER2 negative breast cancer, https://ClinicalTrials.gov/show/NCT04732598

188. Sharp M, Dohme Corp (2018). Study of pembrolizumab (MK-3475) versus placebo in combination with neoadjuvant chemotherapy & adjuvant endocrine therapy in the treatment of early-stage estrogen receptor-positive, human epidermal growth factor receptor 2-negative (ER+/HER2-) breast cancer (MK-3475-756/KEYNOTE-756), https://ClinicalTrials.gov/show/NCT03725059

189. Tannock IF. Have investigators forgotten how to write? Ann Oncol. 2021 Apr;32(4):437–8. https://doi.org/10.1016/j.annonc.2020.12.017.

190. Fundytus A, Booth CM, Tannock IF. How low can you go? PD-L1 expression as a biomarker in trials of cancer immunotherapy. Ann Oncol. 2021;S0923-7534(21):01118–2. https://doi.org/10.1016/j.annonc.2021.03.208.

191. Salgado R, Bellizzi AM, Rimm D, Bartlett JM, Nielsen T, Holger M, et al. How current assay approval policies are leading to unintended imprecision medicine. Ann Oncol. 2021 Apr;32(4):437–8. https://doi.org/10.1016/j.annonc.2020.12.017.

192. Ahmed FS, Gaule P, McGuire J, Patel K, Blenman K, Pusztai L, et al. PD-L1 Protein expression on both tumor cells and macrophages are associated with response to neoadjuvant durvalumab with chemotherapy in triple-negative breast cancer. Clin Cancer Res. 2020;26(20):5456–61.

193. Tang H, Wang Y, Chlewicki LK, Zhang Y, Guo J, Liang W, et al. Facilitating T cell infiltration in tumor microenvironment overcomes resistance to PD-L1 blockade. Cancer Cell. 2016;29(3):285–96.

194. Bassez A, Vos H, van Dyck L, Floris G, Arijs I, Desmedt C, et al. anti-PD1 treatment of patients with breast cancer. Nat Med. 2021; https://doi.org/10.1038/s41591-021-01323-8.

195. Adams S, Loi S, Toppmeyer D, Cescon DW, de Laurentiis M, Nanda R, et al. Pembrolizumab monotherapy for previously untreated, PD-L1-positive, metastatic triple-negative breast cancer: Cohort B of the phase II KEYNOTE-086 study. Ann Oncol. 2019;30(3):405–11.

196. Emens LA, Molinero L, Loi S, Rugo HS, Schneeweiss A, Diéras V, et al. Atezolizumab and nab -Paclitaxel in advanced triple-negative breast cancer: biomarker evaluation of the IMpassion130 study. J Natl Cancer Inst. 2021;

197. Foldi J, Silber A, Reisenbichler E, Singh K, Fischbach N, Persico J, et al. Neoadjuvant durvalumab plus weekly nab-paclitaxel and dose-dense doxorubicin/cyclophosphamide in triple-negative breast cancer. NPJ Breast Cancer. 2021;7(1):9.

198. Emens L, Loi S, Rugo H, Schneeweiss A, Dieras V, Iwata H, et al. IMpassion130: efficacy in immune biomarker subgroup from the global, randomized, double-blind, placebo-controlled, phase III study of atezolizumab + nab-paclitaxel in patients with treatment-naive, locally advanced or metastatic triple-negative breast cancer. Presented at the 2018 San Antonio breast cancer sympsium, San Antonio, TX, 4–7 December 2018.

199. Loi L, Winer E, Lipatov O, Im S, Goncalves A, Cortes J, et al. Relationship between tumor-infiltrating lymphocytes (TILs) and outcomes in the KEYNOTE-119 study of pembrolizumab vs chemotherapy for previously treated metastatic triple-negative breast

cancer (mTNBC). Philadelphia, PA: American Association for Cancer Research; 2020.

200. Loi S, Adams S, Schmid P, Cortes J, Cescon D, Winer E, et al. Relationship between tumor infiltrating lymphocyte levels and response to pembrolizumab in metastatic triple-negative breast cancer: Results from Keynote-086 trial. Presented at the European Society of Medical Oncology (ESMO) 2017 Congress, Madrid, Spain, 8–12 September 2017.

201. Emens LA, Esteva FJ, Beresford M, Saura C, de Laurentiis M, Kim SB, et al. Trastuzumab emtansine plus atezolizumab versus trastuzumab emtansine plus placebo in previously treated, HER2-positive advanced breast cancer (KATE2): a phase 2, multicentre, randomised, double-blind trial. Lancet Oncol. 2020;21(10):1283–95.

202. Loibl S, Untch M, Burchardi N, Huober J, Sinn BV, Blohmer JU, et al. A randomised phase II study investigating durvalumab in addition to an anthracycline taxane-based neoadjuvant therapy in early triple-negative breast cancer: Clinical results and biomarker analysis of study. Ann Oncol. 2019;30:1279–88.

203. Bianchini G, Huang C, Egle D, Bermejo B, Zamagni C, Thill M, et al. Tumour infiltrating lymphocytes (TILs), PD-L1 expression and their dynamics in the NeoTRIPaPDL1 trial. Ann Oncol. 2020;31(Suppl. 4):S1142–215.

204. Dieci MV, Guarneri V, Bisagni G, Tosi A, Musolino A, Spazzapan S, et al. 162MO Neoadjuvant chemotherapy and immunotherapy in Luminal B BC: results of the phase II GIADA trial. Ann Oncol. 2020 Sep;31:S304–5.

205. Khoury T, Peng X, Yan L, Wang D, Nagrale V. Tumor-infiltrating lymphocytes in breast cancer: evaluating interobserver variability, heterogeneity, and fidelity of scoring core biopsies. Am J Clin Pathol. 2018;150(5):441–50.

206. Tramm T, Di Caterino T, Jylling AB, Lelkaitis G, Laenkholm AV, Rago P, et al. Standardized assessment of tumor-infiltrating lymphocytes in breast cancer: an evaluation of inter-observer agreement between pathologists. Acta Oncol. 2018;57(1):90–4.

207. Swisher SK, Wu Y, Castaneda CA, Lyons GR, Yang F, Tapia C, et al. Interobserver agreement between pathologists assessing tumor-infiltrating lymphocytes (TILs) in breast cancer using methodology proposed by the international TILs working group. Ann Surg Oncol. 2016;23(7):2242–8.

208. Amgad M, Stovgaard ES, Balslev E, Thagaard J, Chen W, Dudgeon S, et al. Report on computational assessment of tumor Infiltrating lymphocytes from the international immuno-oncology biomarker working group. NPJ Breast Cancer. 2020;6:16.

209. von Minckwitz G, Schneeweiss A, Loibl S, Salat C, Denkert C, Rezai M, et al. Neoadjuvant carboplatin in patients with triple-negative and HER2-positive early breast cancer (GeparSixto; GBG 66): a randomised phase 2 trial. Lancet Oncol. 2014;15(7):747–56.

210. Dieci MV, Radosevic-Robin N, Fineberg S, van den Eynden G, Ternes N, Penault-Llorca F, et al. Update on tumor-infiltrating lymphocytes (TILs) in breast cancer, including recommendations to assess TILs in residual disease after neoadjuvant therapy and in carcinoma in situ: a report of the International Immuno-Oncology Biomarker Working Group on Breast Cancer. Semin Cancer Biol. 2018;52(Pt 2):16–25.

211. Buisseret L, Desmedt C, Garaud S, Fornili M, Wang X, Van den Eyden G, et al. Reliability of tumor-infiltrating lymphocyte and tertiary lymphoid structure assessment in human breast cancer. Mod Pathol. 2017;30(9):1204–12.

212. Cha YJ, Ahn SG, Bae SJ, Yoon CI, Seo J, Jung WH, et al. Comparison of tumor-infiltrating lymphocytes of breast cancer in core needle biopsies and resected specimens: a retrospective analysis. Breast Cancer Res Treat. 2018;171(2):295–302.

213. Althobiti M, Aleskandarany MA, Joseph C, Toss M, Mongan N, Diez-Rodriguez M, et al. Heterogeneity of tumour-infiltrating lymphocytes in breast cancer and its prognostic significance. Histopathology. 2018;73(6):887–96.

214. Campbell BB, Light N, Fabrizio D, Zatzman M, Fuligni F, de Borja R, et al. Comprehensive analysis of hypermutation in human cancer. Cell. 2017;171(5):1042–1056.e10.

215. Le DT, Durham JN, Smith KN, Wang H, Bartlett BR, Aulakh LK, et al. Mismatch repair deficiency predicts response of solid tumors to PD-1 blockade. Science. 2017;357(6349):409–13.

216. Cheng AS, Leung SCY, Gao D, Burugu S, Anurag M, Ellis MJ, et al. Mismatch repair protein loss in breast cancer: clinicopathological associations in a large British Columbia cohort. Breast Cancer Res Treat. 2020;179(1):3–10.

217. Salgado R, Bellizzi AM, Rimm D, Bartlett JMS, Nielsen T, Holger M, et al. How current assay approval policies are leading to unintended imprecision medicine. Lancet Oncol. 2020;21:1399–401.

218. Litchfield K, Reading JL, Puttick C, Thakkar K, Abbosh C, Bentham R, et al. Meta-analysis of tumor- and T cell-intrinsic mechanisms of sensitization to checkpoint inhibition. Cell. 2021;184(3):596–614.

219. Raskov H, Orhan A, Christensen JP, Gögenur I. Cytotoxic CD8+ T cells in cancer and cancer immunotherapy. Br J Cancer. 2021;124:359–67.

220. Schmidt M, Weyer-Elberich V, Hengstler JG, Heimes AS, Almstedt K, Gerhold-Ay A, et al. Prognostic impact of CD4-positive T cell subsets in early breast cancer: a study based on the FinHer trial patient population. Breast Cancer Res. 2018;20(1):15.

221. Liu S, Lachapelle J, Leung S, Gao D, Foulkes WD, Nielsen TO. CD8 +lymphocyte infiltration is an independent favorable prognostic indicator in basal-like breast cancer. Breast Cancer Res. 2012;14(2):R48.

222. García-Martínez E, Gil GL, Benito AC, González-Billalabeitia E, Conesa MAV, García TG, et al. Tumor-infiltrating immune cell profiles and their change after neoadjuvant chemotherapy predict response and prognosis of breast cancer. Breast Cancer Res. 2014;16(1):488.

223. Oda N, Shimazu K, Naoi Y, Morimoto K, Shimomura A, Shimoda M, et al. Intratumoral regulatory T cells as an independent predictive factor for pathological complete response to neoadjuvant paclitaxel followed by 5-FU/epirubicin/cyclophosphamide in breast cancer patients. Breast Cancer Res Treat. 2012;136(1):107–16.

224. Lee JS, Ruppin E. Multiomics prediction of response rates to therapies to inhibit programmed cell death 1 and programmed cell death 1 ligand 1. JAMA Oncol. 2019;5(11):1614–8.

225. Jiang W, He Y, He W, Wu G, Zhou X, Sheng Q, et al. Exhausted CD8+T cells in the tumor immune microenvironment: new pathways to therapy. Front Immunol. 2021;11:622509.

226. Speiser DE, Ho P-C, Verdeil G. Regulatory circuits of T cell function in cancer. Nat Rev Immunol. 2016;16(10):599–611.

227. Ma X, Xiao L, Liu L, Ye L, Su P, Bi E, et al. CD36-mediated ferroptosis dampens intratumoral CD8+ T cell effector function and impairs their antitumor ability. Cell Metab. 2021;33(5):1001–1012.e5.

228. Gruosso T, Gigoux M, Manem VSK, Bertos N, Zuo D, Perlitch I, et al. Spatially distinct tumor immune microenvironments stratify triple-negative breast cancers. J Clin Investig. 2019;129(4):1785–800.

229. Chen DS, Mellman I. Elements of cancer immunity and the cancer-immune set point. Nature. 2017;541:321–30.

230. Nawaz S, Heindl A, Koelble K, Yuan Y. Beyond immune density: Critical role of spatial heterogeneity in estrogen receptor-negative breast cancer. Mod Pathol. 2015;28(6):766–77.

231. Heindl A, Sestak I, Naidoo K, Cuzick J, Dowsett M, Yuan Y. Relevance of spatial heterogeneity of immune infiltration for predicting risk of recurrence after endocrine therapy of ER+ breast cancer. J Natl Cancer Inst. 2018;110(2)

232. Berben L, Wildiers H, Marcelis L, Antoranz A, Bosisio F, Hatse S, et al. Computerised scoring protocol for identification and quantification of different immune cell populations in breast tumour regions by the use of QuPath software. Histopathology. 2020;77(1):79–91.

233. Berben L, Floris G, Kenis C, Dalmasso B, Smeets A, Vos H, et al. Age-related remodelling of the blood immunological portrait and the local tumor immune response in patients with luminal breast cancer. Clin Transl Immunol. 2020;9(10):e1184.

234. Sobottka B, Pestalozzi B, Fink D, Moch H, Varga Z. Similar lymphocytic infiltration pattern in primary breast cancer and their corresponding distant metastases. OncoImmunology. 2016;5(6):e1153208.

235. Keren L, Bosse M, Marquez D, Angoshtari R, Jain S, Varma S, et al. A structured tumor-immune microenvironment in triple negative breast cancer revealed by multiplexed ion beam imaging. Cell. 2018;174(6):1373–1387.e19.

236. Nederlof I, Horlings HM, Curtis C, Kok M. A high-dimensional window into the micro-environment of triple negative breast cancer. Cancers. 2021;13(2):316.

237. Nederlof I, de Bortoli D, Bareche Y, Nguyen B, de Maaker M, Hooijer GKJ, et al. Comprehensive evaluation of methods to assess overall and cell-specific immune infiltrates in breast cancer. Breast Cancer Res. 2019;21(1):151.

238. de Smet F, Antoranz Martinez A, Bosisio FM. Next-generation pathology by multiplexed immunohistochemistry. Trends Biochem Sci. 2021;46:80–2.

239. Lun XK, Bodenmiller B. Profiling cell signaling networks at single-cell resolution. Mol Cell Proteomics. 2020;19:744–56.

240. Jackson HW, Fischer JR, Zanotelli VRT, Ali HR, Mechera R, Soysal SD, et al. The single-cell pathology landscape of breast cancer. Nature. 2020;578(7796):615–20.

241. Egelston CA, Avalos C, Tu TY, Rosario A, Wang R, Solomon S, et al. Resident memory CD8+ T cells within cancer islands mediate survival in breast cancer patients. JCI Insight. 2019;4(19)

242. Byrne A, Savas P, Sant S, Li R, Virassamy B, Luen SJ, et al. Tissue-resident memory T cells in breast cancer control and immunotherapy responses. Nat Rev Clin Oncol. 2020;17:341–8.

243. Reddy SM, Reuben A, Barua S, Jiang H, Zhang S, Wang L, et al. Poor response to neoadjuvant chemotherapy correlates with mast cell infiltration in inflammatory breast cancer. Cancer Immunol Res. 2019;7(6):1025–35.

244. Carvajal-Hausdorf DE, Patsenker J, Stanton KP, Villarroel-Espindola F, Esch A, Montgomery RR, et al. Multiplexed (18-Plex) measurement of signaling targets and cytotoxic T cells in Trastuzumab-treated patients using imaging mass cytometry. Clin Cancer Res. 2019;25(10):3054–62.

245. Griguolo G, Serna G, Pascual T, Fasani R, Guardia X, Chic N, et al. Immune microenvironment characterisation and dynamics during anti-HER2-based neoadjuvant treatment in HER2-positive breast cancer. NPJ Precis Oncol. 2021;5(1):23.

246. de Angelis C, Nagi C, Hoyt CC, Liu L, Roman K, Wang C, et al. Evaluation of the predictive role of tumor immune infiltrate in patients with HER2-positive breast cancer treated with neoadjuvant anti-HER2 therapy without chemotherapy. Clin Cancer Res. 2020;26(3):738–45.

247. Allam M, Cai S, Coskun AF. Multiplex bioimaging of single-cell spatial profiles for precision cancer diagnostics and therapeutics. NPJ Precis Oncol. 2020;4(1):11.

248. Klauschen F, Müller KR, Binder A, Bockmayr M, Hägele M, Seegerer P, et al. Scoring of tumor-infiltrating lymphocytes: from visual estimation to machine learning. Semin Cancer Biol. 2018;52:151–7.

249. Saltz J, Gupta R, Hou L, Kurc T, Singh P, Nguyen V, et al. Spatial organization and molecular correlation of tumor-infiltrating lymphocytes using deep learning on pathology images. Cell Rep. 2018;23(1):181–93 e7.

250. Basavanhally AN, Ganesan S, Agner S, Monaco JP, Feldman MD, Tomaszewski JE, et al. Computerized image-based detection and grading of lymphocytic infiltration in HER2+ breast cancer histopathology. IEEE Trans Biomed Eng. 2010;57(3):642–53.

251. Acs B, Ahmed FS, Gupta S, Wong PF, Gartrell RD, Sarin Pradhan J, et al. An open source automated tumor infiltrating lymphocyte algorithm for prognosis in melanoma. Nat Commun. 2019;10(1)

252. Chou M, Illa-Bochaca I, Minxi B, Darvishian F, Johannet P, Moran U, et al. Optimization of an automated tumor-infiltrating lymphocyte algorithm for improved prognostication in primary melanoma. Mod Pathol. 2021;34(3):562–71.

253. Yuan Y, Failmezger H, Rueda OM, Ali HR, Gräf S, Chin S-F, et al. Quantitative image analysis of cellular heterogeneity in breast tumors complements genomic profiling. Sci Transl Med. 2012;4(157):157ra43-ra43.

254. Le H, Gupta R, Hou L, Abousamra S, Fassler D, Kurc T, et al. Utilizing automated breast cancer detection to identify spatial distributions of tumor infiltrating lymphocytes in invasive breast cancer. Am J Pathol. 2020;190(7):1491–504.

255. Swiderska-Chadaj Z, Pinckaers H, van Rijthoven M, Balkenhol M, Melnikova M, Oscar G, et al. Convolutional neural networks for lymphocyte detection in immunohistochemically stained whole-slide images MIDL 2018 conference submission2018.

256. Yoon HH, Shi Q, Heying EN, Muranyi A, Bredno J, Ough F, et al. Intertumoral heterogeneity of CD3+ and CD8+ T-cell densities in the microenvironment of DNA mismatch-repair–deficient colon cancers: implications for prognosis. Clin Cancer Res. 2019;25(1):125–33.

257. Corredor G, Wang X, Zhou Y, Lu C, Fu P, Syrigos K, et al. Spatial architecture and arrangement of tumor-infiltrating lymphocytes for predicting likelihood of recurrence in early-stage non–small cell lung cancer. Clin Cancer Res. 2019;25(5):1526–34.

258. Amgad M, Elfandy H, Hussein H, Atteya LA, Elsebaie MAT, Abo Elnasr LS, et al. Structured crowdsourcing enables convolutional segmentation of histology images. Bioinformatics. 2019;35(18):3461–7.

259. Amgad M, Sarkar A, Srinivas C, Redman R, Ratra S, Bechert C, et al. Joint region and nucleus segmentation for characterization of tumor infiltrating lymphocytes in breast cancer. SPIE. 2019;

260. Tizhoosh HR, Pantanowitz L. Artificial intelligence and digital pathology: challenges and opportunities. J Pathol Inform. 2018;9:38.

261. Cui M, Zhang DY. Artificial intelligence and computational pathology. Lab Investig. 2021;101(4):412–22.

Regulation of Tumor Progression and Metastasis by Bone Marrow-Derived Microenvironments

14

Divya Ramchandani, Tyler P. El Rayes, Dingcheng Gao, Nasser K. Altorki, Thomas R. Cox, Janine T. Erler, and Vivek Mittal

Abstract

Activating mutations in driver oncogenes and loss-of-function mutations in tumor suppressor genes contribute to tumor progression and metastasis. Accordingly, therapies targeting key tumor cell intrinsic signaling pathways are being used in clinical trials, and some have met FDA approval. However, these treatments benefit only a small proportion of patients harboring key driver mutations and acquired resistance to these therapies presents a major impediment to effective treatment. More recently, the contribution of the tumor microenvironment (TME) has been an area of active investigation and has begun to pro-

vide critical insights into carcinogenesis. The host stromal cells in the TME co-evolve with tumors and contribute to carcinogenesis in several ways. Among the host cells, bone marrow (BM)-derived cells constitute a significant fraction and directly contribute to proliferation, invasion, intravasation, extravasation, and outgrowth at the metastatic site. While the tumor reprogrammed BM cells constitute attractive targets for anti-cancer therapy, recent studies have also begun to unravel their role as prognostic and predictive molecular markers of the disease.

In this chapter, we will focus on recent advances and emerging concepts of the contribution of BM-derived cells in various steps of primary tumor progression and the metastatic cascade (Fig. 14.1) and discuss future directions in the context of novel diagnostic and therapeutic opportunities.

D. Ramchandani (✉) · N. K. Altorki
Department of Cardiothoracic Surgery, Weill Cornell Medicine, New York, NY, USA

Neuberger Berman Foundation Lung Cancer Center, Weill Cornell Medicine, New York, NY, USA
e-mail: dir2001@med.cornell.edu; nkaltork@med.cornell.edu

T. P. El Rayes
Memorial Sloan Kettering Cancer Center, New York, NY, USA
e-mail: elrayet1@mskcc.org

D. Gao · V. Mittal (✉)
Department of Cardiothoracic Surgery, Weill Cornell Medicine, New York, NY, USA

Neuberger Berman Foundation Lung Cancer Center, Weill Cornell Medicine, New York, NY, USA

Department of Cell and Developmental Biology, Weill Cornell Medicine, New York, NY, USA
e-mail: dig2009@med.cornell.edu; vim2010@med.cornell.edu

T. R. Cox
The Garvan Institute of Medical Research and The Kinghorn Cancer Centre, Darlinghurst, NSW, Australia

St Vincent's Clinical School, Faculty of Medicine, UNSW Sydney, Sydney, NSW, Australia
e-mail: t.cox@garvan.org.au

J. T. Erler
Biotech Research and Innovation Centre (BRIC), University of Copenhagen (UCPH), Copenhagen, Denmark

Take-Home Lessons

- Bone marrow-derived cells contribute to primary tumor growth as well as metastatic progression. These are recruited to primary tumor sites via tumor-secreted factors or via HIF1α in hypoxic tumors. Tumor-associated macrophages, myeloid-derived suppressor cells (MDSCs), endothelial progenitor cells (EPCs), and tumor-associated neutrophils all aid in primary tumor growth via different mechanisms involving immunosuppression, angiogenesis, etc. On the other hand, dendritic cells (DCs) may have both pro-tumorigenic via ENO1 and anti-tumorigenic role via activation of CD4+ and CD8+ T-cells.

- For intravasation, macrophages recruited at primary tumor sites downregulate E-cadherin junctions and trigger actin-rich invadopodia to promote early dis-

© The Author(s), under exclusive license to Springer Nature Switzerland AG 2022
L. A. Akslen, R. S. Watnick (eds.), *Biomarkers of the Tumor Microenvironment*, https://doi.org/10.1007/978-3-030-98950-7_14

semination. Neutrophils aid in the process of intravasation by increasing MMP9 and angiogenesis.

- Platelets are known to promote circulating tumor cells (CTCs) in blood and their metastasis. Clot formation also recruits macrophages, which in turn increase Akt-dependent signaling to promote tumor cell survival. T_{regs} can protect disseminated tumor cells from an immune attack as well. Neutrophils protect CTCs by forming neutrophil extracellular traps (NETs).

- A number of tumor-secreted or BM-derived factors play a role in the formation of premetastatic niche which promotes metastatic outgrowth of tumor cells at secondary sites. Lysyl oxidase secreted from primary tumors modifies ECM at the secondary site to aid in tumor cell colonization. Primary tumor-derived CCL2 also promotes S100A8 and SAA3 secretion from lung endothelial cells that increases vascular permeability to assist in tumor cell colonization. Similarly, macrophages, MDSCs, and neutrophils are recruited at the premetastatic sites to modify the environment at these sites, aid in colonization by tumor cells, promote their survival, support their metabolic needs, and promote metastatic outgrowth.

- Platelets aid in extravasation by promoting adhesion of tumor cells to endothelial cells. Primary tumor-derived G-CSF increases the presence of immunosuppressive G-MDSCs in lungs for metastatic outgrowth. Neutrophils promote metastasis by forming NETs and degrading thrombospondin-1. Different subsets of cancer-associated fibroblasts also enhance metastasis by NOTCH, CXCL12, and TGFβ pathways. Bone microenvironment promotes stemness and plasticity in tumor cells to promote multi-organ metastasis at different sites.

Primary Tumor Growth

The BM contributes significantly to the TME and supports tumor progression and metastasis by regulating angiogenesis, inflammation, and immune suppression. General descriptions of the contribution of the BM-derived TME to tumor growth and metastasis have been covered in several excellent reviews [1–4]. Most solid tumors harbor an immune infiltrate consisting of myeloid and lymphoid cells, whose phenotype and activation status has been shown to change with the stage of malignancy [4]. Hematopoietic stem cells (HSCs) are maintained in the BM compartment and anchored to the endosteal surface by calcium-sensing receptors present on their surface [5]. Major adhesion mechanisms that mediate HSC anchorage in the BM niche include receptor tyrosine kinase TIE2-Angiopoietin-1 (ANG1) interactions [6] and chemokine (C-X-C motif) receptor 4 (CXCR4)-stromal-derived factor-1 (SDF-1) interactions [7]. Furthermore, HSCs also adhere to osteopontin in the bone via β1 integrin [8].

Secreted tumor-specific factors systemically stimulate the quiescent BM compartment, resulting in the expansion, mobilization, and recruitment of BM progenitor cells. For instance, matrix metalloprotease 9 (MMP9) secreted by primary tumors systemically degrades osteopontin [9, 10] and mediates cleavage of SDF-1 [11], thereby releasing BM cells from the bone niche [12]. Similarly, tumor-secreted granulocyte colony-stimulating factor (G-CSF) mobilizes HSCs from the niche by promoting neutrophil elastase-mediated degradation of SDF-1 [13]. The mobilized BM-derived cells are recruited into tumor beds in response to chemoattractants. For instance, SDF-1 secreted by primary tumors recruits CXCR4$^+$ BM-derived cells to the TME [12]. Other tumor-secreted factors such as vascular endothelial growth factor (VEGF) and placental growth factor (PlGF) bind to VEGFR1$^+$ BM cells, while monocyte colony-stimulating factor (M-CSF) recruits monocytes and macrophages [12]. Furthermore, chemokine (C-C motif) ligand 2 (CCL2), also known as monocyte chemotactic protein (MCP-1), was identified as a tumor-derived chemokine that recruits circulating monocytes into the TME, where they undergo differentiation into tumor-associated macrophages (TAMs) [14]. Stromal-derived CCL2/MCP-1 and colony-stimulating factor (CSF1) are also involved in the recruitment of TAMs [15–17]. Additionally, hypoxia-inducible factor 1 alpha (HIF1α) in hypoxic tumors promotes the recruitment of BM-derived myeloid and endothelial progenitor cells (EPCs), which increase the bioavailability of VEGF via their secretion of MMP9, enhancing tumor angiogenesis [18]. Infiltrating BM cells also provide paracrine mitogenic signals to induce proliferation of tumor cells via their secretion of growth factors such as epidermal growth factor (EGF), and cytokines including interleukin-6 (IL-6) and tumor necrosis factor (TNFα) [12]. Colorectal cancer has high VEGFC expression which leads to increased activation of VEGFR3 on cancer-associated macrophages and lymph vessels, important for lymphangiogenesis in colorectal cancer [19].

Macrophages are the most abundant myeloid cells present among the recruited BM-derived cells [20]. Notably, increased macrophage infiltration has been correlated with poor prognosis, as shown in Hodgkin's lymphoma, breast cancer, and lung cancer [21–23]. In ovarian cancer, TAMs mediate an immunosuppressive environment at the primary tumor site, aiding tumor growth and metastasis [24]. These are recruited via an E3 ligase, UBR5, expressed highly by ovarian cancer cells through CCL2/CSF-1 axis [24].

Fig. 14.1 The bone marrow (BM) contributes to primary tumor growth and the metastatic cascade

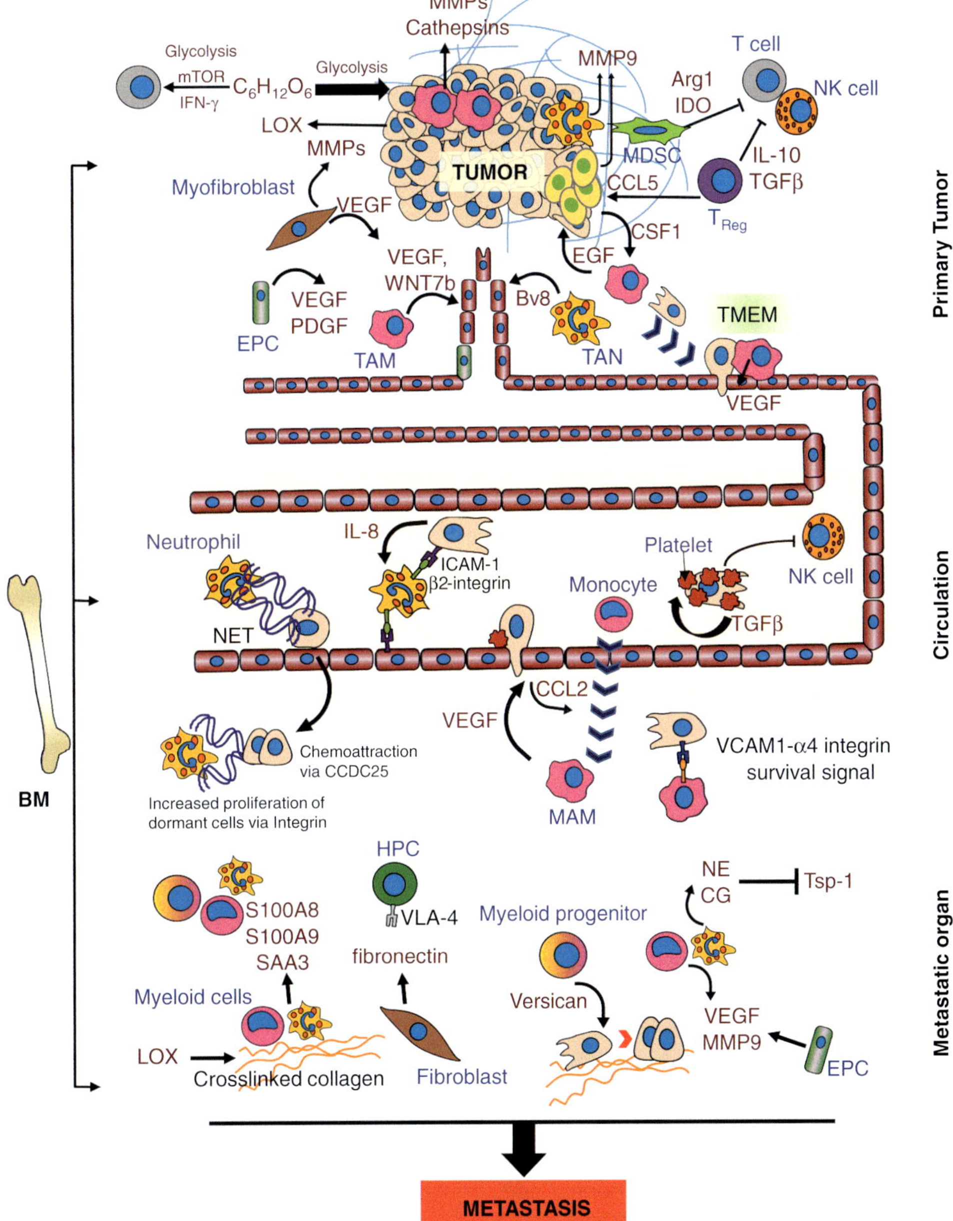

Classically activated macrophages, defined by an M1 phenotype, generate host responses against the growing tumors, whereas "alternatively" activated M2 macrophages, representing "educated" TAMs, are major perpetrators of tumor progression and metastasis. M1 macrophages are characterized by an elevated expression of inducible nitric oxide synthase (iNOS), producing nitric oxide (NO) for effective pathogen killing [25], and the pro-inflammatory cytokine IL-12 [26]. Tumor-derived mediators, such as IL-4, IL-10, IL-13, transforming growth factor beta (TGFβ), and prostaglandin E2 (PGE2) mediate polarization of TAMs toward the tumor-promoting, M2 phenotype [27]. M2 TAMs are characterized by elevated expression of arginase (Arg1) and decreased expression of iNOS - Arg1^{high} iNOS^{low} [28]. M2 TAMs promote immune suppression by expressing high levels of IL-10 and downregulating IL-12 [29]. Paclitaxel has been shown to revert TAMs to an immunocompetent M1 profile in a TLR4-dependent pathway [30]. Interestingly, TAMs have also been shown to promote tumor growth via a key inflammatory mechanism activating the classical complement pathway [31]. Production of C1q by TAMs and C1r, C1s, C4, and C3 by tumor cells leads to the assembly C1 complex and activation of the complement pathway, leading to an immunosuppressive microenvironment and tumor growth in a model of clear-cell renal cell carcinoma [31]. In the same model, mice with deficiency of complement pathway components show decreased tumor growth [31].

M2 TAMs also induce extracellular matrix (ECM) degradation and angiogenesis by producing MMPs and VEGF, respectively [28]. Furthermore, IL-4 secreted by pancreatic tumor cells induces members of the cysteine protease family cathepsins [32, 33] in TAMs, where cathepsin B and S have been shown to promote tumor growth, invasion, and angiogenesis [34]. By contributing to angiogenesis and tumor invasiveness, TAMs ultimately promote metastasis. In the MMTV-PyMT model of breast cancer, genetic ablation of macrophages by CSF1 deletion impairs angiogenesis and suppresses metastasis to the lung, mainly due to the VEGFA-mediated angiogenic action of TAMs [35–37]. Furthermore, deleting an effector of CSF1 signaling, Ets2, in macrophages, induced the expression of antiangiogenic factors thrombospondin 1 (Tsp-1) and Tsp-2 by macrophages, resulting in decreased angiogenesis in PyMT primary tumors and suppression of lung metastasis [38]. Moreover, macrophages promote angiogenesis and metastasis in PyMT primary tumors via their expression of WNT7b [39]. TAMs also associate with newly formed blood vessels induced by EC-derived angiopoietin 2 (ANG2), enhancing angiogenesis and tumor cell dissemination [40]. Primary tumor cells, or tumor cell supernatant, has also been shown to activate TAMs via LAMP2a-PRDX1/CRTC1 leading to enhanced tumor growth [41]. In breast cancer, obesity leads to increase in tumor-infiltrating macrophages, and activation of NLRC4 inflammasome and increased interleukin IL-1β production [42]. IL-1β in turn upregulates angiopoietin-like 4 (ANGPTL4) driving angiogenesis-mediated breast tumor growth [42]. In TNBC, CD169+ macrophages promote tumor growth by inhibiting intratumoral CD8+ T cells, resulting in an upregulation of PD-L1 on macrophages via JAK2/STAT3 signaling pathway [43]. Inhibiting STAT6 downstream of IL-4 and IL-13 inhibits the M2 differentiation of macrophages, thus inhibiting tumor growth and metastasis in an orthotopic 4T1 breast cancer model [44]. Pre-treated gliomas have been found to be infiltrated by blood-derived TAMs with M2 phenotype exhibiting immunosuppressive cytokines (IL10 and TGFB2) and oxidative metabolism [45]. Higher expression of these blood-derived TAM markers but not microglial TAM markers are associated with poor overall survival in these patients [45].

M2 TAMs promote an immune-suppressive TME by producing IL-10, which promotes Th2 cell polarization [14]. In turn, Th2 cells produce IL-4, which in a feedback loop activates M2 TAM polarization [46]. M2 TAMs also secrete CCL22, which recruits regulatory T cells (T_{Reg}) [46]. TAMs also produce TGFβ and process latent TGFβ, releasing its active form [47], and hence reducing T cell cytolytic and antitumor activity [48]. TAMs express programmed death ligand 1 (PD-L1) on their cell surface, which binds the immune inhibitory receptor, programmed death 1 (PD-1), on the surface of T cells, resulting in T cell inactivation and apoptosis [49]. TAMs inhibit T cell growth by depleting arginine in the local microenvironment through expression of Arg1 [50]. A new study recently described that a diet rich in n-3 fatty acids induces significant reactive oxygen species production and macrophage death, inhibiting tumor growth [51].

TAMs also contribute to chemoresistance in the MMTV-PyMT breast cancer model [22], and inhibiting macrophage recruitment using a CSF1R signaling antagonist enhanced the antitumor effect of cytotoxic chemotherapeutics via a CD8+ T cell-dependent mechanism [24]. CCL8 provides a positive regulatory loop between breast cancer cells and TAMs via CSF1 and TNF-α, by enhancing the expression of SIGLEC1 [52]. Interestingly, TAMs that underwent CSF1R signaling blockade failed to elicit CD8+ T cell responses and exhibited reduced immunosuppressive activity [53].

A recently identified cancer-associated fibroblast (CAF) subset expressing CD10 and GPR77 promotes chemoresistance and poor survival in breast and lung cancer patients [54]. GPR77, a C5a receptor, maintains a persistent NF-κB activation in CD10+GPR77+ CAFs and promotes cancer stem cell enrichment and chemoresistance by IL-6 and IL-8 secretion [54]. In colorectal cancer patients, there was a higher proportion of somatic copy number mutations in fibroblasts present in tumors, as compared to adjacent normal tissues and five fibroblast-specific biomarkers: BGN, RCN3, TAGLN, MYL9, and TPM2, were associated with a poor prognosis [55]. Increased granulocyte recruitment to tumors by CAFs is known to limit the efficacy of CSF-1R inhibition [56]. This is because CSF1 in tumor cells reduces granulocyte-specific chemokine expression in CAF which limits their migration to tumors. These findings advocate for combining CSF1R inhibitor with a CXCR2 antagonist [56]. CAFs can also be educated by tumor cells as demonstrated in a pancreatic cancer model with a gain of function mutation in p53 [57]. Tumor cells with mutant p53 increase CAF contractility markers (pMLC, pMYPT1, and ACTA2), which can further increase the invasiveness of cancer cells independent of p53 mutation status in these cells [57]. This crosstalk between CAFs and tumor cells can be interrupted by inhibiting perlecan, thus reducing invasion and metastasis [57].

Myeloid-derived suppressor cells (MDSCs) have been observed in cancer patients and contribute to tumor progression. MDSCs are a heterogeneous population of immature myeloid cells [58, 59], which are activated in response to S100 calcium binding protein A8 (S100A8) and S100A9 pro-inflammatory mediators [60]. MDSCs contribute to tumor immune evasion by suppressing the CD4+ and CD8+ immune response partly via arginase production, by expanding T_{Reg} cells, and by inhibiting the cytolytic activity of natural killer (NK) cells [3, 61]. MDSCs also express the interferon gamma (IFNγ)-inducible enzyme indoleamine 2,3-dioxygenase (IDO), a well-known suppressor of T cell activation [62]. IDO catalyzes tryptophan catabolism, depleting tryptophan from the local microenvironment and blocking T cell activation [63]. IDO expression by MDSCs was found to be STAT3-dependent in breast cancer [64]. Interestingly, in a model of melanoma, tumor-derived IDO was described to recruit and expand MDSCs via a T_{Reg}-dependent mechanism, leading to an immunosuppressive microenvironment [65]. Pancreatic tumor cell-mediated production of IL1β is also known to induce an immunosuppressive environment comprising of M2 macrophages, MDSCs, CD1d^{hi}CD5+ regulatory B cells, and Th17 cells, which leads to reduced infiltration of CD8+ cytotoxic T-cells [66]. Increased emergence of PanINs and PDAC has been also attributed to a decrease in myofibroblast-derived Col1 (type 1 Collagen) [67]. Col1 deletion enhances tumor CXCL5-associated recruitment of CD206+ARG1+MDSCs to suppress CD8+ T-cells [67]. In ovarian carcinoma, a STAT5-dependent increase in AMPKα transcription induced by GM-CSF in MDSCs mediates tumor growth and inhibits antitumor CD8+ T cell immunity [68]. In gliomas, *IDH* mutation leads to lesser T-cell infiltration and are thus immunologically cold tumors [69]. Immune-suppressive effects are also enhanced in the TME by increased competition for glucose between cancer cells and tumor-infiltrating lymphocytes (TILs). Immune checkpoint blockade antibodies against CTLA-4, PD-1, and PD-L1 enhance glycolysis in T-cells, along with mTOR activation and IFNγ production [70, 71]. PD-L1 inhibition on tumor cells also dampens mTOR activity and glycolysis in these cells [70].

Tumor-associated neutrophils (TANs) exert a pro-tumorigenic effect at the primary site, promoting angiogenesis and suppressing immune responses [72–74]. In mice, CD11b$^+$ Gr1$^+$ neutrophils, recruited by primary tumor-derived G-CSF, contribute to refractoriness to anti-VEGF therapy and promote angiogenesis via the expression of *Bombina variegata* peptide 8 (Bv8) [75, 76]. CD11b$^+$ Gr1$^+$ immature myeloid cells recruited to colon and lung tumors promote angiogenesis and vessel maturation via their MMP9 production, increasing VEGF bioavailability, as well as by incorporating into tumor blood vessels [77]. Interestingly, the pro-tumorigenic effects of neutrophils are TGFβ-dependent, whereupon TGFβ blockade, neutrophils switch from the "N2" pro-tumorigenic phenotype to the "N1" anti-tumorigenic phenotype [78]. In the case of dormant tumor cells, stress hormone activated neutrophils release pro-inflammatory S100A8/9, which induces activation of myelo-peroxidase which results in the accumulation of oxidized lipids in neutrophils. These lipids activate FGF pathway in tumor cells to allow them to escape dormancy and form new tumor lesions [79].

Dendritic cells (DCs) are a class of antigen-presenting cells that uptake, process, and present antigens, including tumor-derived antigens, to antigen-specific T cells, resulting in T cell activation and expansion. Mature DCs express CCR7 which is essential for the migration of tumor-derived DCs to tumor draining lymph nodes [80]. In melanoma, tumor-associated DCs do not present tumor antigens and fail to activate T cells [81]. Interestingly, tumor-associated DCs (TADC) in ovarian cancer were found to be immunosuppressive, promoting tumor progression. In multiple myeloma, plasmacytoid DC-expressed enolase 1 (ENO1) suppressed CD8- and NK-cell immunity against multiple myeloma cells [82]. In this context, lipid peroxidation byproducts induce endoplasmic reticulum (ER) stress, activating an ER stress response factor, Xbp1, which reduces the ability of tumor DCs to present antigens and activate T cells [83]. TADC have been recently characterized into three subsets: pre-cDC-derived cDC1s, pre-cDC-derived cDC2s, and monocyte-derived Mo-DCs [84]. Mo-DCs scavenge tumor antigen but do not upregulate CCR7 in tumors and are immunosuppressive [84]. Both cDC1 and cDC2 migrate to lymph nodes, while cDC1 activates CD8+ T-cells and supports Th1 polarization of CD4+T-cells, cDC2s induce Th17 CD4+ T-cell phenotype (cDC2) [80, 84].

In addition to the perivascular contribution of BM-derived hematopoietic cells, BM-derived VEGFR2$^+$ EPCs, recruited to early avascular tumors in response to tumor-derived VEGF, provide an alternative source of endothelial cells, which contributes to neovessel formation of certain tumors in mice and humans [85–88]. The contribution of EPCs to tumor vessel formation has been reported to be variable [89]. However, EPC ablation was associated with angiogenesis inhibition both in primary tumors and metastatic outgrowth [87, 90, 91]. EPCs also contributed to vascular rebound following administration of vascular disrupting agents [92], and chemotherapeutics rapidly induced circulating endothelial progenitor (CEP) mobilization and subsequent tumor homing [93]. Despite these studies, confusion has prevailed due to the extensive variability in EPC contribution to vessel formation in different tumor model systems [64, 89], and some studies have even claimed lack of EPC contribution [94]. However, in addition to vessel incorporation, EPCs have been shown to secrete proangiogenic factors, including VEGF and platelet-derived growth factor (PDGF) [90, 95], suggesting that along with providing stability to nascent vessels, EPCs contribute to vessel recruitment through paracrine mechanisms at a critical early stage of tumor growth. These observations are consistent with other studies demonstrating that paracrine signaling by specific populations of perivascular cells may have significant biological effects. For example, depletion of myeloid cell-derived VEGF caused vessel normalization even when abundant sources of VEGF were present in the TME [96]. Similarly, endothelial cell-autonomous VEGF and not the abundant extracellular VEGF was shown to be critically required for the homeostasis of blood vessels [97].

Furthermore, the BM contributes to myofibroblast populations in the tumor stroma, as shown in a mouse model of pancreatic insulinoma [98, 99]. BM-derived myofibroblasts support angiogenesis in the primary tumor by secreting a host of proangiogenic factors, such as VEGF, basic fibroblast growth factor (bFGF), TGFβ, PDGF, hepatocyte growth factor (HGF), and they remodel the ECM via several MMPs and ADAMs [100]. The BM is also a source of pericytes, cells that support vessel maturation, where BM-derived pericyte progenitor cells are mobilized to remodel the vasculature in tumors [101–104].

Primary Tumor Invasion and Intravasation

In order to metastasize, tumor cells at the primary site invade into the basement membrane, undergo transendothelial migration, and intravasate into circulation. These events are facilitated by BM-derived cells. Cancer cells express EGFR, while TAMs express CSF1R. Secretion of EGF from macrophages stimulates cancer cells to form elongated protrusions for invading into the adjacent matrices and to also produce CSF-1, which, in turn, stimulates TAMs for further production of EGF. Molecular inhibition of either EGF or CSF1 significantly impedes the migratory behavior of both cell types, which further confirms this positive feedback loop [105, 106]. Intratumoral CD4+ T cells in PyMT tumors also induce the expression of EGF in macrophages, via IL-4 [46]. Furthermore, cancer-derived CSF1 signaling through TAM CSF1R activates Wiskott–Aldrich syndrome protein (WASP), promoting macrophage migration and EGF expression [107]. Interestingly, although breast tumor cells that express ErbB3 or the CXCR4 receptor invade in response to the ligands heregulin beta1 (HRGβ1) and SDF-1, respectively, their invasion is still dependent on the EGF-CSF1 paracrine loop, such that blocking this signaling loop results in suppression of invasion in response to other ligands [108]. A causal role for macrophages has been linked to early cancer cell dissemination in HER2+ breast cancer cells. CCL2 secreted by cancer and myeloid cells in premalignant lesions recruits CD206+/Tie2+ macrophages, upregulates Wnt pathway and in turn downregulates E-cadherin junctions in these cancer cells to promote early dissemination and metastasis [109].

Moreover, Mena, the mammalian ortholog of *Drosophila* Enabled (Ena), contributes to cell motility by regulating actin dynamics [110]. Breast cancer cells expressing Mena^{INV}, an invasion-specific isoform, exhibit multicellular streaming and increased intravasation dependent on the EGF-CSF1 paracrine signaling loop between tumor cells and macrophages [111]. Transendothelial migration of breast tumor cells occurs in microanatomical structures known as "Tumor MicroEnvironment of Metastasis" (TMEM) [112]. TMEMs are composed of one TIE2^{high}/VEGF^{high} perivascular macrophage in physical contact with a Mena^{INV}-expressing cancer cell, and an underlying endothelial cell [111–113]. Macrophages induce RhoA GTPase activity in tumor cells, triggering actin-rich invadopodia that allow tumor cell transendothelial migration [114]. Furthermore, transient vascular permeability was observed at the TMEM, where TIE2^{hi} TMEM macrophages secrete VEGFA, causing local loss of vascular junctions, transient permeability, and tumor cell intravasation [112].

In pancreatic cancer, tumor-derived IL-4 induces the expression of the cysteine proteases cathepsin B and cathepsin S in macrophages, which enhance tumor cell invasion and intravasation by altering the extracellular matrix (ECM) [34]. Moreover, an in vitro study suggested that pancreatic cancer cells activate toll-like receptor 4 (TLR4) signaling in macrophages, inducing IL-10 expression and M2 polarization. TAM TLR4/IL-10 signaling promotes epithelial-to-mesenchymal transition (EMT) in tumor cells, characterized by downregulation of E-cadherin, and upregulation of vimentin and Snail, as well as induction of MMP2 and MM9 proteolytic activity, suggesting a mechanism for TAM-driven tumor cell migration [115]. Recently a novel role of Myosin II was discovered. The migratory behavior of rounded-amoeboid like tumor cells is perpetuated by high ROCK-Myosin II expression which drives IL-1α secretion and NF-κB activation, and these rounded tumor cells are found at the leading invasive edge in close proximity to CD206+CD163+ TAMs and vessels to promote tumor progression [116]. High DAB2 (disabled homolog 2 mitogen-responsive phosphoprotein) expression in tumor-infiltrating TAMs is associated with a worse prognosis in patients. DAB2+ TAMs are at the invasive edge of the tumor and assist in tumor cell dissemination by ECM remodeling, integrin recycling, and mechanosensing cues via YAP-TAZ signaling [117]. In hepatocellular carcinoma, cancer-associated fibroblasts (CAFs) via the expression of endosialin on their surface recruit macrophages through CD68 interaction, regulating GAS6 expression in CAFs to mediate M2 polarization in macrophages and tumor growth [118].

Neutrophils recruited by malignant fibrosarcoma and prostate cancer cells enhance angiogenesis and intravasation in primary tumors by secreting MMP9 [119]. In intrahepatic cholangiocarcinoma, neutrophils recruited by tumor-derived CXCL5, a ligand of CXCR2, enhance metastasis [120]. CXCR2 knockout hosts exhibited smaller tumors and reduced metastasis of breast cancer cells, and a decrease in tumor cell proliferation and angiogenesis, coinciding with significantly suppressed recruitment of CD11b+ Gr1+ myeloid cells and F4/80+ macrophages, suggesting a role of the infiltrating pro-inflammatory immune cells in tumor progression and metastasis [121]. Myeloid cells recruited to mammary tumors harboring a Tgfbr2 deletion secrete MMPs and TGFβ1 that mediate tumor cell invasion and metastasis [122].

In a mouse model of colorectal cancer, collective invasion of cancer cells occurs via a paracrine loop between CD34+ immature myeloid cells (iMCs) and tumor cells. Tumor cells secrete CCL9, which recruits CCR1+ iMCs to the invasive front, where they express MMP2 and MMP9 and promote tumor collective migration [123]. Loss of SMAD4 in human colorectal cancer cells leads to an enhanced expression of CXCL1 and CXCL8 in tumor cells, which in turn leads to an increased recruitment of neutrophils via CXCR2 and higher cancer progression [124].

BM-derived mesenchymal stem cells (MSCs) injected subcutaneously with weak metastatic human breast cancer cells enhanced the migration and dissemination of the tumor cells, via the signaling of MSC-derived chemokine CCL5 to its receptor CCR5 on tumor cells [125]. Direct interaction between BM-MSC-derived periostin and CCL2 in B-ALL cells is responsible for increased leukemia burden [126]. Furthermore, myofibroblasts expressing alpha-smooth muscle actin (αSMA) and derived from BM-MSCs secrete MMP13, increasing tumor invasiveness in a model of skin cancer [127].

Tumor Cell Survival in Circulation and Extravasation into Metastatic Organs

Cancer cells from the primary tumor intravasate into the peripheral circulation as circulating tumor cells (CTCs) [128]. Following intravasation, CTCs induce platelet coagulation by secreting thrombin, enabling platelets to shield tumor cells from shear stress encountered in circulation [129]. Platelets also protect tumor cells from the immune activity of NK cells [130, 131]. Platelet depletion or disruption of clot-forming components inhibited metastasis in mouse models [132]. Platelets have also been shown to be a major source of TGFβ1 in the circulation, and platelet-induced EMT enhanced metastasis in vivo [133]. A conditional knockout of PDGFB in platelets has been shown to negatively impact vascular integrity in the tumor microenvironment, thus enhancing hypoxia and EMT in primary tumors, elevating the levels of CTCs and promoting metasta-sis [134].

Clot formation also recruits macrophages, which in turn protect circulating tumor cells. Tumor-initiated clot formation induces the expression of vascular cell adhesion mole-cule 1 (VCAM-1) and vascular adhesion protein 1 (VAP1) on endothelial cells, which recruit macrophages [135]. Macrophages expressing integrin α4 (CD49b) bind to

VCAM-1-expressing tumor cells and propagate AKT-dependent survival signals to them [136]. In colorectal carci-noma (CRC), CD163+ TAMs at the invasive edge regulate EMT, CTC in blood, and metastasis of CRC. TAMs secrete IL-6, activating the JAK2/STAT3 pathway that inhibits miR-506-3p in cancer cells, thus promoting FoxQ2 expression which increases CCL2 secretion to promote the recruitment of macrophages [137]. In TNBC, higher expression of tumor suppressor miR-149 directly targets CSF-1 to inhibit recruit-ment and polarization of M2 macrophages, thus suppressing lung metastasis [138].

CD4+ CD25+ FoxP3+ T_{Reg} cells isolated from lymph nodes of patients with melanoma and from malignant ascites of ovarian cancer patients inhibit CD4+ and CD8+ T cell prolif-eration and cytokine production in vitro [139, 140], suggesting that T_{Reg} cells can protect disseminated cancer cells at the metastatic site from immune attack. Ovarian can-cer stem cells (CSCs) have been found to express CCL5 and recruit T_{reg} through the expression of CCR5 receptor on their surface [141]. This CSC CCL5-T_{reg} CCR5 interaction increases IL-10 and also increases the production of MMP-9 by T_{reg}, aiding with ovarian cancer metastasis [141]. Patients with liver metastasis are known to respond poorly to anti-PD-1 therapy. Recently, the presence of a tumor-specific antigen causing systemic suppression of the immune system and increased activation of T_{regs} and modulation of CD11b+ monocytes was reported [142]. Thus, combining anti-PD-1 with anti-CTLA4 or EZH2 inhibitors to deplete or destabi-lize T_{regs} is considered as a potential approach against liver metastases [142].

The next challenge for CTCs is to exit the circulation and colonize the surrounding tissue of the metastatic organ. The first step of extravasation requires that a CTC properly adheres with the endothelial wall. Tumor-derived IL-8 recruits neutrophils and increases their expression of β2 inte-grin, promoting the interaction between tumor cell intercel-lular adhesion molecule-1 (ICAM-1) and neutrophil β2 integrin [143]. ICAM-1 is also expressed on endothelial cells [129], enabling neutrophils to anchor tumor cells to the endothelium, enhancing extravasation and metastatic foci formation in lungs [143] and liver [144]. Neutrophils also form structures called neutrophil extracellular traps (NETs), composed of extruded DNA and antimicrobial proteases. Neutrophils trap circulating tumor cells in NETs that form in liver and lung capillaries to promote metastasis [145]. NETs have been found to be elevated in invasive esophageal, gas-tric, and lung cancer patients, and shown to regulate disease progression [146]. Using lung and colon cancer murine mod-els, it was observed that inhibiting NETs either using Sivelestat or peptidyl arginine deiminase type IV (PAD4, involved in NET formation) reduced spontaneous lung and liver metastasis in these models [146]. In the blood, circulat-ing tumor cells (CTCs) have been found to be present in association with neutrophils, which help in the cell cycle progression of these tumor cells, followed by an increase in their metastatic potential [147].

Platelets contribute to tumor cell extravasation by promoting the adhesion of tumor cells to ECs at the distant site. In addition to EC P-selectin, platelet-expressed P-selectin promoted lung metastasis of breast cancer and melanoma [148]. CTCs themselves express the selectin ligands sialyl Lewis-a (sLe^a) and sialyl Lewis-x (sLe^x) [149]. These ligands allow tumor cells to adhere to endothelial cell E-selectin and confer increased metastatic potential [150, 151].

Inflammatory monocytes recruited to the premetastatic lungs via the CCL2-CCR2 axis increased tumor cell extravasation from the vasculature into the lung parenchyma by increasing VEGF-induced vessel permeability, resulting in transendothelial migration [152] during breast cancer metastasis to the lungs [153] and colorectal cancer metastasis to the liver [154]. Tumor antigen, CD97, has been shown to stimulate platelet activation via a bidirectional signaling through platelet-derived lysophosphatidic acid (LPA). This increases vascular permeability and transendothelial tumor cell migration [155]. In colon and breast cancer models, platelet-specific receptor for collagen and fibrin, GPVI (glycoprotein VI), interacts with galectin-3 on tumor cells to promote extravasation of tumor cells via ITAM signaling [156]. Tumor cells undergoing EMT and circulating tumor cells express Hsp-47, which has also been shown to increase platelet recruitment and metastatic lung colonization of tumor cells [157].

Tumor Cell Colonization and Initiation of Metastasis in Distant Organs

Metastatic tumors set up a BM-derived microenvironment at the distant site of metastasis, known as the premetastatic niche [158]. This niche functions as a permissive hub for supporting colonization and outgrowth of disseminated tumor cells following extravasation. BM-derived cells at the metastatic site also influence tumor cell tropism and promote metastatic outgrowth.

Contribution of the Premetastatic Niche in Colonization and Initiation of Metastasis

In 1889, Stephen Paget proposed the "seed and soil" hypothesis, in which he suggested that cancer cells, being the "seed," had an affinity for and only colonized organs that were conducive to their growth, or had the proper "soil" [159]. Indeed, in recent years, studies have shown that conducive microenvironments are required for disseminated tumor cells to engraft at distant sites, in agreement with the

"seed and soil" hypothesis. Strikingly, metastatic primary tumors systemically generate bone marrow-derived "premetastatic niches" in distant organs that serve as hubs for supporting future metastases [160].

The first account of the premetastatic niche described that the recruitment of VEGFR1$^+$ hematopoietic progenitor cells to the lungs is necessary for tumor metastasis. In this model, Lewis lung carcinoma and melanoma primary tumors systemically induced the expression of fibronectin in lung fibroblasts, leading to the recruitment of BM-derived VEGFR1$^+$ and CD11b$^+$ myeloid cells to the lungs via their fibronectin receptor, VLA-4 [161]. CD11b$^+$ myeloid cells are also recruited to premetastatic lungs by chemoattractants S100A8 and S100A9, expressed in response to primary tumor-derived VEGFA, TGFβ, and tumor necrosis factor α (TNFα) [162]. The recruited CD11b$^+$ cells in turn express TNFα and TGFβ, which enhance tumor cell metastasis [162]. In addition, serum amyloid A3 (SAA3), induced by S100A8 and S100A9 in lungs, activates NFκB signaling via TLR4 on myeloid cells, potentiating the inflammatory response and accelerating lung metastasis [163]. Furthermore, primary tumor-derived CCL2 signaling through CCR2 on lung endothelial cells induces the secretion of S100A8 and SAA3, which increases vascular permeability, resulting in hyperpermeable foci that attract leukocytes and tumor cells [164]. A novel way to suppress pro-metastatic effects of S100A8 has been utilized in 4T1 model by inhibiting high-fat diet-enhanced premetastatic niche formation [165]. Glycyrrhizic acid prevents Gr1+ myeloid cell migration and S100A8/9 expression by decreasing M1-macrophage population and their CCL2 and TNF-α production leading to modification of premetastatic niche formation and reduction of metastasis [165].

Primary tumor-derived VEGF induces the expression of MMP9 in CD11b$^+$ myeloid cells and endothelial cells in the premetastatic niche [166]. MMP9 in the premetastatic niche releases VEGF from the ECM, promoting angiogenesis [167], and soluble KIT ligand, which further recruits KIT receptor-expressing BM cells [168]. In melanoma metastasis to liver, pro-oncogenic miR-155 decreased levels of its target NFE2L2, a redox regulatory factor, while increasing VEGFA levels in premetastatic liver via pro-oxidative events [169]. In 4T1 models, primary tumor-secreted VEGF was elevated, leading to hyperpermeability of vessels in lungs and reduced levels of tight junction proteins: occluding and ZO-1 [170]. Inhibition of a multifunctional glycoprotein, dipeptidyl peptidase-4, has been shown to accelerate EMT in breast cancer cells and thus their metastasis via induction of CXCL12/CXCR4 and activation of mTOR pathway [171].

Furthermore, hypoxia from primary tumors induces the accumulation of MDSCs in premetastatic lungs, suppressing the cytotoxic function of NK cells [172]. Treatment with epigenetic therapy (azacitidine and entinostat) induces the differentiation of MDSCs into a more-interstitial macrophage-like phenotype by reducing expression of CCR2 and CXCR2, thus disrupting the premetastatic niche [173]. Chronic stress is known to enhance premetastatic niche formation and metastatic colonization of breast cancer cells in lungs via β-adrenergic signaling [174]. β-adrenergic signaling causes an increase in monocytes and macrophages in the premetastatic lungs, which interact with upregulated CCL2 in pulmonary stromal cells, to enhance metastatic colonization [174]. In premetastatic niche, a myeloid-rich, immune-suppressive gene signature is present which enhances metastasis [175]. Recently, this immunosuppressive effect was mitigated using genetically engineered myeloid cells (GEMys) to deliver IL-12 to the secondary site. IL12-GEMy enhanced antigen presentation and T-cell activation at the premetastatic site to reduce metastasis [175].

Lysyl oxidase (LOX), a hypoxia-inducible secreted amine oxidase, is also critical in the generation of premetastatic niches in solid tumor metastasis [176]. Secreted LOX from hypoxic primary breast cancer cells co-localizes with fibronectin in both pulmonary and hepatic premetastatic niches, and crosslinks collagens in the local microenvironment. This modification of the ECM promotes the recruitment of CD11b⁺ BM cells, creating a niche permissive for the colonization of metastasizing tumor cells at these secondary sites [176]. The inhibition of LOX at primary tumors abrogates the establishment of premetastatic niches and decreases metastatic burden in secondary organs. Similarly, the targeting of CD11b⁺ cells restricts the establishment of tumor-supportive premetastatic niches, reducing metastatic burden [176]. In addition, LOX expression and activity during the onset and development of both chemical- and radiation-induced lung and liver fibrosis has been shown to be responsible for fibrosis-enhanced metastasis to these organs. The action of LOX generates tumor cell supportive niches high in fibrillar collagen, which increase seeding, tumor cell persistence, and survival [177]. While the involvement of BM-derived cells was not directly investigated, the changes occurring during fibrosis dramatically recapitulate those observed in premetastatic niche remodeling, suggesting common overlapping mechanisms [178]. More recently, LOX has also been shown to induce the formation of premetastatic osteolytic lesions in the bone. In this case, elevated levels of LOX secreted by hypoxic primary tumors alter the homeostatic balance between osteoclasts and osteoblasts. LOX modulates the BM stroma to drive de novo osteoclastogenesis while decreasing osteoblast proliferation, both in vitro and in vivo. The net result is unbalanced coupling, osteolysis, and premetastatic niche generation within the bone. These LOX-driven premetastatic niches, in turn, support circulating tumor cell colonization and the development of overt bone metastases [179].

In a bladder cancer model, the tumor cell-derived proteoglycan, versican, enhances metastasis to the lungs via a mechanism involving increased lung CCL2 chemokine expression and increased macrophage infiltration [180]. Consistent with these data, the recruitment of CCR2-expressing monocytes and macrophages to the lungs in response to tumor cell-derived and host-derived CCL2 enhances breast tumor metastasis to lungs [153]. In epithelial ovarian cancer, higher expression of miR-590-3p suppressed FOXA2 levels by binding to its 3″ UTR, which increased versican levels to enhance tumor proliferation and metastasis [181]. High versicanV1 expression in HCC promotes metastasis via activation of EGFR-PI3K-AKT pathway [182].

Immature myeloid cells expressing the stem and progenitor cell marker CD117 are involved in premetastatic niche formation [161, 176]. Similarly, mature myeloid cells, such as CD11b⁺ Ly6C⁺ monocytes, are recruited to premetastatic lungs by CCL2, and CD11b⁺ CD68⁺ F4/80⁺ macrophages are recruited by fibrin clots in the premetastatic lungs, where they enhance metastasis of B16 melanoma and breast cancer cells, respectively [183, 184]. Macrophages in the premetastatic niche are derived from circulating BM-derived monocytes, which are recruited via CCL2 [153], and this implies that primary tumor-secreted factors can systemically recruit myeloid progenitors at different stages of differentiation to premetastatic sites, where they differentiate into metastasis-promoting macrophages. Interestingly, primary prostate and breast tumors with a low metastatic potential systemically induce the expression of the antiangiogenic factor Tsp-1 in myeloid cells recruited to the premetastatic lungs [185], indicating that even non-metastatic tumors can modify the microenvironment in distant organs. Recently pro-metastatic effects of chemotherapy, involving taxanes and anthracyclines, were identified that led to primary tumors releasing extracellular vesicles enriched in annexin A6 which promoted NF-κB-dependent endothelial cell activation, CCL2 induction, and Ly6C+CCR2+ monocytes in the premetastatic lungs, followed by overt metastatic outgrowth [186].

Primary tumor-secreted G-CSF recruits Ly6G⁺ neutrophils to premetastatic lungs, where they contribute to the formation of lung metastasis via their expression of Bv8, which promotes tumor cell migration [187]. Interestingly, the CCL2-CCR2 axis was also shown to recruit CCR2⁺ neutrophils to the premetastatic lung [188]. However, instead of promoting metastasis, these neutrophils inhibited the survival of disseminated cells through CCL2-dependent activation of H_2O_2-mediated killing [188]. These results suggest that CCL2 both promotes and blocks metastasis initiation; hence, insights into these processes will be critical for developing anti-metastatic therapies. A novel subset of neutrophils, CD62Ldim, have been found to have stronger adhesion and longer survival [189]. These neutrophils are necessary for the formation of premetastatic niche in lungs in breast cancer models via CXCL12-CXCR4 pathway [189]. Migration of neutrophils to distant tissues to form premetastatic niche was recently identified in the presence of tumors. Bone marrow neutrophils in mice-bearing early-stage tumors have higher OXPHOS and glycolysis, higher ATP production, as well as increased autocrine ATP signaling via purinergic receptors than control neutrophils from non-tumor bearing mice [190]. In osteosarcoma metastasis, tumor-secreted ANGPTL2 stimulates lung epithelial cells to recruit neutrophils to the lungs and form premetastatic niche for osteosarcoma metastasis [191]. Regulators of lipid metabolism, oxysterols, also regulate premetastatic niche in lungs of mice-bearing 4T1 tumors by recruiting neutrophils to the lungs via oxysterol/LXR (nuclear Liver X Receptors-(LXR) α and LXRβ) signaling [192]. Chronic nicotine exposure also increases recruitment of pro-tumor N2-neutrophils to the lungs to form premetastatic niche [193]. This niche promotes STAT3-activated lipocalin 2 (LCN2) release, which has been detected in serum and urine of breast cancer patients and cancer-free women who smoke [193]. Thus, LCN2 can possibly be used as a prognostic biomarker for lung metastasis of breast cancer.

Non-myeloid cells also compose the premetastatic niche. For instance, CD4$^+$ T cells in premetastatic bones increase osteoclastogenesis by secreting receptor activator of nuclear factor-kB ligand (RANKL), thus enhancing the metastasis of breast cancer cells to the bones [194]. Moreover, 4T1 breast cancer cells systemically induce the expression of CCL22 in lung stroma, thereby inducing the recruitment of T$_{Reg}$ cells to premetastatic lungs [195]. A study defining premetastatic niche in tumor draining lymph node using MMTV-PyMT breast cancer model by single-cell RNA sequencing identified that CD4+ and CD8+ T cells have higher angiogenesis pathway genes, upregulated T-reg genes, downregulated IFN and inflammatory gene signatures [196]. The niche in these tumor draining lymph nodes also had upregulation of OXPHOS in fibroblastic reticular cells and genes like *Prdx3*, *Ndufa4*, and *Uqcrb*, demonstrating enhanced ATP consumption, TCA cycle and a metabolic switch to OXPHOS by breast cancer cells [196].

In addition to soluble tumor-derived factors generating the premetastatic niche, exosomes released from primary tumors also induce the mobilization of BM-derived cells which are then recruited to the secondary site to generate the premetastatic niche [197]. Metastatic B16 melanoma cells release exosomes that carry MET, transferring MET to BM progenitors, leading to their recruitment to premetastatic lungs and enhancing metastasis [198]. Bone metastasis of prostate cancer cells was recently found to be dependent on exosome-mediated transfer of pyruvate kinase M2 (PKM2) from prostate cancer cells into bone marrow stromal cells (BMSCs), which then increases CXCL12 production by BMSCs via HIF-1α to mediate bone tropism [199].

Organ Tropism

Correlations have been found between primary tumors and their preferred metastatic destination, and more recent studies have begun to identify mechanism of metastasis organotropism. The tropism, or preferential metastasis, of tumors to specific organs has been shown to be determined in part by cancer cell intrinsic pathways, and as a consequence, gene signatures that mediate organ-specific metastasis have been described [200–202]. However, tumor non-cell-autonomous mechanisms have also been shown to play a necessary role in organ tropism. For example, chemoattractants in metastatic organs are able to recognize cognate chemokine receptors expressed on cancer cells that promote homing. Breast cancer cells expressing CXCR4 and CCR7 migrate toward SDF-1 and CCL21 chemokine gradients, respectively, in metastatic sites [203]. Signaling via CXCR4 and CCR7 mediates actin polymerization and pseudopodia formation, leading to chemotactic responses and invasion [203]. Moreover, blocking CXCR4/SDF-1 signaling suppresses metastasis of breast cancer cells to the lymph nodes and lungs [203]. CXCR4 expression is also required for human epidermal growth factor receptor 2 (HER2)-mediated breast cancer metastasis [204]. In addition to CXCR4 and CCR7, CCR10 expression on melanoma cells confers tropism to the skin [203]. Furthermore, chemokine (C-X3-C motif) receptor 1 (CX3CR1) expression on pancreatic cancer cells mediates their metastasis to chemokine (C-X3-C motif) ligand 1 (CX3CL1)-expressing peripheral neurons [205].

A major step after homing is adhesion of tumor cells at the distant site. During the early steps of pulmonary metastasis, disseminated breast cancer cells arrest in lungs via contacts between tumor α3β1 integrin and laminin 5 expressed on pulmonary vasculature basement membrane [206]. Furthermore, TNFα secreted by primary tumors [162] and by myeloid cells in lungs [207] upregulates the expression of the adhesion molecules E-selectin, P-selectin, and VCAM-1, promoting tumor cell adhesion and migration [3]. TNBC primary tumors increase CD117+ hematopoietic progenitor cells in the bone marrow in the mice compared to luminal primary tumors and control mice [208]. TNBC primary tumors also increase fibronectin, tenascin-c, and periostin in lungs to increase lung metastasis, and the lung-conditioned media from these mice are rich in metastasis proteins like CCL7, FGFR4, GM-CSF, MMP3, TSP-1, and VEGF [208]. A recent study [209] established cell lines derived from circulating tumor cells in breast cancer patients and cultured in vivo. These *ex vivo* cultured cells recapitulated the metastasis phenotypes in mouse models and also identified semaphorin 4D as an important mediator of migration through blood-brain barrier and brain metastasis in breast cancer patients [209]. Breast tumor cells and stroma together create distinct extracellular matrix niches for different organ metastasis [210]. Proteins enriched in CD109, SERPINB1, HCFC1, and cerebellin-1 are prominent in brain metastases, COL4A4 and laminin-121 are rich in lung metastases, and bone marrow metastatic niche is rich in S100A6 and S100A11 [210]. In breast cancer, enhanced expression of POU1F1 transcription factor (or Pit-1) is associated with increased CXCR4 and CXCL12 expression, along with specific breast cancer metastasis to liver and lungs [211].

Primary tumors from multiple organs metastasize to bone. Breast cancer causes osteolytic lesions in bones, stimulating the formation and activity of osteoclasts. These osteolytic lesions cells express CSF1, which activates osteoclasts that break down bone. Breast cancer cells also express parathyroid hormone-related protein (PTHRP) and TNFα, which activate RANKL and inhibit osteoprotegerin synthesis, inducing formation and activity of osteoclasts [212, 213]. In melanoma, inhibition of RANKL reduced metastasis to the bone, but not to other organs [213].

Breast cancer cells that home to the bone express upregulated CXCR4, osteopontin, MMP1, and IL-11 [200]. The bone stroma is rich in SDF-1, the ligand for CXCR4, which may mediate the tropism of the breast cancer cells. Once in the bone, IL-11 activates osteoclasts, and MMP1 releases matrix-sequestered factors, enhancing tumor outgrowth and bone degradation [3]. When bone matrix is degraded, several sequestered factors are released, including insulin-like growth factor 1 (IGF1), TGFβ, and bone morphogenetic proteins (BMPs), which enhance metastatic survival and outgrowth and induce PTHRP synthesis, leading to further bone degradation [212]. This leads to a positive feedback loop of increased bone loss and enhanced metastatic tumor growth. In the case of neuroblastoma that metastasizes to the bone, while some tumors secrete RANKL, others induce IL-6 expression in BM-MSCs. IL-6 activates osteoclasts and is required for bone metastasis [214]. Furthermore, BM-derived IL-6 mediates survival and proliferation of IL-6R$^+$ neuroblastoma cells [215].

Prostate cancer, on the other hand, generates osteoblastic lesions in the bone, characterized by disrupted bone deposition. Prostate metastatic lesions release endothelin 1, TGFβ2, FGF, and BMPs, all of which are osteoblastic and alter bone structure [3]. Moreover, prostate cancer cells also produce urokinase-type plasminogen activator (uPA) and prostate-specific antigen (PSA), which can release growth factors from the bone matrix, enhancing metastatic outgrowth [212].

More recently, tumor-derived exosomes were shown to be implicated in organ-specific metastasis. Exosomes carrying integrins α6β4 and α6β1 directed metastasis to the lungs, while exosomal integrin αvβ5 directed metastasis to the liver, in both cases by inducing the expression of S100 chemoattractants in the target organ [216].

Metastatic Outgrowth

After seeding in the secondary site, metastatic tumors establish vasculature in order to outgrow. This occurs via the production of angiogenic factors, such as VEGFA, and the recruitment of endothelial cells and pericytes. Metastasis-associated macrophages (MAMs) support tumor outgrowth at the metastatic site [152] via a TIE2-dependent mechanism that promotes angiogenesis [40]. On the contrary, a membrane tetraspan molecule, MS4A4A, selectively expressed by macrophage-lineage cells and associated with Dectin-1 in macrophages, is responsible for activation of macrophages and NK cells via Syk-dependent signaling and reactive oxygen species production, to reduce metastasis [217]. In the MMTV-PyMT breast cancer model, BM-derived EPCs are recruited to metastatic lesions, where they incorporate into nascent vessels and contribute to the angiogenic switch, promoting the progression of micrometastases to macrometastases [90]. EPCs express the transcription factor inhibitor of differentiation 1 (ID1), which is required for EPC mobilization and recruitment [90, 91]. Moreover, several proangiogenic genes are upregulated in recruited EPCs, suggesting an additional mechanism whereby EPCs promote angiogenesis and metastatic progression [90].

Furthermore, the contribution of neutrophils to metastatic progression was demonstrated in models of extrinsic lung inflammation, where the neutrophil-secreted serine proteases neutrophil elastase (NE) and cathepsin G (CG) degrade antiangiogenic Tsp-1, coinciding with increased lung metastasis [218]. Furthermore, neutrophils in the premetastatic lungs were shown to expand the metastasis-initiating cell population of breast cancer cells by expressing leukotrienes [219]. Neutrophils also secrete proangiogenic Bv8, which promotes metastatic progression [187].

As in earlier stages of tumor progression, myeloid cells also play a role in metastatic outgrowth. In the MMTV-PyMT breast cancer model, BM-derived CD11b$^+$ Ly6C^{high} myeloid progenitor cells in premetastatic lungs secrete the extracellular matrix protein, versican, which promotes mesenchymal-to-epithelial transition (MET) of metastatic tumor cells via the TGFβ pathway, thereby increasing proliferation and accelerating lung metastatic outgrowth [220]. Primary tumor-secreted G-CSF is known to increase immunosuppressive CD11b+GR1+ MDSCs in the spleen and lungs of a 4T1 breast cancer model. In 4T1 model of metastasis it has been found that presence of orthotopic primary tumor increases (G-) MDSCs, monocytic (M-) MDSCs, macrophages, eosinophils, and NK cells in the lungs [221]. Even upon resection of primary tumor, immunosuppressive G-MDSCs still persist in the lungs, aiding in subsequent metastatic outgrowth. Thus, reduction of G-MDSCs via gemcitabine treatment in addition to primary tumor removal significantly reduces metastasis [221].

Neutrophil accumulation in cancer leads to a worse prognosis in patients and is one of the major reasons for increased cancer metastasis [222]. Interplay between CXCR4 and CXCR2 dictates neutrophil release from the bone marrow, where inhibition of CXCR4 or secretion of CXCL1 and CXCL2 by endothelial cells and megakaryocytes to mediate CXCR2 signaling, promotes neutrophil release into circulation and downstream activity [222]. Neutrophils are known for premetastatic conditioning at secondary sites, T-cell suppression, and promotion of cancer cell survival [223, 224]. In cancer, there is evidence of increased granulopoiesis which enhances neutrophil formation. Obesity has also been shown to increase breast-to-lung metastasis in a GM-CSF- and IL5-dependent manner by causing lung neutrophilia [225]. Weight loss significantly reverses these effects and lowers serum levels of both GM-CSF and IL-5 [225]. Recent evidence also suggests that increased recruitment of neutrophils at the metastatic site via cathepsin C-mediated activation of neutrophil PR3 to increase IL-1β secretion, enhances breast-to-lung metastasis [226]. This increased recruitment also promotes extrusion of their genomic DNA to form NETs via neutrophil-induced reactive oxygen species by NADPH oxidase NOX2 [224], degrading TSP-1 and promoting metastatic outgrowth [226]. Therefore, cathepsin C inhibition via AZD7986 could prove to be an effective strategy for mitigating these effects.

NETs have been shown to promote liver metastasis in early-stage breast cancer patients [227]. In short, NETs in liver or lungs act as a chemoattractant for cancer cells via a transmembrane protein CCDC25 on cancer cells which activates ILK-β-parvin pathway to enhance their motility and thus, metastasis to the secondary sites [227]. Tumor-secreted CXCR1 and CXCR2 ligands also promote NETosis which shields tumor cells from cytotoxic effects of NK cells and lymphocytes [228]. Inhibition of adipose triglyceride lipase activity in neutrophils also promotes breast-to-lung metastasis by increasing lipid storage by these neutrophils in premetastatic lungs [229]. These lipids via macropinocytosis–lysosome pathway are transported to metastasizing tumor cells to enhance their survival and proliferation [229]. Additionally in an obesity model, neutrophils have been shown to regulate transendothelial migration leading to higher extravasation of circulating tumor cells into secondary organs and increased breast cancer metastasis [230]. The increased metastatic potential is due to lowered vascular integrity by neutrophils via MMP9 and LCN2 secretion [230]. Genes like *Ltf* and *Lcn2* were also upregulated in obese mice which led to increased neutrophil ROS production and enhanced NETs to promote extravasation and metastasis [230]. NETs were also shown to convert dormant cancer cells to aggressive lung metastases in vivo in the presence of lung inflammation [231]. Sustained lung inflammation caused elevated NET formation, NET DNA then cleaved laminin by NE and MMP9, causing integrin-mediated FAK/ERK/MLCK/YAP signaling to promote proliferation of dormant cancer cells [231].

A recent study demonstrated that periostin (POSTN) secreted in the lung metastatic niche by stromal αSMA⁺ vimentin (VIM)⁺ fibroblasts was required to maintain cancer stem cells (CSCs) and allow metastatic outgrowth of breast cancer cells by inducing Wnt signaling in the CSCs [232, 233]. Although this study did not determine the exact identity of the fibroblasts secreting POSTN, a previous study had shown that BM-derived MSCs are the source of POSTN [234], suggesting that BM cells in the premetastatic niche could be supporting metastasis by maintaining CSCs via POSTN secretion. In a model of pancreatic cancer, αSMA+ myofibroblasts produce majority of type I collagen (Col1). Deletion of this Col1 leads to spontaneous emergence of PanINs and PDAC, and SOX-9-mediated Cxcl5 upregulation in cancer cells. Cxcl5 causes recruitment of MDSCs and suppression of CD8+ T-cells, thus enhancing PDAC progression [67]. A recent study demonstrated the presence and role of four different cancer-associated fibroblasts in metastatic lymph nodes and how they influence cancer cell invasion. Two myofibroblastic subsets in the lymph node: CAF-S1, enhanced cell invasion by CXCL12 and TGFβ pathways; whereas CAF-S4 enhanced 3-D invasion by NOTCH signaling [235]. CAF-S4 in patient lymph node was also found to correlate with late distant metastases [235].

Recently, studies on metastatic dormancy have identified a mechanism whereby EC-derived Tsp-1 promotes breast cancer dormancy [236]. Interestingly, in another study, metastasis-incompetent primary tumors were shown to induce the expression of Tsp-1 in BM-derived myeloid cells recruited to premetastatic lungs [185], suggesting that myeloid-derived Tsp-1 could be similarly mediating metastatic dormancy.

Clinical Significance, Perspectives, and Future Directions

BM-derived cells contribute to various stages of cancer progression, and given their prevalence in patient tumors, BM-derived cells are being evaluated as prognostic tools and as therapeutic targets. Elevated levels of circulating inflammatory monocytes correlate with a poor prognosis in pancreatic cancer patients [237]. A high preoperative neutrophil to lymphocyte ratio is associated with poor prognosis after resection in NSCLC [238]. In human breast cancer, a high TMEM score, i.e., the number of tumor cell, TAM, and endothelial cell interactions, is correlated with an increased risk of metastasis [239, 240]. Of note, TMEM score predicted the risk of distant metastasis in ER(+)/HER2(−) breast cancer [240]. The increased risk of metastasis observed in patients is consistent with pre-clinical studies showing the role of macrophages in tumor cell egress from the primary site, and intravital imaging revealing the direct contact between perivascular TAMs, endothelial cells, and tumor cells, forming the TMEM [113]. Recently, a correlation between an imbalance in gut microbiota and colorectal cancer (CRC) was found. The imbalance has been shown to upregulate metastasis-related secretory protein cathepsin K (CTSK) in both human CRC samples and mouse models of CRC, leading to a higher expression of M2 TAMs in the stroma, higher CRC metastasis, and a worse clinical prognosis [241]. Thus, making CTSK a novel biomarker and target for CRC.

There is increased translational significance of CSF-1R inhibition in advanced solid tumors. Combination of CSF-1R inhibition with a CD40 agonist led to tumor rejection in multiple solid tumor models [242]. In glioblastoma (GBM), radiotherapy has shown to increase relative abundance of brain-resident microglia and monocyte-derived macrophages which promote recurrence [243]. Pre-clinical models have shown that radiotherapy combined with CSF-1R inhibition is able to effectively overcome this resistance [243]. Inhibiting CSF-1R with PLX3397 has also shown to interfere with the education of TAMs [244] in the GBM tumor microenvironment (depolarizes them from their original M2 state and upregulates M1-like state) [245]. Inhibition of CSF-1R increases the sensitivity of glioma cells to tyrosine kinase inhibitors and improved outcomes in pre-clinical trials [245].

In NSCLC patients, high tumor islet CD68$^+$ macrophage density predicted increased survival, whereas high stromal macrophage density predicted reduced survival [246–248]. Further characterization of macrophage populations revealed that CD68+ M1 macrophages, defined as HLA-DR$^+$ iNOS$^+$ TNFα^+ MRP8/14$^+$, were significantly increased in tumor islets of NSCLC patients with extended survival compared to patients with poor survival, whereas M2 macrophages (CD163$^+$ VEGF$^+$) were reduced [249]. On the other hand, several reports showed a correlation of TAMs with poor prognosis in lung cancer. Adenocarcinoma patients with high CD68$^+$ TAM density had significantly lower 5-year survival rates [250]. Furthermore, CD68$^+$ TAM density correlated with higher tumor expression of the angiogenic factor IL-8, and higher microvessel density, but worse prognosis [251]. CD68$^+$ CD163$^+$ M2-like TAMs were significantly higher in patients whose disease progressed in the presence of EGFR tyrosine kinase inhibitor therapy [23]. M2 TAMs defined as CD204$^+$ were associated with poor outcome [252], and CD206$^+$ TAMs correlated with lymph node metastasis [253].

High levels of IL-10 expression by TAMs were significantly correlated with advanced tumor stage and predicted poor overall survival [254, 255]. Expression of MMP9 and VEGF by CD68$^+$ IL-10^{hi} TAMs correlated with late stage of disease [256]. On the other hand, several studies have failed to find a correlation between macrophage density and NSCLC patient prognosis [27]. In lung cancer, developmental origin of TAMs (tissue-resident vs. CCR2-dependent recruited macrophages) dictates their function, distribution, and response to cancer therapies [257]. In this regard, anti-VEGF therapy combined with chemotherapy reduced both resident- and recruited-TAMs (expressing VEGFR1) without impacting monocyte infiltration and prolonged mouse survival in pre-clinical models [257].

In colorectal cancer higher SPP1 levels and lower mTORC2 activity in TAMs are associated with a worse clinical prognosis [258]. IL-15 receptor alpha chain or hetIL-15 of the heterodimeric cytokine IL-15 treatment in colon and epithelial carcinoma models has shown increased intratumoral accumulation of XCR1+IRF8+CD103+ conventional type 1 dendritic cells (cDC1), with enhanced levels of IFNγ and XCL1, leading to an increased infiltration of CXCR3+ NK and CD8+ T cells in tumors [259]. Thus, enabling tumor immunotherapy approaches to promote effector responses over regulatory lymphocytes to delay tumor growth.

Several therapeutic combinations involving immune checkpoint blockade are being developed as effective antitumor therapeutics. In HCC, a dual anti-PD-1/VEGFR-2 therapy has shown promising effects of inhibiting tumor growth and increasing overall survival in mouse models of cancer by increasing CD8+ T cell activation and infiltration, shifting the M1/M2 ratio of TAMs, reducing T-regs, and reducing CCR2+ monocyte infiltration [241]. A bispecific antibody, A2V, targeting VEGFA and angiopoietin-2 (ANGPT2) enhances recruitment of IFNγ-expressing CD8+ T lymphocytes, with concomitant expression of PD-L1 on tumor endothelial cells in an MMTV pre-clinical model [260]. Thus, supporting the rationale for combining antiangiogenic therapy with immune checkpoint blockade to improve survival.

Immune-suppressive MDSCs, defined as Lin$^-$HLA-DR$^-$CD33$^+$ and CD14$^-$CD11b$^+$CD33$^+$ [261], have been found to be increased in patients with NSCLC and were associated with increased metastasis and a poor response to chemotherapy [262]. Increased levels of circulating and tumor-infiltrating MDSCs were observed in patients with colon cancer and correlated with prognosis and cancer stage [263]. Furthermore, the frequency of circulating monocytic MDSCs predicted patient response to the checkpoint inhibitor ipilimumab (anti-CTLA-4), where patients with low frequencies of MDSCs benefited more from ipilimumab treatment [264]. Glioblastoma patients showed an increase in circulating MDSCs, primarily of granulocytic lineage, that mediated immunosuppressive functions [265]. In patients with breast cancer, an immune signature consisting of CD68^{high}/CD4^{high}/CD8^{low}, denoting the infiltration of the different immune cell types into tumors, significantly correlated with reduced OS [22]. Interestingly, this immune signature predicted OS independently of histopathological grade or receptor status [22].

Another important finding was that the composition of the TME landscape which is complex at the metastatic sites and can be defined by the origin of primary tumors. For instance, melanoma brain metastasis is composed of an abundance of CD4 and CD8 lymphocytes whereas breast cancer brain metastases have a prominence of neutrophils [69]. Even the TME in glioma, a CNS tumor, predominantly is comprised of higher tissue-resident microglia than tumor-infiltrating leukocytes [266]. Brain metastasis presents with the highest frequencies of Tregs, followed by IDH1-wt and IDH1-mutant gliomas [266]. Thus, dictating the differences in the efficacy of immunotherapy.

In addition to their prognostic role, a growing body of literature describing the contribution of the BM-derived microenvironment to tumor progression and metastasis reveals potential therapeutic avenues that bypass the need to target highly mutagenic tumor cells and instead focus on the more genetically stable stromal cells that support the tumor. In that respect, studies targeting BM-derived cells in the TME have shown some promise. For instance, inhibiting the recruitment of TAMs by blocking CSF1R signaling enhanced the cytotoxic effect of standard chemotherapy in a mouse model of breast cancer [22] and increased the efficacy of immunotherapy in a pancreatic cancer model [53]. Tumor refractoriness to anti-VEGF therapy was shown to be dependent on CD11b$^+$ Gr1$^+$ myeloid cell recruitment [73]. Blocking neutrophil recruitment to lungs by administering anti-G-CSF suppressed lung metastasis [187]. Moreover, inhibiting the myeloid cell-secreted angiogenic factor Bv8 reduced primary tumor growth, produced synergistic antitumor effects when combined with anti-VEGF treatment or chemotherapy [76], and reduced lung metastasis [187].

In a model of lung inflammation, deleting the neutrophil proteases NE and CG in the BM compartment significantly suppressed metastatic outgrowth [218], suggesting that targeting neutrophil proteases could present a way to block metastasis. Furthermore, inducing the expression of Tsp-1 by myeloid cells in the lungs by administering a peptide derived from the protein Prosaposin significantly reduced lung metastatic burden [185]. On the other hand, given the immunosuppressive function of MDSCs in cancer, strategies are being developed that promote the differentiation of MDSCs into mature, non-suppressive cells, decrease MDSC levels, or inhibit MDSC function [267]. Pre-clinical studies revealed that all trans retinoic acid (ATRA) induced the differentiation of MDSCs and enhanced T cell antigen-specific immune responses, but only induced an anti-cancer response when combined with a peptide vaccine [58, 268]. Administration of ATRA reduced MDSC levels in metastatic renal cell carcinoma (mRCC) patients that achieved a high plasma concentration of ATRA [269]. Sunitinib, an oral receptor tyrosine kinase inhibitor that targets PDGFR, VEGFR, and c-kit signaling and is FDA-approved for the treatment of advanced RCC, reduces MDSC levels in patients [270] and blocks the expansion of monocytic MDSCs while inducing apoptosis of granulocytic-MDSCs in a mouse model of breast cancer [271]. Furthermore, the immunosuppressive activity of MDSCs was abrogated by the synthetic triterpenoid, CDDO-Me, which upregulated several antioxidant genes and decreased tumor growth in mice [261]. Moreover, CDDO-Me completely blocked the inhibitory function of MDSCs isolated from RCC patients [261].

Another way MDSC function is being targeted is by inhibiting IDO, the rate-limiting enzyme in tryptophan degradation, which leads to suppression of T cell responses [48, 63]. IDO inhibition using 1-methyl-tryptophan (1MT) retarded tumor growth via a T cell-dependent mechanism in mouse models [272–274]. Furthermore, combining 1MT with therapies targeting immune checkpoints on T cells, such as CTLA-4, PD-1/PD-L1, synergizes the antitumor response in a mouse model of melanoma [275]. A recent clinical trial is testing the efficacy of IPI-549, a small molecule PI3Kγ inhibitor, in order to improve the efficacy of immune checkpoint blockade (NCT02637531). This is because resistance to immune checkpoint blockade has been directly correlated to increased infiltration of suppressive myeloid cells in the tumors, which have increased expression of PI3Kγ [276].

Concluding Remarks/Summary

The BM-derived TME constitutes a relatively untapped resource of novel therapeutic targets (Fig. 14.1). A major goal is to target only the "tumor-educated" BM cells and spare normal counterparts so that side effects are drastically reduced. Consistent with this notion, the analysis of enriched stromal compartments derived from human breast cancer revealed gene expression changes associated with cancer progression [277]. Similar analyses have led to the identification of activated stromal transcriptomes and tumor-stroma crosstalk pathways in human [278] and mouse [279] lung cancer. Future studies encompassing genomic, epigenetic, and proteomic analyses have the potential to provide insights into mechanisms that govern activation, expansion, mobilization, and recruitment of specific subsets of BM cells to the tumor bed leading to tumor growth and metastasis.

Key for Fig. 14.1

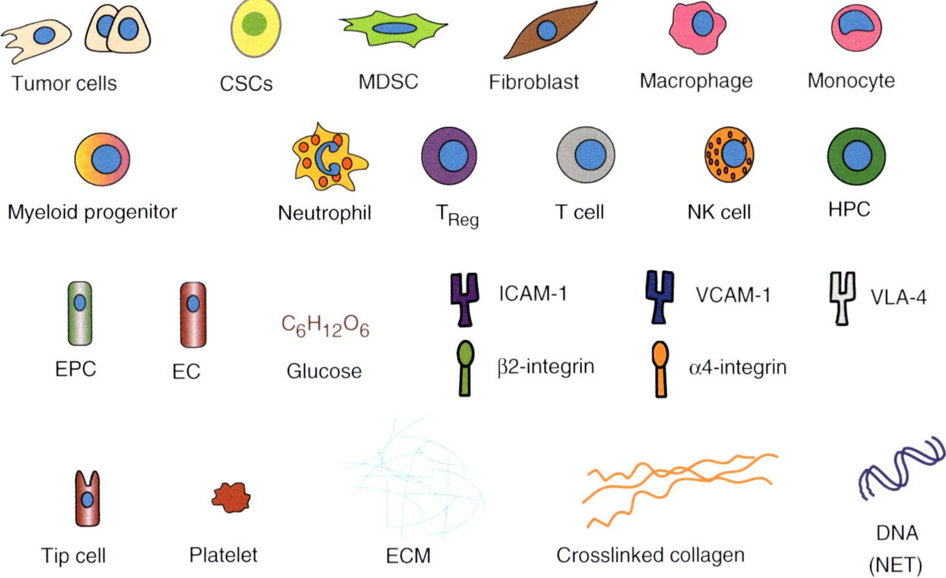

In the primary tumor, TAMs secrete VEGF and WNT7b, to promote angiogenesis, and MMPs and cathepsins, to mediate ECM degradation and tumor cell invasion. TANs secrete Bv8 and MMP9, promoting angiogenesis and ECM degradation. Myofibroblasts can also secrete MMPs and VEGF, contributing to angiogenesis. EPCs secrete angiogenic factors like VEGF and PDGF, generating a paracrine angiogenic signal, in addition to incorporating into nascent vessels. Furthermore, MDSCs suppress the activity of T cells and NK cells by secreting Arg1 and IDO, while T_{Reg} accomplishes immunosuppression by secreting IL-10 and TGFβ. There is a competition for glucose between tumor cells and T-cells. Immune checkpoint blockade is able to increase glycolysis in T-cells and elevate interferon-gamma production. Cancer stem cells (CSCs) recruit T_{regs} to the primary tumor via CCL5. A paracrine loop exists, whereby tumor cells secrete CSF1 to recruit macrophages, which in turn secrete EGF to promote tumor cell migration. Tumor cells, TAMs, and ECs establish the TMEM, where perivascular TAMs secrete VEGF, increasing local permeability and allowing tumor cell intravasation.

In the circulation, tumor cells activate platelet aggregation. Platelets protect tumor cells from shear stress and NK cell attack. Furthermore, platelets promote epithelial-to-mesenchymal transition (EMT) by secreting TGFβ. Platelets promote tumor cell adhesion to blood vessels at the secondary site via P-selectin. Moreover, tumors in circulation recruit neutrophils via IL-8. Neutrophils bridge tumor cells to blood vessels via neutrophil-expressed β2 integrin and tumor cell- and EC-expressed ICAM-1. Neutrophils also trap tumor cells in NETs.

In the metastatic organ, tumor cell-derived CCL2 recruits inflammatory monocytes, which differentiate into MAMs and in turn secrete VEGF to allow tumor cell extravasation. Macrophages also promote tumor cell survival via α4 integrin signaling to VCAM-1 on tumors cells. Tumor-derived factors generate a premetastatic niche, characterized by the recruitment and activation of myeloid cells in response to S100A8 and S100A9 chemokines and SAA3 inflammatory mediator. Myeloid cells are trapped in areas of crosslinked collagen. Increased presence of NETs at the secondary site promotes extravasation and cancer metastasis and can also lead to re-awakening of dormant cells to aggressive metastatic outgrowth. Furthermore, tumor-derived factors induce the secretion of fibronectin in fibroblasts, promoting the recruitment of HPCs via VLA-4. Recruited myeloid progenitor cells induce mesenchymal-to-epithelial transition (MET) via their secretion of versican, promoting metastatic outgrowth. Moreover, macrophages and neutrophils secrete angiogenic factors, and neutrophil serine proteases NE and CG degrade the antiangiogenic factor Tsp-1, enhancing metastatic outgrowth. Finally, recruited EPCs incorporate into the nascent tumor vasculature, and secrete angiogenic factors, inducing the angiogenic switch and contributing to macrometastasis formation.

Abbreviations: Arg1, arginase 1; BM, bone marrow; Bv8, *Bombina variegata* peptide 8; CCL2, chemokine (C-C motif) ligand 2; CCL5, chemokine (C-C motif) ligand 5; CG, cathepsin G; CSC, cancer stem cell; CSF1, colony-stimulating factor 1; ECM, extracellular matrix; EGF, epidermal growth factor; EPC, endothelial progenitor cell; HPC, hematopoietic progenitor cell; ICAM-1, intercellular adhesion molecule-1; IDO, indoleamine 2,3-dioxygenase; IL-8, interleukin-8; IL-10, interleukin-10; MAM, metastasis-associated macrophage; MDSC, myeloid-derived suppressor cell; MMP, matrix metalloprotease; NE, neutrophil elastase; NET, neutrophil extracellular trap; NK, natural killer; PDGF, platelet-derived growth factor; S100A8, S100 calcium binding protein A8; S100A9, S100 calcium binding protein A9; SAA3, serum amyloid A3; TAM, tumor-associated macrophage; TAN, tumor-associated neutrophil; TGFβ, transforming growth factor beta; TMEM, tumor microenvironment of metastasis; T_{Reg}, regulatory T cell; Tsp-1, thrombospondin-1; VCAM-1, vascular cell adhesion molecule-1; VEGF, vascular endothelial growth factor; VLA-4, very late antigen-4; WNT7b, wingless-type MMTV integration site family member 7b

References

1. Murdoch C, et al. The role of myeloid cells in the promotion of tumour angiogenesis. Nat Rev Cancer. 2008;8(8):618–31.
2. Gao D, Mittal V. The role of bone-marrow-derived cells in tumor growth, metastasis initiation and progression. Trends Mol Med. 2009;15(8):333–43.
3. Joyce JA, Pollard JW. Microenvironmental regulation of metastasis. Nat Rev Cancer. 2009;9(4):239–52.
4. Hanahan D, Coussens LM. Accessories to the crime: functions of cells recruited to the tumor microenvironment. Cancer Cell. 2012;21(3):309–22.
5. Adams GB, et al. Stem cell engraftment at the endosteal niche is specified by the calcium-sensing receptor. Nature. 2006;439(7076):599–603.
6. Arai F, et al. Tie2/angiopoietin-1 signaling regulates hematopoietic stem cell quiescence in the bone marrow niche. Cell. 2004;118(2):149–61.
7. Hattori K, Heissig B, Rafii S. The regulation of hematopoietic stem cell and progenitor mobilization by chemokine SDF-1. Leuk Lymphoma. 2003;44(4):575–82.
8. Nilsson SK, et al. Osteopontin, a key component of the hematopoietic stem cell niche and regulator of primitive hematopoietic progenitor cells. Blood. 2005;106(4):1232–9.
9. Kollet O, et al. Osteoclasts degrade endosteal components and promote mobilization of hematopoietic progenitor cells. Nat Med. 2006;12(6):657–64.
10. Takafuji V, et al. An osteopontin fragment is essential for tumor cell invasion in hepatocellular carcinoma. Oncogene. 2007;26(44):6361–71.
11. McQuibban GA, et al. Matrix metalloproteinase activity inactivates the CXC chemokine stromal cell-derived factor-1. J Biol Chem. 2001;276(47):43503–8.
12. Chantrain CF, et al. Bone marrow microenvironment and tumor progression. Cancer Microenviron. 2008;1(1):23–35.
13. Petit I, et al. G-CSF induces stem cell mobilization by decreasing bone marrow SDF-1 and up-regulating CXCR4. Nat Immunol. 2002;3(7):687–94.
14. Allavena P, et al. The inflammatory micro-environment in tumor progression: the role of tumor-associated macrophages. Crit Rev Oncol Hematol. 2008;66(1):1–9.
15. Fujimoto H, et al. Stromal MCP-1 in mammary tumors induces tumor-associated macrophage infiltration and contributes to tumor progression. Int J Cancer. 2009;125(6):1276–84.
16. Priceman SJ, et al. Targeting distinct tumor-infiltrating myeloid cells by inhibiting CSF-1 receptor: combating tumor evasion of antiangiogenic therapy. Blood. 2010;115(7):1461–71.
17. Gao F, et al. Role of inflammation-associated microenvironment in tumorigenesis and metastasis. Curr Cancer Drug Targets. 2014;14(1):30–45.
18. Du R, et al. HIF1alpha induces the recruitment of bone marrow-derived vascular modulatory cells to regulate tumor angiogenesis and invasion. Cancer Cell. 2008;13(3):206–20.
19. Tacconi C, et al. Activation of the VEGFC/VEGFR3 pathway induces tumor immune escape in colorectal cancer. Cancer Res. 2019;79(16):4196–210.
20. Noy R, Pollard JW. Tumor-associated macrophages: from mechanisms to therapy. Immunity. 2014;41(1):49–61.
21. Steidl C, et al. Tumor-associated macrophages and survival in classic Hodgkin's lymphoma. N Engl J Med. 2010;362(10):875–85.
22. DeNardo DG, et al. Leukocyte complexity predicts breast cancer survival and functionally regulates response to chemotherapy. Cancer Discov. 2011;1(1):54–67.
23. Chung FT, et al. Tumor-associated macrophages correlate with response to epidermal growth factor receptor-tyrosine kinase inhibitors in advanced non-small cell lung cancer. Int J Cancer. 2012;131(3):E227–35.
24. Song M, et al. Tumor derived UBR5 promotes ovarian cancer growth and metastasis through inducing immunosuppressive macrophages. Nat Commun. 2020;11(1):6298.
25. Ganster RW, et al. Complex regulation of human inducible nitric oxide synthase gene transcription by Stat 1 and NF-kappa B. Proc Natl Acad Sci U S A. 2001;98(15):8638–43.
26. Krausgruber T, et al. IRF5 promotes inflammatory macrophage polarization and TH1-TH17 responses. Nat Immunol. 2011;12(3):231–8.
27. Quatromoni JG, Eruslanov E. Tumor-associated macrophages: function, phenotype, and link to prognosis in human lung cancer. Am J Transl Res. 2012;4(4):376–89.
28. Redente EF, et al. Tumor progression stage and anatomical site regulate tumor-associated macrophage and bone marrow-derived monocyte polarization. Am J Pathol. 2010;176(6):2972–85.
29. Biswas SK, et al. A distinct and unique transcriptional program expressed by tumor-associated macrophages (defective NF-kappaB and enhanced IRF-3/STAT1 activation). Blood. 2006;107(5):2112–22.
30. Wanderley CW, et al. Paclitaxel reduces tumor growth by reprogramming tumor-associated macrophages to an M1 profile in a TLR4-dependent manner. Cancer Res. 2018;78(20):5891–900.
31. Roumenina LT, et al. Tumor cells hijack macrophage-produced complement C1q to promote tumor growth. Cancer Immunol Res. 2019;7(7):1091–105.
32. Joyce JA, et al. Cathepsin cysteine proteases are effectors of invasive growth and angiogenesis during multistage tumorigenesis. Cancer Cell. 2004;5(5):443–53.
33. Gocheva V, et al. Distinct roles for cysteine cathepsin genes in multistage tumorigenesis. Genes Dev. 2006;20(5):543–56.
34. Gocheva V, et al. IL-4 induces cathepsin protease activity in tumor-associated macrophages to promote cancer growth and invasion. Genes Dev. 2010;24(3):241–55.
35. Lin EY, et al. Colony-stimulating factor 1 promotes progression of mammary tumors to malignancy. J Exp Med. 2001;193(6):727–40.

36. Lin EY, et al. Macrophages regulate the angiogenic switch in a mouse model of breast cancer. Cancer Res. 2006;66(23):11238–46.

37. Lin EY, Pollard JW. Tumor-associated macrophages press the angiogenic switch in breast cancer. Cancer Res. 2007;67(11):5064–6.

38. Zabuawala T, et al. An ets2-driven transcriptional program in tumor-associated macrophages promotes tumor metastasis. Cancer Res. 2010;70(4):1323–33.

39. Yeo EJ, et al. Myeloid WNT7b mediates the angiogenic switch and metastasis in breast cancer. Cancer Res. 2014;74(11):2962–73.

40. Mazzieri R, et al. Targeting the ANG2/TIE2 axis inhibits tumor growth and metastasis by impairing angiogenesis and disabling rebounds of proangiogenic myeloid cells. Cancer Cell. 2011;19(4):512–26.

41. Wang R, et al. Tumor cells induce LAMP2a expression in tumor-associated macrophage for cancer progression. EBioMedicine. 2019;40:118–34.

42. Kolb R, et al. Obesity-associated inflammation promotes angiogenesis and breast cancer via angiopoietin-like 4. Oncogene. 2019;38(13):2351–63.

43. Jing W, et al. Breast cancer cells promote CD169(+) macrophage-associated immunosuppression through JAK2-mediated PD-L1 upregulation on macrophages. Int Immunopharmacol. 2020;78:106012.

44. Binnemars-Postma K, et al. Targeting the Stat6 pathway in tumor-associated macrophages reduces tumor growth and metastatic niche formation in breast cancer. FASEB J. 2018;32(2):969–78.

45. Muller S, et al. Single-cell profiling of human gliomas reveals macrophage ontogeny as a basis for regional differences in macrophage activation in the tumor microenvironment. Genome Biol. 2017;18(1):234.

46. DeNardo DG, et al. CD4(+) T cells regulate pulmonary metastasis of mammary carcinomas by enhancing protumor properties of macrophages. Cancer Cell. 2009;16(2):91–102.

47. Chong H, et al. Immunocytochemical localization of latent transforming growth factor-beta1 activation by stimulated macrophages. J Cell Physiol. 1999;178(3):275–83.

48. Thomas DA, Massague J. TGF-beta directly targets cytotoxic T cell functions during tumor evasion of immune surveillance. Cancer Cell. 2005;8(5):369–80.

49. Kuang DM, et al. Activated monocytes in peritumoral stroma of hepatocellular carcinoma foster immune privilege and disease progression through PD-L1. J Exp Med. 2009;206(6):1327–37.

50. Rodriguez PC, et al. Arginase I production in the tumor microenvironment by mature myeloid cells inhibits T-cell receptor expression and antigen-specific T-cell responses. Cancer Res. 2004;64(16):5839–49.

51. Liu L, et al. Consumption of the fish oil high-fat diet uncouples obesity and mammary tumor growth through induction of reactive oxygen species in protumor macrophages. Cancer Res. 2020;80(12):2564–74.

52. Cassetta L, et al. Human tumor-associated macrophage and monocyte transcriptional landscapes reveal cancer-specific reprogramming, biomarkers, and therapeutic targets. Cancer Cell. 2019;35(4):588–602 e10.

53. Zhu Y, et al. CSF1/CSF1R blockade reprograms tumor-infiltrating macrophages and improves response to T-cell checkpoint immunotherapy in pancreatic cancer models. Cancer Res. 2014;74(18):5057–69.

54. Su S, et al. CD10(+)GPR77(+) cancer-associated fibroblasts promote cancer formation and chemoresistance by sustaining cancer stemness. Cell. 2018;172(4):841–856 e16.

55. Zhou Y, et al. Single-cell multiomics sequencing reveals prevalent genomic alterations in tumor stromal cells of human colorectal cancer. Cancer Cell. 2020;38(6):818–828 e5.

56. Kumar V, et al. Cancer-associated fibroblasts neutralize the anti-tumor effect of CSF1 receptor blockade by inducing PMN-MDSC infiltration of tumors. Cancer Cell. 2017;32(5):654–668 e5.

57. Vennin C, et al. CAF hierarchy driven by pancreatic cancer cell p53-status creates a pro-metastatic and chemoresistant environment via perlecan. Nat Commun. 2019;10(1):3637.

58. Ostrand-Rosenberg S. Immune surveillance: a balance between protumor and antitumor immunity. Curr Opin Genet Dev. 2008;18(1):11–8.

59. Gabrilovich DI, Nagaraj S. Myeloid-derived suppressor cells as regulators of the immune system. Nat Rev Immunol. 2009;9(3):162–74.

60. Sinha P, et al. Proinflammatory S100 proteins regulate the accumulation of myeloid-derived suppressor cells. J Immunol. 2008;181(7):4666–75.

61. Marigo I, et al. Tumor-induced tolerance and immune suppression by myeloid derived suppressor cells. Immunol Rev. 2008;222:162–79.

62. Yu J, et al. Myeloid-derived suppressor cells suppress antitumor immune responses through IDO expression and correlate with lymph node metastasis in patients with breast cancer. J Immunol. 2013;190(7):3783–97.

63. Grohmann U, Fallarino F, Puccetti P. Tolerance, DCs and tryptophan: much ado about IDO. Trends Immunol. 2003;24(5):242–8.

64. Yu J, et al. Noncanonical NF-kappaB activation mediates STAT3-stimulated IDO upregulation in myeloid-derived suppressor cells in breast cancer. J Immunol. 2014;193(5):2574–86.

65. Holmgaard RB, et al. Tumor-expressed IDO recruits and activates MDSCs in a Treg-dependent manner. Cell Rep. 2015;13(2):412–24.

66. Das S, et al. Tumor cell-derived IL1beta promotes desmoplasia and immune suppression in pancreatic cancer. Cancer Res. 2020;80(5):1088–101.

67. Chen Y, et al. Type I collagen deletion in alphaSMA(+) myofibroblasts augments immune suppression and accelerates progression of pancreatic cancer. Cancer Cell. 2021;39(4):548–565 e6.

68. Trillo-Tinoco J, et al. AMPK alpha-1 intrinsically regulates the function and differentiation of tumor myeloid-derived suppressor cells. Cancer Res. 2019;79(19):5034–47.

69. Klemm F, et al. Interrogation of the microenvironmental landscape in brain tumors reveals disease-specific alterations of immune cells. Cell. 2020;181(7):1643–1660 e17.

70. Chang CH, et al. Metabolic competition in the tumor microenvironment is a driver of cancer progression. Cell. 2015;162(6):1229–41.

71. Kaymak I, et al. Immunometabolic interplay in the tumor microenvironment. Cancer Cell. 2021;39(1):28–37.

72. Pekarek LA, et al. Inhibition of tumor growth by elimination of granulocytes. J Exp Med. 1995;181(1):435–40.

73. Shojaei F, et al. Role of Bv8 in neutrophil-dependent angiogenesis in a transgenic model of cancer progression. Proc Natl Acad Sci U S A. 2008;105(7):2640–5.

74. Youn JI, et al. Subsets of myeloid-derived suppressor cells in tumor-bearing mice. J Immunol. 2008;181(8):5791–802.

75. Shojaei F, et al. Tumor refractoriness to anti-VEGF treatment is mediated by CD11b+Gr1+ myeloid cells. Nat Biotechnol. 2007;25(8):911–20.

76. Shojaei F, et al. Bv8 regulates myeloid-cell-dependent tumour angiogenesis. Nature. 2007;450(7171):825–31.

77. Yang L, et al. Expansion of myeloid immune suppressor Gr+CD11b+ cells in tumor-bearing host directly promotes tumor angiogenesis. Cancer Cell. 2004;6(4):409–21.

78. Fridlender ZG, et al. Polarization of tumor-associated neutrophil phenotype by TGF-beta: "N1" versus "N2" TAN. Cancer Cell. 2009;16(3):183–94.

79. Perego M, et al. Reactivation of dormant tumor cells by modified lipids derived from stress-activated neutrophils. Sci Transl Med. 2020;12(572)

80. Wculek SK, et al. Dendritic cells in cancer immunology and immunotherapy. Nat Rev Immunol. 2020;20(1):7–24.

81. Ma Y, et al. Dendritic cells in the cancer microenvironment. J Cancer. 2013;4(1):36–44.

82. Ray A, et al. Preclinical validation of Alpha-Enolase (ENO1) as a novel immunometabolic target in multiple myeloma. Oncogene. 2020;39(13):2786–96.

83. Cubillos-Ruiz JR, et al. ER stress sensor XBP1 controls antitumor immunity by disrupting dendritic cell homeostasis. Cell. 2015;161(7):1527–38.

84. Laoui D, et al. The tumour microenvironment harbours ontogenically distinct dendritic cell populations with opposing effects on tumour immunity. Nat Commun. 2016;7:13720.

85. Lyden D, et al. Impaired recruitment of bone-marrow-derived endothelial and hematopoietic precursor cells blocks tumor angiogenesis and growth. Nat Med. 2001;7(11):1194–201.

86. Peters BA, et al. Contribution of bone marrow-derived endothelial cells to human tumor vasculature. Nat Med. 2005;11(3):261–2.

87. Nolan DJ, et al. Bone marrow-derived endothelial progenitor cells are a major determinant of nascent tumor neovascularization. Genes Dev. 2007;21(12):1546–58.

88. Gao D, et al. Bone marrow-derived endothelial progenitor cells contribute to the angiogenic switch in tumor growth and metastatic progression. Biochim Biophys Acta. 2009;1796(1):33–40.

89. Kerbel RS, et al. Endothelial progenitor cells are cellular hubs essential for neoangiogenesis of certain aggressive adenocarcinomas and metastatic transition but not adenomas. Proc Natl Acad Sci U S A. 2008;105(34):E54. author reply E55

90. Gao D, et al. Endothelial progenitor cells control the angiogenic switch in mouse lung metastasis. Science. 2008;319(5860):195–8.

91. Mellick AS, et al. Using the transcription factor inhibitor of DNA binding 1 to selectively target endothelial progenitor cells offers novel strategies to inhibit tumor angiogenesis and growth. Cancer Res. 2010;70(18):7273–82.

92. Shaked Y, et al. Therapy-induced acute recruitment of circulating endothelial progenitor cells to tumors. Science. 2006;313(5794):1785–7.

93. Shaked Y, et al. Rapid chemotherapy-induced acute endothelial progenitor cell mobilization: implications for antiangiogenic drugs as chemosensitizing agents. Cancer Cell. 2008;14(3):263–73.

94. Purhonen S, et al. Bone marrow-derived circulating endothelial precursors do not contribute to vascular endothelium and are not needed for tumor growth. Proc Natl Acad Sci U S A. 2008;105(18):6620–5.

95. Burchfield JS, Dimmeler S. Role of paracrine factors in stem and progenitor cell mediated cardiac repair and tissue fibrosis. Fibrogenesis Tissue Repair. 2008;1(1):4.

96. Stockmann C, et al. Deletion of vascular endothelial growth factor in myeloid cells accelerates tumorigenesis. Nature. 2008;456(7223):814–8.

97. Lee S, et al. Autocrine VEGF signaling is required for vascular homeostasis. Cell. 2007;130(4):691–703.

98. Direkze NC, et al. Multiple organ engraftment by bone-marrow-derived myofibroblasts and fibroblasts in bone-marrow-transplanted mice. Stem Cells. 2003;21(5):514–20.

99. Direkze NC, et al. Bone marrow contribution to tumor-associated myofibroblasts and fibroblasts. Cancer Res. 2004;64(23):8492–5.

100. Vong S, Kalluri R. The role of stromal myofibroblast and extracellular matrix in tumor angiogenesis. Genes Cancer. 2011;2(12):1139–45.

101. Rajantie I, et al. Adult bone marrow-derived cells recruited during angiogenesis comprise precursors for periendothelial vascular mural cells. Blood. 2004;104(7):2084–6.

102. Song S, et al. PDGFRbeta+ perivascular progenitor cells in tumours regulate pericyte differentiation and vascular survival. Nat Cell Biol. 2005;7(9):870–9.

103. Jodele S, et al. The contribution of bone marrow-derived cells to the tumor vasculature in neuroblastoma is matrix metalloproteinase-9 dependent. Cancer Res. 2005;65(8):3200–8.

104. Lamagna C, Bergers G. The bone marrow constitutes a reservoir of pericyte progenitors. J Leukoc Biol. 2006;80(4):677–81.

105. Wyckoff J, et al. A paracrine loop between tumor cells and macrophages is required for tumor cell migration in mammary tumors. Cancer Res. 2004;64(19):7022–9.

106. Goswami S, et al. Macrophages promote the invasion of breast carcinoma cells via a colony-stimulating factor-1/epidermal growth factor paracrine loop. Cancer Res. 2005;65(12):5278–83.

107. Ishihara D, et al. Wiskott-Aldrich syndrome protein regulates leukocyte-dependent breast cancer metastasis. Cell Rep. 2013;4(3):429–36.

108. Hernandez L, et al. The EGF/CSF-1 paracrine invasion loop can be triggered by heregulin beta1 and CXCL12. Cancer Res. 2009;69(7):3221–7.

109. Linde N, et al. Macrophages orchestrate breast cancer early dissemination and metastasis. Nat Commun. 2018;9(1):21.

110. Gertler F, Condeelis J. Metastasis: tumor cells becoming MENAcing. Trends Cell Biol. 2011;21(2):81–90.

111. Roussos ET, et al. Mena invasive (MenaINV) promotes multicellular streaming motility and transendothelial migration in a mouse model of breast cancer. J Cell Sci. 2011;124(Pt 13):2120–31.

112. Harney AS, et al. Real-time imaging reveals local, transient vascular permeability, and tumor cell intravasation stimulated by TIE2hi macrophage-derived VEGFA. Cancer Discov. 2015;5(9):932–43.

113. Wyckoff JB, et al. Direct visualization of macrophage-assisted tumor cell intravasation in mammary tumors. Cancer Res. 2007;67(6):2649–56.

114. Roh-Johnson M, et al. Macrophage contact induces RhoA GTPase signaling to trigger tumor cell intravasation. Oncogene. 2014;33(33):4203–12.

115. Liu CY, et al. M2-polarized tumor-associated macrophages promoted epithelial-mesenchymal transition in pancreatic cancer cells, partially through TLR4/IL-10 signaling pathway. Lab Invest. 2013;93(7):844–54.

116. Georgouli M, et al. Regional activation of myosin II in cancer cells drives tumor progression via a secretory cross-talk with the immune microenvironment. Cell. 2019;176(4):757–774 e23.

117. Marigo I, et al. Disabled homolog 2 controls prometastatic activity of tumor-associated macrophages. Cancer Discov. 2020;10(11):1758–73.

118. Yang F, et al. Interaction with CD68 and regulation of GAS6 expression by endosialin in fibroblasts drives recruitment and polarization of macrophages in hepatocellular carcinoma. Cancer Res. 2020;80(18):3892–905.

119. Bekes EM, et al. Tumor-recruited neutrophils and neutrophil TIMP-free MMP-9 regulate coordinately the levels of tumor angiogenesis and efficiency of malignant cell intravasation. Am J Pathol. 2011;179(3):1455–70.

120. Zhou SL, et al. CXCL5 contributes to tumor metastasis and recurrence of intrahepatic cholangiocarcinoma by recruiting infiltrative intratumoral neutrophils. Carcinogenesis. 2014;35(3):597–605.

121. Sharma B, et al. Host Cxcr2-dependent regulation of mammary tumor growth and metastasis. Clin Exp Metastasis. 2015;32(1):65–72.

122. Yang L, et al. Abrogation of TGF beta signaling in mammary carcinomas recruits Gr-1+CD11b+ myeloid cells that promote metastasis. Cancer Cell. 2008;13(1):23–35.

123. Kitamura T, et al. SMAD4-deficient intestinal tumors recruit CCR1+ myeloid cells that promote invasion. Nat Genet. 2007;39(4):467–75.

124. Ogawa R, et al. Loss of SMAD4 promotes colorectal cancer progression by recruiting tumor-associated neutrophils via the CXCL1/8-CXCR2 axis. Clin Cancer Res. 2019;25(9):2887–99.

125. Karnoub AE, et al. Mesenchymal stem cells within tumour stroma promote breast cancer metastasis. Nature. 2007;449(7162):557–63.

126. Ma Z, et al. Bone Marrow mesenchymal stromal cell-derived periostin promotes B-ALL progression by modulating CCL2 in leukemia cells. Cell Rep. 2019;26(6):1533–1543 e4.

127. Lecomte J, et al. Bone marrow-derived myofibroblasts are the providers of pro-invasive matrix metalloproteinase 13 in primary tumor. Neoplasia. 2012;14(10):943–51.

128. Maheswaran S, Haber DA. Circulating tumor cells: a window into cancer biology and metastasis. Curr Opin Genet Dev. 2010;20(1):96–9.

129. Reymond N, d'Agua BB, Ridley AJ. Crossing the endothelial barrier during metastasis. Nat Rev Cancer. 2013;13(12):858–70.

130. Palumbo JS, et al. Platelets and fibrin(ogen) increase metastatic potential by impeding natural killer cell-mediated elimination of tumor cells. Blood. 2005;105(1):178–85.

131. Palumbo JS, et al. Tumor cell-associated tissue factor and circulating hemostatic factors cooperate to increase metastatic potential through natural killer cell-dependent and-independent mechanisms. Blood. 2007;110(1):133–41.

132. Camerer E, et al. Platelets, protease-activated receptors, and fibrinogen in hematogenous metastasis. Blood. 2004;104(2):397–401.

133. Labelle M, Begum S, Hynes RO. Direct signaling between platelets and cancer cells induces an epithelial-mesenchymal-like transition and promotes metastasis. Cancer Cell. 2011;20(5):576–90.

134. Zhang Y, et al. Platelet-specific PDGFB ablation impairs tumor vessel integrity and promotes metastasis. Cancer Res. 2020;80(16):3345–58.

135. Ferjancic S, et al. VCAM-1 and VAP-1 recruit myeloid cells that promote pulmonary metastasis in mice. Blood. 2013;121(16):3289–97.

136. Chen Q, Zhang XH, Massague J. Macrophage binding to receptor VCAM-1 transmits survival signals in breast cancer cells that invade the lungs. Cancer Cell. 2011;20(4):538–49.

137. Wei C, et al. Crosstalk between cancer cells and tumor associated macrophages is required for mesenchymal circulating tumor cell-mediated colorectal cancer metastasis. Mol Cancer. 2019;18(1):64.

138. Sanchez-Gonzalez I, et al. miR-149 suppresses breast cancer metastasis by blocking paracrine interactions with macrophages. Cancer Res. 2020;80(6):1330–41.

139. Viguier M, et al. Foxp3 expressing CD4+CD25(high) regulatory T cells are overrepresented in human metastatic melanoma lymph nodes and inhibit the function of infiltrating T cells. J Immunol. 2004;173(2):1444–53.

140. Curiel TJ, et al. Specific recruitment of regulatory T cells in ovarian carcinoma fosters immune privilege and predicts reduced survival. Nat Med. 2004;10(9):942–9.

141. You Y, et al. Ovarian cancer stem cells promote tumour immune privilege and invasion via CCL5 and regulatory T cells. Clin Exp Immunol. 2018;191(1):60–73.

142. Lee JC, et al. Regulatory T cell control of systemic immunity and immunotherapy response in liver metastasis. Sci Immunol. 2020;5(52)

143. Huh SJ, et al. Transiently entrapped circulating tumor cells interact with neutrophils to facilitate lung metastasis development. Cancer Res. 2010;70(14):6071–82.

144. Spicer JD, et al. Neutrophils promote liver metastasis via Mac-1-mediated interactions with circulating tumor cells. Cancer Res. 2012;72(16):3919–27.

145. Cools-Lartigue J, et al. Neutrophil extracellular traps sequester circulating tumor cells and promote metastasis. J Clin Invest. 2013;123(8):3446–58.

146. Rayes RF, et al. Primary tumors induce neutrophil extracellular traps with targetable metastasis promoting effects. JCI Insight. 2019;5

147. Szczerba BM, et al. Neutrophils escort circulating tumour cells to enable cell cycle progression. Nature. 2019;566(7745):553–7.

148. Coupland LA, Chong BH, Parish CR. Platelets and P-selectin control tumor cell metastasis in an organ-specific manner and independently of NK cells. Cancer Res. 2012;72(18):4662–71.

149. Irimura T, et al. Colorectal cancer metastasis determined by carbohydrate-mediated cell adhesion: role of sialyl-LeX antigens. Semin Cancer Biol. 1993;4(5):319–24.

150. Insug O, et al. Role of SA-Le(a) and E-selectin in metastasis assessed with peptide antagonist. Peptides. 2002;23(5):999–1010.

151. Zipin A, et al. Tumor-microenvironment interactions: the fucose-generating FX enzyme controls adhesive properties of colorectal cancer cells. Cancer Res. 2004;64(18):6571–8.

152. Qian B, et al. A distinct macrophage population mediates metastatic breast cancer cell extravasation, establishment and growth. PLoS One. 2009;4(8):e6562.

153. Qian BZ, et al. CCL2 recruits inflammatory monocytes to facilitate breast-tumour metastasis. Nature. 2011;475(7355):222–5.

154. Zhao L, et al. Recruitment of a myeloid cell subset (CD11b/Gr1 mid) via CCL2/CCR2 promotes the development of colorectal cancer liver metastasis. Hepatology. 2013;57(2):829–39.

155. Ward Y, et al. Platelets promote metastasis via binding tumor CD97 leading to bidirectional signaling that coordinates transendothelial migration. Cell Rep. 2018;23(3):808–22.

156. Mammadova-Bach E, et al. Platelet glycoprotein VI promotes metastasis through interaction with cancer cell-derived galectin-3. Blood. 2020;135(14):1146–60.

157. Xiong G, et al. Hsp47 promotes cancer metastasis by enhancing collagen-dependent cancer cell-platelet interaction. Proc Natl Acad Sci U S A. 2020;117(7):3748–58.

158. Peinado H, et al. Pre-metastatic niches: organ-specific homes for metastases. Nat Rev Cancer. 2017;17(5):302–17.

159. Fidler IJ. The pathogenesis of cancer metastasis: the 'seed and soil' hypothesis revisited. Nat Rev Cancer. 2003;3(6):453–8.

160. Psaila B, Lyden D. The metastatic niche: adapting the foreign soil. Nat Rev Cancer. 2009;9(4):285–93.

161. Kaplan RN, et al. VEGFR1-positive haematopoietic bone marrow progenitors initiate the pre-metastatic niche. Nature. 2005;438(7069):820–7.

162. Hiratsuka S, et al. Tumour-mediated upregulation of chemoattractants and recruitment of myeloid cells predetermines lung metastasis. Nat Cell Biol. 2006;8(12):1369–75.

163. Hiratsuka S, et al. The S100A8-serum amyloid A3-TLR4 paracrine cascade establishes a pre-metastatic phase. Nat Cell Biol. 2008;10(11):1349–55.

164. Hiratsuka S, et al. Primary tumours modulate innate immune signalling to create pre-metastatic vascular hyperpermeability foci. Nat Commun. 2013;4:1853.

165. Qiu M, et al. Modulation of intestinal microbiota by glycyrrhizic acid prevents high-fat diet-enhanced pre-metastatic niche formation and metastasis. Mucosal Immunol. 2019;12(4):945–57.

166. Hiratsuka S, et al. MMP9 induction by vascular endothelial growth factor receptor-1 is involved in lung-specific metastasis. Cancer Cell. 2002;2(4):289–300.

167. Bergers G, et al. Matrix metalloproteinase-9 triggers the angiogenic switch during carcinogenesis. Nat Cell Biol. 2000;2(10):737–44.

168. Heissig B, et al. Recruitment of stem and progenitor cells from the bone marrow niche requires MMP-9 mediated release of kit-ligand. Cell. 2002;109(5):625–37.

169. Aksenenko MB, et al. miR-155 overexpression is followed by downregulation of its target gene, NFE2L2, and altered pattern of VEGFA expression in the liver of melanoma B16-bearing mice at the premetastatic stage. Int J Exp Pathol. 2019;100(5-6):311–9.

170. Li R, et al. Primary tumor-secreted VEGF induces vascular hyperpermeability in premetastatic lung via the occludin phosphorylation/ubiquitination pathway. Mol Carcinog. 2019;58(12):2316–26.

171. Yang F, et al. Inhibition of dipeptidyl peptidase-4 accelerates epithelial-mesenchymal transition and breast cancer metastasis via the CXCL12/CXCR4/mTOR axis. Cancer Res. 2019;79(4):735–46.

172. Sceneay J, et al. Primary tumor hypoxia recruits CD11b+/Ly6Cmed/Ly6G+ immune suppressor cells and compromises NK cell cytotoxicity in the premetastatic niche. Cancer Res. 2012;72(16):3906–11.

173. Lu Z, et al. Epigenetic therapy inhibits metastases by disrupting premetastatic niches. Nature. 2020;579(7798):284–90.

174. Chen H, et al. Chronic psychological stress promotes lung metastatic colonization of circulating breast cancer cells by decorating a pre-metastatic niche through activating beta-adrenergic signaling. J Pathol. 2018;244(1):49–60.

175. Kaczanowska S, et al. Genetically engineered myeloid cells rebalance the core immune suppression program in metastasis. Cell. 2021;184(8):2033–2052 e21.

176. Erler JT, et al. Hypoxia-induced lysyl oxidase is a critical mediator of bone marrow cell recruitment to form the premetastatic niche. Cancer Cell. 2009;15(1):35–44.

177. Cox TR, et al. LOX-mediated collagen crosslinking is responsible for fibrosis-enhanced metastasis. Cancer Res. 2013;73(6):1721–32.

178. Cox TR, Erler JT. Molecular pathways: connecting fibrosis and solid tumor metastasis. Clin Cancer Res. 2014;20(14):3637–43.

179. Cox TR, et al. The hypoxic cancer secretome induces pre-metastatic bone lesions through lysyl oxidase. Nature. 2015;522(7554):106–10.

180. Said N, et al. RhoGDI2 suppresses lung metastasis in mice by reducing tumor versican expression and macrophage infiltration. J Clin Invest. 2012;122(4):1503–18.

181. Salem M, et al. miR-590-3p promotes ovarian cancer growth and metastasis via a novel FOXA2-versican pathway. Cancer Res. 2018;78(15):4175–90.

182. Zhangyuan G, et al. VersicanV1 promotes proliferation and metastasis of hepatocellular carcinoma through the activation of EGFR-PI3K-AKT pathway. Oncogene. 2020;39(6):1213–30.

183. van Deventer HW, et al. Circulating fibrocytes prepare the lung for cancer metastasis by recruiting Ly-6C+ monocytes via CCL2. J Immunol. 2013;190(9):4861–7.

184. Gil-Bernabe AM, et al. Recruitment of monocytes/macrophages by tissue factor-mediated coagulation is essential for metastatic cell survival and premetastatic niche establishment in mice. Blood. 2012;119(13):3164–75.

185. Catena R, et al. Bone marrow-derived Gr1+ cells can generate a metastasis-resistant microenvironment via induced secretion of thrombospondin-1. Cancer Discov. 2013;3(5):578–89.

186. Keklikoglou I, et al. Chemotherapy elicits pro-metastatic extracellular vesicles in breast cancer models. Nat Cell Biol. 2019;21(2):190–202.

187. Kowanetz M, et al. Granulocyte-colony stimulating factor promotes lung metastasis through mobilization of Ly6G+Ly6C+ granulocytes. Proc Natl Acad Sci U S A. 2010;107(50):21248–55.

188. Granot Z, et al. Tumor entrained neutrophils inhibit seeding in the premetastatic lung. Cancer Cell. 2011;20(3):300–14.

189. Wang Z, et al. CD62L(dim) neutrophils specifically migrate to the lung and participate in the formation of the pre-metastatic niche of breast cancer. Front Oncol. 2020;10:540484.

190. Patel S, et al. Unique pattern of neutrophil migration and function during tumor progression. Nat Immunol. 2018;19(11):1236–47.

191. Charan M, et al. Tumor secreted ANGPTL2 facilitates recruitment of neutrophils to the lung to promote lung pre-metastatic niche formation and targeting ANGPTL2 signaling affects metastatic disease. Oncotarget. 2020;11(5):510–22.

192. Moresco MA, et al. Enzymatic inactivation of oxysterols in breast tumor cells constraints metastasis formation by reprogramming the metastatic lung microenvironment. Front Immunol. 2018;9:2251.

193. Tyagi A, et al. Nicotine promotes breast cancer metastasis by stimulating N2 neutrophils and generating pre-metastatic niche in lung. Nat Commun. 2021;12(1):474.

194. Monteiro AC, et al. T cells induce pre-metastatic osteolytic disease and help bone metastases establishment in a mouse model of metastatic breast cancer. PLoS One. 2013;8(7):e68171.

195. Olkhanud PB, et al. Breast cancer lung metastasis requires expression of chemokine receptor CCR4 and regulatory T cells. Cancer Res. 2009;69(14):5996–6004.

196. Li YL, et al. Single-cell analysis reveals immune modulation and metabolic switch in tumor-draining lymph nodes. Oncoimmunology. 2020;9(1):1830513.

197. McAllister SS, Weinberg RA. The tumour-induced systemic environment as a critical regulator of cancer progression and metastasis. Nat Cell Biol. 2014;16(8):717–27.

198. Peinado H, et al. Melanoma exosomes educate bone marrow progenitor cells toward a pro-metastatic phenotype through MET. Nat Med. 2012;18(6):883–91.

199. Dai J, et al. Primary prostate cancer educates bone stroma through exosomal pyruvate kinase M2 to promote bone metastasis. J Exp Med. 2019;216(12):2883–99.

200. Kang Y, et al. A multigenic program mediating breast cancer metastasis to bone. Cancer Cell. 2003;3(6):537–49.

201. Nguyen DX, Bos PD, Massague J. Metastasis: from dissemination to organ-specific colonization. Nat Rev Cancer. 2009;9(4):274–84.

202. Obenauf AC, Massague J. Surviving at a distance: organ-specific metastasis. Trends Cancer. 2015;1(1):76–91.

203. Muller A, et al. Involvement of chemokine receptors in breast cancer metastasis. Nature. 2001;410(6824):50–6.

204. Li YM, et al. Upregulation of CXCR4 is essential for HER2-mediated tumor metastasis. Cancer Cell. 2004;6(5):459–69.

205. Marchesi F, et al. The chemokine receptor CX3CR1 is involved in the neural tropism and malignant behavior of pancreatic ductal adenocarcinoma. Cancer Res. 2008;68(21):9060–9.

206. Wang H, et al. Tumor cell alpha3beta1 integrin and vascular laminin-5 mediate pulmonary arrest and metastasis. J Cell Biol. 2004;164(6):935–41.

207. Kim S, et al. Carcinoma-produced factors activate myeloid cells through TLR2 to stimulate metastasis. Nature. 2009;457(7225):102–6.

208. Medeiros B, et al. Triple-negative primary breast tumors induce supportive premetastatic changes in the extracellular matrix and soluble components of the lung microenvironment. Cancers (Basel). 2020;12(1)

209. Klotz R, et al. Circulating tumor cells exhibit metastatic tropism and reveal brain metastasis drivers. Cancer Discov. 2020;10(1):86–103.

210. Hebert JD, et al. Proteomic profiling of the ECM of xenograft breast cancer metastases in different organs reveals distinct metastatic niches. Cancer Res. 2020;80(7):1475–85.

211. Martinez-Ordonez A, et al. Breast cancer metastasis to liver and lung is facilitated by Pit-1-CXCL12-CXCR4 axis. Oncogene. 2018;37(11):1430–44.

212. Mundy GR. Metastasis to bone: causes, consequences and therapeutic opportunities. Nat Rev Cancer. 2002;2(8):584–93.

213. Jones DH, et al. Regulation of cancer cell migration and bone metastasis by RANKL. Nature. 2006;440(7084):692–6.

214. Sohara Y, Shimada H, DeClerck YA. Mechanisms of bone invasion and metastasis in human neuroblastoma. Cancer Lett. 2005;228(1-2):203–9.

215. Ara T, et al. Interleukin-6 in the bone marrow microenvironment promotes the growth and survival of neuroblastoma cells. Cancer Res. 2009;69(1):329–37.

216. Hoshino A, et al. Tumour exosome integrins determine organotropic metastasis. Nature. 2015;527(7578):329–35.

217. Mattiola I, et al. The macrophage tetraspan MS4A4A enhances dectin-1-dependent NK cell-mediated resistance to metastasis. Nat Immunol. 2019;20(8):1012–22.

218. El Rayes T, et al. Lung inflammation promotes metastasis through neutrophil protease-mediated degradation of Tsp-1. Proc Natl Acad Sci U S A. 2015;112(52):16000–5.

219. Wculek SK, Malanchi I. Neutrophils support lung colonization of metastasis-initiating breast cancer cells. Nature. 2015;528(7582):413–7.

220. Gao D, et al. Myeloid progenitor cells in the premetastatic lung promote metastases by inducing mesenchymal to epithelial transition. Cancer Res. 2012;72(6):1384–94.

221. Bosiljcic M, et al. Targeting myeloid-derived suppressor cells in combination with primary mammary tumor resection reduces metastatic growth in the lungs. Breast Cancer Res. 2019;21(1):103.

222. Coffelt SB, Wellenstein MD, de Visser KE. Neutrophils in cancer: neutral no more. Nat Rev Cancer. 2016;16(7):431–46.

223. Kos K, de Visser KE. Neutrophils create a fertile soil for metastasis. Cancer Cell. 2021;39(3):301–3.

224. Nemeth T, Sperandio M, Mocsai A. Neutrophils as emerging therapeutic targets. Nat Rev Drug Discov. 2020;19(4):253–75.

225. Quail DF, et al. Obesity alters the lung myeloid cell landscape to enhance breast cancer metastasis through IL5 and GM-CSF. Nat Cell Biol. 2017;19(8):974–87.

226. Xiao Y, et al. Cathepsin C promotes breast cancer lung metastasis by modulating neutrophil infiltration and neutrophil extracellular trap formation. Cancer Cell. 2021;39(3):423–437 e7.

227. Yang L, et al. DNA of neutrophil extracellular traps promotes cancer metastasis via CCDC25. Nature. 2020;583(7814):133–8.

228. Teijeira A, et al. CXCR1 and CXCR2 chemokine receptor agonists produced by tumors induce neutrophil extracellular traps that interfere with immune cytotoxicity. Immunity. 2020;52(5):856–871 e8.

229. Li P, et al. Lung mesenchymal cells elicit lipid storage in neutrophils that fuel breast cancer lung metastasis. Nat Immunol. 2020;21(11):1444–55.

230. McDowell SAC, et al. Neutrophil oxidative stress mediates obesity-associated vascular dysfunction and metastatic transmigration. Nat Cancer. 2021;2:545–62.

231. Albrengues J, et al. Neutrophil extracellular traps produced during inflammation awaken dormant cancer cells in mice. Science. 2018;361(6409)

232. Malanchi I, et al. Interactions between cancer stem cells and their niche govern metastatic colonization. Nature. 2011;481(7379):85–9.

233. Wang Z, Ouyang G. Periostin: a bridge between cancer stem cells and their metastatic niche. Cell Stem Cell. 2012;10(2):111–2.

234. Coutu DL, et al. Periostin, a member of a novel family of vitamin K-dependent proteins, is expressed by mesenchymal stromal cells. J Biol Chem. 2008;283(26):17991–8001.

235. Pelon F, et al. Cancer-associated fibroblast heterogeneity in axillary lymph nodes drives metastases in breast cancer through complementary mechanisms. Nat Commun. 2020;11(1):404.

236. Ghajar CM, et al. The perivascular niche regulates breast tumour dormancy. Nat Cell Biol. 2013;15(7):807–17.

237. Sanford DE, et al. Inflammatory monocyte mobilization decreases patient survival in pancreatic cancer: a role for targeting the CCL2/CCR2 axis. Clin Cancer Res. 2013;19(13):3404–15.

238. Tomita M, et al. Preoperative neutrophil to lymphocyte ratio as a prognostic predictor after curative resection for non-small cell lung cancer. Anticancer Res. 2011;31(9):2995–8.

239. Robinson BD, et al. Tumor microenvironment of metastasis in human breast carcinoma: a potential prognostic marker linked to hematogenous dissemination. Clin Cancer Res. 2009;15(7):2433–41.

240. Rohan TE, et al. Tumor microenvironment of metastasis and risk of distant metastasis of breast cancer. J Natl Cancer Inst. 2014;106(8)

241. Li R, et al. Gut microbiota-stimulated cathepsin K secretion mediates TLR4-dependent M2 macrophage polarization and promotes tumor metastasis in colorectal cancer. Cell Death Differ. 2019;26(11):2447–63.

242. Hoves S, et al. Rapid activation of tumor-associated macrophages boosts preexisting tumor immunity. J Exp Med. 2018;215(3):859–76.

243. Akkari L, et al. Dynamic changes in glioma macrophage populations after radiotherapy reveal CSF-1R inhibition as a strategy to overcome resistance. Sci Transl Med. 2020;12(552)

244. Kowal J, Kornete M, Joyce JA. Re-education of macrophages as a therapeutic strategy in cancer. Immunotherapy. 2019;11(8):677–89.

245. Yan D, et al. Inhibition of colony stimulating factor-1 receptor abrogates microenvironment-mediated therapeutic resistance in gliomas. Oncogene. 2017;36(43):6049–58.

246. Welsh TJ, et al. Macrophage and mast-cell invasion of tumor cell islets confers a marked survival advantage in non-small-cell lung cancer. J Clin Oncol. 2005;23(35):8959–67.

247. Kim DW, et al. High tumour islet macrophage infiltration correlates with improved patient survival but not with EGFR mutations, gene copy number or protein expression in resected non-small cell lung cancer. Br J Cancer. 2008;98(6):1118–24.

248. Dai F, et al. The number and microlocalization of tumor-associated immune cells are associated with patient's survival time in non-small cell lung cancer. BMC Cancer. 2010;10:220.

249. Ohri CM, et al. Macrophages within NSCLC tumour islets are predominantly of a cytotoxic M1 phenotype associated with extended survival. Eur Respir J. 2009;33(1):118–26.

250. Takanami I, Takeuchi K, Kodaira S. Tumor-associated macrophage infiltration in pulmonary adenocarcinoma: association with angiogenesis and poor prognosis. Oncology. 1999;57(2):138–42.

251. Chen JJ, et al. Up-regulation of tumor interleukin-8 expression by infiltrating macrophages: its correlation with tumor angiogenesis and patient survival in non-small cell lung cancer. Clin Cancer Res. 2003;9(2):729–37.

252. Ohtaki Y, et al. Stromal macrophage expressing CD204 is associated with tumor aggressiveness in lung adenocarcinoma. J Thorac Oncol. 2010;5(10):1507–15.

253. Zhang B, et al. M2-polarized tumor-associated macrophages are associated with poor prognoses resulting from accelerated lymphangiogenesis in lung adenocarcinoma. Clinics (Sao Paulo). 2011;66(11):1879–86.

254. Wang R, et al. Increased IL-10 mRNA expression in tumor-associated macrophage correlated with late stage of lung cancer. J Exp Clin Cancer Res. 2011;30:62.

255. Zeni E, et al. Macrophage expression of interleukin-10 is a prognostic factor in nonsmall cell lung cancer. Eur Respir J. 2007;30(4):627–32.

256. Wang R, et al. Tumor-associated macrophages provide a suitable microenvironment for non-small lung cancer invasion and progression. Lung Cancer. 2011;74(2):188–96.

257. Loyher PL, et al. Macrophages of distinct origins contribute to tumor development in the lung. J Exp Med. 2018;215(10):2536–53.

258. Katholnig K, et al. Inactivation of mTORC2 in macrophages is a signature of colorectal cancer that promotes tumorigenesis. JCI Insight. 2019;4(20)

259. Bergamaschi C, et al. Heterodimeric IL-15 delays tumor growth and promotes intratumoral CTL and dendritic cell accumulation

by a cytokine network involving XCL1, IFN-gamma, CXCL9 and CXCL10. J Immunother Cancer. 2020;8(1)

260. Schmittnaegel M, et al. Dual angiopoietin-2 and VEGFA inhibition elicits antitumor immunity that is enhanced by PD-1 checkpoint blockade. Sci Transl Med. 2017;9(385)

261. Nagaraj S, et al. Anti-inflammatory triterpenoid blocks immune suppressive function of MDSCs and improves immune response in cancer. Clin Cancer Res. 2010;16(6):1812–23.

262. Huang A, et al. Increased CD14(+)HLA-DR (-/low) myeloid-derived suppressor cells correlate with extrathoracic metastasis and poor response to chemotherapy in non-small cell lung cancer patients. Cancer Immunol Immunother. 2013;62(9):1439–51.

263. Zhang B, et al. Circulating and tumor-infiltrating myeloid-derived suppressor cells in patients with colorectal carcinoma. PLoS One. 2013;8(2):e57114.

264. Meyer C, et al. Frequencies of circulating MDSC correlate with clinical outcome of melanoma patients treated with ipilimumab. Cancer Immunol Immunother. 2014;63(3):247–57.

265. Raychaudhuri B, et al. Myeloid-derived suppressor cell accumulation and function in patients with newly diagnosed glioblastoma. Neuro Oncol. 2011;13(6):591–9.

266. Friebel E, et al. Single-cell mapping of human brain cancer reveals tumor-specific instruction of tissue-invading leukocytes. Cell. 2020;181(7):1626–1642 e20.

267. Najjar YG, Finke JH. Clinical perspectives on targeting of myeloid derived suppressor cells in the treatment of cancer. Front Oncol. 2013;3:49.

268. Gabrilovich DI, et al. Mechanism of immune dysfunction in cancer mediated by immature Gr-1+ myeloid cells. J Immunol. 2001;166(9):5398–406.

269. Mirza N, et al. All-trans-retinoic acid improves differentiation of myeloid cells and immune response in cancer patients. Cancer Res. 2006;66(18):9299–307.

270. Ko JS, et al. Sunitinib mediates reversal of myeloid-derived suppressor cell accumulation in renal cell carcinoma patients. Clin Cancer Res. 2009;15(6):2148–57.

271. Ko JS, et al. Direct and differential suppression of myeloid-derived suppressor cell subsets by sunitinib is compartmentally constrained. Cancer Res. 2010;70(9):3526–36.

272. Friberg M, et al. Indoleamine 2,3-dioxygenase contributes to tumor cell evasion of T cell-mediated rejection. Int J Cancer. 2002;101(2):151–5.

273. Muller AJ, et al. Inhibition of indoleamine 2,3-dioxygenase, an immunoregulatory target of the cancer suppression gene Bin1, potentiates cancer chemotherapy. Nat Med. 2005;11(3):312–9.

274. Gu T, et al. Central role of IFNgamma-indoleamine 2,3-dioxygenase axis in regulation of interleukin-12-mediated antitumor immunity. Cancer Res. 2010;70(1):129–38.

275. Holmgaard RB, et al. Indoleamine 2,3-dioxygenase is a critical resistance mechanism in antitumor T cell immunotherapy targeting CTLA-4. J Exp Med. 2013;210(7):1389–402.

276. De Henau O, et al. Overcoming resistance to checkpoint blockade therapy by targeting PI3Kgamma in myeloid cells. Nature. 2016;539(7629):443–7.

277. Allinen M, et al. Molecular characterization of the tumor microenvironment in breast cancer. Cancer Cell. 2004;6(1):17–32.

278. Durrans A, et al. Identification of reprogrammed myeloid cell transcriptomes in NSCLC. PLoS One. 2015;10(6):e0129123.

279. Choi H, et al. Transcriptome analysis of individual stromal cell populations identifies stroma-tumor crosstalk in mouse lung cancer model. Cell Rep. 2015;10(7):1187–201.

The Role of Platelets in the Tumor Microenvironment

15

Qiuchen Guo, Harvey G. Roweth, Kelly E. Johnson, Sandra S. McAllister, Joseph E. Italiano Jr., and Elisabeth M. Battinelli

Abstract

Platelets are small, circulating anuclear cells that have an important and well-defined role in hemostasis and wound healing. Known as the "band-aids of the blood," platelets rapidly activate, aggregate, and release a plethora of growth factors, cytokines, and other biological mediators at sites of vascular damage, thereby forming a clot. Compelling evidence has revealed that tumors can co-opt the normal functions of platelets to advance disease progression and metastasis. We now know that platelets are a key component of the tumor microenvironment and that they promote cancer progression in a myriad of ways. Results from in vitro and in vivo modeling have shown that platelets drive tumor cell invasion and epithelial-to-mesenchymal transition, promote angiogenesis, facilitate intravasation and extravasation of tumor cells, protect circulating tumor cells from shear forces and immune surveillance, and function as long-distance cargo carriers that transmit signals between primary tumors, metastases, and the bone marrow. Platelets have also been reported to have anti-cancer functions by supporting tumor blood vessel normalization and containing anti-angiogenic factors. Therefore, a key challenge to cancer research and treatment remains how to inhibit the pro-tumorigenic effects and/or promote the anti-tumor functions of platelets using conventional and new treatment regimes. In this chapter, we examine the current understanding of the role of platelets in cancer development and progression and explore platelet-targeted therapies as a novel and promising approach to cancer treatment.

Q. Guo · H. G. Roweth · K. E. Johnson · S. S. McAllister
E. M. Battinelli (✉)
Division of Hematology, Department of Medicine, Brigham and Women's Hospital, Boston, MA, USA

Harvard Medical School, Boston, MA, USA
e-mail: qguo1@bwh.harvard.edu; hroweth@bwh.harvard.edu; smcallister1@bwh.harvard.edu; embattinelli@bwh.harvard.edu

J. E. Italiano Jr.
Harvard Medical School, Boston, MA, USA

Vascular Biology Program, Department of Surgery, Boston Children's Hospital, Boston, MA, USA
e-mail: Joseph.Italiano@childrens.harvard.edu

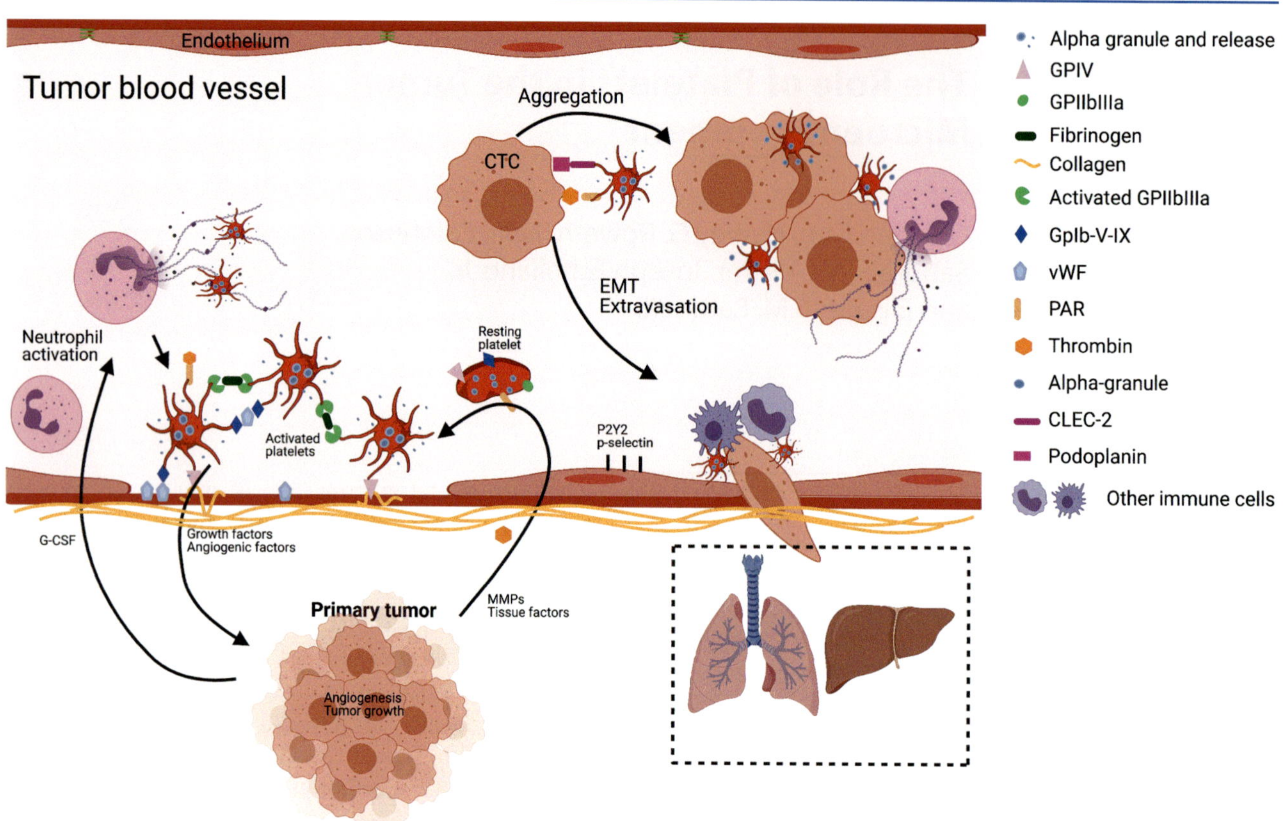

Mechanisms of platelet activation in cancer. Tumor endothelium is often damaged, or "leaky," leading to exposure of underlying collagens and extracellular matrix proteins, which engage glycoproteins on the cell surface of circulating platelets. Platelets activate, undergo a shape change, and release their granular contents. Fibrinogen bridges form between platelets to strengthen their aggregation. Tumors trigger platelet activation and aggregation through a variety of mechanisms, including directly releasing factors to activate platelets and releasing factors activating immune cells such as neutrophils to activate platelets. After tumor cells intravasate into the bloodstream, direct interactions between tumor cells and platelets via ligand/receptor pairing can also lead to platelet activation. Activated platelets can recruit immune cells to tumor clusters and induce tumor cells to undergo epithelial-to-mesenchymal transition, which can be important for tumor cell survival and extravasation. Adapted from "Blood Vessel (Straight, Light Background)," by BioRender.com (2021). Retrieved from https://app.biorender.com/biorender-templates

Take-Home Lessons
- Platelets play an important role in cancer, including the promotion of tumor angiogenesis, growth, invasion, and metastasis.
- Platelets interact with circulating tumor cells (CTCs) and protect CTCs from shear stress and immune surveillance.
- Platelets act as sponges to take up tumor-secreted factors and carry molecular signals to distant locations throughout the body.
- Anti-platelet therapies could have great potential in the treatment of cancer.

Platelets are best understood for their role in thrombosis and hemostasis. These tiny, anuclear circulating cells form clots at sites of vascular damage to initiate the wound healing process. However, we have also learned that platelets are a critical component of the tumor microenvironment (TME) and can profoundly affect tumor progression and metastasis. For example, platelets aid in disseminating tumor cells by protecting them from high shear forces and immune surveillance within the circulation. The resultant tumor cell-platelet aggregates facilitate embolization, promote the adhesion of tumor cells to the vascular endothelium, and release a variety of soluble factors that promote tumor growth and metastasis. Platelets are, by design, carriers of a myriad of cytokines and growth factors, many of which are known to affect disease progression. Cytokines released from activated platelets not only impact the function of tumor cells but also affect other cells in the TME such as endothelial cells, fibroblasts, and immune cells [1–3]. In this chapter, we discuss what is known about the complex cross-talk that occurs between platelets, tumor cells, and other tissue cells in malignancy and highlight features of such communication that may be vulnerable to therapeutic intervention.

Platelet Function

Before exploring the role of platelets in cancer, it is beneficial to review normal physiological platelet function. Platelets are small (1–3 μm), discoid-shaped cell fragments that are released from progenitor cells called megakaryocytes in the bone marrow. Structurally, platelets are anuclear and contain three distinct types of granules: alpha-granules (the most abundant type), dense granules, and lysosomes [4]. Over 300 biologically active factors, including cytokines, adhesion molecules, and coagulation mediators are contained within alpha-granules, which can be selectively released upon platelet activation [5]. Although platelets do not have nuclei, they contain some cytosolic mRNA and translational machinery; hence, protein synthesis can occur to a limited extent [6]. The platelet surface is coated with glycoproteins, adhesion molecules, and signaling receptors, thus enabling them to interact with other cells and to become activated upon contact with agonists such as thrombin, collagen, ADP, thromboxane, and epinephrine [7].

Platelets are often thought of as the "band-aids of the blood" [8]; they prevent blood loss during injury by forming a clot at the site of vascular damage. Damage to the vascular wall causes exposure of subendothelial collagens and von Willebrand factor, which serve to attract circulating platelets by engaging their cell-surface glycoproteins, such as GPIbα, thereby leading to adhesion at the site of damage [9]. Local sources of collagen and thrombin at the wound site initiate platelet activation via GPVI and PAR receptors, respectively, causing platelets to undergo a drastic shape change and to release their granule contents [9]. GPIIbIIIa on the platelet surface is activated, causing fibrinogen binding and allowing for platelet aggregation and the formation of fibrinogen bridges that stabilize the clot [9]. Activated platelets release pro-coagulation factors and serve as a surface for clotting factors to assemble, further strengthening the platelet plug [7].

It is easy to imagine how activation of platelets at inappropriate times or locations could lead to adverse situations. Improper activation and aggregation can lead to the formation of blood clots while the release of growth factors and inflammatory cytokines from alpha-granules can promote atherosclerosis and tumor progression [10]. Indeed, patho-logical platelet function has been shown to occur in a variety of cancer types, and platelets are accepted as key players in a number of the processes underlying disease progression and metastasis.

Identifying a Role for Platelets in Cancer

A link between cancer and abnormal coagulation was first noted in the 1800s when Jean-Baptiste Bouillaud reported a case of deep vein thrombosis occurring in a cancer patient [11]. French physician Armand Trousseau is widely credited as the first person to definitively propose a link between cancer and hypercoagulability of the blood when he noted that patients with cancer were more likely to develop a blood clot than the general population and that blood clots could be predictive of an undiagnosed malignancy [12]. Platelets were specifically implicated in 1872 when a link between elevated platelet count and cancer was reported [13]. Levin and Conley published a detailed examination of thrombocytosis (elevated platelet count) and cancer in the 1960s, finding that thrombocytosis was present in 38% of patients with inoperable tumors [14]. Since then, thrombocytosis has been correlated with poor outcomes in a variety of solid tumor types including cancers of the breast, lung, ovary, colon, kidney, and brain [15–20]. Thrombocytosis is also associated with an increased risk of venous thromboembolism (VTE) in many cancer patients [21]. Cancer patients have a four- to seven-fold greater risk of developing a pulmonary embolism or a deep vein thrombosis than healthy individuals [22].

Is elevated platelet count merely coincidental or do platelets play a direct, active role in cancer progression? To answer that question, Gasic et al. depleted platelets from mice before injecting tumor cells in an experimental murine model of metastasis [23]. Depletion with neuraminidase or anti-platelet serum decreased metastasis, while the infusion of platelet-rich plasma reversed that effect, suggesting that platelets play an active role in cancer progression. Subsequent mouse studies have revealed that disruption of platelet function also reduces metastasis formation; a greater than 50% reduction in metastasis was seen in both GPVI and P-selectin knockout mice [24–27]. Interestingly, metastasis was reduced by 80% in a mouse model of gray platelet syndrome, a disorder in which platelets lack alpha-granules [28] These animal studies verified that platelet activation and alpha-granule release were involved in metastasis.

Taken together, the early observations in cancer patients and experimental mouse models suggested that platelets facilitate metastatic spread. Nevertheless, questions remain about how, mechanistically, platelets influence the metastatic process. Numerous research efforts have focused on answering that question and in this chapter, we highlight research demonstrating the role of platelets at every stage of cancer progression and the metastatic cascade, from the primary tumor site to the tumor cell's journey through the circulation and finally during extravasation and metastatic seeding and growth [29].

Tumor Cell-Induced Platelet Activation and Aggregation

Normally, platelets are only activated at sites of vascular injury and remain inert (resting state) while in transient contact with healthy cells and tissues. However, tumors and their microenvironment are far from normal and have been described as "wounds that never heal" due to persistent inflammation and tissue remodeling [30]. The TME of most solid tumors is conducive to inappropriate platelet activation and thus co-opts platelet function for the tumor's benefit. Activated platelets have been observed within primary tumor tissue in pre-clinical breast cancer models and patient-derived xenografts [31]. Angiogenic vessels associated with tumors are often abnormal and leaky, with gaps between endothelial cells and areas of exposed collagen, allowing platelets entrance and access to tumors [31, 32]. Tumor cells can activate platelets by producing the potent activator, thrombin, and elevated thrombin levels have been observed within the TME of several types of cancer [33–35]. Tumor-derived cathepsin B, matrix metalloproteinase (MMP)-2 and MMP-14 have all been shown to activate platelets and tissue factor (TF) can also be aberrantly released from tumor cells, indirectly activating platelets through the initiation of the coagulation cascade [36, 37]. Direct contact between platelets and tumor cells can also lead to activation; for instance, tumor cell podoplanin or mucins can interact with and activate platelet CLEC-2 and P-selectin, respectively [38–41].

Interactions between platelets and tumor cells either at the primary tumor site or within the circulation often lead to a phenomenon called tumor cell-induced platelet aggregation (TCIPA). TCIPA occurs when tumor cells activate platelets, leading to activation and release of platelet-derived ADP and generation of thromboxane to further trigger aggregation [42–44]. In this process, fibrin is generated, thereby cross-linking tumor cells and platelets, while glycoproteins such as GPIIbIIIa strengthen the platelet–tumor cell aggregates through fibrinogen bridges [45]. Aggregates composed of platelets and tumor cells have been observed within the circulation since the 1970s [46, 47], and tumor cell lines of breast, colon, prostate, lung, and pancreatic origin, to list a few, have been shown to aggregate platelets in vitro [48–51]. These aggregates can be observed in the blood of patients and are implicated in tumor cell immune evasion and embolization [52].

In addition to activation by direct platelet–tumor cell interaction, tumor cells can induce long-range activation of distant platelets. For instance, tumor cells release TF-coated microparticles that can travel through the circulation and may be involved in cancer-associated VTE [53, 54]. Another mechanism of indirect platelet activation can occur when tumor cells secrete granulocyte colony-stimulating factor (G-CSF), causing circulating neutrophils to release platelet-activating neutrophil extracellular traps (NETS) [55, 56].

The cross-talk between platelets and tumor cells that mediates activation and aggregation is thought to be crucial for platelets to support tumor progression. Overall, tumor cells have a diverse arsenal of mechanisms to induce platelet activation, and the specific methods utilized by a particular tumor may depend on the cancer type, stage, or location. For instance, some glioblastoma and pancreatic cell lines release thrombin to induce TCIPA, while MCF-7 breast tumor cells can release MMP-2 or ADP to achieve TCIPA [42, 43, 57, 58]. But regardless of the specific mechanism, activation of platelets seems to be a common phenomenon in cancer progression. In the next sections, we will discuss in detail how activated platelets and platelet–tumor cells aggregates are thought to influence cancer progression.

Platelets in Tumor Growth and Invasion

Platelets are packed with a myriad of biologically active growth factors and cytokines that are critically important during wound healing but can be detrimental when co-opted by tumors. In vitro studies have shown that platelet-derived growth factor (PDGF) and platelet-activating factor (PAF) directly drive tumor cell proliferation [59, 60]. However, the evidence that platelets have a role in influencing the growth of primary tumor proliferation and growth in vivo is limited [59, 60]. A vast body of evidence both in vitro and in vivo suggests that, instead, platelets in the primary TME predominantly influence tumor progression by driving invasion [61, 62].

Platelets promote invasion through a variety of mechanisms. Epithelial-to-mesenchymal transition (EMT) is one process by which tumor cells become invasive. During EMT, tumor cells of epithelial origin lose their cell-to-cell adhesions and polarity, becoming more mobile and developing the characteristics and markers of mesenchymal cells. Platelets were shown to induce the expression of key EMT regulators such as twist, snail, slug, vimentin, and fibronectin while downregulating E-cadherin [63]. Findings from these studies also demonstrated that platelet-derived TGF-β1 drives EMT through activation of the TGF-β1 receptor and NF-κB signaling pathways in the tumor cells, with which they are in direct contact [63, 64]. Furthermore, conditional ablation of platelet TGF-β1 reduced metastasis in mice [63]. While TGF-β1 released from platelets has been identified as the main factor responsible for platelet-induced EMT, hepatocyte growth factor (HGF) and PDGF may contribute to EMT as well [65]. Platelet-derived autotaxin has also been shown to directly induce breast tumor cell migration and invasion [66–68].

Another mechanism by which platelets promote tumor cell invasion is to alter the TME. Simply adding platelets or releasate from activated platelets increases migration and invasion of tumor cells in culture [62]. By releasing MMPs directly into the peritumoral space, platelets could break down the extracellular matrix to enable tumor cell migration [69]. Furthermore, platelets induce MMP expression in other components of the microenvironment including tumor cells and endothelial cells [70–72]. Stromal cells in the TMEs are also influenced by platelet-derived factors as indicated by studies showing that tumor-promoting cancer-associated fibroblasts proliferate and differentiate in response to signals from activated platelets [73, 74].

Platelets Promote Angiogenesis

Angiogenesis is critical for most solid tumors to survive and grow beyond a diameter of 1–2 mm [75]. A role for platelets in tumor angiogenesis was first proposed by Judah Folkman in 1998 and, indeed, platelets are now known to be intimately involved in the angiogenesis process [76]. Platelets are packed with various pro-angiogenic and anti-angiogenic regulators but the net effect of releasates from platelets activated by tumor cells, both in vitro and in vivo, tends to strongly promote endothelial capillary tube formation in vitro, indicating a pro-angiogenic effect [31, 77]. Over 80% of circulating VEGF, a potent pro-angiogenic mediator, is carried within the platelets of both healthy individuals and cancer patients, and VEGF levels within platelets correlate with disease progression [78–80]. In vivo models by depletion of platelets, showed decreased retinal neovascularization, corneal angiogenesis, and tumor angiogenesis [31, 69, 81].

Platelets package different angiogenic mediators into distinct alpha-granules that can be released differentially depending on the specific agonist bioavailability or receptor activation [77]. ADP activation leads to VEGF release and a pro-angiogenic releasate, while activation with thromboxane A_2 causes retention of VEGF and release of the anti-angiogenic protein endostatin, leading to a releasate with net anti-angiogenic effects [77]. Platelet activation via the thrombin receptor PAR1 mediates VEGF release, while stimulation of the PAR4 receptor leads to endostatin release and retention of VEGF [3, 82]. Those studies showed that platelets can make "choices" about which contents to package and release based on the stimulus they receive. Differential packaging of platelets is likely to occur during their production by megakaryocytes. In vitro studies show

megakaryocytes can sort and package contents (e.g., bFGF, VEGF) into distinct alpha-granules that are differentially distributed into platelets [83]. On the contrary, other studies suggest the packaging of proteins with conflicting functions into the alpha-granules could be stochastic [84]. By mathematical analysis of the localization of 15 different human alpha-granule proteins with pro-angiogenic or anti-angiogenic function, a Gaussian distribution indicated random packaging of proteins to individual alpha-granules [84]. However, proteins could also be packaged into distinct zones or with different levels [84, 85], and can be released differentially upon activation by tumor cells to favor tumor angiogenesis.

The promotion of angiogenesis within a tumor by platelets could be due to the basal functions of platelets in physiology. Platelets are the "first responders" to a wound [86], and their degranulation releases factors that initiate clotting, angiogenesis, and immune cell recruitment to facilitate wound repair [87]. By promoting angiogenesis, platelets attempt to preserve the integrity of leaky blood vessels within tumors [81]. On the other hand, platelets could potentially prevent tumor progression by blood vessel normalization. Blood vessel normalization is a therapeutic strategy for cancer, given the synergist efficacy of both anti-VEGF therapy and chemotherapy through normalizing tumor blood vessel structure and maturation to facilitate the uniform administration of anti-cancer therapies to tumors [88]. Platelets may also have important role(s) in blood vessel normalization, where they have been reported to recruit and induce differentiation and maturation of endothelial progenitor cells [89]. Tumors from thrombocytopenic mice showed impaired vessel density and maturation [69]. Specifically, platelets seem to support pericyte coverage in angiogenic vessels and angiopoietin-1 and serotonin released from platelets may promote vessel maturation [69, 90] These data support a paradoxical anti-tumor function of platelets by establishing blood vessel homeostasis. It is possible that the initial purpose of platelet recruitment to the tumor is to repair the leaky tumor blood vessels; however, platelet activation by the TME induces pathological angiogenesis. Therefore, more research is needed to parse the specific signals, conditions, events, and intermediates that favor platelet-induced angiogenesis and vessel stabilization.

In addition to regulating blood vessel integrity, platelets can also act like sponge, taking up molecules from their environment. Angiogenic factors, including VEGF and basic fibroblast growth factor, released by primary tumor are taken up by platelets, stored, trafficked, and delivered to other locations such as distant metastatic sites [91–93]. A study using a murine model of luminal breast cancer demonstrated that platelets sequester angiogenic regulators from the site of an aggressively growing primary tumor and deliver them, via the circulation, to indolent tumors located at distant anatomical sites where these platelets contribute to growth and angiogenesis of the otherwise indolent tumor [31]. Platelet inhibition with aspirin prevented tumor progression, suggesting the potential role of platelets in delivering angiogenic signals from one tumor to the other [31]. Those studies highlight the potential for platelets to serve as long-haul cargo carriers, shuttling signals between distant sites as orchestrated by the tumor.

Mechanisms by which platelets endocytose proteins are active areas of investigation. Platelets from mice lacking expression of dynamin2, vesicle-associated membrane protein-3 or adenosine 5′-diphosphate–ribosylation factor 6 (Arf6) demonstrated decreased fibrinogen uptake, thus implicating those factors as critical for the platelet endocytic machinery [94–96]. Receptor-mediated endocytosis could be an important aspect of platelet function. Platelets from dynamin2 knockout mice showed not only decreased fibrinogen in their alpha-granules, but also dysfunctional responses to stimulation via GPVI [97]. Taken together, these findings imply endocytosis alters both the content and function of platelets. However, little is currently known about the mechanism(s) by which platelets endocytose proteins that favor tumor progression, leaving a critical gap in our knowledge. A deeper understanding of these processes should provide a source of potential therapeutic targets.

Overall, platelets contribute significantly to tumor angiogenesis via a number of mechanisms; they release potent pro-angiogenic factors upon stimulation by tumor cells, they mature and normalize unstable tumor-associated vessels, and they collect angiogenic mediators and deliver them to distant sites, propagating the angiogenic signal from the tumor. Angiogenic neovasculature not only nourishes the tumor but also provides a route for tumor cells to escape into circulation.

Platelet–Tumor Cell Interactions Within Blood Circulation

In order to metastasize, tumor cells need to enter either blood or lymphatic vessels, which serve as conduits for their transport to distant sites. Tumor cells in the blood are often referred to as circulating tumor cells (CTCs) and are a promising predictor of poor prognosis in the clinic. In a large global pooled analysis, breast cancer patients without detectable CTCs at baseline or at follow-up had significantly improved outcomes relative to patients who persistently tested positive for CTCs (47.05 months vs. 17.87 months, hazard ratio = 3.15, $p < 0.0001$) [98].

Hematogenous metastasis is thought to be an inefficient process [99] due to harsh shear stresses and constant immune surveillance faced by tumor cells. It is estimated that the vast majority of tumor cells are destroyed within hours of introduction into circulation, well before they can ever successfully form metastases [100, 101]. As previously discussed, contact between platelets and tumor cells causes heterotypic aggregates to form. Such aggregates can be readily identified in the circulation of cancer patients and in pre-clinical mouse models, they form within minutes of tumor cell introduction into the bloodstream [64]. The mechanical forces exerted on tumor cells in the blood are far greater than those experienced in the TME and are often enough to cause their destruction [102]. Platelets have been shown to provide protection from such forces by coating tumor cells, shielding them from shear stress modeled by plate viscometer [103].

By binding to tumor cells, platelets induce tumor cell alterations that favor their survival. As mentioned in the previous section, platelets can induce tumor cell EMT [63], which is important for gaining tumor cell stemness [104] to support their survival in the non-adherent environment of blood circulation and initiation of new tumor formation in the secondary site to form metastasis [105]. Platelet interactions have also been shown to induce tumor cell expression of immune regulatory factors, such as CCL2 [63], which recruits tumor-associated monocytes and macrophages to suppress immune surveillance in the blood and secondary sites [106]. CTC clearance from the circulation has been shown to be mediated by natural killer (NK) cells [107, 108]. Activated platelets express glucocorticoid-induced tumor necrosis factor receptor ligand (GITRL) on their surface, which binds to the GITR receptor on NKs, leading to inhibition of NK cell activity [109]. Platelets can also inhibit NK cells by downregulation the expression of the NKG2D cell-surface receptor, which is used by NK cells to identify and lyse tumor cells [110]. Furthermore, platelets can protect tumor cells from NK-mediated killing in the blood by transferring MHC class I molecules to the CTC surface [111]. Tumor cells may also avoid lysis in the blood by aberrantly expressing integrins normally found on platelets in a phenomenon known as platelet-mimicry [112, 113].

CTCs have also been found in the blood as clusters. Compared with single CTCs, clustered CTCs are more resistant to apoptosis, have more metastatic potential, and predict poorer prognosis in breast and prostate cancer patients [114]. One way CTC clusters have enhanced survival advantages is by forming homotypic attachments, thereby increasing their resistance to anoikis [115]. Other hypotheses include the notion that CTC clusters are less likely to experience excessive shear force and moreover, larger CTC clusters are more easily trapped in small capillaries of secondary sites [116]. Increased coagulation factors, such as platelet tissue factors F3, F5, and F12, have been found in CTC clusters compared with single CTCs [114], suggesting the platelets that bind to CTC clusters are more activated than those who bind to single CTCs. In a study that analyzed gene expression profiles of CTC clusters and single CTCs, Gene Set Enrichment Analysis revealed that "Hallmark_Coagulation" was the most significantly enriched pathway in CTC clusters compared with single CTCs [117]. Nevertheless, the mechanism(s) underpinning the survival advantages of CTC clusters are still not completely resolved, and the contribution of platelets has yet to be investigated.

Extravasation

Tumors cells must find ways to successfully exit circulation to seed a new metastatic site. Immobile platelet–tumor cell aggregates have been observed in the microvasculature [118, 119] and it was historically assumed that this was a passive process with aggregates simply getting stuck within narrow vessels. We now know that arrest and extravasation are active processes and that platelets are key players in both of them. Platelet surface selectins mediate rolling along the endothelium slowing their velocity in circulation and allowing for further association with endothelial cells. P-selectin on activated platelets interacts with the endothelium while simultaneously mediating binding to tumor cells, thus tethering tumor cells to the endothelium [26, 40]. The importance of P-selectin in this process has been demonstrated in mice through the pharmacological blockade as well as genetic ablation of P-selectin [41]. Platelets can also bind CD97 (adhesion G protein-coupled receptor) on the tumor cell surface, which conducts bidirectional signaling to both platelets and tumor cells during extravasation [120]. The activation of platelets by tumor CD97 leads to platelet ATP release, which disrupts endothelial cell junctions by activating the endothelial $P2Y_2$ nucleotide receptor [121] and binding of platelets to tumor CD97 increases tumor cell invasiveness by Rho activation [120]. Other factors released by platelets including MMP-1, TGF-β, and ADAM12 also facilitate the breakdown of junctions between endothelial cells, allowing tumor cells to cross the now leaky endothelial barrier and enter the surrounding tissue parenchyma [119, 122].

Once disseminated tumor cells have arrived at new metastatic sites, activated platelets promote colonization, angiogenesis, and ship signals to and from distant sites. To quote Yan and Jurasz, "…perhaps a small revision is required to Paget's 'seed and soil' hypothesis of metastasis to include 'seed, soil, and fertilizer', in which platelets take on an unenviable but supportive role of 'fertilizer'" [123]. However, it remains unclear if platelets support tumor cells at secondary sites through the same mechanisms employed at the primary tumor and this question warrants further investigation.

Platelets Coordinate the Systemic Effects of Tumors

As discussed previously, tumors can activate, alter and use platelets to carry molecular signals to distant locations throughout the body, making platelets an integral part of the systemic communication and coordination that occurs in cancer [124–126]. Platelets can propagate messages that serve to mobilize bone marrow progenitors, alter the bone function and even prepare sites to accept future metastases. Tumors recruit bone marrow-derived cells (BMDCs) and endothelial progenitor cells to the TME. Stromal cell-derived factor 1 (SDF-1) and VEGF released from activated platelets have been implicated in mobilizing BMDCs and progenitor cells from the bone marrow [89, 127–129]. Platelets also appear to promote metastasis within the lung by recruiting pro-metastatic granulocytes to platelet–tumor cell aggregates during extravasation through the release of CXCL5 and CXCL7 [64]. Platelets have also been demonstrated to serve as long-range communicators between primary tumors, distant tumors, and the bone marrow, by cooperating with BMDCs to promote the vascularization of distant tumors [31].

Bone remodeling often occurs in the setting of metastatic disease and platelets may mediate this process as well. The presence of primary melanoma or prostate tumor increased bone formation in mice, while platelet depletion reversed this effect [130]. In these two cancer models, platelets traffic tumor-derived MMP-1 and TGF-β to the bone where they promote bone formation. Conversely, platelets are also capable of increasing bone resorption to facilitate bone metastases. In a pre-clinical breast cancer model, platelets promoted osteolytic bone loss by a complex mechanism in which lysophosphatidic acid (LPA) released from activated platelets drove IL (Interleukin)-6 and IL-8 secretion from tumor cells to stimulate bone-destroying osteoclasts [131]. Furthermore, platelets release autotaxin from their alpha-granules, a molecule that catalyzes the production of LPA and guides tumor cells to the bone by interacting with tumor cell αvβ3 integrins [130].

Platelets clearly help orchestrate the complex coordination of events that enable tumors to metastasize. More studies are required to parse the precise role of platelets in the spread of specific tumor types and in the homing of tumor cells to particular sites of metastasis. Additionally, it is necessary to confirm whether similar mechanisms are at play in human patients and, if so, determine whether they are vulnerable to therapeutic intervention (Fig. 15.1).

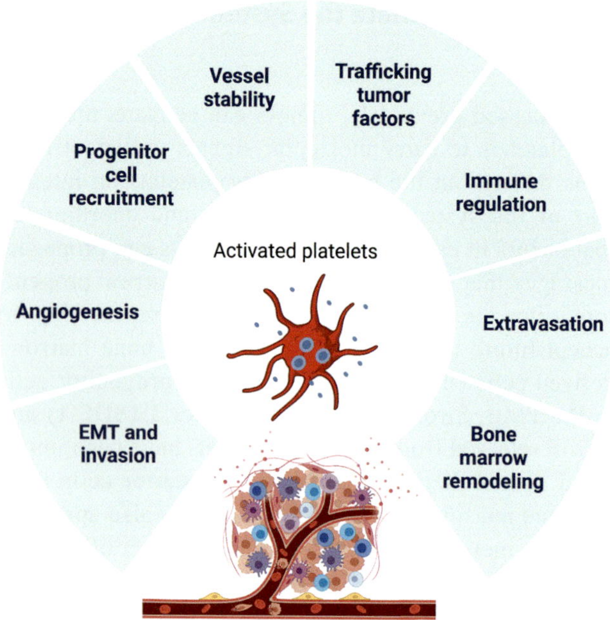

Fig. 15.1 Mechanisms by which platelets promote cancer. Platelets have been found to employ a wide variety of strategies to promote tumor progression and metastasis. Platelets can induce tumor cell EMT to drive tumor cell aggressiveness [63–68], promote angiogenesis [31, 69, 81], impact vessel stability facilitating circulating tumor cell extravasation [64, 120], remodel bone marrow [132–134], and recruit tumor-promoting progenitor cells [89]. In addition, platelets can carry and deliver signals between distant sites including primary and secondary tumors and bone marrow [124–126]. Adapted from "RNA Secondary Structures" and "Tumor microenvironment," by BioRender.com (2021). Retrieved from https://app.biorender.com/biorender-templates

Platelet Microparticles and the Tumor Microenvironment

Recently, interest in platelet-derived microparticles (PMPs) and their potential role in cancer has been growing. PMPs are shed from platelets following activation and consist of membrane-bound proteins and cytoplasmic components [135]. In vitro, PMPs have similar pro-angiogenic and pro-metastatic potential as platelets and increase endothelial cell migration and capillary tube formation as well as promote tumor cell MMP production and invasion through Matrigel [136–138]. PMPs may also transfer membrane receptors and adhesion molecules to the surface of tumor cells, conferring a more invasive phenotype. In vivo, Lewis lung carcinoma cells were more metastatic when coated with PMP prior to injection and, in an ischemia model, the introduction of PMPs increased angiogenesis [139, 140].

Overall, PMPs recapitulate many of the same metastatic and angiogenic effects that are observed with whole platelets. They may potentially provide a mechanism for tumor mimicry, with tumor cells incorporating platelet markers to their cell surface after fusion with PMPs. They may also serve as a way for activated, spent platelets to continue to

play a role in the TME and should be considered when conceptualizing the complex crosstalk that occurs in cancer.

The Role of Platelets in Hematological Malignancies

So far most of our knowledge about the function of platelets in cancer comes from studies of solid tumors, particularly carcinomas. Relatively little is known about the role of platelets in hematological malignancies, and little can be extrapolated from work in solid tumors due to vast differences in the tumorigenesis processes and the TMEs. However, some studies can offer insights.

Unlike cell lines derived from solid tumors, many leukemia cells do not activate platelets and have been shown to inhibit the activation and aggregation of platelets [141–143]. Patients with leukemia often present with thrombocytopenia (low platelet count) and their platelets display lower numbers of dense granules [144, 145]. Conversely, a few AML and CML cell lines can activate and aggregate platelets, and the resulting releasate increases tumor cell proliferation and survival [146–148].

The role of platelets in multiple myeloma (MM) was also investigated. These patients often have elevated soluble P-selectin and thrombopoietin (TPO) levels and are at increased risk of developing VTEs [132–134]. Platelet activation is positively correlated with MM disease progression [149]. Platelets contribute to MM cell proliferation in vitro and tumor engraftment in bone marrow in vivo, potentially by stimulating tumor cell IL-1β production, as IL-1β deletion in tumor cells aborts any platelet-induced effects [149]. Other factors released by platelets that are known to support MM progression include but are not limited to IL-6, SDF-1, and insulin-like growth factor-1 [132–134].

Overall, the role of platelets in hematological malignancies is not well explored. Because thrombocytopenia is a feature of many hematological malignancies, platelets may not be as important as those involved with solid tumors. However, since platelets are shown to be altered in some hematological cancers, it would be wise to examine the interactions of these tumor cells with megakaryocytes, particularly in cancers such as multiple myeloma where the bone marrow serves as a TME. It may be that platelets serve different functions in the different types of hematological cancers and detailed investigations into each type could be beneficial.

Platelets Are Altered in Cancer Patients

Interestingly, platelets isolated from some cancer patients are fundamentally different from those of healthy individuals. Platelets from breast, prostate, lung, and colon cancer patients often display higher baseline activation, suggesting they may be more reactive and have a lower threshold for activation [150–153]. Elevated platelet surface levels of the activation marker P-selectin as well as increased platelet-derived plasma markers such as CD40 ligand, β-thromboglobulin, and soluble P-selectin have been observed in patients with tumors, and these markers tend to correlate with disease progression and poor prognosis [154, 155]. Patients presenting with elevated soluble P-selectin are more than twice as likely to develop a VTE compared to cancer patients with low levels [155].

Platelet contents are also altered in patients; total numbers of alpha-granules are higher, and pro-tumorigenic factors such as VEGF are enriched in platelets from cancer patients compared to those from healthy donors [92, 156]. Platelets from cancer patients also contain altered mRNA transcripts [157] and can be used as a non-invasive liquid biopsy in aiding cancer detection [157–159]. For example, TIMP1 mRNA is upregulated in colorectal cancer patients compared with healthy controls or patients with inflammatory bowel diseases [160]. Tropomyosin 3 mRNA is significantly elevated in breast cancer patients and positively correlated with metastasis [161]. These transcripts could come from two sources: platelets take them up from plasma, which contains tumor cell releasates or tumor cells induce the production of alternative splice variants within platelets. Evidence suggests that mRNAs may be produced and packaged at higher levels at the megakaryocyte level in addition to being taken up from the tumor environment [162].

Thrombocytosis is associated with some specific types of cancer. Lung, colorectal and ovarian cancer are typically the most commonly diagnosed cancers in patients with thrombocytosis [163, 164], but breast cancer patients usually present with normal platelet counts [165]. However, the prognostic effect of thrombocytosis has been found in most types of cancer, including breast, ovarian, lung, and other types of cancers [166]. TPO is the dominant driver of megakaryocyte differentiation and maturation. Pre-clinical studies of ovarian cancer reveal that tumor-derived IL-6 drives TPO production in the liver, leading to a boost in platelet production by megakaryocytes in the bone marrow [167]. IL-6 levels in patients correlate with platelet count, and anti-IL-6 therapy reverses this trend [168, 169]. However, more studies are needed across all tumor types to determine if this mechanism is broadly responsible for tumor-associated thrombocytosis. Another hypothesis posits that tumor cells themselves provide a source of TPO, but this has only been observed in vitro [170]. Other mechanisms that have been proposed are based on reactive thrombocytosis observed in conditions of systemic inflammation. Pro-inflammatory cytokines such as G-CSF, GM-CSF, and IL-1α are often elevated during inflammation as well as cancer progression and have also been implicated in megakaryocyte maturation and platelet production [171–174].

Although an abundance of evidence proves that platelet function, contents, and numbers are altered in cancer patients, we have only begun to understand how that occurs. Studies are needed to elucidate the effect of tumors on megakaryocyte biology and the platelets that result. Understanding the mechanism(s) underlying cancer-associated thrombocytosis remains important, as therapies directed at this process could prevent tumors from generating platelets that favor their progression.

Anti-platelet Therapy and Cancer

Based on their multifaceted role in cancer, platelets are a very attractive therapeutic target. Disrupting the communication between platelets and tumor cells by targeting platelets or tumor cells could theoretically block mechanisms of invasion, EMT, angiogenesis, immunosurveillance escape, and activation of other host cells in the microenvironment and bone marrow to prevent metastasis. Platelet-mimicry, along with many shared surface markers between platelets and tumor cells, suggests that platelet-targeted drugs could also impact the tumor.

Pre-clinical data are quite promising and reveal that targeting several platelet receptors may be an effective approach for limiting cancer progression. Anti-platelet drugs that are currently available for the treatment of cardiovascular disease are now being explored as anti-tumor agents. For example, GPIIbIIIa blockers have been shown to inhibit lung metastasis in a murine model but have not yet been studied in patients with cancer [175]. Clopidogrel and ticagrelor, as P2Y12 antagonists, were used to treat cardiovascular disease, show anti-tumor properties in vivo and in vitro, and can prevent ovarian cancer growth and bone loss in mice [176, 177]. Anti-coagulants including fondaparinux and low molecular weight heparins (LMWH) inhibit tumor cell inducing platelet activation and attenuate the angiogenic potential of platelets in vitro [178]. These drugs make attractive candidates since they are often already given to cancer patients due to their tendency to develop clots. However, clinical data from the use of LMWH in cancer patients show mixed results [179–182]. Large-scale clinical trials are needed to access the efficacy of currently available anti-platelet drugs. What is more, some newly developed platelet-targeting drugs have shown promising efficacy in pre-clinical models of breast cancer. Antisense oligonucleotides that silence hepatic thrombopoietin gene (THPO-ASO) could reduce plasma TPO levels and decrease platelets count by targeting bone marrow megakaryocytes and treatment of THPO-ASO inhibits breast cancer progression in MMTV-

PyMT mouse model [183]. Anti-GPVI therapeutic antibody (JAQ1) has also been shown to reduce metastasis burden in mouse colon and breast cancer models [184]. These data suggest the importance of platelets in cancer progression and finding more efficient and safe methods to target platelets will further improve standard cancer treatment.

Aspirin is perhaps the most intriguing anti-platelet agent that has been studied to date, as aspirin is broadly used with minimal side effects. However, the function of aspirin in cancer treatment remains controversial, with varying efficacies across cancer types, patient cohorts, and study design. Some reports show a beneficial function of aspirin in decreasing cancer risk and death [185, 186]. A long-term epidemiological study revealed that individuals who take aspirin daily are less likely to be diagnosed with cancer and show improved survival if they do develop cancer [187]. Some studies indicate no benefit or even worse prognosis in cancer patients regularly taking aspirin [188–190]. Despite the contradicting results, aspirin is still being extensively studied in cancer research, as it can target both tumor cells and the TME [191]. Better understanding the mechanism of action in both platelets and tumor cells could lead to optimized usage of this drug in some specific types of cancer. The mechanism of action for aspirin's efficacy in cancer was originally thought to be due to decreased inflammation via cyclooxygenase (COX) inhibition. However, the low doses (below 162 mg/day) taken were not enough to prevent inflammation but do cause platelet inhibition through irreversible acetylation of COX-1. Subsequent studies also point to a platelet-based mechanism; platelet inhibition with aspirin diminishes platelet activation, protein release and their ability to induce angiogenesis [77]. Mouse models also confirm that platelet inhibition with aspirin decreases metastasis and improves outcomes [23, 31, 192]. The mechanism of aspirin in inhibiting metastasis has been investigated. Recent studies report that the inhibition of COX-1/thromboxane A_2 pathway of platelets by aspirin decreases platelet–tumor cell aggregation, endothelial activation, and tumor cell–endothelial cell adhesion, which decreased metastasis [193]. Another study shows that aspirin-treated platelets fail to induce IL-8 secretion from tumor cells [194]. Aspirin seems most effective in chemoprevention [195–197], but may also be beneficial if taken in combination with standard treatment to target the tumor and the environment at multiple angles. Further exploring the mechanisms by which aspirin inhibits the tumor promotional function of platelet is critical in the development of drugs that are more specific and efficacious than aspirin but work on the same principle.

Concluding Remarks/Summary

Platelets a now known to be key players in cancer progression and metastasis. These little cells supply the tumor with growth factors and mediators of invasion, provide potent pro-angiogenic regulators and help maintain tumor vessel integrity, protect circulating tumor cells from shear stress and immune attack, and help set up new metastatic niches. Platelets also serve as long-haul cargo carriers, delivering messages to and from the tumor in ways that allow cancer to progress. Such systemic changes also lead to alterations in platelet function, content and number. Overall, research into the role of platelets in cancer has rewarded us with an abundance of novel factors, receptors, and signaling pathways that could serve as powerful new biomarkers, potential therapeutic targets, or even novel drug delivery tools in the fight against cancer.

References

1. Sabrkhany S, Griffioen AW, Oude Egbrink MG. The role of blood platelets in tumor angiogenesis. Biochim Biophys Acta. 2011;1815(2):189–96.
2. Battinelli EM, Hartwig JH, Italiano JE Jr. Delivering new insight into the biology of megakaryopoiesis and thrombopoiesis. Curr Opin Hematol. 2007;14(5):419–26.
3. Italiano JE Jr, Richardson JL, Patel-Hett S, Battinelli E, Zaslavsky A, Short S, et al. Angiogenesis is regulated by a novel mechanism: pro- and antiangiogenic proteins are organized into separate platelet alpha granules and differentially released. Blood. 2008;111(3):1227–33.
4. Blair P, Flaumenhaft R. Platelet alpha-granules: basic biology and clinical correlates. Blood Rev. 2009;23(4):177–89.
5. Coppinger JA, Cagney G, Toomey S, Kislinger T, Belton O, McRedmond JP, et al. Characterization of the proteins released from activated platelets leads to localization of novel platelet proteins in human atherosclerotic lesions. Blood. 2004;103(6):2096–104.
6. Yang H, Lang S, Zhai Z, Li L, Kahr WH, Chen P, et al. Fibrinogen is required for maintenance of platelet intracellular and cell-surface P-selectin expression. Blood. 2009;114(2):425–36.
7. Brass L. Understanding and evaluating platelet function. Hematology Am Soc Hematol Educ Program. 2010;2010:387–96.
8. Italiano JE Jr. Unraveling mechanisms that control platelet production. Semin Thromb Hemost. 2013;39(1):15–24.
9. Li Z, Delaney MK, O'Brien KA, Du X. Signaling during platelet adhesion and activation. Arterioscler Thromb Vasc Biol. 2010;30(12):2341–9.
10. Franco AT, Corken A, Ware J. Platelets at the interface of thrombosis, inflammation, and cancer. Blood. 2015;126(5):582–8.
11. Bouillaud S, Bouillaud J. De l'Obliteration des veines et de son influence sur la formation des hydropisies partielles: consideration sur la hydropisies passive et general. Arch Gen Med. 1823;1:188–204.
12. Trousseau A. Phlegmasia alba dolens. Clin Med Hotel-Dieu Paris. 1865;94–5.

13. Tranum BL, Haut A. Thrombocytosis: platelet kinetics in neoplasia. J Lab Clin Med. 1974;84(5):615–9.
14. Levin J, Conley CL. Thrombocytosis associated with malignant disease. Arch Intern Med. 1964;114:497–500.
15. Gucer F, Moser F, Tamussino K, Reich O, Haas J, Arikan G, et al. Thrombocytosis as a prognostic factor in endometrial carcinoma. Gynecol Oncol. 1998;70(2):210–4.
16. Brown KM, Domin C, Aranha GV, Yong S, Shoup M. Increased preoperative platelet count is associated with decreased survival after resection for adenocarcinoma of the pancreas. Am J Surg. 2005;189(3):278–82.
17. Taucher S, Salat A, Gnant M, Kwasny W, Mlineritsch B, Menzel RC, et al. Impact of pretreatment thrombocytosis on survival in primary breast cancer. Thromb Haemost. 2003;89(6):1098–106.
18. Ikeda M, Furukawa H, Imamura H, Shimizu J, Ishida H, Masutani S, et al. Poor prognosis associated with thrombocytosis in patients with gastric cancer. Ann Surg Oncol. 2002;9(3):287–91.
19. Monreal M, Fernandez-Llamazares J, Pinol M, Julian JF, Broggi M, Escola D, et al. Platelet count and survival in patients with colorectal cancer—a preliminary study. Thromb Haemost. 1998;79(5):916–8.
20. Symbas NP, Townsend MF, El-Galley R, Keane TE, Graham SD, Petros JA. Poor prognosis associated with thrombocytosis in patients with renal cell carcinoma. BJU Int. 2000;86(3):203–7.
21. Simanek R, Vormittag R, Ay C, Alguel G, Dunkler D, Schwarzinger I, et al. High platelet count associated with venous thromboembolism in cancer patients: results from the Vienna Cancer and Thrombosis Study (CATS). J Thromb Haemost JTH. 2010;8(1):114–20.
22. Timp JF, Braekkan SK, Versteeg HH, Cannegieter SC. Epidemiology of cancer-associated venous thrombosis. Blood. 2013;122(10):1712–23.
23. Gasic GJ, Gasic TB, Galanti N, Johnson T, Murphy S. Platelet-tumor-cell interactions in mice. The role of platelets in the spread of malignant disease. Int J Cancer. 1973;11(3):704–18.
24. Jain S, Russell S, Ware J. Platelet glycoprotein VI facilitates experimental lung metastasis in syngenic mouse models. J Thromb Haemost JTH. 2009;7(10):1713–7.
25. Jain S, Zuka M, Liu J, Russell S, Dent J, Guerrero JA, et al. Platelet glycoprotein Ib alpha supports experimental lung metastasis. Proc Natl Acad Sci U S A. 2007;104(21):9024–8.
26. Kim YJ, Borsig L, Varki NM, Varki A. P-selectin deficiency attenuates tumor growth and metastasis. Proc Natl Acad Sci U S A. 1998;95(16):9325–30.
27. Guerrero JA, Bennett C, van der Weyden L, McKinney H, Chin M, Nurden P, et al. Gray platelet syndrome: proinflammatory megakaryocytes and alpha-granule loss cause myelofibrosis and confer metastasis resistance in mice. Blood. 2014;124(24):3624–35.
28. Camerer E, Qazi AA, Duong DN, Cornelissen I, Advincula R, Coughlin SR. Platelets, protease-activated receptors, and fibrinogen in hematogenous metastasis. Blood. 2004;104(2):397–401.
29. Zetter BR. Angiogenesis and tumor metastasis. Annu Rev Med. 1998;49:407–24.
30. Dvorak HF. Tumors: wounds that do not heal. Similarities between tumor stroma generation and wound healing. N Engl J Med. 1986;315(26):1650–9.
31. Kuznetsov HS, Marsh T, Markens BA, Castano Z, Greene-Colozzi A, Hay SA, et al. Identification of luminal breast cancers that establish a tumor-supportive macroenvironment defined by proangiogenic platelets and bone marrow-derived cells. Cancer Discov. 2012;2(12):1150–65.
32. McDonald DM, Baluk P. Significance of blood vessel leakiness in cancer. Cancer Res. 2002;62(18):5381–5.
33. Zacharski LR, Memoli VA, Ornstein DL, Rousseau SM, Kisiel W, Kudryk BJ. Tumor cell procoagulant and urokinase expression in carcinoma of the ovary. J Natl Cancer Inst. 1993;85(15):1225–30.
34. Wojtukiewicz MZ, Zacharski LR, Memoli VA, Kisiel W, Kudryk BJ, Rousseau SM, et al. Malignant melanoma. Interaction with coagulation and fibrinolysis pathways in situ. Am J Clin Pathol. 1990;93(4):516–21.
35. Grossi IM, Fitzgerald LA, Kendall A, Taylor JD, Sloane BF, Honn KV. Inhibition of human tumor cell induced platelet aggregation by antibodies to platelet glycoproteins Ib and IIb/IIIa. Proc Soc Exp Biol Med. 1987;186(3):378–83.
36. Jurasz P, Alonso-Escolano D, Radomski MW. Platelet–cancer interactions: mechanisms and pharmacology of tumour cell-induced platelet aggregation. Br J Pharmacol. 2004;143(7):819–26.
37. Honn KV, Cavanaugh P, Evens C, Taylor JD, Sloane BF. Tumor cell-platelet aggregation: induced by cathepsin B-like proteinase and inhibited by prostacyclin. Science. 1982;217(4559):540–2.
38. Bertozzi CC, Schmaier AA, Mericko P, Hess PR, Zou Z, Chen M, et al. Platelets regulate lymphatic vascular development through CLEC-2-SLP-76 signaling. Blood. 2010;116(4):661–70.
39. Suzuki-Inoue K, Kato Y, Inoue O, Kaneko MK, Mishima K, Yatomi Y, et al. Involvement of the snake toxin receptor CLEC-2, in podoplanin-mediated platelet activation, by cancer cells. J Biol Chem. 2007;282(36):25993–6001.
40. Stone JP, Wagner DD. P-selectin mediates adhesion of platelets to neuroblastoma and small cell lung cancer. J Clin Invest. 1993;92(2):804–13.
41. Ludwig RJ, Boehme B, Podda M, Henschler R, Jager E, Tandi C, et al. Endothelial P-selectin as a target of heparin action in experimental melanoma lung metastasis. Cancer Res. 2004;64(8):2743–50.
42. Boukerche H, Berthier-Vergnes O, Penin F, Tabone E, Lizard G, Bailly M, et al. Human melanoma cell lines differ in their capacity to release ADP and aggregate platelets. Br J Haematol. 1994;87(4):763–72.
43. Alonso-Escolano D, Strongin AY, Chung AW, Deryugina EI, Radomski MW. Membrane type-1 matrix metalloproteinase stimulates tumour cell-induced platelet aggregation: role of receptor glycoproteins. Br J Pharmacol. 2004;141(2):241–52.
44. Pacchiarini L, Zucchella M, Milanesi G, Tacconi F, Bonomi E, Canevari A, et al. Thromboxane production by platelets during tumor cell-induced platelet activation. Invasion Metastasis. 1991;11(2):102–9.
45. Honn KV, Chen YQ, Timar J, Onoda JM, Hatfield JS, Fligiel SE, et al. Alpha IIb beta 3 integrin expression and function in subpopulations of murine tumors. Exp Cell Res. 1992;201(1):23–32.
46. Jones DS, Wallace AC, Fraser EE. Sequence of events in experimental metastases of Walker 256 tumor: light, immunofluorescent, and electron microscopic observations. J Natl Cancer Inst. 1971;46(3):493–504.
47. Sindelar WF, Tralka TS, Ketcham AS. Electron microscopic observations on formation of pulmonary metastases. J Surg Res. 1975;18(2):137–61.
48. Abecassis J, Beretz A, Millon-Collard R, Fricker JP, Eber M, Cazenave JP. In vitro interactions between human breast cancer cells MCF-7 and human blood platelets. Thromb Res. 1987;47(6):693–8.
49. Heinmoller E, Weinel RJ, Heidtmann HH, Salge U, Seitz R, Schmitz I, et al. Studies on tumor-cell-induced platelet aggregation in human lung cancer cell lines. J Cancer Res Clin Oncol. 1996;122(12):735–44.
50. Mitrugno A, Williams D, Kerrigan SW, Moran N. A novel and essential role for FcgammaRIIa in cancer cell-induced platelet activation. Blood. 2014;123(2):249–60.
51. Heinmoller E, Schropp T, Kisker O, Simon B, Seitz R, Weinel RJ. Tumor cell-induced platelet aggregation in vitro by human pancreatic cancer cell lines. Scand J Gastroenterol. 1995;30(10):1008–16.

52. Tsuruo T, Fujita N. Platelet aggregation in the formation of tumor metastasis. Proc Jpn Acad Ser B Phys Biol Sci. 2008;84(6):189–98.

53. Geddings JE, Mackman N. Tumor-derived tissue factor-positive microparticles and venous thrombosis in cancer patients. Blood. 2013;122(11):1873–80.

54. van den Berg YW, Osanto S, Reitsma PH, Versteeg HH. The relationship between tissue factor and cancer progression: insights from bench and bedside. Blood. 2012;119(4):924–32.

55. Fuchs TA, Brill A, Duerschmied D, Schatzberg D, Monestier M, Myers DD Jr, et al. Extracellular DNA traps promote thrombosis. Proc Natl Acad Sci U S A. 2010;107(36):15880–5.

56. Demers M, Krause DS, Schatzberg D, Martinod K, Voorhees JR, Fuchs TA, et al. Cancers predispose neutrophils to release extracellular DNA traps that contribute to cancer-associated thrombosis. Proc Natl Acad Sci U S A. 2012;109(32):13076–81.

57. Haralabopoulos GC, Grant DS, Kleinman HK, Maragoudakis ME. Thrombin promotes endothelial cell alignment in Matrigel in vitro and angiogenesis in vivo. Am J Physiol. 1997;273(1 Pt 1):C239–45.

58. Bastida E, Escolar G, Almirall L, Ordinas A. Platelet activation induced by a human neuroblastoma tumor cell line is reduced by prior administration of ticlopidine. Thromb Haemost. 1986;55(3):333–7.

59. Kim HA, Seo KH, Kang YR, Ko HM, Kim KJ, Back HK, et al. Mechanisms of platelet-activating factor-induced enhancement of VEGF expression. Cell Physiol Biochem. 2011;27(1):55–62.

60. Di Stefano JF, Kirchner M, Dagenhardt K, Hagag N. Activation of cancer cell proteases and cytotoxicity by EGF and PDGF growth factors. Am J Med Sci. 1990;300(1):9–15.

61. Pan S, Hu Y, Hu M, Jian H, Chen M, Gan L, et al. Platelet-derived PDGF promotes the invasion and metastasis of cholangiocarcinoma by upregulating MMP2/MMP9 expression and inducing EMT via the p38/MAPK signalling pathway. Am J Transl Res. 2020;12(7):3577–95.

62. Holmes CE, Levis JE, Ornstein DL. Activated platelets enhance ovarian cancer cell invasion in a cellular model of metastasis. Clin Exp Metastasis. 2009;26(7):653–61.

63. Labelle M, Begum S, Hynes RO. Direct signaling between platelets and cancer cells induces an epithelial-mesenchymal-like transition and promotes metastasis. Cancer Cell. 2011;20(5):576–90.

64. Labelle M, Begum S, Hynes RO. Platelets guide the formation of early metastatic niches. Proc Natl Acad Sci U S A. 2014;111(30):E3053–61.

65. Gotzmann J, Fischer AN, Zojer M, Mikula M, Proell V, Huber H, et al. A crucial function of PDGF in TGF-beta-mediated cancer progression of hepatocytes. Oncogene. 2006;25(22):3170–85.

66. Leblanc R, Lee SC, David M, Bordet JC, Norman DD, Patil R, et al. Interaction of platelet-derived autotaxin with tumor integrin alphaVbeta3 controls metastasis of breast cancer cells to bone. Blood. 2014;124(20):3141–50.

67. van Holten TC, Bleijerveld OB, Wijten P, de Groot PG, Heck AJ, Barendrecht AD, et al. Quantitative proteomics analysis reveals similar release profiles following specific PAR-1 or PAR-4 stimulation of platelets. Cardiovasc Res. 2014;103(1):140–6.

68. Nunes-Xavier CE, Elson A, Pulido R. Epidermal growth factor receptor (EGFR)-mediated positive feedback of protein-tyrosine phosphatase epsilon (PTPepsilon) on ERK1/2 and AKT protein pathways is required for survival of human breast cancer cells. J Biol Chem. 2012;287(5):3433–44.

69. Li R, Ren M, Chen N, Luo M, Deng X, Xia J, et al. Presence of intratumoral platelets is associated with tumor vessel structure and metastasis. BMC Cancer. 2014;14:167.

70. Belloc C, Lu H, Soria C, Fridman R, Legrand Y, Menashi S. The effect of platelets on invasiveness and protease production of human mammary tumor cells. Int J Cancer. 1995;60(3):413–7.

71. Menashi S, He L, Soria C, Soria J, Thomaidis A, Legrand Y. Modulation of endothelial cells fibrinolytic activity by platelets. Thromb Haemost. 1991;65(1):77–81.

72. Alonso-Escolano D, Medina C, Cieslik K, Radomski A, Jurasz P, Santos-Martinez MJ, et al. Protein kinase C delta mediates platelet-induced breast cancer cell invasion. J Pharmacol Exp Ther. 2006;318(1):373–80.

73. Lieubeau B, Garrigue L, Barbieux I, Meflah K, Gregoire M. The role of transforming growth factor beta 1 in the fibroblastic reaction associated with rat colorectal tumor development. Cancer Res. 1994;54(24):6526–32.

74. Shao ZM, Nguyen M, Barsky SH. Human breast carcinoma desmoplasia is PDGF initiated. Oncogene. 2000;19(38):4337–45.

75. Folkman J, Long DM Jr, Becker FF. Growth and metastasis of tumor in organ culture. Cancer. 1963;16:453–67.

76. Pinedo HM, Verheul HM, D'Amato RJ, Folkman J. Involvement of platelets in tumour angiogenesis? Lancet. 1998;352(9142):1775–7.

77. Battinelli EM, Markens BA, Italiano JE Jr. Release of angiogenesis regulatory proteins from platelet alpha granules: modulation of physiologic and pathologic angiogenesis. Blood. 2011;118(5):1359–69.

78. Holmes CE, Huang JC, Pace TR, Howard AB, Muss HB. Tamoxifen and aromatase inhibitors differentially affect vascular endothelial growth factor and endostatin levels in women with breast cancer. Clin Cancer Res. 2008;14(10):3070–6.

79. Peterson JE, Zurakowski D, Italiano JE Jr, Michel LV, Fox L, Klement GL, et al. Normal ranges of angiogenesis regulatory proteins in human platelets. Am J Hematol. 2010;85(7):487–93.

80. Jelkmann W. Pitfalls in the measurement of circulating vascular endothelial growth factor. Clin Chem. 2001;47(4):617–23.

81. Kisucka J, Butterfield CE, Duda DG, Eichenberger SC, Saffaripour S, Ware J, et al. Platelets and platelet adhesion support angiogenesis while preventing excessive hemorrhage. Proc Natl Acad Sci U S A. 2006;103(4):855–60.

82. Ma L, Perini R, McKnight W, Dicay M, Klein A, Hollenberg MD, et al. Proteinase-activated receptors 1 and 4 counter-regulate endostatin and VEGF release from human platelets. Proc Natl Acad Sci U S A. 2005;102(1):216–20.

83. Battinelli EM, Thon JN, Okazaki R, Peters CG, Vijey P, Wilkie AR, et al. Megakaryocytes package contents into separate alpha-granules that are differentially distributed in platelets. Blood Adv. 2019;3(20):3092–8.

84. Kamykowski J, Carlton P, Sehgal S, Storrie B. Quantitative immunofluorescence mapping reveals little functional coclustering of proteins within platelet alpha-granules. Blood. 2011;118(5):1370–3.

85. Pokrovskaya ID, Yadav S, Rao A, McBride E, Kamykowski JA, Zhang G, et al. 3D ultrastructural analysis of alpha-granule, dense granule, mitochondria, and canalicular system arrangement in resting human platelets. Res Pract Thromb Haemost. 2020;4(1):72–85.

86. Menter DG, Kopetz S, Hawk E, Sood AK, Loree JM, Gresele P, et al. Platelet "first responders" in wound response, cancer, and metastasis. Cancer Metastasis Rev. 2017;36(2):199–213.

87. Martinez CE, Smith PC, Palma Alvarado VA. The influence of platelet-derived products on angiogenesis and tissue repair: a concise update. Front Physiol. 2015;6:290.

88. Goel S, Wong AH, Jain RK. Vascular normalization as a therapeutic strategy for malignant and nonmalignant disease. Cold Spring Harb Perspect Med. 2012;2(3):a006486.

89. Langer H, May AE, Daub K, Heinzmann U, Lang P, Schumm M, et al. Adherent platelets recruit and induce differentiation of murine embryonic endothelial progenitor cells to mature endothelial cells in vitro. Circ Res. 2006;98(2):e2–10.

90. Ho-Tin-Noe B, Goerge T, Cifuni SM, Duerschmied D, Wagner DD. Platelet granule secretion continuously prevents intratumor hemorrhage. Cancer Res. 2008;68(16):6851–8.

91. Klement GL, Yip TT, Cassiola F, Kikuchi L, Cervi D, Podust V, et al. Platelets actively sequester angiogenesis regulators. Blood. 2009;113(12):2835–42.

92. Peterson JE, Zurakowski D, Italiano JE Jr, Michel LV, Connors S, Oenick M, et al. VEGF, PF4 and PDGF are elevated in platelets of colorectal cancer patients. Angiogenesis. 2012;15(2):265–73.

93. Kerr BA, Miocinovic R, Smith AK, Klein EA, Byzova TV. Comparison of tumor and microenvironment secretomes in plasma and in platelets during prostate cancer growth in a xenograft model. Neoplasia. 2010;12(5):388–96.

94. Lowenstein CJ. VAMP-3 mediates platelet endocytosis. Blood. 2017;130(26):2816–8.

95. Huang Y, Joshi S, Xiang B, Kanaho Y, Li Z, Bouchard BA, et al. Arf6 controls platelet spreading and clot retraction via integrin alphaIIbbeta3 trafficking. Blood. 2016;127(11):1459–67.

96. Banerjee M, Joshi S, Zhang J, Moncman CL, Yadav S, Bouchard BA, et al. Cellubrevin/vesicle-associated membrane protein-3-mediated endocytosis and trafficking regulate platelet functions. Blood. 2017;130(26):2872–83.

97. Eaton N, Drew C, Wieser J, Munday AD, Falet H. Dynamin 2 is required for GPVI signaling and platelet hemostatic function in mice. Haematologica. 2020;105(5):1414–23.

98. Janni W, Yab T, Hayes D, Cristofanilli M, Bidard F, Ignatiadis M, et al. Clinical utility of repeated circulating tumor cell (CTC) enumeration as early treatment monitoring tool in metastatic breast cancer (MBC)—a global pooled analysis with individual patient data. In: 2020 San Antonio Breast Cancer Symposium 2020; Poster GS4-08.

99. Luzzi KJ, MacDonald IC, Schmidt EE, Kerkvliet N, Morris VL, Chambers AF, et al. Multistep nature of metastatic inefficiency: dormancy of solitary cells after successful extravasation and limited survival of early micrometastases. Am J Pathol. 1998;153(3):865–73.

100. Fidler IJ. Metastasis: quantitative analysis of distribution and fate of tumor emboli labeled with 125 I-5-iodo-2′-deoxyuridine. J Natl Cancer Inst. 1970;45(4):773–82.

101. Fidler IJ. The relationship of embolic homogeneity, number, size and viability to the incidence of experimental metastasis. Eur J Cancer. 1973;9(3):223–7.

102. Brooks DE. The biorheology of tumor cells. Biorheology. 1984;21(1-2):85–91.

103. Egan K, Cooke N, Kenny D. Living in shear: platelets protect cancer cells from shear induced damage. Clin Exp Metastasis. 2014;31(6):697–704.

104. Mani SA, Guo W, Liao MJ, Eaton EN, Ayyanan A, Zhou AY, et al. The epithelial-mesenchymal transition generates cells with properties of stem cells. Cell. 2008;133(4):704–15.

105. Yu M, Bardia A, Wittner BS, Stott SL, Smas ME, Ting DT, et al. Circulating breast tumor cells exhibit dynamic changes in epithelial and mesenchymal composition. Science. 2013;339(6119):580–4.

106. Qian BZ, Li J, Zhang H, Kitamura T, Zhang J, Campion LR, et al. CCL2 recruits inflammatory monocytes to facilitate breast-tumour metastasis. Nature. 2011;475(7355):222–5.

107. Qin Z, Chen J, Zeng J, Niu L, Xie S, Wang X, et al. Effect of NK cell immunotherapy on immune function in patients with hepatic carcinoma: a preliminary clinical study. Cancer Biol Ther. 2017;18(5):323–30.

108. Hanna N, Fidler IJ. Role of natural killer cells in the destruction of circulating tumor emboli. J Natl Cancer Inst. 1980;65(4):801–9.

109. Placke T, Salih HR, Kopp HG. GITR ligand provided by thrombopoietic cells inhibits NK cell antitumor activity. J Immunol. 2012;189(1):154–60.

110. Kopp HG, Placke T, Salih HR. Platelet-derived transforming growth factor-beta down-regulates NKG2D thereby inhibiting natural killer cell antitumor reactivity. Cancer Res. 2009;69(19):7775–83.

111. Placke T, Orgel M, Schaller M, Jung G, Rammensee HG, Kopp HG, et al. Platelet-derived MHC class I confers a pseudonormal phenotype to cancer cells that subverts the antitumor reactivity of natural killer immune cells. Cancer Res. 2012;72(2):440–8.

112. Chen YQ, Trikha M, Gao X, Bazaz R, Porter AT, Timar J, et al. Ectopic expression of platelet integrin alphaIIb beta3 in tumor cells from various species and histological origin. Int J Cancer. 1997;72(4):642–8.

113. Timar J, Tovari J, Raso E, Meszaros L, Bereczky B, Lapis K. Platelet-mimicry of cancer cells: epiphenomenon with clinical significance. Oncology. 2005;69(3):185–201.

114. Aceto N, Bardia A, Miyamoto DT, Donaldson MC, Wittner BS, Spencer JA, et al. Circulating tumor cell clusters are oligoclonal precursors of breast cancer metastasis. Cell. 2014;158(5):1110–22.

115. Yao X, Choudhury AD, Yamanaka YJ, Adalsteinsson VA, Gierahn TM, Williamson CA, et al. Functional analysis of single cells identifies a rare subset of circulating tumor cells with malignant traits. Integr Biol (Camb). 2014;6(4):388–98.

116. Krog BL, Henry MD. Biomechanics of the circulating tumor cell microenvironment. Adv Exp Med Biol. 2018;1092:209–33.

117. Gkountela S, Castro-Giner F, Szczerba BM, Vetter M, Landin J, Scherrer R, et al. Circulating tumor cell clustering shapes DNA methylation to enable metastasis seeding. Cell. 2019;176(1–2):98–112 e14.

118. Malik AB. Pulmonary microembolism. Physiol Rev. 1983;63(3):1114–207.

119. Lewalle JM, Castronovo V, Goffinet G, Foidart JM. Malignant cell attachment to endothelium of ex vivo perfused human umbilical vein. Modulation by platelets, plasma and fibronectin. Thromb Res. 1991;62(4):287–98.

120. Ward Y, Lake R, Faraji F, Sperger J, Martin P, Gilliard C, et al. Platelets promote metastasis via binding tumor CD97 leading to bidirectional signaling that coordinates transendothelial migration. Cell Rep. 2018;23(3):808–22.

121. Schumacher D, Strilic B, Sivaraj KK, Wettschureck N, Offermanns S. Platelet-derived nucleotides promote tumor-cell transendothelial migration and metastasis via P2Y2 receptor. Cancer Cell. 2013;24(1):130–7.

122. Reymond N, d'Agua BB, Ridley AJ. Crossing the endothelial barrier during metastasis. Nat Rev Cancer. 2013;13(12):858–70.

123. Yan M, Jurasz P. The role of platelets in the tumor microenvironment: From solid tumors to leukemia. Biochim Biophys Acta. 2015;1863(3):392–400.

124. Redig AJ, McAllister SS. Breast cancer as a systemic disease: a view of metastasis. J Intern Med. 2013;274(2):113–26.

125. McAllister SS, Weinberg RA. The tumour-induced systemic environment as a critical regulator of cancer progression and metastasis. Nat Cell Biol. 2014;16(8):717–27.

126. Peinado H, Zhang H, Matei IR, Costa-Silva B, Hoshino A, Rodrigues G, et al. Pre-metastatic niches: organ-specific homes for metastases. Nat Rev Cancer. 2017;17(5):302–17.

127. Feng W, Madajka M, Kerr BA, Mahabeleshwar GH, Whiteheart SW, Byzova TV. A novel role for platelet secretion in angiogenesis: mediating bone marrow-derived cell mobilization and homing. Blood. 2011;117(14):3893–902.

128. Stellos K, Langer H, Daub K, Schoenberger T, Gauss A, Geisler T, et al. Platelet-derived stromal cell-derived factor-1 regulates adhesion and promotes differentiation of human CD34+ cells to endothelial progenitor cells. Circulation. 2008;117(2):206–15.

129. Rafii S, Cao Z, Lis R, Siempos II, Chavez D, Shido K, et al. Platelet-derived SDF-1 primes the pulmonary capillary vas-

cular niche to drive lung alveolar regeneration. Nat Cell Biol. 2015;17(2):123–36.

130. Kerr BA, McCabe NP, Feng W, Byzova TV. Platelets govern pre-metastatic tumor communication to bone. Oncogene. 2013;32(36):4319–24.

131. Boucharaba A, Serre CM, Gres S, Saulnier-Blache JS, Bordet JC, Guglielmi J, et al. Platelet-derived lysophosphatidic acid supports the progression of osteolytic bone metastases in breast cancer. J Clin Invest. 2004;114(12):1714–25.

132. Falanga A, Marchetti M, Russo L. Venous thromboembolism in the hematologic malignancies. Curr Opin Oncol. 2012;24(6):702–10.

133. Lemancewicz D, Bolkun L, Mantur M, Semeniuk J, Kloczko J, Dzieciol J. Bone marrow megakaryocytes, soluble P-selectin and thrombopoietic cytokines in multiple myeloma patients. Platelets. 2014;25(3):181–7.

134. Kawano M, Hirano T, Matsuda T, Taga T, Horii Y, Iwato K, et al. Autocrine generation and requirement of BSF-2/IL-6 for human multiple myelomas. Nature. 1988;332(6159):83–5.

135. Hsu J, Gu Y, Tan SL, Narula S, DeMartino JA, Liao C. Bruton's tyrosine kinase mediates platelet receptor-induced generation of microparticles: a potential mechanism for amplification of inflammatory responses in rheumatoid arthritis synovial joints. Immunol Lett. 2013;150(1–2):97–104.

136. Barry OP, Pratico D, Savani RC, FitzGerald GA. Modulation of monocyte-endothelial cell interactions by platelet microparticles. J Clin Invest. 1998;102(1):136–44.

137. Janowska-Wieczorek A, Marquez-Curtis LA, Wysoczynski M, Ratajczak MZ. Enhancing effect of platelet-derived microvesicles on the invasive potential of breast cancer cells. Transfusion. 2006;46(7):1199–209.

138. Dashevsky O, Varon D, Brill A. Platelet-derived microparticles promote invasiveness of prostate cancer cells via upregulation of MMP-2 production. Int J Cancer. 2009;124(8):1773–7.

139. Brill A, Dashevsky O, Rivo J, Gozal Y, Varon D. Platelet-derived microparticles induce angiogenesis and stimulate post-ischemic revascularization. Cardiovasc Res. 2005;67(1):30–8.

140. Janowska-Wieczorek A, Wysoczynski M, Kijowski J, Marquez-Curtis L, Machalinski B, Ratajczak J, et al. Microvesicles derived from activated platelets induce metastasis and angiogenesis in lung cancer. Int J Cancer. 2005;113(5):752–60.

141. Faldt R, Ankerst J, Zoucas E. Inhibition of platelet aggregation by myeloid leukaemic cells demonstrated in vitro. Br J Haematol. 1987;66(4):529–34.

142. Pulte D, Olson KE, Broekman MJ, Islam N, Ballard HS, Furman RR, et al. CD39 activity correlates with stage and inhibits platelet reactivity in chronic lymphocytic leukemia. J Transl Med. 2007;5:23.

143. Jaime-Perez JC, Cantu-Rodriguez OG, Herrera-Garza JL, Gomez-Almaguer D. Platelet aggregation in children with acute lymphoblastic leukemia during induction of remission therapy. Arch Med Res. 2004;35(2):141–4.

144. Gerrard JM, McNicol A. Platelet storage pool deficiency, leukemia, and myelodysplastic syndromes. Leuk Lymphoma. 1992;8(4–5):277–81.

145. Woodcock BE, Cooper PC, Brown PR, Pickering C, Winfield DA, Preston FE. The platelet defect in acute myeloid leukaemia. J Clin Pathol. 1984;37(12):1339–42.

146. Kubota Y, Tanaka T, Ohnishi H, Kitanaka A, Okutani Y, Taminato T, et al. Constitutively activated phosphatidylinositol 3-kinase primes platelets from patients with chronic myelogenous leukemia for thrombopoietin-induced aggregation. Leukemia. 2004;18(6):1127–37.

147. Bruserud O, Foss B, Hervig T. Effects of normal platelets on proliferation and constitutive cytokine secretion by human acute myelogenous leukaemia blasts. Platelets. 1997;8(6):397–404.

148. Velez J, Enciso LJ, Suarez M, Fiegl M, Grismaldo A, Lopez C, et al. Platelets promote mitochondrial uncoupling and resistance to apoptosis in leukemia cells: a novel paradigm for the bone marrow microenvironment. Cancer Microenviron. 2014;7(1–2):79–90.

149. Takagi S, Tsukamoto S, Park J, Johnson KE, Kawano Y, Moschetta M, et al. Platelets enhance multiple myeloma progression via IL-1beta upregulation. Clin Cancer Res. 2018;24(10):2430–9.

150. Ferriere JP, Bernard D, Legros M, Chassagne J, Chollet P, Gaillard G, et al. beta-Thromboglobulin in patients with breast cancer. Am J Hematol. 1985;19(1):47–53.

151. Yazaki T, Inage H, Iizumi T, Koyama A, Kanoh S, Koiso K, et al. Studies on platelet function in patients with prostatic cancer. Preliminary report. Urology. 1987;30(1):60–3.

152. Prisco D, Paniccia R, Coppo M, Filippini M, Francalanci I, Brunelli T, et al. Platelet activation and platelet lipid composition in pulmonary cancer. Prostaglandins Leukot Essent Fatty Acids. 1995;53(1):65–8.

153. Abbasciano V, Bianchi MP, Trevisani L, Sartori S, Gilli G, Zavagli G. Platelet activation and fibrinolysis in large bowel cancer. Oncology. 1995;52(5):381–4.

154. Riedl J, Pabinger I, Ay C. Platelets in cancer and thrombosis. Hamostaseologie. 2014;34(1):54–62.

155. Ay C, Simanek R, Vormittag R, Dunkler D, Alguel G, Koder S, et al. High plasma levels of soluble P-selectin are predictive of venous thromboembolism in cancer patients: results from the Vienna Cancer and Thrombosis Study (CATS). Blood. 2008;112(7):2703–8.

156. Zhuge Y, Zhou JY, Yang GD, Zu DL, Xu XL, Tian MQ, et al. Activated changes of platelet ultra microstructure and plasma granule membrane protein 140 in patients with non-small cell lung cancer. Chin Med J (Engl). 2009;122(9):1026–31.

157. Best MG, Sol N, Kooi I, Tannous J, Westerman BA, Rustenburg F, et al. RNA-Seq of tumor-educated platelets enables blood-based pan-cancer, multiclass, and molecular pathway cancer diagnostics. Cancer Cell. 2015;28(5):666–76.

158. Wurdinger T, In't Veld S, Best MG. Platelet RNA as pan-tumor biomarker for cancer detection. Cancer Res. 2020;80(7):1371–3.

159. Sol N, Wurdinger T. Platelet RNA signatures for the detection of cancer. Cancer Metastasis Rev. 2017;36(2):263–72.

160. Yang L, Jiang Q, Li DZ, Zhou X, Yu DS, Zhong J. TIMP1 mRNA in tumor-educated platelets is diagnostic biomarker for colorectal cancer. Aging (Albany NY). 2019;11(20):8998–9012.

161. Yao B, Qu S, Hu R, Gao W, Jin S, Ju J, et al. Delivery of platelet TPM3 mRNA into breast cancer cells via microvesicles enhances metastasis. FEBS Open Bio. 2019;9(12):2159–69.

162. Zaslavsky A, Baek KH, Lynch RC, Short S, Grillo J, Folkman J, et al. Platelet-derived thrombospondin-1 is a critical negative regulator and potential biomarker of angiogenesis. Blood. 2010;115(22):4605–13.

163. Bailey SE, Ukoumunne OC, Shephard EA, Hamilton W. Clinical relevance of thrombocytosis in primary care: a prospective cohort study of cancer incidence using English electronic medical records and cancer registry data. Br J Gen Pract. 2017;67(659):e405–e13.

164. Zeimet AG, Marth C, Muller-Holzner E, Daxenbichler G, Dapunt O. Significance of thrombocytosis in patients with epithelial ovarian cancer. Am J Obstet Gynecol. 1994;170(2):549–54.

165. Rajkumar A, Szallasi A. Paraneoplastic thrombocytosis in breast cancer. Anticancer Res. 2013;33(10):4545–6.

166. Voutsadakis IA. Thrombocytosis as a prognostic marker in gastrointestinal cancers. World J Gastrointest Oncol. 2014;6(2):34–40.

167. Stone RL, Nick AM, McNeish IA, Balkwill F, Han HD, Bottsford-Miller J, et al. Paraneoplastic thrombocytosis in ovarian cancer. N Engl J Med. 2012;366(7):610–8.

168. Coward J, Kulbe H, Chakravarty P, Leader D, Vassileva V, Leinster DA, et al. Interleukin-6 as a therapeutic target in human ovarian cancer. Clin Cancer Res. 2011;17(18):6083–96.

169. Rossi JF, Negrier S, James ND, Kocak I, Hawkins R, Davis H, et al. A phase I/II study of siltuximab (CNTO 328), an anti-

interleukin-6 monoclonal antibody, in metastatic renal cell cancer. Br J Cancer. 2010;103(8):1154–62.

170. Sasaki Y, Takahashi T, Miyazaki H, Matsumoto A, Kato T, Nakamura K, et al. Production of thrombopoietin by human carcinomas and its novel isoforms. Blood. 1999;94(6):1952–60.

171. Kowanetz M, Wu X, Lee J, Tan M, Hagenbeek T, Qu X, et al. Granulocyte-colony stimulating factor promotes lung metastasis through mobilization of Ly6G+Ly6C+ granulocytes. Proc Natl Acad Sci U S A. 2010;107(50):21248–55.

172. Suzuki A, Takahashi T, Nakamura K, Tsuyuoka R, Okuno Y, Enomoto T, et al. Thrombocytosis in patients with tumors producing colony-stimulating factor. Blood. 1992;80(8):2052–9.

173. Estrov Z, Talpaz M, Mavligit G, Pazdur R, Harris D, Greenberg SM, et al. Elevated plasma thrombopoietic activity in patients with metastatic cancer-related thrombocytosis. Am J Med. 1995;98(6):551–8.

174. Nishimura S, Nagasaki M, Kunishima S, Sawaguchi A, Sakata A, Sakaguchi H, et al. IL-1alpha induces thrombopoiesis through megakaryocyte rupture in response to acute platelet needs. J Cell Biol. 2015;209(3):453–66.

175. Amirkhosravi A, Mousa SA, Amaya M, Blaydes S, Desai H, Meyer T, et al. Inhibition of tumor cell-induced platelet aggregation and lung metastasis by the oral GpIIb/IIIa antagonist XV454. Thromb Haemost. 2003;90(3):549–54.

176. Su X, Floyd DH, Hughes A, Xiang J, Schneider JG, Uluckan O, et al. The ADP receptor P2RY12 regulates osteoclast function and pathologic bone remodeling. J Clin Invest. 2012;122(10):3579–92.

177. Cho MS, Noh K, Haemmerle M, Li D, Park H, Hu Q, et al. Role of ADP receptors on platelets in the growth of ovarian cancer. Blood. 2017;130(10):1235–42.

178. Battinelli EM, Markens BA, Kulenthirarajan RA, Machlus KR, Flaumenhaft R, Italiano JE Jr. Anticoagulation inhibits tumor cell-mediated release of platelet angiogenic proteins and diminishes platelet angiogenic response. Blood. 2014;123(1):101–12.

179. Akl EA, Gunukula S, Barba M, Yosuico VE, van Doormaal FF, Kuipers S, et al. Parenteral anticoagulation in patients with cancer who have no therapeutic or prophylactic indication for anticoagulation. Cochrane Database Syst Rev. 2011;(4):CD006652.

180. Akl EA, Kahale L, Terrenato I, Neumann I, Yosuico VE, Barba M, et al. Oral anticoagulation in patients with cancer who have no therapeutic or prophylactic indication for anticoagulation. Cochrane Database Syst Rev. 2014;7:CD006466.

181. Lyman GH, Khorana AA, Kuderer NM, Lee AY, Arcelus JI, Balaban EP, et al. Venous thromboembolism prophylaxis and treatment in patients with cancer: American Society of Clinical Oncology clinical practice guideline update. J Clin Oncol. 2013;31(17):2189–204.

182. van Doormaal FF, Di Nisio M, Otten HM, Richel DJ, Prins M, Buller HR. Randomized trial of the effect of the low molecular weight heparin nadroparin on survival in patients with cancer. J Clin Oncol. 2011;29(15):2071–6.

183. Shirai T, Revenko AS, Tibbitts J, Ngo ATP, Mitrugno A, Healy LD, et al. Hepatic thrombopoietin gene silencing reduces platelet count and breast cancer progression in transgenic MMTV-PyMT mice. Blood Adv. 2019;3(20):3080–91.

184. Mammadova-Bach E, Gil-Pulido J, Sarukhanyan E, Burkard P, Shityakov S, Schonhart C, et al. Platelet glycoprotein VI promotes metastasis through interaction with cancer cell-derived galectin-3. Blood. 2020;135(14):1146–60.

185. Coyle C, Cafferty FH, Rowley S, MacKenzie M, Berkman L, Gupta S, et al. ADD-ASPIRIN: a phase III, double-blind, placebo controlled, randomised trial assessing the effects of aspirin on disease recurrence and survival after primary therapy in common non-metastatic solid tumours. Contemp Clin Trials. 2016;51:56–64.

186. Holmes MD, Chen WY, Li L, Hertzmark E, Spiegelman D, Hankinson SE. Aspirin intake and survival after breast cancer. J Clin Oncol. 2010;28(9):1467–72.

187. Rothwell PM, Fowkes FG, Belch JF, Ogawa H, Warlow CP, Meade TW. Effect of daily aspirin on long-term risk of death due to cancer: analysis of individual patient data from randomised trials. Lancet. 2011;377(9759):31–41.

188. Frisk G, Ekberg S, Lidbrink E, Eloranta S, Sund M, Fredriksson I, et al. No association between low-dose aspirin use and breast cancer outcomes overall: a Swedish population-based study. Breast Cancer Res. 2018;20(1):142.

189. Cronin-Fenton DP, Heide-Jorgensen U, Ahern TP, Lash TL, Christiansen P, Ejlertsen B, et al. Low-dose aspirin, nonsteroidal anti-inflammatory drugs, selective COX-2 inhibitors and breast cancer recurrence. Epidemiology. 2016;27(4):586–93.

190. Jordan F, Quinn TJ, McGuinness B, Passmore P, Kelly JP, Tudur Smith C, et al. Aspirin and other non-steroidal anti-inflammatory drugs for the prevention of dementia. Cochrane Database Syst Rev. 2020;4:CD011459.

191. Jin MZ, Jin WL. The updated landscape of tumor microenvironment and drug repurposing. Signal Transduct Target Ther. 2020;5(1):166.

192. Futakuchi M, Ogawa K, Sano M, Tamano S, Takeshita F, Shirai T. Suppression of lung metastasis by aspirin but not indomethacin in an in vivo model of chemically induced hepatocellular carcinoma. Jpn J Cancer Res. 2002;93(10):1175–81.

193. Lucotti S, Cerutti C, Soyer M, Gil-Bernabe AM, Gomes AL, Allen PD, et al. Aspirin blocks formation of metastatic intravascular niches by inhibiting platelet-derived COX-1/thromboxane A2. J Clin Invest. 2019;129(5):1845–62.

194. Johnson KE, Ceglowski JR, Roweth HG, Forward JA, Tippy MD, El-Husayni S, et al. Aspirin inhibits platelets from reprogramming breast tumor cells and promoting metastasis. Blood Adv. 2019;3(2):198–211.

195. Thorat MA, Cuzick J. Prophylactic use of aspirin: systematic review of harms and approaches to mitigation in the general population. Eur J Epidemiol. 2015;30(1):5–18.

196. Reimers MS, Bastiaannet E, Langley RE, van Eijk R, van Vlierberghe RL, Lemmens VE, et al. Expression of HLA class I antigen, aspirin use, and survival after a diagnosis of colon cancer. JAMA Intern Med. 2014;174(5):732–9.

197. Cardwell CR, Kunzmann AT, Cantwell MM, Hughes C, Baron JA, Powe DG, et al. Low-dose aspirin use after diagnosis of colorectal cancer does not increase survival: a case-control analysis of a population-based cohort. Gastroenterology. 2014;146(3):700–8 e2.

Neurogenesis in the Tumor Microenvironment

Heidrun Vethe, Ole Vidhammer Bjørnstad, Manuel Carrasco, and Lars A. Akslen

Abstract

The nervous system branches throughout the body in a way similar to the circulatory system, innervates almost all tissues, and regulates normal tissue homeostasis and function. Although it is well known that both the vascular system and the immune system display strong influences on cancer, nerves have often been seen as more silent partners in the tumor microenvironment. However, studies from different tissue types have revealed similarities in how the nervous system regulates normal and neoplastic cellular function. Therefore, neural-cancer crosstalk, both systemically and locally within the tumor microenvironment, is now emerging as a crucial hallmark of cancer initiation, growth, and metastasis.

H. Vethe (✉) · O. V. Bjørnstad · M. Carrasco · L. A. Akslen
Centre for Cancer Biomarkers CCBIO, Department of Clinical Medicine, University of Bergen, Bergen, Norway
e-mail: Heidrun.Vethe@uib.no; Ole.Bjornstad@uib.no; Manuel.Carrasco@uib.no; Lars.Akslen@uib.no

© The Author(s), under exclusive license to Springer Nature Switzerland AG 2022
L. A. Akslen, R. S. Watnick (eds.), *Biomarkers of the Tumor Microenvironment*, https://doi.org/10.1007/978-3-030-98950-7_16

"

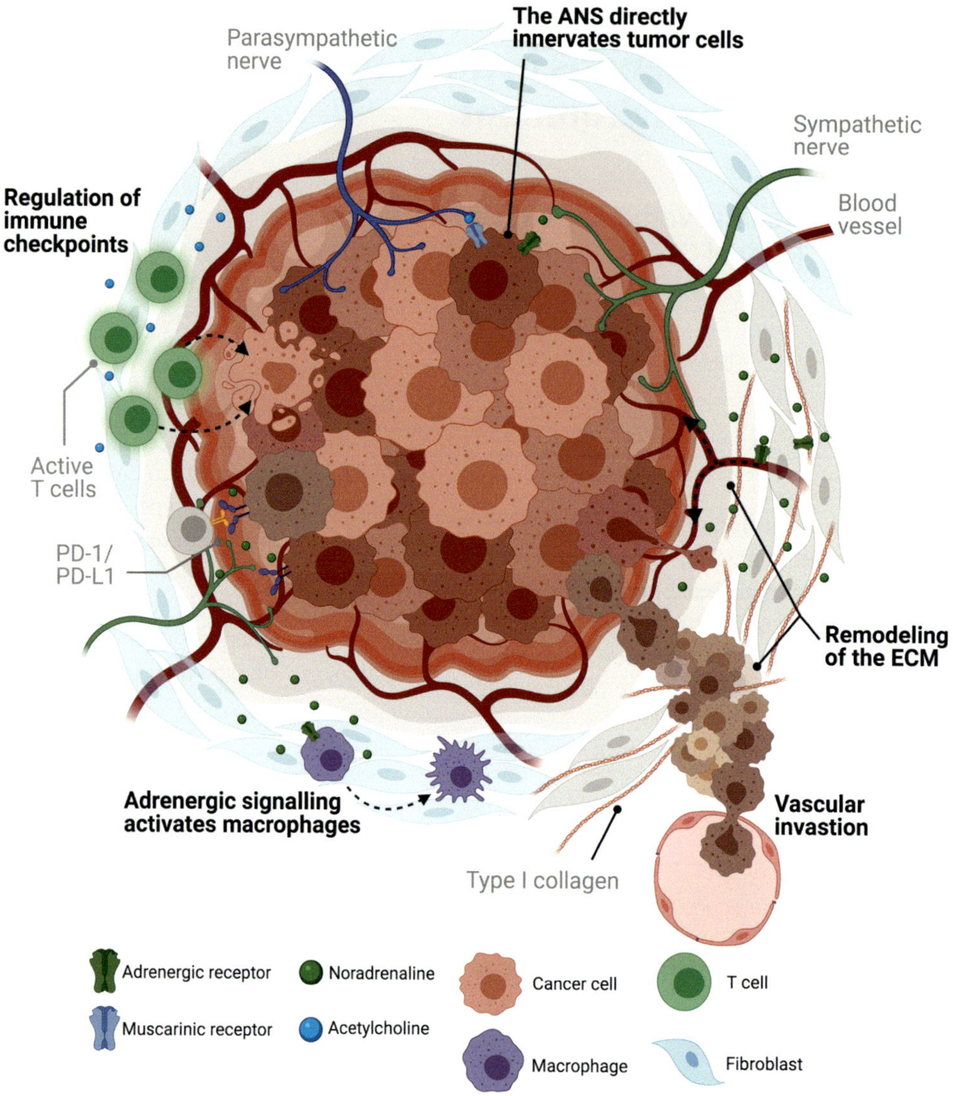

Regulation of the tumor microenvironment mediated by autonomic innervation. The autonomic nervous system (ANS) interacts directly with tumor epithelial cells, along with multiple stromal components in the tumor microenvironment (TME). Remodeling of extracellular matrix components triggered by sympathetic signaling promotes angiogenesis, tumor growth and dissemination. The immune system is another TME component regulated by nerves. Sympathetic nerves stimulate the mobilization of tumor-associated macrophages. The ANS has a dual effect on the expression of immune checkpoints such as PD-1 and PD-L1. The parasympathetic innervation can downregulate these proteins, allowing the immune system to fight malignant cells. Created with BioRender.com

Take-Home Lessons

- Presence of nerves in and around malignant tumors has recently emerged as an important feature of the tumor microenvironment
- Nerve fibers influence cancer growth, spread, therapeutic resistance and prognosis
- The function of different nerve types must be understood in a cancer-specific manner
- Different mechanisms for tumor-nerve interactions have been described, including perineural invasion, axonogenesis, and neo-neurogenesis

Background

The nervous system is involved in physiological processes from organogenesis and growth to tissue homeostasis and repair throughout the body. Similar to these roles, neural elements can also influence the initiation, growth, and metastasis of malignant tumors. This has currently emerged as an expanding and exciting field within cancer research.

The mechanisms underlying peripheral nerve-tumor interactions are largely unexplored. It is not known whether this crosstalk reflects paracrine-signaling events leading to increased neural activity in the local tumor microenvironment (TME), whether nerve-to-cancer cell synapse-like structures are formed, and whether electrical coupling exists outside the central nervous system (CNS) that enable peripheral nerves to interact with cancer cells [1].

It is now known that nerves infiltrate the TME and actively stimulate cancer cell growth and dissemination [2, 3]. This mechanism involves the paracrine release of neurotransmitters [4] into the vicinity of cancer cells and stromal cells to activate corresponding membrane receptors. In addition, the secretion of neurotrophic growth factors by cancer cells drives the outgrowth of nerves in solid tumors. In this way, reciprocal interactions between nerves and cancer cells provide new insights into the cellular and molecular basis of tumorigenesis [4, 5].

Studies in pancreatic [6, 7] and prostate cancer [4] have shown that neurotransmitters and cytokines secreted from nerves can enhance the malignant phenotype of cancer cells, including proliferation, cell survival, and invasiveness. Further, cancer cells secrete neuromodulating signals to induce neuroplasticity, neural invasion, and neuropathic pain sensation [8]. Therefore, reciprocal interactions between nerves and cancer cells cooperate to promote cancer progression.

Tumor-nerve crosstalk may also occur indirectly, by the nervous system regulating other cell types of the TME, e.g., immune cells, endothelial cells, and fibroblasts [9]. This communication may occur locally within the TME or tumor niche, or more systemically through circulating signals that might influence distant pre-metastatic tissue niches.

To better understand the mechanisms by which nerves interact with the TME to drive cancer initiation and progress, we will first review some aspects of developmental biology and regeneration. The parallels between embryonic development and cancer were first considered by Waddington in 1935 [10], linking mechanisms of development or regeneration to uncontrolled tumor growth. Waddington hypothesized that common signaling pathways in regeneration and cancer could provide cues to control cancer progression. Nerve dependence for regeneration and tissue growth was discovered in 1823 (as discussed in Boilly et al. [11]) from studies of salamander limb amputation, demonstrating that innervation was crucial for adult regeneration. The ingrowth of nerves into the blastema (the part of the tissue converted into a zone of undifferentiated progenitors [12]) starts during the early stages of wound healing in the epithelium covering the amputation site. Nerves infiltrate the blastema and recreate the neural networks necessary for regeneration, which is similar to the findings in cancer, indicating that nerves are active participants in tumor progression [11]. This emphasizes the need to investigate links between development, regeneration, and cancer.

Division of the Nervous System

In humans, the nervous system consists of the central nervous system (CNS) and the peripheral nervous system (PNS). The brain and spinal cord constitute the CNS, while the PNS consists of external nerves which connect the rest of the body to the CNS.

Central Nervous System

The CNS consists primarily of the brain and the spinal cord. It is mainly composed of grey and white matter. Grey matter is composed of cell bodies of neurons, glial cells, and capillaries, and it constitutes the outermost layer of the brain. White matter is primarily formed by myelinated axons, with thin elongated cell projections covered in myelin and created by oligodendrocytes [13].

There are two main cell types found within the CNS: neurons and glial cells. Neurons are responsible for the information relay, sensory and motor processing via specialized connections called synapses. The neuron structure varies based on their function, but generally, dendrites on the outer rim of the cell body will receive signals from other nerves. Glial cells, on the other hand, are all non-neuronal supporting cells of the CNS, including astrocytes, oligodendrocytes, microglia, and ependymal cells [14]. These cells are responsible for tissue repair upon damage, creating myelin sheaths around nerve axons, acting as the primary immune defense, and creation and locomotion of the cerebrospinal fluid of the brain, respectively.

Peripheral Nervous System

The peripheral nervous system (PNS) consists of the nerves and ganglia that connect the CNS to the rest of the body. The PNS can be subdivided into three systems: the somatic, the enteric, and the autonomic nervous system. The somatic nervous system is the voluntary division of the PNS and consists of afferent nerves (which transmit the sensory information from the body to the CNS), and efferent nerves (which exit commands from the CNS to the muscles) [15]. The enteric nervous system consists of a mesh-like network of neurons that governs the function of the gastrointestinal tract. It is influenced by the autonomic nervous system (ANS) although it might also be capable of acting independently [16]. The ANS has two branches: the sympathetic nervous system and the parasympathetic nervous system. The ANS acts mainly unconsciously, and innervates and regulates all organs in the body, except skeletal muscle. It is organized as two neurons in series, where the first originates in the CNS and connects the second neuron, which originates in a ganglion in the periphery and innervates the target gland or organ [17].

Autonomic Innervation in Cancer Tissues

A growing body of evidence suggests a link between the ANS and cancer. Multiple studies in animal models and humans have shown that sympathetic and parasympathetic nerves innervate cancer tissues and influence their behavior to promote tumor growth and distant metastasis [18–21]. The fact that the postganglionic neuronal bodies are located relatively close to the target tissues give them the ability to respond to changes in the TME, not only through neurotransmitter secretion, but also through alterations in the transcription or translation and cytoskeletal changes [9]. In addition, the different cells that make up the TME express receptors for sympathetic and parasympathetic neurotransmitters and various neuropeptides and can thereby react to nerve stimulation in ways that affect tumor growth and progression [19, 22–24].

Tumor-Nerve Interactions in the Tumor Microenvironment

Recent advances in genetical engineering and imaging have shed light on the mechanisms of neuronal regulation in cancer. An initial and more straightforward view of nerves affecting tumor proliferation, survival, and migration consider the direct action of neurotransmitters on cancer cells. For example, aberrant innervation of the epithelial cells in the stomach promotes the initiation and progression of gastric cancer [25]. Besides this, there is new evidence indicating that regulation of the TME by the nervous system has a strong impact on the tumor properties and aggressiveness (See Graphic abstract figure):

Angiogenesis is necessary for the availability of nutrients and oxygen in tumors, and therefore, for their expansion and spread. Blood vessels and sympathetic nerves share common patterning cues [26]. In prostate cancer, it has been shown how adrenergic nerves indirectly affect tumor growth by stimulating angiogenesis in the TME [22].

The immune system is another component of the TME highly regulated by the nervous system. By using genetic engineering techniques, the modulation of sympathetic and parasympathetic nerve systems in breast cancer has been shown to affect the expression of immune checkpoints and regulators, including PD-1, PD-L1, and FOXP3, with subsequent impact on antitumor immune response and breast cancer progression [21]. In a different study, sympathetic

nerves were shown to stimulate the mobilization of tumor-associated macrophages that activated a metastatic switch within the primary tumor [27].

Finally, cancer-associated fibroblasts (CAFs), a major component of the TME, have been shown to actively remodel the extracellular matrix (ECM) by producing type I collagen in response to sympathetic stimuli [28]. Such changes in the TME might promote both angiogenesis and neurogenesis, and hence cancer dissemination.

Taken together, nerves interact with both malignant cells and various components of the TME, and this multifaceted nerve-stroma interaction is decisive for tumor growth and dissemination.

Mechanisms of Nerve Involvement in Cancer

Nerve infiltration in TME has recently emerged as a key player in cancer pathogenesis [1, 2, 9], including regulation of cancer initiation, growth, and metastasis. The interaction between cancer cells and nerves is bidirectional and involves trophic factors released by nerves towards both cancer cells and surrounding stromal cells, and cancer cells secrete neurotrophic factors to stimulate nerve infiltration. In combination, the molecular mediators of the tumor-nerve crosstalk represent a dangerous duo that promote tumor-associated neural networks that boosts tumor growth and spread [4, 25, 29].

Perineural invasion was for long the only acknowledged cancer-nerve interaction, but cancer and nerves can also interact via other mechanisms, including axonal outgrowth (sprouting) of pre-existing nerves through a process of axonogenesis, and cancer-stimulated formation of new nerves from neural progenitor cells through the process of neo-neurogenesis [30]. The effects that nerves have on a specific cancer, can vary dependent on tissue type [1].

Perineural Invasion

Perineural invasion (PNI) is a process in which cancer cells invade the perineural space of surrounding nerves and move around them [31], providing a route for metastatic spread along nerves [32] (Fig. 16.1, left). Many cancer types have been observed to attract neural interaction and PNI, at least at advanced disease stages, including gastric cancer [33], lung [34], head and neck [35], pancreas [7], prostate [4], but also breast cancer [36], and PNI is considered an important pathological feature of many tumors that can also be observed in the absence of vascular invasion [31]. Although PNI has been found in many tumor types, the underlying molecular mechanisms by which cancer cells invade perineural

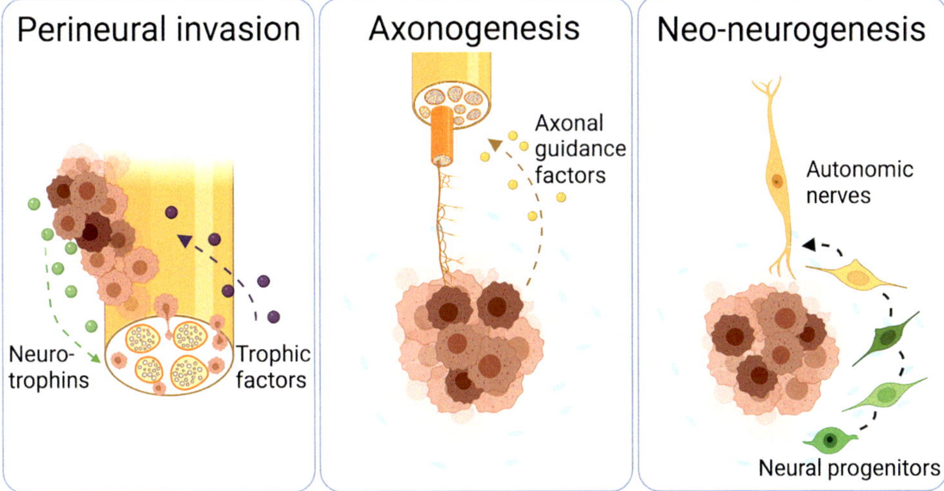

Fig. 16.1 Mechanisms of nerve involvement in cancer. *Perineural invasion* (PNI) (left) is the invasion of cancer cells to the space surrounding nerves. In this process, trophic factors are released by the nerves towards cancer cells, and cancer cells secrete neurotrophic factors to stimulate nerve infiltration. PNI can be used as a route for meta-static spread. *Axonogenesis* (center) is the outgrowth of axons from pre-existing nerves in the TME, stimulated by axonal guidance factors. *Neo-neurogenesis* (right) is the *de novo* formation of functional neurons from neural progenitor cells that are attracted to the TME by unknown mechanisms. Created with BioRender.com

spaces—including which factors are involved—have not been defined and no treatment targeting PNI is currently available.

Axonogenesis

Axonogenesis is a process that involves the outgrowth of pre-existing nerves (Fig. 16.1, center) and which expands tumor-associated nerve networks that generate neural signaling for the regulation of tumorigenesis and metastasis [4, 25]. The process of axonal sprouting shows some parallels with vascular biology [37], where growth factors that direct vessel sprouting, such as axonal guidance molecules, also regulate axonal branching. The process of axonogenesis can therefore be analogous to angiogenesis and lymphangiogenesis (i.e., the development of new lymphatic vessels in tumors) [38]. Adult neurogenesis is a dynamic process that can be stimulated under different pathological and pharmacological settings, such as injury, but is considered limited in normal physiological conditions [39].

Neo-Neurogenesis

Neo-neurogenesis involves the *de novo* production of functional neurons from neural progenitor cells and occurs throughout life (in rodents) in specific regions of the brain, the subgranular zone in the dentate gyrus of the hippocampus, the subventricular zone of the lateral ventricle [39], and to some extent in the striatum [40] and the cerebellum [41].

However, whether neo-neurogenesis also occurs in the adult human brain, is still up for discussion.

Recently, a process of cancer-specific neo-neurogenesis within the TME of prostate cancer was reported [5]. The process was defined as cancer-specific, as regeneration of sympathetic innervation after injury in normal prostate is driven by axonogenesis, without the presence of newly formed nerves [42]. In prostate cancer, neural progenitor cells (arising from the CNS) are abundantly present in the TME, and these progenitors direct the formation of new autonomic nerves in the tumor tissue [5] (Fig. 16.1, right).

This process is explained in a mouse model of prostate cancer, in which cancer development leads to an accumulation of Doublecortin (DCX) expressing neural progenitor cells in the subventricular zone. By cell tracing experiments, these authors were able to trace DCX+ neural progenitors, as these cells enter the circulation by disrupting the blood-brain barrier and migrate to the prostate to innervate the surrounding TME. The process was further associated with cancer-induced differentiation of the neural progenitors towards adrenergic nerves that have been shown to support early stages of prostate tumor development [4]. The mechanism by which the DCX+ neural progenitors are triggered to leave the brain is still unknown, but it is thought that the tumor may produce signals that attract neural progenitor cells, in turn leading to TME remodeling with increased number of cancer-associated autonomic nerves. Removal of neural progenitors from the TME of prostate cancer, significantly inhibited tumor progression in this mouse model.

The findings by Magnon et al. [5] were recently evaluated in a large cohort of prostate cancer patients [43], in which

DCX expression did not differ by disease state, grade or outcome. These findings indicate that further work is needed to define the role of DCX expressing candidate neural progenitor cells in the TME of prostate tumors and other cancer types, and future studies are needed to describe the process of cancer-associated neo-neurogenesis and elucidate the mechanisms for cancer-stimulated targeted differentiation of CNS derived neural progenitors to adrenergic nerves within the TME.

Nerve Involvement in Different Cancer Types

Recent studies have demonstrated neural participation in malignant tumors, evident by the presence of nerve fibers innervating malignant tumors and the TME. Next, we will briefly review data on nerve innervation of gastric, pancreatic, prostate, and breast cancer.

Gastric Cancer

The incidence and mortality rates of non-cardia gastric cancer has been steadily decreasing within the last half century, with large fluctuations dependent on populations [44]. However, even after curative resections, a sizable proportion of patients experience tumor recurrence with poor prognosis. In an attempt to improve patient outcomes, new pathological indicators are being explored, such as neural participation in gastric cancer.

It has been documented that PNI plays a role in cancer progression and dissemination [31]. In a meta-analysis by Zhao et al., the authors found PNI to correlate with more aggressive tumor features, such as a diffuse tumor type, larger tumor size, and tumor metastasis. Notably, the prognostic value of PNI is influenced by the variability introduced by its evaluation process [45].

The enteric nervous system is linked to epithelial homeostasis within the gastrointestinal crypts and signaling between gastric cancer cells and nerves have been reported [46, 47]. Hayakawa et al. demonstrated that the neurotransmitter acetylcholine, from both Doublecortin-like kinase 1 positive tuft cells and nerves, induces neuronal growth factor (NGF) production and expression in gastric epithelial cells. In turn, this overexpression of NGF leads to enteric nerve system expansion and innervation that promote carcinogenesis [25].

The nervous system is known to regulate both stem and progenitor cells of the epithelium, with crosstalk between tumor cells and nerves being evident [48]. This can be seen in tumors inducing active neurogenesis, and nerves in turn stimulate the growing tumor through muscarinic acetylcho-

line receptor activation by the release of acetylcholine, that has been shown to promote cancer progression [49].

Pancreatic Cancer

The pancreas is innervated by sympathetic and parasympathetic nerves [50]. However, in contrast to normal pancreatic tissue, pancreatic ductal adenocarcinoma (PDAC) is characterized by high neuronal activity, marked by high neural density and hypertrophy, thought to be caused by secretion of neurotrophins such as NGF and brain neurotrophic factor (BDNF) [6, 7]. In a recent study, Renz et al., studied the effects of stress as a growth promotor in PDAC, via β-adrenergic signaling [51]. It was found that in the crosstalk between adrenergic signaling and cancer cells, neurotrophins secretion is central to the growth of PDAC. With catecholamine signaling, induced by chronic stress, increased cancer cell secretion of NGF and BDNF has been observed, in turn stimulating axonogenesis through Trk receptors, and creating a positive feedback loop.

PDAC is thought of as a neurotropic cancer, as 70–100% of PDAC patients show PNI [52–54]. PNI in PDAC is associated with a poor prognosis and increased cancer aggressiveness [55]. The high incidence of PNI in PDAC is not clearly understood, but it reflects the strong neurotropic effects of the tumor, and the proximity of the pancreas to multiple neural plexuses might be important [56, 57]. The pain often observed in pancreatic cancers also seems to be related to PNI, as many of the molecular mechanisms involved in this process are also implicated in pain generation, such as NGF, artemin, and granulocyte colony-stimulating factor [6, 7].

The vagus nerve, a major component of the parasympathetic nervous system, has been shown to stimulate the proliferation of pancreatic exocrine cells [58]. In contrast, clinical studies have indicated that vagus nerve signaling might inhibit cancer progression and metastasis [59]. Comparable to what has been shown for stomach cancer, parasympathetic nerve signaling seems to suppress tumorigenesis.

Prostate Cancer

Nerve innervation of the prostate is one of the most studied due to its anatomical distinct neural inputs. Prostate stroma is abundantly innervated by both sympathetic and parasympathetic nerves [60], and PNI has been shown to result in increased tumor growth and spread [61]. In prostate cancer, innervation from newly formed sympathetic nerves contributes to initiation [4], while parasympathetic signaling is important for cancer progression [29].

Magnon et al. were the first to demonstrate the ability of nerves to stimulate prostate cancer progression [4]. In a mouse model of prostate cancer, the authors reported that prostate tumors were infiltrated by sympathetic adrenergic nerves (expressing tyrosine hydroxylase) and parasympathetic cholinergic fibers (expressing vesicular acetylcholine transported (VAChT)). A kinetic analysis of autonomic nerve infiltration, coupled to a measurement of tumor size and metastasis occurrence, suggested that sympathetic nerves stimulated the early stages of cancer progression, while parasympathetic nerves were found to activate cancer cell dissemination at later stages. Potential clinical relevance was evaluated, and the density of sympathetic and parasympathetic nerves was higher in tumors with poor clinical outcomes [4]. In a later study, Mauffrey et al. reported increased expression of DCX+ neural progenitors derived from the CNS in the stroma of prostate cancer, where they are differentiated towards adrenergic neurons that were further associated with tumor aggressiveness, invasion, and recurrence [5].

Breast Cancer

The role of nerve innervation in breast cancer is an understudied phenomenon. Anatomical and histological assessments show that the normal breast is innervated by sympathetic and sensory nerves [62], in which sensory nerves supply the skin and nipple, while sympathetic nerves innervate blood vessels and ducts. The breast is not considered a highly innervated tissue, and from immunohistochemical staining for selected nerve markers in normal breast, nerve fibers are rarely detected, with the exception of nerve bundles [36, 63].

The presence of nerves in the TME of breast tumors have been reported in several studies [36, 63–65], and in breast cancer, axonogenesis has been assumed to be associated with tumor aggressiveness that is driven by NGF production [36, 66]. In a study of over 350 breast cancer tissue specimens [36], tumor-associated nerve fibers (marked by protein gene product 9.5, III beta-tubulin, and neurofilament) correlated with poor differentiation, lymph node metastasis, high clinical staging, and a triple-negative subtype.

As mentioned before, an increasing number of studies are hinting towards a link between autonomic innervation and cancer [9, 18]. Experimental rodent studies suggest that chronic stress accelerates cancer growth and progression via β-adrenergic stimulation, potentially via sympathetic neural mechanisms [27]. Findings from the study suggest activation of the sympathetic nervous system as a regulator of breast cancer metastasis and further proposed antimetastatic treatment targeting the β-adrenergic induction of pro-metastatic gene expression in primary breast cancer. Clinical studies have shown that blocking of β-adrenergic receptors reduces recurrence rates and morbidity in breast cancer patients [67, 68]. In an experimental study of rodents, Kamiya et al. showed the antagonistic innervation of sympathetic and parasympathetic nerves in the breast TME, demonstrating that sympathetic innervation stimulated tumor growth and progression, while parasympathetic innervation had the opposite effect. These findings were further supported by assessment of sympathetic and parasympathetic nerve density in a relatively small sample size of breast cancer patients ($n = 29$), in which a higher density of tumor-associated sympathetic nerves and a lower density of parasympathetic nerve fibers was associated with poor clinical outcome [21].

With regards to the recent findings in prostate cancer, demonstrating that sympathetic and parasympathetic nerves contribute to cancer initiation and progression, and that neural progenitors from the CNS contributes to neo-neurogenesis [4, 5], it will be interesting to study more closely the molecular mechanisms of nerve dependence of breast cancer and the role of different nerve types on tumor progression, and also to search for signals that drive the differentiation of peripheral nerve fibers from CNS derived neural progenitor cells.

The function of a given nerve type must be understood in a context-specific manner, as parasympathetic nerves inhibit growth and progression in PDAC [51], while in the stomach, parasympathetic nerves appear to promote gastric tumorigenesis [25]. Prostate cancer is highly innervated by both sympathetic and parasympathetic nerves, in which both nerve types promote cancer progression [4]. In breast cancer, the recent finding by Kamiya et al. indicates the opposite effect of sympathetic and parasympathetic nerves [21]. Importantly, these studies suggest that nerves may drive opposite effects on different tumor types, by promoting growth in one tissue while inhibiting cancer growth in other organs.

Overview of Nerve Markers

Most nerves in the TME are small fibers or individual axons that require specific neuronal biomarkers to be detected by immunohistochemical staining. In this chapter, we will highlight a few of these neural markers often used in translational cancer studies.

Neurofilament

Neurofilaments are a unique group of cytoskeletal intermediary filaments. The neurofilament triplet proteins—light, medium, and heavy (NF-L, NF-M, and NF-H, respectively)—are neuron-specific (NF-L in breast cancer, Fig. 16.2). In the CNS, the neurofilament triplet proteins have been shown to co-express Internexin-alpha (INA) [69].

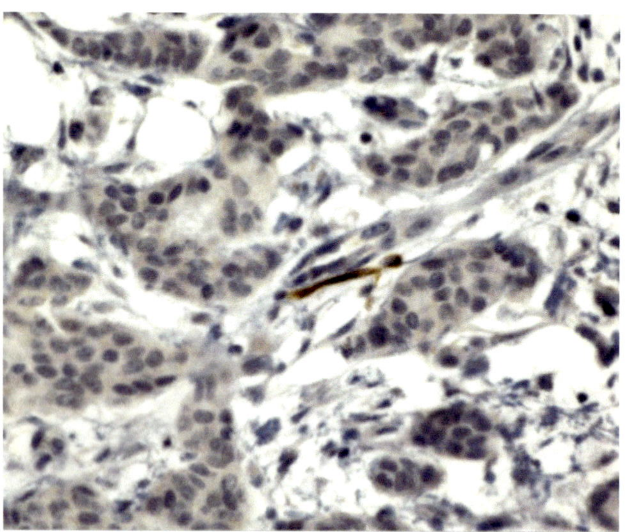

Fig. 16.2 Nerve fibers in breast cancer. IHC for Neurofilament showing isolated nerve fibers (axons) in the stroma (TME) of breast cancer

Neurofilaments are primarily expressed in axons, where they stabilize axonic protrusions [70], which begin with the polymerization of NF-L and INA. The two largest subunits NF-M and NF-H are expressed in more mature and protruded axons. NFs are therefore the main component of the cytoskeleton in mature neurons, with NF-L and INA being expressed earlier than NF-M and NF-H [71].

Class III Beta Tubulin

Microtubules are built by α/β heterodimers, with a linear expression where the α-tubulin is directed towards the rear end of the microtubule and the β-tubulin faces the front [72]. The expression of Class III β-tubulin (βIII-tubulin) is primarily centered around neural crest-derived cells; however, its expression can also be induced in both normal and neoplastic tissues [73, 74]. Classically, βIII-tubulin is an early neuronal marker [75, 76], and recent discoveries suggest βIII-tubulin as a marker for stemness within these cells [77].

Doublecortin

Doublecortin (DCX), is a microtubule-associated protein that aids microtubule stabilization [78]. DCX is a marker associated with neural progenitors and axonal growth cone of migrating central and peripheral neurons [79, 80]. Although DCX is a microtubule-associated protein, it can be demonstrated immunocytochemically in pre-migratory neuroblasts [81].

Autonomic Nerve Markers

In addition to the above-mentioned nerve markers, sympathetic nerves are marked by the expression of tyrosine hydroxylase (TH), and parasympathetic nerves express vesicular acetylcholine transported (VAChT) [4, 21]. TH is present in the CNS and in sympathetic neurons of the PNS, where it functions as the rate-limiting enzyme in the biosynthesis of noradrenaline, in which it catalyzes the conversion of L-tyrosine to L-DOPA [82]. L-DOPA is the precursor for dopamine which is the precursor for neurotransmitters noradrenaline and adrenaline. VAChT is also found in neurons of both the CNS and PNS, where it functions as a neurotransmitter transporter that loads acetylcholine into secretory vesicles [83].

Surgical and Pharmacological Denervation

Retrospective clinical studies have suggested that patients with breast cancer [27, 67, 68], melanoma [84], and prostate [85, 86] cancer that already are taking beta-blockers to treat a pre-existing condition, have lower recurrence rates and morbidity. These results support the idea that reducing stress or suppressing sympathetic activity could be a beneficial adjuvant treatment option for cancer patients [87]; however, the reported impact is relatively small [88]. Administration of beta-blockers in patients would result in a systemic effect, which makes it hard to isolate the true effects on local innervation of tumors.

Similar to regeneration, *in vivo* denervation experiments were important for the discovery of nerve dependence in cancer. Denervation by surgical cutting of afferent nerves, or the local injection of neurotoxic drugs using botulinum toxin or 6-hydroxydopamine, have shown promising results [4, 33]. As demonstrated in mouse models, vagal denervation in gastric cancer involves inhibition of cholinergic signaling and muscarinic receptors [25, 33]. Peripheral nerves consist of groups with different types of nerve fibers such that surgical resection of a peripheral nerve leads to disruption of all the nerve fibers within that nerve. Therefore, the function of a specific nerve type, cannot be studied separately. Potential limitations of experimental denervation therefore include unspecific or incomplete denervation but does not take into account potential cancer-induced nerve regeneration. The effect of different types of nerves on cancer progression remains to be characterized in depth and highlights the need for future studies in different cancer types to study the true importance of cancer-associated neural elements.

Future Perspectives

Nerve fibers were for a long time seen as silent spectators of the TME, but recent studies have demonstrated neural participation in and around malignant tumors, and a new field of research focusing on cancer neuroscience is emerging.

Nerves are difficult to study by regular histology, but big nerve trunks can be seen and constitute the basis for assessing perineural invasion by pathological examination [31]. Although identifying nerves within the TME of different tumors can be similar to looking for needles in a haystack, several studies mentioned earlier have suggested that neural marker density correlates with aggressive tumor features.

The nervous system is among the most complex "organs" and is correspondingly difficult to study *in vivo* and by tissue culture models. Targeting the direct interaction between nervous components and cancer cells requires sophisticated *in vitro* co-culture systems. These experiments can provide useful information about the molecular crosstalk involved. Moreover, a focus on the influence of the nervous system on local stomal cells and remodeling of the TME is needed. Single-cell analysis, lineage tracing, molecular characterization, and neural differentiation profiling will be required to define the mechanisms by which different nerves, and different types of cancer cells, are connected. Precise targeting of tumor-nerve interactions will provide new opportunities for improving outcomes for many tumors.

Within the emerging field of *cancer neuroscience*, many questions still remain to be answered; where do the nerves in the TME of different cancer types come from? through which mechanisms can tumors recruit new nerves? does the density of nerves correlate with more aggressive behavior? are there cancer-specific differences in the mechanisms for nerve dependence? So far, researchers have only investigated the presence and role of nerves in a few cancer types, and the cellular and molecular landscape and significance of cancer-associated nerves will need to be mapped in full detail.

Concluding Remarks/Summary

The presence of nerves in and around malignant tumors has recently emerged as an important feature of the tumor microenvironment. Nerve fibers influence cancer growth, spread, therapeutic resistance, and prognosis. The function of different nerve types must be understood and investigated in a cancer-specific manner. Much remains to be discovered with respect to how the central and peripheral nervous systems influence different solid tumor types and eventually how these interactions can be blocked.

References

1. Monje M, et al. Roadmap for the emerging field of cancer neuroscience. Cell. 2020;181:219–22. https://doi.org/10.1016/j.cell.2020.03.034.
2. Ondicova K, Mravec B. Role of nervous system in cancer aetio-pathogenesis. Lancet Oncol. 2010;11:596–601. https://doi.org/10.1016/S1470-2045(09)70337-7.
3. Jobling P, et al. Nerve-cancer cell cross-talk: a novel promoter of tumor progression. Cancer Res. 2015;75:1777–81. https://doi.org/10.1158/0008-5472.CAN-14-3180.
4. Magnon C, et al. Autonomic nerve development contributes to prostate cancer progression. Science. 2013;341:1236361. https://doi.org/10.1126/science.1236361.
5. Mauffrey P, et al. Progenitors from the central nervous system drive neurogenesis in cancer. Nature. 2019;569:672–8. https://doi.org/10.1038/s41586-019-1219-y.
6. Ceyhan GO, et al. Pancreatic neuropathy results in "neural remodeling" and altered pancreatic innervation in chronic pancreatitis and pancreatic cancer. Am J Gastroenterol. 2009;104:2555–65. https://doi.org/10.1038/ajg.2009.380.
7. Bapat AA, Hostetter G, Von Hoff DD, Han H. Perineural invasion and associated pain in pancreatic cancer. Nat Rev Cancer. 2011;11:695–707. https://doi.org/10.1038/nrc3131.
8. Stopczynski RE, et al. Neuroplastic changes occur early in the development of pancreatic ductal adenocarcinoma. Cancer Res. 2014;74:1718–27. https://doi.org/10.1158/0008-5472.CAN-13-2050.
9. Zahalka AH, Frenette PS. Nerves in cancer. Nat Rev Cancer. 2020;20:143–57. https://doi.org/10.1038/s41568-019-0237-2.
10. Waddington CH. Cancer and the theory of organisers. Nature. 1935;135:606–8. https://doi.org/10.1038/135606a0.
11. Boilly B, Faulkner S, Jobling P, Hondermarck H. Nerve dependence: from regeneration to cancer. Cancer Cell. 2017;31:342–54. https://doi.org/10.1016/j.ccell.2017.02.005.
12. Kragl M, et al. Cells keep a memory of their tissue origin during axolotl limb regeneration. Nature. 2009;460:60–5. https://doi.org/10.1038/nature08152.
13. Nieuwenhuys R, Voogd J, Huijzen C, v. The human central nervous system. 4th ed. Springer; 2008.
14. Jessen KR, Mirsky R. Glial cells in the enteric nervous system contain glial fibrillary acidic protein. Nature. 1980;286:736–7. https://doi.org/10.1038/286736a0.
15. Cuevas J. Reference module in biomedical sciences. Elsevier; 2015.
16. Furness JB. The enteric nervous system and neurogastroenterology. Nat Rev Gastroenterol Hepatol. 2012;9:286–94. https://doi.org/10.1038/nrgastro.2012.32.
17. Catala M, Kubis N. Gross anatomy and development of the peripheral nervous system. Handb Clin Neurol. 2013;115:29–41. https://doi.org/10.1016/B978-0-444-52902-2.00003-5.
18. Cole SW, Nagaraja AS, Lutgendorf SK, Green PA, Sood AK. Sympathetic nervous system regulation of the tumour microenvironment. Nat Rev Cancer. 2015;15:563–72. https://doi.org/10.1038/nrc3978.
19. Faulkner S, Jobling P, March B, Jiang CC, Hondermarck H. Tumor neurobiology and the war of nerves in cancer. Cancer Discov. 2019;9:702–10. https://doi.org/10.1158/2159-8290.CD-18-1398.
20. Hanoun M, Maryanovich M, Arnal-Estape A, Frenette PS. Neural regulation of hematopoiesis, inflammation, and cancer. Neuron. 2015;86:360–73. https://doi.org/10.1016/j.neuron.2015.01.026.

21. Kamiya A, et al. Genetic manipulation of autonomic nerve fiber innervation and activity and its effect on breast cancer progression. Nat Neurosci. 2019;22:1289–305. https://doi.org/10.1038/s41593-019-0430-3.

22. Zahalka AH, et al. Adrenergic nerves activate an angio-metabolic switch in prostate cancer. Science. 2017;358:321–6. https://doi.org/10.1126/science.aah5072.

23. Li J, Tian Y, Wu A. Neuropeptide Y receptors: a promising target for cancer imaging and therapy. Regen Biomater. 2015;2:215–9. https://doi.org/10.1093/rb/rbv013.

24. Hondermarck H, Jobling P. The sympathetic nervous system drives tumor angiogenesis. Trends Cancer. 2018;4:93–4. https://doi.org/10.1016/j.trecan.2017.11.008.

25. Hayakawa Y, et al. Nerve growth factor promotes gastric tumorigenesis through aberrant cholinergic Signaling. Cancer Cell. 2017;31:21–34. https://doi.org/10.1016/j.ccell.2016.11.005.

26. Eichmann A, Brunet I. Arterial innervation in development and disease. Sci Transl Med. 2014;6:252ps259. https://doi.org/10.1126/scitranslmed.3008910.

27. Sloan EK, et al. The sympathetic nervous system induces a metastatic switch in primary breast cancer. Cancer Res. 2010;70:7042–52. https://doi.org/10.1158/0008-5472.CAN-10-0522.

28. Oben JA, Yang S, Lin H, Ono M, Diehl AM. Norepinephrine and neuropeptide Y promote proliferation and collagen gene expression of hepatic myofibroblastic stellate cells. Biochem Biophys Res Commun. 2003;302:685–90. https://doi.org/10.1016/s0006-291x(03)00232-8.

29. Dobrenis K, Gauthier LR, Barroca V, Magnon C. Granulocyte colony-stimulating factor off-target effect on nerve outgrowth promotes prostate cancer development. Int J Cancer. 2015;136:982–8. https://doi.org/10.1002/ijc.29046.

30. Ayala GE, et al. Cancer-related axonogenesis and neurogenesis in prostate cancer. Clin Cancer Res. 2008;14:7593–603. https://doi.org/10.1158/1078-0432.CCR-08-1164.

31. Liebig C, Ayala G, Wilks JA, Berger DH, Albo D. Perineural invasion in cancer: a review of the literature. Cancer. 2009;115:3379–91. https://doi.org/10.1002/cncr.24396.

32. Amit M, Na'ara S, Gil Z. Mechanisms of cancer dissemination along nerves. Nat Rev Cancer. 2016;16:399–408. https://doi.org/10.1038/nrc.2016.38.

33. Zhao CM, et al. Denervation suppresses gastric tumorigenesis. Sci Transl Med. 2014;6:250ra115. https://doi.org/10.1126/scitranslmed.3009569.

34. Yilmaz A, et al. Clinical impact of visceral pleural, lymphovascular and perineural invasion in completely resected non-small cell lung cancer. Eur J Cardiothorac Surg. 2011;40:664–70. https://doi.org/10.1016/j.ejcts.2010.12.059.

35. Scanlon CS, et al. Galanin modulates the neural niche to favour perineural invasion in head and neck cancer. Nat Commun. 2015;6:6885. https://doi.org/10.1038/ncomms7885.

36. Huang D, et al. Nerve fibers in breast cancer tissues indicate aggressive tumor progression. Medicine (Baltimore). 2014;93:e172. https://doi.org/10.1097/MD.0000000000000172.

37. Carmeliet P, Tessier-Lavigne M. Common mechanisms of nerve and blood vessel wiring. Nature. 2005;436:193–200. https://doi.org/10.1038/nature03875.

38. Entschladen F, Palm D, Lang K, Drell TL, t. & Zaenker, K. S. Neoneurogenesis: tumors may initiate their own innervation by the release of neurotrophic factors in analogy to lymphangiogenesis and neoangiogenesis. Med Hypotheses. 2006;67:33–5. https://doi.org/10.1016/j.mehy.2006.01.015.

39. Ming GL, Song H. Adult neurogenesis in the mammalian brain: significant answers and significant questions. Neuron. 2011;70:687–702. https://doi.org/10.1016/j.neuron.2011.05.001.

40. Ernst A, et al. Neurogenesis in the striatum of the adult human brain. Cell. 2014;156:1072–83. https://doi.org/10.1016/j.cell.2014.01.044.

41. Ponti G, Peretto P, Bonfanti L. Genesis of neuronal and glial progenitors in the cerebellar cortex of peripuberal and adult rabbits. PLoS One. 2008;3:e2366. https://doi.org/10.1371/journal.pone.0002366.

42. Kobayashi T, Kihara K, Hyochi N, Masuda H, Sato K. Spontaneous regeneration of the seriously injured sympathetic pathway projecting to the prostate over a long period in the dog. BJU Int. 2003;91:868–72. https://doi.org/10.1046/j.1464-410x.2003.04222.x.

43. Tabrizi S, et al. Doublecortin expression in prostate adenocarcinoma and neuroendocrine Tumors. Int J Radiat Oncol Biol Phys. 2020;108:936–40. https://doi.org/10.1016/j.ijrobp.2020.06.024.

44. Sung H, et al. Global cancer statistics 2020: GLOBOCAN estimates of incidence and mortality worldwide for 36 cancers in 185 countries. CA Cancer J Clin. 2021; https://doi.org/10.3322/caac.21660.

45. Zhao B, et al. Perineural invasion as a predictive factor for survival outcome in gastric cancer patients: a systematic review and meta-analysis. J Clin Pathol. 2020;73:544–51. https://doi.org/10.1136/jclinpath-2019-206372.

46. Gross ER, et al. Neuronal serotonin regulates growth of the intestinal mucosa in mice. Gastroenterology. 2012;143:408–417 e402. https://doi.org/10.1053/j.gastro.2012.05.007.

47. Neal KB, Bornstein JC. Mapping 5-HT inputs to enteric neurons of the Guinea-pig small intestine. Neuroscience. 2007;145:556–67. https://doi.org/10.1016/j.neuroscience.2006.12.017.

48. Lundgren O, Jodal M, Jansson M, Ryberg AT, Svensson L. Intestinal epithelial stem/progenitor cells are controlled by mucosal afferent nerves. PLoS One. 2011;6:e16295. https://doi.org/10.1371/journal.pone.0016295.

49. Mattingly RR, Sorisky A, Brann MR, Macara IG. Muscarinic receptors transform NIH 3T3 cells through a Ras-dependent signalling pathway inhibited by the Ras-GTPase-activating protein SH3 domain. Mol Cell Biol. 1994;14:7943–52. https://doi.org/10.1128/mcb.14.12.7943.

50. Borden MA, Streeter JE, Sirsi SR, Dayton PA. In vivo demonstration of cancer molecular imaging with ultrasound radiation force and buried-ligand microbubbles. Mol Imaging. 2013;12:357–63.

51. Renz BW, et al. Cholinergic signaling via muscarinic receptors directly and indirectly suppresses pancreatic tumorigenesis and cancer stemness. Cancer Discov. 2018;8:1458–73. https://doi.org/10.1158/2159-8290.CD-18-0046.

52. Chen SH, et al. Perineural invasion of cancer: a complex crosstalk between cells and molecules in the perineural niche. Am J Cancer Res. 2019;9:1–21.

53. Ren K, et al. Clinical anatomy of the anterior and posterior hepatic plexuses, including relations with the pancreatic plexus: a cadaver study. Clin Anat. 2020;33:630–6. https://doi.org/10.1002/ca.23470.

54. Mavros MN, Economopoulos KP, Alexiou VG, Pawlik TM. Treatment and prognosis for patients with intrahepatic cholangiocarcinoma: systematic review and meta-analysis. JAMA Surg. 2014;149:565–74. https://doi.org/10.1001/jamasurg.2013.5137.

55. Jurcak N, Zheng L. Signaling in the microenvironment of pancreatic cancer: transmitting along the nerve. Pharmacol Ther. 2019;200:126–34. https://doi.org/10.1016/j.pharmthera.2019.04.010.

56. Stolinski C. Structure and composition of the outer connective tissue sheaths of peripheral nerve. J Anat. 1995;186(Pt 1):123–30.

57. Pour PM, Bell RH, Batra SK. Neural invasion in the staging of pancreatic cancer. Pancreas. 2003;26:322–5. https://doi.org/10.1097/00006676-200305000-00002.

58. Kiba T, et al. Ventromedial hypothalamic lesion-induced vagal hyperactivity stimulates rat pancreatic cell proliferation. Gastroenterology. 1996;110:885–93. https://doi.org/10.1053/gast.1996.v110.pm8608899.

59. De Couck M, Marechal R, Moorthamers S, Van Laethem JL, Gidron Y. Vagal nerve activity predicts overall survival in metastatic pancreatic cancer, mediated by inflammation. Cancer Epidemiol. 2016;40:47–51. https://doi.org/10.1016/j.canep.2015.11.007.

60. McVary KT, et al. Growth of the rat prostate gland is facilitated by the autonomic nervous system. Biol Reprod. 1994;51:99–107. https://doi.org/10.1095/biolreprod51.1.99.

61. Olar A, et al. Biological correlates of prostate cancer perineural invasion diameter. Hum Pathol. 2014;45:1365–9. https://doi.org/10.1016/j.humpath.2014.02.011.

62. Sarhadi NS, Shaw Dunn J, Lee FD, Soutar DS. An anatomical study of the nerve supply of the breast, including the nipple and areola. Br J Plast Surg. 1996;49:156–64. https://doi.org/10.1016/s0007-1226(96)90218-0.

63. Zhao Q, et al. The clinicopathological significance of neurogenesis in breast cancer. BMC Cancer. 2014;14:484. https://doi.org/10.1186/1471-2407-14-484.

64. Tsang WY, Chan JK. Neural invasion in intraductal carcinoma of the breast. Hum Pathol. 1992;23:202–4. https://doi.org/10.1016/0046-8177(92)90247-z.

65. Mitchell BS, Schumacher U, Stauber VV, Kaiserling E. Are breast tumours innervated? Immunohistological investigations using antibodies against the neuronal marker protein gene product 9.5 (PGP 9.5) in benign and malignant breast lesions. Eur J Cancer. 1994;30A:1100–3. https://doi.org/10.1016/0959-8049(94)90465-0.

66. Pundavela J, et al. Nerve fibers infiltrate the tumor microenvironment and are associated with nerve growth factor production and lymph node invasion in breast cancer. Mol Oncol. 2015;9:1626–35. https://doi.org/10.1016/j.molonc.2015.05.001.

67. Barron TI, Connolly RM, Sharp L, Bennett K, Visvanathan K. Beta blockers and breast cancer mortality: a population- based study. J Clin Oncol. 2011;29:2635–44. https://doi.org/10.1200/JCO.2010.33.5422.

68. Melhem-Bertrandt A, et al. Beta-blocker use is associated with improved relapse-free survival in patients with triple-negative breast cancer. J Clin Oncol. 2011;29:2645–52. https://doi.org/10.1200/JCO.2010.33.4441.

69. Yuan A, et al. Alpha-internexin is structurally and functionally associated with the neurofilament triplet proteins in the mature CNS. J Neurosci. 2006;26:10006–19. https://doi.org/10.1523/JNEUROSCI.2580-06.2006.

70. Thyagarajan A, Strong MJ, Szaro BG. Post-transcriptional control of neurofilaments in development and disease. Exp Cell Res. 2007;313:2088–97. https://doi.org/10.1016/j.yexcr.2007.02.014.

71. Wang H, et al. Neurofilament proteins in axonal regeneration and neurodegenerative diseases. Neural Regen Res. 2012;7:620–6. https://doi.org/10.3969/j.issn.1673-5374.2012.08.010.

72. Mariani M, et al. Class III beta-tubulin in normal and cancer tissues. Gene. 2015;563:109–14. https://doi.org/10.1016/j.gene.2015.03.061.

73. Raspaglio G, et al. Hypoxia induces class III beta-tubulin gene expression by HIF-1alpha binding to its 3′ flanking region. Gene. 2008;409:100–8. https://doi.org/10.1016/j.gene.2007.11.015.

74. Raspaglio G, et al. Sox9 and Hif-2alpha regulate TUBB3 gene expression and affect ovarian cancer aggressiveness. Gene. 2014;542:173–81. https://doi.org/10.1016/j.gene.2014.03.037.

75. Blondheim NR, et al. Human mesenchymal stem cells express neural genes, suggesting a neural predisposition. Stem Cells Dev. 2006;15:141–64. https://doi.org/10.1089/scd.2006.15.141.

76. Foudah D, et al. Human mesenchymal stem cells express neuronal markers after osteogenic and adipogenic differentiation. Cell Mol Biol Lett. 2013;18:163–86. https://doi.org/10.2478/s11658-013-0083-2.

77. Draberova E, et al. Class III beta-tubulin is constitutively coexpressed with glial fibrillary acidic protein and nestin in midgestational human fetal astrocytes: implications for phenotypic identity. J Neuropathol Exp Neurol. 2008;67:341–54. https://doi.org/10.1097/NEN.0b013e31816a686d.

78. Ayanlaja AA, et al. Distinct features of doublecortin as a marker of neuronal migration and its implications in cancer cell mobility. Front Mol Neurosci. 2017;10:199. https://doi.org/10.3389/fnmol.2017.00199.

79. Francis F, et al. Doublecortin is a developmentally regulated, microtubule-associated protein expressed in migrating and differentiating neurons. Neuron. 1999;23:247–56. https://doi.org/10.1016/s0896-6273(00)80777-1.

80. Schaar BT, Kinoshita K, McConnell SK. Doublecortin microtubule affinity is regulated by a balance of kinase and phosphatase activity at the leading edge of migrating neurons. Neuron. 2004;41:203–13. https://doi.org/10.1016/s0896-6273(03)00843-2.

81. Sarnat HB. Clinical neuropathology practice guide 5-2013: markers of neuronal maturation. Clin Neuropathol. 2013;32:340–69. https://doi.org/10.5414/NP300638.

82. Kaufman S. Tyrosine hydroxylase. Adv Enzymol Relat Areas Mol Biol. 1995;70:103–220. https://doi.org/10.1002/9780470123164.ch3.

83. Arvidsson U, Riedl M, Elde R, Meister B. Vesicular acetylcholine transporter (VAChT) protein: a novel and unique marker for cholinergic neurons in the central and peripheral nervous systems. J Comp Neurol. 1997;378:454–67.

84. Lemeshow S, et al. Beta-blockers and survival among Danish patients with malignant melanoma: a population-based cohort study. Cancer Epidemiol Biomark Prev. 2011;20:2273–9. https://doi.org/10.1158/1055-9965.EPI-11-0249.

85. Grytli HH, Fagerland MW, Fossa SD, Tasken KA. Association between use of beta-blockers and prostate cancer-specific survival: a cohort study of 3561 prostate cancer patients with high-risk or metastatic disease. Eur Urol. 2014;65:635–41. https://doi.org/10.1016/j.eururo.2013.01.007.

86. Grytli HH, Fagerland MW, Fossa SD, Tasken KA, Haheim LL. Use of beta-blockers is associated with prostate cancer-specific survival in prostate cancer patients on androgen deprivation therapy. Prostate. 2013;73:250–60. https://doi.org/10.1002/pros.22564.

87. Saloman JL, Albers KM, Rhim AD, Davis BM. Can stopping nerves, stop cancer? Trends Neurosci. 2016;39:880–9. https://doi.org/10.1016/j.tins.2016.10.002.

88. Sorensen GV, et al. Use of beta-blockers, angiotensin-converting enzyme inhibitors, angiotensin II receptor blockers, and risk of breast cancer recurrence: a Danish nationwide prospective cohort study. J Clin Oncol. 2013;31:2265–72. https://doi.org/10.1200/JCO.2012.43.9190.

Neuropilins as Cancer Biomarkers: A Focus on Neuronal Origin and Specific Cell Functions

Dakshnapriya Balasubbramanian, Yao Gao, and Diane R. Bielenberg

Abstract

The Neuropilin (NRP) family of type I integral membrane proteins is essential for multiple steps in the metastatic cascade. The dynamic duo of NRP1 and NRP2 act as co-receptors for a multitude of stimulatory growth factors such as VEGF, PGF, HGF, and PDGF. Alternately, NRPs can bind to ligands of the SEMA3 family of chemorepulsive guidance cues. Consequently, these unique receptors can toggle between opposing pro-tumorigenic and anticancer roles. Their location on the cell surface, tissue specificity patterns, and soluble isoforms make them ideal for targeted therapies, diagnostics, and biomarker analysis in cancer. This chapter focuses on the expression of NRPs in neuronal stem cells and malignant tumors of neuronal origin including gliomas and melanomas. The function of each NRP receptor is cell type specific and ligand dependent.

Take-Home Lessons

- Neuropilin-1 and Neuropilin-2 are essential co-receptors for multiple ligands.
- In cancer cells, neuropilins mediate pro-tumorigenic functions of VEGF and HGF.
- However, SEMA3 ligands primarily inhibit tumor progression.
- Neuropilins mediate survival and guidance in neurons, neural crest cells, and melanocytes.
- Increased neuropilin expression correlates with poor prognosis in tumors of neuronal origin such as glioblastoma, medulloblastoma, and melanoma.

D. Balasubbramanian · Y. Gao · D. R. Bielenberg (✉)
Vascular Biology Program, Boston Children's Hospital, Karp Family Research Laboratories, 12.213, Boston, MA, USA

Department of Surgery, Harvard Medical School, Boston, MA, USA
e-mail: diane.bielenberg@childrens.harvard.edu

Introduction to Neuropilins

The Neuropilin (NRP, human; Nrp, mouse) receptors were first discovered as neuronal recognition molecules, hence their name [1]. These type I protein receptors have been intensely studied over the past three decades and are important regulators of diverse processes associated with cancer progression such as growth, migration, invasion, epithelial-to-mesenchymal transition (EMT), and metastasis (reviewed by [2–6]). This receptor family is composed of two homologous proteins, Neuropilin 1 (NRP1) and Neuropilin 2 (NRP2), that share similar domain structures but have unique ligand specificities [7]. The *Nrp1* gene was originally discovered in Xenopus; however, both *Nrp1* and *Nrp2* are highly conserved across many species. Human *NRP1* is located in chromosome 10p11.22, while *NRP2* is found in chromosome 2q33.3 [8]. Both NRP glycoproteins are approximately 130 kilodaltons with 80–90% of the receptor structure oriented outside the cell and a small internal cytoplasmic region with no intrinsic kinase activity (Fig. 17.1).

The extracellular domains of the NRP proteins are essential for mediating disparate ligand binding and dimerization. The N-terminal amino acid sequence of NRP encodes two CUB (complement C1r/C1s, Uegf, Bmp1) motifs called a1 and a2 that mediate binding to the class 3 subfamily of semaphorin (SEMA3) guidance proteins. Following these regions are two coagulation factor 5/8 domains called b1 and b2 that mediate binding to the vascular endothelial growth factor (VEGF) family of angiogenic proteins. Interestingly, crystal structure analyses demonstrate that the NRP a1 domain sits apart from the more tightly packed a2b1b2 domain core [9, 10]. The remaining extracellular region composes the c domain with structural similarity to MAM (meprin, A-5 protein, and mu receptor protein-tyrosine phosphatase). The NRP c domain binds calcium and is thought to mediate adhesion due to its conserved cysteines which likely form disulfide bridges during receptor dimerization [11–14].

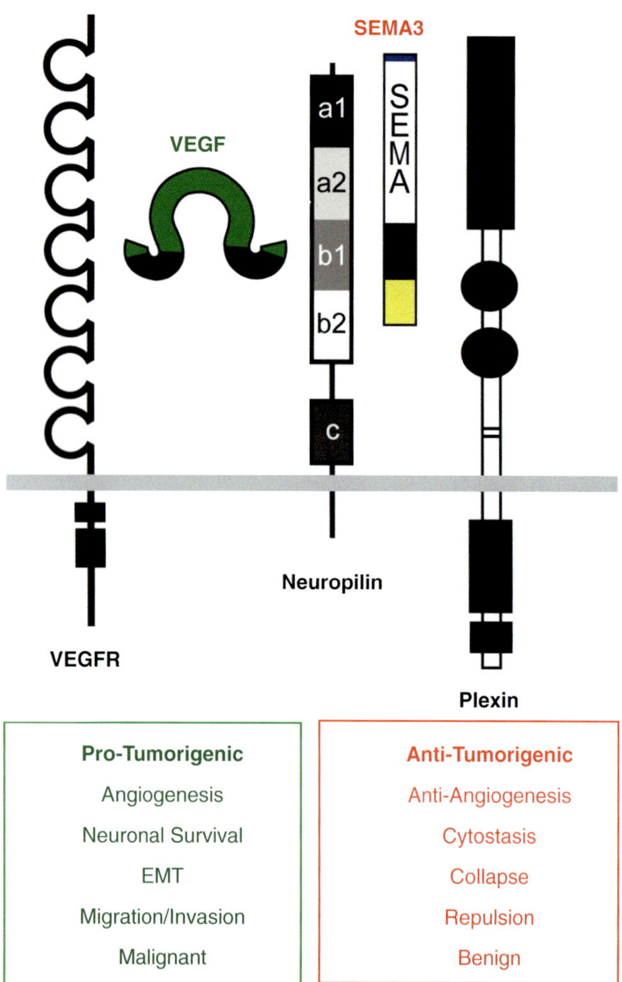

Fig. 17.1 Graphic Abstract. Neuropilins function as essential co-receptors for disparate ligand families and mediate a myriad of diverse functions. In cancer, neuropilins mediate pro-tumorigenic functions primarily through the VEGF and HGF protein families and their cognate receptor tyrosine kinases. On the other hand, SEMA3 ligands bind neuropilins and signal through plexins to attenuate tumor progression

Alternative mRNA splicing of *NRP*s results in multiple isoforms including soluble and transmembrane proteins [15]. The full-length NRP1 isoform consists of 17 exons (923 aa) [16]. Another transmembrane NRP1 isoform (907aa) lacks exon 16, which encodes a region close to the transmembrane domain, yet retains VEGF-binding capacity [17]. The NRP2 receptor exists as four variants: two NRP2a isoforms (926 aa and 931 aa) and two NRP2b isoforms (901 aa and 906 aa) [16, 18]. The cytoplasmic domains of NRP1 and NRP2a are comparable in size and both terminate in the same three amino acids: serine (S), glutamic acid (E), and alanine (A). Conversely, NRP2b has a shorter cytoplasmic region and lacks these terminal amino acids [18]. The S-E-A motif is essential for binding to scaffolding and endocytic pathway proteins that commonly contain a PDZ (PSD95, Dlg1, Zo1) domain. For example, synectin, also called neu-

ropilin interacting protein (NIP) or GAIP interacting protein/C-terminus (GIPC), contains a PDZ domain and binds to the SEA motif of NRP1 or NRP2a [19–21]. NRP2b cannot bind synectin; therefore, the endosomal trafficking of NRP2a and b is presumed to be different but, as yet, is not fully understood.

NRPs can bind to several different types of ligands and mediate diverse processes involved in tumor progression such as angiogenesis, lymphangiogenesis, metastasis, and immune tolerance. However, NRPs do not act alone but rather as a co-receptor complex. In each case, NRP is the ligand-binding partner while another protein transmits the signal to the cytoplasm (Fig. 17.1). As a rule, NRPs do not signal on their own and are not kinases [22–24].

The first proteins discovered to bind to NRP receptors were the SEMA3 family of secreted axonal guidance proteins [18, 25, 26]. There are seven SEMA3 family members named SEMA3A to SEMA3G. Each shares a common 7-bladed β-propeller structure called the "Sema" domain which is homologous to α integrins [27]. SEMA3/NRP binding specificities are complex. All SEMA3 proteins can bind to NRPs via its a1a2 domains with the exception of SEMA3E [28, 29]. Some SEMA3 proteins can bind to either NRP1 or NRP2 such as SEMA3B, C, D, and F, whereas other SEMA3 proteins are specific to only one NRP. For instance, SEMA3A (also called collapsin) binds solely to NRP1 [30, 31], while SEMA3G proprotein prefers NRP2 [32–34]. SEMA3F favors NRP2 with a tenfold higher affinity over NRP1 [18]. Furthermore, SEMA3F cannot functionally signal through NRP1 complexes, suggesting that NRP1 is a decoy receptor for SEMA3F [35]. Upon binding to NRPs, SEMA3 proteins then form a ternary complex with large transmembrane receptors called plexins that transmit the signal into the cell (Fig. 17.1, reviewed by [36, 37]). For instance, SEMA3/NRP leads to the activation of Plexin A1 which inhibits the RhoA pathway and the PI3K pathway [38–40]. The SEMA3-induced downstream depolymerization of f-actin filaments by active cofilin results in a "collapsing" cell phenotype, and cells without actin stress fibers cannot divide, move, or invade.

Alternately, NRPs can bind (via their b1b2 domains) to the angiogenic VEGF protein family members [9, 41–46]. Initially, NRPs were thought to have preference for the heparin-binding isoforms of VEGFA [42, 47, 48], but later studies showed that NRPs bind both $VEGFA_{121}$ and $VEGFA_{165}$ [9, 49, 50], though $VEGFA_{165}$ has a 50× stronger affinity for NRP1 receptor than NRP2 [50]. NRPs form a co-receptor complex with the canonical VEGF receptor tyrosine kinases (RTK) [42, 47, 51, 52]. The domain encoded by exon 4 of VEGFA binds to VEGFR [53], while the region encoded by exon 7/8 binds to NRP [42, 47, 50, 54]. With this dual binding, VEGF acts as a bridge between NRP and VEGFR (Fig. 17.1). After ligand binding and internalization,

VEGF/VEGFR-containing endosomes are trafficked differently depending on the presence of NRPs [55]. In fact, the presence of NRP1 (bound to synectin) causes the receptors to be recycled to the cell surface, thereby prolonging and enhancing VEGF-mediated signaling, whereas lack of NRP results in degradation (reviewed by [56–58]). As such, NRPs are essential for VEGF signaling [59] with Nrp1 important for endothelial tip cell formation [60] and Nrp2 essential for initiating sprout formation from tip cells [61]. Mutant mice studies demonstrate the fundamental role Nrps play in angiogenesis [62–64] and arteriovenous patterning [65].

NRPs have now been shown to bind numerous growth factors including VEGFA, VEGFC, VEGFD, placental growth factor (PGF), platelet-derived growth factor (PDGF), hepatocyte growth factor (HGF), and transforming growth factor beta (TGFβ) [43, 66–72]. These ligands all share common topographical features such as cystine-knots and beta-strands as well as heparin-binding capacity [73]. With each ligand, it is presumed that NRPs form co-receptor complexes with each ligand's cognate RTK. However, NRP (or soluble NRP) can only bind one ligand at a time, and all NRP-specific ligands have some level of competition for one another. For instance, the affinity of NRP1 for $VEGFA_{165}$ and SEMA3A is nearly equal [74] as is the affinity of NRP2 for $VEGFA_{165}$ and SEMA3F [45]; hence, these ligands are competitors. In addition to the complex biochemistry of the NRP receptor pathway, it is also important to fully understand its expression and regulation in various organs and tissues, especially in the setting of cancer, in order to use these molecules as surrogate biomarkers.

Specific Cell Functions of Neuropilins

In the first edition of "Biomarkers of the Tumor Microenvironment: Basic Studies and Practical Applications," our chapter focused on the role of NRPs in carcinoma cells and tumor angiogenesis [24]. The vital role of NRPs in endothelial cells and tumor angiogenesis and lymphangiogenesis has also been extensively reviewed elsewhere [75–77]. In this second edition, we expand on the NRP topic and summarize current knowledge regarding the expression and function of NRPs in various primary cell types including neurons, neural crest cells, and melanocytes as well as in neuronal tumors and melanoma.

Neurons

The establishment of specific, finely organized neural circuits occurs during embryonic development and early postnatal periods and is essential for proper brain functioning. Neurons are generated in spatially controlled proliferative niches and then actively migrate and extend oriented axons to form synaptic connections [78]. For this process, the SEMA3 family of ligands act as repulsive navigation cues located at defined points along the neuronal networks. Subsequent to binding SEMA3 ligands, NRPs engage and activate plexin receptors (Plexin A1–4). Plexin-dependent regulation of cytoskeletal dynamics leads to actin depolymerization at the leading edge and redirection of the growing axon (repulsion from the source of SEMA3). SEMA3A was the first ligand reported to bind NRP1 [25] and is well known for its ability to induce growth cone collapse ex vivo (Fig. 17.2 A-B). In vivo, SEMA3A is known for its role in sympathetic axon guidance and branching of various types of nerves in the central and peripheral nervous systems [79]. SEMA3 signaling steers tangentially migrating neurons, and loss of *Sema3A* or *Nrp1* results in defasciculation and errors

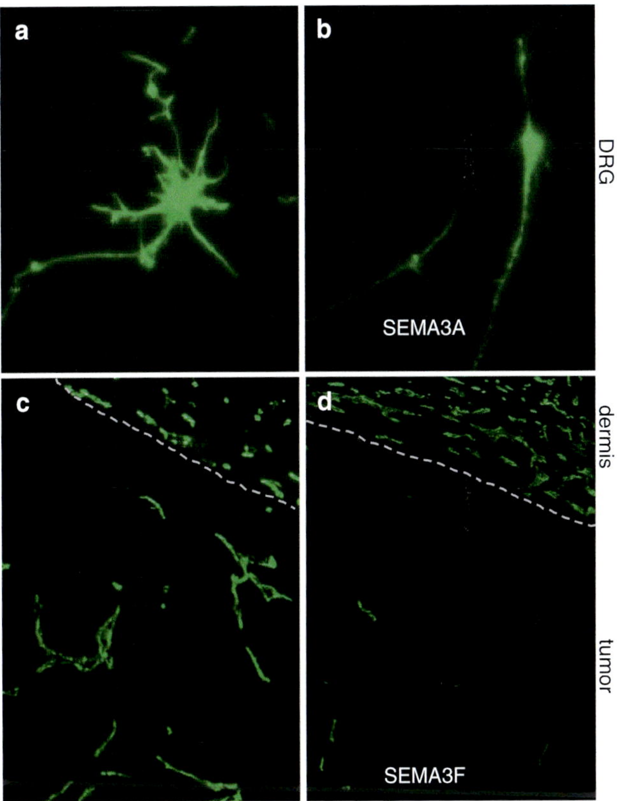

Fig. 17.2 SEMA3 proteins mediate collapse and repulsion. (**a, b**) Dorsal root ganglion (DRG), which express Nrp1, were cultured in vitro +/– SEMA3A protein. Phalloidin staining for f-actin (green color) shows axonal outgrowth in control (**a**) but collapsed growth cones after addition of SEMA3A (**b**). (**c, d**) Human melanoma xenografts were implanted in nude mice. Control tumors (**c**) show massive angiogenesis (CD31 staining, green) from the dermis (top right) into the tumor parenchyma (lower portion of each field), while melanoma overexpressing SEMA3F (**d**) does not. Mouse endothelial cells, which express Nrp2, are repelled from the SEMA3F tumor border (denoted by dotted line), and their migration and invasion are inhibited by SEMA3F resulting in a necrotic and relatively avascular tumor. All images from the Bielenberg Laboratory

in nerve bundling [80, 81]. During corticogenesis, early nervous system development, the migration of neurons out of the ventricular zone is regulated by SEMA3/NRP signaling in mice (reviewed by [2]). Nrp2-expressing neurons are guided by Sema3F into the first intermediate zone, while Nrp1-expressing neurons guided by Sema3A travel farther into the subplate and come to rest in the cortical plate or marginal zone [82]. Intermediate neurons (or interneurons) connect two brain regions to the appropriate layer. Cortical interneuron progenitors originate in the ganglionic eminence (GE) and migrate tangentially around the striatum into the cortex [83]. Sema3A and Sema3F are expressed in the striatum and repel cortical interneurons expressing Nrp1 or Nrp2 [84]. In fact, *Nrp2*-deficient mice demonstrate an excess of neurons that enter the striatum [82]. In contrast, lateral olfactory (LOT) neurons start in the neocortex and migrate perpendicular toward the GE (opposite direction of the cortical intermediate neurons). The spacing of Nrp2-positive LOT neurons along the GE/neocortex border is conducted by Sema3F-induced repulsion from the mantle layer of the GE [85]. Sema3F/Nrp2 also controls sensory innervation of the olfactory bulb [86, 87].

Beyond the central nervous system, the SEMA3/NRP axes affect the spatial patterning of other neuronal progenitors such as gonadotropin-releasing hormone (GnRH) neurons and neural crest cells (NCC). GnRH neurons originate from stem cells in the nasal placode and migrate into the forebrain and hypothalamus [88]. Their journey from nose to brain is guided by Nrp2 as evidenced by twice as many GnRH neurons in the nasal septum and a paucity of GnRH neurons in the hypothalamus of *Nrp2*-deficient mice embryos compared to wildtype embryos [89]. These neurons control reproduction by stimulating the release of gonadotropin from the pituitary gland which, in turn, causes the systemic release of luteinizing hormone and follicle stimulating hormone. *Nrp2*-knockout mice have fertility issues and hypogonadism that may be partially explained by this deficit in GnRH neurons [86, 89, 90].

Neural crest cells (NCC) are transient stem cells unique to vertebrates that give rise to a variety of cell types including neurons, melanocytes, and connective tissues [91]. Early in embryonic development, the neural tube gives rise to various subtypes of NCC: cardiac, trunk, cranial, vagal, or sacral (reviewed by [92]). Defects in cranial NCC migration result in craniofacial malformations, the most common birth defect in humans. In zebrafish, atypical patterning of Sema3F or Sema3G results in aberrant cranial NCC migration [93]. Even in early jawless vertebrates such as the lamprey, Sema3F expression is essential for proper NCC differentiation into ganglia and melanocytes in the head [94]. Anomalous cranial neural crest migration, characterized by connections between NCC streams entering branchial arches 1/2, was seen in mice with deletions of either Sema3F or

Nrp2 [95, 96]. Exogenous expression of soluble NRP-Fc in chick embryos caused NCC to migrate into formerly crest-free zones [97]. Taken together, both NRPs aid in NCC navigation, and without these pathways, the cranial nervous system loses its segmentation and overall function [98]. Trunk NCC are discussed below in detail in the melanocyte section.

Neuronal Tumors

Although NRP expression is downregulated in most tissues after birth [99, 100], many studies have correlated the progression of neuronal tumors (e.g., gliomas, astrocytic tumors, medulloblastomas) with the upregulation of NRP receptors [101–104]. Glioblastoma multiforme (GBM), the most prevalent form of malignant adult brain cancer, is characterized by robust angiogenesis and intratumoral heterogeneity which contributes to its therapeutic resistance [105]. Although GBMs express very high levels of VEGFA, clinical trials incorporating anti-VEGF (bevacizumab) therapy only improved progression-free survival in glioblastoma patients but did not influence overall survival [106, 107]. GBMs have a high recurrence rate that has been partly attributed to the presence of cancer stem-like cells (CSC) within the primary tumor that may be adept at evading current therapies [108]. Although NRPs are frequently expressed in cancer cells, it is rare to find expression of VEGFR2 in cancer cells as it is typically an endothelial-specific marker [99, 109]. However, some highly aggressive cancer cells have been reported to upregulate VEGFR2 [110, 111]. Recent studies have isolated CD133-positive GBM CSC and reported the co-expression of VEGFR2 and NRP1 [112]. As described above (in the Introduction section), NRP1 acts as a co-receptor for VEGF with VEGFR2 to enhance VEGF activity [57]. In GBM CSC, NRP1 promotes the recycling of VEGFR2 back to the cell surface, thereby sustaining and prolonging VEGF-induced effects [112]. Knockdown of NRP1 in human glioma cells led to a concomitant decrease in membranous VEGFR2 levels and increased apoptosis in CSC [112]. In another study, depletion of NRP1 in patient-derived GBM cells reduced the expression of stem cell markers [113]. Silencing *NRP1* in GBM cells including U373, U87MG, A172, and others inhibited proliferation and migration in vitro [112–116] and hindered GBM xenograft growth in vivo to prolong survival in tumor-bearing mice [113]. Novel NRP1-targeting peptides have been used to image gliomas in mice [117] and to repress rat and human glioma growth in vivo [118]. In fact, monoclonal antibodies targeting human NRP1 have also been shown to effectively inhibit glioma cell proliferation and migration in vitro and attenuate the growth of U87 GBM xenografts in immunocompromised mice [119]. Collectively, these studies suggest that targeting NRP in tumor cells, in addition to tumor-associated blood vessels, may prove therapeutically beneficial for neuronal cancers.

In addition to VEGF, other stimulatory ligands have also been reported to signal through NRPs in the tumor microenvironment. HGF is an autocrine growth factor released from glioma cells that signals through the cMET tyrosine kinase receptor, and NRP1 acts as a co-receptor for HGF/cMET [114]. RNA interference of endogenous NRP1 attenuated HGF-stimulated glioma cell growth, blocked p-cMET activation, and prevented downstream activation of p-ERK1/2 and p-BAD (dephosphorylation of BAD is pro-apoptotic) [114]. Intracellularly, p130Cas phosphorylation might be involved in NRP1-mediated HGF and PDGF signaling in glioma cells, as knockdown of NRP1 or p130Cas inhibited the growth factor-induced migration of these cells [120]. More recently, NRP1 was also identified as a receptor for glial cell-derived neurotrophic factor (GDNF), a growth factor that is highly expressed in glioblastoma multiforme. siRNA-mediated silencing of *NRP1* slowed the proliferation rate of glioma cells in response to GDNF [121].

Intense NRP1 expression correlates with decreased overall survival in medulloblastoma patients ($p = 0.0058$) [122]. The NRP ligand, PGF, is secreted from medulloblastoma tumor cells and from surrounding peri-tumoral stromal cells of the cerebellum [122]. NRP1 acts as a co-receptor for PGF/VEGFR1 signaling in endothelial cells [43]. Interestingly, although PGF promotes growth and survival of medulloblastoma cells, only NRP1 inhibition, but not VEGFR1 inhibition, could suppress tumorigenicity and metastasis to spinal cord of D283-MED cells [122]. NRP2 has been implicated in mediating hedgehog signaling, which contributes to medulloblastoma growth. Murine Med1-MB cells in culture showed reduced proliferation upon silencing of *Nrp2*, while *Nrp1* knockdown had little effect [123].

In contrast to the stimulatory ligands of NRPs (VEGFA/C, HGF, PGF), the expression of SEMA3 ligands is negatively correlated with the progression of neuronal tumors. Expression of NRP2 and VEGF-C together ($p = 0.023$) were found to be independent prognostic factors associated with poor survival in human GBM [124], whereas other researchers found SEMA3B ($p = 0.029$) and SEMA3G ($p = 0.016$) expression to associate with prolonged survival [125]. Consistent with these findings, systemic overexpression of SEMA3F (delivered via adenovirus) completely blocked all growth of NRP2-expressing U87MG cells implanted subcutaneously in nude mice [40]. The dramatic antitumor effects of SEMA3F are likely due to direct cytostatic activity in tumor cells as well as indirect effects on tumor angiogenesis. Yet, the local repulsive phenotype of SEMA3 ligands may create problems for invasive brain tumors like GBM. For example, autocrine SEMA3A/NRP1 signaling may promote GBM dispersal and infiltration. GBM cells secrete SEMA3A, and silencing of endogenous SEMA3A inhibits GBM cell

migration [115]. Moreover, SEMA3A decreases cell-substrate adhesion of GBM cells in an NRP1-dependent manner [115]. For anti-angiogenic therapy, monoclonal antibodies to NRP1 have been engineered to block VEGF binding but not SEMA3 binding, with the idea that SEMA3 signaling will also block angiogenesis [126]. However for use in GBM, it may be more effective to block both the a and b domains of NRP to avoid all ligand binding or to target the c domain to interfere with receptor dimerization.

Melanocytes

During embryogenesis, trunk NCC that progress through the dorsolateral route into the ectoderm give rise to melanoblasts, the precursor cells of melanocytes [127]. Similar to cranial and cardiac NCC, the NRP/SEMA3 pathways are critical to the guidance and migration of the trunk NCC [91, 128]. Specifically, NCC in the trunk express the Nrp2 receptor and are repelled by SEMA3F emanating from the posterior-half somite. However, deletion of *Sema3F* or *Nrp2* during this process results in uniform migration of these stem cells and loss of segmentation in their arrangement [96]. Melanoblasts, in turn, differentiate into mature melanocytes or melanocyte stem cells in the skin, hair follicle, and iris [129]. Within the hair follicle, melanocyte stem cells are located in a specialized niche called the bulge, and mature melanocytes are located in the hair bulb where they release pigment into the matrix of the hair shaft [130]. Cutaneous melanocytes represent a minority of cells in the epidermis intermingled among keratinocytes and anchored to the basement membrane in the basal layer. When melanocytes proliferate, they lose adhesion to the basement membrane and weave dendrites through neighboring epithelial cells [131, 132]. The primary function of melanocytes is to provide melanin protein (packaged in melanosomes) to keratinocytes to protect from the DNA-damaging effects of ultraviolet radiation. Keratinocytes help to regulate melanocyte growth via cell:cell interactions and secreted factors [133, 134].

The Nrp2 receptor is strongly expressed in melanocytes, yet its role in these cells is poorly understood. We have previously shown that mouse melanocytes express Nrp2 using *Nrp2*[+/Lacz] reporter mice [99, 100] and now show here, for the first time, melanocytes in the hair follicle of *Nrp2*[+/gfp] mice (Fig. 17.3). *Nrp2*-null mice do not lack melanin or hair; yet, the effect of Nrp2 status on melanocyte number or patterning is unknown. The secretion of SEMA3F from keratinocytes modulates dermal lymphatic networks and lymphedema [135, 136]. Therefore, it is also likely that this SEMA3F production by the superficial keratinocytes may serve to regulate melanocyte positioning within the epidermis or patterning along the basement membrane. In support of this hypothesis, exogenous SEMA3F was shown to inhibit

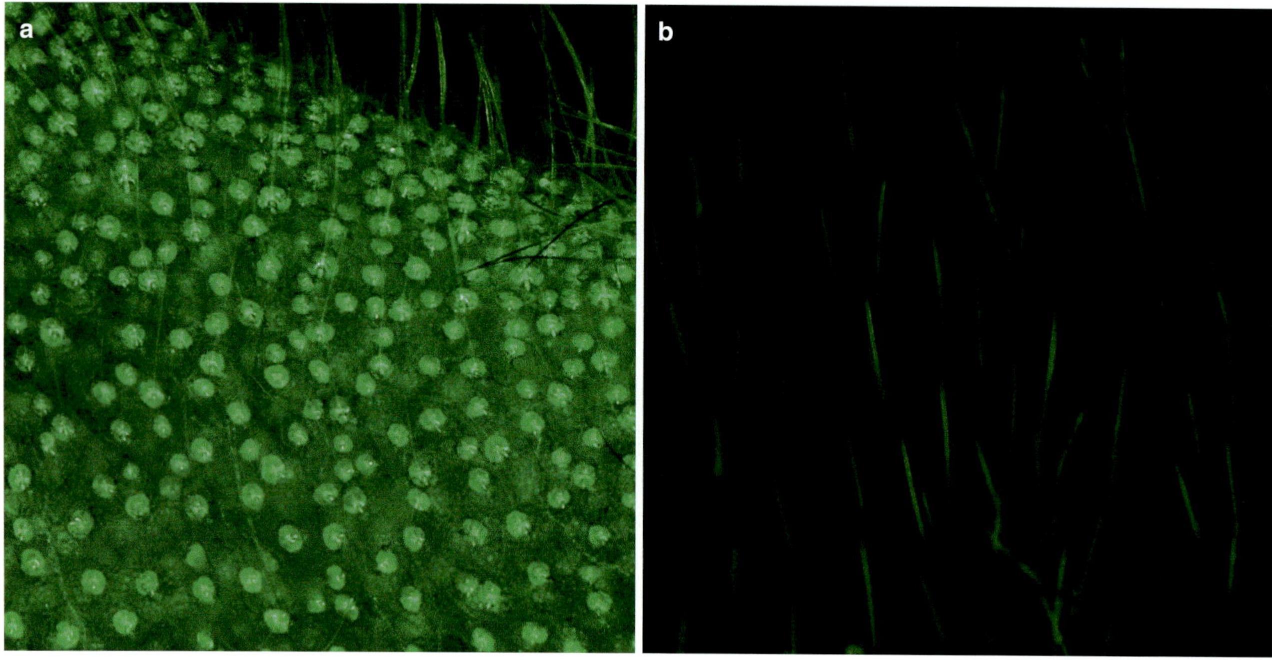

Fig. 17.3 Melanocytes express Nrp2. Fluorescent microscopy localizes Nrp2 (green color) in mouse melanocytes in the hair follicles of mutant *Nrp2+/gfp* mice skin (**a**) but not in wildtype littermates (**b**). Note that hairs are auto-fluorescent in both panels. All images from the Bielenberg Laboratory

p-AKT in primary melanocytes expressing NRP2 and Plexin A1 [40]. Further research is needed to elucidate these mechanisms. In vitro, primary melanocytes cultured in the absence of phorbol ester express Nrp1, VEGFR1, and VEGFR2 [137]. Since keratinocytes constitutively secrete VEGFA [138, 139], it is possible that VEGFA serves as a chemoattractant to melanocytes to induce proliferation or migration via NRP/VEGFR signaling. However, normal mouse melanocytes were not observed to express VEGFR2 in vivo in $VEGFR2^{+/LacZ}$ reporter mice [139].

Melanoma

The growth of melanocytes to form a melanocytic nevus (or mole) is very common in the skin, and the vast majority of all nevi are noncancerous. However, one-third of all melanomas, neuroectodermal neoplasms arising from melanocytes, begin as (dysplastic) nevi that later progress to malignance (recently reviewed by [140, 141]). The mechanisms responsible for this pathologic shift are under intense study but are often associated with activating mutations in the *BRAF* oncogene [142]. In initial stages, called the radial growth phase, melanocytes proliferate and migrate linearly along the basement membrane of the epidermis. Cancers that are caught early in this stage are called melanoma in situ and are not metastatic because there are no blood vessels above the epidermal/dermal border. Albeit in latter stages, melanoma cells begin to grow tangentially—this is called the vertical growth phase [143]. The breach of cells through the epithelial basement membrane is the most critical step in melanoma progression as it frees the cells from the confinement of the epidermis and allows for the potential spread through dermal lymphatic capillaries or blood vessels. The transition from radial to vertical growth correlates with an increase in expression of VEGF and matrix metalloproteinases (MMP) [144–147].

Melanomas account for only 2% of all skin cancers. Yet, shockingly, melanomas are responsible for nearly all skin cancer-related deaths [148]. The neural origin of melanocytes may be one reason that melanomas display the greatest level of cerebral tropism of any cancer and why nearly 50% of end-stage melanoma patients succumb to brain metastasis [149]. Melanoma patient prognosis is correlated with initial tumor staging, degree of ulceration, and lymph node status. The 5-year survival rate is above 95% in tumors with a Breslow thickness (the depth in millimeters of tumor cells beneath the basal layer of epidermis) less than 1 mm but drops precipitously to 60–75% in those with a depth of 2.1–4 mm [150]. Therefore, early detection and accurate biomarkers are urgently needed in this disease. NRP1 and NRP2 have both been shown to correlate with melanoma stage and progression.

Compared to nevi, primary and metastatic human melanoma patient samples have increased NRP1 expression which correlates with poor patient survival [151]. In experimental studies, human melanoma cell lines expressing NRP1 and VEGFR2 showed increased migration after VEGF treatment that resulted in signaling through AKT pathways [152]. But surprisingly, melanomas lacking VEGFR2 still showed NRP1-dependent invasion through extracellular matrix by inducing MMP2 secretion. This phenotype was reversed after *NRP1* silencing and neutralized with NRP1 antibodies [152]. Further evidence linking NRP1 to melanoma aggressive behavior comes from the positive correlation between MMP2 and NRP1 expression in patient biopsies [151]. Mechanistically, NRP1 binds autocrine PGF (in addition to VEGF) in melanoma cells and mediates invasion independently of VEGFR1 [153]. More recently, NRP1 was also linked to PDGF-C-mediated invasion via p130Cas phosphorylation in melanoma cells [154]. In fact, using a Cox proportional hazards regression model (multivariate) from 460 melanotic lesions, NRP1 was found to be an independent prognostic biomarker [151]. Overexpression of SEMA3A, a NRP1 ligand, in B16 mouse melanoma cells inhibited tumorigenicity and metastasis in vivo [155].

Modern melanoma therapies such as vemurafenib (BRAF inhibitor) and ipilimumab (immune checkpoint inhibitor) have caused a 7% annual drop in overall mortality rates from melanoma (from 2013 to 2017) [148]. However, NRP1 expression has been linked to resistance in some therapies. For example, melanoma cells treated with BRAF inhibitors upregulate NRP1 as a means of escape [156]. Galectin-1 (Gal-1), an alternative NRP1 ligand, signals these cells to inhibit p27, a protein involved in cell cycle arrest, and upregulate EGFR. Remarkably, combination therapy using an allosteric inhibitor of Gal-1 and a NRP1 receptor antagonist (EG00229) was able to restore the cells' oncogene addiction and thus their sensitivity to BRAF inhibitors [157].

NRP2 levels increase with melanoma stages of progression with melanocytes<nevi<primary melanoma<metastatic melanoma [158]. In fact, biomarker analysis reveals that high NRP2 levels predict an aggressive phenotype in human melanoma patients [159]. Whereas, RNA interference of *NRP2* slowed human melanoma cell proliferation both in vitro and in xenograft models [159–161]. Recently, NRP2 immunostaining has shown great potential as a diagnostic marker to differentiate between two lesions that are challenging to differentiate: Spitz nevi (benign, low NRP2) and Spitzoid melanoma (cancer, high NRP2) [162, 163].

Lymphatic metastasis occurs early in melanoma (compared to other cancers), and tumor-associated lymphatic vessel area correlates with melanoma progression. In fact, multivariate risk analysis determined that peri-tumoral lymphatic vessel area was more accurate than tumor thickness (Breslow depth) in predicting metastasis to sentinel lymph nodes in primary melanomas [164]. Since melanoma cells highly express NRP2, they can bind and sequester lymphangiogenic proteins such as VEGFA, VEGFC, and VEGFD, thereby chemoattracting lymphatic neovascularization into the tumor microenvironment. Thus, it is no wonder that melanoma xenografts, either from cell lines or patient-derived cells, that express high NRP2 levels predominantly metastasize to draining lymph nodes rather than via hematogenous paths to the lung [165]. Hypoxia represses NRP2 expression in human melanoma cells [166]. Consequently, anti-angiogenic drugs that decrease tumor neovascularization and increase hypoxia within the tumor environment may have additional effects on melanoma cell proliferation via the transcriptional repression of *NRP2*. Preclinical trials targeting NRP2 in melanomas have included the overexpression of soluble NRP2 or SEMA3F [167, 168]. An engineered version of the NRP2 b domain was mutated to preferentially bind VEGFA, MutB-NRP2. In human melanoma models, overexpression of MutB-NRP2 inhibited melanoma tumor growth to a similar level as bevacizumab, whereas the combination of MutB-NRP2 and anti-VEGF significantly enhanced the anti-tumor response [167]. Transfection of SEMA3F into highly metastatic human melanoma cells transformed their phenotype into benign tumors [168]. In fact, SEMA3F completely eradicated metastases in this model, suggesting that *SEMA3F* is a metastasis suppressor gene in addition to a tumor suppressor [168]. Local secretion of SEMA3F from melanoma cells repelled surrounding blood vessels from entering the tumor thereby inhibiting tumor angiogenesis (Fig. 17.2C–D). This SEMA3F-induced reduction in tumor-associated vessels likely contributed to the lack of systemic metastasis [168]. NRP2 monoclonal antibodies inhibited lymphangiogenesis in various preclinical trials but have not yet been tried in melanoma models [169].

Concluding Remarks/Summary

The role of the NRP1-VEGF and NRP2-Sema3F signaling axes has been validated in multiple pre-clinical models. Notably, there have been no severe adverse side effects observed when targeting these pathways either by monoclonal antibodies or recombinant Sema3F. These findings merit further consideration and development of these agents for clinical use either alone or in combination with traditional chemotherapy or immunotherapeutic agents such as checkpoint inhibitors. Moreover, the utility of NRP1 and NRP2 as biomarkers in melanoma and GBM could help to guide strategies regarding therapeutic modalities for these aggressive and difficult to treat tumors.

References

1. Takagi S, Hirata T, Agata K, Mochii M, Eguchi G, Fujisawa H. The A5 antigen, a candidate for the neuronal recognition molecule, has homologies to complement components and coagulation factors. Neuron. 1991;7(2):295–307.

2. Schwarz Q, Ruhrberg C. Neuropilin, you gotta let me know: should I stay or should I go? Cell Adhes Migr. 2010;4(1):61–6.

3. Prud'homme GJ, Glinka Y. Neuropilins are multifunctional coreceptors involved in tumor initiation, growth, metastasis and immunity. Oncotarget. 2012;3(9):921–39.

4. Raimondi C, Ruhrberg C. Neuropilin signalling in vessels, neurons and tumours. Semin Cell Dev Biol. 2013;24(3):172–8.

5. Djordjevic S, Driscoll PC. Targeting VEGF signalling via the neuropilin co-receptor. Drug Discov Today. 2013;18(9–10):447–55.

6. Niland S, Eble JA. Neuropilin: handyman and power broker in the tumor microenvironment. Adv Exp Med Biol. 2020;1223:31–67.

7. Klagsbrun M, Takashima S, Mamluk R. The role of neuropilin in vascular and tumor biology. Adv Exp Med Biol. 2002;515:33–48.

8. Rossignol M, Beggs AH, Pierce EA, Klagsbrun M. Human neuropilin-1 and neuropilin-2 map to 10p12 and 2q34, respectively. Genomics. 1999;57(3):459–60.

9. Appleton BA, Wu P, Maloney J, Yin J, Liang WC, Stawicki S, Mortara K, Bowman KK, Elliott JM, Desmarais W, Bazan JF, Bagri A, Tessier-Lavigne M, Koch AW, Wu Y, Watts RJ, Wiesmann C. Structural studies of neuropilin/antibody complexes provide insights into semaphorin and VEGF binding. EMBO J. 2007;26(23):4902–12.

10. Janssen BJ, Malinauskas T, Weir GA, Cader MZ, Siebold C, Jones EY. Neuropilins lock secreted semaphorins onto plexins in a ternary signaling complex. Nat Struct Mol Biol. 2012;19(12):1293–9.

11. Roth L, Nasarre C, Dirrig-Grosch S, Aunis D, Crémel G, Hubert P, Bagnard D. Transmembrane domain interactions control biological functions of neuropilin-1. Mol Biol Cell. 2008;19(2):646–54.

12. Barton R, Driscoll A, Flores S, Mudbhari D, Collins T, Iovine MK, Berger BW. Cysteines in the neuropilin-2 MAM domain modulate receptor homooligomerization and signal transduction. Biopolymers. 2015;104(4):371–8.

13. Yelland T, Djordjevic S. Crystal structure of the Neuropilin-1 MAM domain: completing the Neuropilin-1 Ectodomain picture. Structure. 2016;24(11):2008–15.

14. Puszko AK, Sosnowski P, Raynaud F, Hermine O, Hopfgartner G, Lepelletier Y, Misicka A. Does cysteine rule (CysR) complete the CendR principle? Increase in affinity of peptide ligands for NRP-1 through the presence of N-terminal cysteine. Biomol Ther. 2020;10(3)

15. Pellet-Many C, Frankel P, Jia H, Zachary I. Neuropilins: structure, function and role in disease. Biochem J. 2008;411(2):211–26.

16. Rossignol M, Gagnon ML, Klagsbrun M. Genomic organization of human neuropilin-1 and neuropilin-2 genes: identification and distribution of splice variants and soluble isoforms. Genomics. 2000;70(2):211–22.

17. Tao Q, Spring SC, Terman BI. Characterization of a new alternatively spliced neuropilin-1 isoform. Angiogenesis. 2003;6(1):39–45.

18. Chen H, Chedotal A, He Z, Goodman CS, Tessier-Lavigne M. Neuropilin-2, a novel member of the neuropilin family, is a high affinity receptor for the semaphorins Sema E and Sema IV but not Sema III. Neuron. 1997;19(3):547–59.

19. Cai H, Reed RR. Cloning and characterization of neuropilin-1-interacting protein: a PSD-95/Dlg/ZO-1 domain-containing protein that interacts with the cytoplasmic domain of neuropilin-1. J Neurosci. 1999;19(15):6519–27.

20. Wang L, Mukhopadhyay D, Xu X. C terminus of RGS-GAIP-interacting protein conveys neuropilin-1-mediated signaling during angiogenesis. FASEB J. 2006;20(9):1513–5.

21. Prahst C, Héroult M, Lanahan AA, Uziel N, Kessler O, Shraga-Heled N, Simons M, Neufeld G, Augustin HG. Neuropilin-1-VEGFR-2 complexing requires the PDZ-binding domain of neuropilin-1. J Biol Chem. 2008;283(37):25110–4.

22. Gaur P, Bielenberg DR, Samuel S, Bose D, Zhou Y, Gray MJ, Dallas NA, Fan F, Xia L, Lu J, Ellis LM. Role of class 3 semaphorins and their receptors in tumor growth and angiogenesis. Clin Cancer Res. 2009;15(22):6763–70.

23. Migliozzi MT, Mucka P, Bielenberg DR. Lymphangiogenesis and metastasis--a closer look at the neuropilin/semaphorin3 axis. Microvasc Res. 2014;96:68–76.

24. Li X, Bielenberg DR. Neuropilin 1 and Neuropilin 2: cancer progression and biomarker analysis. In: Akslen LA, Watnick RS, editors. Biomarkers of the tumor microenvironment: basic studies and practical applications. Switzerland: Springer; 2017. p. 329–49.

25. He Z, Tessier-Lavigne M. Neuropilin is a receptor for the axonal chemorepellent Semaphorin III. Cell. 1997;90(4):739–51.

26. Kolodkin AL, Levengood DV, Rowe EG, Tai YT, Giger RJ, Ginty DD. Neuropilin is a semaphorin III receptor. Cell. 1997;90(4):753–62.

27. Capparuccia L, Tamagnone L. Semaphorin signaling in cancer cells and in cells of the tumor microenvironment--two sides of a coin. J Cell Sci. 2009;122(Pt 11):1723–36.

28. Casazza A, Finisguerra V, Capparuccia L, Camperi A, Swiercz JM, Rizzolio S, Rolny C, Christensen C, Bertotti A, Sarotto I, Risio M, Trusolino L, Weitz J, Schneider M, Mazzone M, Comoglio PM, Tamagnone L. Sema3E-Plexin D1 signaling drives human cancer cell invasiveness and metastatic spreading in mice. J Clin Invest. 2010;120(8):2684–98.

29. Klagsbrun M, Shimizu A. Semaphorin 3E, an exception to the rule. J Clin Invest. 2010;120(8):2658–60.

30. Kolodkin AL, Matthes DJ, Goodman CS. The semaphorin genes encode a family of transmembrane and secreted growth cone guidance molecules. Cell. 1993;75(7):1389–99.

31. Luo Y, Raible D, Raper JA. Collapsin: a protein in brain that induces the collapse and paralysis of neuronal growth cones. Cell. 1993;75(2):217–27.

32. Taniguchi M, Masuda T, Fukaya M, Kataoka H, Mishina M, Yaginuma H, Watanabe M, Shimizu T. Identification and characterization of a novel member of murine semaphorin family. Genes Cells. 2005;10(8):785–92.

33. Kutschera S, Weber H, Weick A, De Smet F, Genove G, Takemoto M, Prahst C, Riedel M, Mikelis C, Baulande S, Champseix C, Kummerer P, Conseiller E, Multon MC, Heroult M, Bicknell R, Carmeliet P, Betsholtz C, Augustin HG. Differential endothelial transcriptomics identifies semaphorin 3G as a vascular class 3 semaphorin. Arterioscler Thromb Vasc Biol. 2011;31(1):151–9.

34. Liu X, Uemura A, Fukushima Y, Yoshida Y, Hirashima M. Semaphorin 3G provides a repulsive guidance cue to lymphatic endothelial cells via Neuropilin-2/PlexinD1. Cell Rep. 2016;17(9):2299–311.

35. Chedotal A, Del Rio JA, Ruiz M, He Z, Borrell V, de Castro F, Ezan F, Goodman CS, Tessier-Lavigne M, Sotelo C, Soriano E. Semaphorins III and IV repel hippocampal axons via two distinct receptors. Development. 1998;125(21):4313–23.

36. Cagnoni G, Tamagnone L. Semaphorin receptors meet receptor tyrosine kinases on the way of tumor progression. Oncogene. 2014;33(40):4795–802.

37. Pascoe HG, Wang Y, Zhang X. Structural mechanisms of plexin signaling. Prog Biophys Mol Biol. 2015;118(3):161–8.

38. Wu KY, Hengst U, Cox LJ, Macosko EZ, Jeromin A, Urquhart ER, Jaffrey SR. Local translation of RhoA regulates growth cone collapse. Nature. 2005;436(7053):1020–4.

39. Shimizu A, Mammoto A, Italiano JE Jr, Pravda E, Dudley AC, Ingber DE, Klagsbrun M. ABL2/ARG tyrosine kinase mediates SEMA3F-induced RhoA inactivation and cytoskeleton collapse in human glioma cells. J Biol Chem. 2008;283(40):27230–8.

40. Nakayama H, Bruneau S, Kochupurakkal N, Coma S, Briscoe DM, Klagsbrun M. Regulation of mTOR signaling by Semaphorin

3F-Neuropilin 2 interactions in vitro and in vivo. Sci Rep. 2015;5:11789.

41. Soker S, Fidder H, Neufeld G, Klagsbrun M. Characterization of novel vascular endothelial growth factor (VEGF) receptors on tumor cells that bind VEGF165 via its exon 7-encoded domain. J Biol Chem. 1996;271(10):5761–7.

42. Soker S, Takashima S, Miao HQ, Neufeld G, Klagsbrun M. Neuropilin-1 is expressed by endothelial and tumor cells as an isoform-specific receptor for vascular endothelial growth factor. Cell. 1998;92(6):735–45.

43. Mamluk R, Gechtman Z, Kutcher ME, Gasiunas N, Gallagher J, Klagsbrun M. Neuropilin-1 binds vascular endothelial growth factor 165, placenta growth factor-2, and heparin via its b1b2 domain. J Biol Chem. 2002;277(27):24818–25.

44. Klagsbrun M, Eichmann A. A role for axon guidance receptors and ligands in blood vessel development and tumor angiogenesis. Cytokine Growth Factor Rev. 2005;16(4–5):535–48.

45. Geretti E, Shimizu A, Kurschat P, Klagsbrun M. Site-directed mutagenesis in the B-neuropilin-2 domain selectively enhances its affinity to VEGF165, but not to semaphorin 3F. J Biol Chem. 2007;282(35):25698–707.

46. Shraga-Heled N, Kessler O, Prahst C, Kroll J, Augustin H, Neufeld G. Neuropilin-1 and neuropilin-2 enhance VEGF121 stimulated signal transduction by the VEGFR-2 receptor. FASEB J. 2007;21(3):915–26.

47. Soker S, Miao HQ, Nomi M, Takashima S, Klagsbrun M. VEGF165 mediates formation of complexes containing VEGFR-2 and neuropilin-1 that enhance VEGF165-receptor binding. J Cell Biochem. 2002;85(2):357–68.

48. Lee CC, Kreusch A, McMullan D, Ng K, Spraggon G. Crystal structure of the human neuropilin-1 b1 domain. Structure. 2003;11(1):99–108.

49. Vander Kooi CW, Jusino MA, Perman B, Neau DB, Bellamy HD, Leahy DJ. Structural basis for ligand and heparin binding to neuropilin B domains. Proc Natl Acad Sci U S A. 2007;104(15):6152–7.

50. Parker MW, Xu P, Li X, Vander Kooi CW. Structural basis for selective vascular endothelial growth factor-A (VEGF-A) binding to neuropilin-1. J Biol Chem. 2012;287(14):11082–9.

51. Gluzman-Poltorak Z, Cohen T, Shibuya M, Neufeld G. Vascular endothelial growth factor receptor-1 and neuropilin-2 form complexes. J Biol Chem. 2001;276(22):18688–94.

52. Neufeld G, Cohen T, Shraga N, Lange T, Kessler O, Herzog Y. The neuropilins: multifunctional semaphorin and VEGF receptors that modulate axon guidance and angiogenesis. Trends Cardiovasc Med. 2002;12(1):13–9.

53. Shibuya M, Ito N, Claesson-Welsh L. Structure and function of vascular endothelial growth factor receptor-1 and -2. Curr Top Microbiol Immunol. 1999;237:59–83.

54. Jia H, Bagherzadeh A, Hartzoulakis B, Jarvis A, Löhr M, Shaikh S, Aqil R, Cheng L, Tickner M, Esposito D, Harris R, Driscoll PC, Selwood DL, Zachary IC. Characterization of a bicyclic peptide neuropilin-1 (NP-1) antagonist (EG3287) reveals importance of vascular endothelial growth factor exon 8 for NP-1 binding and role of NP-1 in KDR signaling. J Biol Chem. 2006;281(19):13493–502.

55. Lanahan A, Zhang X, Fantin A, Zhuang Z, Rivera-Molina F, Speichinger K, Prahst C, Zhang J, Wang Y, Davis G, Toomre D, Ruhrberg C, Simons M. The neuropilin 1 cytoplasmic domain is required for VEGF-A-dependent arteriogenesis. Dev Cell. 2013;25(2):156–68.

56. Zhang X, Simons M. Receptor tyrosine kinases endocytosis in endothelium: biology and signaling. Arterioscler Thromb Vasc Biol. 2014;34(9):1831–7.

57. Kofler NM, Simons M. Angiogenesis versus arteriogenesis: neuropilin 1 modulation of VEGF signaling. F1000Prime Rep. 2015;7:26.

58. Simons M, Gordon E, Claesson-Welsh L. Mechanisms and regulation of endothelial VEGF receptor signalling. Nat Rev Mol Cell Biol. 2016;17(10):611–25.

59. Herzog B, Pellet-Many C, Britton G, Hartzoulakis B, Zachary IC. VEGF binding to NRP1 is essential for VEGF stimulation of endothelial cell migration, complex formation between NRP1 and VEGFR2, and signaling via FAK Tyr407 phosphorylation. Mol Biol Cell. 2011;22(15):2766–76.

60. Fantin A, Vieira JM, Plein A, Denti L, Fruttiger M, Pollard JW, Ruhrberg C. NRP1 acts cell autonomously in endothelium to promote tip cell function during sprouting angiogenesis. Blood. 2013;121(12):2352–62.

61. Dallinga MG, Habani YI, Schimmel AWM, Dallinga-Thie GM, van Noorden CJF, Klaassen I, Schlingemann RO. The role of Heparan sulfate and Neuropilin 2 in VEGFA signaling in human endothelial tip cells and non-tip cells during angiogenesis in vitro. Cell. 2021;10(4)

62. Kitsukawa T, Shimizu M, Sanbo M, Hirata T, Taniguchi M, Bekku Y, Yagi T, Fujisawa H. Neuropilin-semaphorin III/D-mediated chemorepulsive signals play a crucial role in peripheral nerve projection in mice. Neuron. 1997;19(5):995–1005.

63. Kawasaki T, Kitsukawa T, Bekku Y, Matsuda Y, Sanbo M, Yagi T, Fujisawa H. A requirement for neuropilin-1 in embryonic vessel formation. Development. 1999;126(21):4895–902.

64. Takashima S, Kitakaze M, Asakura M, Asanuma H, Sanada S, Tashiro F, Niwa H, Miyazaki Ji J, Hirota S, Kitamura Y, Kitsukawa T, Fujisawa H, Klagsbrun M, Hori M. Targeting of both mouse neuropilin-1 and neuropilin-2 genes severely impairs developmental yolk sac and embryonic angiogenesis. Proc Natl Acad Sci U S A. 2002;99(6):3657–62.

65. Fantin A, Schwarz Q, Davidson K, Normando EM, Denti L, Ruhrberg C. The cytoplasmic domain of neuropilin 1 is dispensable for angiogenesis, but promotes the spatial separation of retinal arteries and veins. Development. 2011;138(19):4185–91.

66. Migdal M, Huppertz B, Tessler S, Comforti A, Shibuya M, Reich R, Baumann H, Neufeld G. Neuropilin-1 is a placenta growth factor-2 receptor. J Biol Chem. 1998;273(35):22272–8.

67. Makinen T, Olofsson B, Karpanen T, Hellman U, Soker S, Klagsbrun M, Eriksson U, Alitalo K. Differential binding of vascular endothelial growth factor B splice and proteolytic isoforms to neuropilin-1. J Biol Chem. 1999;274(30):21217–22.

68. Sulpice E, Plouët J, Bergé M, Allanic D, Tobelem G, Merkulova-Rainon T. Neuropilin-1 and neuropilin-2 act as coreceptors, potentiating proangiogenic activity. Blood. 2008;111(4):2036–45.

69. Glinka Y, Prud'homme GJ. Neuropilin-1 is a receptor for transforming growth factor beta-1, activates its latent form, and promotes regulatory T cell activity. J Leukoc Biol. 2008;84(1):302–10.

70. Ball SG, Bayley C, Shuttleworth CA, Kielty CM. Neuropilin-1 regulates platelet-derived growth factor receptor signalling in mesenchymal stem cells. Biochem J. 2010;427(1):29–40.

71. Pellet-Many C, Frankel P, Evans IM, Herzog B, Jünemann-Ramírez M, Zachary IC. Neuropilin-1 mediates PDGF stimulation of vascular smooth muscle cell migration and signalling via p130Cas. Biochem J. 2011;435(3):609–18.

72. Glinka Y, Stoilova S, Mohammed N, Prud'homme GJ. Neuropilin-1 exerts co-receptor function for TGF-beta-1 on the membrane of cancer cells and enhances responses to both latent and active TGF-beta. Carcinogenesis. 2011;32(4):613–21.

73. Murray-Rust J, McDonald NQ, Blundell TL, Hosang M, Oefner C, Winkler F, Bradshaw RA. Topological similarities in TGF-beta 2, PDGF-BB and NGF define a superfamily of polypeptide growth factors. Structure. 1993;1(2):153–9.

74. Miao HQ, Soker S, Feiner L, Alonso JL, Raper JA, Klagsbrun M. Neuropilin-1 mediates collapsin-1/semaphorin III inhibition of endothelial cell motility: functional competition of col-

lapsin-1 and vascular endothelial growth factor-165. J Cell Biol. 1999;146(1):233–42.

75. Zhao L, Chen H, Lu L, Wang L, Zhang X, Guo X. New insights into the role of co-receptor neuropilins in tumour angiogenesis and lymphangiogenesis and targeted therapy strategies. J Drug Target. 2021;29(2):155–67.

76. Niland S, Eble JA. Neuropilins in the context of tumor vasculature. Int J Mol Sci. 2019;20(3)

77. Lampropoulou A, Ruhrberg C. Neuropilin regulation of angiogenesis. Biochem Soc Trans. 2014;42(6):1623–8.

78. Squarzoni P, Thion MS, Garel S. Neuronal and microglial regulators of cortical wiring: usual and novel guideposts. Front Neurosci. 2015;9:248.

79. Huber AB, Kania A, Tran TS, Gu C, De Marco Garcia N, Lieberam I, Johnson D, Jessell TM, Ginty DD, Kolodkin AL. Distinct roles for secreted semaphorin signaling in spinal motor axon guidance. Neuron. 2005;48(6):949–64.

80. Ulupinar E, Datwani A, Behar O, Fujisawa H, Erzurumlu R. Role of semaphorin III in the developing rodent trigeminal system. Mol Cell Neurosci. 1999;13(4):281–92.

81. Schwarz Q, Waimey KE, Golding M, Takamatsu H, Kumanogoh A, Fujisawa H, Cheng HJ, Ruhrberg C. Plexin A3 and plexin A4 convey semaphorin signals during facial nerve development. Dev Biol. 2008;324(1):1–9.

82. Tamamaki N, Fujimori K, Nojyo Y, Kaneko T, Takauji R. Evidence that Sema3A and Sema3F regulate the migration of GABAergic neurons in the developing neocortex. J Comp Neurol. 2003;455(2):238–48.

83. Marín O, Rubenstein JL. Cell migration in the forebrain. Annu Rev Neurosci. 2003;26:441–83.

84. Marin O, Yaron A, Bagri A, Tessier-Lavigne M, Rubenstein JL. Sorting of striatal and cortical interneurons regulated by semaphorin-neuropilin interactions. Science. 2001;293(5531):872–5.

85. Ito K, Kawasaki T, Takashima S, Matsuda I, Aiba A, Hirata T. Semaphorin 3F confines ventral tangential migration of lateral olfactory tract neurons onto the telencephalon surface. J Neurosci. 2008;28(17):4414–22.

86. Walz A, Rodriguez I, Mombaerts P. Aberrant sensory innervation of the olfactory bulb in neuropilin-2 mutant mice. J Neurosci. 2002;22(10):4025–35.

87. Walz A, Feinstein P, Khan M, Mombaerts P. Axonal wiring of guanylate cyclase-D-expressing olfactory neurons is dependent on neuropilin 2 and semaphorin 3F. Development. 2007;134(22):4063–72.

88. Wray S, Grant P, Gainer H. Evidence that cells expressing luteinizing hormone-releasing hormone mRNA in the mouse are derived from progenitor cells in the olfactory placode. Proc Natl Acad Sci U S A. 1989;86(20):8132–6.

89. Cariboni A, Hickok J, Rakic S, Andrews W, Maggi R, Tischkau S, Parnavelas JG. Neuropilins and their ligands are important in the migration of gonadotropin-releasing hormone neurons. J Neurosci. 2007;27(9):2387–95.

90. Giger RJ, Cloutier JF, Sahay A, Prinjha RK, Levengood DV, Moore SE, Pickering S, Simmons D, Rastan S, Walsh FS, Kolodkin AL, Ginty DD, Geppert M. Neuropilin-2 is required in vivo for selective axon guidance responses to secreted semaphorins. Neuron. 2000;25(1):29–41.

91. Lumb R, Wiszniak S, Kabbara S, Scherer M, Harvey N, Schwarz Q. Neuropilins define distinct populations of neural crest cells. Neural Dev. 2014;9:24.

92. Mayor R, Theveneau E. The neural crest. Development. 2013;140(11):2247–51.

93. Yu HH, Moens CB. Semaphorin signaling guides cranial neural crest cell migration in zebrafish. Dev Biol. 2005;280(2):373–85.

94. York JR, Yuan T, Lakiza O, McCauley DW. An ancestral role for Semaphorin3F-Neuropilin signaling in patterning neural crest within the new vertebrate head. Development. 2018;145(14)

95. Gammill LS, Gonzalez C, Bronner-Fraser M. Neuropilin 2/semaphorin 3F signaling is essential for cranial neural crest migration and trigeminal ganglion condensation. Dev Neurobiol. 2007;67(1):47–56.

96. Gammill LS, Gonzalez C, Bronner-Fraser M. Neuropilin 2/semaphorin 3F signaling is essential for cranial neural crest migration and trigeminal ganglion condensation. J Neurobiol. 2006;67(1):47–56.

97. Osborne NJ, Begbie J, Chilton JK, Schmidt H, Eickholt BJ. Semaphorin/neuropilin signaling influences the positioning of migratory neural crest cells within the hindbrain region of the chick. Dev Dyn. 2005;232(4):939–49.

98. Schwarz Q, Vieira JM, Howard B, Eickholt BJ, Ruhrberg C. Neuropilin 1 and 2 control cranial gangliogenesis and axon guidance through neural crest cells. Development. 2008;135(9):1605–13.

99. Bielenberg DR, Pettaway CA, Takashima S, Klagsbrun M. Neuropilins in neoplasms: expression, regulation, and function. Exp Cell Res. 2006;312(5):584–93.

100. Bielenberg DR, Seth A, Shimizu A, Pelton K, Cristofaro V, Ramachandran A, Zwaans BM, Chen C, Krishnan R, Seth M, Huang L, Takashima S, Klagsbrun M, Sullivan MP, Adam RM. Increased smooth muscle contractility in mice deficient for neuropilin 2. Am J Pathol. 2012;181(2):548–59.

101. Broholm H, Laursen H. Vascular endothelial growth factor (VEGF) receptor neuropilin-1's distribution in astrocytic tumors. APMIS. 2004;112(4–5):257–63.

102. Osada H, Tokunaga T, Nishi M, Hatanaka H, Abe Y, Tsugu A, Kijima H, Yamazaki H, Ueyama Y, Nakamura M. Overexpression of the neuropilin 1 (NRP1) gene correlated with poor prognosis in human glioma. Anticancer Res. 2004;24(2B):547–52.

103. Frankel P, Pellet-Many C, Lehtolainen P, D'Abaco GM, Tickner ML, Cheng L, Zachary IC. Chondroitin sulphate-modified neuropilin 1 is expressed in human tumour cells and modulates 3D invasion in the U87MG human glioblastoma cell line through a p130Cas-mediated pathway. EMBO Rep. 2008;9(10):983–9.

104. Law JW, Lee AY. The role of semaphorins and their receptors in gliomas. J Signal Transduct. 2012;2012:902854.

105. Friedmann-Morvinski D. Glioblastoma heterogeneity and cancer cell plasticity. Crit Rev Oncog. 2014;19(5):327–36.

106. Vredenburgh JJ, Desjardins A, Herndon JE 2nd, Dowell JM, Reardon DA, Quinn JA, Rich JN, Sathornsumetee S, Gururangan S, Wagner M, Bigner DD, Friedman AH, Friedman HS. Phase II trial of bevacizumab and irinotecan in recurrent malignant glioma. Clin Cancer Res. 2007;13(4):1253–9.

107. Chinot OL, Wick W, Mason W, Henriksson R, Saran F, Nishikawa R, Carpentier AF, Hoang-Xuan K, Kavan P, Cernea D, Brandes AA, Hilton M, Abrey L, Cloughesy T. Bevacizumab plus radiotherapy-temozolomide for newly diagnosed glioblastoma. N Engl J Med. 2014;370(8):709–22.

108. Cheray M, Bégaud G, Deluche E, Nivet A, Battu S, Lalloué F, Verdier M, Bessette B. Cancer stem-like cells. In: De Vleeschouwer S, editor. Glioblastoma. Brisbane AU: The Authors; 2017.

109. Yoshida A, Shimizu A, Asano H, Kadonosono T, Kondoh SK, Geretti E, Mammoto A, Klagsbrun M, Seo MK. VEGF-A/NRP1 stimulates GIPC1 and Syx complex formation to promote RhoA activation and proliferation in skin cancer cells. Biol Open. 2015;4(9):1063–76.

110. Migliozzi M, Hida Y, Seth M, Brown G, Kwan J, Coma S, Panigrahy D, Adam RM, Banyard J, Shimizu A, Bielenberg DR. VEGF/VEGFR2 autocrine signaling stimulates metastasis in prostate cancer cells. Curr Angiogen. 2014;3(4):231–44.

111. Hong TM, Chen YL, Wu YY, Yuan A, Chao YC, Chung YC, Wu MH, Yang SC, Pan SH, Shih JY, Chan WK, Yang PC. Targeting neuropilin 1 as an antitumor strategy in lung cancer. Clin Cancer Res. 2007;13(16):4759–68.

112. Hamerlik P, Lathia JD, Rasmussen R, Wu Q, Bartkova J, Lee M, Moudry P, Bartek J Jr, Fischer W, Lukas J, Rich JN, Bartek J. Autocrine VEGF-VEGFR2-Neuropilin-1 signaling promotes glioma stem-like cell viability and tumor growth. J Exp Med. 2012;209(3):507–20.

113. Angom RS, Mondal SK, Wang F, Madamsetty VS, Wang E, Dutta SK, Gulani Y, Sarabia-Estrada R, Sarkaria JN, Quiñones-Hinojosa A, Mukhopadhyay D. Ablation of neuropilin-1 improves the therapeutic response in conventional drug-resistant glioblastoma multiforme. Oncogene. 2020;39(48):7114–26.

114. Hu B, Guo P, Bar-Joseph I, Imanishi Y, Jarzynka MJ, Bogler O, Mikkelsen T, Hirose T, Nishikawa R, Cheng SY. Neuropilin-1 promotes human glioma progression through potentiating the activity of the HGF/SF autocrine pathway. Oncogene. 2007;26(38):5577–86.

115. Bagci T, Wu JK, Pfannl R, Ilag LL, Jay DG. Autocrine semaphorin 3A signaling promotes glioblastoma dispersal. Oncogene. 2009;28(40):3537–50.

116. Li X, Tang T, Lu X, Zhou H, Huang Y. RNA interference targeting NRP-1 inhibits human glioma cell proliferation and enhances cell apoptosis. Mol Med Rep. 2011;4(6):1261–6.

117. Wu HB, Wang Z, Wang QS, Han YJ, Wang M, Zhou WL, Li HS. Use of labelled tLyP-1 as a novel ligand targeting the NRP receptor to image glioma. PLoS One. 2015;10(9):e0137676.

118. Nasarre C, Roth M, Jacob L, Roth L, Koncina E, Thien A, Labourdette G, Poulet P, Hubert P, Crémel G, Roussel G, Aunis D, Bagnard D. Peptide-based interference of the transmembrane domain of neuropilin-1 inhibits glioma growth in vivo. Oncogene. 2010;29(16):2381–92.

119. Chen L, Miao W, Tang X, Zhang H, Wang S, Luo F, Yan J. Inhibitory effect of neuropilin-1 monoclonal antibody (NRP-1 MAb) on glioma tumor in mice. J Biomed Nanotechnol. 2013;9(4):551–8.

120. Evans IM, Yamaji M, Britton G, Pellet-Many C, Lockie C, Zachary IC, Frankel P. Neuropilin-1 signaling through p130Cas tyrosine phosphorylation is essential for growth factor-dependent migration of glioma and endothelial cells. Mol Cell Biol. 2011;31(6):1174–85.

121. Sun S, Lei Y, Li Q, Wu Y, Zhang L, Mu PP, Ji GQ, Tang CX, Wang YQ, Gao J, Gao J, Li L, Zhuo L, Li YQ, Gao DS. Neuropilin-1 is a glial cell line-derived neurotrophic factor receptor in glioblastoma. Oncotarget. 2017;8(43):74019–35.

122. Snuderl M, Batista A, Kirkpatrick ND, Ruiz de Almodovar C, Riedemann L, Walsh EC, Anolik R, Huang Y, Martin JD, Kamoun W, Knevels E, Schmidt T, Farrar CT, Vakoc BJ, Mohan N, Chung E, Roberge S, Peterson T, Bais C, Zhelyazkova BH, Yip S, Hasselblatt M, Rossig C, Niemeyer E, Ferrara N, Klagsbrun M, Duda DG, Fukumura D, Xu L, Carmeliet P, Jain RK. Targeting placental growth factor/neuropilin 1 pathway inhibits growth and spread of medulloblastoma. Cell. 2013;152(5):1065–76.

123. Hayden Gephart MG, Su YS, Bandara S, Tsai FC, Hong J, Conley N, Rayburn H, Milenkovic L, Meyer T, Scott MP. Neuropilin-2 contributes to tumorigenicity in a mouse model of hedgehog pathway medulloblastoma. J Neuro-Oncol. 2013;115(2):161–8.

124. Zhao H, Hou C, Hou A, Zhu D. Concurrent expression of VEGF-C and Neuropilin-2 is correlated with poor prognosis in glioblastoma. Tohoku J Exp Med. 2016;238(2):85–91.

125. Karayan-Tapon L, Wager M, Guilhot J, Levillain P, Marquant C, Clarhaut J, Potiron V, Roche J. Semaphorin, neuropilin and VEGF expression in glial tumours: SEMA3G, a prognostic marker? Br J Cancer. 2008;99(7):1153–60.

126. Pan Q, Chanthery Y, Liang WC, Stawicki S, Mak J, Rathore N, Tong RK, Kowalski J, Yee SF, Pacheco G, Ross S, Cheng Z, Le Couter J, Plowman G, Peale F, Koch AW, Wu Y, Bagri A, Tessier-Lavigne M, Watts RJ. Blocking neuropilin-1 function has an additive effect with anti-VEGF to inhibit tumor growth. Cancer Cell. 2007;11(1):53–67.

127. Serbedzija GN, Fraser SE, Bronner-Fraser M. Pathways of trunk neural crest cell migration in the mouse embryo as revealed by vital dye labelling. Development. 1990;108(4):605–12.

128. Eickholt BJ, Mackenzie SL, Graham A, Walsh FS, Doherty P. Evidence for collapsin-1 functioning in the control of neural crest migration in both trunk and hindbrain regions. Development. 1999;126(10):2181–9.

129. Li A. The biology of melanocyte and melanocyte stem cell. Acta Biochim Biophys Sin Shanghai. 2014;46(4):255–60.

130. Myung P, Ito M. Dissecting the bulge in hair regeneration. J Clin Invest. 2012;122(2):448–54.

131. Danen EH, Jansen KF, Klein CE, Smit NP, Ruiter DJ, van Muijen GN. Loss of adhesion to basement membrane components but not to keratinocytes in proliferating melanocytes. Eur J Cell Biol. 1996;70(1):69–75.

132. Haass NK, Herlyn M. Normal human melanocyte homeostasis as a paradigm for understanding melanoma. J Investig Dermatol Symp Proc. 2005;10(2):153–63.

133. Tang A, Eller MS, Hara M, Yaar M, Hirohashi S, Gilchrest BA. E-cadherin is the major mediator of human melanocyte adhesion to keratinocytes in vitro. J Cell Sci. 1994;107(Pt 4):983–92.

134. Hsu MY, Wheelock MJ, Johnson KR, Herlyn M. Shifts in cadherin profiles between human normal melanocytes and melanomas. J Investig Dermatol Symp Proc. 1996;1(2):188–94.

135. Mucka P, Levonyak N, Geretti E, Zwaans BMM, Li X, Adini I, Klagsbrun M, Adam RM, Bielenberg DR. Inflammation and lymphedema are exacerbated and prolonged by Neuropilin 2 deficiency. Am J Pathol. 2016;186(11):2803–12.

136. Uchida Y, James JM, Suto F, Mukouyama YS. Class 3 semaphorins negatively regulate dermal lymphatic network formation. Biol Open. 2015;4(9):1194–205.

137. Kim EJ, Park HY, Yaar M, Gilchrest BA. Modulation of vascular endothelial growth factor receptors in melanocytes. Exp Dermatol. 2005;14(8):625–33.

138. Detmar M, Yeo KT, Nagy JA, Van de Water L, Brown LF, Berse B, Elicker BM, Ledbetter S, Dvorak HF. Keratinocyte-derived vascular permeability factor (vascular endothelial growth factor) is a potent mitogen for dermal microvascular endothelial cells. J Invest Dermatol. 1995;105(1):44–50.

139. Shahrabi-Farahani S, Wang L, Zwaans BM, Santana JM, Shimizu A, Takashima S, Kreuter M, Coultas L, D'Amore PA, Arbeit JM, Akslen LA, Bielenberg DR. Neuropilin 1 expression correlates with differentiation status of epidermal cells and cutaneous squamous cell carcinomas. Lab Investig. 2014;94(7):752–65.

140. Leonardi GC, Falzone L, Salemi R, Zanghì A, Spandidos DA, McCubrey JA, Candido S, Libra M. Cutaneous melanoma: from pathogenesis to therapy (review). Int J Oncol. 2018;52(4):1071–80.

141. Kodet O, Kučera J, Strnadová K, Dvořánková B, Štork J, Lacina L, Smetana K Jr. Cutaneous melanoma dissemination is dependent on the malignant cell properties and factors of intercellular crosstalk in the cancer microenvironment (review). Int J Oncol. 2020;57(3):619–30.

142. Damsky WE, Bosenberg M. Melanocytic nevi and melanoma: unraveling a complex relationship. Oncogene. 2017;36(42):5771–92.

143. Laga AC, Murphy GF. Cellular heterogeneity in vertical growth phase melanoma. Arch Pathol Lab Med. 2010;134(12):1750–7.

144. Väisänen A, Tuominen H, Kallioinen M, Turpeenniemi-Hujanen T. Matrix metalloproteinase-2 (72 kD type IV collagenase) expression occurs in the early stage of human melanocytic tumour progression and may have prognostic value. J Pathol. 1996;180(3):283–9.

145. Hofmann UB, Westphal JR, Van Muijen GN, Ruiter DJ. Matrix metalloproteinases in human melanoma. J Invest Dermatol. 2000;115(3):337–44.

146. Streit M, Detmar M. Angiogenesis, lymphangiogenesis, and melanoma metastasis. Oncogene. 2003;22(20):3172–9.

147. Rajabi P, Neshat A, Mokhtari M, Rajabi MA, Eftekhari M, Tavakoli P. The role of VEGF in melanoma progression. J Res Med Sci. 2012;17(6):534–9.

148. Siegel RL, Miller KD, Jemal A. Cancer statistics, 2020. CA Cancer J Clin. 2020;70(1):7–30.

149. Tawbi HA, Boutros C, Kok D, Robert C, McArthur G. New era in the management of melanoma brain metastases. Am Soc Clin Oncol Educ Book. 2018;38:741–50.

150. Puckett Y, Wilson AM, Farci F, Thevenin C. Melanoma Pathology, in StatPearls2021, ©. Treasure Island FL: StatPearls Publishing LLC; 2021.

151. Lu J, Cheng Y, Zhang G, Tang Y, Dong Z, McElwee KJ, Li G. Increased expression of neuropilin 1 in melanoma progression and its prognostic significance in patients with melanoma. Mol Med Rep. 2015;12(2):2668–76.

152. Ruffini F, D'Atri S, Lacal PM. Neuropilin-1 expression promotes invasiveness of melanoma cells through vascular endothelial growth factor receptor-2-dependent and -independent mechanisms. Int J Oncol. 2013;43(1):297–306.

153. Pagani E, Ruffini F, Antonini Cappellini GC, Scoppola A, Fortes C, Marchetti P, Graziani G, D'Atri S, Lacal PM. Placenta growth factor and neuropilin-1 collaborate in promoting melanoma aggressiveness. Int J Oncol. 2016;48(4):1581–9.

154. Ruffini F, Levati L, Graziani G, Caporali S, Atzori MG, D'Atri S, Lacal PM. Platelet-derived growth factor-C promotes human melanoma aggressiveness through activation of neuropilin-1. Oncotarget. 2017;8(40):66833–48.

155. Chakraborty G, Kumar S, Mishra R, Patil TV, Kundu GC. Semaphorin 3A suppresses tumor growth and metastasis in mice melanoma model. PLoS One. 2012;7(3):e33633.

156. Rizzolio S, Cagnoni G, Battistini C, Bonelli S, Isella C, Van Ginderachter JA, Bernards R, Di Nicolantonio F, Giordano S, Tamagnone L. Neuropilin-1 upregulation elicits adaptive resistance to oncogene-targeted therapies. J Clin Invest. 2018;128(9):3976–90.

157. Rizzolio S, Corso S, Giordano S, Tamagnone L. Autocrine signaling of NRP1 ligand Galectin-1 elicits resistance to BRAF-targeted therapy in melanoma cells. Cancers (Basel). 2020;12(8)

158. Rossi M, Tuck J, Kim OJ, Panova I, Symanowski JT, Mahalingam M, Riker AI, Alani RM, Ryu B. Neuropilin-2 gene expression correlates with malignant progression in cutaneous melanoma. Br J Dermatol. 2014;171(2):403–8.

159. Rushing EC, Stine MJ, Hahn SJ, Shea S, Eller MS, Naif A, Khanna S, Westra WH, Jungbluth AA, Busam KJ, Mahalingam M, Alani RM. Neuropilin-2: a novel biomarker for malignant melanoma? Hum Pathol. 2012;43(3):381–9.

160. Stine MJ, Wang CJ, Moriarty WF, Ryu B, Cheong R, Westra WH, Levchenko A, Alani RM. Integration of genotypic and phenotypic screening reveals molecular mediators of melanoma-stromal interaction. Cancer Res. 2011;71(7):2433–44.

161. Moriarty WF, Kim E, Gerber SA, Hammers H, Alani RM. Neuropilin-2 promotes melanoma growth and progression in vivo. Melanoma Res. 2016;26(4):321–8.

162. Wititsuwannakul J, Mason AR, Klump VR, Lazova R. Neuropilin-2 as a useful marker in the differentiation between Spitzoid malignant melanoma and Spitz nevus. J Am Acad Dermatol. 2013;68(1):129–37.

163. Eisenstein A, Panova IP, Chung HJ, Goldberg LJ, Zhang Q, Lazova R, Bhawan J, Busam KJ, Symanowski JT, Alani RM, Ryu B. Quantitative assessment of neuropilin-2 as a simple and sensitive diagnostic assay for spitzoid melanocytic lesions. Melanoma Res. 2018;28(1):71–5.

164. Dadras SS, Lange-Asschenfeldt B, Velasco P, Nguyen L, Vora A, Muzikansky A, Jahnke K, Hauschild A, Hirakawa S, Mihm MC, Detmar M. Tumor lymphangiogenesis predicts melanoma metastasis to sentinel lymph nodes. Mod Pathol. 2005;18(9):1232–42.

165. Huang R, Andersen LMK, Rofstad EK. Metastatic pathway and the microvascular and physicochemical microenvironments of human melanoma xenografts. J Transl Med. 2017;15(1):203.

166. Coma S, Shimizu A, Klagsbrun M. Hypoxia induces tumor and endothelial cell migration in a semaphorin 3F- and VEGF-dependent manner via transcriptional repression of their common receptor neuropilin 2. Cell Adhes Migr. 2011;5(3):266–75.

167. Geretti E, van Meeteren LA, Shimizu A, Dudley AC, Claesson-Welsh L, Klagsbrun M. A mutated soluble neuropilin-2 B domain antagonizes vascular endothelial growth factor bioactivity and inhibits tumor progression. Mol Cancer Res. 2010;8(8):1063–73.

168. Bielenberg DR, Hida Y, Shimizu A, Kaipainen A, Kreuter M, Kim CC, Klagsbrun M. Semaphorin 3F, a chemorepulsant for endothelial cells, induces a poorly vascularized, encapsulated, nonmetastatic tumor phenotype. J Clin Invest. 2004;114(9):1260–71.

169. Caunt M, Mak J, Liang WC, Stawicki S, Pan Q, Tong RK, Kowalski J, Ho C, Reslan HB, Ross J, Berry L, Kasman I, Zlot C, Cheng Z, Le Couter J, Filvaroff EH, Plowman G, Peale F, French D, Carano R, Koch AW, Wu Y, Watts RJ, Tessier-Lavigne M, Bagri A. Blocking neuropilin-2 function inhibits tumor cell metastasis. Cancer Cell. 2008;13(4):331–42.

The Role of AXL Receptor Tyrosine Kinase in Cancer Cell Plasticity and Therapy Resistance

18

Maria L. Lotsberg, Kjersti T. Davidsen,
Stacey D'Mello Peters, Gry S. Haaland, Austin Rayford,
James B. Lorens, and Agnete S. T. Engelsen

Abstract

Therapy resistance continues to confound all available cancer therapies, including immune checkpoint inhibitors. The astonishing heterogeneity and plasticity of cancers limit long-term therapeutic benefit, and recent insights into the epigenetic heterogeneity of cancers have emphasized a need to address the underlying mechanisms driving cancer cell plasticity. Epithelial-to-mesenchymal transition (EMT)-related trans-differentiation programs are prevalent in aggressive tumors displaying a drug-resistant, invasive, and immune evasive phenotype. Novel therapeutically actionable targets are needed in order to disable tumor plasticity mechanisms. AXL receptor tyrosine kinase has a remarkably broad association with aggressive and therapy-resistant cancers and has emerged as a promising therapeutic target. Recent research has revealed that AXL is not a traditional oncogenic driver as first envisioned, but rather AXL is involved in regulating cancer cell plasticity related to the EMT program. This new knowledge has provided a framework to understand the role of AXL-mediated signal transduction in cancer. Accordingly, a growing number of studies have demonstrated that AXL signaling is required to maintain cancer cell plasticity and resistance to cytotoxic and targeted anti-cancer agents, as well as immune checkpoint inhibition. Several AXL-targeting agents are currently being explored in clinical trials dedicated to reverse the plasticity-mediated resistance mechanisms and potentiate current anti-cancer treatments. In this chapter, we aim to explore the unique roles of the AXL receptor tyrosine kinase in cancer cell plasticity and therapeutic resistance and discuss the alternative ways of targeting AXL in clinical trials.

Maria L. Lotsberg and Kjersti T. Davidsen contributed equally to this publication.

M. L. Lotsberg · K. T. Davidsen · S. D'Mello Peters
G. S. Haaland · A. Rayford · J. B. Lorens · A. S. T. Engelsen (✉)
Department of Biomedicine, Centre for Cancer Biomarkers
CCBIO, Norwegian Center of Excellence, Faculty of Medicine,
University of Bergen, Bergen, Norway
e-mail: agnete.engelsen@uib.no

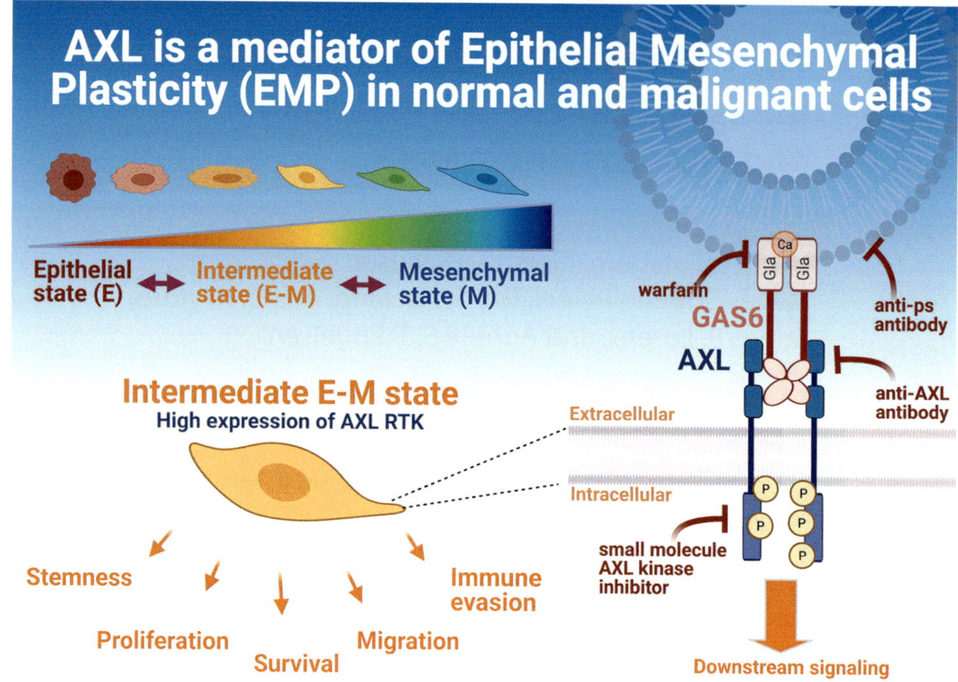

AXL is a mediator of Epithelial Mesenchymal Plasticity (EMP) in normal and malignant cells.

Abbreviations

AML	Acute myeloid leukemia
BMDSC	Bone marrow-derived stem cells
CML	Chronic myeloid leukemia
DKK3	Dickkopf-homologue 3
ECM	Extracellular matrix
EGFR	Epidermal growth factor receptor/ErbB-1
EMT	Epithelial-to-mesenchymal transition
EMP	Epithelial-to-mesenchymal plasticity
GAS6	Growth arrest specific 6
GIST	Gastrointestinal stromal tumors
HER2	Human epidermal growth factor receptor 2/ErbB-2
HER3	Human epidermal growth factor receptor 3/ErbB-3
HGF	Hepatocyte growth factor
HIF1α	Hypoxia-inducible factor 1α
HNSCC	Head- and neck-squamous cell carcinoma
HUVECs	Human umbilical vein endothelial cells
MET	Mesenchymal-to-epithelial transition
MMPs	Matrix metalloproteinases
NSCLC	Non-small cell lung cancer
PS	Phosphatidyl serine
RTK	Receptor tyrosine kinase
SCC	Squamous cell carcinoma
TK	Tyrosine kinase
TKI	Tyrosine kinase inhibitor
TNBC	Triple negative breast cancer
VEGF	Vascular endothelial growth factor
VEGFR	Vascular endothelial growth factor receptor
VSMC	Vascular smooth muscle cells

Take-Home Lessons

- Epithelial-mesenchymal plasticity (EMP) is a term used to describe the ability of cells to respond to microenvironmental clues by adopting different phenotypes along the epithelial to mesenchymal spectrum.
- EMP is an important feature for the maintenance of homeostasis in epithelial tissues, and hallmarks of EMP are frequently found to be hijacked by malignant epithelial cells (carcinoma cells).
- The receptor tyrosine kinase AXL has been identified as a mediator of EMP in normal and malignant epithelial cells. AXL is frequently upregulated in solid and liquid malignancies and correlated with poor prognosis, and a mediator of immune evasion and resistance to various cytotoxic and targeted therapies.
- The receptor tyrosine kinase AXL represents a promising therapeutic target for drug-resistant and immune evasive cancers, and several small molecule AXL inhibitors are currently in clinical development.

Introduction

Cancer remains a leading cause of morbidity and mortality worldwide, and more than half of adults born after 1960 are expected to be diagnosed with cancer at some point during their lifetime [1]. Our understanding of the molecular basis of cancer has evolved remarkably during the past two decades, and massive parallel sequencing endeavors performed by The Cancer Genome Atlas program, the International Cancer Genome Consortium, and numerous individual investigators have identified a broad range of recurrent genetic mutations and structural rearrangements driving tumorigenesis. In concert with this, the pharmaceutical industry has developed a wide range of molecularly targeted therapeutics. However, despite this progress, most cancer patients with advanced disease do not experience durable clinical responses [2]. A recent study estimated that only about 9% of patients with metastatic cancer are eligible for a genome-targeted drug, and only 5% will actually benefit from the therapy [3].

The astonishing heterogeneity and plasticity of cancers limits long-term therapeutic benefit [4, 5]. The overall landscape of inter-tumor and intratumor heterogeneity comprises both genetic and epigenetic components evolving from the founding clone. In concert with genomic instability, the breakdown of normal tissue structure during malignant progression exposes cancer cells to numerous biophysical challenges, nutritional deprivation, and a hostile non-native microenvironment comprising different matrix proteins and a variety of stromal cells. How this mutational landscape influences reciprocal tumor-stroma interactions is less well understood. The tumor microenvironment triggers adaptive, cellular plasticity programs related to stem cell differentiation and trans-differentiation, characteristic of adult tissue homeostasis and repair. This endows cancer cells with a remarkable phenotypic and functional flexibility engendering malignant attributes of stemness, invasiveness, chemotherapeutic resistance, immune evasion, metastasis, and poor prognosis. Thus, the confounding reality for anti-cancer drug development is the heterogeneity and plasticity of tumors [6]. Hence, delineating the molecular mechanisms necessary to induce and sustain cellular plasticity and how the resulting phenotypic diversity contributes to therapy resistance represents an urgent unmet need in oncology [7]. The receptor tyrosine kinase AXL has been identified as a mediator of epithelial phenotypic plasticity mediating normal epithelial homeostasis as well as immune evasion and therapy resistance in malignant epithelial (carcinoma) cells. AXL is also expressed on various immune cell subsets and serves as a negative regulator of antitumor inflammation, which is becoming increasingly critical to reinvigorate in the context of immunotherapy. In this chapter, we aim to explain the particular activation of AXL receptor tyrosine kinase and explore the unique role of AXL in mediating cancer cell plasticity and how this relates to therapy resistance.

Epithelial Phenotypic Plasticity of Cancer Cells

Malignant tumors are appropriately considered "quasi-organs" [8], an abnormal tissue comprising cancer cell hierarchies and a dynamic microenvironment consisting of stromal cells, including fibroblasts, endothelial cells, and various immune cells, and a reactive extracellular matrix. The cells of the tumor microenvironment interact tightly with the body's healthy cells and organs, and upon instructions from the malignant cells, the tumor microenvironment is transformed into the immune-suppressive and cancer-supportive niche required to allow further expansion of the malignant cells. Within this shifting landscape of developing cancers, the cancer cell population also displays a significant phenotypic variation [9]. These acquired phenotypic plasticity of the malignant cells are in part attributed to the activation of cellular plasticity programs governing normal embryonic development, wound healing, and adult organ homeostasis [10]. For example, carcinomas, which are epithelial-derived tumors, encompass nearly 80% of human malignancies and display a remarkable phenotypic diversity reflective of the normal epithelial cell hierarchies, and such a cellular hierarchy provides the cancer cells with a repertoire of cellular functions similar to those required to form and maintain adult organs [11–13].

This epithelial cell plasticity is engendered by the epithelial-to-mesenchymal transition (EMT) program, a complex embryonic trans-differentiation program where non-motile, polarized epithelial cells within cohesive planar barrier-cell sheets lose their apical-basal polarity, remodulate their cytoskeleton and degrade their cell–cell junctions to convert into solitary migratory mesenchymal cells with enhanced cell survival attributes [14–16]. Cells that have undergone EMT may also be reverted to a more epithelial state through the reverse transition, mesenchymal-to-epithelial transition (MET). Importantly, EMT is not an on or off switch, but rather considered as a continuum of cell states along an epithelial to mesenchymal axis. Cells that are able to adopt mixed or intermediate epithelial-mesenchymal phenotypes on this axis are considered to harbor the highest potential to transit between the states [16]. This ability to transit between the epithelial-mesenchymal states along the EMT spectrum is referred to as epithelial-to-mesenchymal plasticity (EMP) [16]. EMP is regulated by several dedicated developmental transcription factors that act in concert with epigenetic mechanisms including DNA methylation, histone modifications, and microRNAs to affect the expression of hundreds of genes in concert [17]. Interestingly, the stability of the EMT states vary in different biological contexts, and epithelial plasticity has been shown to be governed largely by microenvironmental cues from the local "niche" comprising growth factors, cytokines, extracellular matrix (ECM), oxygen tension, and tensile forces that control cellular signal transduction systems [16, 18].

The process of EMT is well established as a critical component of successful embryonic development [19]. EMT regulators also induce epithelial plasticity during mammary gland development and recent evidence suggests that EMT-related gene expression is a primary component of adult mammary epithelial stem cells [20]. Epithelial-mesenchymal plasticity is apparent in adult epithelial cell hierarchies mediating conversions between stem-like and more differentiated progeny [21, 22]. It has been shown that induction of EMT in differentiated adult epithelial cells may induce stem cell traits consistent with dedifferentiation [23, 24]. This indicates that aspects of the embryonic EMT gene program have been assimilated into the adult epithelial cell hierarchies to mediate cell state conversions. We have recently shown that the receptor tyrosine kinase AXL, is a driver of EMP and stemness in normal mammary gland tissue and also in breast cancer [25]. This serves to illustrate the fact that carcinoma cells have the ability to assume an intermediate or hybrid EMT state along an epithelial to mesenchymal continuum providing an expanded functional repertoire [26]. Phenotypic plasticity within tumors is considered the main source of stem cell-like traits driving tumor initiation capacity and drug resistance, underpinning recurrence and metastasis [7]. EMT gene signatures correlating with stem cell-like traits were shown to predict poor patient survival in several malignancies [27, 28]. The EMT transcriptional program was initially associated with drug resistance and later invasiveness and metastasis. Induction of cancer cell plasticity is critical for the invasive behavior of malignant carcinoma and blockade of EMT can inhibit metastasis [29]. Epithelial plasticity in the metastatic microenvironment allows metastatic cells to suppress cell migration while enhancing stem cell traits during metastatic site colonization to re-establish cellular hierarchies [13, 30]. In this respect, metastatic cells resemble multipotent epithelial progenitors found in adult epithelial cell hierarchies.

While initial lineage-tracing experiments failed to confirm a major role for EMP in metastatic dissemination, these studies concluded that EMT is required for resistance to chemotherapy and accumulating data support a role for hybrid epithelial–mesenchymal phenotypes in metastasis [31–33]. The ability to dynamically switch between different phenotypic cellular states is closely linked to acquired drug resistance [34]. Cancer cells that can readily alter gene expression programs and assume new phenotypes in response to thera-

peutic challenges are more likely to survive. This dynamic nature of tumor plasticity has important clinical implications for the design of anti-cancer therapeutic strategies, and the identification of novel druggable therapeutic targets that can impact the fundamental mechanisms underpinning cellular plasticity is crucial to overcome acquired therapy resistance [35]. In this context, the receptor tyrosine kinase AXL has emerged as a promising opportunity to target tumor cell plasticity [25].

AXL Activation and Signaling

AXL belongs to the TAM family of receptor tyrosine kinases (RTKs), comprising three family members: Tyro3, AXL, and Mer. The TAM family of RTKs share a common unique molecular structure and a role as homeostatic mediators in various tissues. The TAM family was one of the latest to evolve and one of the last to be identified. The late development of this tyrosine kinase family underscores the important role of the TAM family members as immune regulators and mediators of tissue homeostasis [36]. TAM family RTKs are activated by the ligands Growth arrest specific 6 (GAS6) and Protein S [36]. GAS6 has the highest affinity for AXL, while Protein S is a ligand for Tyro3 and Mer. Vitamin K-dependent Y-carboxylation on the N-terminal Gla domain of both ligands is essential for optimal kinase activation [37].

GAS6 interacts with AXL through a high-affinity and low-affinity Ig2 binding interface on the receptor's extracellular region (Fig. 18.1).

GAS6 has high affinity (Kd 50–600 pM) for the extracellular domain of AXL. GAS6 binds to phosphatidyl serine (PS) exposed on the outer leaflet of membranes such as enveloped viruses and apoptotic cells through a Ca2+ dependent interaction with the N-terminal gamma-carboxylated Gla domain. Binding of membrane-bound GAS6 likely facilitates AXL receptor activation via induced proximity [37–39]. Interestingly, a report suggests the existence of an ancestral Gla-RTK, highly homologous to the Gla domain of GAS6 and whose receptor kinase domain is highly homologous to AXL, indicating a ligand role for PS [40]. Indeed, recent models combining quantitative experiments with mathematical modeling have shown that AXL functions as a spatial localization sensor of PS on cell membranes and vesicles [41].

Ligand-independent AXL activation may also occur in the context of AXL overexpression in malignant cells. Data on heterodimerization and transactivation across TAM receptors have also been reported, and heterodimerization with receptors from other RTK families will be described in greater detail below when we discuss the role of AXL in resistance to targeted therapies (section "AXL RTK in Resistance to Molecularly Targeted Therapies"). Since AXL activation is not required for AXL-mediated cell

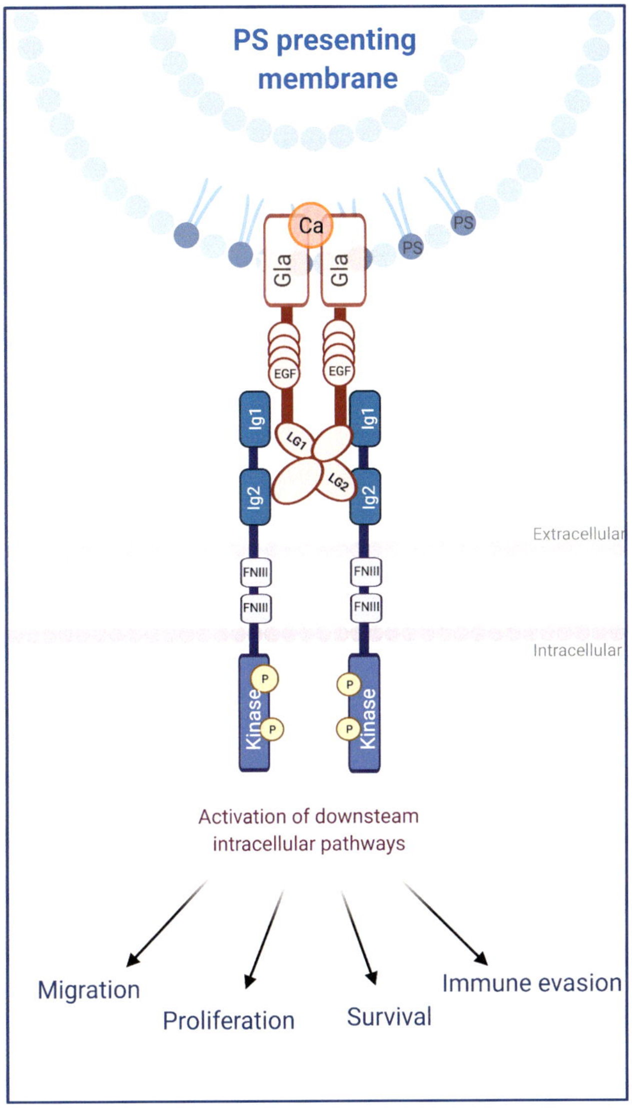

Fig. 18.1 GAS6 mediated AXL activation. The AXL receptor tyrosine kinase is activated by a single protein ligand GAS6. GAS6 binds phosphatidylserine-containing membranes via an N-terminal vitamin K-dependent GLA (gamma-carboxyglutamic acid) domain, and the AXL receptor through its C-terminal LG-domains. This unique activation mechanism results in autophosphorylation of tyrosines on the AXL kinase domain and downstream signaling. Figure created with BioRender.com

aggregation, this mechanism of activation is likely different from ligand-dependent activation. In addition, other factors influencing AXL function include posttranslational modifications such as glycosylation and ubiquitination [42]. GAS6 activation of AXL has been associated with varying cellular functions in different cell types, including growth, proliferation, migration, aggregation, and survival, through different downstream signal transduction pathways. For a comprehensive review of AXL activation and downstream signaling see [36].

AXL Is Associated with a Wide Range of Malignancies and Poor Clinical Outcomes

As briefly mentioned above, AXL overexpression is correlated with a remarkably wide range of solid tumor types and myeloid malignancies. In spite of a dearth of substantiated AXL activating mutations or genetic amplifications, transcriptional up-regulation and increased ligand-induced or ligand-independent activation is more frequently associated with neoplasia [43, 44]. For most of the studies examining the correlation between AXL and malignant disease progression, the AXL activation status has not been examined. AXL was first isolated and described as a putative oncogene from two patients with chronic myeloid leukemia (CML) in 1988 [43, 45, 46] (see [47] for review). During the ensuing three decades, AXL expression was found to be associated with most cancer types (Table 18.1), and linked to poorer prognosis in several cancer forms [48–50]. Table 18.1 provides an overview of the correlation of AXL with poor outcomes in the different cancer forms.

The Role of AXL in Cancer Cell Plasticity

Although gene mutations or genetic amplifications are commonly detected amongst receptor tyrosine kinases that act as oncogenic drivers, there are few reports of mutations and amplifications of AXL [43, 44]. Considering the prevalence of AXL in cancer, this indicates that maintaining AXL signaling dynamics in tumors is important and that the role of AXL in malignant progression may be incompatible with constitutive overexpression/activation. Congruently, a study by Del Pozo Martin and colleagues showed that constitutive AXL overexpression specifically led to reduced metastatic capacity as increased growth was detected in the primary tumor, supporting the idea that downregulation of AXL is important during colonization [51].

Thus, AXL may be particularly important in settings requiring adaptive survival to altered or foreign microenvironments, such as during tumor dissemination and metastatic colonization or during therapeutic intervention [52, 53]. Carcinoma metastases often exhibit histo-pathological traits similar to the primary tumor, and lack a mesenchymal phenotype, supporting the hypothesis that re-establishment of an epithelial phenotype via MET is required for successful colonization at the metastatic site [54–56]. Recent results indicate that MET may not be an absolute requirement for the outgrowth of metastases at distant sites, but rather depends on the specific organ site [57]. This is consistent with measurable gene expression differences between metastases recovered from different organs that also maintain plasticity traits required for establishment of cellular hierarchies [13].

Table 18.1 A summary of publications linking AXL expression to various cancer forms and poor prognosis

Malignancies	Up-regulation	Human tumor samples	Poor prognosis	Independent prognostic factor
Astrocytic brain tumors	[76, 138–142]	[76, 140–142]	[76]	[76]
Breast cancer	[49, 143–155]	[49, 146–154, 156]	[49, 152]	[49]
Gallbladder cancer	[157]	[157]	[157]	
GI cancers:				
– Colon cancer	[52, 158–162]	[160, 161]	[160]	
– Esophageal cancer	[84, 163–165]	[84, 164, 165]	[164, 165]	
– Gastric cancer	[166–168]	[166–168]	[168]	
Gynecological cancers:				
– Ovarian cancer	[63, 113, 169–173]	[63, 113, 169–173]	[169, 170, 172]	[169]
– Uterine cancer	[174–177]	[174–177]	[176]	
HCC	[178–182]	[179, 182]	[179, 182]	[179, 182]
HNSCC	[85, 90, 102, 183–185]	[85, 184–186]	[85, 184, 186]	[184]
Leukemias:				
– AML	[48, 187–189]	[48, 187–189]	[48, 187]	[48, 187]
– CLL	[190–193]	[190–193]		
– CML	[43, 62, 189, 194]	[43, 189, 194]		
Melanoma	[108, 109, 195–198]	[109, 198]		
Mesothelioma	[199–203]	[199, 202, 203]	[199, 203]	[199]
NSCLC	[28, 50, 52, 59, 77, 95, 101, 158, 202, 204–211]	[50, 59, 77, 95, 202, 207–211]	[95, 206, 207, 210, 211]	[210]
LCNEC	[202]			
Pancreatic cancer	[53, 64, 65, 212]	[53, 65, 212]	[53, 65]	[53]
Sarcomas:				
– Ewing Sarcoma	[213]	[213]	[213]	
– Kaposis sarcoma	[214]	[214]		
– Liposarcoma	[215, 216]	[215, 216]	[215]	[215]
– Osteosarcoma	[217–220]	[217]	[217]	[217]
– Undifferentiated pleomorphic sarcoma	[221]	[221]	[221]	
Skin SCC	[222, 223]	[222, 223]		
Salivary Adenoid Cystic Carcinomas	[224]	[224]		
Thyroid cancer	[225–229]	[225, 226, 228, 229]	[229]	
Urological cancers:				
– Bladder cancer	[230–232]	[230]		
– Prostate cancer	[233–236]	[234, 236]		
– RCC	[70, 237–241]	[237–241]	[70, 239]	[239]

Abbreviations: *AML* Acute myeloid leukemia, *CLL* Chronic lymphatic leukemia, *CML* Chronic myeloid leukemia, *GI* Gastrointestinal, *HCC* Hepatocellular carcinoma, *HNSCC* Head- and Neck-squamous cell carcinoma, *LCNEC* Large cell neuroendocrine cancer, *NSCLC* Non-small cell lung cancer, *RCC* Renal cell carcinoma, *SCC* Squamous cell carcinoma

Indeed, in a cohort of breast cancer patients, we noted that AXL expression was higher in the metastatic lesions when compared to their matched biopsy samples from the primary tumor site, suggesting that maintained cellular plasticity is required in the evolving metastatic lesions [49].

The demonstration that AXL expression induced by EMT transcription factors including SLUG, SNAIL, TWIST, and ZEB2 is required for metastasis in breast cancer models solidified the notion of AXL signaling as a regulator of plasticity during malignant progression [49, 58]. This unique relationship between AXL and EMT was further demonstrated in several different cancers [28, 59–64]. Inhibition of AXL signaling affects EMT transcription levels and reverses tumor plasticity features in carcinoma cells [64–66].

A comprehensive proteomic analysis of different EMT signaling states revealed key changes in different cell signaling pathways [67]. Using distinct epithelial metastable EMT versus "epigenetically-fixed" mesenchymal lung tumor cells from an isogenic background, this systems-view study highlights the metastable (hybrid or intermediate) EMT state in which the cancer cells are not epigenetically fixed, as is the case with the most aggressive and therapy-resistant cancer cells. This is congruent with separate reports that used transcriptional analyses [26]. During EMT, Epidermal Growth Factor Receptor (EGFR), Insulin-like Growth Factor 1 Receptor (IGF1R), and c-MET phosphorylation are reduced, indicating a loss of signaling via these receptors. Concomitantly, pro-survival IL11/IL6-JAK2-STAT and

AXL/TYRO3/PDGFR/FGFR signaling were increased. Phosphorylated AXL was correlated with acquisition of EMT-related plasticity. This study further demonstrated that AXL was specifically up-regulated and activated upon EMT-induction by SNAIL in a non-small cell lung cancer (NSCLC) cell system [67]. These emerging signaling landscapes associated with the metastable (hybrid or intermediate) EMT-state provide a novel avenue for future targeting strategies against aggressive and therapy-resistant cancer cells and suggest a prominent role for AXL signaling as a therapeutic target.

AXL-Related Tumor-Stroma Crosstalk

A paper by Jokela and colleagues applied microarrays of robotically printed combinatorial microenvironments of known composition (ME arrays) to examine the effect of different microenvironmental contexts on the expression of AXL and cKIT markers in an isogenic human mammary epithelial cell (HMEC) progression series [68]. The authors hypothesized that specific combinations of microenvironment constituents would induce expression of these plasticity markers in a non-sporadic manner, and identified key microenvironmental factors, including osteopontin, IL-8, collagen Type VI α3, significantly upregulated cKIT and AXL, and these factors were shown by RNA *in situ* hybridization to co-localize in normal and malignant breast cancer tissues [68]. A greater diversity of combinatorial microenvironments induced cKIT and AXL expression in the tumorigenic cells compared to the normal or immortal cells of the isogenic HMEC progression series, suggesting a reduced perception of microenvironment specificity in the malignant cells [68]. These results support the notion that specific microenvironments could impose reprogramming and drive drug-tolerant cellular phenotypes. AXL has been identified as a driver of epithelial plasticity in normal and malignant mammary epithelia, and represents a promising therapeutic target for preventing plasticity-mediated acquired drug resistance [25, 68].

In the environment of a tumor, the conditions are often hypoxic compared to the surrounding tissue. Hypoxia has been shown to play an important role as a driver of intratumor genetic and non-genetic heterogeneity and greatly affects the composition of the tumor immune microenvironment [69]. Hypoxia will increase the expression of Hypoxia-inducible factor 1α (HIF1α) which in turn promotes increased AXL transcription [70]. Indeed, AXL expression is prevalent in myeloid leukemia where it has been shown to play a key role in mediating cytokine crosstalk with the hypoxic bone marrow niche. A study from Ben-Batalla and colleagues [48] demonstrated that acute myeloid leukemia (AML) cells educated bone marrow-derived stem cells (BMDSCs) to secrete GAS6, which then mediated proliferation of AXL-positive AML cells and induced therapy resistance [48]. A recent paper by Yttersian-Sletta and colleagues showed that AXL overexpression in a preclinical model of triple-negative breast cancer (TNBC) was induced by hypoxia, and experimental Hyperbaric-Oxygen Therapy (HBOT) significantly reduced expression of AXL in this tumor model [71, 72].

AXL is not only regulated by the microenvironment, but rather this communication is a two-way crosstalk where AXL also regulates factors in the tumor microenvironment. Malignant tumors may gain the ability to invade surrounding tissues. In order to achieve this hallmark, the cancer cells must gain the capacity to produce matrix-degrading enzymes, including Matrix metalloproteinases (MMPs). MMP-9 is a type IV collagenase, which degrades type IV collagen, an important component of the basement membrane and the extracellular matrix. It has been shown that AXL induces transcriptional upregulation of MMP-9 through the MAP kinase pathway [73].

An early indication that AXL is not exclusively a driver of tumor cell proliferation came as the result of a functional genetic screen to identify regulators of cell migration in response to gradients of extracellular matrix components, also known as haptotactic cell migration [74]. Strikingly, dominant-negative regulators of both the GAS6 ligand and AXL receptor were isolated in this screen and independently validated by gene silencing via RNA interference. These results suggest that GAS6-AXL signaling mediates pro-invasive microenvironmental cues consistent with the role of AXL in regulating tumor plasticity and metastasis.

A recent study from Martin *et al* [51] showed that metastatic mammary carcinoma cells require AXL to maintain a mesenchymal phenotype and metastasis initiating capacity in the lung, consistent with previous reports [49, 66]. Notably, AXL signaling in lung metastatic mammary carcinoma cells is required for activation of cancer-associated fibroblasts (CAFs) and secretion of thrombospondin 2. Importantly, these CAFs exert a reciprocal effect on carcinoma cell plasticity by downregulating AXL expression and reverting the carcinoma cells into a more proliferative epithelial phenotype. This demonstrates key role for dynamic AXL signaling in mediating tumor-stromal crosstalk in the metastatic niche.

AXL also plays a role in regulating angiogenesis [74, 75]. Studies show that AXL expression is present not only in tumor cells but also in surrounding vascular cells of tumors [76, 77]. Vascular smooth muscle cells (VSMC) express GAS6, and exogenous application of GAS6 stimulates proliferation and mobility of VSMC [78]. AXL influences angiogenesis through modulation of signaling, via angiopoietin/Tie2 and Dickkopf-homologue 3 (DKK3) pathways [52]. AXL knockdown together with anti-vascular endothelial growth factor (anti-VEGF) therapy blocks in vitro tube formation compared to anti-VEGF therapy alone [52].

Furthermore, a report by Ruan et al shows that AXL is essential for VEGF-A mediated activation of PI3K/Akt [79]. Notably AXL knockdown in human umbilical vein endothelial cells (HUVECs) impaired regenerative blood vessel formation in an in vivo tissue engineering model [74], while a similar effect was observed with pharmacological AXL inhibition of angiogenesis in corneal micropocket and tumor models [58, 74], supporting a role of AXL in angiogenesis.

AXL RTK in Resistance to Cytotoxic Therapies

AXL was identified as one of several genes up-regulated in ovarian cancer cell lines with acquired resistance to cisplatin [80]. Since this initial observation, high AXL expression has been established as prevalent feature of therapy-resistant cancers, and AXL-mediated signaling is thus suggested as a key regulator of acquired resistance to anti-cancer agents of various classes (Table 18.2). The role of AXL in therapy resistance was initially attributed to the enhanced anti-apoptotic signaling apparent in several different cancer systems. AXL is a potent activator of the PI3K-pathway [81], and activation of PI3K and subsequently AKT and NF-κB pathways have been correlated with increased expression of multiple anti-apoptotic proteins (e.g. BCL-2, BCL-XL, and PUMA) and inactivation of pro-apoptotic factors such as caspase-3 [48, 82]. Also, the inhibitory interaction between BAD and BCL-2 and BCL-XL will be blocked due to AKT-mediated phosphorylation of BAD. The cumulative effect will be prevention of apoptosis and increased cellular survival signaling [47, 82].

Overexpression of the plasma membrane efflux pump P-glycoprotein (P-gp) is a common cause of multidrug resistance in cancer cells. In adriamycin-paclitaxel-vincristine-resistant breast cancer and CML cell lines, AXL and P-gp are co-upregulated, and siRNA knockdown of AXL results in decreased P-gp expression and decreased resistance to these agents both in vitro and in vivo [83]. Drug-resistant AXL-overexpressing cell lines are also more invasive in vitro, and this can be diminished by AXL silencing [83]. AXL expression also blocks apoptosis by inhibiting c-ABL/p73 signaling in response to DNA damage in p53 deficient esophageal adenocarcinoma cells [84]. In pancreatic cancer, AXL down-regulation increases apoptosis following gamma-radiation in vitro, as measured by PARP-cleavage [53]. In head- and neck squamous cell carcinoma, AXL inhibition sensitizes AXL expressing cells to gamma radiation, with data indicating that AXL mediates DNA double-strand break repair. In HNSCC xenograft and PDX models, intrinsically radioresistant tumors have high AXL expression and phosphorylation [85]. Inhibition of AXL in putative cancer stem cell populations sensitizes these inherently chemo-resistant cells to

Table 18.2 AXL in resistance to cytotoxic therapy

Treatment	Malignancy	Reference
Radiation:	HNSCC	[85, 242]
	Pancreatic cancer	[53]
Platinum compounds: - Cisplatin - Carboplatin	AML	[243]
	Astrocytoma	[139]
	Esophageal adenocarcinoma	[84]
	HNSCC	[85]
	Neuroblastoma	[244]
	NSCLC	[60, 77]
	Ovarian cancer	[80, 173]
Anthracyclins: - Doxorubicin	AML	[243]
	Breast cancer	[83]
	CML	[83]
	NSCLC	[77, 245, 246]
	Skin cancer (SCC)	[86]
Alkylating agents: - Temozolomide	Astrocytoma	[139]
Tubulin inhibitors: Taxanes: - Paclitaxel - Docetaxel	Breast cancer (TNBC)	[83, 87, 88]
	CML	[83]
	NSCLC	[60, 88, 246]
	Prostate cancer	[247]
	Uterine cancer	[177]
	Ovarian cancer	[248]
- Vinca alkaloids: - Vincristine	Breast cancer	[83]
	CML	[83]
	Neuroblastoma	[244]
	NSCLC	[246]
Topoisomerase inhibitors: - Etoposide	AML	[243]
	Breast cancer	[87]
	NSCLC	[77]
	Skin cancer (SCC)	[86]
Antimetabolites: - Fluorouracil - Gemcitabine	Breast cancer (TNBC)	[147]
	Colon cancer	[249]
	Pancreatic cancer	[212, 248, 250]
Histone deacetylase inhibitors - Panobinostat	Astrocytic brain tumors (diffuse intrinsic pontine glioma)	[142]

Abbreviations: *AML* acute myeloid leukemia, *BCSC* breast cancer stem cells, *CML* chronic myeloid leukemia, *HNSCC* Head- and Neck-squamous cell carcimoma, *NSCLC* non-small cell lung cancer, *SCC* squamous cell carcinoma, *TNBC* triple-negative breast cancer

cytotoxic chemotherapy, suggesting a role for AXL in protecting stem-like populations of cells [86, 87].

An analysis of 643 human cancer cell lines found a strong correlation between AXL expression and a mesenchymal, drug-resistant phenotype. Mesenchymal NSCLC cells are more resistant to chemotherapeutic agents, and AXL inhibition with the small molecule inhibitor bemcentinib was shown to sensitize cross-resistant EGFR-mutated NSCLC cells to taxanes as well as other antimitotic agents, such as aurora kinase inhibitors, that activate the mitotic spindle checkpoint. Co-treatment resulted in de-phosphorylation of cyclin-dependent kinase-1 (CDC2), which regulates mitotic entry [88]. Acquisition of resistance to cisplatin was shown to impair sensitivity to subsequent gefitinib treatment through induction of EMT, and AXL was found to be responsible for increased motility of cisplatin-resistant cells [89].

AXL RTK in Resistance to Molecularly Targeted Therapies

Up-regulation of AXL has been demonstrated more recently to be a key mechanism of acquired drug resistance to molecularly targeted anti-cancer therapies, including several compounds directed towards the ErbB family of RTKs, including Epidermal Growth Factor Receptor (EGFR), Human Epidermal Growth Factor Receptor 2 (HER2/ErbB-2) and Human Epidermal Growth Factor Receptor 3 (HER3/ErbB-3). In addition to regulating phenotypic plasticity, AXL has also been reported to heterodimerize with other RTKs and thereby diversify downstream signal transduction to circumvent molecularly targeted kinase inhibitors [90, 91].

The Role of AXL in Resistance to ErbB Family Targeted Therapy

NSCLC tumors with EGFR-activating mutations are currently treated with EGFR small-molecule tyrosine kinase inhibitors (EGFR-TKI) such as gefitinib and erlotinib. Although initially effective, acquired resistance to these targeted agents represents a significant obstacle to clinical efficacy. Several explanations have been postulated to explain the lack of response to EGFR-targeted therapy, including mutations in the binding sites of the drug target, as well as secondary effector mutations affecting downstream signaling molecules in the EGFR-activated pathway [92]. In addition to secondary mutations in EGFR (T790M) and up-regulation of the c-MET kinase, secondary alterations that are both druggable, the presence of AXL has been shown to limit the response to EGFR-targeted inhibitors in NSCLC [59]. Additionally, EMT was recognized several years ago as an important mechanism of non-mutational resistance to EGFR inhibitors [93]. EMT signatures derived from patient samples and cell lines with EGFR TKI resistance highlight a potential role for AXL [28], and independent estimates establish AXL expression in approximately 50% of NSCLC samples which in turn is correlated with advanced stages and poor clinical outcome [50, 94, 95].

In an analysis of matched human samples before and after EGFR TKI treatment, AXL was found to be up-regulated in 20% of the resistant specimens [59]. AXL expression and activation have also been detected in NSCLC tumors with EGFR TKI-resistance mutations [59, 94, 96]. In acquired resistance to third-generation mutant-selective EGFR TKIs, resistant cells displayed an EMT gene signature and high expression of AXL [97]. A study using the cell line H820 harboring both the T790M mutation and c-MET amplification validated AXL overexpression as an important contributor to EGFR-TKI resistance [98]. Furthermore, in cancers displaying primary/innate resistance, high AXL expression was detected in 22% of the tumors [99]. Analysis of HCC827 NSCLC xenograft tumors with in vivo acquired resistance to EGFR-inhibitor erlotinib showed AXL up-regulation was present in 88% of tumors [59]. Importantly, AXL knockdown effectively reversed erlotinib resistance in this system.

EGFR is frequently overexpressed in triple-negative breast cancer (TNBC), but a response to EGFR inhibitors in this aggressive, inherently chemo-resistant disease is lacking. TBNC often expresses high levels of AXL [88], and AXL has been found to be trans-activated by EGFR through a physical clustering interaction, leading to downstream signaling diversification that impacts migration and proliferation in response to EGF [91]. It has been shown across several cancer cell lines (breast, colon, tongue, liver, kidney) that EGFR resistance is mediated through Hepatocyte Growth Factor (HGF)/c-MET signaling. EGFR is inactivated by HGF/c-MET. This leads to resistance to EGFR inhibition and facilitates the interaction of EGFR with alternative receptors, including AXL [100]. Reduced degradation of AXL has also recently been identified as a mechanism for gefitinib-induced AXL overexpression [101].

EGFR is targeted in the clinic by the anti-EGFR antibody cetuximab, but both primary/innate and acquired resistance are common [92]. AXL expression and activation were shown to be increased in cetuximab-resistant cell lines and xenograft tumors from NSCLC and HNSCC. Inhibition of AXL signaling with the AXL kinase inhibitor bemcentinib decreases proliferation, migration, and invasion and increases sensitivity to cetuximab in AXL expressing HNSCC cell lines. AXL and EGFR are physically associated in resistant cells and tumors, and overexpression of AXL confers resistance to cetuximab in vitro. Furthermore, EGFR directly regulates the expression of AXL mRNA through MAPK signaling and the transcription factor c-JUN [85, 102].

In breast cancer, AXL was identified as a resistance mechanism to the HER2- inhibitor lapatinib by mass spectrometry-based peptide sequencing of a protein detected by a phosphotyrosine-specific antibody in cell lines with acquired lapatinib resistance. Silencing of AXL by siRNA and inhibition of AXL using a small molecule inhibitor of c-MET, VEGFR, and AXL restored sensitivity to the HER2 targeting agents lapatinib and trastuzumab [61].

The Role of AXL in Resistance to c-Kit/PDGFR/Bcr-Abl Inhibitors

Gastrointestinal stromal tumors (GIST) are driven by c-KIT and/or αPDGFR-mutations and respond to the c-KIT/PDGFR/BCR-ABL inhibitor imatinib. A kinase switch from c-KIT to AXL was identified as a novel mechanism of resistance in imatinib-resistant cell lines as well as patient samples [103]. The presence of AXL up-regulation was confirmed by immunohistochemistry of human patient samples, and inhibition with the dual AXL/c-MET inhibitor amuvatinib acted synergistically with imatinib, erlotinib, and the covalent EGFR and HER2 inhibitor afatinib in a panel of GIST-cell lines [104]. Pan-genomic microarrays of CML cell lines with acquired resistance to BCR-ABL inhibitors found increased expression of AXL [105] as a possible mechanism of resistance, and AXL knockdown re-sensitized the imatinib-resistant CML cells [62]. Furthermore, resistance to second-generation BCR-ABL inhibitors, like nilotinib, has been shown to be promoted by a tyrosine kinase (TK) network where AXL and non-receptor TKs SYK and LYN form a complex, and these tyrosine kinases were verified to be up-regulated in nilotinib-resistant tumor cells from CML patients [106]. The ubiquitin ligase CBL was identified as crucial in regulating the expression of these TKs by regulating their degradation. Interestingly, AXL induced resistance in the absence of kinase activity, indicating a scaffolding role in this model [107].

The Role of AXL in Resistance to MAPK and PI3K Pathway Inhibitors

AXL is overexpressed in a subset of malignant melanomas lacking the microphthalmia-associated transcription factor (MITF), and correlates with a more invasive phenotype [108]. Cell lines sensitive to MAPK pathway inhibitors strongly express MITF, and intrinsically resistant lines show low MITF expression and high expression of AXL [109]. However, extrinsic overexpression of MITF can increase resistance to BRAF and MEK inhibitors, and in acquired resistance to BRAF and ERK inhibitor in vitro, resistant cells divide into two types: one which maintains high MITF expression upon resistance, and another where MITF expression is lost. These findings were supported by the same pattern in human melanoma samples. The resistant cells that maintained high MITF expression were not cross-resistant to MEK or ERK inhibition, while the resistant cells that lost MITF expression were cross-resistant to a full panel of MAPK pathway inhibitors. The cells that lost MITF were more invasive and displayed hallmarks of EMT. Cells with endogenous low MITF expression were intrinsically resistant to BRAF, MEK, and ERK inhibition. AXL was again confirmed to be inversely correlated with MITF, and consistently up-regulated in cell lines that lost MITF expression

during acquired resistance to BRAF inhibition. Targeting AXL with the small-molecule AXL inhibitor bemcentinib increased sensitivity to MAPK-pathway inhibition in resistant cells [110].

A recent study by Elkabets and colleagues showed that head and neck and esophageal squamous cell carcinomas refractory to PI3Kα inhibition express AXL [90]. AXL dimerization with EGFR results in PLCγ-PKC signaling and subsequent PI3K/AKT-independent mTOR activation. Importantly, inhibition of AXL kinase activity by bemcentinib reverses PI3Kα-inhibitor resistance.

For the majority of pancreatic cancer patients, mutated KRAS is a key oncogenic driver, and targeting KRAS directly has so far not been feasible. Targeting the downstream signaling pathways by combined PI3K and MEK inhibitors have yielded high toxicity [111], and MEK inhibition lacks clinical benefit in KRAS-driven tumors. Inhibition of MEK1 drives activation of the PI3K-AKT-mTOR pathway through feedback loops with the recruitment of AXL, PDGFRa, and ErbB receptors EGFR, HER2, and HER3. However, inhibition of any single RTK activated by MEK inhibition was shown in a KRAS-mutated mouse model to have no additional benefit, and to achieve antitumor effects all RTKs activated by MEK inhibition had to be targeted simultaneously [112]. Whether such an approach can be tolerated clinically remains to be explored. In ovarian cancer, simultaneous activation of multiple RTKs have also been established in cell lines and patient samples, and inhibition of AXL, EGFR, HER2, and c-MET by HSP90-inhibitors led to inactivation of these receptors, which inhibited proliferation to a greater extent than single RTK inhibition [113].

Taken together, AXL is up-regulated in response to cytotoxic chemotherapy as well as targeted therapies, and is up-regulated under challenging microenvironmental conditions like serum starvation [48], acidification [114], oxidative stress [115, 116], and laminar shear stress [117]. This suggests that AXL serves a broad function in protecting cells under particularly challenging conditions.

In several in vitro studies, drug-tolerant persister cells characterized by transient phenotypic alterations have been observed in culture upon treatment [118–120]. Single-cell sequencing and protein expression assays of melanoma cell lines and patient samples revealed that these rare 'jackpot' cells expressed markers of therapy resistance and epithelial phenotypic plasticity, including AXL, EGFR, NGFR, FGFR1, and WNT5A. Prior to treatment, the jackpot cells were detected at frequencies of 1:50–1:500, and the frequency increased dramatically compared to more differentiated populations expressing, *e.g.*, MITF and SOX10 upon therapeutic intervention and development of resistant clones [118–120]. In their study, Tirosh and colleagues dissected the multicellular ecosystems of malignant melanoma by single-cell RNA sequencing and provided strong evidence for the involvement of AXL as well as AXL-related genes

(AXL *signature*) in acquired resistance to both BRAF inhibitor (vemurafenib) and MEK inhibitor (Trametinib) [120].

AXL in Resistance to Immunotherapy

Immune checkpoint blockade (ICB) represents a paradigm shift in cancer treatment and accumulating evidence suggests that EMP of cancer cells is also a critical determinant of acquired resistance to immune checkpoint blockade (ICB) [121, 122].

In a cohort of patients with metastatic urothelial cancer treated with a PD-1 inhibitor, nivolumab, wang et al., were able to demonstrate that in patients with T-cell infiltrated tumors, higher EMT/stroma-related gene expression was associated with lower response rates and shorter progression-free and overall survival. Taken together their findings suggest a stroma-mediated source of immune resistance in urothelial cancer and provide rationale for co-targeting PD-1 and EMT/stromal elements [123]. A retrospective study by Thompson et al. analyzed transcriptional profiles from pre-treatment tumor samples of 52 chemotherapy-refractory advanced NSCLC patients treated with anti-PD1/PD-L1 therapy. Gene signatures of tumor inflammation and EMT were shown to predict responses to ICB with high accuracy. Patients whose tumors responded to ICB had higher scores in an inflammatory gene signature or a more epithelial phenotype [124]. A study by Terry and colleagues found that AXL expression in the mesechymal clones of primary NSCLC cells correlated with increased cancer cell–intrinsic resistance to both natural killer (NK)–and cytotoxic T lymphocyte (CTL)–mediated killing. Targeting AXL by a small molecule inhibitor sensitized the cancer cells to immune cell-mediated cytotoxicity. These results revealed an AXL-mediated immune-escape regulatory pathway, suggest AXL as a candidate biomarker for resistance to NK and CTL immunity, and support AXL targeting to optimize immune response in NSCLC [125, 126].

A recent paper from Lotsberg and colleagues showed that AXL expression is associated with a high pre-mortem autophagic flux in EGFR mutated NSCLC, and when targeted by the small molecule AXL inhibitor bemcentinib, an immunogenic form of cell death was induced, characterized by the externalization of calreticulin (CALR), secretion of HMGB1 and ATP into the extracellular space [127]. This finding is significant as immunogenic cell death has been shown to mediate immune cell infiltration and the onset of the cancer immunity cycle. This indicates that AXL inhibition could thus be particularly beneficial also in the EGFR mutant tumors, that respond poorly to immune checkpoint inhibition [128, 129] Thus, EMP represents a promising therapeutic avenue within the overarching strategy to reactivate an interrupted cancer immunity cycle and establish a robust immune response against the cancer cells. Several

pre-clinical trials support the feasibility of this approach [130, 131], and the hypothesis is currently being tested in clinical trials.

AXL-Targeted Agents in Preclinical Development and Clinical Trials

AXL can be targeted therapeutically in several ways (Fig. 18.2). The anti-coagulant warfarin, a drug that has been used clinically for more than 50 years for the prevention of thrombosis, blocks gamma-carboxylation of GAS6 that is

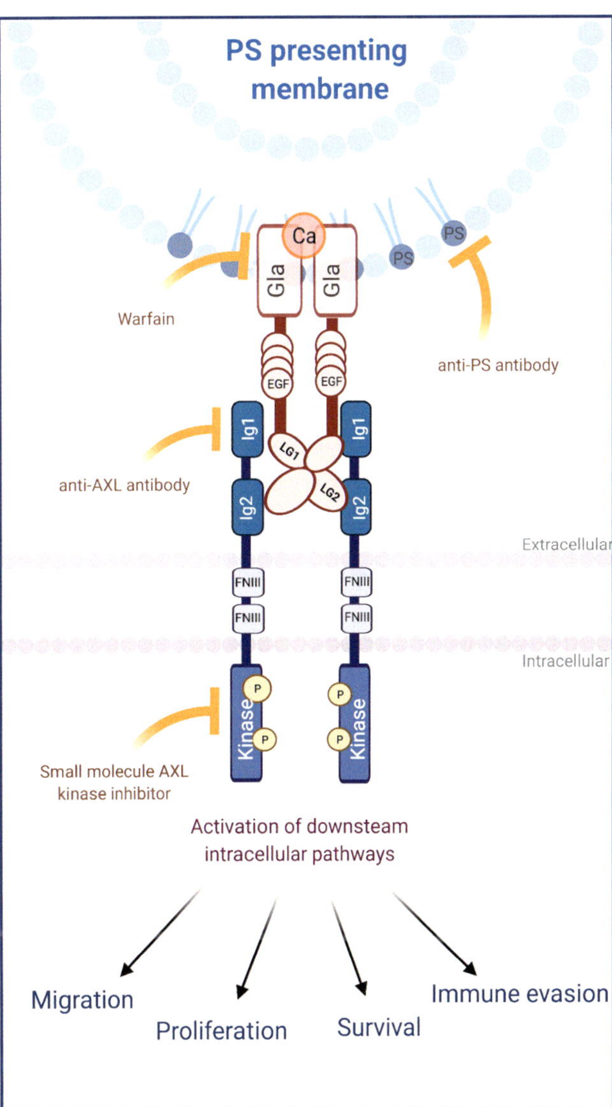

Fig. 18.2 Therapeutic targeting of AXL-mediated signaling. AXL signaling can be targeted at several levels including blocking of GAS6-PS interactions with anti-PS antibodies, inhibition of GAS6 post-translational gamma-carboxylation with vitamin K antagonists (e.g., warfarin), disruption of the GAS6-AXL interaction with compounds or antibodies that recognize epitopes within the AXL Ig-like domain, or by AXL-targeted small molecule kinase inhibitors. Figure created with BioRender.com

necessary to effectuate the ligand-induced activation of AXL. Warfarin acts by reducing the functional vitamin K reserves in the body, and thus reduce the vitamin K-dependent activation of numerous clotting factors, as well as the TAM receptor ligands GAS6 and ProteinS, since gamma-carboxylation of these factors and ligands are vitamin K dependent. Since the 1960s there have been reports that warfarin exerts anti-cancer effects [132]. In a study of pancreatic ductal adenocarcinoma (PDAC) GAS6-dependent AXL activation was inhibited in two ways, first by low-dose of warfarin, sufficient to inhibit gamma-carboxylation of GAS6 but not affect coagulation, and secondly by specific small molecule AXL-targeted agents. Inhibiting GAS6 dependent AXL activation in this PDAC model efficiently blocked the tumor-stroma crosstalk mediated progression and spread of pancreatic cancer in vitro and in vivo. The authors concluded that GAS6-induced AXL signaling is a critical driver of pancreatic cancer plasticity and progression, and suggest that inhibition by low-dose warfarin or other AXL-targeted agents may improve outcome in patients with AXL-overexpressing PDAC [64]. Kirane and colleagues demonstrate that the molecular mechanism underlying the antitumor effects of warfarin are unrelated to its effect on coagulation, but due to the inhibition of the AXL receptor tyrosine kinase on tumor cells [64]. These findings are supported by a large register-based cohort study, with a cohort comprising 1,2 million persons aged 53–82 years, utilizing the Norwegian National Registry, the cancer registry of Norway, and the Norwegian prescription database. This study showed lower cancer incidence in warfarin users compared to non-users, both for total cancer cases and for most of the major cancer forms such as prostate and lung [133].

The accumulating evidence supporting the involvement of AXL RTK activity as a key mediator of therapeutic resistance has spurred interest in developing AXL targeting agents for clinical translation [134, 135]. A complete overview of current clinical trials evaluating AXL inhibition for various malignancies can be found at *clinicaltrials.gov*. The majority of these are small-molecule kinase inhibitors originally identified as potent c-MET inhibitors. Bemcentinib (formerly known as BGB324, R428) was the first small molecule inhibitor specifically developed to target AXL kinase currently to enter clinical trials [136]. Several companies report ongoing preclinical development of selective AXL inhibitors. The results from ongoing trials with specific AXL inhibitors are of particular interest to provide proof-of-principle evidence for the clinical efficacy of AXL inhibition in the therapy-resistant setting.

AXL as a Biomarker

The role of AXL as an independent prognostic biomarker has been discussed in detail above and is summarized in Table 18.1. The role of AXL as biomarker of resistance to cytotoxic therapies and targeted therapies are summarized in Tables 18.2 and 18.3. Furthermore, high AXL protein expression in a malignant tissue does not necessarily imply high AXL-mediated signaling in the carcinoma cells, as AXL may also be expressed on numerous stromal and immune cell compartments of the malignant tissue. A few ongoing studies have addressed this issue by quantification of AXL expression of malignant cells and stromal cells separately, and the correlation to prognosis or therapy response can be calculated on the cancer cell score, stromal cell score, or combined score. This information may be particularly useful for evaluating the role of AXL as a biomarker for resistance to immune checkpoint blockade. Most clinical studies performed have not stratified patients according to their EMT score or AXL expression.

Soluble AXL (sAXL) is formed when the receptor's extracellular domain is cleaved by metalloproteases and represents an additional modality of AXL-mediated signaling and regulation. Increased serum sAXL has been suggested as a biomarker of response to AXL-targeted therapies (reviewed in: [42, 137]).

Concluding Remarks/Summary and Future Perspectives

Despite the steady introduction of improved molecularly targeted compounds and tailored treatment regimens, innate and acquired therapy resistance remains a confounding reality for cancer patients and a significant obstacle to successful cancer therapy. Cellular plasticity is increasingly recognized as a major mediator of therapy resistance and metastatic dissemination of cancer cells, although the underlying molecular mechanisms are still largely unexplored. The AXL receptor tyrosine kinase has emerged as a prominent mediator of cellular plasticity, and, as summarized in this chapter, up-regulation and activation of AXL RTK has been shown in a wide range of both solid and liquid malignancies with a poor prognosis. Accumulating evidence has demonstrated AXL overexpression and activation as a central mechanism of acquired resistance to both cytotoxic and molecularly targeted therapies, and more recently as part of signatures of cancers with innate resistance to immunotherapy by immune checkpoint blockade. The recently discovered role of AXL

Table 18.3 AXL in resistance to targeted therapeutics

Target	Drug	Malignancy	Reference
ADI-PEG20	Arginine depleting enzyme	Melanoma	[251]
ALK	Crizotinib	NSCLC	[252, 253]
ALK^{F1174L}	TAE684, ceritinib	Neuroblastoma	[254]
ATR	VX-970/M6620/berzosertib VE-822	NSCLC LCNEC Melanoma	[202, 255]
BCR-ABL	Imatinib, Nilotinib Ponatinib	CML	[62, 106, 107, 194]
BTK	Ibrutinib TP-4216	CLL	[193, 256]
CHK1/2	AZD7762	Melanoma	[255]
c-KIT	Imatinib	GIST	[103, 104]
EGFR	EGFR-TKI (erlotinib, gefitinib)	NSCLC (EGFR mutated)	[28, 59, 60, 98, 99, 101, 206, 209, 257]
		NSCLC (EGFR wildtype)	[60, 246]
		Breast cancer (TNBC)	[91, 258]
		HNSCC	[186]
		Colon cancer	[100]
		Liver cancer	[100]
		Tongue cancer	[100]
	Irreversible EGFR-TKI (rociletinib/CO-1686, Osimertinib/AZD9291)	NSCLC	[97, 208, 211, 259, 260]
	Cetuximab	HNSCC	[85, 102, 242]
		NSCLC	[102, 261]
		Colon cancer	[262]
FLT3	PKC412, Quizartinib/AC220	AML	[263, 264]
HER2	Lapatinib, trastuzumab	Breast cancer, including TNBC	[61, 265]
		Ovarian cancer	[265]
		Esophageal cancer	[266]
	Sapitinib, Afatinib (EGFR/HER2/HER3- inhibitor)	Breast cancer	[267]
		Gastric cancer	[268]
IGF-IR	MAB39 (IGF-IR-blocking Ab)	Rhabdomyosarcoma	[269]
MAPK pathway in BRAFV600E	BRAF inhibitors (PLX4720, vemurafenib, dabrafenib) MEK inhibitors (AZD6244/selumetinib, trametinib)	Melanoma	[109, 110, 118, 120, 198, 270]
	ERK inhibitor (SCH772684)	Glioma	[271]
MEK	MEK1 inhibitor	Pancreatic cancer	[112]
		Melanoma (NRAS mutated)	[198]
PARP	Olaparib	NSCLC TNBC HNSCC	[272]
PI3Kα	Alpelisib/BYL719	Esophageal SCC	[90, 185]
		HNSCC	[90, 185, 273]
TRAIL	Recombinant TRAIL	Esophageal adenocarcinoma	[274]
VEGF	Bevacizumab	Colon cancer	[275]
	Anti- VEGF	Breast cancer	[60]
		NSCLC	[60]
	Axitinib	RCC	[241, 276]
Multi-kinase inhibitors	Sunitinib, Pazopanib (VEGFR, PDGFR, c-KIT, FGFR)	RCC	[241, 276, 277]

Abbreviations: *AML* acute myeloid leukemia, *CML* chronic myeloid leukemia, *GIST* gastrointestinal stromal tumors, *HNSCC* head- and neck-squamous cell carcinoma, *LCNEC* Large cell neuroendocrine carcinoma, *NSCLC* non-small cell lung cancer, *RCC* renal cell carcinoma, *SCC* Squamous cell carcinoma, *TNBC* triple negative breast cancer as a stem cell regulator in epithelial tissues, could perhaps also serve to provide an explanation for the particular regulation of AXL activation. Due to its role as a mediator of cancer cell plasticity, AXL is an exceptionally promising molecular target for contemporary treatment regimens under evaluation in ongoing clinical trials with specific AXL inhibitors.

Acknowledgments Parts of the text, tables, and figure was published in the first edition of "Biomarkers of the Tumor Microenvironment: Basic Studies and Practical applications" (ISBN 978-3-319-39145-8). The contents are reprinted in this updated version of the book chapter with permission from the publisher: Springer Nature.

Conflict of interest statement: J.B.L. is the founder of BerGenBio ASA. The remaining authors declare no potential conflicts of interest.

References

1. Ahmad AS, Ormiston-Smith N, Sasieni PD. Trends in the lifetime risk of developing cancer in Great Britain: comparison of risk for those born from 1930 to 1960. Br J Cancer. 2015;112(5):943–7.

2. Pazarentzos E, Bivona TG. Adaptive stress signaling in targeted cancer therapy resistance. Oncogene. 2015;34(45):5599–606.

3. Marquart J, Chen EY, Prasad V. Estimation of the percentage of US patients with cancer who benefit from genome-driven oncology. JAMA Oncol. 2018;4(8):1093–8.

4. Junttila MR, de Sauvage FJ. Influence of tumour microenvironment heterogeneity on therapeutic response. Nature. 2013;501(7467):346–54.

5. Meacham CE, Morrison SJ. Tumour heterogeneity and cancer cell plasticity. Nature. 2013;501(7467):328–37.

6. !!! INVALID CITATION !!! [3, 4].

7. Ye X, Weinberg RA. Epithelial-mesenchymal plasticity: a central regulator of cancer progression. Trends Cell Biol. 2015;25(11):675–86.

8. Egeblad M, Nakasone ES, Werb Z. Tumors as organs: complex tissues that interface with the entire organism. Dev Cell. 2010;18(6):884–901.

9. Polyak K. Tumor heterogeneity confounds and illuminates: a case for Darwinian tumor evolution. Nat Med. 2014;20(4):344–6.

10. Easwaran H, Tsai HC, Baylin SB. Cancer epigenetics: tumor heterogeneity, plasticity of stem-like states, and drug resistance. Mol Cell. 2014;54(5):716–27.

11. Nieto MA. The ins and outs of the epithelial to mesenchymal transition in health and disease. Annu Rev Cell Dev Biol. 2011;27:347–76.

12. Nieto MA. Epithelial plasticity: a common theme in embryonic and cancer cells. Science. 2013;342(6159):1234850.

13. Lawson DA, Bhakta NR, Kessenbrock K, Prummel KD, Yu Y, Takai K, et al. Single-cell analysis reveals a stem-cell program in human metastatic breast cancer cells. Nature. 2015;526(7571):131–5.

14. Hay ED. The mesenchymal cell, its role in the embryo, and the remarkable signaling mechanisms that create it. Dev Dyn. 2005;233(3):706–20.

15. Pinto CA, Widodo E, Waltham M, Thompson EW. Breast cancer stem cells and epithelial mesenchymal plasticity - implications for chemoresistance. Cancer Lett. 2013;341(1):56–62.

16. Yang J, Antin P, Berx G, Blanpain C, Brabletz T, Bronner M, et al. Guidelines and definitions for research on epithelial-mesenchymal transition. Nat Rev Mol Cell Biol. 2020;21(6):341–52.

17. Thiery JP, Sleeman JP. Complex networks orchestrate epithelial-mesenchymal transitions. Nat Rev Mol Cell Biol. 2006;7(2):131–42.

18. Sun Y, Chen CS, Fu J. Forcing stem cells to behave: a biophysical perspective of the cellular microenvironment. Annu Rev Biophys. 2012;41:519–42.

19. Hay ED. An overview of epithelio-mesenchymal transformation. Acta Anat (Basel). 1995;154(1):8–20.

20. Rios AC, Fu NY, Lindeman GJ, Visvader JE. In situ identification of bipotent stem cells in the mammary gland. Nature. 2014;506(7488):322–7.

21. Phillips S, Prat A, Sedic M, Proia T, Wronski A, Mazumdar S, et al. Cell-state transitions regulated by SLUG are critical for tissue regeneration and tumor initiation. Stem Cell Rep. 2014;2(5):633–47.

22. Phillips S, Kuperwasser C. SLUG: Critical regulator of epithelial cell identity in breast development and cancer. Cell Adh Migr. 2014;8(6):578–87.

23. Mani SA, Guo W, Liao MJ, Eaton EN, Ayyanan A, Zhou AY, et al. The epithelial-mesenchymal transition generates cells with properties of stem cells. Cell. 2008;133(4):704–15.

24. Guo W, Keckesova Z, Donaher JL, Shibue T, Tischler V, Reinhardt F, et al. Slug and Sox9 cooperatively determine the mammary stem cell state. Cell. 2012;148(5):1015–28.

25. Engelsen AST, Wnuk-Lipinska K, Bougnaud S, Pelissier Vatter FA, Tiron C, Villadsen R, et al. AXL is a driver of stemness in normal mammary gland and breast cancer. iScience. 2020;23(11):101649.

26. Tan TZ, Miow QH, Miki Y, Noda T, Mori S, Huang RY, et al. Epithelial-mesenchymal transition spectrum quantification and its efficacy in deciphering survival and drug responses of cancer patients. EMBO Mol Med. 2014;6(10):1279–93.

27. Blick T, Hugo H, Widodo E, Waltham M, Pinto C, Mani SA, et al. Epithelial mesenchymal transition traits in human breast cancer cell lines parallel the CD44(hi/)CD24 (lo/-) stem cell phenotype in human breast cancer. J Mammary Gland Biol Neoplasia. 2010;15(2):235–52.

28. Byers LA, Diao L, Wang J, Saintigny P, Girard L, Peyton M, et al. An epithelial-mesenchymal transition gene signature predicts resistance to EGFR and PI3K inhibitors and identifies Axl as a therapeutic target for overcoming EGFR inhibitor resistance. Clin Cancer Res. 2013;19(1):279–90.

29. Talbot LJ, Bhattacharya SD, Kuo PC. Epithelial-mesenchymal transition, the tumor microenvironment, and metastatic behavior of epithelial malignancies. Int J Biochem Mol Biol. 2012;3(2):117–36.

30. Ocana OH, Corcoles R, Fabra A, Moreno-Bueno G, Acloque H, Vega S, et al. Metastatic colonization requires the repression of the epithelial-mesenchymal transition inducer Prrx1. Cancer Cell. 2012;22(6):709–24.

31. Zheng X, Carstens JL, Kim J, Scheible M, Kaye J, Sugimoto H, et al. Epithelial-to-mesenchymal transition is dispensable for metastasis but induces chemoresistance in pancreatic cancer. Nature. 2015;527(7579):525–30.

32. Fischer KR, Durrans A, Lee S, Sheng J, Li F, Wong ST, et al. Epithelial-to-mesenchymal transition is not required for lung metastasis but contributes to chemoresistance. Nature. 2015;527(7579):472–6.

33. Williams ED, Gao D, Redfern A, Thompson EW. Controversies around epithelial-mesenchymal plasticity in cancer metastasis. Nat Rev Cancer. 2019;19(12):716–32.

34. Brabletz T. To differentiate or not--routes towards metastasis. Nat Rev Cancer. 2012;12(6):425–36.

35. Aparicio LA, Blanco M, Castosa R, Concha A, Valladares M, Calvo L, et al. Clinical implications of epithelial cell plasticity in cancer progression. Cancer Lett. 2015;366(1):1–10.

36. Graham DK, DeRyckere D, Davies KD, Earp HS. The TAM family: phosphatidylserine sensing receptor tyrosine kinases gone awry in cancer. Nat Rev Cancer. 2014;14(12):769–85.

37. Lew ED, Oh J, Burrola PG, Lax I, Zagorska A, Traves PG, et al. Differential TAM receptor-ligand-phospholipid interactions delimit differential TAM bioactivities. Elife. 2014;3

38. Hasanbasic I, Rajotte I, Blostein M. The role of gamma-carboxylation in the anti-apoptotic function of gas6. J Thromb Haemost. 2005;3(12):2790–7.

39. Zhang Y, Wolf-Yadlin A, Ross PL, Pappin DJ, Rush J, Lauffenburger DA, et al. Time-resolved mass spectrometry of tyrosine phosphorylation sites in the epidermal growth factor receptor signaling network reveals dynamic modules. Mol Cell Proteomics. 2005;4(9):1240–50.

40. Wang CP, Yagi K, Lin PJ, Jin DY, Makabe KW, Stafford DW. Identification of a gene encoding a typical gamma-carboxyglutamic acid domain in the tunicate Halocynthia roretzi. J Thromb Haemost. 2003;1(1):118–23.

41. Meyer AS, Zweemer AJ, Lauffenburger DA. The AXL receptor is a sensor of ligand spatial heterogeneity. Cell Syst. 2015;1(1):25–36.

42. Korshunov VA. Axl-dependent signalling: a clinical update. Clin Sci (Lond). 2012;122(8):361–8.

43. O'Bryan JP, Frye RA, Cogswell PC, Neubauer A, Kitch B, Prokop C, et al. Axl, a transforming gene isolated from primary human myeloid leukemia cells, encodes a novel receptor tyrosine kinase. Mol Cell Biol. 1991;11(10):5016–31.

44. Verma A, Warner SL, Vankayalapati H, Bearss DJ, Sharma S. Targeting Axl and Mer kinases in cancer. Mol Cancer Ther. 2011;10(10):1763–73.

45. Liu E, Hjelle B, Bishop JM. Transforming genes in chronic myelogenous leukemia. Proc Natl Acad Sci U S A. 1988;85(6):1952–6.

46. Janssen JW, Schulz AS, Steenvoorden AC, Schmidberger M, Strehl S, Ambros PF, et al. A novel putative tyrosine kinase receptor with oncogenic potential. Oncogene. 1991;6(11):2113–20.

47. Linger RM, Keating AK, Earp HS, Graham DK. TAM receptor tyrosine kinases: biologic functions, signaling, and potential therapeutic targeting in human cancer. Adv Cancer Res. 2008;100:35–83.

48. Ben-Batalla I, Schultze A, Wroblewski M, Erdmann R, Heuser M, Waizenegger JS, et al. Axl, a prognostic and therapeutic target in acute myeloid leukemia mediates paracrine crosstalk of leukemia cells with bone marrow stroma. Blood. 2013;122(14):2443–52.

49. Gjerdrum C, Tiron C, Hoiby T, Stefansson I, Haugen H, Sandal T, et al. Axl is an essential epithelial-to-mesenchymal transition-induced regulator of breast cancer metastasis and patient survival. Proc Natl Acad Sci U S A. 2010;107(3):1124–9.

50. Shieh YS, Lai CY, Kao YR, Shiah SG, Chu YW, Lee HS, et al. Expression of axl in lung adenocarcinoma and correlation with tumor progression. Neoplasia. 2005;7(12):1058–64.

51. Del Pozo Martin Y, Park D, Ramachandran A, Ombrato L, Calvo F, Chakravarty P, et al. Mesenchymal cancer cell-stroma crosstalk promotes niche activation, epithelial reversion, and metastatic colonization. Cell Rep. 2015;13(11):2456–69.

52. Li Y, Ye X, Tan C, Hongo JA, Zha J, Liu J, et al. Axl as a potential therapeutic target in cancer: role of Axl in tumor growth, metastasis and angiogenesis. Oncogene. 2009;28(39):3442–55.

53. Song X, Wang H, Logsdon CD, Rashid A, Fleming JB, Abbruzzese JL, et al. Overexpression of receptor tyrosine kinase Axl promotes tumor cell invasion and survival in pancreatic ductal adenocarcinoma. Cancer. 2011;117(4):734–43.

54. Thiery JP. Epithelial-mesenchymal transitions in tumour progression. Nat Rev Cancer. 2002;2(6):442–54.

55. Tam WL, Weinberg RA. The epigenetics of epithelial-mesenchymal plasticity in cancer. Nat Med. 2013;19(11):1438–49.

56. Kalluri R, Weinberg RA. The basics of epithelial-mesenchymal transition. J Clin Invest. 2009;119(6):1420–8.

57. Obenauf AC, Massague J. Surviving at a distance: organ-specific metastasis. Trends Cancer. 2015;1(1):76–91.

58. Holland SJ, Pan A, Franci C, Hu Y, Chang B, Li W, et al. R428, a selective small molecule inhibitor of Axl kinase, blocks tumor spread and prolongs survival in models of metastatic breast cancer. Cancer Res. 2010;70(4):1544–54.

59. Zhang Z, Lee JC, Lin L, Olivas V, Au V, LaFramboise T, et al. Activation of the AXL kinase causes resistance to EGFR-targeted therapy in lung cancer. Nat Genet. 2012;44(8):852–60.

60. Ye X, Li Y, Stawicki S, Couto S, Eastham-Anderson J, Kallop D, et al. An anti-Axl monoclonal antibody attenuates xenograft tumor growth and enhances the effect of multiple anticancer therapies. Oncogene. 2010;29(38):5254–64.

61. Liu L, Greger J, Shi H, Liu Y, Greshock J, Annan R, et al. Novel mechanism of lapatinib resistance in HER2-positive breast tumor cells: activation of AXL. Cancer Res. 2009;69(17):6871–8.

62. Dufies M, Jacquel A, Belhacene N, Robert G, Cluzeau T, Luciano F, et al. Mechanisms of AXL overexpression and function in Imatinib-resistant chronic myeloid leukemia cells. Oncotarget. 2011;2(11):874–85.

63. Rankin EB, Fuh KC, Taylor TE, Krieg AJ, Musser M, Yuan J, et al. AXL is an essential factor and therapeutic target for metastatic ovarian cancer. Cancer Res. 2010;70(19):7570–9.

64. Kirane A, Ludwig KF, Sorrelle N, Haaland G, Sandal T, Ranaweera R, et al. Warfarin blocks Gas6-Mediated Axl activation required for pancreatic cancer epithelial plasticity and metastasis. Cancer Res. 2015;75(18):3699–705.

65. Koorstra JB, Karikari CA, Feldmann G, Bisht S, Rojas PL, Offerhaus GJ, et al. The Axl receptor tyrosine kinase confers an adverse prognostic influence in pancreatic cancer and represents a new therapeutic target. Cancer Biol Ther. 2009;8(7):618–26.

66. Vuoriluoto K, Haugen H, Kiviluoto S, Mpindi JP, Nevo J, Gjerdrum C, et al. Vimentin regulates EMT induction by Slug and oncogenic H-Ras and migration by governing Axl expression in breast cancer. Oncogene. 2011;30(12):1436–48.

67. Thomson S, Petti F, Sujka-Kwok I, Mercado P, Bean J, Monaghan M, et al. A systems view of epithelial-mesenchymal transition signaling states. Clin Exp Metastasis. 2011;28(2):137–55.

68. Jokela TA, Engelsen AST, Rybicka A, Pelissier Vatter FA, Garbe JC, Miyano M, et al. Microenvironment-induced non-sporadic expression of the AXL and cKIT receptors are related to epithelial plasticity and drug resistance. Front Cell Dev Biol. 2018;6:41.

69. Terry S, Engelsen AST, Buart S, Elsayed WS, Venkatesh GH, Chouaib S. Hypoxia-driven intratumor heterogeneity and immune evasion. Cancer Lett. 2020;492:1–10.

70. Rankin EB, Fuh KC, Castellini L, Viswanathan K, Finger EC, Diep AN, et al. Direct regulation of GAS6/AXL signaling by HIF promotes renal metastasis through SRC and MET. Proc Natl Acad Sci U S A. 2014;111(37):13373–8.

71. Yttersian Sletta K, Tveitaras MK, Lu N, Engelsen AST, Reed RK, Garmann-Johnsen A, et al. Oxygen-dependent regulation of tumor growth and metastasis in human breast cancer xenografts. PLoS One. 2017;12(8):e0183254.

72. Moen I, Stuhr LE. Hyperbaric oxygen therapy and cancer--a review. Target Oncol. 2012;7(4):233–42.

73. Tai KY, Shieh YS, Lee CS, Shiah SG, Wu CW. Axl promotes cell invasion by inducing MMP-9 activity through activation of NF-kappaB and Brg-1. Oncogene. 2008;27(29):4044–55.

74. Holland SJ, Powell MJ, Franci C, Chan EW, Friera AM, Atchison RE, et al. Multiple roles for the receptor tyrosine kinase axl in tumor formation. Cancer Res. 2005;65(20):9294–303.

75. Melaragno MG, Fridell YW, Berk BC. The Gas6/Axl system: a novel regulator of vascular cell function. Trends Cardiovasc Med. 1999;9(8):250–3.

76. Hutterer M, Knyazev P, Abate A, Reschke M, Maier H, Stefanova N, et al. Axl and growth arrest-specific gene 6 are frequently overexpressed in human gliomas and predict poor prognosis

in patients with glioblastoma multiforme. Clin Cancer Res. 2008;14(1):130–8.

77. Linger RM, Cohen RA, Cummings CT, Sather S, Migdall-Wilson J, Middleton DH, et al. Mer or Axl receptor tyrosine kinase inhibition promotes apoptosis, blocks growth and enhances chemosensitivity of human non-small cell lung cancer. Oncogene. 2013;32(29):3420–31.

78. Fridell YW, Villa J Jr, Attar EC, Liu ET. GAS6 induces Axl-mediated chemotaxis of vascular smooth muscle cells. J Biol Chem. 1998;273(12):7123–6.

79. Ruan GX, Kazlauskas A. Axl is essential for VEGF-A-dependent activation of PI3K/Akt. EMBO J. 2012;31(7):1692–703.

80. Macleod K, Mullen P, Sewell J, Rabiasz G, Lawrie S, Miller E, et al. Altered ErbB receptor signaling and gene expression in cisplatin-resistant ovarian cancer. Cancer Res. 2005;65(15):6789–800.

81. Weinger JG, Gohari P, Yan Y, Backer JM, Varnum B, Shafit-Zagardo B. In brain, Axl recruits Grb2 and the p85 regulatory subunit of PI3 kinase; in vitro mutagenesis defines the requisite binding sites for downstream Akt activation. J Neurochem. 2008;106(1):134–46.

82. Goruppi S, Ruaro E, Varnum B, Schneider C. Gas6-mediated survival in NIH3T3 cells activates stress signalling cascade and is independent of Ras. Oncogene. 1999;18(29):4224–36.

83. Zhao Y, Sun X, Jiang L, Yang F, Zhang Z, Jia L. Differential expression of Axl and correlation with invasion and multidrug resistance in cancer cells. Cancer Invest. 2012;30(4):287–94.

84. Hong J, Peng D, Chen Z, Schdev V, Belkhiri A. ABL regulation by AXL promotes cisplatin resistance in esophageal cancer. Cancer Res. 2013;73(1):331–40.

85. Brand TM, Iida M, Stein AP, Corrigan KL, Braverman CM, Coan JP, et al. AXL Is a logical molecular target in head and neck squamous cell carcinoma. Clin Cancer Res. 2015;21(11):2601–12.

86. Cichon MA, Szentpetery Z, Caley MP, Papadakis ES, Mackenzie IC, Brennan CH, et al. The receptor tyrosine kinase Axl regulates cell-cell adhesion and stemness in cutaneous squamous cell carcinoma. Oncogene. 2014;33(32):4185–92.

87. Asiedu MK, Beauchamp-Perez FD, Ingle JN, Behrens MD, Radisky DC, Knutson KL. AXL induces epithelial-to-mesenchymal transition and regulates the function of breast cancer stem cells. Oncogene. 2014;33(10):1316–24.

88. Wilson C, Ye X, Pham T, Lin E, Chan S, McNamara E, et al. AXL inhibition sensitizes mesenchymal cancer cells to antimitotic drugs. Cancer Res. 2014;74(20):5878–90.

89. Kurokawa M, Ise N, Omi K, Goishi K, Higashiyama S. Cisplatin influences acquisition of resistance to molecular-targeted agents through epithelial-mesenchymal transition-like changes. Cancer Sci. 2013;104(7):904–11.

90. Elkabets M, Pazarentzos E, Juric D, Sheng Q, Pelossof RA, Brook S, et al. AXL mediates resistance to PI3Kalpha inhibition by activating the EGFR/PKC/mTOR axis in head and neck and esophageal squamous cell carcinomas. Cancer Cell. 2015;27(4):533–46.

91. Meyer AS, Miller MA, Gertler FB, Lauffenburger DA. The receptor AXL diversifies EGFR signaling and limits the response to EGFR-targeted inhibitors in triple-negative breast cancer cells. Sci Signal. 2013;6(287):ra66.

92. Rosland GV, Engelsen AS. Novel points of attack for targeted cancer therapy. Basic Clin Pharmacol Toxicol. 2015;116(1):9–18.

93. Thomson S, Buck E, Petti F, Griffin G, Brown E, Ramnarine N, et al. Epithelial to mesenchymal transition is a determinant of sensitivity of non-small-cell lung carcinoma cell lines and xenografts to epidermal growth factor receptor inhibition. Cancer Res. 2005;65(20):9455–62.

94. Wu Z, Bai F, Fan L, Pang W, Han R, Wang J, et al. Coexpression of receptor tyrosine kinase AXL and EGFR in human primary lung adenocarcinomas. Hum Pathol. 2015;46(12):1935–44.

95. Ishikawa M, Sonobe M, Nakayama E, Kobayashi M, Kikuchi R, Kitamura J, et al. Higher expression of receptor tyrosine kinase Axl, and differential expression of its ligand, Gas6, predict poor survival in lung adenocarcinoma patients. Ann Surg Oncol. 2013;20(Suppl 3):S467–76.

96. Yoshida T, Zhang G, Smith MA, Lopez AS, Bai Y, Li J, et al. Tyrosine phosphoproteomics identifies both codrivers and cotargeting strategies for T790M-related EGFR-TKI resistance in non-small cell lung cancer. Clin Cancer Res. 2014;20(15):4059–74.

97. Walter AO, Sjin RT, Haringsma HJ, Ohashi K, Sun J, Lee K, et al. Discovery of a mutant-selective covalent inhibitor of EGFR that overcomes T790M-mediated resistance in NSCLC. Cancer Discov. 2013;3(12):1404–15.

98. Rho JK, Choi YJ, Kim SY, Kim TW, Choi EK, Yoon SJ, et al. MET and AXL inhibitor NPS-1034 exerts efficacy against lung cancer cells resistant to EGFR kinase inhibitors because of MET or AXL activation. Cancer Res. 2014;74(1):253–62.

99. Kim GW, Song JS, Choi CM, Rho JK, Kim SY, Jang SJ, et al. Multiple resistant factors in lung cancer with primary resistance to EGFR-TK inhibitors confer poor survival. Lung Cancer. 2015;88(2):139–46.

100. Gusenbauer S, Vlaicu P, Ullrich A. HGF induces novel EGFR functions involved in resistance formation to tyrosine kinase inhibitors. Oncogene. 2013;32(33):3846–56.

101. Bae SY, Hong JY, Lee HJ, Park HJ, Lee SK. Targeting the degradation of AXL receptor tyrosine kinase to overcome resistance in gefitinib-resistant non-small cell lung cancer. Oncotarget. 2015;6(12):10146–60.

102. Brand TM, Iida M, Stein AP, Corrigan KL, Braverman CM, Luthar N, et al. AXL mediates resistance to cetuximab therapy. Cancer Res. 2014;74(18):5152–64.

103. Mahadevan D, Cooke L, Riley C, Swart R, Simons B, Della Croce K, et al. A novel tyrosine kinase switch is a mechanism of imatinib resistance in gastrointestinal stromal tumors. Oncogene. 2007;26(27):3909–19.

104. Mahadevan D, Theiss N, Morales C, Stejskal AE, Cooke LS, Zhu M, et al. Novel receptor tyrosine kinase targeted combination therapies for imatinib-resistant gastrointestinal stromal tumors (GIST). Oncotarget. 2015;6(4):1954–66.

105. Grosso S, Puissant A, Dufies M, Colosetti P, Jacquel A, Lebrigand K, et al. Gene expression profiling of imatinib and PD166326-resistant CML cell lines identifies Fyn as a gene associated with resistance to BCR-ABL inhibitors. Mol Cancer Ther. 2009;8(7):1924–33.

106. Gioia R, Leroy C, Drullion C, Lagarde V, Etienne G, Dulucq S, et al. Quantitative phosphoproteomics revealed interplay between Syk and Lyn in the resistance to nilotinib in chronic myeloid leukemia cells. Blood. 2011;118(8):2211–21.

107. Gioia R, Tregoat C, Dumas PY, Lagarde V, Prouzet-Mauleon V, Desplat V, et al. CBL controls a tyrosine kinase network involving AXL, SYK and LYN in nilotinib-resistant chronic myeloid leukaemia. J Pathol. 2015;237(1):14–24.

108. Sensi M, Catani M, Castellano G, Nicolini G, Alciato F, Tragni G, et al. Human cutaneous melanomas lacking MITF and melanocyte differentiation antigens express a functional Axl receptor kinase. J Invest Dermatol. 2011;131(12):2448–57.

109. Konieczkowski DJ, Johannessen CM, Abudayyeh O, Kim JW, Cooper ZA, Piris A, et al. A melanoma cell state distinction influences sensitivity to MAPK pathway inhibitors. Cancer Discov. 2014;4(7):816–27.

110. Muller J, Krijgsman O, Tsoi J, Robert L, Hugo W, Song C, et al. Low MITF/AXL ratio predicts early resistance to multiple targeted drugs in melanoma. Nat Commun. 2014;5:5712.

111. Shimizu T, Tolcher AW, Papadopoulos KP, Beeram M, Rasco DW, Smith LS, et al. The clinical effect of the dual-targeting strategy involving PI3K/AKT/mTOR and RAS/MEK/ERK

111. pathways in patients with advanced cancer. Clin Cancer Res. 2012;18(8):2316–25.
112. Pettazzoni P, Viale A, Shah P, Carugo A, Ying H, Wang H, et al. Genetic events that limit the efficacy of MEK and RTK inhibitor therapies in a mouse model of KRAS-driven pancreatic cancer. Cancer Res. 2015;75(6):1091–101.
113. Jiao Y, Ou W, Meng F, Zhou H, Wang A. Targeting HSP90 in ovarian cancers with multiple receptor tyrosine kinase coactivation. Mol Cancer. 2011;10:125.
114. D'Arcangelo D, Gaetano C, Capogrossi MC. Acidification prevents endothelial cell apoptosis by Axl activation. Circ Res. 2002;91(7):e4–12.
115. Konishi A, Aizawa T, Mohan A, Korshunov VA, Berk BC. Hydrogen peroxide activates the Gas6-Axl pathway in vascular smooth muscle cells. J Biol Chem. 2004;279(27):28766–70.
116. Huang JS, Cho CY, Hong CC, Yan MD, Hsieh MC, Lay JD, et al. Oxidative stress enhances Axl-mediated cell migration through an Akt1/Rac1-dependent mechanism. Free Radic Biol Med. 2013;65:1246–56.
117. D'Arcangelo D, Ambrosino V, Giannuzzo M, Gaetano C, Capogrossi MC. Axl receptor activation mediates laminar shear stress anti-apoptotic effects in human endothelial cells. Cardiovasc Res. 2006;71(4):754–63.
118. Shaffer SM, Dunagin MC, Torborg SR, Torre EA, Emert B, Krepler C, et al. Rare cell variability and drug-induced reprogramming as a mode of cancer drug resistance. Nature. 2017;546(7658):431–5.
119. Torre E, Dueck H, Shaffer S, Gospocic J, Gupte R, Bonasio R, et al. Rare cell detection by single-cell RNA sequencing as guided by single-molecule RNA FISH. Cell Syst. 2018;6(2):171–9 e5.
120. Tirosh I, Izar B, Prakadan SM, Wadsworth MH 2nd, Treacy D, Trombetta JJ, et al. Dissecting the multicellular ecosystem of metastatic melanoma by single-cell RNA-seq. Science. 2016;352(6282):189–96.
121. Lotsberg ML, Rayford AJ, Thiery JP, Belleggia G, D'Mello Peters S, Lorens JB, Chouaib S, Terry S, Engelsen AST. Decoding cancer's camouflage: epithelial-mesenchymal plasticity in resistance to immune checkpoint blockade. Cancer Drug Resist. 2020;3
122. Nishino M, Ramaiya NH, Hatabu H, Hodi FS. Monitoring immune-checkpoint blockade: response evaluation and biomarker development. Nat Rev Clin Oncol. 2017;14(11):655–68.
123. Wang L, Saci A, Szabo PM, Chasalow SD, Castillo-Martin M, Domingo-Domenech J, et al. EMT- and stroma-related gene expression and resistance to PD-1 blockade in urothelial cancer. Nat Commun. 2018;9(1):3503.
124. Thompson JC, Hwang WT, Davis C, Deshpande C, Jeffries S, Rajpurohit Y, et al. Gene signatures of tumor inflammation and epithelial-to-mesenchymal transition (EMT) predict responses to immune checkpoint blockade in lung cancer with high accuracy. Lung Cancer. 2020;139:1–8.
125. Terry S, Abdou A, Engelsen AST, Buart S, Dessen P, Corgnac S, et al. AXL targeting overcomes human lung cancer cell resistance to NK- and CTL-mediated cytotoxicity. Cancer Immunol Res. 2019;7(11):1789–802.
126. Chouaib S, Janji B, Tittarelli A, Eggermont A, Thiery JP. Tumor plasticity interferes with anti-tumor immunity. Crit Rev Immunol. 2014;34(2):91–102.
127. Lotsberg ML, Wnuk-Lipinska K, Terry S, Tan TZ, Lu N, Trachsel-Moncho L, et al. AXL targeting abrogates autophagic flux and induces immunogenic cell death in drug-resistant cancer cells. J Thorac Oncol. 2020;15(6):973–99.
128. Garg AD, Agostinis P. Editorial: immunogenic cell death in cancer: from benchside research to bedside reality. Front Immunol. 2016;7:110.
129. Chen DS, Mellman I. Oncology meets immunology: the cancer-immunity cycle. Immunity. 2013;39(1):1–10.
130. Guo Z, Li Y, Zhang D, Ma J. Axl inhibition induces the anti-tumor immune response which can be further potentiated by PD-1 blockade in the mouse cancer models. Oncotarget. 2017;8(52):89761–74.
131. Boshuizen J, Pencheva N, Krijgsman O, D'Empaire Altimari D, Garrido Castro P, de Bruijn B, et al. Cooperative targeting of immunotherapy-resistant melanoma and lung cancer by an AXL-targeting antibody-drug conjugate and immune checkpoint blockade. Cancer Res. 2021;81(7):1775–87.
132. Bobek V, Kovarik J. Antitumor and antimetastatic effect of warfarin and heparins. Biomed Pharmacother. 2004;58(4):213–9.
133. Haaland GS, Falk RS, Straume O, Lorens JB. Association of warfarin use with lower overall cancer incidence among patients older than 50 years. JAMA Intern Med. 2017;177(12):1774–80.
134. Myers SH, Brunton VG, Unciti-Broceta A. AXL inhibitors in cancer: a medicinal chemistry perspective. J Med Chem. 2015;59:3593–608.
135. Feneyrolles C, Spenlinhauer A, Guiet L, Fauvel B, Dayde-Cazals B, Warnault P, et al. Axl kinase as a key target for oncology: focus on small molecule inhibitors. Mol Cancer Ther. 2014;13(9):2141–8.
136. Sheridan C. First Axl inhibitor enters clinical trials. Nat Biotechnol. 2013;31(9):775–6.
137. Merilahti JAM, Elenius K. Gamma-secretase-dependent signaling of receptor tyrosine kinases. Oncogene. 2019;38(2):151–63.
138. Cheng P, Phillips E, Kim SH, Taylor D, Hielscher T, Puccio L, et al. Kinome-wide shRNA screen identifies the receptor tyrosine kinase AXL as a key regulator for mesenchymal glioblastoma stem-like cells. Stem Cell Reports. 2015;4(5):899–913.
139. Keating AK, Kim GK, Jones AE, Donson AM, Ware K, Mulcahy JM, et al. Inhibition of Mer and Axl receptor tyrosine kinases in astrocytoma cells leads to increased apoptosis and improved chemosensitivity. Mol Cancer Ther. 2010;9(5):1298–307.
140. Vajkoczy P, Knyazev P, Kunkel A, Capelle HH, Behrndt S, von Tengg-Kobligk H, et al. Dominant-negative inhibition of the Axl receptor tyrosine kinase suppresses brain tumor cell growth and invasion and prolongs survival. Proc Natl Acad Sci U S A. 2006;103(15):5799–804.
141. Yen SY, Chen SR, Hsieh J, Li YS, Chuang SE, Chuang HM, et al. Biodegradable interstitial release polymer loading a novel small molecule targeting Axl receptor tyrosine kinase and reducing brain tumour migration and invasion. Oncogene. 2015;
142. Meel MH, de Gooijer MC, Metselaar DS, Sewing ACP, Zwaan K, Waranecki P, et al. Combined Therapy of AXL and HDAC Inhibition Reverses Mesenchymal Transition in Diffuse Intrinsic Pontine Glioma. Clin Cancer Res. 2020;26(13):3319–32.
143. Meric F, Lee WP, Sahin A, Zhang H, Kung HJ, Hung MC. Expression profile of tyrosine kinases in breast cancer. Clin Cancer Res. 2002;8(2):361–7.
144. Zhang YX, Knyazev PG, Cheburkin YV, Sharma K, Knyazev YP, Orfi L, et al. AXL is a potential target for therapeutic intervention in breast cancer progression. Cancer Res. 2008;68(6):1905–15.
145. Neve RM, Chin K, Fridlyand J, Yeh J, Baehner FL, Fevr T, et al. A collection of breast cancer cell lines for the study of functionally distinct cancer subtypes. Cancer Cell. 2006;10(6):515–27.
146. Berclaz G, Altermatt HJ, Rohrbach V, Kieffer I, Dreher E, Andres AC. Estrogen dependent expression of the receptor tyrosine kinase axl in normal and malignant human breast. Ann Oncol. 2001;12(6):819–24.
147. Li Y, Jia L, Liu C, Gong Y, Ren D, Wang N, et al. Axl as a downstream effector of TGF-beta1 via PI3K/Akt-PAK1 signaling pathway promotes tumor invasion and chemoresistance in breast carcinoma. Tumour Biol. 2015;36(2):1115–27.

148. Ren D, Li Y, Gong Y, Xu J, Miao X, Li X, et al. Phyllodes tumor of the breast: role of Axl and ST6GalNAcII in the development of mammary phyllodes tumors. Tumour Biol. 2014;35(10):9603–12.

149. Wang X, Saso H, Iwamoto T, Xia W, Gong Y, Pusztai L, et al. TIG1 promotes the development and progression of inflammatory breast cancer through activation of Axl kinase. Cancer Res. 2013;73(21):6516–25.

150. Nalwoga H, Ahmed L, Arnes JB, Wabinga H, Akslen LA. Strong expression of hypoxia-inducible factor-1alpha (HIF-1alpha) is associated with Axl expression and features of aggressive tumors in african breast cancer. PLoS One. 2016;11(1):e0146823.

151. Dine JL, O'Sullivan CC, Voeller D, Greer YE, Chavez KJ, Conway CM, et al. The TRAIL receptor agonist drozitumab targets basal B triple-negative breast cancer cells that express vimentin and Axl. Breast Cancer Res Treat. 2016;155(2):235–51.

152. Wu X, Zahari MS, Ma B, Liu R, Renuse S, Sahasrabuddhe NA, et al. Global phosphotyrosine survey in triple-negative breast cancer reveals activation of multiple tyrosine kinase signaling pathways. Oncotarget. 2015;6(30):29143–60.

153. Di Benedetto A, Mottolese M, Sperati F, Ercolani C, Di Lauro L, Pizzuti L, et al. Association between AXL, hippo transducers, and survival outcomes in male breast cancer. J Cell Physiol. 2017;232(8):2246–52.

154. Zajac O, Leclere R, Nicolas A, Meseure D, Marchio C, Vincent-Salomon A, et al. AXL controls directed migration of mesenchymal triple-negative breast cancer cells. Cells. 2020;9(1)

155. Kosok M, Alli-Shaik A, Bay BH, Gunaratne J. Comprehensive proteomic characterization reveals subclass-specific molecular aberrations within triple-negative breast cancer. iScience. 2020;23(2):100868.

156. Ahmed L, Nalwoga H, Arnes JB, Wabinga H, Micklem DR, Akslen LA. Increased tumor cell expression of Axl is a marker of aggressive features in breast cancer among African women. APMIS. 2015;123(8):688–96.

157. Li M, Lu J, Zhang F, Li H, Zhang B, Wu X, et al. Yes-associated protein 1 (YAP1) promotes human gallbladder tumor growth via activation of the AXL/MAPK pathway. Cancer Lett. 2014;355(2):201–9.

158. Mudduluru G, Ceppi P, Kumarswamy R, Scagliotti GV, Papotti M, Allgayer H. Regulation of Axl receptor tyrosine kinase expression by miR-34a and miR-199a/b in solid cancer. Oncogene. 2011;30(25):2888–99.

159. Mudduluru G, Vajkoczy P, Allgayer H. Myeloid zinc finger 1 induces migration, invasion, and in vivo metastasis through Axl gene expression in solid cancer. Mol Cancer Res. 2010;8(2):159–69.

160. Dunne PD, McArt DG, Blayney JK, Kalimutho M, Greer S, Wang T, et al. AXL is a key regulator of inherent and chemotherapy-induced invasion and predicts a poor clinical outcome in early-stage colon cancer. Clin Cancer Res. 2014;20(1):164–75.

161. Martinelli E, Martini G, Cardone C, Troiani T, Liguori G, Vitagliano D, et al. AXL is an oncotarget in human colorectal cancer. Oncotarget. 2015;6(27):23281–96.

162. Craven RJ, Xu LH, Weiner TM, Fridell YW, Dent GA, Srivastava S, et al. Receptor tyrosine kinases expressed in metastatic colon cancer. Int J Cancer. 1995;60(6):791–7.

163. Paccez JD, Duncan K, Vava A, Correa RG, Libermann TA, Parker MI, et al. Inactivation of GSK3beta and activation of NF-kappaB pathway via Axl represents an important mediator of tumorigenesis in esophageal squamous cell carcinoma. Mol Biol Cell. 2015;26(5):821–31.

164. Hector A, Montgomery EA, Karikari C, Canto M, Dunbar KB, Wang JS, et al. The Axl receptor tyrosine kinase is an adverse prognostic factor and a therapeutic target in esophageal adenocarcinoma. Cancer Biol Ther. 2010;10(10):1009–18.

165. Hong J, Abid F, Phillips S, Salaria SN, Revetta FL, Peng D, et al. Co-overexpression of AXL and c-ABL predicts a poor prognosis in esophageal adenocarcinoma and promotes cancer cell survival. J Cancer. 2020;11(20):5867–79.

166. Sawabu T, Seno H, Kawashima T, Fukuda A, Uenoyama Y, Kawada M, et al. Growth arrest-specific gene 6 and Axl signaling enhances gastric cancer cell survival via Akt pathway. Mol Carcinog. 2007;46(2):155–64.

167. Wu CW, Li AF, Chi CW, Lai CH, Huang CL, Lo SS, et al. Clinical significance of AXL kinase family in gastric cancer. Anticancer Res. 2002;22(2B):1071–8.

168. Bae CA, Ham IH, Oh HJ, Lee D, Woo J, Son SY, et al. Inhibiting the GAS6/AXL axis suppresses tumor progression by blocking the interaction between cancer-associated fibroblasts and cancer cells in gastric carcinoma. Gastric Cancer. 2020;23(5):824–36.

169. Chen PX, Li QY, Yang Z. Axl and prostasin are biomarkers for prognosis of ovarian adenocarcinoma. Ann Diagn Pathol. 2013;17(5):425–9.

170. Rea K, Pinciroli P, Sensi M, Alciato F, Bisaro B, Lozneanu L, et al. Novel Axl-driven signaling pathway and molecular signature characterize high-grade ovarian cancer patients with poor clinical outcome. Oncotarget. 2015;6(31):30859–75.

171. Sun W, Fujimoto J, Tamaya T. Coexpression of Gas6/Axl in human ovarian cancers. Oncology. 2004;66(6):450–7.

172. Kanlikilicer P, Ozpolat B, Aslan B, Bayraktar R, Gurbuz N, Rodriguez-Aguayo C, et al. Therapeutic targeting of AXL receptor tyrosine kinase inhibits tumor growth and intraperitoneal metastasis in ovarian cancer models. Mol Ther Nucleic Acids. 2017;9:251–62.

173. Tian M, Chen XS, Li LY, Wu HZ, Zeng D, Wang XL, et al. Inhibition of AXL enhances chemosensitivity of human ovarian cancer cells to cisplatin via decreasing glycolysis. Acta Pharmacol Sin. 2020;

174. Sun WS, Fujimoto J, Tamaya T. Coexpression of growth arrest-specific gene 6 and receptor tyrosine kinases Axl and Sky in human uterine endometrial cancers. Ann Oncol. 2003;14(6):898–906.

175. Sun WS, Fujimoto J, Tamaya T. Clinical implications of coexpression of growth arrest-specific gene 6 and receptor tyrosine kinases Axl and Sky in human uterine leiomyoma. Mol Hum Reprod. 2003;9(11):701–7.

176. Divine LM, Nguyen MR, Meller E, Desai RA, Arif B, Rankin EB, et al. AXL modulates extracellular matrix protein expression and is essential for invasion and metastasis in endometrial cancer. Oncotarget. 2016;7(47):77291–305.

177. Palisoul ML, Quinn JM, Schepers E, Hagemann IS, Guo L, Reger K, et al. Inhibition of the receptor tyrosine kinase AXL restores paclitaxel chemosensitivity in uterine serous cancer. Mol Cancer Ther. 2017;16(12):2881–91.

178. Lee HJ, Jeng YM, Chen YL, Chung L, Yuan RH. Gas6/Axl pathway promotes tumor invasion through the transcriptional activation of Slug in hepatocellular carcinoma. Carcinogenesis. 2014;35(4):769–75.

179. Reichl P, Dengler M, van Zijl F, Huber H, Fuhrlinger G, Reichel C, et al. Axl activates autocrine transforming growth factor-beta signaling in hepatocellular carcinoma. Hepatology. 2015;61(3):930–41.

180. Tsou AP, Wu KM, Tsen TY, Chi CW, Chiu JH, Lui WY, et al. Parallel hybridization analysis of multiple protein kinase genes: identification of gene expression patterns characteristic of human hepatocellular carcinoma. Genomics. 1998;50(3):331–40.

181. Xu J, Jia L, Ma H, Li Y, Ma Z, Zhao Y. Axl gene knockdown inhibits the metastasis properties of hepatocellular carcinoma via PI3K/Akt-PAK1 signal pathway. Tumour Biol. 2014;35(4):3809–17.

182. Liu J, Wang K, Yan Z, Xia Y, Li J, Shi L, et al. Axl expression stratifies patients with poor prognosis after hepatectomy for hepatocellular carcinoma. PLoS One. 2016;11(5):e0154767.

183. Lee CH, Liu SY, Chou KC, Yeh CT, Shiah SG, Huang RY, et al. Tumor-associated macrophages promote oral cancer progression through activation of the Axl signaling pathway. Ann Surg Oncol. 2014;21(3):1031–7.

184. Lee CH, Yen CY, Liu SY, Chen CK, Chiang CF, Shiah SG, et al. Axl is a prognostic marker in oral squamous cell carcinoma. Ann Surg Oncol. 2012;19(Suppl 3):S500–8.

185. Badarni M, Prasad M, Balaban N, Zorea J, Yegodayev KM, Joshua BZ, et al. Repression of AXL expression by AP-1/JNK blockage overcomes resistance to PI3Ka therapy. JCI Insight. 2019;5

186. Giles KM, Kalinowski FC, Candy PA, Epis MR, Zhang PM, Redfern AD, et al. Axl mediates acquired resistance of head and neck cancer cells to the epidermal growth factor receptor inhibitor erlotinib. Mol Cancer Ther. 2013;12(11):2541–58.

187. Rochlitz C, Lohri A, Bacchi M, Schmidt M, Nagel S, Fopp M, et al. Axl expression is associated with adverse prognosis and with expression of Bcl-2 and CD34 in de novo acute myeloid leukemia (AML): results from a multicenter trial of the Swiss Group for Clinical Cancer Research (SAKK). Leukemia. 1999;13(9):1352–8.

188. Park IK, Mishra A, Chandler J, Whitman SP, Marcucci G, Caligiuri MA. Inhibition of the receptor tyrosine kinase Axl impedes activation of the FLT3 internal tandem duplication in human acute myeloid leukemia: implications for Axl as a potential therapeutic target. Blood. 2013;121(11):2064–73.

189. Neubauer A, Fiebeler A, Graham DK, O'Bryan JP, Schmidt CA, Barckow P, et al. Expression of axl, a transforming receptor tyrosine kinase, in normal and malignant hematopoiesis. Blood. 1994;84(6):1931–41.

190. Boysen J, Sinha S, Price-Troska T, Warner SL, Bearss DJ, Viswanatha D, et al. The tumor suppressor axis p53/miR-34a regulates Axl expression in B-cell chronic lymphocytic leukemia: implications for therapy in p53-defective CLL patients. Leukemia. 2014;28(2):451–5.

191. Ghosh AK, Secreto C, Boysen J, Sassoon T, Shanafelt TD, Mukhopadhyay D, et al. The novel receptor tyrosine kinase Axl is constitutively active in B-cell chronic lymphocytic leukemia and acts as a docking site of nonreceptor kinases: implications for therapy. Blood. 2011;117(6):1928–37.

192. Ghosh AK, Secreto CR, Knox TR, Ding W, Mukhopadhyay D, Kay NE. Circulating microvesicles in B-cell chronic lymphocytic leukemia can stimulate marrow stromal cells: implications for disease progression. Blood. 2010;115(9):1755–64.

193. Sinha S, Boysen JC, Chaffee KG, Kabat BF, Slager SL, Parikh SA, et al. Chronic lymphocytic leukemia cells from ibrutinib treated patients are sensitive to Axl receptor tyrosine kinase inhibitor therapy. Oncotarget. 2018;9(98):37173–84.

194. Ben-Batalla I, Erdmann R, Jorgensen H, Mitchell R, Ernst T, von Amsberg G, et al. Axl blockade by BGB324 inhibits BCR-ABL tyrosine kinase inhibitor-sensitive and -resistant chronic myeloid leukemia. Clin Cancer Res. 2017;23(9):2289–300.

195. Tworkoski K, Singhal G, Szpakowski S, Zito CI, Bacchiocchi A, Muthusamy V, et al. Phosphoproteomic screen identifies potential therapeutic targets in melanoma. Mol Cancer Res. 2011;9(6):801–12.

196. van Ginkel PR, Gee RL, Shearer RL, Subramanian L, Walker TM, Albert DM, et al. Expression of the receptor tyrosine kinase Axl promotes ocular melanoma cell survival. Cancer Res. 2004;64(1):128–34.

197. Kim JE, Leung E, Baguley BC, Finlay GJ. Heterogeneity of expression of epithelial-mesenchymal transition markers in melanocytes and melanoma cell lines. Front Genet. 2013;4:97.

198. Boshuizen J, Koopman LA, Krijgsman O, Shahrabi A, van den Heuvel EG, Ligtenberg MA, et al. Cooperative targeting of melanoma heterogeneity with an AXL antibody-drug conjugate and BRAF/MEK inhibitors. Nat Med. 2018;24(2):203–12.

199. Pinato DJ, Mauri FA, Lloyd T, Vaira V, Casadio C, Boldorini RL, et al. The expression of Axl receptor tyrosine kinase influences the tumour phenotype and clinical outcome of patients with malignant pleural mesothelioma. Br J Cancer. 2013;108(3):621–8.

200. Ou WB, Corson JM, Flynn DL, Lu WP, Wise SC, Bueno R, et al. AXL regulates mesothelioma proliferation and invasiveness. Oncogene. 2011;30(14):1643–52.

201. Ou WB, Hubert C, Corson JM, Bueno R, Flynn DL, Sugarbaker DJ, et al. Targeted inhibition of multiple receptor tyrosine kinases in mesothelioma. Neoplasia. 2011;13(1):12–22.

202. Ramkumar K, Stewart CA, Cargill KR, Della Corte CM, Wang Q, Shen L, et al. AXL inhibition induces DNA damage and replication stress in non-small cell lung cancer cells and promotes sensitivity to ATR inhibitors. Mol Cancer Res. 2020;

203. Song W, Wang H, Lu M, Ni X, Bahri N, Zhu S, et al. AXL inactivation inhibits mesothelioma growth and migration via regulation of p53 expression. Cancers (Basel). 2020;12(10)

204. Chen JJ, Peck K, Hong TM, Yang SC, Sher YP, Shih JY, et al. Global analysis of gene expression in invasion by a lung cancer model. Cancer Res. 2001;61(13):5223–30.

205. Wimmel A, Glitz D, Kraus A, Roeder J, Schuermann M. Axl receptor tyrosine kinase expression in human lung cancer cell lines correlates with cellular adhesion. Eur J Cancer. 2001;37(17):2264–74.

206. Wang Y, Xia H, Zhuang Z, Miao L, Chen X, Cai H. Axl-altered microRNAs regulate tumorigenicity and gefitinib resistance in lung cancer. Cell Death Dis. 2014;5:e1227.

207. Qu XH, Liu JL, Zhong XW, Li XI, Zhang QG. Insights into the roles of hnRNP A2/B1 and AXL in non-small cell lung cancer. Oncol Lett. 2015;10(3):1677–85.

208. Taniguchi H, Yamada T, Wang R, Tanimura K, Adachi Y, Nishiyama A, et al. AXL confers intrinsic resistance to osimertinib and advances the emergence of tolerant cells. Nat Commun. 2019;10(1):259.

209. Nonagase Y, Takeda M, Azuma K, Hayashi H, Haratani K, Tanaka K, et al. Tumor tissue and plasma levels of AXL and GAS6 before and after tyrosine kinase inhibitor treatment in EGFR-mutated non-small cell lung cancer. Thorac Cancer. 2019;10(10):1928–35.

210. de Miguel-Perez D, Bayarri-Lara CI, Ortega FG, Russo A, Moyano Rodriguez MJ, Alvarez-Cubero MJ, et al. Post-surgery circulating tumor cells and AXL overexpression as new poor prognostic biomarkers in resected lung adenocarcinoma. Cancers (Basel). 2019;11(11)

211. Koopman LA, Terp MG, Zom GG, Janmaat ML, Jacobsen K, Gresnigt-van den Heuvel E, et al. Enapotamab vedotin, an AXL-specific antibody-drug conjugate, shows preclinical antitumor activity in non-small cell lung cancer. JCI Insight. 2019;4(21)

212. D'Errico G, Alonso-Nocelo M, Vallespinos M, Hermann PC, Alcala S, Garcia CP, et al. Tumor-associated macrophage-secreted 14-3-3zeta signals via AXL to promote pancreatic cancer chemoresistance. Oncogene. 2019;38(27):5469–85.

213. Fleuren ED, Hillebrandt-Roeffen MH, Flucke UE, Te Loo DM, Boerman OC, van der Graaf WT, et al. The role of AXL and the in vitro activity of the receptor tyrosine kinase inhibitor BGB324 in Ewing sarcoma. Oncotarget. 2014;5(24):12753–68.

214. Liu R, Gong M, Li X, Zhou Y, Gao W, Tulpule A, et al. Induction, regulation, and biologic function of Axl receptor tyrosine kinase in Kaposi sarcoma. Blood. 2010;116(2):297–305.

215. Hoffman A, Ghadimi MP, Demicco EG, Creighton CJ, Torres K, Colombo C, et al. Localized and metastatic myxoid/round cell liposarcoma: clinical and molecular observations. Cancer. 2013;119(10):1868–77.

216. Peng T, Zhang P, Liu J, Nguyen T, Bolshakov S, Belousov R, et al. An experimental model for the study of well-differentiated and dedifferentiated liposarcoma; deregulation of targetable tyrosine kinase receptors. Lab Invest. 2011;91(3):392–403.

217. Han J, Tian R, Yong B, Luo C, Tan P, Shen J, et al. Gas6/Axl mediates tumor cell apoptosis, migration and invasion and predicts the clinical outcome of osteosarcoma patients. Biochem Biophys Res Commun. 2013;435(3):493–500.

218. Nakano T, Tani M, Ishibashi Y, Kimura K, Park YB, Imaizumi N, et al. Biological properties and gene expression associated with metastatic potential of human osteosarcoma. Clin Exp Metastasis. 2003;20(7):665–74.

219. Zhang Y, Tang YJ, Man Y, Pan F, Li ZH, Jia LS. Knockdown of AXL receptor tyrosine kinase in osteosarcoma cells leads to decreased proliferation and increased apoptosis. Int J Immunopathol Pharmacol. 2013;26(1):179–88.

220. Tian R, Xie X, Han J, Luo C, Yong B, Peng H, et al. miR-199a-3p negatively regulates the progression of osteosarcoma through targeting AXL. Am J Cancer Res. 2014;4(6):738–50.

221. Roland CL, May CD, Watson KL, Al Sannaa GA, Dineen SP, Feig R, et al. Analysis of clinical and molecular factors impacting oncologic outcomes in undifferentiated pleomorphic sarcoma. Ann Surg Oncol. 2016;23(7):2220–8.

222. Papadakis ES, Cichon MA, Vyas JJ, Patel N, Ghali L, Cerio R, et al. Axl promotes cutaneous squamous cell carcinoma survival through negative regulation of pro-apoptotic Bcl-2 family members. J Invest Dermatol. 2011;131(2):509–17.

223. Green J, Ikram M, Vyas J, Patel N, Proby CM, Ghali L, et al. Overexpression of the Axl tyrosine kinase receptor in cutaneous SCC-derived cell lines and tumours. Br J Cancer. 2006;94(10):1446–51.

224. Ferrarotto R, Mitani Y, McGrail DJ, Li K, Karpinets TV, Bell D, et al. Proteogenomic analysis of salivary adenoid cystic carcinomas defines molecular subtypes and identifies therapeutic targets. Clin Cancer Res. 2021;27(3):852–64.

225. Avilla E, Guarino V, Visciano C, Liotti F, Svelto M, Krishnamoorthy G, et al. Activation of TYRO3/AXL tyrosine kinase receptors in thyroid cancer. Cancer Res. 2011;71(5):1792–804.

226. Ito M, Nakashima M, Nakayama T, Ohtsuru A, Nagayama Y, Takamura N, et al. Expression of receptor-type tyrosine kinase, Axl, and its ligand, Gas6, in pediatric thyroid carcinomas around chernobyl. Thyroid. 2002;12(11):971–5.

227. Tanaka K, Nagayama Y, Nakano T, Takamura N, Namba H, Fukada S, et al. Expression profile of receptor-type protein tyrosine kinase genes in the human thyroid. Endocrinology. 1998;139(3):852–8.

228. Ito T, Ito M, Naito S, Ohtsuru A, Nagayama Y, Kanematsu T, et al. Expression of the Axl receptor tyrosine kinase in human thyroid carcinoma. Thyroid. 1999;9(6):563–7.

229. Collina F, La Sala L, Liotti F, Prevete N, La Mantia E, Chiofalo MG, et al. AXL Is a novel predictive factor and therapeutic target for radioactive iodine refractory thyroid cancer. Cancers (Basel). 2019;11(6)

230. Kim YW, Yun SJ, Jeong P, Kim SK, Kim SY, Yan C, et al. The c-MET network as novel prognostic marker for predicting bladder cancer patients with an increased risk of developing aggressive disease. PLoS One. 2015;10(7):e0134552.

231. Yeh CY, Shin SM, Yeh HH, Wu TJ, Shin JW, Chang TY, et al. Transcriptional activation of the Axl and PDGFR-alpha by c-Met through a ras- and Src-independent mechanism in human bladder cancer. BMC Cancer. 2011;11:139.

232. Sayan AE, Stanford R, Vickery R, Grigorenko E, Diesch J, Kulbicki K, et al. Fra-1 controls motility of bladder cancer cells via transcriptional upregulation of the receptor tyrosine kinase AXL. Oncogene. 2012;31(12):1493–503.

233. Mishra A, Wang J, Shiozawa Y, McGee S, Kim J, Jung Y, et al. Hypoxia stabilizes GAS6/Axl signaling in metastatic prostate cancer. Mol Cancer Res. 2012;10(6):703–12.

234. Paccez JD, Vasques GJ, Correa RG, Vasconcellos JF, Duncan K, Gu X, et al. The receptor tyrosine kinase Axl is an essential regulator of prostate cancer proliferation and tumor growth and represents a new therapeutic target. Oncogene. 2013;32(6):689–98.

235. Sainaghi PP, Castello L, Bergamasco L, Galletti M, Bellosta P, Avanzi GC. Gas6 induces proliferation in prostate carcinoma cell lines expressing the Axl receptor. J Cell Physiol. 2005;204(1):36–44.

236. Shiozawa Y, Pedersen EA, Patel LR, Ziegler AM, Havens AM, Jung Y, et al. GAS6/AXL axis regulates prostate cancer invasion, proliferation, and survival in the bone marrow niche. Neoplasia. 2010;12(2):116–27.

237. Chung BI, Malkowicz SB, Nguyen TB, Libertino JA, McGarvey TW. Expression of the proto-oncogene Axl in renal cell carcinoma. DNA Cell Biol. 2003;22(8):533–40.

238. Dalgin GS, Holloway DT, Liou LS, DeLisi C. Identification and characterization of renal cell carcinoma gene markers. Cancer Inform. 2007;3:65–92.

239. Gustafsson A, Martuszewska D, Johansson M, Ekman C, Hafizi S, Ljungberg B, et al. Differential expression of Axl and Gas6 in renal cell carcinoma reflecting tumor advancement and survival. Clin Cancer Res. 2009;15(14):4742–9.

240. Yu H, Liu R, Ma B, Li X, Yen HY, Zhou Y, et al. Axl receptor tyrosine kinase is a potential therapeutic target in renal cell carcinoma. Br J Cancer. 2015;113(4):616–25.

241. Zhou L, Liu XD, Sun M, Zhang X, German P, Bai S, et al. Targeting MET and AXL overcomes resistance to sunitinib therapy in renal cell carcinoma. Oncogene. 2015;

242. McDaniel NK, Iida M, Nickel KP, Longhurst CA, Fischbach SR, Rodems TS, et al. AXL mediates cetuximab and radiation resistance through tyrosine 821 and the c-ABL kinase pathway in head and neck cancer. Clin Cancer Res. 2020;26(16):4349–59.

243. Hong CC, Lay JD, Huang JS, Cheng AL, Tang JL, Lin MT, et al. Receptor tyrosine kinase AXL is induced by chemotherapy drugs and overexpression of AXL confers drug resistance in acute myeloid leukemia. Cancer Lett. 2008;268(2):314–24.

244. Li Y, Wang X, Bi S, Zhao K, Yu C. Inhibition of Mer and Axl receptor tyrosine kinases leads to increased apoptosis and improved chemosensitivity in human neuroblastoma. Biochem Biophys Res Commun. 2015;457(3):461–6.

245. Lay JD, Hong CC, Huang JS, Yang YY, Pao CY, Liu CH, et al. Sulfasalazine suppresses drug resistance and invasiveness of lung adenocarcinoma cells expressing AXL. Cancer Res. 2007;67(8):3878–87.

246. Wu F, Li J, Jang C, Wang J, Xiong J. The role of Axl in drug resistance and epithelial-to-mesenchymal transition of non-small cell lung carcinoma. Int J Clin Exp Pathol. 2014;7(10):6653–61.

247. Lin JZ, Wang ZJ, De W, Zheng M, Xu WZ, Wu HF, et al. Targeting AXL overcomes resistance to docetaxel therapy in advanced prostate cancer. Oncotarget. 2017;8(25):41064–77.

248. Kariolis MS, Miao YR, Diep A, Nash SE, Olcina MM, Jiang D, et al. Inhibition of the GAS6/AXL pathway augments the efficacy of chemotherapies. J Clin Invest. 2017;127(1):183–98.

249. Heckmann D, Maier P, Laufs S, Li L, Sleeman JP, Trunk MJ, et al. The disparate twins: a comparative study of CXCR4 and CXCR7 in SDF-1alpha-induced gene expression, invasion and chemosensitivity of colon cancer. Clin Cancer Res. 2014;20(3):604–16.

250. Ludwig KF, Du W, Sorrelle NB, Wnuk-Lipinska K, Topalovski M, Toombs JE, et al. Small-molecule inhibition of Axl targets tumor immune suppression and enhances chemotherapy in pancreatic cancer. Cancer Res. 2018;78(1):246–55.

251. Tsai WB, Long Y, Park JR, Chang JT, Liu H, Rodriguez-Canales J, et al. Gas6/Axl is the sensor of arginine-auxotrophic response in targeted chemotherapy with arginine-depleting agents. Oncogene. 2016;35(13):1632–42.

252. Kim HR, Kim WS, Choi YJ, Choi CM, Rho JK, Lee JC. Epithelial-mesenchymal transition leads to crizotinib resistance in H2228

lung cancer cells with EML4-ALK translocation. Mol Oncol. 2013;7(6):1093–102.

253. Nakamichi S, Seike M, Miyanaga A, Chiba M, Zou F, Takahashi A, et al. Overcoming drug-tolerant cancer cell subpopulations showing AXL activation and epithelial-mesenchymal transition is critical in conquering ALK-positive lung cancer. Oncotarget. 2018;9(43):27242–55.

254. Debruyne DN, Bhatnagar N, Sharma B, Luther W, Moore NF, Cheung NK, et al. ALK inhibitor resistance in ALK-driven neuroblastoma is associated with AXL activation and induction of EMT. Oncogene. 2015;

255. Flem-Karlsen K, McFadden E, Omar N, Haugen MH, Oy GF, Ryder T, et al. Targeting AXL and the DNA damage response pathway as a novel therapeutic strategy in melanoma. Mol Cancer Ther. 2020;19(3):895–905.

256. Sinha S, Boysen J, Nelson M, Secreto C, Warner SL, Bearss DJ, et al. Targeted Axl inhibition primes chronic lymphocytic Leukemia B cells to apoptosis and shows synergistic/additive effects in combination with BTK inhibitors. Clin Cancer Res. 2015;21(9):2115–26.

257. Ji W, Choi CM, Rho JK, Jang SJ, Park YS, Chun SM, et al. Mechanisms of acquired resistance to EGFR-tyrosine kinase inhibitor in Korean patients with lung cancer. BMC Cancer. 2013;13:606.

258. Su CM, Chang TY, Hsu HP, Lai HH, Li JN, Lyu YJ, et al. A novel application of E1A in combination therapy with EGFR-TKI treatment in breast cancer. Oncotarget. 2016;7(39):63924–36.

259. Namba K, Shien K, Takahashi Y, Torigoe H, Sato H, Yoshioka T, et al. Activation of AXL as a preclinical acquired resistance mechanism against osimertinib treatment in EGFR-mutant non-small cell lung cancer cells. Mol Cancer Res. 2019;17(2):499–507.

260. Okura N, Nishioka N, Yamada T, Taniguchi H, Tanimura K, Katayama Y, et al. ONO-7475, a novel AXL inhibitor, suppresses the adaptive resistance to initial EGFR-TKI treatment in EGFR-mutated non-small cell lung cancer. Clin Cancer Res. 2020;26(9):2244–56.

261. Brand TM, Iida M, Corrigan KL, Braverman CM, Coan JP, Flanigan BG, et al. The receptor tyrosine kinase AXL mediates nuclear translocation of the epidermal growth factor receptor. Sci Signal. 2017;10(460)

262. Hu S, Dai H, Li T, Tang Y, Fu W, Yuan Q, et al. Broad RTK-targeted therapy overcomes molecular heterogeneity-driven resistance to cetuximab via vectored immunoprophylaxis in colorectal cancer. Cancer Lett. 2016;382(1):32–43.

263. Park IK, Mundy-Bosse B, Whitman SP, Zhang X, Warner SL, Bearss DJ, et al. Receptor tyrosine kinase Axl is required for resistance of leukemic cells to FLT3-targeted therapy in acute myeloid leukemia. Leukemia. 2015;29(12):2382–9.

264. Dumas PY, Naudin C, Martin-Lanneree S, Izac B, Casetti L, Mansier O, et al. Hematopoietic niche drives FLT3-ITD acute myeloid leukemia resistance to quizartinib via STAT5-

and hypoxia-dependent upregulation of AXL. Haematologica. 2019;104(10):2017–27.

265. Torka R, Penzes K, Gusenbauer S, Baumann C, Szabadkai I, Orfi L, et al. Activation of HER3 interferes with antitumor effects of Axl receptor tyrosine kinase inhibitors: suggestion of combination therapy. Neoplasia. 2014;16(4):301–18.

266. Hsieh MS, Yang PW, Wong LF, Lee JM. The AXL receptor tyrosine kinase is associated with adverse prognosis and distant metastasis in esophageal squamous cell carcinoma. Oncotarget. 2016;7(24):36956–70.

267. Creedon H, Gomez-Cuadrado L, Tarnauskaite Z, Balla J, Canel M, MacLeod KG, et al. Identification of novel pathways linking epithelial-to-mesenchymal transition with resistance to HER2-targeted therapy. Oncotarget. 2016;7:11539–52.

268. Yoshioka T, Shien K, Takeda T, Takahashi Y, Kurihara E, Ogoshi Y, et al. Acquired resistance mechanisms to afatinib in HER2-amplified gastric cancer cells. Cancer Sci. 2019;110(8):2549–57.

269. Huang F, Hurlburt W, Greer A, Reeves KA, Hillerman S, Chang H, et al. Differential mechanisms of acquired resistance to insulin-like growth factor-i receptor antibody therapy or to a small-molecule inhibitor, BMS-754807, in a human rhabdomyosarcoma model. Cancer Res. 2010;70(18):7221–31.

270. Zuo Q, Liu J, Huang L, Qin Y, Hawley T, Seo C, et al. AXL/AKT axis mediated-resistance to BRAF inhibitor depends on PTEN status in melanoma. Oncogene. 2018;37(24):3275–89.

271. Yao TW, Zhang J, Prados M, Weiss WA, James CD, Nicolaides T. Acquired resistance to BRAF inhibition in BRAFV600E mutant gliomas. Oncotarget. 2017;8(1):583–95.

272. Balaji K, Vijayaraghavan S, Diao L, Tong P, Fan Y, Carey JP, et al. AXL inhibition suppresses the DNA damage response and sensitizes cells to PARP inhibition in multiple cancers. Mol Cancer Res. 2017;15(1):45–58.

273. Ruicci KM, Meens J, Plantinga P, Stecho W, Pinto N, Yoo J, et al. TAM family receptors in conjunction with MAPK signalling are involved in acquired resistance to PI3Kalpha inhibition in head and neck squamous cell carcinoma. J Exp Clin Cancer Res. 2020;39(1):217.

274. Hong J, Belkhiri A. AXL mediates TRAIL resistance in esophageal adenocarcinoma. Neoplasia. 2013;15(3):296–304.

275. Burbridge MF, Bossard CJ, Saunier C, Fejes I, Bruno A, Leonce S, et al. S49076 is a novel kinase inhibitor of MET, AXL, and FGFR with strong preclinical activity alone and in association with bevacizumab. Mol Cancer Ther. 2013;12(9):1749–62.

276. Xiao Y, Zhao H, Tian L, Nolley R, Diep AN, Ernst A, et al. S100A10 is a critical mediator of GAS6/AXL-induced angiogenesis in renal cell carcinoma. Cancer Res. 2019;79(22):5758–68.

277. Qu L, Ding J, Chen C, Wu ZJ, Liu B, Gao Y, et al. Exosome-transmitted lncARSR promotes sunitinib resistance in renal cancer by acting as a competing endogenous RNA. Cancer Cell. 2016;29(5):653–68.

Modeling the Tumor Microenvironment in Patient-Derived Xenografts: Challenges and Opportunities

Katrin Kleinmanns, Christiane Helgestad Gjerde, Anika Langer, Vibeke Fosse, Elvira García de Jalón, Calum Leitch, Mihaela Popa, Pascal Gelebart, and Emmet McCormack

Abstract

The development of targeted and personalized therapies for cancer patients has underlined the need for more advanced preclinical animal models to facilitate and favor clinical translation. Patient-derived xenografts (PDXs) allow for the preservation of patient tumor architecture and intra-tumor heterogeneity and have emerged as a powerful tool in preclinical cancer research to identify predictive and therapeutic biomarkers. In addition, PDXs facilitate the investigation of biomarker-driven treatment approaches as avatars for personalized medicine. Orthotopic engraftment promotes the establishment of the patient tumor in its physiological tumor niche, allowing investigation of the stromal contribution to treatment response, as well as the opportunity to study spontaneous metastasis from the primary tumor. The successful engraftment of a human immune system in so-called humanized PDX mice is a further evolution of the model system permitting tumor-immune cell interactions and investigation of the impact of immune components on therapeutic efficacy. However, while orthotopic humanized PDX models afford novel opportunities for biomarker discovery and therapy development, the complete human tumor microenvironment is not fully represented in these systems. Therefore, this review will critically investigate the strengths and limitations of PDXs in personalized cancer research, and discuss how more clinically relevant animal models can realize new opportunities in the development of novel therapeutics.

K. Kleinmanns (✉) · C. H. Gjerde · A. Langer · V. Fosse
C. Leitch · M. Popa · P. Gelebart
University of Bergen, Department of Clinical Science, Centre for Cancer Biomarkers CCBIO, Bergen, Norway
e-mail: katrin.kleinmanns@uib.no; christiane.gjerde@uib.no; anika.langer@avencell.com; Vibeke.Fosse@uib.no; Calum.Leitch@uib.no; Mihaela.Popa@uib.no; Pascal.Gelebart@uib.no

E. G. de Jalón
University of Bergen, Department of Clinical Science, Centre for Cancer Biomarkers CCBIO, Bergen, Norway

Department of Chemistry and Centre for Pharmacy, Bergen, Norway
e-mail: Elvira.Vioegra@uib.no

E. McCormack
University of Bergen, Department of Clinical Science, Centre for Cancer Biomarkers CCBIO, Bergen, Norway

Department of Clinical Science, Centre for Pharmacy, Bergen, Norway

Department of Clinical Science, Vivarium, Bergen, Norway
e-mail: emmet.mc.cormack@uib.no

Graphic figure. Created with BioRender.com

Take-Home Lessons

- Advances in the generation of more severely immunocompromised mouse strains improved the development of patient-derived xenograft (PDX) models for solid and hematological malignancies.
- PDX models preserve the genetic landscape and phenotypic traits, including intra-tumor heterogeneity, and are therefore considered a precious tool for drug and biomarker development.
- Heterogenous orthotopic PDXs enable modeling of metastasis and investigation of tumor-TME interactions as well as sensitivity and resistance to therapies.
- For clinical translatability, the critical role of the TME and the mouse-originated TME components needs to be considered, including non-malignant cells (e.g., immune cells, fibroblasts, endothelial cells, adipocytes) as well as non-cellular elements (e.g., extracellular matrix and physiological microenvironment).
- Progress has been made in developing PDX models with a functional human immune system, indicated by activated lymphocytes, immune cell infiltration, and immune-dependent response to immune checkpoint inhibition.
- To monitor tumor growth and treatment efficacy in advanced PDX models, fluorescence and PET-based imaging serve as tools for non-invasive in vivo monitoring, while post-mortem ex vivo single-cell analysis tools are valuable to uncover mechanisms of sensitivity and resistance to applied therapies.

expansion of cancer and can influence the tumor behavior in relation to growth, metastasis, dormancy, and therapy response [7–10]. Immune cells are one of the most well-characterized TME components, and a plethora of studies report the interactions between cancer cells and host immune cells [11–15]. The recent discovery of immune checkpoint inhibitors has shown that targeting the TME represents an important therapeutic opportunity for the treatment of cancers [16, 17]. Checkpoint inhibitors have also highlighted that human immune cells have a broad function in supporting cancer development and counteracting drug treatment [18–21]. With an abundance of evidence describing the role of the TME in cancer, it seems clear that this component must be better integrated into diseases models. The development of new cancer therapies has been impeded by a lack of animal models that can mimic tumor heterogeneity, replicate the role of the TME in drug response and predict the efficacy of new drugs in humans [22–24]. As such, there is an urgent need for more robust preclinical models that generate accurate and predictive data to identify and validate biomarkers [25]. Patient-derived xenograft (PDX) models are generally considered one of the most relevant in vivo models utilized in preclinical cancer research. PDX models, generated by transplanting surgically-derived tumors into immunodeficient mice, have been developed for many malignancies. The first objective of these PDXs was to recapitulate the intra- and inter-tumor heterogeneity to better predict response to therapy. However, one of the limitations of using these models resides in the incomplete presence, or even total absence, of several components of the TME. In the following paragraphs, we will elaborate on the challenges and opportunities related to the development of PDX models integrating key human TME components in order to offer a better evaluation of novel therapeutics.

The Tumor Microenvironment

Tumors are heterogeneous cell populations of malignant and non-malignant cells that are infiltrated by an array of resident cells, blood vessels, and lymphatics, in addition to various surrounding growth factors and proteins [1]. The tumor microenvironment (TME) can be broadly defined as the non-malignant cells and non-cellular elements [2, 3] (Fig. 19.1). The non-malignant cells may include immune cells, vascular cells, fibroblasts, and adipocytes. Non-cellular elements comprise the extracellular matrix (ECM), a scaffold of proteins and proteoglycans, and physiological factors of the extracellular milieu. Tumors have the potential to induce physiological changes in the TME, such as countering conditions of low pH and hypoxia, illustrating the dynamic relationship that exists between the different components of the TME [4–6]. The TME has a key role in the development and

History of PDX Models

Since the eighteenth century researchers have attempted to study human cancer by developing animal models and by the twentieth century, mice emerged as the most common animal model [26]. Mice are genetically similar to humans, sharing >90% of their genes, but also provide practical advantages due to their small size and short lifecycles enabling large scale experiments and fast analysis of phenotypes generated by genetic manipulation [27]. An important milestone in the use of mice for cancer research was the development of inbred, genetically identical mice. Cohorts of mice carrying the same genetic background allowed researchers to perform experiments without the confounding influence of biological variation [28] (Fig. 19.2).

In order to successfully engraft and study human tumors, the murine immune system must be suppressed. The first to

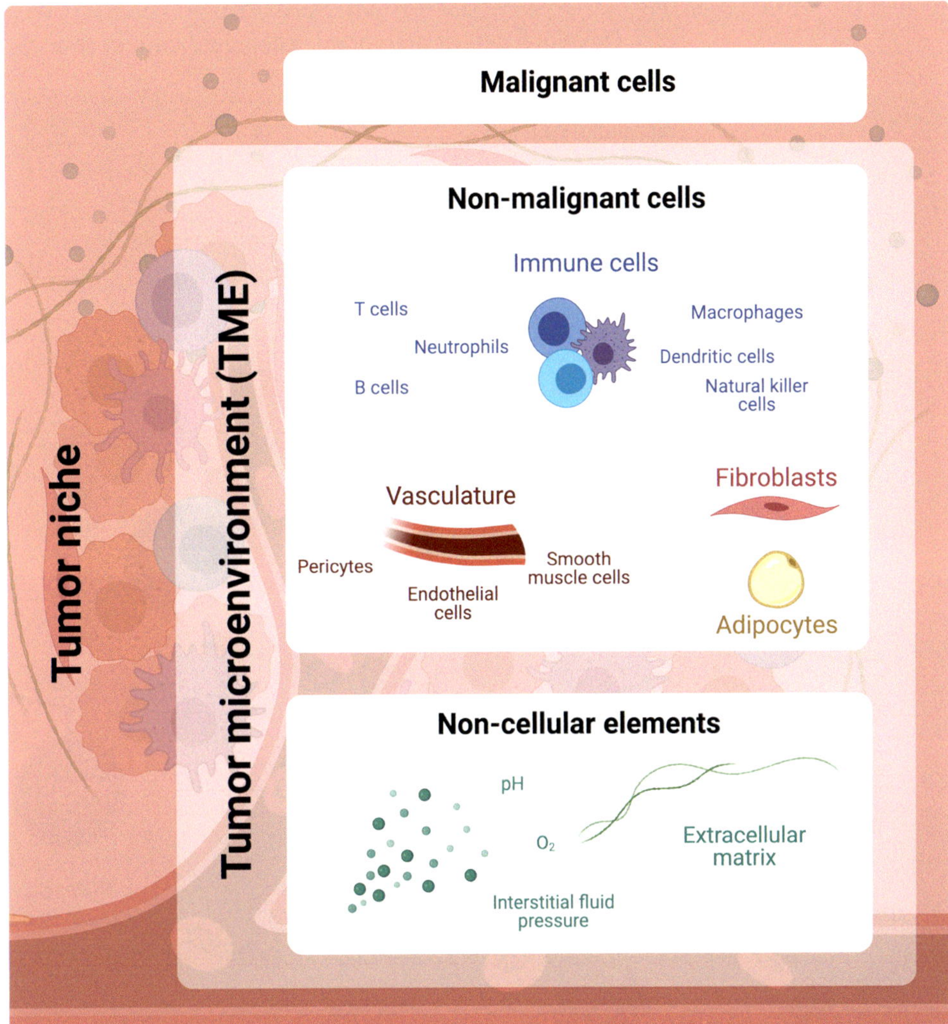

Fig. 19.1 The interplay between the components of the tumor niche determines tumor growth and response to therapy. The tumor niche comprises the malignant tumor cells and the tumor microenvironment (TME). Modeling the complete TME in preclinical models is challenging but creates the opportunity to study and evaluate new treatment regimes. Created with BioRender.com

succeed was Helene Toolan in 1951, who was able to grow human tumor cells in x-irradiated mice and rats [29]. She later discovered that the addition of the immunosuppressive drug cortisone increased cancer cell proliferation in the mice [30]. Initial models struggled with low engraftment rates but were greatly improved with the development of immunocompromised mouse strains [31] (Fig. 19.2). Athymic (nude) mice lacking functional T cells were first used for PDX from hematological cancers in 1969 [32, 33]. Later Fiebig and colleagues established PDX models with 34 tumors of different origins in nude mice and were able to show comparable response to chemotherapeutic agents in mice and patients [34]. Over the last decades more severely immunocompromised mouse strains have been developed which further increase tumor engraftment. Non-obese diabetic severe combined immunodeficiency (NOD-*scid*) mice lack functional T cells and B cells and have multiple defects in innate immunity [35]. The next breakthrough in the development of immunodeficient mice came from the discovery of the IL-2Rγ mutation. The defect of

IL-2Rγ causes a complete lack of T, B, and natural killer (NK) cell activity and a longer lifespan from 37 to 90 weeks in NOD.Cg-Prkdc^{scid}Il2rg^{tm1Wjl}/Sz (NSG) mice as compared with NOD-*scid* [28, 36–38]. Increased murine immunodeficiency improves tumor growth and allows the development of a human immune system in so-called humanized mice. The injection of human hematopoietic stem cells (HSC) in NSG mice to generate humanized mice results in increased engraftment and favorable differentiation of HSCs into lymphocytes, NK cells, myeloid cells, and dendritic cells (DCs) when compared to NOD-scid mice [37]. Additional immunocompromised mouse strains have been generated since, such as NSG-SGM and M(I)STRG, which have been engineered to express supraphysiological concentrations of human cytokines to favor the engraftment and development of acute myeloid leukemia (AML) PDX models [39, 40]. The supraphysiological cytokine concentration further supports the maturation and frequency of functional NK cells, regulatory T cells (Tregs), and myeloid cells in humanized models [41, 42].

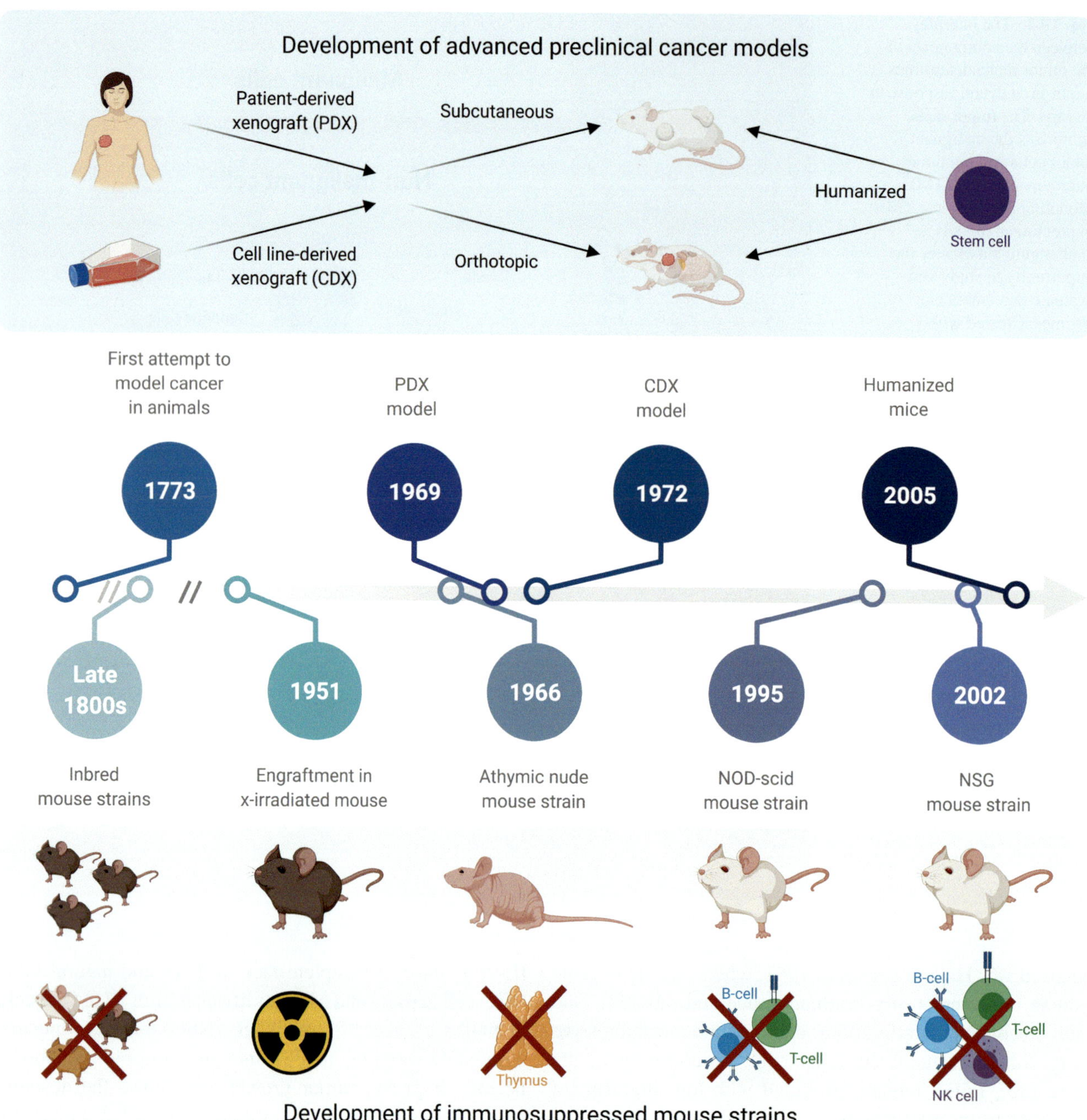

Fig. 19.2 The history of PDX models: Development of immunosuppressed mouse strains (lower panel) improved the development and engraftment rate of advanced preclinical cancer models (upper panel). Created with BioRender.com

PDX Models

Insights into the pathophysiology of cancer have demonstrated the importance of inter- and intra-tumor heterogeneity and the critical role of the TME. Genomic comparison of cancer cell lines and patient tumor samples has demonstrated substantial variability and even the loss of key molecular traits, highlighting that cell line-derived xenograft (CDX) models are not fully representative of the human paradigm [43]. This has generated a shift in translational research away from models focusing solely on efficacy toward the development of more sophisticated preclinical models. PDXs provide a more robust approach to disease modeling as they can preserve the genetic landscape and phenotypic traits such as intra-tumor heterogeneity, and are able to predict therapy response of the primary patient sample [44–46]. As such, PDX models are a precious tool for drug and biomarker development but can be limited by low engraftment rates and prolonged disease latency. In some cases, prolonged disease latency challenges the validity of the models as mice can develop human tissue lymphomas if the patient was exposed to the Epstein-Barr virus [47]. Furthermore, systematic studies have reported inconsistencies between the original patient samples and retrieved PDX tissues from the mouse at the genomic level [48, 49]. However, large investigations have also found that the genetic and epigenetic fidelity were generally preserved in PDX models [50–54]. These apparent discrepancies of tumor heterogeneity representation between the different studies highlight the need for a systematic approach to the establishment of PDX models and ex vivo validation. Standardization of the methodology and validation procedures could ensure better reproducibility and improved translation to clinical practice. The complexity of maintaining such a high degree of molecular annotation has led to the development of large-scale collaborative PDX networks, such as the EurOPDX consortium, the US National Cancer Institute (NCI) repository of patient-derived models, the Public Repository of Xenografts (PRoXe), the Children's Oncology Group (COG) cell culture and xenograft repository, the Pediatric Preclinical Testing Consortium (PPTC), and the Novartis Institutes for Biomedical Research PDX Encyclopedia (NIBR PDXE) [44]. Another limitation of PDX models relates to their immunodeficient status, which limits the evaluation of the human immunological response toward cancer development and therapeutic efficacy. To overcome this issue, various methodologies are employed to generate a competent human immune system. The humanized PDX models offer a degree of immune reconstitution, which will be further discussed in detail below.

PDX Models of Solid Cancers

In solid cancers, PDX models are generated by implanting sectioned patient tumor fragments or freshly prepared cell suspensions into immunodeficient mice, ectopically (usually subcutaneously) or orthotopically, to mimic tumor growth in its site of origin [45, 46]. One advantage of subcutaneous (s.c.) PDX engraftments is that they allow for easy tumor growth measurement in response to treatment, but these models rarely produce metastasis. In contrast, endogenous metastases can occur when patient tumors are implanted through orthotopic engraftment. Orthotopic PDXs can be technically challenging to generate and often require high technical skills and non-invasive imaging modalities for monitoring [55, 56]. However, orthotopic models offer a more clinically relevant representation of the tumor in situ and the possibility to interrogate the TME contribution in response to therapy. One drawback of PDX models relates to the fact that the human TME components are gradually replaced by murine-derived ECM, fibroblasts, lymphatic,

blood vessels, and adipocytes, leading to decreased human tumor-TME interactions [57]. The time and frequency of the replacement of human endothelial cells and fibroblasts in growing xenograft tumors seems to be dependent on the tumor type and mouse strain [58–60]. It is important to note that the murine TME induces species-specific interactions that can alter some physical properties, such as the interstitial fluid pressure (IFP), which may in turn generate interference in the clinical evaluation of drug response, delivery, and efficacy [61]. Leaky and disorganized blood vessels and compression of lymphatics contribute to an increased IFP [62] that can hinder the delivery, and therefore efficacy, of targeted therapies, chemotherapeutic agents, and immunotherapies [63, 64]. Moreover, steep pressure gradients (PG) in the tumor periphery push fluid into the surrounding tissues, facilitating the transport of growth factors and cancer cells, which promotes tumor growth and metastasis. PG have also been shown to reduce retention time and homogenous distribution of drugs in tumors [65]. A study by Blomme et al. investigated the impact of mouse TME components on the metabolic activity and found no difference in metabolic signatures even after complete replacement of the human stroma [66]. This is an important finding, as it may indicate a human-like TME phenotype. Thus, despite the preservation of heterogeneity in PDX models, the human TME components continuously degrade as the tumor grows and undergoes serial passaging, and this impact of murine TME components on the human tumor biology has yet to be fully elucidated.

Hematological PDX Models

The bone marrow (BM) comprises osteoclasts, osteoblasts, cartilage tissue, blood vessels, adipocytes, endothelial cells, mesenchymal stem cells (MSC) and the immune cells (including the HSC), and constitute the unique TME of leukemic hematological cancers [67]. Therefore, the preferred route of engraftment, to model leukemia or multiple myeloma, is by direct injection into the bloodstream or BM of immunocompromised mice. The engraftment rate is influenced by both the primary source material and the mouse strain used to model the disease [68, 69]. Of the different strains available, the most commonly used are the NSG and the NOG (NOD.Cg-Prkdc^{scid} Il2rg^{tm1Sug}/Jic) mice [70, 71]. In order to achieve higher levels of human cells engraftment in hematological malignancies, conditioning, i.e., myeloablation via irradiation or chemotherapy, is often required. This procedure will annihilate the host's immune cells, generating a space for the donor graft in the BM niche. However, the conditioning can induce damage to the hemato-lymphoid system, gastrointestinal tract, neural and muscle tissues, and may influence response to therapy. To alleviate these artifacts, new NSG strains carrying *c-kit* loss-of-function alleles (NSG$^{W/V}$ and NSG^{W41}) were developed and shown to be free of the associated side effects produced by conditioning regiments. Moreover, these strains have impaired HSCs development, and thereby allow a competitive advantage for transplanted human cells [72, 73].

PDX engraftment has proven to be highly successful for acute leukemia and enables evaluation of the response of leukemic stem cells to drug therapy and drug resistance [45, 74]. In contrast, the engraftment of human samples from non-acute hematologic malignancies, such as myelodysplastic syndrome (MDS), myeloproliferative neoplasms and chronic myelomonocytic leukemia (CMML), remains very challenging. The recent introduction of the NSG-SGM3 strain, characterized by the constitutive expression of human stem cell factor (SCF), granulocyte-monocyte-colony-stimulating factor (GM-CSF) and interleukin-3 (IL3), was designed to improve myeloid cell differentiation and proliferation [39]. In comparison to NSG, the use of NSG-SGM3 gave rise to robust cell engraftment for almost all patient cases evaluated. However, in CMML secondary recipients failed to engraft or presented low levels of human cells in the BM [75]. Serial transplantation was only achieved by transducing patient cells with the human oncogene *Meningioma 1 (MN1)*, indicating that this strain was still not the most suitable at creating a favorable environment for CMML cells to grow [76]. PDX modeling of AML was further developed through the use of a bone-marrow-like structure, referred to as ossicle. This structure was created by in situ differentiation of human MSCs implanted subcutaneously in NSG or NSG-SGM3 mice. Intra-ossicle transplantation of AML cells showed a superior engraftment rate in comparison to previously used models. Moreover, the system demonstrated the ability to engraft patient cells that were previously shown to never engraft in mice [77]. Thus, advances in the development of (1) immunodeficient mice with constitutive human cytokine expression, (2) BM myeloablation, and (3) the generation of human-like BM structures, have increased the engraftment rate of orthotopic hematological PDX models, which is a critical step toward proper drug assessment in animal models.

Strategies to Model TME in PDXs

PDX models are increasingly utilized in clinical decision making; as PDX population "xenopatient" trials for therapeutic screening, as co-clinical avatar studies in individual patients, and for biomarker discovery. While co-clinical trials have shown that drug sensitivity can be correlated between patients and corresponding PDXs [54], it is important to note that not all components of the human TME are captured in the PDX model. In the new era of cancer therapy,

an increasing emphasis is placed on drug combinations and TME-modulating targeted therapies, such as angiogenesis inhibitors and immune checkpoint inhibitors. Therefore, it is crucial to develop clinically relevant PDX models that fully incorporate the TME. Several approaches are being exploited to integrate the TME components into the modeling of PDXs. The following paragraphs will discuss the different routes used to humanize the TME.

Immune System and Immunotherapies: Humanized PDX Models

The absence of a human immune system in traditional PDX models limits the evaluation of novel drugs, and especially the testing of immunotherapeutics. Substantial efforts have been devoted to generate humanized PDX models incorporating a human immune system, through co-transplantation of human HSCs, in order to identify combination therapies, predictive biomarkers, define biologically active doses and evaluate safety. The immune component of the TME harbors cells from both the adaptive and the innate immune system. The presence of CD8$^+$ cytotoxic T cells in the TME has been associated with good prognostic outcomes [11, 78–81]. The CD4$^+$ T cells present in the TME are mostly composed of the T helper cells (Th-1) and the Treg populations. The Th-1 cells stimulate an immune anti-tumor microenvironment by promoting the activation of the CD8$^+$ T cells through the secretion of IFN-γ and has been associated with a favorable outcome in some solid cancers [82–86]. On the other hand, Tregs participate in the establishment of an immune-suppressive microenvironment by promoting cancer cell growth through the release of growth factors and inhibiting cells involved in adaptive (CD8$^+$) or innate immunity (NK cells) [87–91]. The tumor-specific cytotoxic T cell response is induced by DCs that can be divided into conventional (cDC) and plasmacytoid (pDC) [92–94]. Another major component of innate immunity are macrophages. The tumor-associated macrophages (TAMs) can be found in the TME where they can represent up to 50% of the tumor in some forms of cancer [95–98]. The TAMs can be classified into two main categories; [99] the pro-inflammatory M1 phenotypes and the immune-suppressive M2 phenotypes [100]. Despite the anti-tumor activity of the M1 population [101], TAM presence in the TME is associated with a poor outcome as the TME favors the presence of the M2 subtype [101, 102]. TAMs secrete vascular endothelial growth factor (VEGF) that can promote angiogenesis [99, 103] and induce immune suppression of T cells [104]. Overall, the composition, frequency, and activation status of tumor-promoting (i.e., immune-suppressing) cells such as M2 or Treg, and tumor-suppressing (i.e., immune-stimulating) cells such as CD8$^+$ T cells, not only have prognostic value for many solid cancers but can also be used to predict the response to targeted immune-modulating therapy [105, 106]. The development of an "immunoscore" has been proposed, along with current available biomarkers, to improve the treatment regime at diagnosis for cancer patients [107]. Therefore, human immune cells need to be represented and functional in PDX models to efficiently evaluate novel drugs.

Different strategies are exploited to support the differentiation, growth, and functionality of immune cell subsets in immunodeficient mice [38, 39, 108]. Factors that influence the immune cell reconstitution include niche space, injection route (intrahepatic, intracardiac, or intravenous), cell source (umbilical cord blood, BM or fetal liver), and mouse strain [40, 109]. NSG-SGM3 (SCF, GM-CSF, IL-3) and MI(S) TRG (additionally encoding for macrophage colony-stimulating factor [M-CSF] and thrombopoietin) human transgene knock-in models increase the frequency and maturation of monocytes, granulocytes, and natural killer cells through species-specific cytokine signaling [39, 40, 42]. Other drawbacks of models which obstruct hematopoiesis are (1) the impaired formation of lymphoid organs and lymph node structures, entailed by the gamma chain deficiency in immunodeficient mouse strains, (2) HLA mismatch and (3) the complexity of the BM microenvironment [37, 109]. As a result, cell subsets; in particular granulocytes, myeloid cells, platelets, and erythrocytes, are underrepresented as well as the functionality of lymphoid NK, B and T cells may be impaired in available humanized models [110, 111]. NK cells belong to the innate immune response and have the ability to kill tumor cells without previous sensitization and are highly effective at killing circulating cancer cells [112, 113]. However, it has been shown that HSCs engrafted in NSG mice support the development of functional T and B cells with cytotoxic activity [37]. Interestingly, the data suggest that thymic lymphopoiesis may occur in the NSG mouse thymus, mediated by mouse thymic epithelial cells [37, 110].

Consequently, humanized PDX models have been established for several different tumor types and used in preclinical validation of immunotherapy [42, 114–118]. In a humanized PDX of colorectal cancer, the treatment with the PD-1 inhibitor nivolumab resulted in inhibition of tumor growth coupled with increased levels of INF-γ producing intertumoral CD8+ T cells [115]. The treatment efficacy of a PD-1 targeting monoclonal antibody pembrolizumab in humanized lung, sarcoma, and triple-negative breast cancer PDX models showed that the tumor growth response to immune checkpoint inhibitors is dependent on CD8 T+ cells, PD-L1+ cells and interestingly the characteristics of the HSC donor [116]. The response rate to immune checkpoint inhibitors is low and the only biomarkers currently available are high mutational tumor burden, CD8+ T cell infiltration, and PD-L1 expression status in the tumor [119]. However, the HSC donor-dependent immune response in humanized breast cancer PDX models highlights that the response to immune checkpoint inhibitors is not only dependent on the TME, but also on the patient's immune system. T cell involvement in the TME can be mainly split into three distinct immune phenotypes. The first phenotype is characterized by the infiltration of T cells into the tumor [120–122]. Alternatively, the tumor is surrounded by, but not infiltrated with T cells. These two phenotypes are also called "hot tumors," given that the presence of T cells is the hallmark of an active immune response against cancer [10]. The third phenotype describes the total absence of T cells in the TME. Such non-immunogenic malignancies are also referred to as "cold tumors" [10, 123]. The differentiation of "cold" and "hot" tumors highlights the need for personalized immunotherapy with regards to the immune phenotype, and models that are able to recapitulate that concept [124]. The predictive value of the immune phenotype is a powerful tool in the rising field of personalized medicine, which may enable the identification of combination therapies for heterogenous tumors. The humanized PDX model provides a preclinical tool to mimic human tumor-immune system interactions and unravel further predictive biomarkers.

Modeling the TME in 3D

In addition to advanced PDX models, a variety of 3D culture models have emerged that attempt to bridge the gap between simplified 2D cell culture models and complex in vivo animal models [125]. Most of them consider the interaction of tumor cells and TME; however, they differ in the extent of cellular and non-cellular TME components. A crucial factor that dominates 3D culture approaches is the ECM. The ECM is the structural component of the TME, which provides the essential physical scaffold for the cellular components, but also mediates biochemical and biomechanical cues that are required for tissue morphogenesis, differentiation, and homeostasis [126]. The ECM network, which is composed of macromolecules like collagen, fibronectin, laminin and enzymes, functions as a reservoir for cytokines and chemokines. Thereby, ECM is an essential factor of the TME, exerting crucial functions in tumor development by (1) its biophysical characteristics including topography, stiffness, molecular density and tension and (2) its mediated dynamic crosstalk between cells through growth factors, chemokines, and integrins.

Cultures of 3D cell aggregates, called spheroids, have been developed for many different cancer types and are frequently employed to mimic human tumors and drug screenings [127–129]. While spheroids show some degree of relevance for drug testing, they still have a huge 2D interface and lack important components of the ECM [130]. Significant efforts are being made to integrate TME components into tumor spheroid cultures [131], and one of the most studied cell types are cancer-associated fibroblasts (CAFs). These cells are of diverse origin and can arise from, among others, endothelial cells, adipocytes, and BM MSCs [132]. CAFs are activated fibroblasts with proliferative properties, the ability to secrete growth factors and promote ECM formation that confers a tumor-promoting microenvironment for the cancer cells [133, 134]. The presence of CAFs in the TME is often associated with a poor prognosis in serval forms of cancer [135–137]. However, recent studies differentiate between various different CAF subtypes with pro- or anti-tumoral effects [134, 138, 139].

Other 3D culture approaches use engineered 3D environments, whereby the tumor cell behavior is highly dependent on the biophysical properties of the selected ECM [140]. This could be circumvented by the use of decellularized scaffolds from the tissue of interest [141]. This approach is quite similar to the culture of fresh tissue slices but has the advantage of flexibility (e.g., cell types added, stiffness) to fit specific research questions [142]. Decellularized scaffolds can be re-populated with various different cell types and offer the possibility to generate fully vascularized and perfused preclinical models [143], maintained within a bioreactor [144, 145]. Moreover, decellularized scaffolds used as matrix for tumor formation have been shown to be feasible models for drug testing [146]. Other approaches, such as organ-on-a-chip models containing microfluidics and 3D bio-printing are more complex systems that need bioengineering expertise but offer high specialization and a high control of the 3D architecture [147, 148]. Standardization of these models is still in progress, but their application should afford valuable research opportunities. The implementation of such innovative 3D platforms into basic research and preclinical studies will improve clinical translatability and ultimately facilitate the development of novel mono- or combination therapies in general and personalized medicine. Novel 3D culture approaches and classical PDX models may complement each other since none of these models will fit all purposes. 3D culture models used prior to animal models have the potential to reduce the number of animals needed and its combined used (i.e., engraftment of 3D culture into mice) may pave the way to more advanced animal models that will integrate more efficiently the different components of the TME.

In Vivo Evaluation of PDX Models: Non-invasive Imaging

As PDX models are improved to better represent human TME it will become increasingly important to develop a repertoire of technologies capable of tracing disease evolution in these models. In orthotopic PDX models, the patient's tumor is implanted in the physiological environment of the organ of origin and can give rise to metastatic disease thus providing an important platform to validate therapeutics in this setting. To enable disease progression monitoring longitudinally, and examine drug efficacy in orthotopic PDX models, sensitive non-invasive imaging techniques are required. While bioluminescence imaging is the most frequently used technique for luciferase positive cell line models, fluorescence optical imaging (FLI) and multimodal positron emission tomography in combination with computed tomography or with magnetic resonance imaging (PET/CT or PET/MRI) are most commonly used to monitor disease progression and therapeutic efficacy in PDX models.

Fluorescence Imaging

FLI employs fluorophores as contrast agents, preferably in the near-infrared (NIR) range (650–900 nm), which allows for deeper tissue penetration and reduced tissue autofluorescence compared to the visible light spectrum (400–650 nm) [149]. By conjugating a fluorophore to a biomarker targeting the malignant cells or the TME, non-invasive FLI can facilitate specific detection of xenografting, tumor growth and metastatic spread, as well as response to treatment [150, 151]. Specific targeting of a biomarker overexpressed in the tumor enhances the tumor-to-background (TBR) fluorescence contrast [152]. Different types of ligands are used in FLI, such as antibodies, small molecules, engineered antibody fragments and peptides that present with different properties influencing binding affinity, pharmacokinetics, stability, and safety [152]. The most widely used ligands are monoclonal antibodies, as a wide variety of targeted therapies are antibody-based and therefore already available (e.g., trastuzumab, bevacizumab) [153].

One of the most clinically advanced imaging biomarkers targets the folate receptor alpha (FRα) [154–156]. Fluorescently labeled small molecules, antibodies and nanoparticles targeting FRα demonstrated specific accumulation in ovarian cancer xenografts but also aided the identification of infiltrated FRβ+ activated macrophages in tumor tissues and lymph nodes [157]. This result also indicates that unspecific binding needs to be considered in the design and development of new FLI conjugates, to avoid the detection of healthy tissue when targeting primarily the cancer cells. The cell surface protein CD24 is another promising biomarker to image ovarian cancer PDX models. CD24 is expressed at a low level in healthy tissue and is almost ubiquitously overexpressed in ovarian cancer, suggesting favorable fluorescence contrast [158–160]. Interestingly, CD24 is also overexpressed in 68% of other solid tumors, suggesting its broad applicability as a tumor imaging ligand [159]. Non-invasive FLI using CD24 conjugated to the NIR fluorophore Alexa Fluor 680 (AF680) has demonstrated a strong potential to longitudinally follow the metastatic disease and monitor treatment response to standard of care chemotherapy in orthotopic xenograft models [151]. The conjugation of CD24 to the higher emitting NIR dye Alexa Fluor 750 (AF750) allowed real-time FLI and enabled better contrast with reduced autofluorescence in five ovarian PDX models, presenting with heterogenous CD24 expression (Fig. 19.3A) [56]. The epithelial cell adhesion molecule (EpCAM) is highly expressed in epithelial carcinomas, including endometrial, ovarian, head and neck, colon, and breast [150, 161] and is another promising target for PDX FLI. The NIR dye AF680 conjugated to the monoclonal antibody EpCAM allowed identification of tumor growth and evaluation of the treatment response to a targeted treatment regimen using trastuzumab, a monoclonal antibody targeting the human epidermal growth factor 2 (HER2), in HER2-expressing orthotopic endometrial carcinoma PDX models [150]. This approach emphasizes the use of PDX models as avatars for personalized medicine to identify efficient treatment regimens that can be monitored longitudinally in vivo by noninvasive FLI. Additionally, EpCAM-targeted (IRDye 800CW) FLI allowed monitoring of disease progression in colorectal, breast, head, and neck orthotopic cancer xenograft models [162]. In 2014, a BCL-2 inhibitor was tested in AML PDX models, showing distinctive response efficacies among different patients, highlighting the power of heterogenous models [163]. Disease tumor burden in AML PDX mice was determined post mortem by human anti-CD45 flow cytometry. Alternatively, disease progression in AML PDX models can be monitored by anti-CD45 AF680 FLI in vivo (Fig. 19.3B). Inhibition of tumor growth in AML PDX models treated with a combination of Ara-C and daunorubicin was demonstrated by longitudinal FLI accompanied with reduced human leukemic stem cell burden in the BM identified by single cell flow cytometry post mortem [164]. An FLI technique using a multiplexing antibody cocktail approach (anti-CD45, -HLA ABC, -CD13, or -CD33 conjugated to AF680) demonstrated a superior efficacy, in comparison to the use of a single antibody, for the early detection of cancer cells and metastasis [164].

As discussed above, imaging biomarkers targeting proteins expressed by tumor cells have been successfully employed to monitor the disease burden in various PDX models of different cancer types. However, molecular imaging markers of the TME also exist and may be similarly exploited. ECM proteins and physiological non-cellular elements, such as hypoxia and pH changes, vasculature and integrins are well described [165]. Solid malignant tumors gradually outgrow their oxygen and nutrients supply via native blood vessels. This leads to hypoxia and acidosis, two

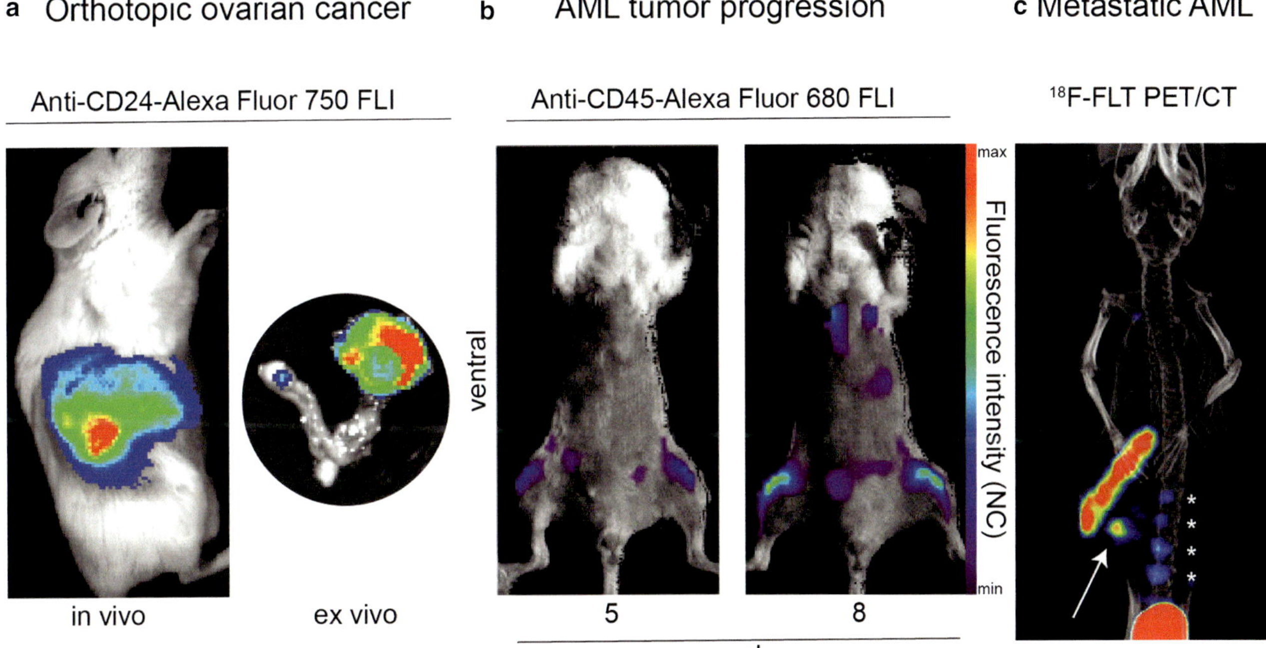

Fig. 19.3 Imaging modalities to image PDX models. (**a**) Fluorescence imaging (FLI) of orthotopic ovarian cancer PDX models 48 h after intravenous injection of a monoclonal antibody conjugated to the contrast agent Alexa Fluor 750. Primary tumor in the left ovary and metastatic spread in the abdominal cavity. (**b**) Longitudinal FLI in orthotopic AML PDX model at week 5 and 8. Metastatic progression can be observed using an anti-CD45-AlexaFluor 680 conjugate 24 hours after injection. **c**) PET/CT imaging with 18F-FLT depicts BM infiltration (*) and infiltration of malignant cells to the ovary (white arrow) in an AML PDX model

key features of the TME that promote tumor progression and therapy resistance [166]. Hypoxia leads to increased expression of hypoxia-inducible factor 1 alpha that in turn alters cellular metabolism to support tumor cell survival, growth and proliferation in the absence of oxygen [167]. In regions of deep hypoxia, oxidative phosphorylation is prevented and cancer cell metabolism shifts to glycolysis. This leads to an increase in the release of lactate and protons that decrease the pH of the extracellular compartment resulting in tissue acidosis [168]. One commonly applied strategy in optical FLI is the use of activatable contrast agents that utilize the physiological change in the TME to increase the contrast between malignant and healthy tissue [169]. The fluorescence of activatable contrast agents is quenched and can be restored after activation by tumor-specific enzymes or an acidic pH in the TME, which avoids off-target fluorescence and increases the TBR [170]. The γ-glutamyltranspeptidase (GGT) is highly abundant in many cancer types. An activatable fluorescent contrast agent targeting GGT allowed rapid and sensitive detection of small tumor deposits in metastatic ovarian xenografts [171]. An improved design of the GGT-activated fluorescent probe was applied in pancreatic PDX models leading to a long-lasting specific signal in the tumor tissue [172]. All these different FLI imaging techniques have proven to be a great set of tools to identify the efficacy of treatment regimens and to monitor disease development in vivo.

PET/CT and PET/MRI Imaging

While optical FLI is a key modality to monitor response to therapies in preclinical research, a major drawback to its application is the limited tissue penetration depth of light (5–7 mm) [173]. PET/CT and PET/MRI circumvent this limitation, allowing simultaneous anatomic and molecular imaging and are frequently used to assess the tumor response to therapy in patients. PET employs radiotracers that have unlimited penetration depth to provide molecular information, whereas CT and MRI provide 3D anatomic images based on the attenuation of X-rays by tissue or on the different relaxation times of magnetic particles. PET/CT can be exploited preclinically, especially for the quantitative assessment of probe pharmacokinetics. ^{18}F-Fluorodeoxyglucose (^{18}F-FDG, glucose analog) and ^{18}F-fluorothymidine (^{18}F-FLT, nucleoside analog) report metabolic activity, viability and proliferation of cancer cells, respectively, and are commonly used PET tracers in PDX tumor evaluation (Fig. 19.3C) [174]. In an orthotopic endometrial PDX model, ^{18}F-FDG and ^{18}F-FLT were successfully used to monitor tumor growth and detect disease spread [174]. The applicability of ^{18}F-FLT was also demonstrated in a metastatic AML PDX model allowing the visualization of an established secondary tumor in the ovary (Fig. 19.3C). In orthotopic xenograft models of colorectal cancer, ^{18}F-FLT PET metabolic imaging allowed to monitor response to targeted therapy, suggesting its suitability for quantitative drug efficacy studies [175]. In addition, the high glucose metabolism observed in lung cancer patients correlated with a high ^{18}F-FDG tracer uptake in the corresponding PDX models and demonstrates its clinical prognostic value [176, 177]. ^{18}F-FDG-PET was exploited to investigate the metabolic activity in four generations of passaged orthotopic colorectal PDX models to assess the impact of murine TME replacement. Interestingly, stable tracer uptake in colorectal PDXs across all generations was demonstrated [66]. While ^{18}F-FLT uptake is believed to be specific for tumor tissue, some technical and physiologic factors, such as inflammation, alter the ^{18}F-FDG tracer uptake, making molecular targeted PET/CT imaging approaches more appealing [178]. ^{89}Zr-M9346A, a radiolabeled anti-FRα PET tracer, proved useful to evaluate the expression of FRα in triple-negative breast cancer PDXs, providing a screening tool for consecutive treatment with the FRα targeting antibody-drug conjugate Mirvetuximab soravtansine [179]. ^{89}Zr-C4, a radiotracer targeting both mouse and human PD-L1, allowed to determine PD-L1 expression in a clinically relevant lung PDX model derived from an immunotherapy responder in vivo. The quantitative assessment of changes in PD-L1 biomarker expression in response to standard of care treatment can be used for immune checkpoint inhibitor stratifications [180]. In conclusion, PET/CT and PET/MRI allow simultaneous detection of anatomical structures and deeply located tumor lesions. The adoption of these imaging modalities for validation of treatment responses in relevant PDX models is expected to translate into an improved selection of relevant drugs and shorter bench-to-bedside transitions of these drugs, while aiding the clinical translation of molecular imaging probes and technologies.

Ex Vivo Verification of PDX Models: Single-Cell Technologies

To effectively interrogate the TME in PDX models beyond imaging, new and emerging molecular technologies must be harnessed to study complex, chimeric tissues containing a variety of cell types. Single-cell analysis has revolutionized cancer research and affords novel opportunities for understanding cancer cells-TME relationship [181] (Fig. 19.4).

Mass cytometry is a powerful technique used to analyze single cells stained with antibodies conjugated to stable metal isotopes. Unlike conventional fluorescence flow

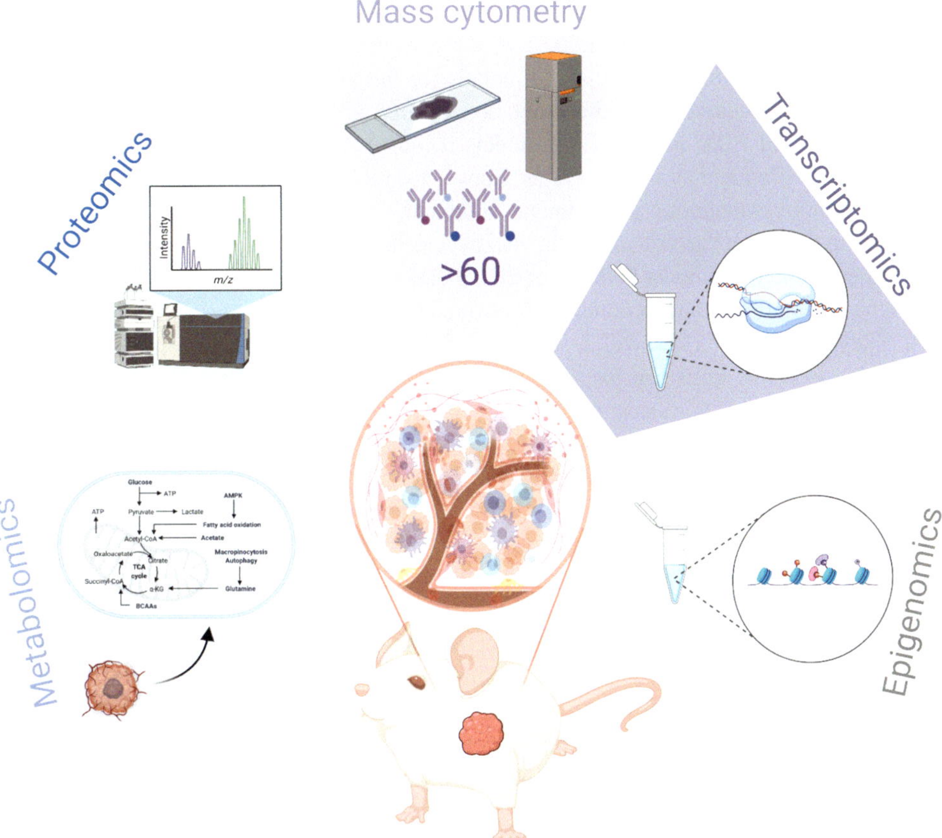

Fig. 19.4 Ex vivo single-cell analysis technologies provide unique opportunities to uncover mechanisms of sensitivity and resistance to applied therapies in PDX models of cancer. Created with BioRender.com

cytometry, mass cytometry is unburdened by issues of spectral overlap and currently enables the analysis of 60 protein markers simultaneously [182, 183]. Imaging mass cytometry (IMC) further develops the principle of analyzing metal-conjugated antibodies but uses tissue sections as a source material [184]. Small regions of tissue sections are ablated, thereby conserving the structure and localization of cells, enabling to study the interaction of cells within the TME. Subsequent analysis is performed using computer-generated recreations to produce high-dimensional images [185].

Single-cell transcriptomics is performed to quantify gene expression in thousands of individual cells simultaneously [186]. Fundamental to the technique is the isolation of single cells and subsequent amplification of cDNA. Simple qPCR-based studies assessing only a few selected genes were first performed almost 30 years ago [187]. However, in the last decade, technological innovations in robotic microfluidics, amplification and sequencing technologies, and the development of sophisticated computational platforms have transformed the scale of single-cell transcriptomic studies [188]. Single-cell RNA-seq performed in over 200,000 individual stromal cells isolated from a variety of solid cancer types revealed a common gene expression signature likely to be important for generating TME supporting cancer development [189]. Similar studies should be performed in tissues

harvested from PDX models to improve engraftment and verify the suitability and clinical relevance of the models being developed.

The transformative technologies harnessed in the development of single-cell transcriptomics have also supported the development of single-cell protocols for assessing other cellular phenotypes, such as epigenomics, proteomics, and metabolomics. Characterization of single cells on multiple parameters reveals that seemingly identical cell types may vary significantly in regard to cell state. Single-cell analysis of mouse HSCs revealed clone-specific functional heterogeneity corresponding to epigenetic configuration, while transcription patterns remained unchanged [190]. A deeper characterization of individual cell states in host animal tissue (e.g., NSG-SGM mice) and engrafted cancer tissues can vastly improve PDX models and our understanding of their associated TME. It seems clear that single-cell technologies have the capacity to significantly enhance our understanding of PDX models and the role of TME in cancer. Like patients, PDX models and associated TME are comprised of heterogenous cell populations, where bulk analysis of tissues may conceal cell-type-specific patterns of gene expression or protein activity. An integrated application of single-cell technologies can provide novel research opportunities to better understand the role of TME in cancer progression and therapy development.

Concluding Remarks/Summary

PDXs are currently the best preclinical models for the discovery of new biomarkers and the evaluation of drug efficacy. Humanized PDX mice, animal models reconstituted with a human immune system, serve as a powerful tool to evaluate immune-modulatory treatment approaches. The response to treatment can be assessed in vivo by non-invasive fluorescence and multimodal PET/CT or PET/MRI imaging, and novel predictive biomarkers can be discovered by single-cell analysis ex vivo. However, despite the advantages of preserving genomic traits and inter-patient tumor heterogeneity, humanized PDX models fail to fully represent the TME as most non-malignant cells and non-cellular elements are replaced over time by mouse counterparts. The impact of murine TME for the successful evaluation of therapies in these advanced preclinical animal models is not yet fully understood. Given our increasing understanding of how the TME influences cancer progression and therapeutic intervention, the future lies in the development of preclinical models capable of integrating and investigating the human TME. Therefore, a better representation of human-originating TME needs to be accomplished to improve the preclinical evaluation of personalized medicine.

References

1. Ayres F, Zuffo M, Rangayyan R, Boag G, Valente M. Estimation of the tissue composition of the tumour mass in neuroblastoma using segmented CT images. Med Biol Eng Comput. 2004;42(3):366–77.
2. Valkenburg KC, de Groot AE, Pienta KJ. Targeting the tumour stroma to improve cancer therapy. Nat Rev Clin Oncol. 2018;15(6):366–81.
3. Ansell SM, Vonderheide RH. Cellular composition of the tumor microenvironment. Am Soc Clin Oncol Educ Book. 2013;33(1):e91–e7.
4. Barriga V, Kuol N, Nurgali K, Apostolopoulos V. The complex interaction between the tumor micro-environment and immune checkpoints in breast cancer. Cancers. 2019;11(8):1205.
5. Seager RJ, Hajal C, Spill F, Kamm RD, Zaman MH. Dynamic interplay between tumour, stroma and immune system can drive or prevent tumour progression. Convergent Sci Phys Oncol. 2017;3(3):034002.
6. Annaratone L, Cascardi E, Vissio E, Sarotto I, Chmielik E, Sapino A, et al. The multifaceted nature of tumor microenvironment in breast carcinomas. Pathobiology. 2020;87(2):1–18.
7. Arneth B. Tumor microenvironment. Medicina. 2020;56(1):15.
8. Baghban R, Roshangar L, Jahanban-Esfahlan R, Seidi K, Ebrahimi-Kalan A, Jaymand M, et al. Tumor microenvironment complexity and therapeutic implications at a glance. Cell Commun Signal. 2020;18:1–19.
9. Hinshaw DC, Shevde LA. The tumor microenvironment innately modulates cancer progression. Cancer Res. 2019;79(18):4557–66.
10. Duan Q, Zhang H, Zheng J, Zhang L. Turning cold into hot: firing up the tumor microenvironment. Trends Cancer 2020.
11. Gonzalez H, Hagerling C, Werb Z. Roles of the immune system in cancer: from tumor initiation to metastatic progression. Genes Dev. 2018;32(19–20):1267–84.
12. Gajewski T, Schreiber H, Fu Y. Defective IFN production can reduce cross priming while targeting tumor tissues with type I IFN can bridge innate and adaptive immune responses. Nat Immunol. 2013;14(10):1014–22.
13. Pitt J, Marabelle A, Eggermont A, Soria J-C, Kroemer G, Zitvogel L. Targeting the tumor microenvironment: removing obstruction to anticancer immune responses and immunotherapy. Ann Oncol. 2016;27(8):1482–92.
14. Katsuta E, Rashid OM, Takabe K. Clinical relevance of tumor microenvironment: immune cells, vessels, and mouse models. Hum Cell. 2020;1–8
15. Whiteside TL. The role of immune cells in the tumor microenvironment. The link between inflammation and cancer. Springer; 2006. p. 103–24.
16. Joyce JA. Therapeutic targeting of the tumor microenvironment. Cancer Cell. 2005;7(6):513–20.
17. Dominiak A, Chełstowska B, Olejarz W, Nowicka G. Communication in the cancer microenvironment as a target for therapeutic interventions. Cancers. 2020;12(5):1232.
18. Hirata E, Sahai E. Tumor microenvironment and differential responses to therapy. Cold Spring Harb Perspect Med. 2017;7(7):a026781.
19. Son B, Lee S, Youn H, Kim E, Kim W, Youn B. The role of tumor microenvironment in therapeutic resistance. Oncotarget. 2017;8(3):3933.
20. Li Z-W, Dalton WS. Tumor microenvironment and drug resistance in hematologic malignancies. Blood Rev. 2006;20(6):333–42.
21. Benavente S, Sánchez-García A, Naches S, LLeonart ME, Lorente J. Therapy-induced modulation of the tumor microenvironment: new opportunities for cancer therapies in Front Oncol 2020;10:2169.
22. Polson AG, Fuji RN. The successes and limitations of preclinical studies in predicting the pharmacodynamics and safety of cell-surface-targeted biological agents in patients. Br J Pharmacol. 2012;166(5):1600–2.
23. Van Norman GA. Limitations of animal studies for predicting toxicity. Clin Trials 2019.
24. Seyhan AA. Lost in translation: the valley of death across preclinical and clinical divide–identification of problems and overcoming obstacles. Translat Med Commun. 2019;4(1):1–19.
25. Tentler JJ, Tan AC, Weekes CD, Jimeno A, Leong S, Pitts TM, et al. Patient-derived tumour xenografts as models for oncology drug development. Nat Rev Clin Oncol. 2012;9(6):338–50.
26. Faguet GB. A brief history of cancer: age-old milestones underlying our current knowledge database. Int J Cancer. 2015;136(9):2022–36.
27. Bailey M, Christoforidou Z, Lewis MC. The evolutionary basis for differences between the immune systems of man, mouse, pig and ruminants. Vet Immunol Immunopathol. 2013;152(1–2):13–9.
28. Decker WK, da Silva RF, Sanabria MH, Angelo LS, Guimarães F, Burt BM, et al. Cancer immunotherapy: historical perspective of a clinical revolution and emerging preclinical animal models. Front Immunol. 2017;8:829.
29. Toolan HW. Successful subcutaneous growth and transplantation of human tumors in X-irradiated laboratory animals. Proc Soc Exp Biol Med. 1951;77(3):572–8.
30. Toolan HW. Growth of human tumors in cortisone-treated laboratory animals: the possibility of obtaining permanently transplantable human tumors. Cancer Res. 1953;13(4–5):389–94.
31. Van Duyne R, Pedati C, Guendel I, Carpio L, Kehn-Hall K, Saifuddin M, et al. The utilization of humanized mouse models for the study of human retroviral infections. Retrovirology. 2009;6:76.
32. Kelland LR. Of mice and men: values and liabilities of the athymic nude mouse model in anticancer drug development. Eur J Cancer. 2004;40(6):827–36.

33. Rygaard J, Povlsen CO. Heterotransplantation of a human malignant tumour to "Nude" mice. Acta Pathol Microbiol Scand. 1969;77(4):758–60.

34. Fiebig HH, Schuchhardt C, Henss H, Fiedler L, Löhr GW. Comparison of tumor response in nude mice and in the patients. Behring Inst Mitt. 1984;74:343–52.

35. Shultz LD, Schweitzer PA, Christianson SW, Gott B, Schweitzer IB, Tennent B, et al. Multiple defects in innate and adaptive immunologic function in NOD/LtSz-scid mice. J Immunol. 1995;154(1):180–91.

36. Yoshida GJ. Applications of patient-derived tumor xenograft models and tumor organoids. J Hematol Oncol. 2020;13(1):4.

37. Shultz LD, Lyons BL, Burzenski LM, Gott B, Chen X, Chaleff S, et al. Human lymphoid and myeloid cell development in NOD/LtSz-scid IL2R null mice engrafted with mobilized human hemopoietic stem cells. J Immunol. 2005;174(10):6477–89.

38. Pearson T, Greiner D, Shultz L. Humanized SCID mouse models for biomedical research. Humanized Mice. 2008:25–51.

39. Wunderlich M, Chou FS, Link KA, Mizukawa B, Perry RL, Carroll M, et al. AML xenograft efficiency is significantly improved in NOD/SCID-IL2RG mice constitutively expressing human SCF, GM-CSF and IL-3. Leukemia. 2010;24(10):1785–8.

40. Saito Y, Ellegast JM, Rafiei A, Song Y, Kull D, Heikenwalder M, et al. Peripheral blood CD34+ cells efficiently engraft human cytokine knock-in mice. Blood. 2016;128(14):1829–33.

41. Willinger T, Rongvaux A, Strowig T, Manz MG, Flavell RA. Improving human hemato-lymphoid-system mice by cytokine knock-in gene replacement. Trends Immunol. 2011;32(7):321–7.

42. Rongvaux A, Willinger T, Martinek J, Strowig T, Gearty SV, Teichmann LL, et al. Development and function of human innate immune cells in a humanized mouse model. Nat Biotechnol. 2014;32(4):364–72.

43. Warren A, Chen Y, Jones A, Shibue T, Hahn WC, Boehm JS, et al. Global computational alignment of tumor and cell line transcriptional profiles. Nat Commun. 2021;12(1):22.

44. Byrne AT, Alferez DG, Amant F, Annibali D, Arribas J, Biankin AV, et al. Interrogating open issues in cancer precision medicine with patient-derived xenografts. Nat Rev Cancer. 2017;17(4):254–68.

45. Hidalgo M, Amant F, Biankin AV, Budinská E, Byrne AT, Caldas C, et al. Patient-derived xenograft models: an emerging platform for translational cancer research. Cancer Discov. 2014;4(9):998–1013.

46. Gengenbacher N, Singhal M, Augustin HG. Preclinical mouse solid tumour models: status quo, challenges and perspectives. Nat Rev Cancer. 2017;17(12):751–65.

47. Shi J, Li Y, Jia R, Fan X. The fidelity of cancer cells in PDX models: characteristics, mechanism and clinical significance. Int J Cancer. 2020;146(8):2078–88.

48. Collins AT, Lang SH. A systematic review of the validity of patient derived xenograft (PDX) models: the implications for translational research and personalised medicine. PeerJ. 2018;6:e5981.

49. Ben-David U, Ha G, Tseng YY, Greenwald NF, Oh C, Shih J, et al. Patient-derived xenografts undergo mouse-specific tumor evolution. Nat Genet. 2017;49(11):1567–75.

50. Richter-Pechanska P, Kunz JB, Bornhauser B, von Knebel DC, Rausch T, Erarslan-Uysal B, et al. PDX models recapitulate the genetic and epigenetic landscape of pediatric T-cell leukemia. EMBO Mol Med. 2018;10(12)

51. Tomar T, de Jong S, Alkema NG, Hoekman RL, Meersma GJ, Klip HG, et al. Genome-wide methylation profiling of ovarian cancer patient-derived xenografts treated with the demethylating agent decitabine identifies novel epigenetically regulated genes and pathways. Genome Med. 2016;8(1):107.

52. Woo XY, Giordano J, Srivastava A, Zhao ZM, Lloyd MW, de Bruijn R, et al. Conservation of copy number profiles during engraftment and passaging of patient-derived cancer xenografts. Nat Genet. 2021;53(1):86–99.

53. Mer AS, Ba-Alawi W, Smirnov P, Wang YX, Brew B, Ortmann J, et al. Integrative pharmacogenomics analysis of patient-derived xenografts. Cancer Res. 2019;79(17):4539–50.

54. Koga Y, Ochiai A. Systematic review of patient-derived xenograft models for preclinical studies of anti-cancer drugs in solid tumors. Cell. 2019;8(5):418.

55. Helland O, Popa M, Vintermyr OK, Molven A, Gjertsen BT, Bjorge L, et al. First in-mouse development and application of a surgically relevant xenograft model of ovarian carcinoma. PLoS One. 2014;9(3):e89527.

56. Kleinmanns K, Fosse V, Davidson B, de Jalón EG, Tenstad O, Bjørge L, et al. CD24-targeted intraoperative fluorescence image-guided surgery leads to improved cytoreduction of ovarian cancer in a preclinical orthotopic surgical model. EBioMedicine. 2020;56:102783.

57. Delitto D, Pham K, Vlada AC, Sarosi GA, Thomas RM, Behrns KE, et al. Patient-derived xenograft models for pancreatic adenocarcinoma demonstrate retention of tumor morphology through incorporation of murine stromal elements. Am J Pathol. 2015;185(5):1297–303.

58. Scott CL, Becker MA, Haluska P, Samimi G. Patient-derived xenograft models to improve targeted therapy in epithelial ovarian cancer treatment. Front Oncol. 2013;3:295.

59. Hylander BL, Punt N, Tang H, Hillman J, Vaughan M, Bshara W, et al. Origin of the vasculature supporting growth of primary patient tumor xenografts. J Transl Med. 2013;11(1):1–14.

60. Bankert RB, Balu-Iyer SV, Odunsi K, Shultz LD, Kelleher RJ Jr, Barnas JL, et al. Humanized mouse model of ovarian cancer recapitulates patient solid tumor progression, ascites formation, and metastasis. PLoS One. 2011;6(9):e24420.

61. Williams JA. Using PDX for preclinical cancer drug discovery: the evolving field. J Clin Med. 2018;7(3):41.

62. Jain RK, Martin JD, Stylianopoulos T. The role of mechanical forces in tumor growth and therapy. Annu Rev Biomed Eng. 2014;16(1):321–46.

63. Jain RK. Normalizing tumor microenvironment to treat cancer: bench to bedside to biomarkers. J Clin Oncol. 2013;31(17):2205–18.

64. Jain RK. Antiangiogenesis strategies revisited: from starving tumors to alleviating hypoxia. Cancer Cell. 2014;26(5):605–22.

65. Mitchell MJ, Jain RK, Langer R. Engineering and physical sciences in oncology: challenges and opportunities. Nat Rev Cancer. 2017;17(11):659–75.

66. Blomme A, Van Simaeys G, Doumont G, Costanza B, Bellier J, Otaka Y, et al. Murine stroma adopts a human-like metabolic phenotype in the PDX model of colorectal cancer and liver metastases. Oncogene. 2018;37(9):1237–50.

67. Bianco P, Riminucci M, Gronthos S, Robey PG. Bone marrow stromal stem cells: nature, biology, and potential applications. Stem Cells. 2001;19(3):180–92.

68. Okada S, Vaeteewoottacharn K, Kariya R. Application of highly immunocompromised mice for the establishment of patient-derived xenograft (PDX) models. Cell. 2019;8(8)

69. Gelebart P, Popa M, McCormack E. Xenograft models of primary acute myeloid leukemia for the development of imaging strategies and evaluation of novel targeted therapies. Curr Pharm Biotechnol. 2016;17(1):42–51.

70. Ito M, Hiramatsu H, Kobayashi K, Suzue K, Kawahata M, Hioki K, et al. NOD/SCID/gamma(c)(null) mouse: an excellent recipient mouse model for engraftment of human cells. Blood. 2002;100(9):3175–82.

71. Chijiwa T, Kawai K, Noguchi A, Sato H, Hayashi A, Cho H, et al. Establishment of patient-derived cancer xenografts in immunodeficient NOG mice. Int J Oncol. 2015;47(1):61–70.

72. McIntosh BE, Brown ME. No irradiation required: the future of humanized immune system modeling in murine hosts. Chimerism. 2015;6(1–2):40–5.

73. Almosailleakh M, Schwaller J. Murine models of acute myeloid Leukaemia. Int J Mol Sci. 2019;20(2).

74. Li L, Osdal T, Ho Y, Chun S, McDonald T, Agarwal P, et al. SIRT1 activation by a c-MYC oncogenic network promotes the maintenance and drug resistance of human FLT3-ITD acute myeloid leukemia stem cells. Cell Stem Cell. 2014;15(4):431–46.

75. Zhang Y, He L, Selimoglu-Buet D, Jego C, Morabito M, Willekens C, et al. Engraftment of chronic myelomonocytic leukemia cells in immunocompromised mice supports disease dependency on cytokines. Blood Adv. 2017;1(14):972–9.

76. Kloos A, Mintzas K, Winckler L, Gabdoulline R, Alwie Y, Jyotsana N, et al. Effective drug treatment identified by in vivo screening in a transplantable patient-derived xenograft model of chronic myelomonocytic leukemia. Leukemia. 2020;34(11):2951–63.

77. Reinisch A, Thomas D, Corces MR, Zhang X, Gratzinger D, Hong WJ, et al. A humanized bone marrow ossicle xenotransplantation model enables improved engraftment of healthy and leukemic human hematopoietic cells. Nat Med. 2016;22(7):812–21.

78. Gooden MJ, de Bock GH, Leffers N, Daemen T, Nijman HW. The prognostic influence of tumour-infiltrating lymphocytes in cancer: a systematic review with meta-analysis. Br J Cancer. 2011;105(1):93–103.

79. Chen Y, Zhao B, Wang X. Tumor infiltrating immune cells (TIICs) as a biomarker for prognosis benefits in patients with osteosarcoma. BMC Cancer. 2020;20(1):1022.

80. Zhang S, Zeng Z, Liu Y, Huang J, Long J, Wang Y, et al. Prognostic landscape of tumor-infiltrating immune cells and immune-related genes in the tumor microenvironment of gastric cancer. Aging (Albany NY). 2020;12(18):17958–75.

81. St Paul M, Ohashi PS. The roles of CD8(+) T cell subsets in anti-tumor immunity. Trends Cell Biol. 2020;30(9):695–704.

82. Bevan MJ. Helping the CD8(+) T-cell response. Nat Rev Immunol. 2004;4(8):595–602.

83. van der Leun AM, Thommen DS, Schumacher TN. CD8(+) T cell states in human cancer: insights from single-cell analysis. Nat Rev Cancer. 2020;20(4):218–32.

84. Jin YW, Hu P. Tumor-infiltrating CD8 T cells predict clinical breast cancer outcomes in young women. Cancers (Basel). 2020;12(5)

85. So YK, Byeon SJ, Ku BM, Ko YH, Ahn MJ, Son YI, et al. An increase of CD8(+) T cell infiltration following recurrence is a good prognosticator in HNSCC. Sci Rep. 2020;10(1):20059.

86. Naito Y, Saito K, Shiiba K, Ohuchi A, Saigenji K, Nagura H, et al. CD8+ T cells infiltrated within cancer cell nests as a prognostic factor in human colorectal cancer. Cancer Res. 1998;58(16):3491–4.

87. Paluskievicz CM, Cao X, Abdi R, Zheng P, Liu Y, Bromberg JS. T regulatory cells and priming the suppressive tumor microenvironment. Front Immunol. 2019;10:2453.

88. Ohue Y, Nishikawa H. Regulatory T (Treg) cells in cancer: can Treg cells be a new therapeutic target? Cancer Sci. 2019;110(7):2080–9.

89. Saleh R, Elkord E. FoxP3(+) T regulatory cells in cancer: prognostic biomarkers and therapeutic targets. Cancer Lett. 2020;490:174–85.

90. Whiteside TL. FOXP3+ Treg as a therapeutic target for promoting anti-tumor immunity. Expert Opin Ther Targets. 2018;22(4):353–63.

91. Vignali DA, Collison LW, Workman CJ. How regulatory T cells work. Nat Rev Immunol. 2008;8(7):523–32.

92. Ma Y, Aymeric L, Locher C, Kroemer G, Zitvogel L. The dendritic cell-tumor cross-talk in cancer. Curr Opin Immunol. 2011;23(1):146–52.

93. Lin A, Schildknecht A, Nguyen LT, Ohashi PS. Dendritic cells integrate signals from the tumor microenvironment to modulate immunity and tumor growth. Immunol Lett. 2010;127(2):77–84.

94. Di Blasio S, van Wigcheren GF, Becker A, van Duffelen A, Gorris M, Verrijp K, et al. The tumour microenvironment shapes dendritic cell plasticity in a human organotypic melanoma culture. Nat Commun. 2020;11(1):2749.

95. Vitale I, Manic G, Coussens LM, Kroemer G, Galluzzi L. Macrophages and metabolism in the tumor microenvironment. Cell Metab. 2019;30(1):36–50.

96. Cassetta L, Fragkogianni S, Sims AH, Swierczak A, Forrester LM, Zhang H, et al. Human tumor-associated macrophage and monocyte transcriptional landscapes reveal cancer-specific reprogramming, biomarkers, and therapeutic targets. Cancer Cell. 2019;35(4):588–602 e10.

97. Gentles AJ, Newman AM, Liu CL, Bratman SV, Feng W, Kim D, et al. The prognostic landscape of genes and infiltrating immune cells across human cancers. Nat Med. 2015;21(8):938–45.

98. Wagner J, Rapsomaniki MA, Chevrier S, Anzeneder T, Langwieder C, Dykgers A, et al. A single-cell atlas of the tumor and immune ecosystem of human breast cancer. Cell. 2019;177(5):1330–45 e18.

99. Yang M, McKay D, Pollard JW, Lewis CE. Diverse functions of macrophages in different tumor microenvironments. Cancer Res. 2018;78(19):5492–503.

100. Cassetta L, Pollard JW. Targeting macrophages: therapeutic approaches in cancer. Nat Rev Drug Discov. 2018;17(12):887–904.

101. Mantovani A, Marchesi F, Malesci A, Laghi L, Allavena P. Tumour-associated macrophages as treatment targets in oncology. Nat Rev Clin Oncol. 2017;14(7):399–416.

102. Wenes M, Shang M, Di Matteo M, Goveia J, Martin-Perez R, Serneels J, et al. Macrophage metabolism controls tumor blood vessel morphogenesis and metastasis. Cell Metab. 2016;24(5):701–15.

103. Roma-Lavisse C, Tagzirt M, Zawadzki C, Lorenzi R, Vincentelli A, Haulon S, et al. M1 and M2 macrophage proteolytic and angiogenic profile analysis in atherosclerotic patients reveals a distinctive profile in type 2 diabetes. Diab Vasc Dis Res. 2015;12(4):279–89.

104. Lai YS, Wahyuningtyas R, Aui SP, Chang KT. Autocrine VEGF signalling on M2 macrophages regulates PD-L1 expression for immunomodulation of T cells. J Cell Mol Med. 2019;23(2):1257–67.

105. Curiel TJ, Coukos G, Zou L, Alvarez X, Cheng P, Mottram P, et al. Specific recruitment of regulatory T cells in ovarian carcinoma fosters immune privilege and predicts reduced survival. Nat Med. 2004;10(9):942–9.

106. Galon J, Costes A, Sanchez-Cabo F, Kirilovsky A, Mlecnik B, Lagorce-Pagès C, et al. Type, density, and location of immune cells within human colorectal tumors predict clinical outcome. Science. 2006;313(5795):1960–4.

107. Bruni D, Angell HK, Galon J. The immune contexture and Immunoscore in cancer prognosis and therapeutic efficacy. Nat Rev Cancer. 2020;20(11):662–80.

108. McIntosh BE, Brown ME, Duffin BM, Maufort JP, Vereide DT, Slukvin II, et al. Nonirradiated NOD, B6. SCID Il2rγ−/− KitW41/ W41 (NBSGW) mice support multilineage engraftment of human hematopoietic cells. Stem Cell Rep. 2015;4(2):171–80.

109. Brehm MA, Cuthbert A, Yang C, Miller DM, DiIorio P, Laning J, et al. Parameters for establishing humanized mouse models to study human immunity: analysis of human hematopoietic stem cell engraftment in three immunodeficient strains of mice bearing the IL2rγnull mutation. Clin Immunol. 2010;135(1):84–98.

110. Ishikawa F, Yasukawa M, Lyons B, Yoshida S, Miyamoto T, Yoshimoto G, et al. Development of functional human blood

and immune systems in NOD/SCID/IL2 receptor {gamma} chain(null) mice. Blood. 2005;106(5):1565–73.

111. Wege AK, Ernst W, Eckl J, Frankenberger B, Vollmann-Zwerenz A, Mannel DN, et al. Humanized tumor mice--a new model to study and manipulate the immune response in advanced cancer therapy. Int J Cancer. 2011;129(9):2194–206.

112. Terren I, Orrantia A, Vitalle J, Zenarruzabeitia O, Borrego F. NK cell metabolism and tumor microenvironment. Front Immunol. 2019;10:2278.

113. Larsen SK, Gao Y, Basse PH. NK cells in the tumor microenvironment. Crit Rev Oncog. 2014;19(1–2):91–105.

114. Liu WN, Fong SY, Tan WWS, Tan SY, Liu M, Cheng JY, et al. Establishment and characterization of humanized mouse NPC-PDX model for testing immunotherapy. Cancers. 2020;12(4):1025.

115. Capasso A, Lang J, Pitts TM, Jordan K, Lieu C, Davis S, et al. Characterization of immune responses to anti-PD-1 mono and combination immunotherapy in hematopoietic humanized mice implanted with tumor xenografts. J Immunother Cancer. 2019;7(1):37.

116. Wang M, Yao LC, Cheng M, Cai D, Martinek J, Pan CX, et al. Humanized mice in studying efficacy and mechanisms of PD-1-targeted cancer immunotherapy. FASEB J. 2018;32(3):1537–49.

117. Wang Z, Sun K, Xiao Y, Feng B, Mikule K, Ma X, et al. Niraparib activates interferon signaling and potentiates anti-PD-1 antibody efficacy in tumor models. Sci Rep. 2019;9(1):1–12.

118. Ashizawa T, Iizuka A, Nonomura C, Kondou R, Maeda C, Miyata H, et al. Antitumor effect of programmed death-1 (PD-1) blockade in humanized the NOG-MHC double knockout mouse. Clin Cancer Res. 2017;23(1):149–58.

119. Gibney GT, Weiner LM, Atkins MB. Predictive biomarkers for checkpoint inhibitor-based immunotherapy. Lancet Oncol. 2016;17(12):e542–e51.

120. Lanitis E, Dangaj D, Irving M, Coukos G. Mechanisms regulating T-cell infiltration and activity in solid tumors. Ann Oncol 2017;28(suppl_12):xii18–32.

121. Labani-Motlagh A, Ashja-Mahdavi M, Loskog A. The tumor microenvironment: a milieu hindering and obstructing antitumor immune responses. Front Immunol. 2020;11:940.

122. Swann JB, Smyth MJ. Immune surveillance of tumors. J Clin Invest. 2007;117(5):1137–46.

123. Bonaventura P, Shekarian T, Alcazer V, Valladeau-Guilemond J, Valsesia-Wittmann S, Amigorena S, et al. Cold tumors: a therapeutic challenge for immunotherapy. Front Immunol. 2019;10:168.

124. Galon J, Bruni D. Approaches to treat immune hot, altered and cold tumours with combination immunotherapies. Nat Rev Drug Discov. 2019;18(3):197–218.

125. Di Modugno F, Colosi C, Trono P, Antonacci G, Ruocco G, Nisticò P. 3D models in the new era of immune oncology: focus on T cells, CAF and ECM. J Exp Clin Cancer Res. 2019;38(1):1–14.

126. Frantz C, Stewart KM, Weaver VM. The extracellular matrix at a glance. J Cell Sci. 2010;123(24):4195–200.

127. Simian M, Bissell MJ. Organoids: a historical perspective of thinking in three dimensions. J Cell Biol. 2017;216(1):31–40.

128. Dart A. Organoid diversity. Nat Rev Cancer. 2018;18(7):404–5.

129. Tuveson D, Clevers H. Cancer modeling meets human organoid technology. Science. 2019;364(6444):952–5.

130. Driehuis E, Kretzschmar K, Clevers H. Establishment of patient-derived cancer organoids for drug-screening applications. Nat Protoc. 2020;15(10):3380–409.

131. Yuki K, Cheng N, Nakano M, Kuo CJ. Organoid models of tumor immunology. Trends Immunol. 2020.

132. Tao L, Huang G, Song H, Chen Y, Chen L. Cancer associated fibroblasts: an essential role in the tumor microenvironment. Oncol Lett. 2017;14(3):2611–20.

133. Liao Z, Tan ZW, Zhu P, Tan NS. Cancer-associated fibroblasts in tumor microenvironment - accomplices in tumor malignancy. Cell Immunol. 2019;343:103729.

134. Liu T, Han C, Wang S, Fang P, Ma Z, Xu L, et al. Cancer-associated fibroblasts: an emerging target of anti-cancer immunotherapy. J Hematol Oncol. 2019;12(1):1–15.

135. Kawase A, Ishii G, Nagai K, Ito T, Nagano T, Murata Y, et al. Podoplanin expression by cancer associated fibroblasts predicts poor prognosis of lung adenocarcinoma. Int J Cancer. 2008;123(5):1053–9.

136. Underwood TJ, Hayden AL, Derouet M, Garcia E, Noble F, White MJ, et al. Cancer-associated fibroblasts predict poor outcome and promote periostin-dependent invasion in oesophageal adenocarcinoma. J Pathol. 2015;235(3):466–77.

137. Zhao X, Ding L, Lu Z, Huang X, Jing Y, Yang Y, et al. Diminished CD68(+) cancer-associated fibroblast subset induces regulatory T-cell (Treg) infiltration and predicts poor prognosis of oral squamous cell carcinoma patients. Am J Pathol. 2020;190(4):886–99.

138. Sidaway P. Fibroblast subtypes alter the microenvironment Nat Rev Clin Oncol 2018;15(5):265-.

139. Pereira BA, Vennin C, Papanicolaou M, Chambers CR, Herrmann D, Morton JP, et al. CAF subpopulations: a new reservoir of stromal targets in pancreatic cancer. Trends Cancer. 2019;5(11):724–41.

140. Benton G, Kleinman HK, George J, Arnaoutova I. Multiple uses of basement membrane-like matrix (BME/Matrigel) in vitro and in vivo with cancer cells. Int J Cancer. 2011;128(8):1751–7.

141. Genovese L, Zawada L, Tosoni A, Ferri A, Zerbi P, Allevi R, et al. Cellular localization, invasion, and turnover are differently influenced by healthy and tumor-derived extracellular matrix. Tissue Eng Part A. 2014;20(13–14):2005–18.

142. Misra S, Moro CF, Del Chiaro M, Pouso S, Sebestyén A, Löhr M, et al. Ex vivo organotypic culture system of precision-cut slices of human pancreatic ductal adenocarcinoma. Sci Rep. 2019;9(1):1–16.

143. Groeber F, Engelhardt L, Lange J, Kurdyn S, Schmid FF, Rücker C, et al. A first vascularized skin equivalent as an alternative to animal experimentation. ALTEX-Alternat Anim Exp. 2016;33(4):415–22.

144. Groeber F, Kahlig A, Loff S, Walles H, Hansmann J. A bioreactor system for interfacial culture and physiological perfusion of vascularized tissue equivalents. Biotechnol J. 2013;8(3):308–16.

145. Schuerlein S, Schwarz T, Krziminski S, Gätzner S, Hoppensack A, Schwedhelm I, et al. A versatile modular bioreactor platform for tissue engineering. Biotechnol J. 2017;12(2):1600326.

146. Sensi F, D'Angelo E, Piccoli M, Pavan P, Mastrotto F, Caliceti P, et al. Recellularized colorectal cancer patient-derived scaffolds as in vitro pre-clinical 3D model for drug screening. Cancers. 2020;12(3):681.

147. Skardal A, Shupe T, Atala A. Organoid-on-a-chip and body-on-a-chip systems for drug screening and disease modeling. Drug Discov Today. 2016;21(9):1399–411.

148. Knowlton S, Onal S, Yu CH, Zhao JJ, Tasoglu S. Bioprinting for cancer research. Trends Biotechnol. 2015;33(9):504–13.

149. Owens EA, Lee S, Choi J, Henary M, Choi HS. NIR fluorescent small molecules for intraoperative imaging. Wiley Interdiscip Rev Nanomed Nanobiotechnol. 2015;7(6):828–38.

150. Fonnes T, Strand E, Fasmer KE, Berg HF, Espedal H, Sortland K, et al. Near-infrared fluorescent imaging for monitoring of treatment response in endometrial carcinoma patient-derived xenograft models. Cancers. 2020;12(2):370.

151. Kleinmanns K, Bischof K, Anandan S, Popa M, Akslen LA, Fosse V, et al. CD24-targeted fluorescence imaging in patient-derived xenograft models of high-grade serous ovarian carcinoma. EBioMedicine. 2020.

152. Joshi BP, Wang TD. Targeted optical imaging agents in cancer: focus on clinical applications. Contrast Media Mol Imaging. 2018;2018:2015237.

153. Hernot S, van Manen L, Debie P, Mieog JSD, Vahrmeijer AL. Latest developments in molecular tracers for fluorescence image-guided cancer surgery. Lancet Oncol. 2019;20(7):e354–e67.

154. Hekman MCH, Boerman OC, Bos DL, Massuger L, Weil S, Grasso L, et al. Improved intraoperative detection of ovarian cancer by folate receptor alpha targeted dual-modality imaging. Mol Pharm. 2017;14(10):3457–63.

155. Mahalingam SM, Kularatne SA, Myers CH, Gagare P, Norshi M, Liu X, et al. Evaluation of novel tumor-targeted near-infrared probe for fluorescence-guided surgery of cancer. J Med Chem. 2018;61(21):9637–46.

156. Song J, Zhang N, Zhang L, Yi H, Liu Y, Li Y, et al. IR780-loaded folate-targeted nanoparticles for near-infrared fluorescence image-guided surgery and photothermal therapy in ovarian cancer. Int J Nanomedicine. 2019;14:2757.

157. Hoogstins CE, Tummers QR, Gaarenstroom KN, de Kroon CD, Trimbos JB, Bosse T, et al. A novel tumor-specific agent for intraoperative near-infrared fluorescence imaging: a translational study in healthy volunteers and patients with ovarian cancer. Clin Cancer Res. 2016;22(12):2929–38.

158. Kleinmanns K, Fosse V, Bjørge L, McCormack E. The emerging role of CD24 in cancer theranostics—a novel target for fluorescence image-guided surgery in ovarian cancer and beyond. J Pers Med. 2020;10(4):255.

159. Lee J-H, Kim S-H, Lee E-S, Kim Y-S. CD24 overexpression in cancer development and progression: a meta-analysis. Oncol Rep. 2009;22(5):1149–56.

160. Davidson B. CD24 is highly useful in differentiating high-grade serous carcinoma from benign and malignant mesothelial cells. Hum Pathol. 2016;58:123–7.

161. Went PT, Lugli A, Meier S, Bundi M, Mirlacher M, Sauter G, et al. Frequent EpCam protein expression in human carcinomas. Hum Pathol. 2004;35(1):122–8.

162. van Driel PB, Boonstra MC, Prevoo HA, van de Giessen M, Snoeks TJ, Tummers QR, et al. EpCAM as multi-tumour target for near-infrared fluorescence guided surgery. BMC Cancer. 2016;16(1):884.

163. Pan R, Hogdal LJ, Benito JM, Bucci D, Han L, Borthakur G, et al. Selective BCL-2 inhibition by ABT-199 causes on-target cell death in acute myeloid leukemia. Cancer Discov. 2014;4(3):362–75.

164. McCormack E, Mujić M, Osdal T, Bruserud Ø, Gjertsen BT. Multiplexed mAbs: a new strategy in preclinical time-domain imaging of acute myeloid leukemia. Blood J Am Soc Hematol. 2013;121(7):e34–42.

165. Abadjian M-CZ, Edwards WB, Anderson CJ. Imaging the tumor microenvironment. In: Tumor immune microenvironment in cancer progression and cancer therapy. Springer; 2017. p. 229–57.

166. Apte S, Chin FT, Graves EE. Molecular imaging of hypoxia: strategies for probe design and application. Curr Org Synth. 2011;8(4):593–603.

167. Nakazawa MS, Keith B, Simon MC. Oxygen availability and metabolic adaptations. Nat Rev Cancer. 2016;16(10):663–73.

168. Corbet C, Feron O. Tumour acidosis: from the passenger to the driver's seat. Nat Rev Cancer. 2017;17(10):577–93.

169. Kobayashi H, Choyke PL. Target-cancer-cell-specific activatable fluorescence imaging probes: rational design and in vivo applications. Accounts Chem Res. 2011;44(2):83–90.

170. Olson MT, Ly QP, Mohs AM. Fluorescence guidance in surgical oncology: challenges, opportunities, and translation. Mol Imaging Biol. 2019;21(2):200–18.

171. Urano Y, Sakabe M, Kosaka N, Ogawa M, Mitsunaga M, Asanuma D, et al. Rapid cancer detection by topically spraying a γ-glutamyltranspeptidase–activated fluorescent probe. Sci Transl Med 2011;3(110):110ra9-ra9.

172. Obara R, Kamiya M, Tanaka Y, Abe A, Kojima R, Kawaguchi T, et al. γ-Glutamyltranspeptidase (GGT)-activatable fluorescence probe for durable tumor imaging. Angew Chem. 2020.

173. Alam IS, Steinberg I, Vermesh O, van den Berg NS, Rosenthal EL, van Dam GM, et al. Emerging intraoperative imaging modalities to improve surgical precision. Mol Imaging Biol. 2018;20(5):705–15.

174. Haldorsen IS, Popa M, Fonnes T, Brekke N, Kopperud R, Visser NC, et al. Multimodal imaging of orthotopic mouse model of endometrial carcinoma. PLoS One. 2015;10(8):e0135220.

175. McKinley ET, Smith RA, Zhao P, Fu A, Saleh SA, Uddin MI, et al. 3′-deoxy-3′-18F-fluorothymidine PET predicts response to V600EBRAF-targeted therapy in preclinical models of colorectal cancer. J Nucl Med. 2013;54(3):424–30.

176. Valtorta S, Moro M, Prisinzano G, Bertolini G, Tortoreto M, Raccagni I, et al. Metabolic evaluation of non–small cell lung cancer patient–derived xenograft models using 18F-FDG PET: a potential tool for early therapy response. J Nucl Med. 2017;58(1):42–7.

177. Pastorino U, Landoni C, Marchianò A, Calabrò E, Sozzi G, Miceli R, et al. Fluorodeoxyglucose uptake measured by positron emission tomography and standardized uptake value predicts long-term survival of CT screening detected lung cancer in heavy smokers. J Thorac Oncol. 2009;4(11):1352–6.

178. Wolf G, Abolmaali N. Preclinical molecular imaging using PET and MRI. Mol Imaging Oncol. 2013:257–310.

179. Heo GS, Detering L, Luehmann HP, Primeau T, Lee Y-S, Laforest R, et al. Folate receptor α-targeted 89Zr-M9346A Immuno-PET for image-guided intervention with Mirvetuximab Soravtansine in triple-negative breast cancer. Mol Pharm. 2019;16(9):3996–4006.

180. Truillet C, Oh HLJ, Yeo SP, Lee C-Y, Huynh LT, Wei J, et al. Imaging PD-L1 expression with ImmunoPET. Bioconjug Chem. 2018;29(1):96–103.

181. de Vries NL, Mahfouz A, Koning F, de Miranda N. Unraveling the complexity of the cancer microenvironment with multidimensional genomic and cytometric technologies. Front Oncol. 2020;10:1254.

182. Bandura DR, Baranov VI, Ornatsky OI, Antonov A, Kinach R, Lou X, et al. Mass cytometry: technique for real time single cell multitarget immunoassay based on inductively coupled plasma time-of-flight mass spectrometry. Anal Chem. 2009;81(16):6813–22.

183. Hartmann FJ, Bendall SC. Immune monitoring using mass cytometry and related high-dimensional imaging approaches. Nat Rev Rheumatol. 2020;16(2):87–99.

184. Giesen C, Wang HA, Schapiro D, Zivanovic N, Jacobs A, Hattendorf B, et al. Highly multiplexed imaging of tumor tissues with subcellular resolution by mass cytometry. Nat Methods. 2014;11(4):417–22.

185. Baharlou H, Canete NP, Cunningham AL, Harman AN, Patrick E. Mass cytometry imaging for the study of human diseases—applications and data analysis strategies. Front Immunol. 2019;10.

186. Aldridge S, Teichmann SA. Single cell transcriptomics comes of age. Nat Commun 2020;11(1):1–4.

187. Eberwine J, Yeh H, Miyashiro K, Cao Y, Nair S, Finnell R, et al. Analysis of gene expression in single live neurons. Proc Natl Acad Sci. 1992;89(7):3010–4.

188. Svensson V, Vento-Tormo R, Teichmann SA. Exponential scaling of single-cell RNA-seq in the past decade. Nat Protoc. 2018;13(4):599–604.

189. Qian J, Olbrecht S, Boeckx B, Vos H, Laoui D, Etlioglu E, et al. A Pan-cancer blueprint of the heterogeneous tumour microenvironment revealed by single-cell profiling. bioRxiv. 2020.

190. Yu VW, Yusuf RZ, Oki T, Wu J, Saez B, Wang X, et al. Epigenetic memory underlies cell-autonomous heterogeneous behavior of hematopoietic stem cells. Cell. 2017;168(5):944.

Use of Imaging Mass Cytometry in Studies of the Tissue Microenvironment

Ida Herdlevær, Lucia Lisa Petrilli, Fatime Qosaj,
Maria Vinci, Dario Bressan, and Sonia Gavasso

Abstract

Techniques for analysis of tissues, such as immunofluorescence, immunohistochemistry and flow cytometry-based approaches for analysis of cell suspensions, have allowed the characterization of single cells within heterogeneous cell populations. However, the limitations in the number of parameters that can be simultaneously assessed have hampered advances in understanding complex tissue systems. The advent of single-cell mass cytometry, cytometry by time of flight (CyTOF), which uses metal-tagged antibodies, has made it possible to overcome these constraints as CyTOF allows the detection of a large number of cell markers in parallel. A more recently developed technique, imaging mass cytometry (IMC), has pushed the boundaries even further. By combining the transformational power of mass spectrometry with tissue-based approaches, the IMC allows for high-dimensional analysis of tissues with spatial resolution. However, different challenges must be faced to fully exploit the capabilities of IMC. Here, we provide an overview of IMC, covering the basic principles of the technology, the types of tissues used, marker selection, and antibody panel design. This technical discussion is followed by specific examples of applications of IMC to breast cancer tissues, paediatric brain tumours, and paraneoplastic cerebellar degeneration with a focus on our own research. Computational tools used to analyze the resulting multi-parametric data are also addressed.

Take-Home Lessons

- Imaging mass cytometry (IMC) combines traditional immunohistochemistry with laser ablation and mass cytometry (CyTOF); to enable the detection of up to 40 markers simultaneously.
- The multiplexing capabilities of IMC are made possible by replacing the detection system commonly employed in fluorescence assays or brightfield IHC with stable metal isotope reporters. Metals are conjugated to the antibodies of interest by means of metal-chelating polymer chains.
- Comprehensively capturing and understanding the heterogeneity of tissue microenvironments reaches far beyond the molecular and cellular diversity, requiring the 'architectural' design of tissues to also be profiled.
- IMC feasibly and practically permits a comprehensive and rich examination of breast tumours by first, preserving the tissue architecture, and second, capturing a wide array of biologically relevant markers; this, coupled to genomic and transcriptomic profiles presents a powerful approach for studying breast tumours.

Ida Herdlevær, Lucia Lisa Petrilli, Fatime Qosaj, Maria Vinci, Dario Bressan and Sonia Gavasso contributed equally with all other contributors.

I. Herdlevær · S. Gavasso (✉)
Department of Neurology, Haukeland University Hospital, Bergen, Norway

Department of Clinical Medicine, University of Bergen, Bergen, Norway

Neuro-SysMed, Department of Neurology, Haukeland University Hospital, Bergen, Norway
e-mail: ida.viktoria.herdlever@helse-bergen.no;
sonia.gavasso@helse-bergen.no

L. L. Petrilli · M. Vinci
Department of Onco-Haematology, Gene and Cell Therapy, Bambino Gesù Children's Hospital-IRCCS, Rome, Italy
e-mail: lucialisa.petrilli@opbg.net; maria.vinci@opbg.net

F. Qosaj · D. Bressan
CRUK Cambridge Institute, University of Cambridge, Li Ka Shing Centre, Cambridge, UK
e-mail: Fatime.Qosaj@cruk.cam.ac.uk;
Dario.Bressan@cruk.cam.ac.uk

© The Author(s), under exclusive license to Springer Nature Switzerland AG 2022
L. A. Akslen, R. S. Watnick (eds.), *Biomarkers of the Tumor Microenvironment*, https://doi.org/10.1007/978-3-030-98950-7_20

- Paediatric high-grade gliomas (pHGG) are very heterogeneous brain tumours affecting children and young adults for which only tiny biopsies are available. The understanding of the cell actors involved in the tumour network and the decoding of the molecular mechanisms existing between them, is critical for the identification of specific biomarkers useful for better patient stratification, as well as for the discovery of new molecular targets that could lead to the development of innovative therapeutic strategies. Such challenging goals can be achieved by exploiting the potential of the IMC approach that, by analyzing tumour tissue sections in situ, at single-cell level, allows the dissection of tumour heterogeneity with sub-cellular resolution.
- IMC can be used to study immune cells in different brain regions from patients with the neurodegenerative disease paraneoplastic cerebellar degeneration (PCD), to unravel the disease mechanisms.

Immunofluorescence and Immunohistochemistry

Immunofluorescence (IF) and immunohistochemistry (IHC) approaches involve the use of antibodies to detect specific antigens such as proteins and their modifications within tissues. The primary antibody–antigen reaction is visualized directly or indirectly by a label detectable via light microscopy. A direct approach entails a single labelling protocol step in which the primary antibody is labelled, whilst the indirect approach is a multi-step process in which the label antibody is the secondary antibody. In both methods, the use of different fluorescent dyes facilitates the detection of multiple antigens within a given tissue sample.

Fluorescence-based IHC was first described in 1941, when Albert Coons and colleagues used a fluorophore-conjugated antibody to localize bacteria in infected tissue [1, 2]. Though a popular approach, the method had drawbacks. First, some tissues were prone to autofluorescence, and, second, the fluorescent staining fades with time. Thus, alternative approaches were developed. In the 1960s, a method for labelling antibodies with the enzyme peroxidase was developed precluding the need to attach fluorophores to the primary or secondary antibody. The reaction product was detected with 3,3′-diaminobenzidine and hydrogen peroxide. A brown coloured precipitate was formed at the reaction site and nickel salt could be added to produce different-coloured reaction products, allowing for labelling of multiple antigens. Investigators later succeeded in developing the peroxidase anti-peroxidase (PAP) technique. In this approach, the

tissue is first incubated with a primary antibody, followed by a secondary antibody, and completed with the enzyme-labelled PAP antibody. This and the alkaline phosphatase-anti-alkaline phosphatase complex approaches were the most sensitive methods available up to the 1980s.

Until the 1970s, these techniques were mainly applied for research purposes, but the clinical value was becoming apparent, prompting the shift towards using formalin-fixed paraffin-embedded tissues (FFPE) instead of frozen samples. The main advantages of applying IHC or IF to fixed tissues included increased 'shelf life' and better-preserved tissue morphology [3]. By the 1980s, immunoperoxidase staining of fixed tissues became the preferred method due to higher sensitivity. However, with the advent of more permanent, sensitive, and brighter fluorophores and the development of more powerful confocal microscopes, this changed. Both techniques are now widespread and commonly used to study a wide scope of biological processes including infections, neurodegenerative disorders, brain trauma, and tumour pathology.

Although the multiplexing capability of immuno-based staining is steadily growing as a result of technical advancements and the increasing repertoire of fluorophores, the physical overlap of the emission spectra of fluorescent dyes greatly limits the number of targets that can be measured simultaneously. Understanding complex tissue biology requires a high-resolution view, cell by cell, which necessitates single-cell multiplexed imaging technologies [4–6].

The Emergence of Imaging Mass Cytometry

Since its introduction in 2009, single-cell mass cytometry (CyTOF) has become a powerful, widely used technique enabling the simultaneous detection of around 40 cellular targets within heterogeneous samples in suspension [7]. Multiplexed antibody labelling is made possible by replacing fluorescent probes commonly employed in fluorescence assays with stable metal isotope reporters. Metals, primarily from the lanthanide series, are conjugated to the antibodies of interest by means of metal-chelating polymer chains [7–9]. The non-overlapping atomic masses of these metals and their isotopes allow, in theory, for simultaneous detection of over 100 antibodies co-labelled in a single cell [8, 10]. The heavy isotopes used are rare metals not naturally found in biological samples, thus almost completely removing the background signal and mitigating concerns commonly associated with fluorescent probes and autofluorescence, which affect antibody detection and quantification [11, 12].

Once stained with a panel of metal-labelled antibodies, cells in suspension are nebulized into single droplets and injected into the mass cytometer. Upon atomization and ionization in the inductively coupled plasma, the cloud of elemental ions passes through a quadrupole where high-abundance low-mass elements are removed and the remaining high-mass metal tags are detected and quantified in the time-of-flight (TOF) mass spectrometer. The data is then computationally formatted into single-cell standard flow cytometry (FCS) files [7–9, 13].

Single-cell mass cytometry, like flow cytometry, requires cells to be in suspension for analysis. Therefore, tissues must be dissociated into single cells by mechanical and/or enzymatic methods that may lead to skewed tissue cell type composition and phenotypes. In addition to the risk of losing cell types of interest that may be more sensitive to the selected dissociation protocol or the over-representation of some cell types, the protocols can lead to loss of epitopes for both cell-surface and intracellular features of interest [4]. Despite these issues, the in-depth profiling of single cells within heterogeneous samples such as blood or dissociated tissues, such as tumours, with single-cell resolution has revolutionized the exploration of systems biology and its complexity.

Suspension mass cytometry lacks spatial resolution, a key factor for understanding tissue biology, as cell location and interactions among cells are of crucial importance. In 2014, imaging mass cytometry (IMC), a new imaging method that extended the multiplex capabilities of CyTOF to tissue analysis, was introduced [14]. IMC enables the analysis of adherent cells and tissue sections with subcellular resolution (500–1000 nm) by coupling mass cytometry with IHC and laser ablation. Tissue processing in IMC is similar to conventional IHC and can be performed on frozen or formalin-fixed tissues [14–16]. Like suspension mass cytometry, the antibodies are conjugated to metal tags, and currently, 37 metal tags are available for multiplexing. The noteworthy problem of tissue autofluorescence when working with FFPE or postmortem tissues is circumvented in IMC [17].

In IMC, tissue sections are stained with the metal-labelled antibody cocktail. In the Hyperion Imaging system, the stained tissue slides are then ablated by a fixed laser, 1 μm spot per pulse, while the tissue is moved to the next spot with predetermined coordinates. Each ablated tissue spot forms a plume, a cloud that contains tissue and metal-tagged antibodies bound to their epitopes. Every plume, spot by spot, is introduced into the Helios mass cytometer, and the metal tags are detected using CyTOF technology (Fig. 20.1). The digitized data output files used to generate images.

IMC provides the possibility of monitoring surface antigens to identify cell phenotypes, intracellular proteins and their modifications to analyze signalling pathways, cell viability features and enzymatic activity reporters. The cell nuclei are identified by DNA intercalator and/or antibodies against histone. An additional layer can be added by measuring mRNA [18]. Of note, agents used in medical treatments such as some forms of cisplatin in cancer and gadolinium in brain imaging can be detected in cells if their masses are within the atomic mass range of the mass spectrometer (75–209 kDa). The detection of therapeutic agents can be leveraged to study their distribution within tissues [14, 19]. If not expected, these agents cause erratic results illustrating the importance of patient history.

A Practical Guide: IMC Panel Curation, Validation, and Optimization Pipeline

IMC is a powerful tool and has great potential in basic mechanistic research and pathology. Similar to mass and flow cytometry approaches, antibody panel design is a challenge, and curation, validation, and optimization of antibodies are crucial [20]. This is particularly true for non-human tissue as the current repertoire of commercially available, fully validated metal-labelled antibodies is largely limited to human targets. Here, we outline a workflow that can be used to facilitate robust and thorough curation of an IMC antibody panel that is applicable across various tissue types and processing methods.

Tissue Samples

FFPE tissue sections, tissue cryosections, or cells immobilized on glass slides can be stained for IMC, following protocols similar to those used for IHC or IF [21]. FFPE processing is the standard method for archiving tissues in most clinical settings. Any patient-derived tissue, including surgical specimens and autopsy tissue samples, even stored for several years, can be analyzed by IMC. Thus, IMC can be used to carry out retrospective studies on historical patient sample cohorts. Moreover, this technology is particularly powerful in cases where a lot of information needs to be collected on tiny and rare biopsy samples.

The IMC protocol requires the selection of specific regions of interest (ROIs); this is often done with the guidance of a pathologist. When selecting tissue areas to be analyzed, time and cost issues must be considered. The pathologist will carefully evaluate tissue (often stained with haematoxylin and eosin (H&E)) under a microscope and identify ROIs (e.g. neoplastic areas, heterogeneous areas, infiltrating cell aggregates) or regions to avoid (e.g. necrotic areas), thus allowing the IMC analysis to be tailored to a research question or be exploratory in nature. It is important to consider which tissue sections will be used for H&E staining and pathology annotation, if this is performed. H&E staining is known to reduce the ability of a tissue to be stained with metal-conjugated antibodies, unless the stain is removed. For this purpose, staining and annotation are often performed on serial sections collected from the same FFPE

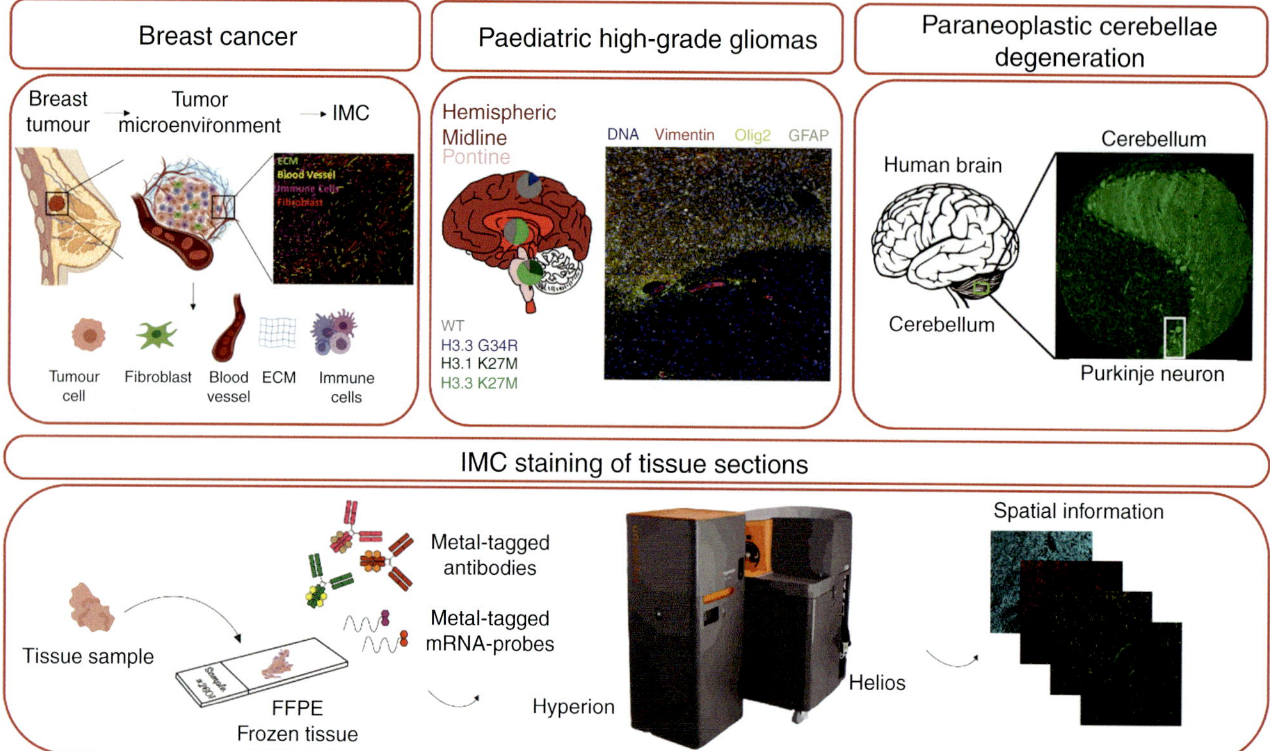

Fig. 20.1 **IMC workflow.** *Top left*: The tumour microenvironment (TME) of breast cancers exhibits prominent tumour heterogeneity. The TME entails a heterogeneous population of both tumour cells and stromal components, the latter containing a plethora of cellular and noncellular constituents including, but not limited to: fibroblasts, blood vessels, extracellular matrix, and immune cells. Within the TME, blood vessels are present and supply surrounding tumour cells with nutrients and oxygen, supporting their continued survival. IMC spatial mapping of a breast tumour derived from a mouse reveals the heterogeneous nature of these various stromal components. *Top middle*: Illustration of human brain depicting the different locations and the histone driver mutations characteristic of paediatric high-grade glioma (pHGG). A representative image of a diffuse intrinsic pontine glioma (DIPG) autopsy tissue section obtained by IMC displays the expression of Vimentin (red), Olig2 (yellow) and GFAP (green), and cell nuclei in blue. *Top right*: Illustration of the human brain and a tissue section of the cerebellum obtained by IMC. Purkinje neurons (green), fan-shaped cells in the cerebellum (green), are lost in patients with paraneoplastic cerebellar degeneration. *Bottom left:* Tissue slides, with FFPE- or cryotissue sections, are stained with a cocktail of metal-tagged antibodies commercially available or custom conjugated in-house. *Bottom middle:* Regions of interest (ROI) of the tissue section, selected based on the specific scientific question and with the guidance of a pathologist, are analyzed using the Hyperion Imaging System composed of both the Hyperion imager and the Helios module for cell suspension. After ablation by a laser, the cloud of tissue and isotopes are atomized, ionized and analyzed using the CyTOF mass spectrometer. *Bottom right:* Masses are identified and quantified, and data are integrated with spatial information, generating a high-dimensional image that can be visualized using different tools. High-dimensional data can also be retrieved and exported for further downstream analysis

or frozen block immediately before or after the one undergoing IMC processing, so that the histological features identified by the pathologist are largely conserved in the IMC section.

FFPE sections must be subjected to antigen retrieval steps, as is done for IHC, in order to remove the crosslinks formed by formalin fixation and to make epitopes accessible for antibody binding. Since the antigen retrieval can be performed by boiling tissue in a buffer with a pH ranging from 3 to 10, it is necessary that all the antibodies included in the panel perform well under the same retrieval condition. Antibody incubation time and temperature must be optimized to ensure proper antibody binding. In recent publications, two sequential stainings, one at room temperature for 5 h and the other at 4 °C overnight, were successfully used to capture optimal working conditions for two sets of antibodies [22].

Features and Probes

IMC is a biased platform and requires that the user defines the plethora of cell features to be spatially mapped through a rigorous selection process to ensure that the panel of epitopes analyzed meets the biological goals and to facilitate effective analysis of the resulting spatial maps. Selecting features can be demanding, especially if the pathway or process to be probed lacks known markers. In addition to the literature, it is advised to peruse molecular data such as transcriptomic and proteomic profiles. For example, the molecular fingerprints of perturbed cells subjected to single-cell transcriptomics can be utilized to guide the selection of a set of markers that enable direct and comprehensive elucidation of relevant targets in situ. Specific microglia markers, for example, were identified through a comprehensive transcriptomic study that led to the discovery of proteins such as P2Y12 that were able to distinguish microglia from macrophages [23].

Once a set of features of interest are defined, the subsequent step in the pipeline is to carefully select appropriate antibody clones. The hefty price of antibodies and the time required for validating them reinforces the need for a strict selection process. Clonality encompasses the first consideration. Monoclonal antibodies exhibit greater specificity than polyclonal antibodies. Polyclonal antibodies target numerous epitopes and generally have higher affinity, but are inherently more prone to nonspecific binding [24]. The artifacts that may result from use of polyclonal antibodies must be carefully accounted for in downstream analysis; therefore, monoclonal antibodies are preferred over polyclonal types. The second consideration is the buffer used for the storage of the antibody. Ideally, the buffer should be carrier-free (i.e. without bovine serum albumin (BSA) and glycerol). Glycerol primarily interferes with concentration measurements of the final conjugated product, whereas BSA may directly impede the conjugation, greatly reducing the product yield. In many cases, BSA in up to 0.1% of the original antibody formulation, is tolerated. Echoing common practice in standard IHC methods, the selected antibody should be tested on similarly processed samples (i.e. FFPE or frozen) with an additional consideration of the optimal epitope unmasking method. With the recent advent of in situ technologies it is recommended to choose antibodies that have been validated using the same antigen retrieval method required for the test samples. Using metal-conjugated antibodies allows analysis over a year after the staining procedure due to the high stability, based on our own observations. A plethora of commercially available metal-tagged IMC antibodies are currently commercially available. The list of available antibodies is constantly increasing, with many coupled to different metals to further facilitate the customization of panels. However, if the antibody of interest is not available in a metal-tagged format, the primary antibody can be purchased from any other vendor and conjugated in-house. Conjugation can be performed in less than 5 h using conjugation kits sold by Fluidigm that include the metal of choice and a polymer that allows metal–antibody binding. In some cases, other metals (different from the ones supplied by Fluidigm) can be conjugated to the polymer. Metal with divalent ionic forms are working best

for this (personal communication, Bodenmiller Laboratory). However, this non-canonical conjugation should be tried with great caution as there is a risk of producing antibodies bearing too much metal, which could damage the mass cytometer's detectors.

Metal–Antibody Pairing

The IMC platform outperforms fluorophore-based in situ methods in terms of the number of features that can be probed simultaneously, whilst largely mitigating the crosstalk between channels. Though IMC is devoid of physical overlap of the emission spectra, which is an issue with fluorescent dyes, predictable spillover between the lanthanide metals does occur and can be avoided through careful panel design and antibody titration and/or downstream compensation [25, 26]. Titration and validation strategies will identify potential issues caused by mass impurities of isotopes of the same metal used in the same panel and by abundance sensitivity in the m+/−1 channel and unspecific binding issue [7, 20, 27–29]. A compensation algorithm can computationally correct spillover signals and is applicable to both suspension mass cytometry and IMC. However, removing signals due to nonspecific binding remains a challenge. Handling of spillovers post acquisition improves the flexibility of antibody-metal pairing, increases the data quality, and streamlines the panel development pipeline. In longitudinal clinical samples, for example from patients undergoing cancer treatments, many features and expression levels may be affected and unexpected spillover issues may occur that can be resolved by compensation for the signal after data acquisition by acquiring a compensation matrix or using ad hoc-developed R packages [25].

Although metals used in IMC are naturally rare, and therefore not present in commonly used laboratory reagents, it is important to avoid external contaminants arising from common sources of heavy metals such as glass or metal-containing solutions. Therefore, the use of plastic equipment is preferred in all steps of the protocol and when preparing the instrument for sample acquisition.

Antibody Validation

Appropriate antibody validation ensures that the conjugation process successfully labels each antibody without impeding specificity. Ensuring that the labelling protocol preserves this specificity is a multi-step process that commonly starts with an IF staining using the pre-conjugated antibody. The metal conjugated antibody is then tested on the tissue of interest with a fluorescent or metal-tagged secondary antibody by IF or IMC, respectively. Validating the final conjugated product, however, requires more comprehensive approaches.

Tissue microarrays (TMA), consisting of paraffin blocks in which hundreds of separate tissue cores are arranged in a grid, have proven to be immensely powerful resources in IMC analysis as use of the TMA format drastically increases the throughput and efficiency, and reduces batch variabilities. Within a single TMA, replicates of both positive and negative controls can be acquired in a single run, ensuring sample quality and reproducibility.

Spillover is not only grounded in metal crosstalk. In fact, antibodies themselves may be the source of background signal, which, if particularly high, may extend into adjacent channels. This is likely due to nonspecific binding and/or use of a high working concentration. Thus, titration experiments should ideally be performed prior to analysis to prevent this type of signal. One granular approach to address antibody-derived channel crosstalk is to strategically position antibodies in such a way that the source of spillover is easily discernible. For example, one may want to conjugate metals that are detected in adjacent channels to anti-E-cadherin, which targets a membrane-localized protein, and anti-Ki-67, which targets a nuclear-bound protein, rather than two membrane-bound targets. This method is largely reserved for small-scale panels or exhaustive panels that have sets of 'essential' markers. Another clever technique, primarily useful for larger scale panels, is to test the panel for spillovers by leaving m+/−1 channels and channels of the same metal isotopes open. 'Empty' channels that pick up signals are indicative of spillover from neighbouring channels, giving the user a quick yet comprehensive identification of the extent and source of channel bleed-through.

Applications of IMC

The ability to provide a system-level analysis of a complex biological niche is now possible with IMC. In the following sections, we will describe how we have applied IMC in our own work with discussions of issues faced. We start with breast cancer, which in recent years has become a hot topic in the IMC field, as exemplified by the wealth of research covered in this chapter in addition to ours. IMC has been employed to study tumour heterogeneity and, coupled with various 'omics' approaches, has facilitated a rich, comprehensive, and highly multiplexed interrogation of the dynamic tumour microenvironment. IMC has also helped illuminate poorly studied biological processes, such as vascular mimicry.

The application of IMC to paediatric high-grade gliomas (pHGG) is also presented. pHGGs are very heterogeneous brain tumours affecting children and young adults for which only tiny biopsies are available. Using IMC, these precious samples can now be fully explored. IMC experiments have revealed features of the microenvironments of these tumours

and may lead to the discovery of new targets and biomarkers of clinical relevance.

The final project discussed involves the study of microglia in paraneoplastic cerebellar degeneration (PCD). Microglia are the resident immune cells of the central nervous system, show high heterogeneity throughout the brain, and change phenotypic character upon activation [30]. We have studied PCD post-mortem brain tissue sections by IMC to allow for high-dimensional phenotyping of microglia and to distinguish them from infiltrating macrophages.

Spatial Mapping of the Breast Cancer Tumour Microenvironment with IMC

The tumour microenvironment (TME) is an intricate and complex niche system in which tumour cells and the cellular and noncellular components of the stromal compartment coexist and interact. The TME encompasses all non-neoplastic constituents of a tumour including fibroblasts, endothelial cells, and the extracellular matrix [31]. There is a significant degree of heterogeneity across patient tumours and within an individual tumour [32]. In primary tumours, this heterogeneity may present spatially with numerous anatomically distinct, molecularly unique cellular populations or as a 'ubiquitous' set of driver mutations with a differential distribution of additional somatic alterations [33]. Heterogeneity is driven by the continuous exposure of the TME to intrinsic signalling and/or external perturbations that can induce dynamic remodelling of the tumour landscape [31, 34, 35]. The impact of molecular, phenotypic and histological diversification across the tumour topography has clinical relevance [36–40], highlighting the need for a better understanding of the 'ecological' context of the tumour and its impact on therapeutic response.

In pre-invasive, ductal carcinoma in situ breast cancers, histological analysis revealed heterogeneous nuclear grading and differential expression of relevant biomarkers within individual tumours, likely corresponding to the plethora of distinct micro niches present in the TME even at this early stage of tumourigenesis [41]. Dynamic contrast material-enhanced magnetic resonance imaging of locally advanced breast cancers identified three distinct intratumour subregions that were characterized by poor, moderate, or marked perfusion that served as markers indicative of recurrence-free survival [42]. The heterogeneous nature of the vasculature and subsequent perfusion directly reflects the diverse hypoxia patterns exhibited across the tumour [43]. The amalgamation of these studies suggests a fundamental role of tumour heterogeneity in dictating tumour growth, progression, and clinical outcome.

Within the tumultuous TME, tumour cells employ numerous stealthy mechanisms to coerce stromal cells to co-opt 'pro-tumourigenic' activities, which enable tumour cells to wreak havoc, ensure their survival, and facilitate therapeutic evasion [44, 45]. Interaction and 'collaboration' are demonstrated across the broader stromal spectrum. For instance, integrin-expressing tumour-associated macrophages (TAMs) bind breast cancer cells that express the adhesion molecule VCAM1 in the lungs, aiding seeding and metastatic growth in environments enriched with leukocytes [46]. TAMs may also safeguard breast cancer cells from paclitaxel chemotherapy by impeding therapy-induced tumour cell death mediated cathepsins or proteins involved in lysosomal degradation. Co-administration of a cathepsin inhibitor with paclitaxel slowed tumour growth in transgenic mice induced with MMTV-PyMT[1] breast cancer cells. Cancer-associated fibroblasts also play important roles in the TME by remodelling of the extracellular matrix, communicating with both cancer cells and immune cells, and releasing growth factors and cytokines that promote tumour cell activation and survival [47, 48]. The pervasive tumour-promoting role of fibroblasts is reinforced by their response to external perturbations, such as anti-angiogenic therapies, which includes an upregulation of hypoxia-related genes and secreted factors, subsequently obstructing therapy and promoting angiogenesis [49]. It is now clear that stromal cells orchestrate an overwhelming number of 'pro-tumour' responses, underscoring the importance of understanding the granularity of the TME. Many biological features and processes within the TME are topological in nature, such as the distribution of these various stromal cell types across the tumour landscape, their interactions with tumour cells, necessitating the use of state-of-the-art spatial technologies to better understand tumour heterogeneity.

The spatial heterogeneity of the TME has been mapped using a variety of IHC and digital pathology techniques [50]. Though such methods remain crucial for diagnostic and prognostic clinical applications, they do not allow multiplexing and are not amenable to high throughput, prominent drawbacks in in situ protein expression analysis. As the community of researchers is becoming increasingly aware of the complexity of the TME and its imperative role in clinical response, the desire for technologies that capture the molecular fingerprints of individual cells whilst placing them into a spatial context is at an ultimate high.

The structure of the breast tumour ecosystem is largely driven by dynamic interactions between tumour and stromal cells [36, 51, 52]. This was neatly exemplified in an extensive suspension CyTOF study, which utilized an antibody panel primarily targeting the stromal immune repertoire, coupled to transcriptome sequencing to profile human breast cancers across all clinical subtypes [53]. The resulting large-scale, single-cell atlas revealed varying T cell landscapes across different tumour grades, with high-grade tumours dis-

playing a more prominent immunosuppressive environment. A subset of estrogen receptor-positive breast cancer patients, not previously thought to exhibit immunogenicity, displayed distinct immune cell types, prompting speculation that these patients might benefit from immunotherapy.

Though the clinical implications of these single-cell tumour maps are far-reaching, a strong caveat of suspension mass cytometry is the need to dissociate tumours into a single-cell suspension. This technical aspect may induce alterations in surface markers and skew downstream analysis, and, more importantly, obliterates all spatial information, which is needed to illuminate tumour–stroma interactions. The spatial heterogeneity of tumour marker expression in breast cancer biopsies has recently been demonstrated using multiplexed ion beam imaging (MIBI), another platform under the umbrella of spatial proteomics [15, 54]. Though MIBI permits higher resolution imaging than IMC, it lacks the remarkable multiplexing capacity inherent to IMC and is further limited by the matrix required for sample embedding. This further underlines imaging mass cytometry's inherent advantages for the elucidation of tumour ecosystems. This has been demonstrated across numerous studies, which have utilized multiplexed IMC panels to study the TME of breast cancers.

One of the first studies to do so identified cellular phenotypes and TME landscapes across a cohort of 49 human breast tumours [55]. Analysis of IMC images and the corresponding single-cell data facilitated the classification of 20 distinct phenotype clusters, which varied across tumour types. Through the implementation of neighbourhood analysis, communities of interacting cells were identified. For example, proliferative and hypoxic tumour cells were found 'neighbouring' CD68[+] macrophages, likely reflecting of an interactive tumour–stroma organization. Subsequently, analysis of specific cell–cell interactions across tumour histological grades revealed that high-grade tumours exhibit a distinct 'social network' containing hypoxic cells and interacting stromal cells. Although clinical validation was beyond the scope of the work, the study achieved two goals: it provided a proof-of-principle that IMC enables a rich analysis of cellular phenotypes and interactions, whilst highlighting the power of switching between spatial and single-cell data to probe the cellular features and organization of the TME.

Multiplexed spatial mapping has also been utilized to elucidate the immune microenvironment in a cohort of HER2[+] breast cancer patients who relapsed following treatment with trastuzumab, an antibody-based therapeutic that binds the extracellular domain of the HER2 receptor [56, 57]. Previous research had suggested that better outcomes were achieved with a combination of adjuvant chemotherapy and trastuzumab in patients with tumours exhibiting similar levels of HER2 extracellular and intracellular domains, whilst the converse was seen in patients with lower levels of the extracellular domain [58]. These studies, however, primarily

---

[1]MMTV-PyMT = mouse mammary tumour virus-polyoma middle tumour-antigen.

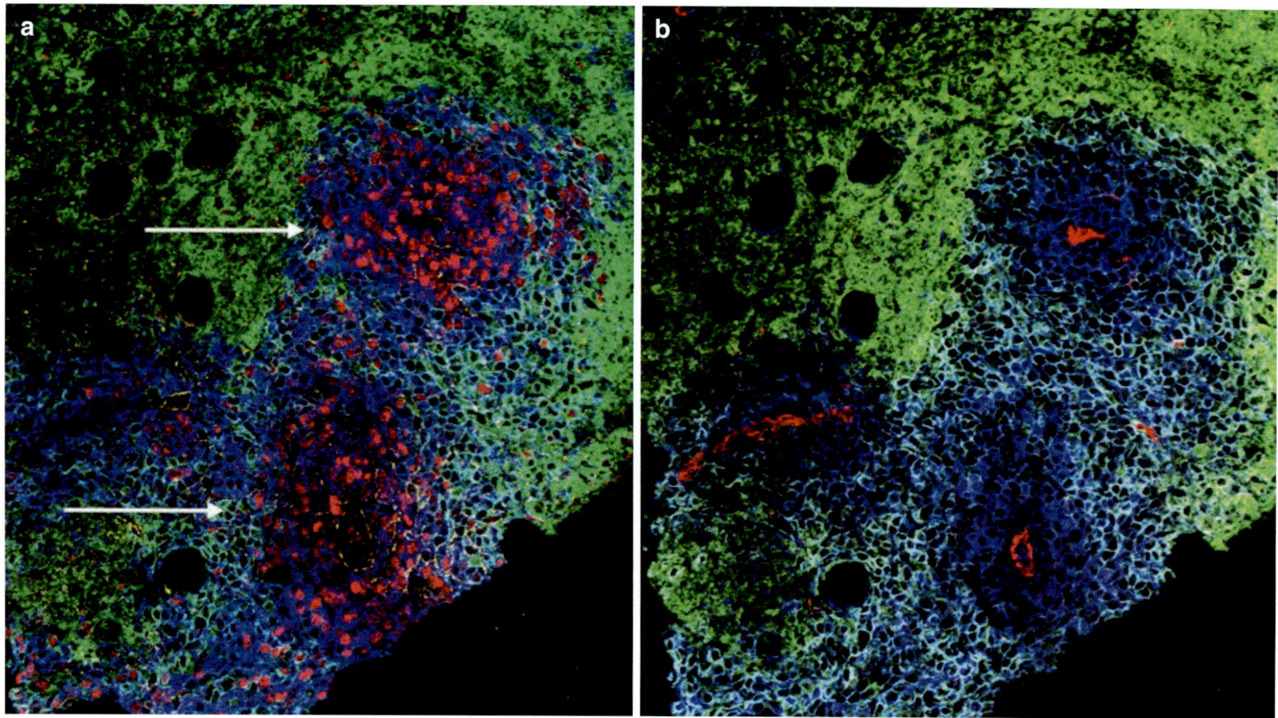

Fig. 20.2 IMC of a mouse-derived TNBC sample reveals features and cell types of the TME. IMC reveals (**a**) 'pockets' of proliferating cells (red; arrows), surrounded by hypoxia (green) and (**b**) heterogeneous morphological features of CD31-expressing blood vessel structures (red), with CD44-positive mesenchymal cells (blue) within close proximity

relied on IF and were therefore limited to very few markers. To address this limitation, an 18-marker IMC antibody panel targeting HER2 signalling was established. This panel was first used to corroborate previous findings before identifying correlations between HER2 domains and other cell types, by targeting related epitopes simultaneously. Tumour cells with relatively higher levels of the extracellular domain were found to be within a closer distance to CD8+ T cells, as compared to those with higher levels of the intracellular domain. In this study, IMC enabled the immune repertoire and cellular communities to be robustly interrogated.

Highly multiplexed IMC spatial profiles, tethered to large volumes of genomic data, have enabled comprehensive analyses of TME heterogeneity across genomically stratified tumour subtypes, by defining the stromal repertoire and characterizing cell–cell interactions [59]. An in-depth analysis of human breast cancer samples from the METABRIC cohort[2] [32], arranged in TMAs, was performed using a 37-plex panel of antibodies that allowed detection of epithelial-derived tumour, stromal, and immune cells of the TME. Genomically unstable basal-like tumours, as well as other subtypes defined by *TP53* mutations, revealed an enrichment of myofibroblasts, T cells, and macrophages and a hypoxia-prone microenvironment, which has previously been shown to be a potential culprit of tumour resistance to anti-angiogenic therapies [60]. Furthermore, tumours with greater genomic instability exhibited a higher percentage of CD68+ fibroblasts, proliferating epithelial cells, and macrophages. An enrichment of fibroblasts impeded immune cell interactions, an observation in agreement with previous research implicating fibroblasts in immune exclusion [61]. This work culminated in the identification and characterization of the TME in breast cancers as a spectrum, each defined by distinct spatial patterns of stromal cells, primarily in reference to the immune repertoire, and which may help rationalize differential responses to immunotherapies.

The spatial diversity of the immune landscape of breast cancers was probed in a separate study using a modified IMC protocol, which simultaneously captured both proteins and transcripts [18]. This analysis showed that cells expressing high levels of the immunomodulator *CXCL10* interact significantly with each other and form local clusters, or niches, within the TME. There is a correlation between the frequency of T cells and cells highly expressing *CXCL10* within the stroma, aligning with the role of CXCL10 as a T cell chemoattractant [18, 62]. Similar 'pockets' of proliferating tumour cells have also been observed in IMC data generated from mouse-derived triple-negative breast cancer (TNBC) tumours (Fig. 20.2A). Integrating genomic data with IMC

---

[2]METABRIC cohort = Molecular Taxonomy of Breast Cancer International Consortium; ten subtypes or integrative clusters of breast cancer identified through an integrated analysis of genomic and transcriptomic data.

revealed characteristic cellular compositions, defined by different patterns of stromal enrichment and cell–cell interactions, across genomically distinct subtypes, underscoring the utility of IMC in study of the heterogeneous TME and the benefit of coalescing IMC with other modalities.

Recently, a 35-plex antibody panel was developed to quantify clinically relevant molecular targets in breast tumours. Analysis of 289 human breast cancers better define the multicellular landscape of the tumours and more thoroughly refine histopathology-based subtypes [63]. Noticeable differences in the expression of clinically relevant markers were observed across different subtypes of breast cancer. For example, a cohort of triple-negative breast cancer (TNBC) tumours were further stratified into subgroups, each characterized by differential marker expression and distinct clinical outcomes; those lacking luminal epithelial markers and expressing higher levels of either hypoxic, proliferative, or basal markers were associated with poor clinical outcome. Neighbourhood analysis, utilized to isolate interacting phenotypes, revealed that both, T cells and proliferative tumour cells neighbour endothelial cells, potentially foreshadowing an intravasation event. IMC also enabled the characterization of the tumour architecture into one of two interaction 'signatures': one in which the tumour and stroma are demarcated and compartmentalized, and the other in which the stroma-tumour interface is heterogeneous and therefore 'interactive'. Among the (TNBC) clusters identified, the stromal environments varied from macrophage to T cell-enriched, while others were predominantly occupied by epithelial cells with very little stroma. Corroborating these findings, Ali et al. demonstrated that communities exhibiting a greater presence of fibroblasts were associated with fewer interacting immune cells, reinforcing their role in suppressing immune response [59].

Although IMC on its own is an immensely powerful technology, a recent study demonstrated the benefits of integrating IMC with its sister technology CyTOF, to further characterize phenotypic heterogeneity in patient-derived tumour xenografts (PDTXs) [64]. Cellular phenotypes previously masked in genomic and transcriptomic analyses were illuminated via mass cytometry, using a panel of 33 breast cancer-related antibodies, including cell type-specific and signalling markers. Analysis of the mass cytometry data revealed 13 Cell-Clusters (CCs), 11 of which were of human epithelial tumour cell origin. IMC was subsequently used to spatially map these CCs in 8 PDTX models, using a panel of 10 antibodies that overlapped with the mass cytometry panel; the datasets revealed a distinct spatial distribution and organization of cell phenotypes within the models.

Spatial heterogeneity encompasses niches characterized by both distinct physiological features and diverse cell types, which are influenced by selective pressures present in the TME including changes in oxygen levels, disruptions to tumour perfusion, induction of an immune response, perturbation of signalling pathways via drug inhibitors, and aberrant pH levels that may lead to systemic acidosis [40]. At the ecosystem level, this includes extreme fluctuations in oxygen supply, especially as solid tumours increase in volume and their cores become hypoxic. Variable hypoxia expression across the TME is driven by several factors: microvessel density, extent of vessel permeability and leakiness, and the metabolic activity of cells within these regions [65]. Irregular tumour blood supply has been attributed to weakened chemotherapy response, and its sporadic nature is exemplified in IMC images of a TNBC mouse tumour (Fig. 20.2B). Capturing the dynamic vasculature and its changes across tumour progression is possible with IMC.

IMC is now being utilized in conjugation with other 'omics' technologies to elucidate a biological phenomenon referred to as vasculogenic mimicry (VM), described as the unique ability of tumour cells to create and physically line blood vessels. Often referred to as 'pseudo' blood vessels, VM networks have been postulated to be functional and therefore perfused with blood and thus may drive metastatic disease [63]. A wealth of evidence suggests that VM networks are present across a multitude of solid cancers, and a recent report linking VM with evasion of anti-angiogenic therapies underscores the clinical relevance of these networks [64]. However, the field generally lacks empirical data which directly demonstrates the biological importance of VM in tumour biology and therapeutic response.

In recent work in our laboratory we have coupled IMC to large-scale single-cell imaging and transcriptomics to capture the dynamic and complex nature of VM-driven tumours, in order to understand how tumour cells 'masquerade' as endothelial cells. The data generated were used to identify important VM-related features and markers, which were subsequently fed back into the IMC panel. Unlike most other spatial proteomics methods, IMC facilitates a comprehensive and robust investigation of the vast TME. Whilst capturing the expression and spatial profiles of VM markers, the multiplexing capabilities of IMC enable components of the stromal repertoire to be simultaneously probed, including endothelial cells and immune cells, both of which are believed to have a role in VM. To our knowledge, this study is the first to approach this mysterious biological phenomenon from an IMC and large-scale, 'omics' perspective.

Collectively, IMC has permitted comprehensive and high-resolution, single-cell stratification of histologically defined breast cancer subtypes, identifying a plethora of cellular phenotypes, the communities they inhabit, their interactions within the TME landscape, and, of utmost importance, the relationships of these features to disease outcome. The application of IMC, in conjunction with other 'omics' technologies is enabling the study of biological pathways and processes that cannot be directly analyzed with other proteomics approaches, underscoring the profound potential of IMC. The work highlighted here exemplifies the direct applicability of IMC to spatially map tumour ecosystems, in breast cancer and beyond, and highlighting the implications of the spatial dimension on therapy outcome.

IMC Offers a New Lens for Studies of Heterogeneity in Paediatric High-Grade Glioma

Among the central nervous system (CNS) neoplasms, paediatric high-grade gliomas (pHGGs) are the most aggressive tumours, accounting for about 10% of all CNS cancers in the paediatric population from 0 to 19 years [66] with an incidence of approximately 1 in 100,000 individuals [66, 67] and a median overall survival of 9–15 months [68]. pHGGs are a diverse group of tumour entities that differ by the age of onset, clinicopathological features, anatomical location of the tumour, and histology and molecular status [69].

pHGGs can occur anywhere in the CNS: about 47% arise in the cerebral hemispheres; approximately 31% occur in the brainstem, with most cases in the pons, and others in the midbrain and medulla; and about 22% are found in midline regions such as thalamus, cerebellum, spinal cord, and ventricles [69]. The pontine tumours have been classically called diffuse intrinsic pontine glioma (DIPG); these tumours are highly diffuse with unique radiological features [70]. Due to their location, not all pHGGs can be surgically removed. In particular, the pontine tumours are inoperable. This has drastically impeded molecular characterization, and only recently, controlled biopsy [71, 72] and autopsy [73–76] protocols have been adopted, allowing the collection of tumour samples and analysis.

The availability of these precious samples has enabled important molecular studies that have contributed to the definition of mutational subgroups in association with the presence of recurrent mutations in genes encoding histone variants [77, 78] such as H3.3 K27M, most strongly associated with midline (59.7%) and brainstem tumours (63%), H3.1/H3.2 K27M associated with pontine tumours (21.4%), and the H3.3 G34R/V arising in a subgroup of the hemispheric pHGG tumours (16.4%) [69]. The H3 K27M mutations are often associated with other driver mutations in genes such as *TP53* and *PPM1D* or *ACVR1* and *PI3KR1* [79, 80]. The H3.3 G34R/V mutations are associated with mutations in *TP53*, *ATRX*, and *PDGFRA* [69]. Moreover, studies that combined DNA sequencing, RNA sequencing, and methylation profiling have further contributed to the identification of additional pHGG subgroups with wild-type histones including *BRAF*-mutant tumours in hemispheric and midline locations, *IDH1*-mutant tumours in the hemispheric location of older children [69], and *ALK, NTRK1-3, ROS1,*

and *MET* gene fusions observed in tumours arising in 0–4 year-old children with good outcomes [81, 82].

The identification of such molecular subgroups has also had an impact on the classification of these tumours by the World Health Organization (WHO), prompting them to introduce a new tumour entity in 2016, the diffuse midline glioma (DMG) H3 K27M. For the first time, this classification takes both the mutation and histological and pathological features into account. It is expected that additional entities will be reviewed by the WHO with an expected shift towards more molecular pathology. From a histological point of view, pHGG presents characteristic features such as hypercellularity, nuclear atypia, and high mitotic activity with or without microvascular proliferation and necrosis. pHGG are classified by the WHO according to a grading of malignancy as either Grade III (anaplastic astrocytoma) or Grade IV (glioblastoma multiforme, GBM), meaning that they are highly malignant tumours [82]. Given the highly heterogeneous nature of pHGG, a clear histological grading cannot always be assigned, with some tumours presenting features of different grades within the same tumour [83–85].

A high degree of intra-tumour heterogeneity is evident at genetic, epigenetic, and phenotypic levels in pHGGs [84, 86–89]. Interestingly, for GBM and DIPG, distinct heterogeneous clones isolated from the same tumour have been shown using co-culture systems and in orthotopic mouse models to work as a functional network, cooperating to result in more aggressive phenotypes [84, 89]. Moreover, single-cell RNA-seq studies have added additional layers of information about the biology of these tumours, in particular their cells of origin and potential therapeutic targets [90, 91].

Recently the CyTOF single-cell approach has been utilized to characterize the phenotypic and functional heterogeneity of glioblastoma stem cells from freshly dissociated tumour specimens and the derived cell cultures [92]. CyTOF has also revealed T cell infiltration in paediatric glioma, which shows this is higher in low-grade glioma than pHGG, though in low-grade glioma T cell infiltration can be variable and depends on specific tumour subtypes [85]. CyTOF was also used to monitor the immune systems of DMG and DIPG patients in a clinical study [93], and, coupled to machine learning, CyTOF single-cell mass cytometry can stratify GBM patient survival [94].

CyTOF analyses of single-cell suspensions cannot provide spatial-topographical information. This element, together with a comprehensive picture of cell type composition and relationships, is provided by IMC. The multiplexing power of IMC will more finely elucidate the cell–cell interactions taking place between different cell populations coexisting within the same tumour [84, 87] as well as between glioma cells and other elements of the TME such as, for example, the neuronal cells [95, 96].

The application of IMC can be particularly useful for the analysis of precious biopsy tissue samples, in particular for the brainstem tumours, for which often little material is available for diagnostic purposes. Our lab is applying the IMC to pHGG tissue samples collected from different areas of the same tumour and/or at different time points during the course of the disease. By doing so, we are able to map these tumours through space and time. We collaborate with a neuropathologist to select ROIs on FFPE tissue slices, for the identification of neoplastic areas and exclusion of necrotic spots (Fig. 20.3A). We have established IMC protocols for pHGG tissue samples for a number of metal-tag antibodies that recognize, among other epitopes, structural elements of the brain TME such as collagen-I (for identification of components of the extracellular matrix), CD31 and α-SMA (for identification of vascular structures), and Ki-67 (for identification of proliferating cells). Interestingly, in the example shown in Fig. 20.3B, Ki-67 is expressed only in one area of the selected ROI, even though the entire area is neoplastic, confirming the heterogeneous nature of these tumours.

The most challenging part of applying IMC to the study of brain tumour tissues is the need to build a unique panel of metal-tagged antibodies that, in addition to common phenotypic markers for which commercially antibodies are already available, also includes custom conjugated antibodies to identify specific pHGG tumour features, such as the expression of mutant histone proteins (H3 K27M and H3.3 G34R) and the loss of the trimethylation on H3 K27. These diagnostic markers for specific pHGG subgroups are utilized in routine histopathological assessment of FFPE tissue samples. Thus, we are working on the validation of custom-conjugated antibodies that can be used in IMC to specifically identify these unique pHGG features.

IMC Enables the Investigation of Functions of Microglia in Paraneoplastic Cerebellar Degeneration

Paraneoplastic neurologic syndromes are rare immune-mediated, neurodegenerative diseases characterized by the presence of onconeural antibodies directed against antigens expressed ectopically by cancer cells and endogenously by neurons [97]. PCD is one of the most common paraneoplastic neurologic syndromes. Patients with PCD develop severe cerebellar ataxia. Diagnosis is supported by the detection of onconeural antibodies in serum and cerebrospinal fluid [98]. The most frequently detected PCD-associated antibody is anti-Yo, and it is most commonly associated with gynaecological or breast cancers [99, 100]. Anti-Yo binds to the cerebellar degeneration-related antigens CDR2 and CDR2L, localized in the cell nucleus and cytoplasm, respectively, in cerebellar Purkinje neurons [101]. This binding causes neu-

ronal dysfunction and Purkinje neuron death and leads to gradual loss of motor control in PCD patients [102, 103]. As with many other paraneoplastic syndromes, the role of immune cells in PCD pathogenesis is not well established. The extensive loss of Purkinje neurons observed in PCD patients is thought to be caused by parenchymal infiltration of cytotoxic CD8+ T cells, microglia activation, and a direct damaging effect of Yo antibodies [103–105]. Production of antibodies and activation of cytotoxic T cells against onco-neuronal antigens expressed in the associated gynaecological cancer is a common finding and a prerequisite for the immune response [104, 106, 107].

Microglia are the resident immune cells of the central nervous system and are involved in host defence mechanisms against pathogens and in homeostasis during development, adulthood, and ageing [108]. Microglia perform three essential functions: sensing environmental changes, physiological housekeeping that promotes normal operations, and defence against modified-self and harmful non-self-agents [108]. Microglia cell numbers, activation state, subcellular structures, and localization vary depending on the anatomical region. IHC results obtained from mouse brains show higher microglia density in the hippocampus, olfactory bulb, basal ganglia, and substantia nigra and lower density in the fibre tracts, cerebellum, and brainstem [109, 110]. As the phenotypic changes in rodent models are not detected in humans, Böttcher et al. performed a study of human microglia heterogeneity and phenotypic characteristics using multiplexed single-cell mass cytometry [30]. Use of two panels consisting of 32 and 35 markers allowed for high-dimensional immune phenotyping of microglia and peripheral immune cells from different brain regions, blood, and cerebrospinal fluid from several donors. Eight phenotypic markers were found to be important when distinguishing microglia subsets: CD11c, CD206, CD45, CD64, CD68, CX3CR1, HLA-DR, and IRF8 [30]. Despite the low microglia density in the cerebellum, these cells are involved in regulating the survival of Purkinje neurons and have a high sensitivity to homeostatic disruption during cerebral disease or injury [111, 112]. Microglia undergo large changes in gene expression during ageing [113], and cerebellar microglia have been found to be more sensitive to ageing than microglia in other brain regions [114]. Still, microglia dynamics in the cerebellum and its role in PCD pathogenesis is largely unknown.

IHC and IF are suitable methods to study the tissue morphology and expression of a limited number of markers simultaneously. Thus, we performed a pilot project including the most commonly used microglia markers, CD11c, HLA-DR, and IBA-1. Despite gaining new and insightful information regarding the localization of microglia in various brain tissues from PCD patients, it was difficult to study the function and effect of these cells on pathogenesis in part due to the fact that microglia and immune cells, such as mac-

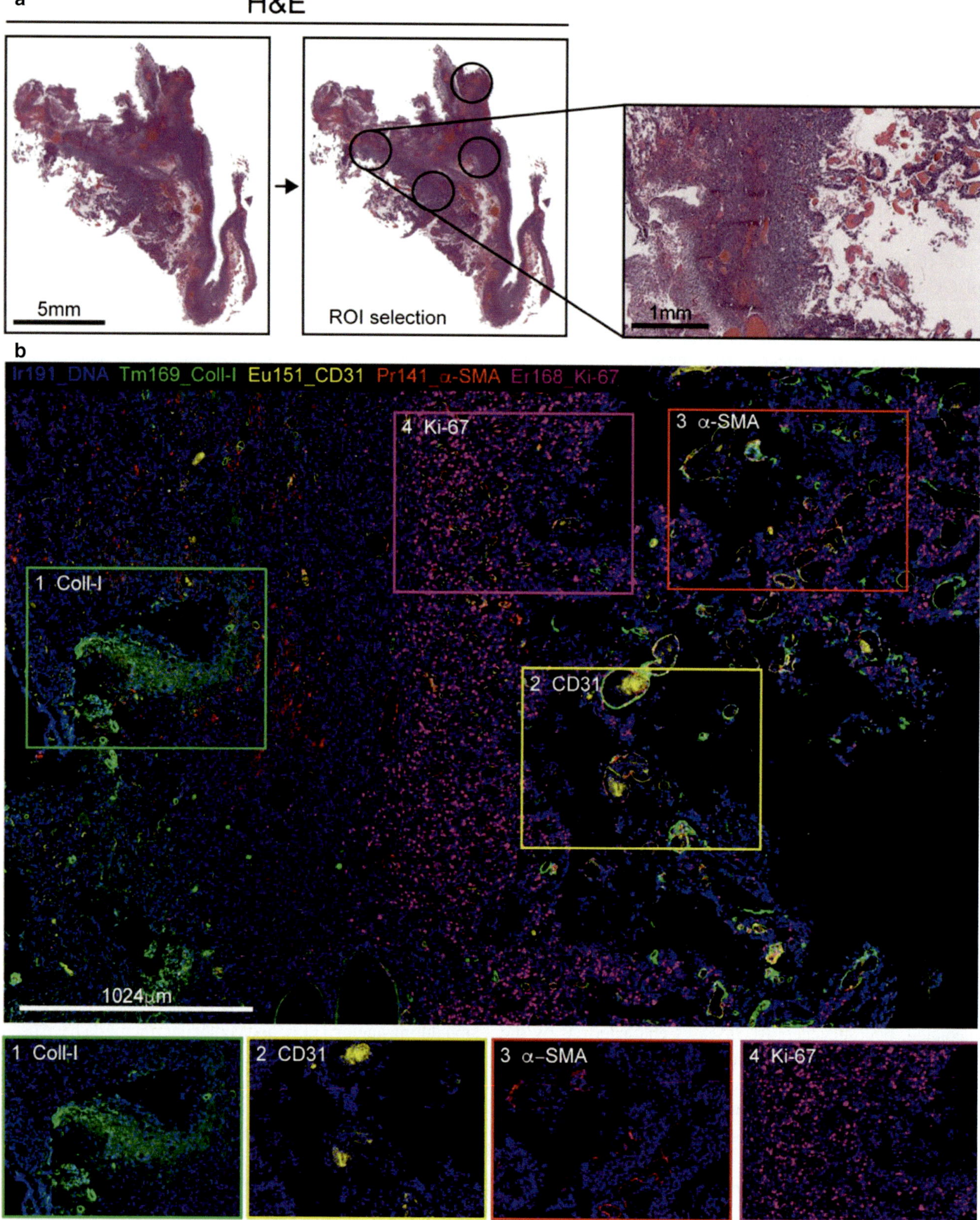

Fig. 20.3 **Imaging mass cytometry analysis of pHGG tumour tissue.** (**a**) Representative image of an H&E stained pHGG FFPE tissue slice with four different areas, circled in black, selected by a neuropathologist, to be scanned with the Hyperion imaging system. The higher power magnification image on the right corresponds to the ROI analyzed by IMC and displayed in panel B. (**b**) Representative image of the ROI with regions displaying the expression of (1) collagen-I (green), (2) CD31 (yellow), (3) α-SMA (red), and (4) Ki-67 as overlay or in individual channels. DNA (blue) is also shown

rophages, monocytes and dendritic cells, originate from myeloid stem cells and thus share numerous molecular markers [115]. Therefore, when studying the presence, distribution, and function of immune cells in complex tissues, more advanced techniques are required. The development of IMC enabled us to overcome this challenge and to distinguish closely related cell types, obtain information on their localization, and map cellular interactions [14]. We developed a 36-antibody panel to study the role of microglia and other immune cells in PCD pathogenesis. Preliminary data confirm that Purkinje neurons, identified by the marker calbindin, are lost in PCD patients (Fig. 20.4). In addition, our findings suggest that there is a degeneration of microglia in PCD patients, illustrated by the loss of microglia in the Purkinje neuron layer of the cerebellum. The main challenges of this project are related to data analysis and interpretation. The data processing is complex and requires advanced software, especially when studying irregularly shaped cells, such as microglia. Our approach involves pixel analysis and cell segmentation using Python and Ilastik, respectively. Data analysis is described in more detail in the next section.

Analysis of IMC Data

Imaging mass cytometry produces stunning images. However, to produce biological insight, such images must be processed and analyzed to yield quantitative data on the spatial expression profiles of the markers detected. This is a thread common to all histology, but it is much more relevant for highly multiplexed methods such as IMC, where a human eye, even that of a trained pathologist, can hardly grasp the multi-dimensional data produced by the imaging protocol.

Almost all of the currently available pipelines for the analysis of IMC data, and other similar imaging methods, share a common structure: images are first segmented in order to extract the areas corresponding to individual cells (or, in some cases, to subcellular compartments such as the nucleus and cytoplasm), and then an integrated value corresponding to the expression of a given marker for each cell is determined. Subsequently, the cell-level data are used to identify cell types and states, detect expression changes within or across samples, and calculate a variety of spatial measurements that can be ultimately correlated with a biological process.

Segmentation

Segmentation is perhaps the most critical step of IMC analysis, since any biological insight deriving from the analysis of cell-level data relies on the assumption that cells are correctly defined. Image segmentation is very complex, but there has recently been a focus on this issue due to the diffusion of large-scale microscopy and in situ biological analysis technologies. A detailed review of segmentation methods is beyond the scope of this chapter (for a review see [116]), but we will describe some strategies that have been successfully employed, or are being currently tested, for the processing of IMC datasets.

The first, and conceptually simplest segmentation pipeline relies on intensity-based thresholding. In this process, pixels of the images corresponding to one or more markers in the IMC dataset (usually the ones including the iridium nuclear counterstain) are defined as 'object' or 'background' based on an intensity threshold, and contiguous 'object' pixels are grouped together to define cells. Given that signal intensity can vary across a section (e.g., due to gradients in the diffusion or penetration of the antibodies and dyes), it is crucial to perform pre-filtering steps to homogenize signal and remove background. The threshold value can also be calculated dynamically for different regions of the image (a process known as adaptive thresholding). Although intensity-based thresholding methods are very sensitive to inhomogeneity in signal intensity, IMC does not suffer from illumination variation across the field of view as fluorescence microscopy does (since it does not use illumination, and the laser power tends to be stable over the course of a single ablation). Therefore, this method can sometimes be applied to IMC data with good results and very fast processing times compared to other strategies [64]. The processing time is important when the areas to segment are very large, for instance, whole histological slides.

An alternative method, which is at the base of the popular IMC analysis pipeline developed by the laboratory of Bernd Bodenmiller (currently the only analysis pipeline officially supported by Fluidigm), is based on pixel classification using a random forest algorithm implemented in the *Ilastik* package [116]. Here, the user manually defines a small number of areas of the image as belonging to a given number of classes (e.g. 'membrane', 'nucleus' and 'background'). The algorithm then uses data from the raw images from all channels, as well as a number of enhancements and filters, including blurring and edge detection, to compute probability maps in which the intensity of each pixel corresponds to its likelihood of belonging to any of the categories. These maps are usually independent of intensity variation and can be used to identify single cells with more precision than intensity-based thresholding since information from many more channels is used to define the classification.

Since cells in most cases touch each other, a key step in all segmentation methods is the division of cell 'clumps' into individual entities. The de facto standard for this is the watershed algorithm, which identifies separation lines by treating the grayscale profile of the clumps as an elevation map, with

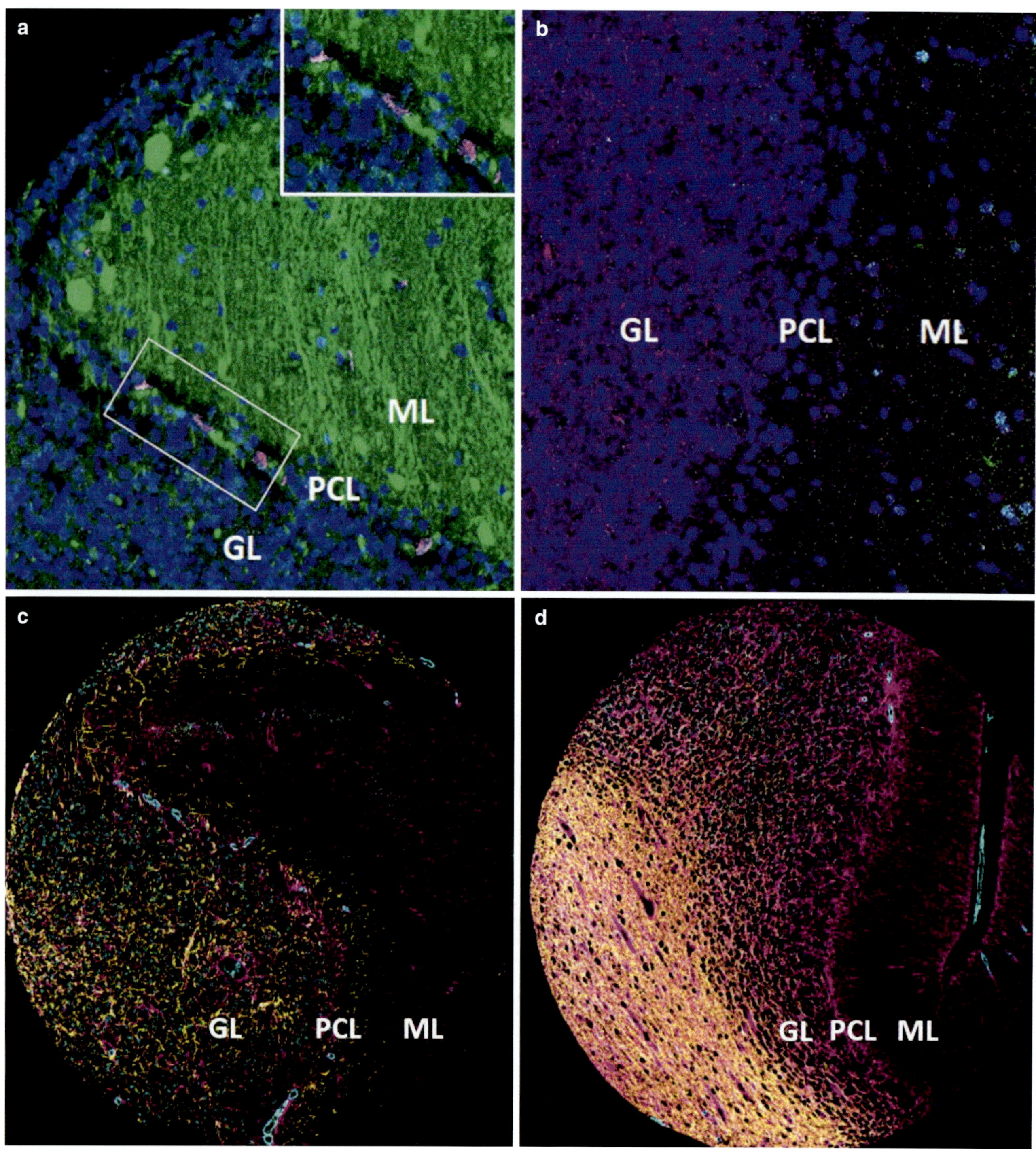

Fig. 20.4 Preliminary images of microglia in human cerebellum obtained using IMC. Detection of Purkinje neurons (green), microglia (magenta), and nuclei (blue) in human cerebellum tissue with a 1-mm core size from (**a**) a healthy individual and (**b**) a PCD patient. Overview of smooth-muscle actin (cyan), the astrocyte marker GFAP (magenta) and the dendritic cell marker CD11c (yellow) in core sections from the same healthy individual (**c**) and PCD patient (**d**). GL, granular layer; PL, Purkinje neuron layer; ML, molecular layer

the centre of cells corresponding to expanding pools of liquid and cell–cell boundaries corresponding to the lines where the liquids from different pools collide. In most cases, this process can be greatly improved by combining a nuclear segmentation with a membrane one, using the predicted nuclei as seed points and the membrane signal as boundary for the watershed algorithm.

In the last few years, the advent of deep learning methods has revolutionized many areas of biological data analysis. Image analysis is not an exception, and several public initiatives and competitions have sought to spur the application of these novel strategies to the problem of segmentation [117]. Among other methods, U-NET convolutional neural networks have emerged as a promising option, outperforming most other systems when a sufficiently large dataset is used to train the model [117]. Recently a generalized version of the U-NET network, combined with an improved declumping algorithm based on gradient flow tracking, was used to develop the *cellpose* package [118]. These methods have not yet been applied to IMC data segmentation. However, once the models have been trained with a sufficient amount of pre-segmented IMC data, they have better speed and accuracy than other segmentation methods.

Any segmentation method ultimately produces a set of segmentation masks, matching each pixel of the dataset to a specific object. Depending on how many markers are used in the process, such masks can correspond only to the nucleus of each cell or to the entire cell area. In almost all cases, the nucleus is significantly easier to segment than the cell membrane, due to its relatively regular shape and to the availability of DNA intercalators that stain all nuclei; in contrast, a universal membrane stain has not been identified. Given that a vast number of protein markers are expressed in the cytoplasm or membrane, however, it is very important that the whole cellular area is included in the segmentation mask.

Whatever the method used to segment an IMC dataset, it is of crucial importance that the accuracy of the results is carefully evaluated. The risk of mis-identification of cells resulting in misguided biological conclusions is very high. As an example, cell clumps or doublets could appear as a new population of cells with a marker expression profile intermediate between two or more cell types. This could be mistaken as a discovery of a new cell class with novel hybrid features, whereas in fact it would just represent a processing error. It is very important, therefore, that a subset of the segmentation masks is carefully examined by the user after overlay on the raw data. Another measure of segmentation errors that is often used is the percentage of 'impossible' cells, defined as segmented cells expressing a combination of markers extremely unlikely to be biologically co-occurring in the same cell, but likely to be present in cells located in close proximity. For instance, a 'cell' expressing both immune markers and epithelial markers would likely be a segmentation error. A similar strategy can be used to disaggregate mass cytometry data from the same sample (or a closely related one) as 'ground truth', since the cell dissociation produces bona fide single cells that should in theory include all the cell types that are detected in the IMC dataset. It should be noted that no segmentation will ever be 100% precise. The main objective, therefore, should be to estimate the fraction of errors and consider it carefully when interpreting the results of an experiment.

Analysis of Cell-Level Data

Once segmentation has been performed, an IMC dataset can be converted into a catalogue of cell objects, each associated with a vector of marker abundance measurements. At this step of the process, the analysis must consider (1) interchannel compensation, (2) normalization within the sample, and (3) normalization across samples. Even though mass cytometry does not suffer from significant cross-talk between channels, a small amount of signal can "bleed" between contiguous mass bands due to imprecisions in the time-of-flight detection of the ion cloud or to the presence of trace isotope variants in the metals used to tag antibodies. It is therefore important that a compensation matrix is obtained for each antibody panel [28] and applied, if needed, to the intensity profile of each pixel. Depending on the method used to integrate the signal of each marker over the cell area, the abundance value extracted for each cell can correlate with the cell size and confuse downstream analysis. It is therefore important to consider the normalization of the abundance values on a case-by-case basis. The abundance values can be transformed or left as they are. Transformations can be useful to accentuate differences across cells and to compress the dynamic range in order to assist with visualization. The transformation used in most CyTOF and IMC work is the hyperbolic arcsine (arcsinh). Finally, if multiple samples have to be compared, it is important to consider methods to normalize signals across different IMC acquisitions and to account for differences in detector voltage and laser power. Currently, no standardized solution exists for this, but several options have been proposed, including using adhesive tape 'calibration targets' coated with a thin layer of metal isotopes to calibrate the acquisition parameters and production of a tissue standard that can be cut and incorporated during data acquisition (e.g. by producing a tissue microarray for FFPE samples) and used as a stable reference for signal intensity.

Once normalization and feature extraction is completed, the user is finally presented with a final single-cell spatial dataset that can be mined for biological insight. The breadth of potential analyses and operations that can be performed on this sort of data is beyond the scope of this chapter, but here it is perhaps useful to cover some of the main steps of dataset processing that are likely to be included in most applications.

Dimensional reduction is a crucial step in the analysis of most high-dimensional datasets. Principal component analysis is the chief method used for this and is still at the basis of most computations. However, in recent years, two other methods have proven to be very effective in displaying the complexity of both single-cell RNA-seq data and CyTOF data: t-stochastic network embedding [118] and uniform manifold approximation and projection [119]. A full description of the advantages and disadvantages of the two methods is beyond the scope of this review, but in general, UMAP offers the advantage of a faster processing time, as well as a better preservation of the global data structure and gradients of marker expression (i.e. distance between clusters can be said to be more meaningful as a measure of expression difference in UMAP than in t-SNE). Another fundamental analysis step is the identification of cell populations based on unbiased clustering of the data. Whereas traditional hierarchical clustering methods (e.g. *k*-means clustering) work reasonably well if the number of cell populations is expected, graph-based methods (e.g. Phenograph or the Louvain algorithm [119]) have been used more frequently for IMC datasets with good success. In most cases, the aim of clustering is to identify cell groups and assign all cells belonging to them to known biological cell types and states by inspecting their marker expression; this is referred to as phenotyping. Typical applications for phenotyping involve calculation of the abundance of a given cell type in a sample or in specific areas of a sample or determination of spatial relationships of one cell type to another, parameters that can change significantly in response to both physiological and pathological events. Another use is detecting differential expression of markers between different cell types or states or between cells from the same population that are located in different spatial locations.

Many statistical frameworks are available to calculate the significance of marker expression changes, although few of them have been specifically developed for IMC data. Care should be taken to not use tools designed for single-cell RNA expression for IMC analysis, as the assumptions of the model and the underlying data distributions are very different. For instance, statistical models based on sequencing reads or UMI (usually used for single cell sequencing data), which normally follow a zero-inflated negative binomial distribution, should not be used to normalize IMC signals, which are intensity-based, or to compute differential expression. In most cases, simpler statistical models and tests, often inherited from the flow cytometry or histology field, perform best.

One particular procedure that can only be performed on IMC data, or similar spatial 'omics data, is unbiased neighbourhood analysis [53]. This analysis measures the frequency of interaction between cell populations based on their physical proximity. For each cell in the dataset, neighbours are defined as other cells within a defined distance. A permutation test is then used to estimate whether cells belonging to one cluster are more or less likely (compared to a random distribution) to be in close proximity to each other. Neighbourhood analysis has been shown to detect features (e.g. the association between immune cells and tumour cells) that correlate with cancer sub-type and outcome [57].

Software Packages

Currently, no integrated solution exists for the analysis of IMC datasets, although some tools that allow most of the key steps of the analysis to be performed in a relatively simple and integrated way are emerging. The Bodenmiller lab has developed a pipeline based on the Python programming language, the Ilastik pixel-classification software mentioned above, and the Cellprofiler package [120] for segmentation, de-clumping, and feature extraction. The same group also released a set of viewers for IMC datasets (Histocat++, Histocat 3D) [121] that can be used to perform some degree of segmentation processing.

Post-segmentation, the main integrated package for IMC dataset analysis is Histocat [53], which enables dimensional reduction, physical space and parameter space (marker 2D and 3D plot) visualization, clustering, and neighbourhood analysis in a user-friendly interface. An alternative, which often gives the user more control, is to analyze the data directly using the R or Python programming languages. Both ecosystems include modules designed to work with single-cell multi-parametric data (*SingleCellExperiment* for R and *Anndata* for Python), as well as a plethora of single-cell analysis tools. An important caveat is that most of these tools have been designed to operate on RNA-seq datasets and therefore care should be taken when applying these algorithms to IMC data. The Bodenmiller laboratory is making an effort to release modules specifically dedicated to the processing of IMC data such as *cytomapper* for R and dedicated visualization tools such as *napari-imc*.

Alternative Technologies

This chapter is focused on IMC, but IMC is just one of an increasing number of methods available for highly multiplexed protein imaging. Broadly, these can be divided into mass spectrometry-based and fluorescence-based approaches and into cyclical staining/clearing methods or all-at-once detection methods. IMC is an example of an all-at-once method using true multiplexing to detect many different channels at once. This multiplexing is possible due to the extremely high discriminating power of mass spectrometry, which is capable of differentiating isotopes differing by just one atomic mass. Another all-at-once method is MIBI [122], now commercially available through IonPath. MIBI has a higher spatial resolution than IMC but requires more data processing and, at the time of this writing, is not as widely adopted or well supported as IMC. Both IMC and MIBI have upper boundaries to the number of channels that can be imaged based on the number of different, commercially available, non-radioactive isotopes in the mass detection window of the mass spectrometer. A conceptually similar method, where all the antibodies are bound to the sample at once, but detection is performed in cycles of fluorescent imaging, is CODEX [123], a system distributed by Akoya Biosciences. In this technology, antibodies are conjugated to double-stranded DNA oligonucleotides that are specifically ligated to fluorescent tags according to a combinatorial scheme. There is, in theory, no limit to the number of antibodies that can be evaluated using CODEX, though of course the acquisition time proportionally increases with each additional antibody detected.

On the other end of the spectrum are methods based on cycles of antibody binding. One such approach is the 4i technology developed by the Pelkmans laboratory. In the 4i approach, antibodies are bound and stripped from tissues in cycles under mild conditions [124]. This technique is more damaging to the tissue than CODEX. During 4i, the tissue becomes progressively less intact with each cycle of restaining, but 4i has the crucial advantage of being compatible with native antibodies: it does not require special conjugations or instruments and therefore presents a lower barrier of entry for new users. A similar alternative has been commercialized by Miltenyi Biotech with the MACSima platform.

Concluding Remarks/Summary and Future Perspectives

Imaging mass cytometry has incredible potential to revolutionize the way many biological questions are approached and to have a lasting impact in many fields of biology where spatial analysis is relevant including some areas where it has not seen a lot of use so far. Yet, even with all its potential, IMC can be made much more powerful if it were integrated as part of an ecosystem of analysis methods to produce multi-modal datasets.

One of the biggest limitations of IMC is its slow speed of acquisition. A full histological slide can take up to 4 days to image, thus limiting the application of this technique to large-scale studies unless small samples or core biopsies are used. A potential solution to this issue is to use different technologies to pre-screen large libraries of sections and prioritize regions of interest for highly multiplexed imaging. The last decade has seen the appearance of a variety of microscopy techniques (including light sheet microscopy, serial two-photon tomography, and others) capable of imaging whole organs in a matter of hours or days. In parallel, whole-slide scanners have reached a speed sufficient to image hundreds of slides at a time. If some limited combination of markers (IHC antibodies and/or histological stainings) could be used to identify regions of interest with the help of a pathologist or, in the future, automated artificial intelligence classification tools, only a fraction of the sample would need to be routed to IMC for deep analysis, allowing studies to leverage the power of this technology on much wider and more relevant sample sets. An obvious caveat here is that, the smaller the sub-section selected for analysis, the higher the risk to interrogate just a fraction of the tissue heterogeneity present in the sample. Before any pre-selection strategy is used, a series of studies should be conducted to verify at which spatial scales (i.e. cellular, microscopic, or macroscopic) the heterogeneity is present and biologically relevant. Financial considerations should also be included.

Another limitation of mass cytometry is that the number of markers that can be multiplexed, even though much higher than previously possible, is still somewhat limited. In comparison, some of the genomics techniques that have recently become available allow the detection and quantification of hundreds, or even thousands, of different genes in single cells, both post-dissociation (DROP-Seq, 10X Chromium, CEL-seq) and in situ (merFISH, seqFISH, spatial transcriptomics, Slide-Seq). In some cases, hundreds of antibodies can be detected together with RNA transcripts on disaggregated cells (CITE-Seq). Although the sample types used by these techniques are sometimes different from those compatible with the IMC, it should be possible (and it is indeed being done in some of our laboratories) to design a study to perform IMC and other spatial 'omics measurements at the same time. Provided that the methods overlap by a significant number of markers, it should be possible to integrate these datasets and assign the cells detected by IMC to one of the cell types or states identified by the other methods, effectively leveraging different technologies to produce a coherent model with the potential to be biologically informative. Techniques such as CITE-seq and single-cell RNA-seq will be good starting points to define protein markers unique, or specific, to certain cell classes, which can then be optimized and included in IMC panels.

Acknowledgements MV is a Children with Cancer UK Fellow (grant 16-234) and acknowledges Children with Cancer UK and The Cure Starts Now, Fondazione Heal and Banca D´Italia for supporting this study. LLP acknowledges Fondazione AIRC. MV and LLP are grateful to Dr. Angela Mastronuzzi (Head of Neuro-Oncology Unit, OPBG), Dr. Andrea Carai (Oncological Neurosurgery Unit, OPBG), and Dr. Sabrina Rossi (Pathology Lab, OPBG) for clinical and pathological assessment of the DIPG case and the patient family. DB and FQ are funded by a CRUK 'Grand Challenge' grant (A24042), DB acknowledges the entire IMAXT project team and in particular the staff of the University of Cambridge Institute of Astronomy for the work performed on IMC data analysis and Dr. Bernd Bodenmiller and his laboratory, at the University of Zurich, for the many discussions and suggestions in implementing mass cytometry.

SG and IH would like to thank senior research technician, Bendik Nordanger, at the Department of Clinical Medicine, University of Bergen for his support in preparing PCD post-mortem TMA, and Head Engineer at the Core Facility for Flow Cytometry, Jørn Skavland, Department of Clinical Science, University of Bergen, for his technical support. Research grants from Torbjørg Hauges legacy supported this study. SG and IH are funded by NeuroSys-Med and Helse Vest.

References

1. Coons AH. The demonstration of pneumococcal antigen in tissues by the use of fluorescent antibody. J Immunol. 1942;45:159.

2. Coons AH, Creech HJ, Jones RN. Immunological properties of an antibody containing a fluorescent group. Proc Soc Exp Biol Med. 1941;47(2):200–2.

3. Macrea ER. Immunology II: immunohistochemistry: roots and review. Lab Med. 1999;30(12):787–90.

4. de Vries NL, et al. Unraveling the complexity of the cancer microenvironment with multidimensional genomic and cytometric technologies. Front Oncol. 2020;10:1254.

5. O'Donnell EA, Ernst DN, Hingorani R. Multiparameter flow cytometry: advances in high resolution analysis. Immune Netw. 2013;13(2):43–54.

6. Futamura K, et al. Novel full-spectral flow cytometry with multiple spectrally-adjacent fluorescent proteins and fluorochromes and visualization of in vivo cellular movement. Cytometry A. 2015;87(9):830–42.

7. Bandura DR, et al. Mass cytometry: technique for real time single cell multitarget immunoassay based on inductively coupled plasma time-of-flight mass spectrometry. Anal Chem. 2009;81(16):6813–22.

8. Ornatsky O, et al. Highly multiparametric analysis by mass cytometry. J Immunol Methods. 2010;361(1–2):1–20.

9. Bendall SC, et al. Single-cell mass cytometry of differential immune and drug responses across a human hematopoietic continuum. Science. 2011;332(6030):687–96.

10. Bendall SC, et al. Single-cell trajectory detection uncovers progression and regulatory coordination in human B cell development. Cell. 2014;157(3):714–25.

11. Chang Q, et al. Single-cell measurement of the uptake, intratumoral distribution and cell cycle effects of cisplatin using mass cytometry. Int J Cancer. 2015;136(5):1202–9.

12. Chang Q, et al. Biodistribution of cisplatin revealed by imaging mass cytometry identifies extensive collagen binding in tumor and normal tissues. Sci Rep. 2016;6:36641.

13. Atkuri KR, Stevens JC, Neubert H. Mass cytometry: a highly multiplexed single-cell technology for advancing drug development. Drug Metab Dispos. 2015;43(2):227–33.

14. Giesen C, et al. Highly multiplexed imaging of tumor tissues with subcellular resolution by mass cytometry. Nat Methods. 2014;11(4):417–22.

15. Angelo M, et al. Multiplexed ion beam imaging of human breast tumors. Nat Med. 2014;20(4):436–42.

16. Keren L, et al. MIBI-TOF: a multiplexed imaging platform relates cellular phenotypes and tissue structure. Sci Adv. 2019;5(10):eaax5851.

17. Davis AS, et al. Characterizing and diminishing autofluorescence in formalin-fixed paraffin-embedded human respiratory tissue. J Histochem Cytochem. 2014;62(6):405–23.

18. Schulz D, et al. Simultaneous multiplexed imaging of mRNA and proteins with subcellular resolution in breast cancer tissue samples by mass cytometry. Cell Syst. 2018;6(1):25–36.e5.

19. Bolognesi MM, et al. Multiplex staining by sequential immunostaining and antibody removal on routine tissue sections. J Histochem Cytochem. 2017;65(8):431–44.

20. Gullaksen SE, et al. Titrating complex mass cytometry panels. Cytometry A. 2019;95(7):792–6.

21. Chang Q, Ornatsky O, Hedley D. Staining of frozen and formalin-fixed, paraffin-embedded tissues with metal-labeled antibodies for imaging mass cytometry analysis. Curr Protoc Cytom. 2017;82:12.47.1–8.

22. Ijsselsteijn ME, et al. A 40-marker panel for high dimensional characterization of cancer immune microenvironments by imaging mass cytometry. Front Immunol. 2019;10:2534.

23. Butovsky O, et al. Identification of a unique TGF-β-dependent molecular and functional signature in microglia. Nat Neurosci. 2014;17(1):131–43.

24. Lipman NS, et al. Monoclonal versus polyclonal antibodies: distinguishing characteristics, applications, and information resources. ILAR J. 2005;46(3):258–68.

25. Chevrier S, et al. Compensation of signal spillover in suspension and imaging mass cytometry. Cell Syst. 2018;6(5):612–620.e5.

26. Bringeland GH, et al. Optimization of receptor occupancy assays in mass cytometry: standardization across channels with QSC beads. Cytometry A. 2019;95(3):314–22.

27. Takahashi C, et al. Mass cytometry panel optimization through the designed distribution of signal interference. Cytometry A. 2017;91(1):39–47.

28. Fernández-Zapata C, et al. The use and limitations of single-cell mass cytometry for studying human microglia function. Brain Pathol. 2020;30(6):1178–91.

29. Ornatsky OI, et al. Development of analytical methods for multiplex bio-assay with inductively coupled plasma mass spectrometry. J Anal At Spectrom. 2008;23(4):463–9.

30. Böttcher C, et al. Human microglia regional heterogeneity and phenotypes determined by multiplexed single-cell mass cytometry. Nat Neurosci. 2019;22(1):78–90.

31. Junttila MR, de Sauvage FJ. Influence of tumour microenvironment heterogeneity on therapeutic response. Nature. 2013;501(7467):346–54.

32. Curtis C, et al. The genomic and transcriptomic architecture of 2,000 breast tumours reveals novel subgroups. Nature. 2012;486(7403):346–52.

33. Dagogo-Jack I, Shaw AT. Tumour heterogeneity and resistance to cancer therapies. Nat Rev Clin Oncol. 2018;15(2):81–94.

34. Anderson AR, et al. Tumor morphology and phenotypic evolution driven by selective pressure from the microenvironment. Cell. 2006;127(5):905–15.

35. Gerlinger M, et al. Intratumor heterogeneity and branched evolution revealed by multiregion sequencing. N Engl J Med. 2012;366(10):883–92.

36. Marusyk A, Almendro V, Polyak K. Intra-tumour heterogeneity: a looking glass for cancer? Nat Rev Cancer. 2012;12(5):323–34.

37. Rye IH, et al. Intratumor heterogeneity defines treatment-resistant HER2+ breast tumors. Mol Oncol. 2018;12(11):1838–55.

38. Yuan Y, Spatial heterogeneity in the tumor microenvironment. Cold Spring Harb Perspect Med. 2016;6(8).

39. Andor N, et al. Pan-cancer analysis of the extent and consequences of intratumor heterogeneity. Nat Med. 2016;22(1):105–13.

40. Gillies RJ, Verduzco D, Gatenby RA. Evolutionary dynamics of carcinogenesis and why targeted therapy does not work. Nat Rev Cancer. 2012;12(7):487–93.

41. Allred DC, et al. Ductal carcinoma in situ and the emergence of diversity during breast cancer evolution. Clin Cancer Res. 2008;14(2):370–8.

42. Wu J, et al. Intratumoral spatial heterogeneity at perfusion MR imaging predicts recurrence-free survival in locally advanced breast cancer treated with neoadjuvant chemotherapy. Radiology. 2018;288(1):26–35.

43. Carmona-Bozo JC, et al. Hypoxia and perfusion in breast cancer: simultaneous assessment using PET/MR imaging. Eur Radiol. 2021;31(1):333–44.

44. Egeblad M, Nakasone ES, Werb Z. Tumors as organs: complex tissues that interface with the entire organism. Dev Cell. 2010;18(6):884–901.

45. Bergers G, Hanahan D. Modes of resistance to anti-angiogenic therapy. Nat Rev Cancer. 2008;8(8):592–603.

46. Chen Q, Zhang XH, Massagué J. Macrophage binding to receptor VCAM-1 transmits survival signals in breast cancer cells that invade the lungs. Cancer Cell. 2011;20(4):538–49.

47. Sahai E, et al. A framework for advancing our understanding of cancer-associated fibroblasts. Nat Rev Cancer. 2020;20(3):174–86.
48. Luga V, et al. Exosomes mediate stromal mobilization of autocrine Wnt-PCP signaling in breast cancer cell migration. Cell. 2012;151(7):1542–56.
49. Loges S, Schmidt T, Carmeliet P. Mechanisms of resistance to anti-angiogenic therapy and development of third-generation anti-angiogenic drug candidates. Genes Cancer. 2010;1(1):12–25.
50. Heindl A, Nawaz S, Yuan Y. Mapping spatial heterogeneity in the tumor microenvironment: a new era for digital pathology. Lab Investig. 2015;95(4):377–84.
51. Quail DF, Joyce JA. Microenvironmental regulation of tumor progression and metastasis. Nat Med. 2013;19(11):1423–37.
52. Kalluri R. The biology and function of fibroblasts in cancer. Nat Rev Cancer. 2016;16(9):582–98.
53. Wagner J, et al. A single-cell atlas of the tumor and immune ecosystem of human breast cancer. Cell. 2019;177(5):1330–1345. e18.
54. Keren L, et al. A structured tumor-immune microenvironment in triple negative breast cancer revealed by multiplexed ion beam imaging. Cell. 2018;174(6):1373–1387.e19.
55. Schapiro D, et al. histoCAT: analysis of cell phenotypes and interactions in multiplex image cytometry data. Nat Methods. 2017;14(9):873–6.
56. Carvajal-Hausdorf DE, et al. Multiplexed (18-plex) measurement of signaling targets and cytotoxic T cells in trastuzumab-treated patients using imaging mass cytometry. Clin Cancer Res. 2019;25(10):3054–62.
57. McKeage K, Perry CM. Trastuzumab: a review of its use in the treatment of metastatic breast cancer overexpressing HER2. Drugs. 2002;62(1):209–43.
58. Carvajal-Hausdorf DE, et al. Measurement of domain-specific HER2 (ERBB2) expression may classify benefit from trastuzumab in breast cancer. J Natl Cancer Inst. 2015;107(8)
59. Ali HR, et al. Imaging mass cytometry and multiplatform genomics define the phenogenomic landscape of breast cancer. Nat Cancer. 2020;1(2):163–75.
60. Pàez-Ribes M, et al. Antiangiogenic therapy elicits malignant progression of tumors to increased local invasion and distant metastasis. Cancer Cell. 2009;15(3):220–31.
61. Barrett RL, Puré E. Cancer-associated fibroblasts and their influence on tumor immunity and immunotherapy. elife. 2020;9
62. Taub DD, Longo DL, Murphy WJ. Human interferon-inducible protein-10 induces mononuclear cell infiltration in mice and promotes the migration of human T lymphocytes into the peripheral tissues and human peripheral blood lymphocytes-SCID mice. Blood. 1996;87(4):1423–31.
63. Jackson HW, et al. The single-cell pathology landscape of breast cancer. Nature. 2020;578(7796):615–20.
64. Georgopoulou D, et al. Landscapes of cellular phenotypic diversity in breast cancer xenografts and their impact on drug response. Nat Commun. 2021;12(1):1998.
65. Serganova I, et al. Tumor hypoxia imaging. Clin Cancer Res. 2006;12(18):5260–4.
66. Patil N, et al. Epidemiology of brainstem high-grade gliomas in children and adolescents in the United States, 2000–2017. Neuro Oncol. 2021;23(6):990–8.
67. Jones C, Baker SJ. Unique genetic and epigenetic mechanisms driving paediatric diffuse high-grade glioma. Nat Rev Cancer. 2014;14(10)
68. Jones C, Perryman L, Hargrave D. Paediatric and adult malignant glioma: close relatives or distant cousins? Nat Rev Clin Oncol. 2012;9(7):400–13.
69. Mackay A, et al. Integrated molecular meta-analysis of 1,000 pediatric high-grade and diffuse intrinsic pontine glioma. Cancer Cell. 2017;32(4):520–537.e5.
70. Leach JL, et al. MR imaging features of diffuse intrinsic pontine glioma and relationship to overall survival: report from the international DIPG registry. Neuro-Oncology. 2020;22(11):1647–57.
71. Puget S, et al. Biopsy in a series of 130 pediatric diffuse intrinsic pontine gliomas. Childs Nerv Syst. 2015;31(10):1773–80.
72. Carai A, et al. Robot-assisted stereotactic biopsy of diffuse intrinsic pontine glioma: a single-center experience. World Neurosurg. 2017;101:584–8.
73. Broniscer A, et al. Prospective collection of tissue samples at autopsy in children with diffuse intrinsic pontine glioma. Cancer. 2010;116(19):4632–7.
74. Angelini P, et al. Post mortem examinations in diffuse intrinsic pontine glioma: challenges and chances. J Neuro-Oncol. 2011;101(1):75–81.
75. Caretti V, et al. Implementation of a multi-institutional diffuse intrinsic pontine glioma autopsy protocol and characterization of a primary cell culture. Neuropathol Appl Neurobiol. 2013;39(4):426–36.
76. Brandon JC, et al. Emphysematous cholecystitis: pitfalls in its plain film diagnosis. Gastrointest Radiol. 1988;13(1):33–6.
77. Wu G, et al. Somatic histone H3 alterations in pediatric diffuse intrinsic pontine gliomas and non-brainstem glioblastomas. Nat Genet. 2012;44(3):251–3.
78. Schwartzentruber J, et al. Driver mutations in histone H3.3 and chromatin remodelling genes in paediatric glioblastoma. Nature. 2012;482(7384):226–31.
79. Taylor KR, et al. Recurrent activating ACVR1 mutations in diffuse intrinsic pontine glioma. Nat Genet. 2014;46(5):457–61.
80. Nikbakht H, et al. Spatial and temporal homogeneity of driver mutations in diffuse intrinsic pontine glioma. Nat Commun. 2016;7:11185.
81. Clarke M, et al. Infant high-grade gliomas comprise multiple subgroups characterized by novel targetable gene fusions and favorable outcomes. Cancer Discov. 2020;10(7):942–63.
82. Ceglie G, et al. Infantile/congenital high-grade gliomas: molecular features and therapeutic perspectives. Diagnostics (Basel). 2020;10(9)
83. Buczkowicz P, et al. Histopathological spectrum of paediatric diffuse intrinsic pontine glioma: diagnostic and therapeutic implications. Acta Neuropathol. 2014;128(4):573–81.
84. Vinci M, et al. Functional diversity and cooperativity between subclonal populations of pediatric glioblastoma and diffuse intrinsic pontine glioma cells. Nat Med. 2018;24(8):1204–15.
85. Robinson MH, et al. Subtype and grade-dependent spatial heterogeneity of T-cell infiltration in pediatric glioma. J Immunother Cancer. 2020;8(2)
86. Salloum R, et al. Characterizing temporal genomic heterogeneity in pediatric high-grade gliomas. Acta Neuropathol Commun. 2017;5(1):78.
87. Hoffman M, et al. Intratumoral genetic and functional heterogeneity in pediatric glioblastoma. Cancer Res. 2019;79(9):2111–23.
88. Castel D, et al. Transcriptomic and epigenetic profiling of 'diffuse midline gliomas, H3 K27M-mutant' discriminate two subgroups based on the type of histone H3 mutated and not supratentorial or infratentorial location. Acta Neuropathol Commun. 2018;6(1):117.
89. Pericoli G, et al. Integration of multiple platforms for the analysis of multifluorescent marking technology applied to pediatric GBM and DIPG. Int J Mol Sci. 2020;21(18)
90. Filbin MG, et al. Developmental and oncogenic programs in H3K27M gliomas dissected by single-cell RNA-seq. Science. 2018;360(6386):331–5.
91. Chen CCL, et al. Histone H3.3G34-mutant interneuron progenitors co-opt PDGFRA for gliomagenesis. Cell. 2020;183(6):1617–1633.e22.

92. Galdieri L, et al. Defining phenotypic and functional heterogeneity of glioblastoma stem cells by mass cytometry. JCI Insight. 2021;6(4):e128456.

93. Mueller S, et al. Mass cytometry detects H3.3K27M-specific vaccine responses in diffuse midline glioma. J Clin Invest. 2020;130(12):6325–37.

94. Leelatian N, et al. Unsupervised machine learning reveals risk stratifying glioblastoma tumor cells. elife. 2020;9

95. Venkatesh HS, et al. Neuronal activity promotes glioma growth through Neuroligin-3 secretion. Cell. 2015;161(4):803–16.

96. Venkatesh HS, et al. Electrical and synaptic integration of glioma into neural circuits. Nature. 2019;573(7775):539–45.

97. Raspotnig M, et al. Cerebellar degeneration-related proteins 2 and 2-like are present in ovarian cancer in patients with and without Yo antibodies. Cancer Immunol Immunother. 2017;66(11):1463–71.

98. Herdlevær, I., et al., Paraneoplastic cerebellar degeneration: the importance of including CDR2L as a diagnostic marker. Neurol Neuroimmunol Neuroinflamm. 2021;8(2).

99. Peterson K, et al. Paraneoplastic cerebellar degeneration. I. a clinical analysis of 55 anti-Yo antibody-positive patients. Neurology. 1992;42(10):1931–7.

100. Kråkenes T, et al. CDR2L is the major Yo antibody target in paraneoplastic cerebellar degeneration. Ann Neurol. 2019;86(2):316–21.

101. Herdlevaer I, et al. Localization of CDR2L and CDR2 in paraneoplastic cerebellar degeneration. Annals Clin Transl Neurol. 2020;7(11):2231–42.

102. Schubert M, et al. Paraneoplastic CDR2 and CDR2L antibodies affect Purkinje cell calcium homeostasis. Acta Neuropathol. 2014;128(6):835–52.

103. Greenlee JE, et al. Anti-Yo antibody uptake and interaction with its intracellular target antigen causes Purkinje cell death in rat cerebellar slice cultures: a possible mechanism for paraneoplastic cerebellar degeneration in humans with gynecological or breast cancers. PLoS One. 2015;10(4):e0123446.

104. Storstein A, Krossnes BK, Vedeler CA. Morphological and immunohistochemical characterization of paraneoplastic cerebellar degeneration associated with Yo antibodies. Acta Neurol Scand. 2009;120(1):64–7.

105. Yshii L, et al. Neurons and T cells: understanding this interaction for inflammatory neurological diseases. Eur J Immunol. 2015;45(10):2712–20.

106. Darnell RB, Posner JB. Paraneoplastic syndromes involving the nervous system. N Engl J Med. 2003;349(16):1543–54.

107. Monstad SE, et al. Yo antibodies in ovarian and breast cancer patients detected by a sensitive immunoprecipitation technique. Clin Exp Immunol. 2006;144(1):53–8.

108. Hickman S, et al. Microglia in neurodegeneration. Nat Neurosci. 2018;21(10):1359–69.

109. Tan Y-L, Yuan Y, Tian L. Microglial regional heterogeneity and its role in the brain. Mol Psychiatry. 2020;25(2):351–67.

110. Lawson LJ, et al. Heterogeneity in the distribution and morphology of microglia in the normal adult mouse brain. Neuroscience. 1990;39(1):151–70.

111. Stowell RD, et al. Cerebellar microglia are dynamically unique and survey Purkinje neurons in vivo. Dev Neurobiol. 2018;78(6):627–44.

112. Tay TL, et al. A new fate mapping system reveals context-dependent random or clonal expansion of microglia. Nat Neurosci. 2017;20(6):793–803.

113. Soreq L, et al. Major shifts in glial regional identity are a transcriptional hallmark of human brain aging. Cell Rep. 2017;18(2):557–70.

114. Grabert K, et al. Microglial brain region-dependent diversity and selective regional sensitivities to aging. Nat Neurosci. 2016;19(3):504–16.

115. Ransohoff RM, Cardona AE. The myeloid cells of the central nervous system parenchyma. Nature. 2010;468:253.

116. Vicar T, et al. Cell segmentation methods for label-free contrast microscopy: review and comprehensive comparison. BMC Bioinf. 2019;20(1):360.

117. Ronneberger O, Fischer P, Brox T. U-Net: Convolutional Networks for Biomedical Image Segmentation 2015. arXiv:1505.04597.

118. van der Maaten L, Hinton G. Viualizing data using t-SNE. J Mach Learn Res. 2008;9:2579–605.

119. McInnes L, Healy J, Melville J. UMAP: Uniform Manifold Approximation and Projection for Dimension Reduction. 2018. arXiv:1802.03426.

120. Carpenter AE, et al. CellProfiler: image analysis software for identifying and quantifying cell phenotypes. Genome Biol, 2006;7(10):R100.

121. Kuett L, Catena R, Özcan A, et al. Three-dimensional imaging mass cytometry for highly multiplexed molecular and cellular mapping of tissues and the tumor microenvironment. Nat Cancer. 2022;3:122–33.

122. Ptacek J, et al. Multiplexed ion beam imaging (MIBI) for characterization of the tumor microenvironment across tumor types. Lab Invest. 2020;100(8):1111–23.

123. Goltsev Y, et al. Deep profiling of mouse splenic architecture with CODEX multiplexed imaging. Cell. 2018;174(4):968–81.e15.

124. Gut G, Herrmann MD, Pelkmans L. Multiplexed protein maps link subcellular organization to cellular states. Science. 2018;361(6401):468.

Artificial Intelligence in Studies of Malignant Tumours

21

André Pedersen, Ingerid Reinertsen, Emiel A. M. Janssen, and Marit Valla

Abstract

With the introduction of digital pathology and artificial intelligence (AI)-based methods, we may be facing a new era in cancer diagnostics and prognostication. AI can assist pathologists in labour-intensive tasks and potentially discover new features currently not detected and characterized in routine diagnostics. As entire digital histopathological sections can be included in the analysis, AI can be used both to study the epithelial component of a tumour and the microenvironment. Most state-of-the-art AI approaches used for image analysis utilize multi-step pipelines. AI-based methods have shown promising results in a wide range of clinically relevant tasks. It is, however, important to be aware of some challenges and limitations, such as the lack of generalizability of AI-based models, and the importance of understanding the reason behind a conclusion.

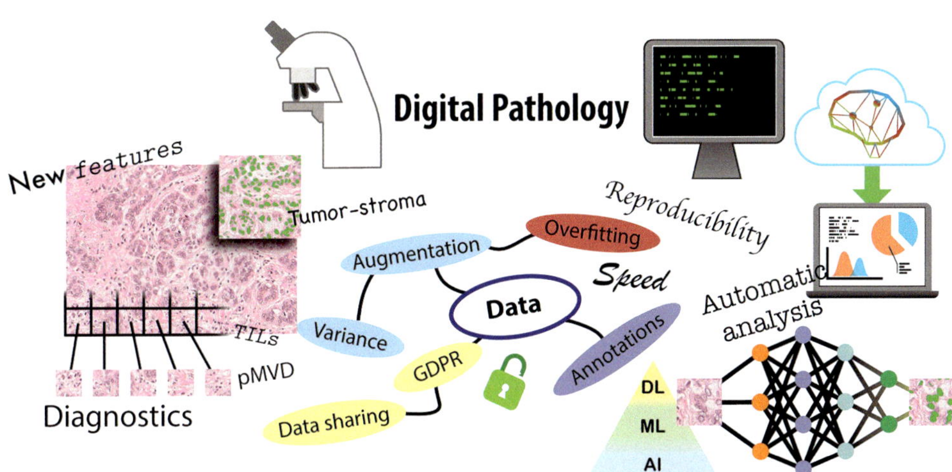

Digital Pathology

A. Pedersen · M. Valla (✉)
Norwegian University of Science and Technology, Trondheim, Norway
e-mail: andre.pedersen@ntnu.no; marit.valla@ntnu.no

I. Reinertsen
SINTEF, Trondheim, Norway
e-mail: ingerid.reinertsen@sintef.no

E. A. M. Janssen
Stavanger University Hospital/University of Stavanger, Stavanger, Norway
e-mail: emilius.adrianus.maria.janssen@sus.no

L. A. Akslen, R. S. Watnick (eds.), *Biomarkers of the Tumor Microenvironment*, https://doi.org/10.1007/978-3-030-98950-7_21

> **Take-Home Lessons**
> - Digital pathology and artificial intelligence (AI) represent a new era in cancer diagnostics
> - Most state-of-the-art AI approaches utilize multi-step pipelines
> - AI has shown promising results for many clinically relevant tasks
> - AI can discover new clinically relevant features in digital histopathological slides
> - Challenges of using AI in digital pathology include lack of generalizability of the derived models

Pathology laboratories are challenged by a continuous increase in the number of diagnostic biopsies received each year. The inclusion of new biomarkers has made cancer diagnostics more complex, and inter- and intra-observer variation remain challenges in the histologic assessment of cancers [1, 2]. With the introduction of digital pathology and artificial intelligence (AI)-based methods, we may be facing a new era in cancer diagnostics and prognostication. Using AI, and with more powerful computers and graphics processing units (GPUs), there is a large potential for new discoveries and higher efficiency in the analysis of histopathological slides. AI-based methods can assist pathologists in labour-intensive tasks prone to inter- and intra-observer variation and potentially discover features currently not characterized in routine diagnostics. To further underline this potential, AI has been named the third revolution in pathology, following implementation of immunohistochemistry (IHC) in the 80s and 90s (first revolution), and molecular pathology in the following decades (second revolution) [3].

AI is the ability of a computer program to perform tasks that are commonly associated with intelligent beings, and in particular the ability to learn from experience. Machine learning (ML) is a subfield within AI (Fig. 21.1) where mathematical methods are used to iteratively improve the performance of the algorithm[1] in detecting patterns in data without being explicitly programmed. These methods have outperformed humans at increasingly complex tasks [4–7] and are widely used in numerous applications such as smartphones, autonomous cars, and advertising. In the assessment of digital histopathological sections, machine learning permits unbiased extraction of subtle, but reproducible features and patterns, some of which may not be immediately recognized by humans. In the Cancer Metastases in Lymph Nodes Challenge 2016, deep learning algorithms outperformed a

---

[1]Algorithm: A finite list of computer-implemented instructions and rules a computer needs to solve a specific task.

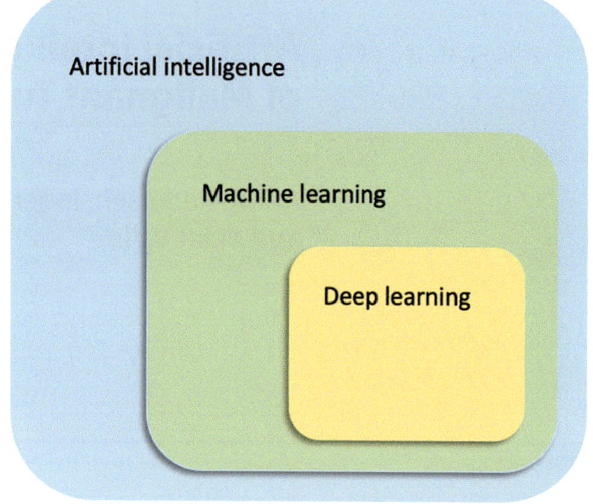

Fig. 21.1 The difference between artificial intelligence, machine learning, and deep learning

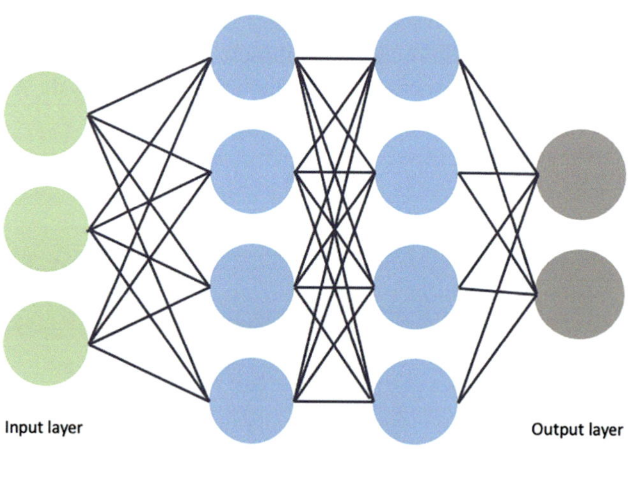

Fig. 21.2 Structure of a neural network

panel of 11 pathologists working under time constraints designed to mimic routine pathology workflow [2].

The machine learning methods most commonly used today are artificial neural networks. These networks are loosely inspired by the neural networks of the human brain. Similar to biological neural networks, artificial neural networks consist of neurons that receive input from one or several other neurons. The output (result) is a function of the inputs. Apart from this conceptual high-level similarity, biological and artificial neural networks have few resemblances. In deep learning, the artificial neurons are typically organized in several layers (Fig. 21.2). In general, networks with many layers (deep networks) can solve more complex tasks than networks with few layers.

For image analysis in general and for medical image analysis in particular, deep learning based on convolutional neu-

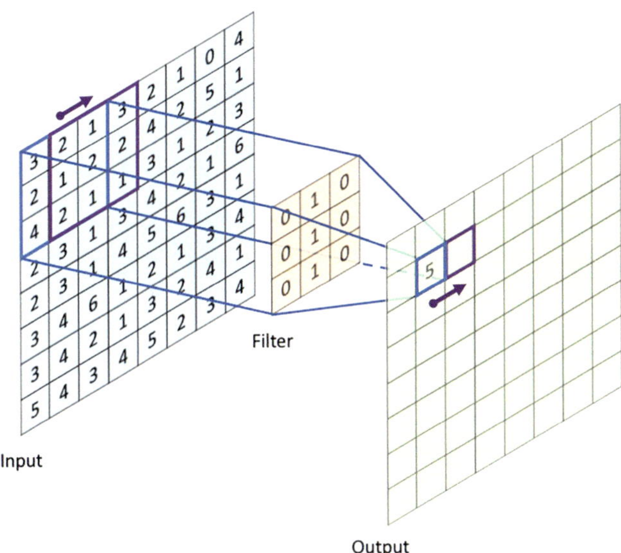

Fig. 21.3 Convolutional operations inside a convolutional neural network

ral networks (CNNs) have become the methodology of choice. The term CNN indicates that the network performs a mathematical operation called a convolution[2] (Fig. 21.3). The most widely used deep learning approach for training neural networks in medical imaging is supervised learning, where the network is presented with labelled examples of the task at hand. This could be histopathological images with annotations of specific structures such as nuclei, or images that are linked to information regarding molecular markers or prognosis. During training, the model must learn to weight the different input data to make a decision (prediction) that corresponds with the desired output or ground truth (e.g. prognosis). The network will thus learn to identify features in the data that are indicative of good and poor prognosis. The ability to learn important features directly from data is particularly interesting in applications such as automatic interpretation of histopathological slides, where only a limited number of features are characterized by the pathologist during routine histopathological evaluation. The resulting trained AI-model is consequently directly dependent on the data in the training data set and may be unable to handle cases that are not sufficiently represented in the training data. This could be rare cases, unusual morphology or contrast, or different resolution. It is therefore important to use a training data set that includes the full expected variability regarding different morphological features, scanners, staining, and

resolution. For proper and unbiased evaluation after training, the AI-based model must be tested on independent and unseen data.

A major challenge in the development and validation of AI-based models is availability of data. As described above, large amounts of data that cover the expected variance are needed to develop models that generalize well. In medicine, open, annotated data sets suitable for machine learning are still limited, and they contain considerably fewer cases than data sets of natural images [8]. High-quality annotations performed by medical experts are laborious to make and as such difficult to obtain. Furthermore, privacy laws and regulations make data sharing challenging. Also, large, well curated, and annotated data sets have a business value that may limit free distribution. However, it has been shown that the diagnosis from the routine pathology report can also be used directly as the only label for training [9]. Using this approach, pathology laboratories have enormous amounts of labelled data that may be used for the development of AI-based models. As these models can only be as good as their training data, data availability is key to obtain accurate and robust models with high external validity.

State-of-the-Art Analysis of Histopathological Images

Due to the large size of histopathological images, it is necessary to subdivide the image into smaller patches[3] prior to image analysis. Such patches can be made with or without overlap. To solve tasks, such as detection or segmentation of cell nuclei or prediction of prognosis, each patch can be assessed individually. This is referred to as a patch-wise method (Fig. 21.4). The result can be visualized as a heatmap, where each small square in the heatmap represents the result of an individual patch. Then, a final prediction for the entire whole slide image (WSI) can be made from calculating a histogram[4] and defining the overall prediction as the most common occurrence in the histogram/heatmap. The histogram is an example of a feature extraction method.

Using a heatmap comprising several patch-wise results as the input to a machine learning method has some disadvantages. The approach is often computationally expensive. Furthermore, sine results obtained from multiple, individual, small patches, low-resolution/high-level features are not

---

[2]Convolution: A mathematical operation that performs filtering of input data, using a predefined filter function or kernel. An example could be to blur an image or extract edge information.

[3]Patch: A subregion of an image. It is also commonly referred to as a *tile*.

[4]Histogram: A method used to extract the frequency of different values.

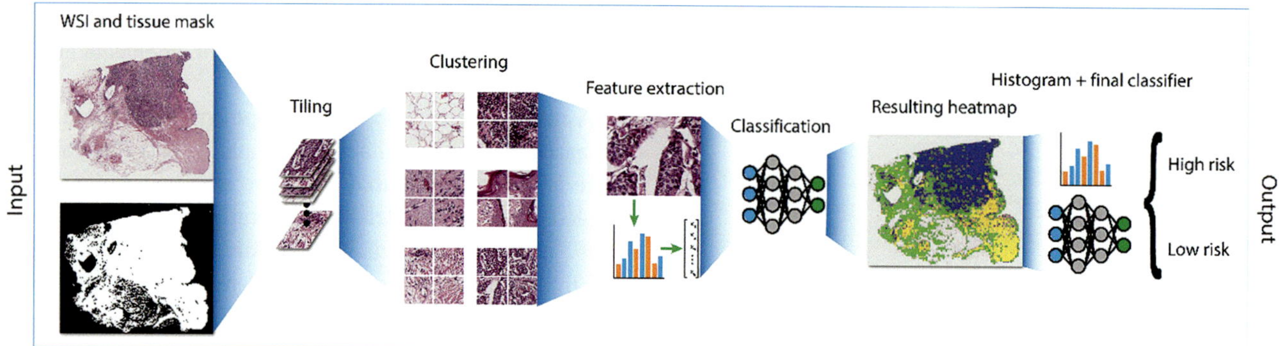

Fig. 21.4 Patch-wise approach for prediction of prognosis in a histopathological section from a breast cancer tumour

used to make the initial prediction. To solve the task, it may be necessary to include information from both high and low resolution. The histogram is an example of a low-level feature. High-level features could be specific types of edges or patterns in an image.

In traditional machine learning, artificial neural networks are used to classify images, using a predefined method/algorithm that extracts features from the image. Today, the most common approach is to use CNNs. During training, CNNs learn to solve a task by identifying features that are relevant to solve the task at hand. A typical CNN classifier comprises two components: an encoder and a classifier head. The encoder is trained to extract relevant information (features) from the image. The classifier head then uses these features to solve the task, similarly to traditional neural networks.

To perform segmentation, that is to classify individual pixels[5] of an image, it is common to use a decoder instead of a classifier head. The decoder learns to transform the features extracted by the encoder to produce a segmentation. The most popular encoder–decoder neural network is called U-Net [10]. The U-Net architecture can be used directly, or it can be modified to perform segmentation of different objects and structures in an image [11–15]. In traditional machine learning, pixels with similar morphology can be assembled into what is referred to as a superpixel using a predefined algorithm. A classifier is then trained to classify each superpixel independently, for instance, using traditional methods such as ordinary neural networks, support vector machines (SVMs) [16], or random forests (RFs) [17]. These methods usually require labelled data to produce a segmentation. The superpixel method [18] is robust and works well on smaller data sets [19–21]. There are also other segmentation algorithms such as watershed [22], region growing [23], and level set [24]. The latter three are traditional algorithms that do not require training data. Provided that sufficient, labelled train-

ing data are available, CNNs usually outperform these traditional methods in image recognition tasks.

When using CNNs for image analysis, overfitting may be a challenge, especially when the amount of training data is limited. By overfitting, we mean that the network is trained to memorize the training data, but the resultant AI-based model does not generalize well to new data. The risk of overfitting is higher when all sections are stained in the same laboratory, and when a single scanner is used. To avoid or reduce overfitting, methods to expand or control the network or training scheme are commonly used, one of which is data augmentation. With data augmentation, the data set is expanded by producing artificial copies of the original data. An example could be to rotate the images with varying angles, or to adjust the colour components of an image, a method called colour augmentation. As different laboratories have different staining and scanning procedures, it may be necessary to use data augmentation to develop models that are more likely to generalize to data sets from other laboratories. An alternative to colour augmentation is stain normalization. In the latter method, colours are normalized across the different WSIs in the data set, for instance, by using the stainings of one patch or one WSI as reference. Using colour augmentation or stain normalization, slide colour becomes less important. Several studies show improved generalizability of AI-models after using stain normalization and/or colour augmentation [25–27].

Data augmentation alone does not necessarily compensate for missing variance in the training data set, and it may be necessary to include new samples. Another solution is to use a model that was pretrained on another data set, before introducing it to the training data set. Thus, instead of training the model from scratch, the weights of the pretrained model are modified to suit the current task and data set. This approach is called fine-tuning. Ideally, the pretrained model should be developed based on similar data. However, the most common approach is to use a model that was pretrained on natural images. ImageNet is a large data set containing more than 14 million images

---

[5]Pixel: The smallest addressable region in an image. The size of a pixel is defined by the resolution.

and 1000 classes[6] [8]. ImageNet is not composed of medical images, but due to the large number of images and classes included, the generated models may be suitable for solving other tasks. In the Grand Challenge on BreAst Cancer Histology images (BACH), all top competing teams used fine-tuning, with models that were originally trained on images from ImageNet [28].

Due to the large size and heterogeneity of WSIs, patches can be sorted based on a morphological criterion. For instance, if tumours in a training data set are dominated by stromal tissue, the generated model may not perform well on sections with more epithelial tissue. Thus, it is common to perform clustering [29–31] of patches to sort the patches into natural groups based on morphological similarities using a predefined criterion. Clustering is an unsupervised method, as the models are trained without labels. During training, the model can then be forced to focus on all clusters, instead of just the most common ones. Using clustering, different tissue types may be automatically labelled, thus avoiding laborious annotation work. However, it is challenging to control which groups in the data the clustering method finds the most natural.

Several attempts have been made to improve the CNN architectures or training procedures [28, 32, 33]. A current state of the art for assessment of histopathological images is multiple instance learning (MIL) [34, 35]. In MIL, not all patches are given the same ground truth label as the WSI. Instead, a label is given to a set of patches and the network learns to solve a task by identifying the patches within the set that are relevant to solve the task. Using this approach, the network may identify relevant features currently not included in the pathologist's routine assessment. MIL is commonly used in classification tasks such as histological grading of a tumour [36, 37]. It is an example of a semi-supervised method, as it learns to solve a task without assigning labels to each patch explicitly during training. However, this approach generally requires more data, compared to supervised methods, as training is less controlled.

AI and the Microenvironment

Most prognostic cancer studies focus on molecular alterations in epithelial cells. However, it is well established that the tumour microenvironment also plays an important role in cancer development [38]. Information regarding immune cell infiltration, angiogenesis, and stromal changes are not always included in the histopathological reporting of cancers. Including such information would further increase

pathologists' workload. In many cancers, such as breast cancer, biomarker status is used for treatment decisions [39–41]. However, most biomarkers reflect molecular changes in the epithelial cancer cells, and thus comprise only a fraction of the information that is found in a histopathological section [42]. Using AI, the whole histopathological section can be included in the analysis, thus incorporating both epithelial cancer cells and surrounding stromal tissue. Using this approach, it may be possible to identify new, clinically relevant features.

As the market for digital pathology is increasing, more stakeholders are getting involved in the development of tools that may be useful for diagnostic pathology. Such tools vary from simple slide viewers and annotation tools to complex algorithms that recognize and count mitoses in whole slides from breast cancer [43].

Tumour Infiltrating Lymphocytes

In urothelial bladder cancer, several authors have looked into the prognostic and predictive information of tumour infiltrating lymphocytes (TILs) showing that an increased level of TILs is associated with better overall survival [44]. Unfortunately, a consensus on how to score TILs in urothelial cancer does not exist. In order to get more specific data on the composition of the immune cell infiltrate, IHC T-cell markers like CD3, CD4, and CD8 have been used and analysed with or without image analyses [45–49]. For some of these markers, an increase in number correlates with non-recurrent disease. However, a comparison between studies is difficult since different markers and scoring methods have been used, and different patient groups have been included.

To standardize TIL assessment, an automatic method for separating urothelium from the surrounding stromal and muscular tissue could be of value [50]. Overlaying the results of such a model on IHC slides might result in more accurate and standardized TIL scores, as the cells can be counted in the urothelium or stroma only. Furthermore, such models may be used to detect infiltration of tumour cells in the stromal and muscular layer. This is important for staging of bladder cancer. Hosseini et al. recently published a detailed, organ-independent database containing 36 different tissue types to enable development of deep learning-based models for tissue segmentation [51]. More location specific IHC scores could be provided by using such databases in the digital assessment of IHC slides.

CNN-based models were used for detection and quantification of intratumoural lymphocytes in IHC images from breast, prostate, and colon cancer [52]. Using a machine learning-based approach, intratumoural and stromal lymphocytes were separately quantified in IHC-stained sections [53]. When compared to visual inspection by a pathologist, concordance was moderate. Based on features extracted

---

[6]Class: A predefined type of object or structure in a data sample. A set of images of cats and a set of images of dogs could be labelled with two different classes, one for each animal. Then a *classifier* may be trained to distinguish between images of the different classes/animals.

from the tumour immune microenvironment, patients were regrouped into five subgroups. One of these subgroups was associated with poor prognosis.

An international working group published a report on computational assessment of TILs [54]. By computational assessment, scoring can be differentiated into different scales (number per area stroma/number per number of tumour cells/TIL cluster size/TIL cluster morphology), and efficiency can be improved since pathologists can confirm predictions that are automatically generated by an algorithm. Published algorithms are still at a research stage and not yet implemented in diagnostic pathology. Clinically validated cut-offs need to be established in the same way as for other biomarkers before implementation [55]. For localized colorectal cancer, Immunoscore, a digital scoring system for CD3+ and CD8+ T-cells is included in the European Society for Medical Oncology (ESMO) clinical practice guidelines for clinical decision making [56]. Adding machine learning to the Immunoscore analysis workflow reduced analysis time [57], thus illustrating the great potential for the use of machine learning in pathology.

The clinical success of immunotherapy in several cancers is driving the need for new prognostic and predictive assays. Our understanding of the composition and interactions of the immune response needs to be expanded as well. Machine learning can help by integrating quantitative analyses and spatial information.

Saltz et al. used sections from The Cancer Genome Atlas (TCGA) to analyse the composition and spatial organization of TILs [58]. By computational staining, they used CNNs to identify lymphocyte-infiltrated regions in digitized haematoxylin–eosin (HE)-stained sections, producing TIL maps. The composition of the TIL maps varied across tumour types, prognostic groups, and molecular subtypes.

AbdulJabbar et al. combined multiregion exome and RNA-sequencing (RNA-seq) data with spatial histology for different cell types (cancer cells, lymphocytes, stromal cells such as fibroblasts and endothelial cells, and other cells such as macrophages, pneumocytes, and nonidentifiable cells) in non-small cell lung cancer. The cells were mapped by deep learning [59]. They developed a deep learning-based pipeline to spatially profile immune cell infiltration (triplex CD4/CD8/FOXP3 IHC) and discovered tumour topological determinants of immunosuppression, which they validated in a cohort of patients with lung adenocarcinoma. Tumours with many cold regions had higher risk of relapse in both cohorts. The cold tumour regions had more extensive physical contact between cancer and stromal cells, suggesting a stroma-modulated inhibition of immune responses.

Bailly et al. used data generated by digital analysis of IHC sections and ran these through a machine learning algorithm [60]. The authors identified eleven different cancer associated fibroblasts (CAF) patterns in pancreatic cancer.

Combining these data with spatial data from TILs could be highly informative and might give better insights into whether CAFs play a key role in the recruitment or exclusion of immune cells near the tumour.

Angiogenesis

Several studies have demonstrated that vascular proliferation is a prognostic factor in cancer [61–65]. It can be assessed by manual quantification of microvessel density (MVD), proliferating MVD (pMVD), and vascular proliferation index, the latter defined as pMVD/MVD [62–64, 66]. Such manual quantifications are time consuming, and currently not included in routine diagnostic pathology.

In 2009, Mete et al. proposed a method for automatic quantification of angiogenesis in liver cancer biopsies [67]. Using DBSCAN[7] on digital images, both morphologic and spatial features were included. Other studies have shown that AI-based classifiers [68–70] and deep learning [71–73] can be used for automatic identification and quantification of vessels in tumours, and that this information can be used for prognostic predictions. Nalisnik et al. used an interactive machine learning-based system called HistomicsML to identify and characterize vessels in gliomas. The vascular phenotypes were used to predict grade, molecular subtypes, and prognosis [74].

Other Stromal Features

Assuming that stromal–epithelial interactions contribute to cancer development and progression, Bejnordi et al. used deep learning to focus on the extracellular matrix stroma only [75]. By training deep learning-based models with manually annotated WSIs, they were able to separate invasive breast cancer from non-cancer. They found that tumour-associated stroma was highly correlated to grade 3 ductal carcinoma in situ, and ductal carcinoma in situ associated with an invasive component. Northey et al. recently showed that collagen-rich, stiff stroma increases breast cancer risk [76]. Zhao et al. used deep learning to calculate the tumour–stromal ratio (TSR) in colorectal cancer and showed significant differences in overall survival between cancers with low and high TSR [77]. Kather et al. used deep learning to segment tissue components in HE-stained slides from colorectal cancers, and used some of the stromal components to establish a new prognostic marker called the deep stroma score [78].

---

[7]DBSCAN: A density-based algorithm for discovering clusters in large spatial databases with noise. An unsupervised machine learning method for performing clustering.

A review from 2018 suggested a combination of computational morphogenesis and digital pathology to generate digital timelines through carcinogenesis by including epithelial cells and the TME [79]. Such decision support systems can be created using tissue types where successive phases of carcinogenesis and tumour progression are known, e.g., progression from normal to EIN to cancer in the endometrium, or from normal to polyp to cancer in the colon.

AI and Prognosis in Cancer

Several studies have examined the prognostic capabilities of AI-based models. When using AI in the interpretation of digital slides, both the epithelial cancer cells and the surrounding tissue can be taken into account. Thus, AI-based methods have the potential to discover new features that are not currently assessed by pathologists. Other data of relevance for prognosis can also be included in the AI-model, such as information on molecular biomarkers, age, grade, and stage [80, 81]. AI-based prognostication allows for automatic assessment and thus potentially more reproducible results.

Machine learning can be used both to predict the molecular properties of a tumour and prognosis [42]. Using an end-to-end approach, where the histopathological images were directly linked to prognostic information, multivariate analysis showed that an AI-based model could be used to predict prognosis in colorectal cancer [82]. In the paper by Skrede et al., the tissue surrounding the tumour was not included in the prognostic predictions. In another study, tissue microarrays from colorectal cancers were used for prognostic predictions, including only one 1 mm tissue core from each patient. The generated AI-based model was superior to pathologists' stratification of patients into low- and high-risk groups [83]. Turkki et al. predicted outcome in breast cancer using TMAs [84]. In their pipeline they used a pretrained encoder for feature extraction and an SVM for classification. They showed that machine learning methods can identify prognostic features in tumour images without domain knowledge. Thus, algorithms can extract features for prognostication that can complement the established prognostic factors in breast cancer. Meier et al. showed that AI-based prognostic predictions improved when both HE and IHC on TMAs from the same patients were used [81].

Machine learning algorithms combining images from both HE and IHC slides, separated breast cancers into low- and high-risk groups with accuracies comparable to mRNA-based molecular assays [72]. Several papers have shown that machine learning/deep learning based on histopathological slides can provide additional prognostic information in breast cancer [85], non-small cell lung cancer [86], and brain cancer [80].

While numerous studies have shown the potential of using AI-based methods for prognostic prediction for a single cancer type, Wulczyn et al. [87] showed that a single CNN model can predict prognosis for ten different cancer types. In their pipeline they used image features and patient-specific features such as age and gender. The model was able to distinguish short/long survival and cancer stage in five out of ten and seven out of ten cancer types, respectively.

A popular approach, especially when the data set is small, is to improve overall model performance by training and using multiple models in one single pipeline [28]. This is commonly referred to as ensembling. Increased runtime is a challenge using this approach. In the BACH challenge, most of the top competing teams did not perform ensembling [28]. A similar conclusion was reached by Yao et al. [88]. They compared deep learning to traditional machine learning approaches, where predefined features were used, and found that results improved with a deep learning approach. They were able to predict survival without any preselected region of interest (ROI) or annotations, by using multiple instance learning. Over time other studies have shown the same [31, 87, 88].

Courtiol et al. [89] used a deep learning-based pipeline for prognostic prediction of mesothelioma and found that stromal areas were important for prognostication. Mobadersany et al. [80] found that oedema in histopathological sections from low-grade gliomas and glioblastomas was important for prognostication, thus confirming findings from radiological studies [90]. Further studies focusing on understanding the computer models could pave way for new research hypotheses and ultimately lead to the discovery of novel prognostic markers.

Challenges and Limitations Using AI in Pathology

The use of AI in pathology has shown promising results. Nevertheless, it is important to be aware of the limitations, challenges, and potential pitfalls. The main challenge in the field is access to sufficiently large, high-quality data sets with expert annotations. The data sets used for training need to be large enough to cover the true variability in the patient population, but also variability due to different staining protocols and scanners. If the data set is not representative of this variability, the resulting model will perform poorly on new data. Using small data sets, the model might memorize the data set entirely, i.e., overfit to the training data, instead of learning to solve the task. There is also a risk that the model will learn the wrong features that happen to be correlated with the task at hand in the training data set. For instance, in a study aiming to develop an AI-based model for prognostic predictions of histopathological cancer sections, an artefact that is overrepresented in the poor prognosis group in the training data set, may be interpreted as a sign of poor prognosis. Validation on new, independent test data sets is therefore important to verify external validity of the model's performance.

In applications of AI for medical image analysis, most models are trained on manually annotated or labelled data, using supervised learning. The manual annotation process is time consuming and requires expert knowledge. Large data sets with expert annotations are thus difficult, time consuming, and expensive to obtain, and may represent high commercial value. Privacy rules and regulations, such as the GDPR in Europe, may also limit the re-use and sharing of data. A good data management plan and obtention of consents and approvals well in advance before data collection and annotation enable re-use and sharing of data and thus more efficient use of research resources and possibly faster progress.

Machine learning models in general, and deep neural networks in particular perform well in numerous contexts, but the generated models are often difficult or impossible to interpret directly [91, 92]. In medicine, the reason behind a given prediction or decision is particularly important and should not be left to a black box. Thus, the AI-models need to output an explanation that can be interpreted, understood, and verified by the clinician. Explainable AI (XAI) has become an increasingly active field of research over the past years and will be crucial for clinical acceptance and large-scale deployment of AI-based tools in digital pathology and medicine in general. If AI-based models are applied to histopathological cancer sections for prediction of prognosis, a first approach is to trace the result back to the section to highlight the decisive regions of the tumour. These regions can then be examined by the pathologist to confirm that the conclusion is plausible. There are several XAI methods for image data, signal data, and numerical data, e.g. shap [93], lime [94], and grad-CAM [95]. These methods can point to the regions in the image that were most important for the conclusion or show how each input of a numerical vector was weighted. However, these networks cannot output a concise explanation for the decision. There are also traditional machine learning methods with explainability integrated in the model, such as decision trees [96].

Another challenge with AI-based methods, especially CNNs, is that they are often computationally expensive. In a typical routine clinical context, results need to be computed fast using medium to low-end computers. By using a central server, the analysis is less dependent on local hardware as long as the Internet speed is satisfactory. This solution is especially beneficial when financial resources are limited. Commercial server-based solutions like Philips IntelliSite Open Pathology platform [97], Cytomine [98], and Aiforia [99] have been developed. Furthermore, free-to-use, open-source software like QuPath [100], Orbit [101], and FastPathology [102] can be used to test AI-based solutions, or develop custom models and/or pipelines, intended for histopathological sections. The latter three software are usually run on local hardware. Before AI-based models can be implemented in the clinic, thorough clinical validation must be performed.

Concluding Remarks/Summary and Future Perspectives

Most state-of-the-art AI approaches used for image analysis utilize multi-step pipelines. Such pipelines typically include colour augmentation and/or stain normalization, patch generation, automatic patch sorting (e.g. clustering), and feature extraction using either a pretrained ImageNet model directly, a fine-tuned pretrained model, or a CNN that is trained from scratch. Using a classifier, patch-wise predictions and a final conclusive prediction for the whole WSI can be made.

AI-based methods have shown promising results in a wide range of clinically relevant tasks, and with the implementation of digital pathology, AI may have a role in diagnostic pathology in the future. It is, however, important to be aware of some challenges, such as the lack of generalizability of AI-based models, and the importance of understanding the reason behind a conclusion. Furthermore, pathologists are not technologists, and vice versa, and incorporating digital pathology and AI-based methods into the diagnostic workflow may be a significant challenge. The AI revolution is especially challenging because of the simultaneous revolution within molecular pathology. Perhaps the solution for the modern pathology laboratory would be to strengthen cross disciplinary diagnostic work, including new professions to enable implementation of AI-based models in the future.

References

1. Chung YR, Jang MH, Park SY, Gong G, Jung WH. Korean breast pathology Ki-67 study G. Interobserver variability of Ki-67 measurement in breast cancer. J Pathol Transl Med. 2016;50(2):129–37.
2. Ehteshami Bejnordi B, Veta M, Johannes van Diest P, van Ginneken B, Karssemeijer N, Litjens G, et al. Diagnostic assessment of deep learning algorithms for detection of lymph node metastases in women with breast cancer. JAMA. 2017;318(22):2199–210.
3. Salto-Tellez M, Maxwell P, Hamilton P. Artificial intelligence-the third revolution in pathology. Histopathology. 2019;74(3):372–6.
4. Ardila D, Kiraly AP, Bharadwaj S, Choi B, Reicher JJ, Peng L, et al. End-to-end lung cancer screening with three-dimensional deep learning on low-dose chest computed tomography. Nat Med. 2019;25(6):954–61.
5. McKinney SM, Sieniek M, Godbole V, Godwin J, Antropova N, Ashrafian H, et al. International evaluation of an AI system for breast cancer screening. Nature. 2020;577(7788):89–94.
6. Silver D, Hubert T, Schrittwieser J, Antonoglou I, Lai M, Guez A, et al. Mastering Chess and Shogi by Self-Play with a General

Reinforcement Learning Algorithm. arXiv preprint arXiv. 2017:1712.01815.

7. Senior AW, Evans R, Jumper J, Kirkpatrick J, Sifre L, Green T, et al. Improved protein structure prediction using potentials from deep learning. Nature. 2020;577(7792):706–10.

8. Stanford Vision Lab. Imagenet [cited 2021 02.15]. Available from: http://www.image-net.org/.

9. Campanella G, Hanna MG, Geneslaw L, Miraflor A, Werneck Krauss Silva V, Busam KJ, et al. Clinical-grade computational pathology using weakly supervised deep learning on whole slide images. Nat Med. 2019;25(8):1301–9.

10. Ronneberger O, Fischer P, Brox T. U-net: convolutional networks for biomedical image segmentation. International conference on medical image computing and computer-assisted intervention. 9351. Cham: Springer; 2015. p. 234–41.

11. Oskal KRJ, Risdal M, Janssen EAM, Undersrud ES, Gulsrud TO. A U-net based approach to epidermal tissue segmentation in whole slide histopathological images. SN Appl Sci. 2019;1(7):672.

12. Schmitz R, Madesta F, Nielsen M, Werner R, Rösch T. Multi-scale fully convolutional neural networks for histopathology image segmentation: from nuclear aberrations to the global tissue architecture. arXiv preprint arXiv. 2019;1909.10726.

13. Dong N, Kampffmeyer M, Liang X, Wang Z, Dai W, Xing E. Reinforced auto-zoom net: towards accurate and fast breast cancer segmentation in whole-slide images. Deep learning in medical image analysis and multimodal learning for clinical decision support. Cham: Springer; 2018. p. 317–25.

14. Mehta S, Mercan E, Bartlett J, Weave D, Elmore J, Shapiro L. Y-Net: joint segmentation and classification for diagnosis of breast biopsy images. In: International conference on medical image computing and computer-assisted intervention. Cham: Springer; 2018. p. 893–901.

15. Priego-Torres BM, Sanchez-Morillo D, Fernandez-Granero MA, Garcia-Rojo M. Automatic segmentation of whole-slide H&E stained breast histopathology images using a deep convolutional neural network architecture. Expert Syst Appl. 2020;151:113387.

16. Cortes C, Vapnik V. Support-vector networks. Chem Biol Drug Des. 2009;297:273–97.

17. Ho TK. Random decision forests. In: Proceedings of 3rd International Conference on Document Analysis and Recognition, Montreal, Quebec, Canada; 1995. p. 278–82.

18. Ren M, editor. Learning a classification model for segmentation. In: Proceedings Ninth IEEE International Conference on Computer Vision; 2003. 13–16 Oct. 2003.

19. Xing F, Yang L. Robust nucleus/cell detection and segmentation in digital pathology and microscopy images: a comprehensive review. IEEE Rev Biomed Eng. 2016;9:234–63.

20. Hansen S, Kuttner S, Kampffmeyer M, Markussen T-V, Sundset R, Øen SK, et al. Unsupervised supervoxel-based lung tumor segmentation across patient scans in hybrid PET/MRI. Expert Syst Appl. 2021;167:114244.

21. Bejnordi BE, Litjens G, Hermsen M, Karssemeijer N, van der Laak JA. A multi-scale superpixel classification approach to the detection of regions of interest in whole slide histopathology images. In: SPIE Medical Imaging 2015. 9420: International Society for Optics and Photonics; 2015. p. 94200H.

22. Beucher S, Lantuéjoul C. Use of Watersheds in Contour Detection. In: International workshop on image processing, real-time edge and motion detection. 1979.

23. Zucker SW. Region growing: childhood and adolescence. Comput Graph Image Proc. 1976;5(3):382–99.

24. Osher S, Sethian JA. Fronts propagating with curvature-dependent speed: algorithms based on Hamilton-Jacobi formulations. J Comput Phys. 1988;79(1):12–49.

25. Bianconi F, Kather JN, Reyes-Aldasoro CC. Evaluation of colour pre-processing on patch-based classification of H&E-stained images. In: Reyes-Aldasoro CC, Janowczyk A, Veta M, Bankhead P, Sirinukunwattana K, editors. European congress on digital pathology. Cham: Springer; 2019. p. 56–64.

26. Tellez D, Litjens G, Bándi P, Bulten W, Bokhorst J-M, Ciompi F, et al. Quantifying the effects of data augmentation and stain color normalization in convolutional neural networks for computational pathology. Med Image Anal. 2019;58:101544.

27. Bankhead P, Fernandez JA, McArt DG, Boyle DP, Li G, Loughrey MB, et al. Integrated tumor identification and automated scoring minimizes pathologist involvement and provides new insights to key biomarkers in breast cancer. Lab Investig. 2018;98(1):15–26.

28. Aresta G, Araújo T, Kwok S, Chennamsetty SS, Safwan M, Alex V, et al. BACH: grand challenge on breast cancer histology images. Med Image Anal. 2019;56:122–39.

29. Karim M, Beyan O, Zappa A, Costa I, Rebholz-Schuhman D, Cochez M, et al. Deep learning-based clustering approaches for bioinformatics. Brief Bioinform. 2020;22:393–415.

30. Chenni W, Herbi H, Babaie M, Tizhoosh HR. Patch clustering for representation of histopathology images. European congress on digital pathology. Cham: Springer; 2019. p. 28–37.

31. Abbet C, Zlobec I, Bozorgtabar B, Thiran J-P. Divide-and-rule: self-supervised learning for survival analysis in colorectal cancer. In: Martel AL, Abolmaesumi P, Stoyanov D, Mateus D, Zuluaga MA, Zhou SK, et al., editors. International conference on medical image computing and computer-assisted intervention. Cham: Springer; 2020. p. 480–9.

32. Li MWL, Wiliem A, Zhao K, Zhang T, Lovell B. Deep instance-level hard negative mining model for histopathology images. In: International conference on medical image computing and computer-assisted intervention, vol. 11764. Cham: Springer; 2019. p. 514–22.

33. Tomita N, Abdollahi B, Wei J, Ren B, Suriawinata A, Hassanpour S. Finding a Needle in the Haystack: Attention-Based Classification of High Resolution Microscopy Images. arXiv preprint arXiv. 2018:1811.08513.

34. Ilse M, Tomczak J, Welling M. Attention-based deep multiple instance learning. In: International conference on machine learning: PMLR; 2018. p. 2127–2136.

35. Keeler J, Rumelhart D, Leow WK. Integrated Segmentation and Recognition of Hand-Printed Numerals: Microelectronics and Computer Technology Corporation; 1991.

36. Sudharshan PJ, Petitjean C, Spanhol F, Oliveira L, Heutte L, Honeine P. Multiple instance learning for histopathological breast cancer image classification. Expert Syst Appl. 2018;117:103–11.

37. Wang S, Zhu Y, Yu L, Chen H, Lin H, Wan X, et al. RMDL: recalibrated multi-instance deep learning for whole slide gastric image classification. Med Image Anal. 2019;58:101549.

38. Hanahan D, Weinberg RA. Hallmarks of cancer: the next generation. Cell. 2011;144(5):646–74.

39. Lakhani SR, Ellis IO, Schnitt SJ, Tan PH, van de Vijver MJ, editors. WHO classification of Tumours of the breast. 4th ed. Lyon: International Agency for Research on Cancer (IARC); 2012.

40. Coates AS, Winer EP, Goldhirsch A, Gelber RD, Gnant M, Piccart-Gebhart M, et al. Tailoring therapies-improving the management of early breast cancer: St Gallen international expert consensus on the primary therapy of early breast cancer 2015. Ann Oncol. 2015;26(8):1533–46.

41. Parker JS, Mullins M, Cheang MC, Leung S, Voduc D, Vickery T, et al. Supervised risk predictor of breast cancer based on intrinsic subtypes. J Clin Oncol. 2009;27(8):1160–7.

42. Beck AH, Sangoi AR, Leung S, Marinelli RJ, Nielsen TO, van de Vijver MJ, et al. Systematic analysis of breast cancer morphology uncovers stromal features associated with survival. Sci Transl Med 2011;3(108):108ra13.

43. Balkenhol MCA, Tellez D, Vreuls W, Clahsen PC, Pinckaers H, Ciompi F, et al. Deep learning assisted mitotic counting for breast cancer. Lab Investig. 2019;99(11):1596–606.

44. Huang HS, Su HY, Li PH, Chiang PH, Huang CH, Chen CH, et al. Prognostic impact of tumor infiltrating lymphocytes on patients with metastatic urothelial carcinoma receiving platinum based chemotherapy. Sci Rep. 2018;8(1):7485.

45. Wang B, Wu S, Zeng H, Liu Z, Dong W, He W, et al. CD103+ tumor infiltrating lymphocytes predict a favorable prognosis in urothelial cell carcinoma of the bladder. J Urol. 2015;194(2):556–62.

46. Sharma P, Shen Y, Wen S, Yamada S, Jungbluth AA, Gnjatic S, et al. CD8 tumor-infiltrating lymphocytes are predictive of survival in muscle-invasive urothelial carcinoma. Proc Natl Acad Sci U S A. 2007;104(10):3967–72.

47. Krpina K, Babarovic E, Dordevic G, Fuckar Z, Jonjic N. The association between the recurrence of solitary nonmuscle invasive bladder cancer and tumor infiltrating lymphocytes. Croat Med J. 2012;53(6):598–604.

48. Zhu X, Ma LL, Ye T. Expression of CD4(+)CD25(high) CD127(low/−) regulatory T cells in transitional cell carcinoma patients and its significance. J Clin Lab Anal. 2009;23(4):197–201.

49. Parodi A, Traverso P, Kalli F, Conteduca G, Tardito S, Curto M, et al. Residual tumor micro-foci and overwhelming regulatory T lymphocyte infiltration are the causes of bladder cancer recurrence. Oncotarget. 2016;7(6):6424–35.

50. Wetteland R, Engan K, Eftestøl T, Kvikstad V, Janssen EAM. A multiscale approach for whole-slide image segmentation of five tissue classes in urothelial carcinoma slides. Technol Cancer Res Treat. 2020;19:1–15.

51. Hosseini MS, Chan L, Tse G, Tang M, Deng J, Norouzi S, et al. Atlas of digital pathology: a generalized hierarchical histological tissue type-annotated database for deep learning. In: Proceedings of the IEEE/CVF Conference on Computer Vision and Pattern Recognition; 2019. p. 11747–11756.

52. Evangeline IK, Precious JG, Pazhanivel N, Kirubha SPA. Automatic detection and counting of lymphocytes from immunohistochemistry cancer images using deep learning. J Med Biol Eng. 2020;40(5):735–47.

53. Yoo SP, Park HE, Kim JH, Wen X, Jeong S, Cho NY, et al. Whole-slide image analysis reveals quantitative landscape of tumor-immune microenvironment in colorectal cancers. Clin Cancer Res. 2020;26(4):870–81.

54. Amgad M, Stovgaard ES, Balslev E, Thagaard J, Chen W, Dudgeon S, et al. Report on computational assessment of tumor infiltrating lymphocytes from the international Immuno-oncology biomarker working group. Npj Breast Cancer. 2020;6(1)

55. Baak JPA. The framework of pathology: good laboratory practice by quantitative and molecular methods. J Pathol. 2002;198(3):277–83.

56. Galon J, Costes A, Sanchez-Cabo F, Kirilovsky A, Mlecnik B, Lagorce-Pagès C, et al. Type, density, and location of immune cells within human colorectal tumors predict clinical outcome. Science. 2006;313(5795):1960–4.

57. Benchaaben A, Guimaraes M, Prestat E, Kassambara A, Filah IM, Laugé C, et al. Immunoscore workflow enhanced by Artificial Intelligence (Poster) 2020 [cited 2021 02.15]. Available from: https://www.haliodx.com/fileadmin/pdf/Poster_AACR_2020_AI_200605.pdf.

58. Saltz J, Gupta R, Hou L, Kurc T, Singh P, Nguyen V, et al. Spatial organization and molecular correlation of tumor-infiltrating lymphocytes using deep learning on pathology images. Cell Rep. 2018;23(1):181–93.e7.

59. AbdulJabbar K, Raza SEA, Rosenthal R, Jamal-Hanjani M, Veeriah S, Akarca A, et al. Geospatial immune variability illuminates differential evolution of lung adenocarcinoma. Nat Med. 2020;26(7):1054–62.

60. Bailly AL DC, Filahi M, Martirosyan A, Kassambara A, Perbost R, Girardi H, Sbarrato T, Fieschi J. Unravelling the mystery of Cancer Associated Fibroblasts (CAFs) populations in the tumor microenvironment by fully automated sequential chromogenic multiplex assay (Poster) 2020 [cited 2021 02.15]. Available from: https://www.haliodx.com/fileadmin/pdf/Poster_CAF__AACR2020.pdf.

61. Kruger K, Stefansson IM, Collett K, Arnes JB, Aas T, Akslen LA. Microvessel proliferation by co-expression of endothelial nestin and Ki-67 is associated with a basal-like phenotype and aggressive features in breast cancer. Breast. 2013;22(3):282–8.

62. Arnes JB, Stefansson IM, Straume O, Baak JP, Lonning PE, Foulkes WD, et al. Vascular proliferation is a prognostic factor in breast cancer. Breast Cancer Res Treat. 2012;133(2):501–10.

63. Stefansson IM, Salvesen HB, Akslen LA. Vascular proliferation is important for clinical progress of endometrial cancer. Cancer Res. 2006;66(6):3303–9.

64. Gravdal K, Halvorsen OJ, Haukaas SA, Akslen LA. Proliferation of immature tumor vessels is a novel marker of clinical progression in prostate cancer. Cancer Res. 2009;69(11):4708–15.

65. Ramnefjell M, Aamelfot C, Aziz S, Helgeland L, Akslen LA. Microvascular proliferation is associated with aggressive tumour features and reduced survival in lung adenocarcinoma. J Pathol Clin Res. 2017;3(4):249–57.

66. Weidner N, Semple JP, Welch WR, Folkman J. Tumor angiogenesis and metastasis--correlation in invasive breast carcinoma. N Engl J Med. 1991;324(1):1–8.

67. Mete M, Hennings L, Spencer HJ, Topaloglu U. Automatic identification of angiogenesis in double stained images of liver tissue. BMC Bioinf. 2009;10(11):S13.

68. Kather JN, Marx A, Reyes-Aldasoro CC, Schad LR, Zöllner FG, Weis C-A. Continuous representation of tumor microvessel density and detection of angiogenic hotspots in histological whole-slide images. Oncotarget. 2015;6(22):19163–76.

69. Chantrain CF, DeClerck YA, Groshen S, McNamara G. Computerized quantification of tissue vascularization using high-resolution slide scanning of whole tumor sections. J Histochem Cytochem. 2003;51(2):151–8.

70. van Niekerk CG, van der Laak JA, Börger ME, Huisman HJ, Witjes JA, Barentsz JO, et al. Computerized whole slide quantification shows increased microvascular density in pT2 prostate cancer as compared to normal prostate tissue. Prostate. 2009;69(1):62–9.

71. Yi F, Yang L, Wang S, Guo L, Huang C, Xie Y, et al. Microvessel prediction in H&E Stained Pathology Images using fully convolutional neural networks. BMC Bioinf. 2018;19(1):64.

72. Basavanhally A, Feldman M, Shih N, Mies C, Tomaszewski J, Ganesan S, et al. Multi-field-of-view strategy for image-based outcome prediction of multi-parametric estrogen receptor-positive breast cancer histopathology: comparison to oncotype DX. J Pathol Inform. 2011;2:S1.

73. Fraz MM, Khurram SA, Graham S, Shaban M, Hassan M, Loya A, et al. FABnet: feature attention-based network for simultaneous segmentation of microvessels and nerves in routine histology images of oral cancer. Neural Comput & Applic. 2020;32(14):9915–28.

74. Nalisnik M, Amgad M, Lee S, Halani SH, Velazquez Vega JE, Brat DJ, et al. Interactive phenotyping of large-scale histology imaging data with HistomicsML. Sci Rep. 2017;7(1):14588.

75. Bejnordi BE, Mullooly M, Pfeiffer RM, Fan S, Vacek PM, Weaver DL, et al. Using deep convolutional neural networks to identify and classify tumor-associated stroma in diagnostic breast biopsies. Mod Pathol. 2018;31(10):1502–12.

76. Northey JJ, Barrett AS, Acerbi I, Hayward M-K, Talamantes S, Dean IS, et al. Stiff stroma increases breast cancer risk by inducing the oncogene ZNF217. J Clin Invest. 2020;130(11):5721–37.

77. Zhao K, Li Z, Yao S, Wang Y, Wu X, Xu Z, et al. Artificial intelligence quantified tumour-stroma ratio is an independent predictor for overall survival in resectable colorectal cancer. EBioMedicine. 2020;61:103054.

78. Kather JNKJ, Charoentong P, Luedde T, Herpel E, Weis C-A, Gaiser T, Marx A, Valous NA, Ferber D, Jansen L, Reyes-Aldasoro CC, Zörnig I, Jäger D, Brenner H, Chang-Claude J, Hoffmeister M, Halama N. Predicting survival from colorectal cancer histology slides using deep learning: a retrospective multicenter study. PLoS Med. 2019;16(1):e1002730.

79. Siregar P, Julen N, Hufnagl P, Mutter GL. Computational morphogenesis – embryogenesis, cancer research and digital pathology. Biosystems. 2018;169–170:40–54.

80. Mobadersany P, Yousefi S, Amgad M, Gutman DA, Barnholtz-Sloan JS, Velazquez Vega JE, et al. Predicting cancer outcomes from histology and genomics using convolutional networks. Proc Natl Acad Sci U S A. 2018;115(13):E2970–E9.

81. Meier A, Nekolla K, Hewitt LC, Earle S, Yoshikawa T, Oshima T, et al. Hypothesis-free deep survival learning applied to the tumour microenvironment in gastric cancer. J Pathol Clin Res. 2020;6(4):273–82.

82. Skrede OJ, De Raedt S, Kleppe A, Hveem TS, Liestol K, Maddison J, et al. Deep learning for prediction of colorectal cancer outcome: a discovery and validation study. Lancet. 2020;395(10221):350–60.

83. Bychkov D, Linder N, Turkki R, Nordling S, Kovanen PE, Verrill C, et al. Deep learning based tissue analysis predicts outcome in colorectal cancer. Sci Rep. 2018;8(1):3395.

84. Turkki R, Byckhov D, Lundin M, Isola J, Nordling S, Kovanen PE, et al. Breast cancer outcome prediction with tumour tissue images and machine learning. Breast Cancer Res Treat. 2019;177(1):41–52.

85. Chen JM, Qu AP, Wang LW, Yuan JP, Yang F, Xiang QM, et al. New breast cancer prognostic factors identified by computer-aided image analysis of HE stained histopathology images. Sci Rep. 2015;5:10690.

86. Yu KH, Zhang C, Berry GJ, Altman RB, Re C, Rubin DL, et al. Predicting non-small cell lung cancer prognosis by fully automated microscopic pathology image features. Nat Commun. 2016;7:12474.

87. Wulczyn E, Steiner DF, Xu Z, Sadhwani A, Wang H, Flament-Auvigne I, et al. Deep learning-based survival prediction for multiple cancer types using histopathology images. PLoS One. 2020;15(6):e0233678.

88. Yao J, Zhu X, Jonnagaddala J, Hawkins N, Huang J. Whole slide images based cancer survival prediction using attention guided deep multiple instance learning networks. Med Image Anal. 2020;65:101789.

89. Courtiol P, Maussion C, Moarii M, Pronier E, Pilcer S, Sefta M, et al. Deep learning-based classification of mesothelioma improves prediction of patient outcome. Nat Med. 2019;25(10):1519–25.

90. Wu CX, Lin GS, Lin ZX, Zhang JD, Liu SY, Zhou CF. Peritumoral edema shown by MRI predicts poor clinical outcome in glioblastoma. World J Surg Oncol. 2015;13:97.

91. Samek W, Binder A, Montavon G, Lapuschkin S, Muller KR. Evaluating the visualization of what a deep neural network has learned. IEEE Trans Neural Netw Learn Syst. 2017;28(11):2660–73.

92. Montavon G, Samek W, Müller K-R. Methods for interpreting and understanding deep neural networks. Digital Signal Proc. 2018;73:1–15.

93. Lundberg SM, Lee SI. A Unified Approach to Interpreting Model Predictions. arXiv preprint arXiv. 2017:1705.07874.

94. Ribeiro M, Singh S, Guestrin C. "Why Should I Trust You?": Explaining the Predictions of Any Classifier; 2016. 97–101 p.

95. Selvaraju RR, Cogswell M, Das A, Vedantam R, Parikh D, Batra D. Grad-CAM: Visual Explanations from Deep Networks via Gradient-Based Localization. Proceedings of the IEEE international conference on computer vision; 2017. p. 618–26.

96. Quinlan JR. Induction of Decision Trees: CiteCeerX; 1986 [cited 2021 02.15]. Available from: http://citeseerx.ist.psu.edu/viewdoc/similar?doi=10.1.1.167.3624&type=cc.

97. Philips IntelliSite Pathology Solution 2021 [cited 2021 02.15]. Available from: https://www.philips.no/healthcare/resources/landing/philips-intellisite-pathology-solution.

98. Marée R, Rollus L, Stévens B, Hoyoux R, Louppe G, Vandaele R, et al. Collaborative analysis of multi-gigapixel imaging data using Cytomine. Bioinformatics (Oxford, England). 2016;32(9):1395–401.

99. Aiforia [cited 2021 02.15]. Available from: https://www.aiforia.com/.

100. Bankhead P, Loughrey MB, Fernandez JA, Dombrowski Y, McArt DG, Dunne PD, et al. QuPath: open source software for digital pathology image analysis. Sci Rep. 2017;7(1):16878.

101. Stritt M, Stalder A, Vezzali E. Orbit image analysis: an open-source whole slide image analysis tool. PLoS Comput Biol. 2020;16(2):e1007313.

102. Pedersen A, Valla M, Bofin A, Frutos J, Reinertsen I, Smistad E. FastPathology: An open-source platform for deep learning-based research and decision support in digital pathology. arXiv preprint arXiv. 2020:2011.06033.

Clinical Applications: Organ Related Studies of Biomarkers and Therapy

The Tumor and Its Microenvironment as Complementary Sources of Cancer Biomarkers

Roopali Roy, Emily Man, Rama Aldakhlallah, Emma Rashes, and Marsha A. Moses

Abstract

The continuing success of the field of cancer research in elucidating the mechanisms that regulate solid tumor development, growth, and progression has provided an extraordinary opportunity to leverage this information to develop novel traditional and precision medicines for a variety of human cancers. Within this context, the discovery and validation of sensitive, accurate, and readily translatable cancer biomarkers have never been more essential. The expanding utility of such biomarkers includes, but is not limited to, risk assessment, early detection, determination of cancer status and stage, monitoring therapeutic efficacy, development of resistance and patient stratification and selection among other uses. Until relatively recently, it has been the tumor epithelial compartment that has been the focus and the source of the majority of cancer biomarkers despite the critical role of the tumor microenvironment (TME) in influencing cancer outcome. Here, we intentionally focus on the TME as a source of biomarkers for a wide variety of human cancers. We comprehensively review the key biological components of the TME and their importance in human cancers, we present and extensively discuss the validated TME-derived biomarkers to date including their applications and sample sources and we provide up-to-date information with respect to their current clinical status.

Take-Home Lessons

- Biomarkers are measurable in body fluids and tissues and serve as indicators of health and disease status.
- Common cancer biomarkers include proteins, nucleic acids, metabolites, lipids, extracellular vesicles/exosomes, microRNAs, immune cells and others.
- Biomarkers from solid tumors and the surrounding tumor microenvironment (TME) can serve as diagnostic, prognostic, and predictive tools for cancer.
- The complex TME affects tumor biology, development, progression, therapeutic response and resistance and may be a useful target for both cancer diagnostics and therapy.
- Clinical applications of markers from the tumor and its TME extend across early detection, risk assessment, patient stratification, recurrence prediction and therapeutic efficacy.

Introduction

The field of biomarker medicine has been foundational to the development of successful cancer therapeutics, diagnostics, and prognostics. Multiple approaches to biomarker discovery and validation continue to be utilized and have been extensively reviewed by our group and others [1–5]. As noted above, there are several unmet biomarker needs with respect to cancer detection and subsequent treatment including early and accurate disease detection, risk assessment, reliable monitoring of therapeutic efficacy and resistance and the ability to determine which patient populations will most benefit from a particular therapy, among other uses.

Emily Man and Rama Aldakhlallah contributed equally.

R. Roy · M. A. Moses (✉)
Vascular Biology Program, Boston Children's Hospital, Boston, MA, USA

Department of Surgery, Harvard Medical School and Boston Children's Hospital, Boston, MA, USA
e-mail: roopali.roy@childrens.harvard.edu;
marsha.moses@childrens.harvard.edu

E. Man · R. Aldakhlallah · E. Rashes
Vascular Biology Program, Boston Children's Hospital, Boston, MA, USA

L. A. Akslen, R. S. Watnick (eds.), *Biomarkers of the Tumor Microenvironment*, https://doi.org/10.1007/978-3-030-98950-7_22

The important contribution of the TME to the development of cancer diagnostics and prognostics has been, to date, overshadowed by that of biomarkers derived from the tumor epithelium despite the fact that it is now well recognized that the complex microenvironment of solid tumors plays a crucial role in cancer development and progression. The TME is a dynamic and complex system composed of a variety of components that are produced and/or are recruited by the cancer cells during tumor progression. These components include the tumor vasculature, immune cells, fibroblasts, adipocytes, extracellular matrix (ECM) components, and a variety of secreted factors (Fig. 22.1). The TME affects solid tumor biology, development and progression, as well as therapeutic response and resistance. For these reasons, an appreciation of the TME is essential to our understanding of tumor development and progression as well to the identification of novel

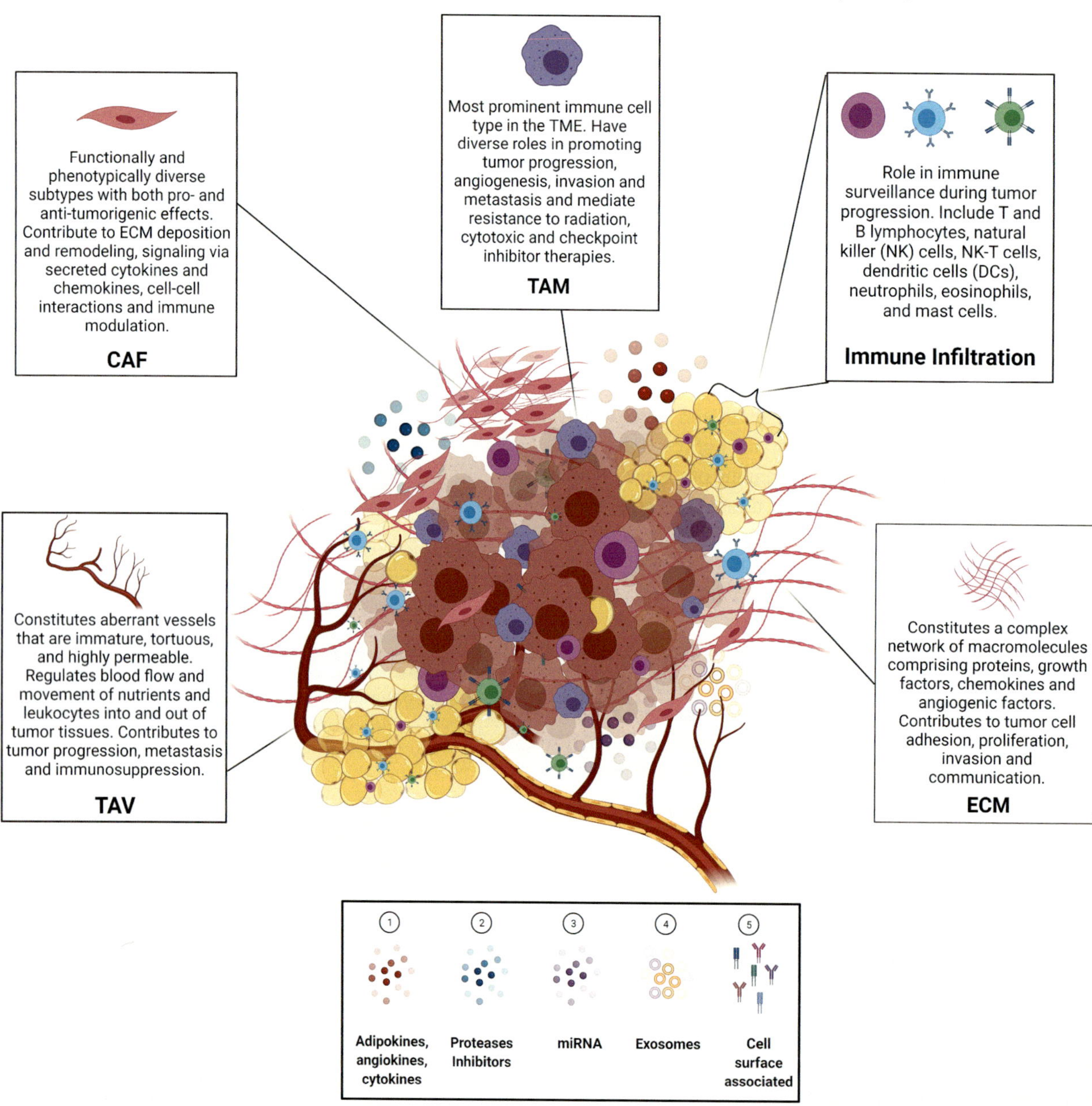

Fig. 22.1 The TME is a dynamic system containing a variety of components that are recruited and/or produced by the cancer cells during tumor establishment and maintenance including blood vessels (tumor vasculature; TAV), immune cells (Immune Infiltration), fibroblasts (CAF), adipocytes, extracellular matrix (ECM) components and regulators and a variety of secreted factors. The complex TME of solid tumors plays a crucial role in cancer development, progression and in modulating therapeutic responses and resistance mechanisms. Created with Biorender.com

and effective methods of cancer diagnosis and therapy. In addition, the targeting of the TME, its cellular components as well as TME-associated biomarkers represents potential therapeutic benefits for cancer patients as well.

The clinical necessity of accurate and easily translatable cancer biomarkers of all types is indisputable and the growing number of potential biomarker candidates associated with the TME, complemented by those derived from the tumor epithelium, hold the promise for early cancer detection, more instructive accurate monitoring of therapeutic efficacy and resistance and a number of other required elements of successful cancer diagnostics and prognostics. In this Chapter, we have provided a comprehensive overview of the predominant biological components of the TME with respect to their importance in human cancers and we present and extensively discuss current, validated TME-derived biomarkers across a large number of cancer types along with their sample sources, their potential clinical applications and the current status of those that have reached the stage of FDA clinical trial validation.

Fibroblasts

Cancer-associated fibroblasts (CAF) are key components of the TME and have diverse functions that include ECM deposition and remodeling, signaling, cell-cell interactions and immune modulation. CAFs can be phenotypically and functionally diverse with distinct subtypes that may have both pro- or anti-tumorigenic functions [6]. Soluble secreted factors from CAFs can influence tumor progression. For example, vascular endothelial growth factor (VEGF) expression by stromal cells has been shown to drive tumor angiogenesis [7]. Cytokines and chemokines produced by CAFs can also affect a range of immune cells such as leukocytes, T cells and macrophages and may exert both immunosuppressive or immunopromoting effects [8]. CAFs, therefore, may serve as both a source of biomarkers for cancer detection and prognosis as well as represent potential targets for therapeutic anticancer strategies.

Endothelium

The endothelium plays an important role in tumor initiation, progression, and metastasis. In normal tissues, an organized and efficient vascular endothelium regulates blood flow and the bidirectional movement of nutrients and leukocytes. In proliferating tumors, an overexpression of a variety of proangiogenic factors leads to the development of a distinct tumor-associated vasculature (TAV) characterized by disorganized aberrant vascular networks, immature and tortuous vessels and increased permeability [9–13]. Within the hypoxic,

nutrient-deprived TME of a rapidly growing tumor, increased autophagy of the dysfunctional endothelial cells lining the blood vessels may further promote a pathological angiogenic cascade [14]. The TAV plays a significant role in tumor cell intravasation, an important component of metastasis and may also promote immunoevasion by actively suppressing the recruitment, adhesion, and activity of T cells to the tumor [15]. These unique features of the TAV have made it an attractive target of selective therapeutic intervention for a variety of cancers.

Immune Infiltration

Immune infiltration of tumors has been reported to contribute to the prediction of clinical outcomes. For several types of cancer, the composition of tumor-infiltrating immune cells (TIICs) can serve as novel targets for therapy as well as being important biomarkers for monitoring therapeutic response [16], predicting risk of recurrence and informing patient survival [17, 18]. TIIC include macrophages, T and B lymphocytes, natural killer (NK) cells, NK-T cells, dendritic cells (DCs), neutrophils, eosinophils, and mast cells.

Macrophages are the most prominent immune cell type in the TME and have diverse functions linked to cancer development, progression, and angiogenesis [19–21]. Tumor-associated macrophages (TAM) can augment, mediate and/or antagonize the antitumor activity of radiation therapy, cytotoxic agents, and checkpoint inhibitors [22]. TAMs have been shown to induce tumor angiogenesis [23–25] and support tumor migration, invasion, and proliferation through the production of various molecules, such as VEGF [26, 27]. Studies have also revealed that macrophages can assist circulating cancer cells in extravasating to distant sites, leading to metastases [28].

Extracellular Matrix (ECM)

The extracellular matrix (ECM) plays a key role in cancer development and progression and constitutes a versatile scaffold composed of a network of proteins such as glycosaminoglycans, fibrous proteins such as collagen, laminin, fibronectin, elastin, growth factors, angiogenic factors and chemokines that interact with cell surface receptors [29]. Importantly, the ECM influences tumor cell adhesion, proliferation, migration, and communication [19, 30]. The ECM is characterized by its biochemical composition as well as biophysical characteristics including topography, density, and elasticity. The ECM undergoes remodeling by tumor cells, CAFs, and other component cells of the TME as well as factors such as matrix metalloproteinases (MMPs) to release chemokines, growth and angiogenic factors to modify and support the TME [1, 2, 31–34]. The ECM of both the stromal and epithelial compartments of a tumor is modified by the activity of ECM-degrading proteases such the MMPs and ADAMs (A Disintegrin And Metalloprotease), which themselves are controlled by their endogenous inhibitors, the tissue inhibitors of metalloproteinases (TIMP) along with other factors [35–38].

Cancer Diagnostics and Prognostics

Here, we review the current status of biomarkers from the tumor and the tumor microenvironment (TME) with respect to cancer diagnosis, prognosis, disease progression, and therapeutic efficacy (Table 22.1). Studies have been included here if their sample numbers studied were $n = 50$ or greater with the exception of cancers where published sample sizes were limited as a function of lower prevalence of disease.

Breast Cancer

Breast cancer (BC) is the most common cancer in women in the USA (seer.cancer.gov) as well as globally [166]. In the early stages of breast cancer, cancer cells localize within the breast tissue and the tumors are identified as being "in situ"

(e.g., ductal carcinoma in situ). Subsequently, in more advanced stages, cancer cells invade into the neighboring tissues and lymph nodes and, at the most malignant stage, metastasize to distant organs, such as bone, lung, and brain. Early detection and subtype-specific therapy for BC can significantly improve patient prognosis, with >90% 5-yr survival rates being observed for patients diagnosed with Stage I and II BC (seer.cancer.gov). However, survival is considerably lower for Stage IV disease (~26%) or for certain BC subtypes, ~77% for triple-negative breast cancer (TNBC) and ~75% for Her2+ BC, respectively [167]. Mammography and MRI approaches are the current gold standard for BC detection, however, the sensitivity and specificity of mammography can be low for young women and women with dense breast tissue [168]. Therefore, novel and effective methods of BC diagnosis and prognosis are urgently needed. We have previously reviewed the potential of MMP/ADAM biomarkers for the detection of BC [1, 2, 73]. Here we will focus on biomarkers originating from the breast tumor and its TME (Table 22.1).

While BC is not considered to be highly immunogenic, the impact of the immune landscape of the TME on BC progression is currently an intense area of investigation. High levels of tumor-infiltrating lymphocytes (TILs) are most commonly found in HER2+ and TNBC tumors and are associated with a good prognosis and response to the anti-HER2

Table 22.1 Biomarkers of the tumor and its microenvironment

Cancer	Application	Biomarker	Sample Type	References
Breast	Prognostic	ADAM12, MMP-9	Tissue, urine	[2, 39–41]
		MMP-9	Tissue, serum	[42]
		CD68, CD163, MMP-9	Tissue	[43]
		PD-L1, CD8	Tissue	[44]
		TIL	Tissue	[45–47]
	Diagnostic	MMP-9, MMP-9/NGAL	Urine	[1, 48, 49]
		MMP-7, MMP-26, CA15-3	Plasma	[50]
		miR-99a-5p	Plasma	[51]
	Predictive	miR-18b, miR-103, miR-107, miR-652	Serum	[52]
Lung	Prognostic	*EGFR, BRAF-ALK, ROS1-RTK*	Tissue	[53]
	Diagnostic	TP63, keratin 5, CECAM6, SFTPB	Serum	[54]
		NSE	Serum	[55]
		CYFRA21-1	Plasma	[56]
	Predictive	IL-18	Serum	[57]
		ProGRP	Tissue	[58]
		LKB1	Tissue	[59]
Prostate	Prognostic	MMP-1, MMP-9, TIMP-2	Tissue	[2, 60]
		MMP-2, MMP-7, MMP-11	Serum	[61–63]
		ADAM15	Tissue	[64]
		Cav-1	Tissue	[65, 66]
		miR-205	Tissue	[67]
		IL-6, IL-8, TNF-α, CCL2	Serum	[68–70]
	Diagnostic	MMP-2, VEGF	Serum	[1, 48, 71, 72]
		β2M, PGA3, MUC3	Urine	[3, 73, 74]
		ADAM12	Serum, urine	[75]
		AR, PR	Tissue	[76]
		ASPN	Tissue	[77]
		SFRP4	Tissue	[78]

Table 22.1 (continued)

Cancer	Application	Biomarker	Sample Type	References
Pancreatic	Prognostic	Cav-1, FASN	Tissue	[79, 80]
		ADAM12	Tissue, serum, urine	[81–83]
	Diagnostic	VEGF	Blood	[84]
		MMP-7, CCN2, IGFBP2, TSP-2, sICAM1, TIMP-1, PLG	Plasma	[85]
		TFPI, TNC-FNII-C, CA19-9	Plasma	[86]
		LIF	Tissue, serum	[87]
		miR-3940/miR-8069	Urine	[88]
		MMP-2, TIMP-1	Urine	[2, 89]
		LYVE-1, REG1B, TFF1	Urine	[90]
Ovarian	Prognostic	TEM8	Tissue	[91]
		S100A1	Tissue	[92]
		YKL-40	Serum	[93]
	Diagnostic	MMP-2, MMP-9, NGAL	Urine, ascitic fluid	[2, 94, 95]
		ADAM17, ADAM12	Tissue, serum	[96–99]
		VEGF	Serum	[100]
		HE4	Serum, plasma	[101–104]
	Predictive	IL-6	Tissue, plasma	[105, 106]
		NLR	Blood	[107]
Liver	Prognostic	VASP	Tissue	[108]
		MMP-9	Tissue	[109]
		ST2	Serum	[110]
		VEGFR-1	Tissue	[111]
		GPC3, AFP	Cytoplasm	[112]
		MDK	Serum	[113]
		miR-18b	Tissue	[114]
	Diagnostic	GPC3, AFP	Cytoplasm	[112]
		miR-92a-3p, miR-107, miR-3126-5p	Tissue	[115]
	Predictive	VASP	Tissue	[109]
		MMP-2, MMP-9	Tissue	[109]
		sVEGFR-1, VEGF, bFGF, CD3, CD4, Treg, CD56, IL-6, s-MET	Plasma	[116]
		VEGF, Ang-2, bFGF	Plasma	[117]
		FGF19	Tissue	[118]
		MDK	Serum	[113]
		miR-18b, miR-92a-3p, miR-107, miR-3126-5p	Tissue	[114, 115]
Gastric	Prognostic	PAK6	Tissue	[119]
		ADAMTS-2	Tissue	[120]
		COL12A1	Tissue	[121]
		CD163	Tissue	[122]
		KLK10	Urine	[123]
	Diagnostic	MMP-9/NGAL, MMP-9, ADAM12	Urine	[124]
		TFF1, ADAM12, *H. pylori*	Urine	[125]
		miR-6807-5p, miR-6856-5p, *H. pylori*	Urine	[126]
		FAP-α	Tissue	[119]
	Predictive	Ki-67, TS, COX2, ERCC1, P21	Tissue	[119]
Kidney	Prognostic	TuM2PK	Plasma	[127]
		TGF-α, VEGFR-2, TNF-RII	Plasma	[128]
		CXCL7	Plasma	[129]
		CAIX	Tissue	[130, 131]
		MVD	Tissue	[132]
	Predictive	Ang-2, MMP-2	Serum, plasma	[127, 133, 134]
		MMP-9	Serum	[135]
		IL-8, IL-9, IL-2Rα, PDGF-AA, TNF-RI, TNF-α	Plasma	[128]
		CXCL10	Serum, plasma	[128, 133]

(continued)

Table 22.1 (continued)

Cancer	Application	Biomarker	Sample Type	References
Brain	Prognostic	OPN	Tissue, serum, plasma	[136]
		miR-340-5p, CD163, POSTN, LIBP1, HMGA-2	Tissue	[137]
		MMP-2, MMP-9, MMP-2/TIMP-1	Tissue, blood, cytoplasm	[138–140]
		AREG	Serum	[141]
	Diagnostic	BMP2, HSP70, CXC, CXCL10	Serum	[142]
		CD163, CD70, CD3	Tissue	[143]
	Predictive	MMP-9	Tissue	[138]
Brain (Pediatric)	Prognostic	CTC	Blood, CSF	[144]
	Diagnostic	MMP-2, MMP-9, MMP-9/NGAL, VEGF	Tissue, urine, CSF	[144, 145]
		bFGF, TIMP-3	Urine	[146]
		Neogenin, netrin-1	Urine	[147]
		Netrin-1, bFGF, MMP-3, TIMP-1	Urine	[148]
	Predictive	MMP-9, TIMP-1, MMP-13	Urine	[148]
Neuroblastoma (Pediatric)	Prognostic	*MYCN*	Blood	[149]
		USP17L5, SLC25A5, POF1B, RND3, KLC4, SLC12A1	Genetic	[150]
		Cell-free DNA	Plasma	[151, 152]
		TH, PHOX2B, DCX	Blood, bone marrow	[153]
		miR-29c, miR-342-3p, let-7b	Plasma	[154, 155]
		Catecholamines, VMA, HVA	Urine	[156]
		LDH, ferritin	Serum	[156, 157]
		NSE	Serum	[158]
	Predictive	*MYCN,* ALK, TrkB, GD2	Genetic	[159]
Wilms' Tumor (Pediatric)	Prognostic	Gain of 1q	Genetic	[160–162]
		Loss of 14q	Genetic	[160]
		11p15 loss of heterozygosity, *WT1* mutation	Genetic	[163]
		IL-6, STAT3	Tissue	[164]
	Predictive	PHB	Urine	[165]

Note: Studies were included if sample numbers were $n = 50$ or greater with the exception of cancers where published sample sizes were limited as a function of lower prevalence of disease

therapy, Trastuzumab [45–47]. For TNBC patients treated with nab-Paclitaxel (Abraxane) + Atezolizumab, programmed death-ligand 1 (PD-L1) expression on immune cells and tumor cells of both primary and metastatic BC have been reported to be linked to progression-free survival (PFS) and overall survival (OS) benefit [44]. Intratumoral CD8 expression and TIL positivity also predicted improved outcome in this study, suggesting that patients with a richer immune TME have a clinical benefit from this combination therapy [44]. TAMs are gaining interest as biomarkers of BC prognosis and therapeutic response. Immunofluorescence detection of the TAM markers CD68, CD163, and MMP-9 in two independent BC cohorts indicated that all three markers were expressed in TNBC. While CD68 positivity correlated with poor OS for TNBC, increased expression of CD163 in TAMs was associated with improved OS in the same group [43]. Interestingly, MMP-9 TAM expression was associated with worse OS in ER-positive but not ER-negative BC [43], suggesting that TAM-targeted therapies may be beneficial in the former group.

MicroRNAs (miRNAs) are a class of small noncoding RNA that can regulate gene expression and are known to be dysregulated at all stages of BC. Liquid biopsy-based detec-tion of both cell-free and extracellular vesicle (EV)-associated miRNA may serve as biomarkers for the early detection, prognosis and therapy response for BC [169–171]. Plasma levels of miR-99a-5p were reported to be significantly higher in BC patients compared to healthy controls and demonstrated good diagnostic potential for early BC (Stage I and II) [51]. A four-miRNA serum signature (miR-18b, miR-103, miR-107, and miR-652) was associated with recurrence and reduced OS in TNBC patients [52], suggesting that this high-risk signature score may serve as a predictor of the presence of TNBC. Importantly, circulating miRNAs are currently being studied in multiple clinical trials as biomarkers for BC screening, early diagnosis and as sentinels of therapeutic efficacy for patients undergoing neo-adjuvant treatment (clinicaltrials.gov).

MMPs are expressed by both tumor cells and stromal cells within the TME and are critical for tumor progression and metastasis [38, 172–174]. Plasma levels of MMP-7 and MMP-26 combined with the standard marker for BC, cancer antigen 15-3 (CA15-3), provided the highest diagnostic specificity for advanced BC (Stage III and IV), indicating that combined assessment of these circulating markers can improve the diagnostic utility of CA15-3 in determining disease progression [50]. Monitoring serum levels as well as immunohistochemistry (IHC) staining of tumors for MMP-9 expression during neoadjuvant chemotherapy for TNBC indicated that a decrease in MMP-9 levels after treatment was significantly associated with pathological complete response (PCR) in patients, illustrating the utility of MMP-9 detection to identify the subgroups of TNBC patients that are most likely to benefit from therapy [42]. We have previously reported that MMP-9 and MMP-9/NGAL complex [48, 49] and ADAM12 [39] are significantly upregulated in the urine of BC patients and may serve as predictive biomarkers of BC status and stage. We have also demonstrated that multiplexed analyses of urinary MMP-9 and ADAM12 can predict which patients are at an increased risk of developing BC [40]. ADAM12 expression in BC tissues has been reported to be closely related to Ki67 (cellular proliferation marker) and HER2 status in ER-positive tumors and high ADAM12 levels were reported to be associated with shorter OS [41]. In terms of translating these markers for use in BC management, MMPs, in particular, based on our work and others, MMP-2 and MMP-9 are currently or have been investigated in over forty FDA-approved clinical trials as biomarkers of therapeutic efficacy of a variety of BC therapies (clinicaltrials.gov).

Lung Cancer

Lung cancer (LC) is the second most commonly diagnosed malignancy of men and women and has the highest cancer-related mortality (seer.cancer.gov) [175]. LC comprises two major histological types: small cell (SCLC) and non-small cell lung cancer (NSCLC). In particular, NSCLC is the most prevalent form of lung cancer with a dismal 5-yr prognosis of ~15% [175]. Despite recent advances in surgery, radiation, chemotherapy, and targeted therapies, LC prognosis remains poor due to delayed diagnosis and the presence of locally advanced and metastatic disease [176]. Identification of NSCLC molecular subtypes including tumors with activating EGFR mutations, *BRAF-ALK* gene fusions and *ROS1-RTK* fusions have enabled targeted therapies that can improve OS in patients with metastatic disease [53]. However, these targeted therapies benefit only ~20% of LC patients and while initially effective may lead to eventual therapy resistance [53], underscoring the crucial importance of novel biomarkers for the diagnosis and prognosis of LC. We have previously reviewed the potential of MMP/ADAM biomarkers for the detection of LC [73], and here we will focus on biomarkers from the LC tumor and the TME (Table 22.1).

The TME plays a central role in the initiation and progression of primary lung cancers and is recognized as a viable target for anti-cancer therapies [177]. A panel of 4 exosomal mRNAs, including TP63, keratin 5, CEA cell adhesion molecule 6 (CECAM6) and surfactant protein B (SFTPB), iso-

lated from the serum of LC patients has been reported to provide improved specificity and sensitivity compared to the individual mRNAs to differentiate between adenocarcinoma and squamous carcinoma, two subtypes of NSCLC [54]. The serum concentration of neuron-specific enolase (NSE) a glycolytic enzyme, was reported to be significantly higher in LC patients with bone metastasis compared to those without bone lesions [55], suggesting that NSE may be used to identify bone metastasis during primary LC diagnoses. Circulating cytokeratin 19 fragments (CYFRA21-1) levels have been reported to be an independent prognostic factor for all stages of LC as well as an indicator of metastasis [56]. The prognostic significance of blood CYFRA21-1 levels is currently being investigated via clinical trials to predict OS in NSCLC patients (clinicaltrials.gov).

Serum-based biomarkers from the tumor and the TME may also be used to determine prognosis or to monitor therapeutic efficacy in LC. For example, serum IL-18 has been reported to be an early biomarker for tumor response to Atezolizumab (anti-PD-L1) in NSCLC therapy [57]. Levels of progastrin-releasing peptide (ProGRP), which regulates gastric acid secretion, were shown to be elevated in most patients with SCLC and could aid in the diagnosis of suspicious lung nodules [58, 178], which is important for determining optimal treatment strategy. In addition, for LC patients with elevated baseline ProGRP levels, a reduction in ProGRP after chemotherapy has been reported to represent a lack of disease progression for SCLC suggesting that serum ProGRP may be useful in monitoring response to chemotherapy and might provide valuable prognostic information [58]. Liver kinase B1 (LKB1) is a key sensor for metabolic stress of the TME and is upregulated in hypoxia and during glucose deprivation, conditions that may arise during tumor anti-angiogenic therapy. LKB1 has been reported to be a potential predictive marker of sensitivity to Bevacizumab (Avastin) therapy for advanced NSCLC patients [59]. Moderate to intense LKB1 IHC staining of lung tumors was associated with lower risk of patient death, whereas negative LKB1 lung tissue staining correlated with the lack of clinical benefit from Bevacizumab treatment [59].

Manipulating the immune response to target tumor cells has revolutionized LC treatment resulting in prolonged OS in a subset of patients. Biomarkers such as PD-L1, tumor mutational burden and TILs in the TME may all serve as markers of response to immunotherapy in LC patients and have been extensively reviewed in the literature [179, 180]. A prognostic immune gene signature composed of 40 unique genes has been reported to be able to stratify low- and high-risk patients in terms of estimating OS in nonsquamous NSCLC [181]. A high immune score analyzed via PDL-1 IHC of tumors, and the presence of several immune cell types belonging to the adaptive immune system may also be predictive of prognosis after surgery for lung adenocarcinoma patients [182].

Prostate Cancer

Prostate cancer (PCa) is one of the most common malignancies in men and is associated with a high mortality rate when disease progresses to metastasis and acquires androgen and therapeutic resistance [3, 183]. Current prognostic factors of PCa include the Gleason score and prostate-specific antigen (PSA) which is secreted from prostate epithelial cells. However, serum levels of PSA are elevated in both benign and malignant prostate growth conditions resulting in limited sensitivity and specificity for PCa detection. Therefore, patients often have to rely on invasive prostate biopsies for a precise diagnosis. This highlights a clinical need for more accurate PCa biomarkers that differentiate between benign prostatic conditions and PCa. We have previously reported that MMPs, TIMPs, and other non-invasive biomarkers can predict the presence of early PCa as well as distinguish between PCa and benign prostatic hypertrophy (BPH) [2, 3, 73, 74]. Here we will focus on biomarkers from prostate tumors and the surrounding TME (Table 22.1).

Our group has reported that urinary MMP-2 and VEGF levels were significantly higher in PCa patients compared to age and sex-matched healthy controls and could aid in diagnosis and prediction of therapeutic response [1, 48, 71, 72]. We have also reported that elevated urinary levels of β_2 microglobulin (β2M), pepsinogen A3 (PGA3), and mucin 3 (MUC3) can distinguish between PCa and BPH [73, 74]. A meta-analysis has demonstrated that MMP-2 expression in tumor tissues of PCa patients was significantly higher compared to that in prostatic tissues of BPH patients and was also significantly associated with Gleason score and PCa clinical stage [61]. IHC studies have demonstrated that elevated expression of MMP-1 and MMP-9 in prostate tumor tissue was associated with better disease-free survival (DFS) [60]. Interestingly, the expression of TIMP-2, which inhibits MMP activity and may modulate endothelial cell proliferation and angiogenesis [35, 37], was upregulated in the normal adjacent tissues of PCa patients and was also associated with DFS [60]. Serum levels of MMP-7 have been reported to be significantly higher in PCa patients with metastatic disease, but there were no differences between patients with local disease and healthy controls [62]. MMP-11 has been shown to be strongly correlated with Gleason score, pathologic tumor stage, and shorter survival and as well as being associated with poor prognosis [63]. Several MMPs and their inhibitors are currently being investigated as biomarkers of therapeutic efficacy in FDA-approved clinical trials (clinical trials.gov). Additionally, ADAM family members have been reported to be significantly elevated in PCa patients compared to healthy controls. For example, increased ADAM15 expression in PCa tumor tissues was linked to high Gleason grade, advanced pathological tumor stage, positive nodal stage, surgical resection margin and PSA recurrence [64].

ADAM12 levels in serum and urine were significantly increased in patients with PCa compared to healthy controls, suggesting that ADAM12 might be a potential biomarker of PCa [75].

PCa tumor cells produce several inflammatory factors, which modify the TME and contribute to tumor cell growth, survival, invasion, and progression. Increased serum levels of IL-6, IL-8, tumor necrosis factor (TNF-α), and C-C Motif Chemokine Ligand 2 (CCL2) have been reported to be associated with accelerated progression and poor prognosis in PCa [68–70]. Importantly, cytokines including various interleukins, TNF-α, and other factors such as VEGF are being evaluated in clinical trials as biomarkers for a variety of therapeutic strategies for PCa (clinicaltrials.gov). Caveolin-1 (Cav-1) expression in PCa stroma has been reported to be inversely correlated with disease progression [65, 66]. Studies have shown that low stromal Cav-1 expression was associated with poor disease-specific survival (DSS), increased Gleason score and reduced relapse-free survival (RFS) [65, 66]. Furthermore, stromal expression of Cav-1 was found to be highest in non-malignant tissue [65]. These findings suggest that reduced stromal Cav-1 levels in the TME may contribute to cancer progression and may serve as a useful prognostic marker for PCa.

PCa markers originating in the TME have also been investigated in relation to the Gleason score. While progesterone receptor (PR) was expressed only in prostate stromal cells, androgen receptor (AR) and estrogen receptor (ER) were expressed in both epithelial and stromal cells. Interestingly, significant decreases have been reported in the expression of AR in tumor tissues (Gleason score 8) when compared with normal prostate tissues [76]. ER and AR-targeted therapies for PCa have been extensively studied in clinical trials (clinicaltrials.gov).

CAFs and other stromal cells in the TME have been reported to express asporin (ASPN), which regulates transforming growth factor β (TGFβ) and fibroblast growth factor 2 (FGF2) activity [184, 185]. ASPN expression in stroma was assessed by IHC and was significantly increased in tumors compared with benign prostate samples and correlated with biochemical recurrence or relapse following cancer treatment [77]. Secreted frizzled-related protein 4 (SFRP4), which regulates Wnt signaling, is upregulated in prostate tumors and has been reported to be associated with disease recurrence, poor prognosis and PCa aggressiveness. In a microarray study of PCa tissues, SFRP4 expression was also reported to be linked to high Gleason grade, lymph node metastasis, and a positive surgical margin [78], suggesting SFRP4 might have prognostic utility in specific types of PCa.

Another potential biomarker for PCa, miR-205, is a tumor suppressor and has been reported to be downregulated in PCa epithelium compared to adjacent normal tissues [67].

High expression of miR-205 in the normal epithelium of PCa patients was independently associated with biochemical relapse, and therefore, miR-205 may serve as a prognostic biomarker for PCa. In prostate tumors, miR-205 correlated positively with angiogenesis-related markers such as platelet-derived growth factor (PDGF)-D, PDGF-B, VEGF-A, VEGF-C, and VEGFR-2. A number of other microRNAs are currently being investigated as biomarkers for therapeutic response in PCa clinical trials (clinicaltrials.gov).

Pancreatic Cancer

Pancreatic cancer (PC) is a lethal malignancy associated with an extremely poor prognosis due to a combination of late diagnosis, frequent recurrence and resistance to current therapeutic modalities [167] (seer.cancer.gov). The majority (~82%) of PC patients present with regional or distant metastases at initial diagnosis making complete resection impossible, thereby leaving patients to rely predominantly on conventional chemotherapeutic options [186, 187], which results in drastically reduced patient survival (5-yr, ~10%). A lack of specific symptoms makes PC difficult to diagnose. Unfortunately, the only approved clinical PC biomarker, CA19-9, [188, 189] has moderate sensitivity and specificity for detecting PC [189–191], and in particular, a very low sensitivity for the detection of early PC [188, 192].

For these compelling reasons, there exists an intense interest in the development of accurate biomarkers for PC that can better detect disease and guide therapy. PC has a particularly active tumor TME characterized by desmoplastic fibrotic stroma, an abundant ECM, poor effector T cell infiltration and other immune-suppressive features. We have previously reviewed the potential of MMP/ADAM biomarkers for the detection of PC [2]. Here we will focus on biomarkers from the PC tumor and the TME (Table 22.1). CAFs have a crucial function in driving PC progression through paracrine interactions. Cav-1, a scaffolding protein, is expressed by fibroblasts of the desmoplastic PC stroma but not by stromal cells of the normal pancreas [79] and the co-expression of Cav-1 and fatty acid synthase (FASN) is reported to correlate with histologic grade and advanced tumor stage as well as lower survival in PC patients [79]. Loss of stromal Cav-1 expression was found to be associated with PC TNM stages, lymph node and distant metastasis and could predict poor clinical outcome for PC patients [80].

ADAM12 was reported to be upregulated in pancreatic CAFs compared to fibroblasts from normal pancreatic tissues [81] and is considered to be a marker of activated stroma. An analysis of patient tumors and serum samples from the Phase II MPACT trial found that high ADAM12 levels were significantly associated with poor outcome for PC patients [82]. Low ADAM12 levels associated with lon-

ger survival for PC patients who received nab-Paclitaxel (Abraxane) [82], suggesting that ADAM12 is a circulating biomarker for stromal activation with both prognostic and therapeutic significance. Ongoing clinical trials are assessing the relative abundance of stroma in metastatic PC tumor tissues and stromal markers such as ADAM12, in tissues and blood as a predictor of response to treatment and survival in PC patients (clinicaltrials.gov). We have previously reported that urinary ADAM12 levels could serve as significant independent predictor for distinguishing pancreatic ductal adenocarcinoma (PDAC) and pancreatic neuroendocrine tumors (pNET) patients from healthy controls [83]. Patient survival stratified by urinary ADAM12 levels indicated a significantly shorter OS for PDAC patients with high ADAM12 levels compared to patients with lower urinary ADAM12 [83]. We have reported that urinary levels of MMP-2 and its endogenous inhibitor TIMP-1 are significant independent predictors to distinguish PDAC patients from healthy controls [89]. Combined analysis of urinary MMP-2 and TIMP-1 resulted in a markedly improved accuracy [89] over using CA19-9 alone [193], the currently utilized biomarker for PDAC. In addition, urinary MMP-2 may predict the presence of pNET tumors, whereas TIMP-1 levels may differentiate between PDAC and pNET patient groups [89]. In an ongoing clinical trial, MMP-9 levels in pancreatic cyst fluid are being analyzed in patients with high-risk intraductal papillary mucinous neoplasm (IPMN) lesions who are at an increased risk of radiographic progression to PDAC (clinicaltrials.gov). Ongoing trials are also investigating the blood levels of MMP-7 and MMP-9 as surrogate markers of therapeutic efficacy for combined PRI-724 + Gemcitabine and proton beam therapies for PC patients, respectively (clinicaltrials.gov). VEGF is overexpressed in PC and reported to be a useful marker for poor prognosis in PC [194]. VEGF levels in portal blood were associated with tumor grade and correlate with tumor size for patients with PDAC [84]. Soluble stroma-based markers have also been investigated as potential biomarkers for PDAC. A biomarker panel of stroma-related proteins such as MMP-7, cellular communication network factor 2 (CCN2), insulin-like growth factor binding protein 2 (IGFBP2), thrombospondin-2 (TSP-2), soluble ICAM1 (sICAM1), TIMP-1, and plasminogen precursor (PLG) were evaluated in plasma samples and were reported to discriminate PDAC from healthy controls and from chronic pancreatitis [85].

Detection of early and localized PDAC has been shown to increase the 5-yr survival of PC patients to ~43% (Stage II) and ~50% (Stage I) from ~10.8% (5-yr overall survival) [195]. A 29-biomarker serum signature has been shown to discriminate between patients with Stage I and II PDAC from healthy controls and was subsequently validated in an independent case-control cohort [196]. Similarly, a plasma panel including tissue factor pathway inhibitor (TFPI), tenascin C (TNC-FNII-C) and CA19-9 improved upon CA19-9 alone in discriminating early-stage PDAC compared to healthy controls as well as distinguishing early-stage PDAC from patients with benign pancreatic conditions such as diabetes and chronic pancreatitis [86]. PDAC is associated with pathogenic modifications to the peripheral nervous system that elevate metastatic capacity. IL6-related stem cell–promoting factor (LIF) has been reported to support PDAC-associated neural remodeling and is upregulated in PC tumor tissues compared to the healthy pancreas [87]. Compared to serum from patients with benign pancreatic conditions or healthy controls, the sera from PDAC patients contained elevated LIF levels which correlated with intratumoral nerve density, suggesting that LIF could be a candidate biomarker and a therapeutic target for PDAC-associated neural remodeling [87].

PC-derived exosomes have been explored for their potential application as cancer biomarkers [197, 198]. The miR-3940-5p/miR-8069 ratio was found to be elevated in the urinary exosomes of PDAC patients with early-stage disease [88] compared to that of healthy controls or chronic pancreatitis patients and when combined with CA19-9, were shown to be a useful tool for the diagnosis of PDAC [88]. A 3-protein (LYVE-1, REG1B, and TFF1) urinary biomarker panel has been reported to distinguish Stage I and II PDAC from healthy controls and when combined with plasma CA19-9, this panel achieved an increased accuracy [90, 199]. This 3-biomarker urine panel was recently combined with a logistic regression model to create the algorithm PancRISK score, which provided high sensitivity and specificity for the stratification of patients into normal or elevated risk categories [200]. The PancRISK score is being suggested for use in surveillance of individuals with a family history or genetic background for PC or at an increased risk due to benign diseases of the pancreas [200].

Ovarian Cancer

Epithelial ovarian cancer (OC) is the leading cause of death among women with gynecologic cancers. Despite advances in surgery and chemotherapy, 5-yr survival rates for OC have not significantly improved over the past few decades (seer.cancer.gov). The most common subtypes of OC include serous carcinomas, endometriosis carcinomas, mucinous carcinomas and clear cell carcinomas. Elevated serum levels of CA125 are widely used to detect OC. However, many patients with early-stage OC and a subset of patients with advanced OC have CA125 levels within the normal range (~35 U/mL), such that these women are left without reliable diagnostic biomarkers to detect OC status. We have previously reported that urinary MMP-2, MMP-9, and lipocalin-2 (NGAL) significantly discriminated between OC patients with normal CA125 levels compared to healthy controls and could represent an important predictor of the presence of OC in the ~30% of women for whom no reliable diagnostic test exists [2, 94]. Grounded in some of this work, several MMPs have been investigated as biomarkers of therapeutic efficacy in clinical trials for OC patients (clinicaltrials.gov). MMP-9 expression was significantly higher in the EVs isolated from the ascites of high-grade serous OC patients compared to patients with benign liver cirrhosis, suggesting the potential of this EV population to serve as a biomarker for high-grade serous OC [95]. Several members of the ADAMs family, specifically ADAM17, ADAM12, and ADAM9 are highly expressed in early and advanced OC tissues [96–99]. ADAM17 is a sheddase for activated leukocyte cell adhesion molecule (sALCAM) whose serum levels were found to be elevated in OC patients compared to healthy controls [97]. ADAM12 serum levels were associated with shorter PFS, OS, and tumor lymphatic and vascular invasion in an aggressive subtype of high-grade serous OC [98]. Finally, mutations in ADAMTS (A disintegrin and metalloproteinase with thrombospondin motifs) members have been significantly associated with an improved OS as well as PFS in OC patients without BRCA1/2 mutations [201].

Serum levels of CA125 and VEGF were reported to be significantly higher in patients with OC than in healthy controls [100]. In this study, the combination of CA125 and VEGF improved the specificity and sensitivity of detection of early-stage OC and was suggested to be more efficacious than CA125 alone. Similarly, the combination of human epididymis protein 4 (HE4) and CA125 has been shown to improve the sensitivity, specificity, and diagnostic power compared to CA125 alone [101] and has been reported to be increased in the serum of patients with OC compared with benign disease and healthy controls [102–104]. Elevated serum levels of HE4 and CA125 in patients with OC were also associated with worse PFS [103, 104]. The neutrophil-to-lymphocyte ratio (NLR) has been reported as a potential predictive marker of OC in patients with normal CA125 levels, and the combination of NLR and CA125 had greater specificity than CA125 alone [107].

Several potential biomarkers have been identified in the TME of OC. IL-6 signaling plays a significant role in carcinogenesis across a variety of solid tumors, including OC and is expressed by ovarian tumor and stromal cells. IHC staining of IL-6 was reported to be significantly higher in malignant tumors and was associated with shorter PFS in OC [105]. IL-6 has also been reported to be predictive of a therapeutic advantage of Bevacizumab for PFS and OS compared with the placebo group [106]. IL-6 in addition to other interleukins and VEGF have been investigated as predictive biomarkers in clinical trials for OC (clinicaltrials.gov).

Tumor endothelial marker 8 (TEM8) is highly expressed in the OC TME and is associated with poor prognosis and tumor-associated angiogenesis. Expression of TEM8 was elevated in the malignant tumor tissues and the borderline tumor tissues with atypical epithelial proliferation compared to normal ovarian tissues and was significantly associated with the International Federation of Gynecology and Obstetrics (FIGO) stages, lymph node metastasis, and poor prognosis in OC patients [91]. S100 calcium-binding protein A1 (S100A1) is a calcium-binding protein belonging to the family of S100 proteins that are reported to be implicated in the crosstalk between tumor cells and stroma and is highly expressed in OC tissues [202]. Compared with healthy fallopian tubes and ovarian tissues, S100A1 expression was significantly increased in OC tissues and correlated with lymph node metastasis, FIGO stage and tumor grade [92]. The chitinase-like glycoprotein, YKL-40, is secreted by various cell types including tumor cells and TAMs in the TME and may represent a novel marker for OC. Preoperative YKL-40 serum levels in early-stage OC were significantly elevated compared with healthy controls [93]. YKL-40 serum levels were also reported to be significantly associated with stage and worse prognosis [93].

Liver Cancer

Liver cancer is the sixth most diagnosed cancer as well as the third leading cause of cancer-related death worldwide (GLOBOCAN)(gco.iarc.fr). Hepatocellular carcinoma (HCC) is the most common primary malignant liver tumor in the USA (seer.cancer.gov). Although screening for liver disease has increased over time, insufficient diagnostic and monitoring tools and the lack of consistent screening limits treatment options for patients. Early diagnosis is essential to improve OS for HCC patients and provide better treatment options [203]. Curative treatments are available for patients with early-stage diagnosis, which has in turn increased HCC survival rates by ~70% [204]. Developing and identifying robust diagnostic and prognostic markers is essential for the early detection of HCC and for predicting clinical outcomes. Here we discuss biomarkers of the liver tumor and its TME that play a role in the diagnostic, prognostic, and therapeutic efficacy in HCC patients (Table 22.1). Vasodilator-stimulated phosphorylation (VASP) is a regulator of actin cytoskeleton and cell migration, and has been reported to be overexpressed in HCC and is indicative of poor prognosis as it promoted aggressive phenotype and metastasis [109]. Although VASP was reported to be an independent factor in predicting survival of HCC patients, the downstream effect of VASP overexpression resulted in upregulated MMP-2 and MMP-9 levels, which were associated with increased migration and invasion of HCC cells in these studies [109]. Upregulated expression of ADAMTS5 in tumor tissues has been reported to be associated with poor prognosis and worse OS for HCC patients [108]. A recent

study demonstrated a correlation between angiogenic and immune biomarkers of the liver TME and time of progression (TTP) during combination Sorafenib and FOLFOX treatment in HCC patients [116]. Shorter TTP was found to be associated with high plasma levels of sVEGFR-1, VEGF, bFGF, circulating CD3+, CD3+CD4+Treg and CD56 for Sorafenib treatment alone. There was an increase in CD56, IL-6 and soluble Met (s-Met) plasma levels for the combination treatment suggesting that these markers may be useful to monitor therapeutic efficacy for HCC [116]. Similarly, circulating biomarkers have been evaluated as sentinels of therapeutic efficacy for Cediranib (panVEGFR RTK inhibitor) in HCC patients [117]. Increased plasma levels of VEGF, angiopoietin-2 (Ang-2) and bFGF were associated with poor outcome, whereas an increase in IFN-γ was significantly associated with longer PFS in this study [117], suggesting that proangiogenic and inflammatory factors may serve as potential biomarkers of anti-VEGF therapy in HCC [117]. Currently, MMPs, chemokines, and immune infiltrates are being investigated via clinical trials as tools to monitor clinical efficacy and response to different treatment interventions for HCC such as Axitinib, Lenvatinib, and Nivolumab (clinicaltrials.gov).

ST2 is a member of the interleukin-1 receptor family, and is the receptor for IL-33. While serum IL-33 levels remained unchanged, soluble ST2 was a significant predictor of OS in HCC [110]. Fibroblast growth factor 19 (FGF19) was significantly associated with larger tumor size and higher score according to the Barcelona Clinic Liver Cancer staging (BCLC) system. FGF19 can be an effective predictor of early recurrence and poor prognosis of HCC, which makes it a potential preventive target for HCC patients [118]. In a study designed to assess the clinicopathological features associated with progression and poor differentiation, strong expression of VEGFR-1 in HCC patient tissues was reported to be a prognosticator factor for RFS and OS. This study concluded that after curative resections, high expression of VEGFR-1 in HCC tissues resulted in diminished RFS and OS [111]. Glypican-3 (GPC3), an oncofetal protein, is overexpressed in ~84% of HCC tissues, where it was found to be mainly localized in the cytoplasm. High expression of GPC3 was found to correlate with multiple tumors, high serum alpha-fetoprotein (AFP) levels, and late TNM stage. High GPC3 expression was an independent risk factor for both tumor recurrence and OS in HCC patients who have normal AFP levels and has been reported to be a prognostic biomarker and a good predictor for differing clinical outcomes for HCC patients [112]. Midkine (MDK) is a heparin-binding growth factor involved in cell growth and invasion during HCC progression. MDK levels have been shown to be elevated in patients with early-stage HCC as well as those with untreated or recurrent HCC. In addition, serum MDK has better diagnostic performance in the detection of HCC in AFP negative HCC [113].

In HCC cell lines from human tissue samples, miR-18b overexpression has been associated with tumor progression, metastatic potential and a poor prognosis for HCC. miR-18b downregulated its target gene trinucleotide repeat containing 6B (TNRC6B) and the decreased TNRC6B expression in turn promoted the metastatic potential of HCC cells [114]. A panel of four serum miRNAs (miR-16-2-3p, 92a-3p, 107, and 3126-5p) were analyzed as potential biomarkers for the early detection of HCC. Logistic regression analysis identified three miRNAs (miR-92a-3p, 107, and 3126-5p) to be significantly changed in early-stage HCC patients. The combination of the 3-miRNA panel and AFP allowed for a better and more effective way in identifying the early stages of HCC in low-AFP level patients compared to the healthy patients [115]. Multiple clinical trials have investigated the high expression of FGF19, VEGFR-1, GPC3 in HCC patients as biomarkers to monitor the therapeutic efficacy of targeted therapies. Other current clinical trials have utilized the usefulness of combining biomarkers with AFP for early detection and therapy surveillance of HCC (clinicaltrials.gov).

Gastric Cancer

Gastric Cancer (GC) represents a global health concern as it is the fifth most frequently diagnosed cancer and the third leading cause of cancer-related mortality worldwide (GLOBOCAN)(gco.iarc.fr) [205]. Characterized as having a highly aggressive nature, it is often diagnosed at an advanced stage when the gastric wall tumor invasion and metastasis have already occurred [206]. The standard treatment for early-stage GC is endoscopic resection which has fewer complications and provides a much better life quality for GC patients compared to partial or total gastrectomy procedures typically used to treat more advanced stage GC [206]. Biomarker-based stratification of Stage II or III GC patients who could benefit from adjuvant chemotherapy is currently needed [207]. For example, 5-Fluorouracil (5-Fu) and Oxaliplatin are commonly used for GC management, however, the administration of such drugs to all Stage II and III GC patients is ineffective [208], since many patients relapse after this initial treatment with acquired resistance to the 5-Fu based chemotherapy [208]. For these reasons, a more accurate diagnostic method is needed to correctly classify patients who may be sensitive to 5-Fu chemotherapy and to provide more effective treatment options. The expression of cyclin-dependent kinase inhibitor (p21)-activated kinase 6 (PAK6) was reported to correlate with an aggressive phenotype in GC patients as well as chemoresistance to 5-Fu chemotherapy [119]. Chemotherapy score, a support vector machine (CS-SVM) classifier, is used to distinguish subgroups of Stage II and III GC patients [119]. The addition of Ki-67, thymidylate synthase (TS), cyclooxygenase 2 (COX2), excision repair cross-complementing gene 1 (ERCC1), and P21 to the chemotherapy score has been reported to effectively identify a small subset of GC patients that would benefit from 5-Fu chemotherapy [119]. With the increased understanding of the relationship between biomarkers and disease, many of these markers have been investigated as potential therapeutic and monitoring targets in clinical trials. COX2 inhibition has been used in clinical trials as a therapeutic target as well as to measure treatment prognosis and response (clinicaltrials.gov). In addition, current clinical trials are evaluating Ki-67, TS, ERCC1, and p21 as biomarkers of clinical outcomes and treatment response for GC (clinicaltrials.gov).

MMPs have been found to be elevated in patients with GC compared to healthy controls. Urinary levels of MMP-9/NGAL complex and ADAM12 were significantly elevated in the GC patients compared with healthy controls [124]. IHC of GC tissues demonstrated significant upregulation of MMP-9, lipocalin-2, and ADAM12 expression compared with adjacent normal tissues [124]. Additionally, urinary kallikrein 10 (uKLK10) was significantly elevated in inoperable GC compared to operable GC patients and uKLK10 levels were positively associated with tumor stage and GC progression [123]. Interestingly, both the high urinary levels and increased pathological expression of KLK10 were associated with shorter DFS in this study [123].

Urinary trefoil factor 1 (TFF1) and ADAM12 have been reported to be independent diagnostic biomarkers for GC as well. A panel combining TFF1, ADAM12, *and Helicobacter pylori* (*H. pylori*) was reported to significantly distinguish between healthy controls and GC patients with excellent accuracy [125]. A similar panel of markers including urinary miR-6807-5p, miR-6856-5p, and *H. pylori* indicated excellent accuracy in distinguishing between healthy patients and Stage I GC patients [126]. ADAMTS-2 is a procollagen enzyme and a member of the larger ADAMTS family. ADAMTS-2 expression was higher in GC cells and CAFs compared to normal gastric tissues and was reported to be associated with OS [120].

Collagen type XII α1 chain (*COL12A1*) is a member of the fibril-associated collagen family and has a tumor-promoting role in human cancer making it a potential prognostic indicator as well as therapeutic targeting candidate. Elevated expression of COL12A1 levels, through immunoreactivity scoring, has been associated with GC invasiveness, clinical metastasis and aggressive clinical features [121].

TAMs play a significant role in tumor progression and angiogenesis. Based on the analysis of infiltrating TAMs in the stroma and tumor margins, increased CD163+ TAMs were associated with tumor progression and depth of invasion in GC [122]. Fibroblast activation protein alpha (FAP-α) expression has been reported to be upregulated in GC tumor tissues of patients with adverse clinical-pathological characteristics, diffuse histological subtypes, advanced pathological stage and poor survival [119].

Kidney Cancer

Renal cell carcinoma (RCC) is the most common type of kidney cancer and encompasses several subtypes. The most common subtype (~70% of cases) is clear cell RCC (ccRCC). Although the standard of care for ccRCC has improved significantly over the past few decades with the emergence of new treatments [209], there remains a need for biomarkers to detect RCC, monitor resistance, and predict therapeutic efficacy of these treatments. Several cytokines and angiogenic factors in the plasma of patients with non-ccRCC have been identified as potential prognostic markers. Ang-2 is expressed by the tumor endothelium and has been reported to be elevated in the plasma of patients with advanced RCC compared to those with benign disease [127]. Higher preoperative plasma levels of Ang-2 were also associated with shorter DFS [133]. Elevated preoperative levels of Ang-2 and M2 Pyruvate kinase (TuM2PK), a dimeric form of the M2 isoform of pyruvate kinase implicated in oncogenesis and overexpressed in tumor cells, were correlated with increased tumor size and advanced grade [127], suggesting potential clinical value for the detection of RCC. Ang-2 is currently being investigated as a potential biomarker for therapeutic response in a clinical trial for advanced solid renal tumors (clinicaltrials.gov).

Several studies have identified biomarkers originating from the TME as predictors of therapeutic response in kidney cancer (Table 22.1). Serum Ang-2 and MMP-2 were identified as relevant baseline biomarkers of Sunitinib activity in advanced RCC. Lower Ang-2 and higher MMP-2 pretreatment serum levels were significantly associated with therapeutic response and are potential baseline efficacy markers for Sunitinib treatment in advanced RCC [134]. Elevated serum levels of MMP-9 before BNC105P monotherapy of patients with ccRCC were associated with improved PFS [135]. In addition, high plasma levels of IL-8, PDGF-AA, TGF-α, and VEGFR-2 were independently associated with reduced OS; whereas high plasma levels of IL-2 receptor alpha (IL-2Rα) chain, TNF-RI, TNF-RII, and TNF-α were associated with reduced PFS in addition to OS in RCC [128]. IL-8, IL-9, IL-2Rα, PDGF-AA, TNF-RI and TNF-α were also associated with poor response to Sunitinib treatment [128]. TGFs and TNFs are secreted by macrophages and inflammatory cells in the TME. C-X-C motif chemokine ligand 10 (CXCL10), a chemokine with known anti-angiogenic and immune-stimulatory properties, has been shown to enhance T cell and NK-cell activity, and may be a prognostic biomarker of RCC. CXCL10 serum and plasma levels increased during Sunitinib and Sorafenib treatment, and higher baseline levels were associated with worse OS and DFS [128, 133]. Another chemokine, CXCL7, is involved in inflammation and angiogenesis and generates autocrine and paracrine loops that impact the TME. Metastatic ccRCC patients with CXCL7 plasma levels above the baseline of 250 ng/ml had significantly longer PFS [129], suggesting that baseline plasma levels of CXCL7 may predict the therapeutic efficacy of Sunitinib or other anti-angiogenic drugs targeting the VEGF/VEGFR axis in RCC. Tissue biomarker carbonic anhydrase IX (CAIX) is a transmembrane enzyme induced by hypoxia that has also been proposed to have prognostic value for RCC. Expression of CAIX in RCC tissue has been reported to be inversely associated with tumor stage, tumor grade, and worse DSS, PFS, and OS [130, 131], suggesting that renal tissue CAIX expression may have prognostic utility in RCC. Importantly, MMP-2 and MMP-9 as well as IL-6, IL-2, CAIX, and chemokines have been or are currently being investigated as biomarkers in clinical trials for response to treatment for RCC (clinicaltrials.gov).

Microvessel density (MVD) is a commonly used measurement of tumor angiogenesis. High MVD in primary RCC nephrectomy tissues was significantly associated with improved OS [132]. High MVD also correlated with lower prognostic factor Fuhrman grade, clear cell histology, and absence of necrosis but not with gender, age, sarcomatoid features, lymphovascular invasion, or tumor size, suggesting high MVD may be indicative of better prognosis of RCC [132]. MVD is also being explored as a RCC biomarker for therapeutic efficacy in ongoing clinical trials (clinicaltrial.gov).

Brain Cancer

Brain and central nervous system (CNS) cancers are the tenth leading cause of mortality for adults in the USA and survival rates decrease with age (www.cancer.nets). The main brain tumor types are gliomas which include astrocytomas, oligodendrogliomas, brain stem gliomas along with non-glioma tumors such as meningiomas, primary CNS lymphomas, and medulloblastomas [210]. Gliomas are the most common primary intracranial malignant tumors in adults with a high recurrence rate [211]. Astrocytomas are diagnosed in adults as infiltrating tumors that spread to surrounding tissue in the brain and originate from the astrocytes that form the supportive tissue of the brain [211]. Glioblastoma is a form of high-grade astrocytoma that arises with no prior clinical history of precursor neoplasia or abnormal growth of tissue [212].

The expression of MMP-2 and MMP-9 has been demonstrated to correlate with tumor grade of primary and recurrent gliomas, making them key players in the progression and invasiveness of tumors [138, 139]. Overexpression of membrane-associated MMP-2 correlated with tumor grade and OS in glioblastoma and astrocytoma compared to normal brain tissue [140]. Multiplexing MMP-2 and TIMP-1 resulted in a positive correlation between the two proteins allowing for a stronger prognostic impact [140]. The benefits of these markers specifically MMP-2 and MMP-9 have been shown in a number of current clinical trials along with neuro-imaging to evaluate disease status and therapeutic efficacy (clinicaltrials.gov).

Amphiregulin (AREG), which stimulates cell growth, survival, and migration, is upregulated in the serum of patients with glioma and has been shown to associate with a worse survival prognosis [141]. Osteopontin (OPN) mediates cancer progression and regulates processes such as immune response, cell adhesion and migration. OPN levels have been reported to be higher in tissue, plasma, and serum in high-grade glioma patients compared to those with low-grade glioma and is related to OS [136]. Another study has reported that multiplexing bone morphogenic protein 2 (BMP2), heat shock 70-kDA protein (HSP70) and CXCL10 resulted in better specificity and sensitivity to accurately distinguish between GBM patients and healthy controls [142]. miRNAs expressed by the TME in glioblastoma have been shown to be involved in disease progression and may prove to be important biomarkers of this disease. For example, the downregulation of the miR-340-5p has been correlated with the density of TAMs which are associated with poor prognosis. Additionally, patients with low miR-340-5p expression, high CD163, periostin (POSTN), LIBP1 and high mobility group A (HMGA-2) levels were associated with a poor prognosis and shorter OS [137]. In terms of the immunological markers, GBM patients exhibited, in tissue, a decreased expression of CD163 and CD70 while CD3 immunoreactivity increased in tumor cells and blood vessels [143].

To monitor the efficacy of Bevacizumab treatment in patients with recurrent GBM, a new approach was developed termed "TME mapping." This approach consists of multiparametric magnetic resonance imaging (MRI) along with methods to visualize oxygen metabolism in the TME. TME mapping allowed for the classification of five different TME compartments and has been used to monitor the tumor biology and treatment efficacy for GBM [213].

Pediatric Cancers

In this section, we will discuss biomarkers for pediatric brain cancer, neuroblastoma and Wilms' tumor (Table 22.1) as they are among the most common pediatric solid tumors.

Brain Cancer

Brain cancer is the most common solid tumor in pediatric patients with one of the highest mortality rates. The highest rates of pediatric BC are found in the USA with an incidence rate of between 1.15 to 5.14 cases per 100,000 children [214]. We have previously reported the significant upregulation of MMP-2, MMP-9, MMP-9/NGAL complex, and VEGF in urine of patients with brain tumors. MMP activity was reduced after surgery, demonstrating that MMPs can be both diagnostic markers and markers of tumor recurrence. We confirmed that these proteins originate in the brain tumor tissues as elevated MMPs were observed in cerebrospinal fluid (CSF) and brain tumor tissue [145, 215]. Other urinary biomarkers such as bFGF and TIMP-3 have been reported as successful diagnostic markers in detecting juvenile pilocytic astrocytoma (JPA) with high accuracy [146]. MMPs, VEGF, bFGF, thrombospondin, TNF-α, IL-12 and IL-8 in blood and urine have been investigated as CNS tumor biomarkers in clinical trials for radiation therapy (clinicaltrials.gov). Additionally, neogenin and netrin-1 have been identified as urinary biomarkers for diffuse intrinsic pontine glioma (DIPG), a pediatric brain tumor representing a major clinical challenge [147]. Urinary biomarkers were evaluated in a pediatric brain tumor consortium (PBTC) clinical trial of Veliparib and radiation therapy followed by Veliparib and Temozolomide (TMZ) in DIPG patients. High levels of netrin-1, bFGF, MMP-3, and TIMP-1 could distinguish DIPG patients compared to healthy controls [148]. Additionally, in the same study other biomarkers significantly predicted survival (MMP-9), progression-free survival (TIMP-1) and correlation with baseline tumor volume (MMP-13) [148]. Circulating tumor cells (CTCs) have also been detected in blood and CSF samples and could be useful markers for tumor surveillance [144]. CTCs in CSF may be used to determine tumor staging in both adult and pediatric brain cancers [216]. Diagnosis of brain cancer is currently heavily reliant on radiographic studies where sedation is required for the pediatric population [215]. Therefore, biomarker discovery and validation would lead to better diagnostic tools as well as a reduction in the use of sedation and its risks [144, 215].

Neuroblastoma

Neuroblastoma (NB) is the second most common solid tumor in pediatric patients. One in 100,000 children in the USA is diagnosed with NB each year (seer.cancer.gov). NB develops from neural crest cells and is a cancer of the peripheral sympathetic nervous system, typically found within the adrenal medulla. Therapeutics for NB are currently chosen based on tumor gene expression, disease stage and age. Therapeutic targets include *MYCN*, anaplastic lymphoma kinase (ALK), tropomyosin receptor kinase B (TrkB) and disialoganglioside (GD2), a surface antigen in NB tumor cells [159]. *MYCN* oncogene amplification is currently the most powerful prognostic biomarker known in NB. Circulating *MYCN* concentration in the blood of NB patients has been reported to decrease after chemotherapy treatment [149]. It has been reported that there was a significant difference in the TME of *MYCN*-amplified (*MYCN* -A) and non-amplified (*MYCN* -NA) NB tumors, differing in the levels of stromal inflammatory cells and immunosuppressive activity [154]. Importantly, *MYCN*, ALK, TrkB, and GD2 are currently being investigated as therapeutic targets in clinical trials for pediatric NB (clinicaltrials.gov). For NB, expression of two genes *USP17L5* and *SLC25A5* in tumor tissues has been reported to correlate with low OS in patients with an older diagnostic age [150]. In the same study, expression of four genes, including *POF1B*, *RND3*, *KLC4*, and *SLC12A1*, was reported to be upregulated in patients with a younger age at diagnosis and correlated with a higher OS [150]. Plasma cell-free DNA was found to be a marker of tumor burden [151] and prognosis in NB [152]. Elevated levels of mRNAs including tyrosine hydroxylase (TH), PHOX2B, and doublecortin (DCX) in bone marrow and peripheral blood at diagnosis strongly predicted worse event-free survival (EFS) and OS in patients with Stage 4 NB [153].

MicroRNA from EVs originating from the TME is important for tumor cell communication in NB and have the potential to serve as biomarkers of tumor aggressiveness and therapy response for NB [154]. Exosomal miRNA expression has been reported to be a prognostic marker for high-risk NB patients and correlated with disease aggression. A 3-exosomal miRNA signature (miR-29c, miR-342-3p, let-7b) was identified that could predict EFS and differentiate between good and poor responders to induction chemotherapy for NB [155]. Urinary metabolites, such as catecholamines, vanillylmandelic acid (VMA), and homovanillic acid (HVA), were first recognized as NB biomarkers in the 1970s. At diagnosis, VMA and HVA levels were upregulated in ~90–95% of NB patients and a low VMA/HVA ratio indicated poor prognosis [156]. Various serum proteins such as lactate dehydrogenase (LDH), neuron-specific enolase (NSE), and ferritin were also recognized as biomarkers for NB. Serum NSE has been reported to be a useful marker for advanced NB, wherein elevated NSE levels were associated with a poor outcome in patients and returned to normal after therapy [158]. NB tumor burden has been estimated by tracking serum LDH levels in patients [156]. For NB patients >18 months of age with metastatic disease, serum LDH and ferritin levels have been shown to be significant predictors of EFS and OS [157]. Ferritin is a useful prognostic biomarker for NB since tumor cells express glycosylated ferritin, whereas healthy cells secrete non-glycosylated ferritin. Serum ferritin has been reported to distinguish between NB disease stages with significantly higher levels present in Stage IV (metastases to bone) patients compared to Stage IVS (metastases to liver, skin, or bone marrow but not to bone) NB patients [156]. LDH and ferritin have both been studied in clinical trials as pediatric NB biomarkers for predicting treatment success (clinicaltrials.gov).

Wilms' Tumor

Wilms' tumor (WT) is the fourth most common pediatric cancer [217]. Renal tumors afflict 600 pediatric patients per year in the USA, and ~90% of these patients have WT [218]. Long-term survival rates for WT are over 90%, however, ~50% of patients who relapse ultimately die from this disease. With more effective prognostic biomarkers, the identification of patients who have a greater chance of relapse would facilitate earlier and perhaps more aggressive treatment as would the identification of patients with a greater chance of survival who might be treated with less aggressive treatment with lower morbidity [218]. Multiple studies have linked the gain of chromosome 1q to worse EFS and OS in tumor subsets of patients with intermediate-risk localized disease or non-anaplastic localized disease making this a good prognostic biomarker for WT [160, 161]. Additionally, gain of 1q was significantly correlated with an increased risk of recurrence in WT with absence of anaplasia, i.e., favorable histology WT [162]. Loss of chromosome 14q was also found to be related to worse EFS in WT [160]. 11p15 loss of heterozygosity and *WT1* mutation were both significantly related to relapse in very low-risk Wilms tumors weighing <550 gm and were classified as Stage I favorable histology WTs in children younger than 24 months of age (patients who do not undergo chemotherapy). All patients with the *WT1* mutation also had 11p15 loss of heterozygosity [163]. A correlation has been noted between tumor progression and prognosis and IL-6 and signal transducer and activator of transcription 3 (STAT3) expression in WT [164]. IL-6 and STAT3 were reported to be upregulated in invasive and metastatic WT compared to non-invasive and non-metastatic WT. IL-6 expression was correlated with DFS and OS, whereas STAT3 was correlated with DFS alone [164]. Prohibitin (PHB), a protein that regulates cellular proliferation has been reported to be a predictive marker for tumor stage in WT. Urinary PHB levels were significantly upregulated in patients with recurrent disease and might therefore serve as a WT marker. PHB might also serve as an important biomarker of drug resistance given that the overexpression of PHB limited mitochondrial apoptosis and led to resistance to certain chemotherapy drugs [165].

Concluding Remarks/Summary

The studies reviewed above highlight the importance of the TME as a rich source of viable biomarkers for a wide variety of human cancers and support a renewed effort to exploit this important tumor component as a potentially powerful theranostic target.

Acknowledgements The authors gratefully acknowledge the support of the NIH R21 CA253051, the Breast Cancer Research Foundation, the Karp Family Foundation, the Goodman and Kaplan Families, the Michael B. Rukin Charitable Foundation, and the Brad and Tracy Stevens Family Foundation.

References

1. Yang J, Roy R, Jedinak A, Moses MA. Mining the Human Proteome: Biomarker Discovery for Human Cancer and Metastases. Cancer J. 2015;21(4):327–36.

2. Roy R, Morad G, Jedinak A, Moses MA. Metalloproteinases and their roles in human cancer. Anat Rec (Hoboken). 2020;303(6):1557–72.

3. Jedinak A, Loughlin KR, Moses MA. Approaches to the discovery of non-invasive urinary biomarkers of prostate cancer. Oncotarget. 2018;9(65):32534–50.

4. Sohel MMH. Circulating microRNAs as biomarkers in cancer diagnosis. Life Sci. 2020;248:117473.

5. Srivastava S, Wagner PD. The early detection research network: a national infrastructure to support the discovery, development, and validation of cancer biomarkers. Cancer Epidemiol Prev Biomark. 2020;29(12):2401–10.

6. Liu T, Han C, Wang S, Fang P, Ma Z, Xu L, et al. Cancer-associated fibroblasts: an emerging target of anti-cancer immunotherapy. J Hematol Oncol. 2019;12(1):1–15.

7. Ito T, Ishii G, Chiba H, Ochiai A. The VEGF angiogenic switch of fibroblasts is regulated by MMP-7 from cancer cells. Oncogene. 2007;26(51):7194–203.

8. Sahai E, Astsaturov I, Cukierman E, DeNardo DG, Egeblad M, Evans RM, et al. A framework for advancing our understanding of cancer-associated fibroblasts. Nat Rev Cancer. 2020;20(3):174–86.

9. Folkman J. Tumor angiogenesis: a possible control point in tumor growth. Ann Intern Med. 1975;82(1):96–100.

10. Huang J, Guo P, Moses MA. Rationally designed antibody drug conjugates targeting the breast cancer-associated endothelium. ACS Biomater Sci Eng. 2019;6(5):2563–9.

11. Dvorak HF. Vascular permeability factor/vascular endothelial growth factor: a critical cytokine in tumor angiogenesis and a potential target for diagnosis and therapy. J Clin Oncol. 2002;20(21):4368–80.

12. Nagy JA, Benjamin L, Zeng H, Dvorak AM, Dvorak HF. Vascular permeability, vascular hyperpermeability and angiogenesis. Angiogenesis. 2008;11(2):109–19.

13. Majidpoor J, Mortezaee K. Angiogenesis as a hallmark of solid tumors-clinical perspectives. Cell Oncol. 2021:1–23.

14. Schaaf MB, Houbaert D, Mece O, Agostinis P. Autophagy in endothelial cells and tumor angiogenesis. Cell Death Differ. 2019;26(4):665–79.

15. Schaaf MB, Garg AD, Agostinis P. Defining the role of the tumor vasculature in antitumor immunity and immunotherapy. Cell Death Dis. 2018;9(2):115.

16. Zhang SC, Hu ZQ, Long JH, Zhu GM, Wang Y, Jia Y, et al. Clinical implications of tumor-infiltrating immune cells in breast cancer. J Cancer. 2019;10(24):6175–84.

17. Pages F, Galon J, Dieu-Nosjean MC, Tartour E, Sautes-Fridman C, Fridman WH. Immune infiltration in human tumors: a prognostic factor that should not be ignored. Oncogene. 2010;29(8):1093–102.

18. Stoll G, Zitvogel L, Kroemer G. Immune infiltrate in cancer. Aging (Albany NY). 2015;7(6):358–9.

19. Arneth B. Tumor microenvironment. Medicina (Kaunas) 2019;56(1).

20. Ngambenjawong C, Gustafson HH, Pun SH. Progress in tumor-associated macrophage (TAM)-targeted therapeutics. Adv Drug Deliv Rev. 2017;114:206–21.

21. Noy R, Pollard JW. Tumor-associated macrophages: from mechanisms to therapy. Immunity. 2014;41(1):49–61.

22. Mantovani A, Marchesi F, Malesci A, Laghi L, Allavena P. Tumour-associated macrophages as treatment targets in oncology. Nat Rev Clin Oncol. 2017;14(7):399–416.

23. Ono M, Torisu H, Fukushi J-i, Nishie A, Kuwano M. Biological implications of macrophage infiltration in human tumor angiogenesis. Cancer Chemother Pharmacol. 1999;43(1):S69–71.

24. Sunderkötter C, Steinbrink K, Goebeler M, Bhardwaj R, Sorg C. Macrophages and angiogenesis. J Leukoc Biol. 1994;55(3):410–22.

25. Chen Y, Song Y, Du W, Gong L, Chang H, Zou Z. Tumor-associated macrophages: an accomplice in solid tumor progression. J Biomed Sci. 2019;26(1):78.

26. Hughes R, Qian BZ, Rowan C, Muthana M, Keklikoglou I, Olson OC, et al. Perivascular M2 macrophages stimulate tumor relapse after chemotherapy. Cancer Res. 2015;75(17):3479–91.

27. Osterberg N, Ferrara N, Vacher J, Gaedicke S, Niedermann G, Weyerbrock A, et al. Decrease of VEGF-A in myeloid cells attenuates glioma progression and prolongs survival in an experimental glioma model. Neuro-Oncology. 2016;18(7):939–49.

28. Qian BZ, Pollard JW. Macrophage diversity enhances tumor progression and metastasis. Cell. 2010;141(1):39–51.

29. Eble JA, Niland S. The extracellular matrix in tumor progression and metastasis. Clin Exp Metastasis. 2019;36(3):171–98.

30. Walker C, Mojares E, Del Rio Hernandez A. Role of extracellular matrix in development and cancer progression. Int J Mol Sci. 2018;19(10).

31. Fang J, Shing Y, Wiederschain D, Yan L, Butterfield C, Jackson G, et al. Matrix metalloproteinase-2 is required for the switch to the angiogenic phenotype in a tumor model. Proc Natl Acad Sci. 2000;97(8):3884–9.

32. Yan L, Borregaard N, Kjeldsen L, Moses MA. The high molecular weight urinary matrix metalloproteinase (MMP) activity is a complex of gelatinase B/MMP-9 and neutrophil gelatinase-associated lipocalin (NGAL): modulation of MMP-9 activity by NGAL. J Biol Chem. 2001;276(40):37258–65.

33. Balkwill FR, Capasso M, Hagemann T. The tumor microenvironment at a glance. J Cell Sci. 2012;125(Pt 23):5591–6.

34. Roy R, Yang J, Moses MA. Matrix metalloproteinases as novel biomarkers and potential therapeutic targets in human cancer. J Clin Oncol. 2009;27(31):5287.

35. Fernández CA, Butterfield C, Jackson G, Moses MA. Structural and functional uncoupling of the enzymatic and angiogenic inhibitory activities of tissue inhibitor of metalloproteinase-2 (TIMP-2): loop 6 is a novel angiogenesis inhibitor. J Biol Chem. 2003;278(42):40989–95.

36. Moses MA. The regulation of neovascularization by matrix metalloproteinases and their inhibitors. Stem Cells. 1997;15(3):180–9.

37. Fernandez CA, Roy R, Lee S, Yang J, Panigrahy D, Van Vliet KJ, et al. The anti-angiogenic peptide, loop 6, binds insulin-like growth factor-1 receptor. J Biol Chem. 2010;285(53):41886–95.

38. Shimoda M, Ohtsuka T, Okada Y, Kanai Y. Stromal metalloproteinases: crucial contributors to the tumor microenvironment. Pathol Int. 2021;71(1):1–14.

39. Roy R, Wewer UM, Zurakowski D, Pories SE, Moses MA. ADAM 12 cleaves extracellular matrix proteins and correlates with cancer status and stage. J Biol Chem. 2004;279(49):51323–30.

40. Pories SE, Zurakowski D, Roy R, Lamb CC, Raza S, Exarhopoulos A, et al. Urinary metalloproteinases: noninvasive biomarkers for breast cancer risk assessment. Cancer Epidemiol Prev Biomark. 2008;17(5):1034–42.

41. Ma B, Ma Q, Jin C, Wang X, Zhang G, Zhang H, et al. ADAM12 expression predicts clinical outcome in estrogen receptor-positive breast cancer. Int J Clin Exp Pathol. 2015;8(10):13279.

42. Wang R-X, Chen S, Huang L, Shao Z-M. Predictive and prognostic value of matrix metalloproteinase (MMP)-9 in neoadjuvant chemotherapy for triple-negative breast cancer patients. BMC Cancer. 2018;18(1):1–8.

43. Pelekanou V, Villarroel-Espindola F, Schalper KA, Pusztai L, Rimm DL. CD68, CD163, and matrix metalloproteinase 9 (MMP-9) co-localization in breast tumor microenvironment predicts survival differently in ER-positive and-negative cancers. Breast Cancer Res. 2018;20(1):1–10.

44. Emens LA, Molinero L, Loi S, Rugo HS, Schneeweiss A, Diéras V, et al. Atezolizumab and nab-paclitaxel in advanced triple-negative breast cancer: biomarker evaluation of the IMpassion130 study. JNCI: J Natl Cancer Inst 2020;113(8):1005–16.

45. Okabe M, Toh U, Iwakuma N, Saku S, Akashi M, Kimitsuki Y, et al. Predictive factors of the tumor immunological microenvironment for long-term follow-up in early stage breast cancer. Cancer Sci. 2017;108(1):81–90.

46. Loi S, Michiels S, Salgado R, Sirtaine N, Jose V, Fumagalli D, et al. Tumor infiltrating lymphocytes are prognostic in triple negative breast cancer and predictive for trastuzumab benefit in early breast cancer: results from the FinHER trial. Ann Oncol. 2014;25(8):1544–50.

47. Salgado R, Denkert C, Demaria S, Sirtaine N, Klauschen F, Pruneri G, et al. The evaluation of tumor-infiltrating lymphocytes (TILs) in breast cancer: recommendations by an international TILs working group 2014. Ann Oncol. 2015;26(2):259–71.

48. Moses MA, Wiederschain D, Loughlin KR, Zurakowski D, Lamb CC, Freeman MR. Increased incidence of matrix metalloproteinases in urine of cancer patients. Cancer Res. 1998;58(7):1395–9.

49. Fernández CA, Yan L, Louis G, Yang J, Kutok JL, Moses MA. The matrix metalloproteinase-9/neutrophil gelatinase-associated lipocalin complex plays a role in breast tumor growth and is present in the urine of breast cancer patients. Clin Cancer Res. 2005;11(15):5390–5.

50. Piskór BM, Przylipiak A, Dąbrowska E, Sidorkiewicz I, Niczyporuk M, Szmitkowski M, et al. Plasma concentrations of Matrilysins MMP-7 and MMP-26 as diagnostic biomarkers in breast cancer. J Clin Med. 2021;10(7):1436.

51. Garrido-Cano I, Constâncio V, Adam-Artigues A, Lameirinhas A, Simón S, Ortega B, et al. Circulating miR-99a-5p expression in plasma: a potential biomarker for early diagnosis of breast cancer. Int J Mol Sci. 2020;21(19):7427.

52. Sahlberg KK, Bottai G, Naume B, Burwinkel B, Calin GA, Børresen-Dale A-L, et al. A serum microRNA signature predicts tumor relapse and survival in triple-negative breast cancer patients. Clin Cancer Res. 2015;21(5):1207–14.

53. Mayekar MK, Bivona TG. Current landscape of targeted therapy in lung cancer. Clin Pharmacol Ther. 2017;102(5):757–64.

54. Cao B, Wang P, Gu L, Liu J. Use of four genes in exosomes as biomarkers for the identification of lung adenocarcinoma and lung squamous cell carcinoma. Oncol Lett 2021;21(4):1-.

55. Zhou Y, Chen W-Z, Peng A-F, Tong W-L, Liu J-M, Liu Z-L. Neuron-specific enolase, histopathological types, and age as risk factors for bone metastases in lung cancer. Tumor Biol. 2017;39(7):1010428317714194.

56. Zhang L, Liu D, Li L, Pu D, Zhou P, Jing Y, et al. The important role of circulating CYFRA21-1 in metastasis diagnosis and prognostic value compared with carcinoembryonic antigen and neuron-specific enolase in lung cancer patients. BMC Cancer. 2017;17(1):1–14.

57. Netterberg I, Li CC, Molinero L, Budha N, Sukumaran S, Stroh M, et al. A PK/PD analysis of circulating biomarkers and their relationship to tumor response in atezolizumab-treated non-small cell lung cancer patients. Clin Pharmacol Therap. 2019;105(2):486–95.

58. Muley T, Zhang X, Holdenrieder S, Korse CM, Zhi X-y, Molina R, et al. A continuous responder algorithm to optimize clinical management of small-cell lung cancer with progastrin-releasing peptide as a simple blood test. Tumor Biol 2020;42(9):1010428320958603.

59. Bonanno L, De Paoli A, Zulato E, Esposito G, Calabrese F, Favaretto A, et al. LKB1 expression correlates with increased survival in patients with advanced non–small cell lung cancer treated with chemotherapy and bevacizumab. Clin Cancer Res. 2017;23(13):3316–24.

60. Ozden F, Saygin C, Uzunaslan D, Onal B, Durak H, Aki H. Expression of MMP-1, MMP-9 and TIMP-2 in prostate carcinoma and their influence on prognosis and survival. J Cancer Res Clin Oncol. 2013;139(8):1373–82.

61. Xie T, Dong B, Yan Y, Hu G, Xu Y. Association between MMP-2 expression and prostate cancer: a meta-analysis. Biomed Rep. 2016;4(2):241–5.

62. Szarvas T, Becker M, Vom Dorp F, Meschede J, Scherag A, Bankfalvi A, et al. Elevated serum matrix metalloproteinase 7 levels predict poor prognosis after radical prostatectomy. Int J Cancer. 2011;128(6):1486–92.

63. Nonsrijun N, Mitchai J, Brown K, Leksomboon R, Tuamsuk P. Overexpression of matrix metalloproteinase 11 in Thai prostatic adenocarcinoma is associated with poor survival. Asian Pac J Cancer Prev. 2013;14(5):3331–5.

64. Burdelski C, Fitzner M, Hube-Magg C, Kluth M, Heumann A, Simon R, et al. Overexpression of the a disintegrin and metalloproteinase ADAM15 is linked to a small but highly aggressive subset of prostate cancers. Neoplasia. 2017;19(4):279–87.

65. Ayala G, Morello M, Frolov A, You S, Li R, Rosati F, et al. Loss of caveolin-1 in prostate cancer stroma correlates with reduced relapse-free survival and is functionally relevant to tumour progression. J Pathol. 2013;231(1):77–87.

66. Hammarsten P, Dahl Scherdin T, Hagglof C, Andersson P, Wikstrom P, Stattin P, et al. High Caveolin-1 expression in tumor stroma is associated with a favourable outcome in prostate cancer patients managed by watchful waiting. PLoS One. 2016;11(10):e0164016.

67. Nordby Y, Richardsen E, Ness N, Donnem T, Patel HRH, Busund LT, et al. High miR-205 expression in normal epithelium is associated with biochemical failure - an argument for epithelial crosstalk in prostate cancer? Sci Rep. 2017;7(1):16308.

68. Nakashima J, Tachibana M, Horiguchi Y, Oya M, Ohigashi T, Asakura H, et al. Serum interleukin 6 as a prognostic factor in patients with prostate cancer. Clin Cancer Res. 2000;6(7):2702–6.

69. Sharma J, Gray KP, Harshman LC, Evan C, Nakabayashi M, Fichorova R, et al. Elevated IL-8, TNF-alpha, and MCP-1 in men with metastatic prostate cancer starting androgen-deprivation therapy (ADT) are associated with shorter time to castration-resistance and overall survival. Prostate. 2014;74(8):820–8.

70. Archer M, Dogra N, Kyprianou N. Inflammation as a driver of prostate cancer metastasis and therapeutic resistance. Cancers (Basel). 2020;12(10).

71. Chan LW, Moses MA, Goley E, Sproull M, Muanza T, Coleman CN, et al. Urinary VEGF and MMP levels as predictive markers of 1-year progression-free survival in cancer patients treated with radiation therapy: a longitudinal study of protein kinetics throughout tumor progression and therapy. J Clin Oncol. 2004;22(3):499–506.

72. Roy R, Louis G, Loughlin KR, Wiederschain D, Kilroy SM, Lamb CC, et al. Tumor-specific urinary matrix metalloproteinase fingerprinting: identification of high molecular weight urinary matrix metalloproteinase species. Clin Cancer Res. 2008;14(20):6610–7.

73. Jia D, Roy R, Moses MA. MMPs in Biology and Medicine. Matrix metalloproteinase biology. 2015:183.

74. Jedinak A, Curatolo A, Zurakowski D, Dillon S, Bhasin MK, Libermann TA, et al. Novel non-invasive biomarkers that distinguish between benign prostate hyperplasia and prostate cancer. BMC Cancer. 2015;15(1):1–9.

75. Bilgin Dogru E, Dizdar Y, Aksit E, Ural F, Sanli O, Yasasever V. EMMPRIN and ADAM12 in prostate cancer: preliminary results of a prospective study. Tumour Biol. 2014;35(11):11647–53.

76. Gevaert T, Van Eycke YR, Vanden Broeck T, Van Poppel H, Salmon I, Rorive S, et al. Comparing the expression profiles of steroid hormone receptors and stromal cell markers in prostate cancer at different Gleason scores. Sci Rep. 2018;8(1):14326.

77. Rochette A, Boufaied N, Scarlata E, Hamel L, Brimo F, Whitaker HC, et al. Asporin is a stromally expressed marker associated with prostate cancer progression. Br J Cancer. 2017;116(6):775–84.

78. Bernreuther C, Daghigh F, Moller K, Hube-Magg C, Lennartz M, Lutz F, et al. Secreted frizzled-related protein 4 (SFRP4) is an independent prognostic marker in prostate cancers lacking TMPRSS2: ERG fusions. Pathol Oncol Res. 2020;26(4):2709–22.

79. Witkiewicz AK, Nguyen K, Dasgupta A, Kennedy EP, Yeo CJ, Lisanti MP, et al. Co-expression of fatty acid synthase and caveolin-1 in pancreatic ductal adenocarcinoma: implications for tumor progression and clinical outcome. Cell Cycle. 2008;7(19):3021–5.

80. Shan T, Lu H, Ji H, Li Y, Guo J, Chen X, et al. Loss of stromal caveolin-1 expression: a novel tumor microenvironment biomarker that can predict poor clinical outcomes for pancreatic cancer. PLoS One. 2014;9(6):e97239.

81. Yu J, Walter K, Omura N, Hong S-M, Young A, Li A, et al. Unlike pancreatic cancer cells pancreatic cancer associated fibroblasts display minimal gene induction after 5-aza-2'-deoxycytidine. PLoS One. 2012;7(9):e43456.

82. Veenstra V, Damhofer H, Waasdorp C, van Rijssen L, van de Vijver M, Dijk F, et al. ADAM12 is a circulating marker for stromal activation in pancreatic cancer and predicts response to chemotherapy. Oncogenesis. 2018;7(11):1–11.

83. Roy R, Dagher A, Zurakowski D, Kulke M, Moses MA. Abstract A53: ADAM12 contributes to the malignant potential of pancreatic cancer and may serve as a non-invasive biomarker for its detection. AACR; 2016.

84. Hogendorf P, Durczynski A, Kumor A, Strzelczyk J. Pancreatic head carcinoma and vascular endothelial growth factor (VEGF-A) concentration in portal blood: its association with cancer grade, tumor size and probably poor prognosis. Arch Med Sci. 2014;10(2):288–93.

85. Resovi A, Bani MR, Porcu L, Anastasia A, Minoli L, Allavena P, et al. Soluble stroma-related biomarkers of pancreatic cancer. EMBO Mol Med. 2018;10(8).

86. Balasenthil S, Huang Y, Liu S, Marsh T, Chen J, Stass SA, et al. A plasma biomarker panel to identify surgically resectable early-stage pancreatic cancer. JNCI: J Natl Cancer Inst. 2017;109(8):djw341.

87. Bressy C, Lac S, Nigri J, Leca J, Roques J, Lavaut M-N, et al. LIF drives neural remodeling in pancreatic cancer and offers a new candidate biomarker. Cancer Res. 2018;78(4):909–21.

88. Yoshizawa N, Sugimoto K, Tameda M, Inagaki Y, Ikejiri M, Inoue H, et al. miR-3940-5p/miR-8069 ratio in urine exosomes is a novel diagnostic biomarker for pancreatic ductal adenocarcinoma. Oncol Lett. 2020;19(4):2677–84.

89. Roy R, Zurakowski D, Wischhusen J, Frauenhoffer C, Hooshmand S, Kulke M, et al. Urinary TIMP-1 and MMP-2 levels detect the presence of pancreatic malignancies. Br J Cancer. 2014;111(9):1772–9.

90. Radon TP, Massat NJ, Jones R, Alrawashdeh W, Dumartin L, Ennis D, et al. Identification of a three-biomarker panel in urine for early detection of pancreatic adenocarcinoma. Clin Cancer Res. 2015;21(15):3512–21.

91. Wang CX, Xiong HF, Wang S, Wang J, Nie X, Guo Q, et al. Overexpression of TEM8 promotes ovarian cancer progression via Rac1/Cdc42/JNK and MEK/ERK/STAT3 signaling pathways. Am J Transl Res. 2020;12(7):3557–76.

92. Tian T, Li X, Hua Z, Ma J, Liu Z, Chen H, et al. S100A1 promotes cell proliferation and migration and is associated with lymph node metastasis in ovarian cancer. Discov Med. 2017;23(127):235–45.

93. Dupont J, Tanwar MK, Thaler HT, Fleisher M, Kauff N, Hensley ML, et al. Early detection and prognosis of ovarian cancer using serum YKL-40. J Clin Oncol. 2004;22(16):3330–9.

94. Coticchia CM, Yang J, Moses MA. Ovarian cancer biomarkers: current options and future promise. J Natl Compr Cancer Netw. 2008;6(8):795–802.

95. Reiner AT, Tan S, Agreiter C, Auer K, Bachmayr-Heyda A, Aust S, et al. EV-associated MMP9 in high-grade serous ovarian cancer is preferentially localized to annexin V-binding EVs. Dis Markers. 2017;2017:9653194.

96. Yagi H, Miyamoto S, Tanaka Y, Sonoda K, Kobayashi H, Kishikawa T, et al. Clinical significance of heparin-binding epidermal growth factor-like growth factor in peritoneal fluid of ovarian cancer. Br J Cancer. 2005;92(9):1737–45.

97. Carbotti G, Orengo AM, Mezzanzanica D, Bagnoli M, Brizzolara A, Emionite L, et al. Activated leukocyte cell adhesion molecule soluble form: a potential biomarker of epithelial ovarian cancer is increased in type II tumors. Int J Cancer. 2013;132(11):2597–605.

98. Cheon DJ, Li AJ, Beach JA, Walts AE, Tran H, Lester J, et al. ADAM12 is a prognostic factor associated with an aggressive molecular subtype of high-grade serous ovarian carcinoma. Carcinogenesis. 2015;36(7):739–47.

99. Ueno M, Shiomi T, Mochizuki S, Chijiiwa M, Shimoda M, Kanai Y, et al. ADAM9 is over-expressed in human ovarian clear cell carcinomas and suppresses cisplatin-induced cell death. Cancer Sci. 2018;109(2):471–82.

100. Robati M, Ghaderi A, Mehraban M, Shafizad A, Nasrolahi H, Mohammadianpanah M. Vascular endothelial growth factor (VEGF) improves the sensitivity of CA125 for differentiation of epithelial ovarian cancers from ovarian cysts. Arch Gynecol Obstet. 2013;288(4):859–65.

101. Kristjansdottir B, Levan K, Partheen K, Sundfeldt K. Diagnostic performance of the biomarkers HE4 and CA125 in type I and type II epithelial ovarian cancer. Gynecol Oncol. 2013;131(1):52–8.

102. Lakshmanan M, Kumar V, Chaturvedi A, Misra S, Gupta S, Akhtar N, et al. Role of serum HE4 as a prognostic marker in carcinoma of the ovary. Indian J Cancer. 2019;56(3):216–21.

103. Sandri MT, Bottari F, Franchi D, Boveri S, Candiani M, Ronzoni S, et al. Comparison of HE4, CA125 and ROMA algorithm in women with a pelvic mass: correlation with pathological outcome. Gynecol Oncol. 2013;128(2):233–8.

104. Hamed EO, Ahmed H, Sedeek OB, Mohammed AM, Abd-Alla AA, Abdel Ghaffar HM. Significance of HE4 estimation in com-

parison with CA125 in diagnosis of ovarian cancer and assessment of treatment response. Diagn Pathol. 2013;8:11.

105. Coward J, Kulbe H, Chakravarty P, Leader D, Vassileva V, Leinster DA, et al. Interleukin-6 as a therapeutic target in human ovarian cancer. Clin Cancer Res. 2011;17(18):6083–96.

106. Alvarez Secord A, Bell Burdett K, Owzar K, Tritchler D, Sibley AB, Liu Y, et al. Predictive blood-based biomarkers in patients with epithelial ovarian cancer treated with carboplatin and paclitaxel with or without bevacizumab: results from GOG-0218. Clin Cancer Res. 2020;26(6):1288–96.

107. Zhang H, Huo Q, Huang L, Cheng Y, Liu Y, Bao H. Neutrophil-to-lymphocyte ratio in ovarian cancer patients with low CA125 concentration. Biomed Res Int. 2019;2019:8107906.

108. Li C, Xiong Y, Yang X, Wang L, Zhang S, Dai N, et al. Lost expression of ADAMTS5 protein associates with progression and poor prognosis of hepatocellular carcinoma. Drug Des Devel Ther. 2015;9:1773–83.

109. Liu Z, Wang Y, Dou C, Xu M, Sun L, Wang L, et al. Hypoxia-induced up-regulation of VASP promotes invasiveness and metastasis of hepatocellular carcinoma. Theranostics. 2018;8(17):4649–63.

110. Bergis D, Kassis V, Ranglack A, Koeberle V, Piiper A, Kronenberger B, et al. High serum levels of the Interleukin-33 receptor soluble ST2 as a negative prognostic factor in hepatocellular carcinoma. Transl Oncol. 2013;6(3):311–8.

111. Li T, Zhu Y, Qin CY, Yang Z, Fang A, Xu S, et al. Expression and prognostic significance of vascular endothelial growth factor receptor 1 in hepatocellular carcinoma. J Clin Pathol. 2012;65(9):808–14.

112. Fu SJ, Qi CY, Xiao WK, Li SQ, Peng BG, Liang LJ. Glypican-3 is a potential prognostic biomarker for hepatocellular carcinoma after curative resection. Surgery. 2013;154(3):536–44.

113. Vongsuvanh R, van der Poorten D, Iseli T, Strasser SI, McCaughan GW, George J. Midkine increases diagnostic yield in AFP negative and NASH-related hepatocellular carcinoma. PLoS One. 2016;11(5):e0155800.

114. Murakami Y, Tamori A, Itami S, Tanahashi T, Toyoda H, Tanaka M, et al. The expression level of miR-18b in hepatocellular carcinoma is associated with the grade of malignancy and prognosis. BMC Cancer. 2013;13:99.

115. Zhang Y, Li T, Qiu Y, Zhang T, Guo P, Ma X, et al. Serum microRNA panel for early diagnosis of the onset of hepatocellular carcinoma. Medicine (Baltimore). 2017;96(2):e5642.

116. Goyal L, Zheng H, Abrams TA, Miksad R, Bullock AJ, Allen JN, et al. A phase II and biomarker study of sorafenib combined with modified FOLFOX in patients with advanced hepatocellular carcinoma. Clin Cancer Res. 2019;25(1):80–9.

117. Zhu AX, Ancukiewicz M, Supko JG, Sahani DV, Blaszkowsky LS, Meyerhardt JA, et al. Efficacy, safety, pharmacokinetics, and biomarkers of cediranib monotherapy in advanced hepatocellular carcinoma: a phase II study. Clin Cancer Res. 2013;19(6):1557–66.

118. Hyeon J, Ahn S, Lee JJ, Song DH, Park CK. Expression of fibroblast growth factor 19 is associated with recurrence and poor prognosis of hepatocellular carcinoma. Dig Dis Sci. 2013;58(7):1916–22.

119. Jiang Y, Liu W, Li T, Hu Y, Chen S, Xi S, et al. Prognostic and predictive value of p21-activated kinase 6 associated support vector machine classifier in gastric cancer treated by 5-fluorouracil/oxaliplatin chemotherapy. EBioMedicine. 2017;22:78–88.

120. Jiang C, Zhou Y, Huang Y, Wang Y, Wang W, Kuai X. Overexpression of ADAMTS-2 in tumor cells and stroma is predictive of poor clinical prognosis in gastric cancer. Hum Pathol. 2019;84:44–51.

121. Jiang X, Wu M, Xu X, Zhang L, Huang Y, Xu Z, et al. COL12A1, a novel potential prognostic factor and therapeutic target in gastric cancer. Mol Med Rep. 2019;20(4):3103–12.

122. Park JY, Sung JY, Lee J, Park YK, Kim YW, Kim GY, et al. Polarized CD163+ tumor-associated macrophages are associated with increased angiogenesis and CXCL12 expression in gastric cancer. Clin Res Hepatol Gastroenterol. 2016;40(3):357–65.

123. Shimura T, Ebi M, Yamada T, Yamada T, Katano T, Nojiri Y, et al. Urinary kallikrein 10 predicts the incurability of gastric cancer. Oncotarget. 2017;8(17):29247–57.

124. Shimura T, Dagher A, Sachdev M, Ebi M, Yamada T, Yamada T, et al. Urinary ADAM12 and MMP-9/NGAL complex detect the presence of gastric cancer. Cancer Prev Res. 2015;8(3):240–8.

125. Shimura T, Dayde D, Wang H, Okuda Y, Iwasaki H, Ebi M, et al. Novel urinary protein biomarker panel for early diagnosis of gastric cancer. Br J Cancer. 2020;123(11):1656–64.

126. Iwasaki H, Shimura T, Yamada T, Okuda Y, Natsume M, Kitagawa M, et al. A novel urinary microRNA biomarker panel for detecting gastric cancer. J Gastroenterol. 2019;54(12):1061–9.

127. Gayed BA, Gillen J, Christie A, Pena-Llopis S, Xie XJ, Yan J, et al. Prospective evaluation of plasma levels of ANGPT2, TuM2PK, and VEGF in patients with renal cell carcinoma. BMC Urol. 2015;15:24.

128. Bilen MA, Zurita AJ, Ilias-Khan NA, Chen HC, Wang X, Kearney AY, et al. Hypertension and circulating cytokines and angiogenic factors in patients with advanced non-clear cell renal cell carcinoma treated with sunitinib: results from a phase II trial. Oncologist. 2015;20(10):1140–8.

129. Dufies M, Giuliano S, Viotti J, Borchiellini D, Cooley LS, Ambrosetti D, et al. CXCL7 is a predictive marker of sunitinib efficacy in clear cell renal cell carcinomas. Br J Cancer. 2017;117(7):947–53.

130. Samberkar S, Rajandram R, Mun KS, Samberkar P, Danaee M, Zulkafli IS. Carbonic anhydrase IX immunohistochemistry has potential to predict renal cell carcinoma outcomes: a systematic review and meta-analyses. Malays J Pathol. 2019;41(3):233–42.

131. Zhao Z, Liao G, Li Y, Zhou S, Zou H, Fernando S. Prognostic value of carbonic anhydrase IX immunohistochemical expression in renal cell carcinoma: a meta-analysis of the literature. PLoS One. 2014;9(11):e114096.

132. Jilaveanu LB, Puligandla M, Weiss SA, Wang XV, Zito C, Flaherty KT, et al. Tumor microvessel density as a prognostic marker in high-risk renal cell carcinoma patients treated on ECOG-ACRIN E2805. Clin Cancer Res. 2018;24(1):217–23.

133. Xu W, Puligandla M, Manola J, Bullock AJ, Tamasauskas D, McDermott DF, et al. Angiogenic factor and cytokine analysis among patients treated with adjuvant VEGFR TKIs in resected renal cell carcinoma. Clin Cancer Res. 2019;25(20):6098–106.

134. Motzer RJ, Hutson TE, Hudes GR, Figlin RA, Martini JF, English PA, et al. Investigation of novel circulating proteins, germ line single-nucleotide polymorphisms, and molecular tumor markers as potential efficacy biomarkers of first-line sunitinib therapy for advanced renal cell carcinoma. Cancer Chemother Pharmacol. 2014;74(4):739–50.

135. Pal S, Azad A, Bhatia S, Drabkin H, Costello B, Sarantopoulos J, et al. A phase I/II trial of BNC105P with everolimus in metastatic renal cell carcinoma. Clin Cancer Res. 2015;21(15):3420–7.

136. Zhao M, Xu H, Liang F, He J, Zhang J. Association of osteopontin expression with the prognosis of glioma patient: a meta-analysis. Tumour Biol. 2015;36(1):429–36.

137. Liu Y, Li X, Zhang Y, Wang H, Rong X, Peng J, et al. An miR-340-5p-macrophage feedback loop modulates the progression and tumor microenvironment of glioblastoma multiforme. Oncogene. 2019;38(49):7399–415.

138. Zhou W, Yu X, Sun S, Zhang X, Yang W, Zhang J, et al. Increased expression of MMP-2 and MMP-9 indicates poor prognosis in glioma recurrence. Biomed Pharmacother. 2019;118:109369.

139. Könnecke H, Bechmann I. The role of microglia and matrix metalloproteinases involvement in neuroinflammation and gliomas. Clin Dev Immunol. 2013.

140. Ramachandran RK, Sorensen MD, Aaberg-Jessen C, Hermansen SK, Kristensen BW. Expression and prognostic impact of matrix metalloproteinase-2 (MMP-2) in astrocytomas. PLoS One. 2017;12(2):e0172234.

141. Urbanaviciute R, Skauminas K, Skiriute D. The evaluation of AREG, MMP-2, CHI3L1, GFAP, and OPN serum combined value in astrocytic glioma patients' diagnosis and prognosis. Brain Sci. 2020;10(11).

142. Elstner A, Stockhammer F, Nguyen-Dobinsky TN, Nguyen QL, Pilgermann I, Gill A, et al. Identification of diagnostic serum protein profiles of glioblastoma patients. J Neuro-Oncol. 2011;102(1):71–80.

143. Rahman M, Kresak J, Yang C, Huang J, Hiser W, Kubilis P, et al. Analysis of immunobiologic markers in primary and recurrent glioblastoma. J Neuro-Oncol. 2018;137(2):249–57.

144. Madlener S, Gojo J. Liquid biomarkers for pediatric brain tumors: biological features, advantages and perspectives, J Pers Med. 2020;10(4).

145. Smith ER, Manfredi M, Scott RM, Black PM, Moses MA. A recurrent craniopharyngioma illustrates the potential usefulness of urinary matrix metalloproteinases as noninvasive biomarkers: case report. Neurosurgery. 2007;60(6):E1148–9. discussion E9

146. Pricola Fehnel K, Duggins-Warf M, Zurakowski D, McKee-Proctor M, Majumder R, Raber M, et al. Using urinary bFGF and TIMP3 levels to predict the presence of juvenile pilocytic astrocytoma and establish a distinct biomarker signature. J Neurosurg Pediatr. 2016;18(4):396–407.

147. Sesen J, Driscoll J, Shah N, Moses-Gardner A, Luiselli G, Alexandrescu S, et al. Neogenin is highly expressed in diffuse intrinsic pontine glioma and influences tumor invasion. Brain Res. 2021;1762:147348.

148. Baxter PA, Su JM, Onar-Thomas A, Billups CA, Li XN, Poussaint TY, et al. A phase I/II study of veliparib (ABT-888) with radiation and temozolomide in newly diagnosed diffuse pontine glioma: a pediatric brain tumor consortium study. Neuro-Oncology. 2020;22(6):875–85.

149. Combaret V, Audoynaud C, Iacono I, Favrot MC, Schell M, Bergeron C, et al. Circulating MYCN DNA as a tumor-specific marker in neuroblastoma patients. Cancer Res. 2002;62(13):3646–8.

150. Diviney A, Chobrutskiy BI, Zaman S, Blanck G. An age-based, RNA expression paradigm for survival biomarker identification for pediatric neuroblastoma and acute lymphoblastic leukemia. Cancer Cell Int. 2019;19:73.

151. Wang X, Wang L, Su Y, Yue Z, Xing T, Zhao W, et al. Plasma cell-free DNA quantification is highly correlated to tumor burden in children with neuroblastoma. Cancer Med. 2018.

152. Chicard M, Boyault S, Colmet Daage L, Richer W, Gentien D, Pierron G, et al. Genomic copy number profiling using circulating free tumor DNA highlights heterogeneity in neuroblastoma. Clin Cancer Res. 2016;22(22):5564–73.

153. Viprey VF, Gregory WM, Corrias MV, Tchirkov A, Swerts K, Vicha A, et al. Neuroblastoma mRNAs predict outcome in children with stage 4 neuroblastoma: a European HR-NBL1/SIOPEN study. J Clin Oncol. 2014;32(10):1074–83.

154. Blavier L, Yang RM, DeClerck YA. The tumor microenvironment in neuroblastoma: new players, new mechanisms of interaction and new perspectives. Cancers (Basel). 2020;12(10).

155. Morini M, Cangelosi D, Segalerba D, Marimpietri D, Raggi F, Castellano A, et al. Exosomal microRNAs from longitudinal liquid biopsies for the prediction of response to induction chemotherapy in high-risk neuroblastoma patients: a proof of concept SIOPEN study. Cancers (Basel). 2019;11(10).

156. Trigg RM, Shaw JA, Turner SD. Opportunities and challenges of circulating biomarkers in neuroblastoma. Open Biol. 2019;9(5):190056.

157. Morgenstern DA, Potschger U, Moreno L, Papadakis V, Owens C, Ash S, et al. Risk stratification of high-risk metastatic neuroblastoma: a report from the HR-NBL-1/SIOPEN study. Pediatr Blood Cancer. 2018;65(11):e27363.

158. Zeltzer PM, Marangos PJ, Evans AE, Schneider SL. Serum neuron-specific enolase in children with neuroblastoma. Relationship to stage and disease course. Cancer. 1986;57(6):1230–4.

159. Pastor ER, Mousa SA. Current management of neuroblastoma and future direction. Crit Rev Oncol Hematol. 2019;138:38–43.

160. Segers H, van den Heuvel-Eibrink MM, Williams RD, van Tinteren H, Vujanic G, Pieters R, et al. Gain of 1q is a marker of poor prognosis in Wilms' tumors. Genes Chromosomes Cancer. 2013;52(11):1065–74.

161. Chagtai T, Zill C, Dainese L, Wegert J, Savola S, Popov S, et al. Gain of 1q as a prognostic biomarker in Wilms tumors (WTs) treated with preoperative chemotherapy in the International Society of Paediatric Oncology (SIOP) WT 2001 trial: a SIOP renal Tumours biology consortium study. J Clin Oncol. 2016;34(26):3195–203.

162. Gratias EJ, Jennings LJ, Anderson JR, Dome JS, Grundy P, Perlman EJ. Gain of 1q is associated with inferior event-free and overall survival in patients with favorable histology Wilms tumor: a report from the children's oncology group. Cancer. 2013;119(21):3887–94.

163. Perlman EJ, Grundy PE, Anderson JR, Jennings LJ, Green DM, Dome JS, et al. WT1 mutation and 11P15 loss of heterozygosity predict relapse in very low-risk wilms tumors treated with surgery alone: a children's oncology group study. J Clin Oncol. 2011;29(6):698–703.

164. Zhang LJ, Liu W, Gao YM, Qin YJ, Wu RD. The expression of IL-6 and STAT3 might predict progression and unfavorable prognosis in Wilms' tumor. Biochem Biophys Res Commun. 2013;435(3):408–13.

165. Ortiz MV, Ahmed S, Burns M, Henssen AG, Hollmann TJ, MacArthur I, et al. Prohibitin is a prognostic marker and therapeutic target to block chemotherapy resistance in Wilms' tumor. JCI Insight 2019;4(15).

166. Sharma R. Global, regional, national burden of breast cancer in 185 countries: evidence from GLOBOCAN 2018. Breast Cancer Res Treat. 2021;187(2):557–67.

167. Miller KD, Nogueira L, Mariotto AB, Rowland JH, Yabroff KR, Alfano CM, et al. Cancer treatment and survivorship statistics, 2019. CA Cancer J Clin. 2019;69(5):363–85.

168. Roganovic D, Djilas D, Vujnovic S, Pavic D, Stojanov D. Breast MRI, digital mammography and breast tomosynthesis: comparison of three methods for early detection of breast cancer. Bosn J Basic Med Sci. 2015;15(4):64.

169. Nassar FJ, Nasr R, Talhouk R. MicroRNAs as biomarkers for early breast cancer diagnosis, prognosis and therapy prediction. Pharmacol Ther. 2017;172:34–49.

170. Ozawa PMM, Jucoski TS, Vieira E, Carvalho TM, Malheiros D, Ribeiro EMdSF. Liquid biopsy for breast cancer using extracellular vesicles and cellfree microRNAs as biomarkers. Transl Res. 2020;223:40–60.

171. Morad G, Moses MA. Brainwashed by extracellular vesicles: the role of extracellular vesicles in primary and metastatic brain tumour microenvironment. J Extracell Vesic. 2019;8(1):1627164.

172. Deryugina EI, Quigley JP. Matrix metalloproteinases and tumor metastasis. Cancer Metastasis Rev. 2006;25(1):9–34.

173. MacDougall JR, Matrisian LM. Contributions of tumor and stromal matrix metalloproteinases to tumor progression, invasion and metastasis. Cancer Metastasis Rev. 1995;14(4):351–62.

174. Roy R, Zhang B, Moses MA. Making the cut: protease-mediated regulation of angiogenesis. Exp Cell Res. 2006;312(5):608–22.
175. Siegel RL, Miller KD, Jemal A. Cancer statistics, 2018. CA Cancer J Clin. 2018;68(1):7–30.
176. Herbst RS, Morgensztern D, Boshoff C. The biology and management of non-small cell lung cancer. Nature. 2018;553(7689):446–54.
177. Altorki NK, Markowitz GJ, Gao D, Port JL, Saxena A, Stiles B, et al. The lung microenvironment: an important regulator of tumour growth and metastasis. Nat Rev Cancer. 2019;19(1):9–31.
178. Molina R, Augé JM, Bosch X, Escudero JM, Viñolas N, Marrades R, et al. Usefulness of serum tumor markers, including progastrin-releasing peptide, in patients with lung cancer: correlation with histology. Tumor Biol. 2009;30(3):121–9.
179. Bodor JN, Boumber Y, Borghaei H. Biomarkers for immune checkpoint inhibition in non-small cell lung cancer (NSCLC). Cancer. 2020;126(2):260–70.
180. Bianco A, Perrotta F, Barra G, Malapelle U, Rocco D, De Palma R. Prognostic factors and biomarkers of responses to immune checkpoint inhibitors in lung cancer. Int J Mol Sci. 2019;20(19):4931.
181. Li B, Cui Y, Diehn M, Li R. Development and validation of an individualized immune prognostic signature in early-stage nonsquamous non-small cell lung cancer. JAMA Oncol. 2017;3(11):1529–37.
182. Öjlert ÅK, Halvorsen AR, Nebdal D, Lund-Iversen M, Solberg S, Brustugun OT, et al. The immune microenvironment in non-small cell lung cancer is predictive of prognosis after surgery. Mol Oncol. 2019;13(5):1166–79.
183. Siegel RL, Miller KD, Jemal A. Cancer statistics, 2017. CA Cancer J Clin. 2017;67(1):7–30.
184. Awata T, Yamada S, Tsushima K, Sakashita H, Yamaba S, Kajikawa T, et al. PLAP-1/Asporin positively regulates FGF-2 activity. J Dent Res. 2015;94(10):1417–24.
185. Kizawa H, Kou I, Iida A, Sudo A, Miyamoto Y, Fukuda A, et al. An aspartic acid repeat polymorphism in asporin inhibits chondrogenesis and increases susceptibility to osteoarthritis. Nat Genet. 2005;37(2):138–44.
186. Li D, Xie K, Wolff R, Abbruzzese JL. Pancreatic cancer. Lancet. 2004;363(9414):1049–57.
187. Borazanci E, Dang CV, Robey RW, Bates SE, Chabot JA, Von Hoff DD. Pancreatic cancer: "a riddle wrapped in a mystery inside an enigma". Clin Cancer Res. 2017;23(7):1629–37.
188. Steinberg W. The clinical utility of the CA 19-9 tumor-associated antigen. Am J Gastroenterol. 1990;85(4):350–5.
189. Goggins M. Molecular markers of early pancreatic cancer. J Clin Oncol. 2005;23(20):4524–31.
190. Yeo TP, Hruban RH, Leach SD, Wilentz RE, Sohn TA, Kern SE, et al. Pancreatic cancer. Curr Probl Cancer. 2002;26(4):176–275.
191. Ozkan H, Kaya M, Cengiz A. Comparison of tumor marker CA 242 with CA 19-9 and carcinoembryonic antigen (CEA) in pancreatic cancer. Hepato-Gastroenterology. 2003;50(53):1669–74.
192. Goggins M. Identifying molecular markers for the early detection of pancreatic neoplasia. Semin Oncol. 2007;34(4):303–10.
193. Sandblom G, Granroth S, Rasmussen IC. TPS, CA 19-9, VEGF-A, and CEA as diagnostic and prognostic factors in patients with mass lesions in the pancreatic head. Ups J Med Sci. 2008;113(1):57–64.
194. Pistol-Tanase C, Raducan E, Dima SO, Albulescu L, Alina I, Marius P, et al. Assessment of soluble angiogenic markers in pancreatic cancer. 2008;2(5):447–55.
195. Matsuno S, Egawa S, Fukuyama S, Motoi F, Sunamura M, Isaji S, et al. Pancreatic cancer registry in Japan: 20 years of experience. Pancreas. 2004;28(3):219–30.
196. Mellby LD, Nyberg AP, Johansen JS, Wingren C, Nordestgaard BG, Bojesen SE, et al. Serum biomarker signature-based liquid biopsy for diagnosis of early-stage pancreatic cancer. J Clin Oncol. 2018;36(28):2887.
197. Jin H, Wu Y, Tan X. The role of pancreatic cancer-derived exosomes in cancer progress and their potential application as biomarkers. Clin Transl Oncol. 2017;19(8):921–30.
198. Madhavan B, Yue S, Galli U, Rana S, Gross W, Müller M, et al. Combined evaluation of a panel of protein and miRNA serum-exosome biomarkers for pancreatic cancer diagnosis increases sensitivity and specificity. Int J Cancer. 2015;136(11):2616–27.
199. Debernardi S, O'Brien H, Algahmdi AS, Malats N, Stewart GD, Plješa-Ercegovac M, et al. A combination of urinary biomarker panel and PancRISK score for earlier detection of pancreatic cancer: a case–control study. PLoS Med. 2020;17(12):e1003489.
200. Blyuss O, Zaikin A, Cherepanova V, Munblit D, Kiseleva EM, Prytomanova OM, et al. Development of PancRISK, a urine biomarker-based risk score for stratified screening of pancreatic cancer patients. Br J Cancer. 2020;122(5):692–6.
201. Liu Y, Yasukawa M, Chen K, Hu L, Broaddus RR, Ding L, et al. Association of somatic mutations of ADAMTS genes with chemotherapy sensitivity and survival in high-grade serous ovarian carcinoma. JAMA Oncol. 2015;1(4):486–94.
202. Chen H, Xu C, Jin Q, Liu Z. S100 protein family in human cancer. Am J Cancer Res. 2014;4(2):89–115.
203. Dimitroulis D, Damaskos C, Valsami S, Davakis S, Garmpis N, Spartalis E, et al. From diagnosis to treatment of hepatocellular carcinoma: an epidemic problem for both developed and developing world. World J Gastroenterol. 2017;23(29):5282–94.
204. Choi DT, Kum HC, Park S, Ohsfeldt RL, Shen Y, Parikh ND, et al. Hepatocellular carcinoma screening is associated with increased survival of patients with cirrhosis. Clin Gastroenterol Hepatol. 2019;17(5):976–87 e4.
205. Bray F, Ferlay J, Soerjomataram I, Siegel RL, Torre LA, Jemal A. Global cancer statistics 2018: GLOBOCAN estimates of incidence and mortality worldwide for 36 cancers in 185 countries. CA Cancer J Clin. 2018;68(6):394–424.
206. Song Z, Wu Y, Yang J, Yang D, Fang X. Progress in the treatment of advanced gastric cancer. Tumour Biol. 2017;39(7):1010428317714626.
207. Jiang Y, Xie J, Huang W, Chen H, Xi S, Han Z, et al. Tumor immune microenvironment and chemosensitivity signature for predicting response to chemotherapy in gastric cancer. Cancer Immunol Res. 2019;7(12):2065–73.
208. Noh SH, Park SR, Yang HK, Chung HC, Chung IJ, Kim SW, et al. Adjuvant capecitabine plus oxaliplatin for gastric cancer after D2 gastrectomy (CLASSIC): 5-year follow-up of an open-label, randomised phase 3 trial. Lancet Oncol. 2014;15(12):1389–96.
209. Duda DG. Molecular biomarkers of response to antiangiogenic therapy for cancer. ISRN Cell Biol 2012;2012.
210. Perkins A, Liu G. Primary brain tumors in adults: diagnosis and treatment. Am Fam Physician. 2016;93(3):211–7.
211. Mesfin FB, Al-Dhahir MA. Gliomas. Treasure Island (FL): StatPearls; 2021.
212. Caren H, Pollard SM, Beck S. The good, the bad and the ugly: epigenetic mechanisms in glioblastoma. Mol Asp Med. 2013;34(4):849–62.
213. Stadlbauer A, Roessler K, Zimmermann M, Buchfelder M, Kleindienst A, Doerfler A, et al. Predicting glioblastoma response to bevacizumab through MRI biomarkers of the tumor microenvironment. Mol Imaging Biol. 2019;21(4):747–57.
214. Subramanian S, Ahmad T. Childhood brain tumors. Treasure Island (FL): StatPearls; 2021.

215. Smith ER, Zurakowski D, Saad A, Scott RM, Moses MA. Urinary biomarkers predict brain tumor presence and response to therapy. Clin Cancer Res. 2008;14(8):2378–86.

216. Le Rhun E, Seoane J, Salzet M, Soffietti R, Weller M. Liquid biopsies for diagnosing and monitoring primary tumors of the central nervous system. Cancer Lett. 2020;480:24–8.

217. Leslie SW, Sajjad H, Murphy PB. Wilms tumor. Treasure Island (FL): StatPearls; 2021.

218. Cone EB, Dalton SS, Van Noord M, Tracy ET, Rice HE, Routh JC. Biomarkers for Wilms tumor: a systematic review. J Urol. 2016;196(5):1530–5.

Gene Expression Signatures of the Tumor Microenvironment: Relation to Tumor Phenotypes and Progress in Breast Cancer

Elisabeth Wik, Lise M. Ingebriktsen, and Lars A. Akslen

Abstract

Cancer cell invasion and progression to metastasis have been extensively studied. There is not one all-inclusive model that encompasses the complete picture of the different conditions and pathways operating in human tumors. Application of gene expression signatures is one way of mining the complex tumor landscape and has been proposed to represent a robust method to reflect the many signaling systems.

This chapter gives an update on gene expression signature studies related to breast cancer progress, with particular focus on the supporting stroma. Several signature studies indicate that a combination of extracellular remodeling, activated vascular biology, immune responses, and metabolic reprogramming, in part adipocyte-related, takes place during breast cancer progression. Stromal alterations are likely to be exploited for novel biomarkers and com-

panion treatment targets. Some basic methodological aspects and recent developments are highlighted.

potentially being a powerful resource for identifying markers of the complex biological processes taking place in cancer.

- Interactions between vascular processes, immune responses, cancer-associated adipocytes, and extracellular remodeling appear to be critically important features of tumor subtypes and their associated outcomes, as reflected in composite signature biomarkers.
- Identifying genes and proteins with known functions, differentially expressed between subgroups, may provide improved understanding of the biological differences between tumor phenotypes.
- Gene networks analyses, by means of gene set enrichment analyses and mRNA data paralleling protein–protein interaction analyses, provide increased biological understanding of complex large-scale data.

Take-Home Lessons

- Global gene expression data may better reflect the complexity of cancer biology as compared to the detection of single gene or protein alterations,

Introduction

And above all, watch with glittering eyes the whole world around you because the greatest secrets are always hidden in the most unlikely places. Those who don't believe in magic will never find it.—Roald Dahl (1916–1990)

Tumor cell invasion and metastasis are multistep processes that are detrimental to the organ in which they occur. The route to cancer dissemination is suggested by distinct steps; local infiltration, intravasation, and transport of cancer cells in the lymphatic or hematogenous systems, followed by extravasation of tumor cells from the vessels into the tissue parenchyma (or niche) of the new site where micrometastases may form and grow to macroscopic lesions [1, 2]. The English surgeon Stephen Paget postulated "the seed and soil hypothesis" in 1889, suggesting that tumor cells (denoted

E. Wik (✉)
Department of Clinical Medicine, Centre for Cancer Biomarkers CCBIO, University of Bergen, Bergen, Norway

Department of Pathology, Haukeland University Hospital, Bergen, Norway
e-mail: elisabeth.wik@uib.no

L. M. Ingebriktsen
Department of Clinical Medicine, Centre for Cancer Biomarkers CCBIO, University of Bergen, Bergen, Norway
e-mail: lise.ingebriktsen@uib.no

L. A. Akslen
Centre for Cancer Biomarkers CCBIO, Department of Clinical Medicine, University of Bergen, Bergen, Norway
e-mail: lars.akslen@gades.uib.no

"seeds") have affinity for specific tissue environments (denoted "soil") in certain organs [3]. Literally, Paget sedded a hypothesis followed by many researchers studying cancer invasion and the metastatic process over the next century.

Before setting off on the invasion-metastasis cascade, it is crucial that tumor cells fulfill prerequisites such as the ability to detach and move from the original colony, with unlimited proliferative potential, and a capacity to evade from destruction [4]. The underlying effectors in the invasion-metastasis cascade are suggested to be classified as *metastasis initiating*, *metastasis progressing* and *metastasis virulent* [5]. Metastasis-initiating genes generate a supportive environment that facilitates tumor infiltration to surrounding tissue. Expression of such genes, in the epithelial cells or the microenvironmental compartments, may promote angiogenesis, vascular invasion, epithelial-mesenchymal transition (EMT), and evasion from immune destruction with important implications to the processes involved in cancer metastasis.

The microenvironment is regarded to play a crucial role both in embryonic organ development and in cancer invasion, two processes with several similar features [6]. Cellular and molecular interactions between the epithelial cells and the microenvironment and between elements within the microenvironment also take place in functional differentiation of the normal mammary tissue. Exploiting the normal microenvironment programs, by a form of "hacking" these pathways, is suggested as potential ways of promoting cancer invasion [7]. This may be reversely exploited when targeting the metastatic processes in the therapy setting, exemplified by a study on a xenograft model of breast cancer, identifying neutrophils within the lung microenvironment supporting metastatic initiation and as drivers of establishing lung metastases [8]. Thus, inhibiting the enzyme Alox5 abolished the pro-metastatic neutrophil activity in the lung microenvironment and reduced the occurrence and growth of lung metastases.

Genes supporting *metastasis progression* promote extravasation and survival of the cancer cells outside of their original environment [5]. Cancer cells that have entered the circulation may subsequently extravasate and infiltrate distant organs. When entering such new environment, cancer cells are required to adapt rapidly for colonization to occur, where the disseminated cancer cells reside in their new microenvironment and grow into macro-metastases. Specific cancer cell gene expression has been implicated to direct organ-specific tropism. One example is the expression of IL-11, which facilitates breast cancer metastases to the bone [9]. The establishment of a "receptive" environment at the future metastatic location before the colonization of tumor cells (the *pre-metastatic niche*) is suggested as a mechanistic model explaining metastatic organotropism [10]. Cancer-specific factors released from the primary tumor promote changes in the future metastatic microenvironment before the tumor cells arrive to this location. Also, bone marrow cells may migrate to the pre-metastatic niche in response to the systemically released factors, facilitating the environment for the cancer cells to "thrive" [11, 12].

The tumor microenvironment is increasingly focused in cancer research, both in pre-invasive lesions, primary tumors, pre-metastatic niches, as well as in the metastatic lesions. The tumor microenvironment components have been regarded as genetically more stable than the tumor cells. This is an important factor that renders the stromal components a strategic focus when searching targets for cancer therapy.

Since the discovery of cell signaling, researchers have debated how to best reflect alterations of pathways and levels of pathway activation in different model systems. One major trend in cancer research has been to undertake relatively simple approaches (*e.g.,* measuring one protein or one specific mutation) when searching for markers of deregulated pathways as prognostic and predictive markers. A simplified approach to the complex and unstable cancer biology likely contributes to the lack of biomarker and treatment effects when translating the research findings to the clinical setting.

Global gene expression data may have a stronger potential to reflect the complexity of cancer biology as compared to the detection of single-gene alterations and may be a powerful platform for identifying markers for the complex biological processes taking place in the tumors. When taking the global expression profiles into account, we somehow compensate for the lack of knowledge regarding "the complete picture" of specific signaling pathways and their phenotypic consequences, including potential compensatory mechanisms derived from their deregulation.

From the beginning of this century, gene expression arrays have been increasingly applied in translational cancer research. Some of the first array studies demonstrated that gene expression data could identify known and novel cancer subclasses, with similarities in terms of biological behavior [13, 14]. In addition to identifying molecular phenotypes in various cancer types [15–18], transcriptional alterations have proven to be powerful tools for creating classifiers predicting cancer recurrences [19–22], and to identify alterations in functional pathways, suggesting relevant targets for therapy [23].

Improved Understanding of Cancer Biologic Processes

Oncogenic and non-oncogenic alterations underlie and support the cancer biological processes leading to cancer progress and metastatic disease. High-throughput techniques such as DNA microarrays and RNA sequencing measure the expression of a multitude of genes in one single experiment. This enables multi-faceted views on the phenotypes being studied and provides information about associations between complex gene expression alterations and the phenotypes.

In the era of global gene expression studies, two landmark reports in the field introduced the potential of exploring biological function via studies of gene expression alterations [24, 25]. By studying how the gene expression pattern changed when altering the conditions from fermentation to aerobic metabolism in the yeast *Saccharomyces cerevisiae*, deRisi and colleagues characterized this metabolic reprogramming at a functional genetic and biochemical level [24], and they were amongst the pioneers in applying large-scale gene expression data to biological questions. deRisi also demonstrated how gene expression patterns change according to deletion or overexpression of specific transcription factors, proposing application of DNA gene expression microarrays for examination of the "signature pattern" accompanying such molecular alterations. deRisi stated: *"Perhaps the greatest challenge now is to develop efficient methods for organizing, distributing, interpreting, and extracting insights from the large volumes of data these experiments will provide"* [24]. And he was right: although such "global analyses" have assisted in some of the major progresses made in translational cancer research, the issues deRisi raised are still major challenges when translating "omics" data and analysis output into biological relevant information.

Hughes and colleagues published one of the earliest reports considering the signaling complexity when relating gene expression data to genetic and phenotypic alterations [25]. The functions of uncharacterized genes were identified through mapping of gene expression alterations induced by specific gene deletions to transcriptional profiles of known perturbations. A few years later, Huang and colleagues demonstrated that the expression pattern from several genes, included in a "metagene," characterized and predicted the neoplasm classes under study [26]. These studies were amongst the "precursor studies" to the many reports on gene expression signatures that followed the next decade. Several studies have since been conducted, supporting the assertion that multigene markers better reflect the complexity in the signaling of multiple pathways [27–29], as demonstrated by Huang et al. for *MYC* and *HRAS* pathways [26].

Gene Expression Signatures as Biomarkers

The Biomarkers Definition Working Group defines a biomarker as*: "A characteristic that is objectively measured and evaluated as an indicator of normal biologic processes, pathogenic processes, or pharmacologic responses to a therapeutic intervention."* [30]. D. Hanahan and R.A. Weinberg describe in their "Hallmarks of Cancer" reviews, the tumor biologic processes and enabling characteristics that are essential for tumor initiation and progression to take place [31, 32]. Gene expression signatures might reflect such hallmark characteristics of a tumor, including specific biological processes—and may as such function as biomarkers. Gene expression signature studies have assisted in identifying targets for therapy, suggested as prognostic and predictive markers for specific cancer therapies.

Bild and colleagues integrated early on gene expression profiles and oncogenic alterations, identifying metagenes— gene signatures—reflecting activation levels of, for example, *MYC* and *RAS* signaling pathways [27]. The identified signatures are is associated with patient outcomes, demonstrating a prognostic effect of these metagenes. Bild suggested that oncogenic signatures may reflect the oncogenic phenotype and point to tumor biological processes underlying the phenotypic alterations. Moreover, measures of pathway deregulation in this study were linked to therapy response for drugs targeting components of the specific pathways. In this manner, Bild suggested a potential for gene expression signatures also as markers guiding therapy selection.

Lamb and colleagues defined in one of their Connectivity Map papers "the ultimate objective of biomedical research:" *To connect human diseases with the genes that underlie them and drugs that treat them* [33]. He regarded this *"a daunting task"* but aimed for a solution. The Connectivity Map tool was developed, aiming to reveal functional connections in diseases and linking these to genetic perturbations and drug actions [33]. As part of this endeavor, a reference bank of gene expression signatures derived from the effects on cultured human cells treated with small molecules (*e.g.,* approved drugs and other bioactive compounds) was established. Bioinformatic analyses were integrated into a publicly available (online) tool, making it possible to match any other signature (also the "homemade" ones) to the drug signatures, thereby enabling researchers to pattern-match the specific gene expression profiles under study with gene expression profiles reflecting effects of the small molecules tested as part of the Connectivity Map database [33, 34]. In the primary publication of the Connectivity Map, the authors demonstrated this tool as a powerful resource to link gene expression patterns to functional effects, bio-physiological processes, and targets for therapy in various diseases. However, the Connectivity Map is suggested as a hypothesis-generating tool, and the importance of validating the findings in other model systems is stressed by the authors. In 2017, Subramanian and coworkers published a 1000-fold expanded Connectivity Map version, assessing each perturbation by RNA sequencing of selected 1000 genes, providing 1.3 million perturbation-linked gene expression profiles freely available for the scientific community (https://clue.io) [35].

Gene Expression Signatures in Breast Cancer

Since the gene expression microarray methodology entered the cancer research field, many breast cancer gene expression signatures have been published. Perou, Sørlie and colleagues explored global gene expression data in breast cancer and identified molecular classes [16]. These were further demonstrated with clinical relevance in follow-up studies [17, 36]. In the same decade, van't Veer described a *"poor prognosis gene expression signature"* [20]. Subsequently, gene expression signatures like MammaPrint, OncotypeDx, PAM50, and the Genomic Grade Index (GGI) have been approved by the FDA, and have demonstrated prognostic value for breast cancer patients—overall and within subgroups (*e.g.,* stage I/II, ER-positive breast cancer in postmenopausal women, for the Oncotype DX).

These early signatures were primarily derived as part of a whole section tissue approach, extracting RNA from bulk tumor tissue, with epithelial and stromal cells intermixed. Enrichment of the epithelial component of the tissue samples was promoted, implying lower expression signal from the stromal cells as compared to the epithelial component [37]. For prognostication, adding data about the specific stromal components could add important information. Increased knowledge about the microenvironment, its heterogeneity between tumor subtypes and the epithelial-microenvironmental interactions will likely assist in improving personalized diagnostics and treatment strategies (Fig. 23.1).

Gene Expression Signatures Reflecting the Tumor Microenvironment

As the role of the tumor stroma became a "hot topic" in discussions of the mechanisms for cancer progression, researchers advanced to some extent from bulk tissue gene expression approaches to focusing on specific tumor compartments (Fig. 23.2). Gene expression changes related to the tumor microenvironment (TME) in cancer have been increasingly studied in many types of cancer. Cell-specific alterations (*e.g.,* gene expression changes in immune cells, endothelial cells, cancer-associated fibroblasts, adipocytes) have been described and gene signatures generated, partly as pure prognostic metagenes, partly reflecting cell subsets and cancer biologic processes in the tumor compartments. Deconvolution of bulk gene expression data, a form of "computational dissection," into information about cell type or compartments, and accompanying counts or expression profiles, came into play a few years ago [39, 40], adding to the methodological approaches applied when deciphering TME data from whole tissue gene expression information.

Microenvironmental or stromal signatures might help elucidate biological processes critical for the progression of cancer, and may thereby improve the vision of the still quite blurred understanding of tumor progression and development of metastatic disease. In the following sections of this chapter, selected thematic groups of gene expression signatures are elucidated, reflecting biological processes and acting as prognosticators and predictors of therapy response.

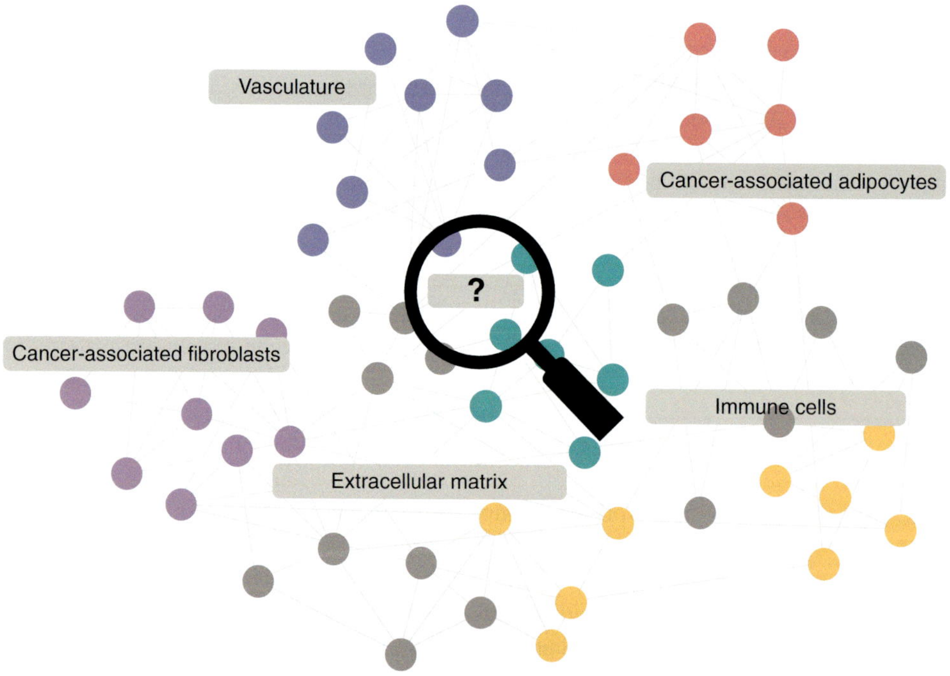

Fig. 23.1 The figure illustrates the networks between genes expressed in the tumor microenvironment, and also how the topics and subheadings presented in this chapter are connected. *Figure by Lise M. Ingebriktsen*

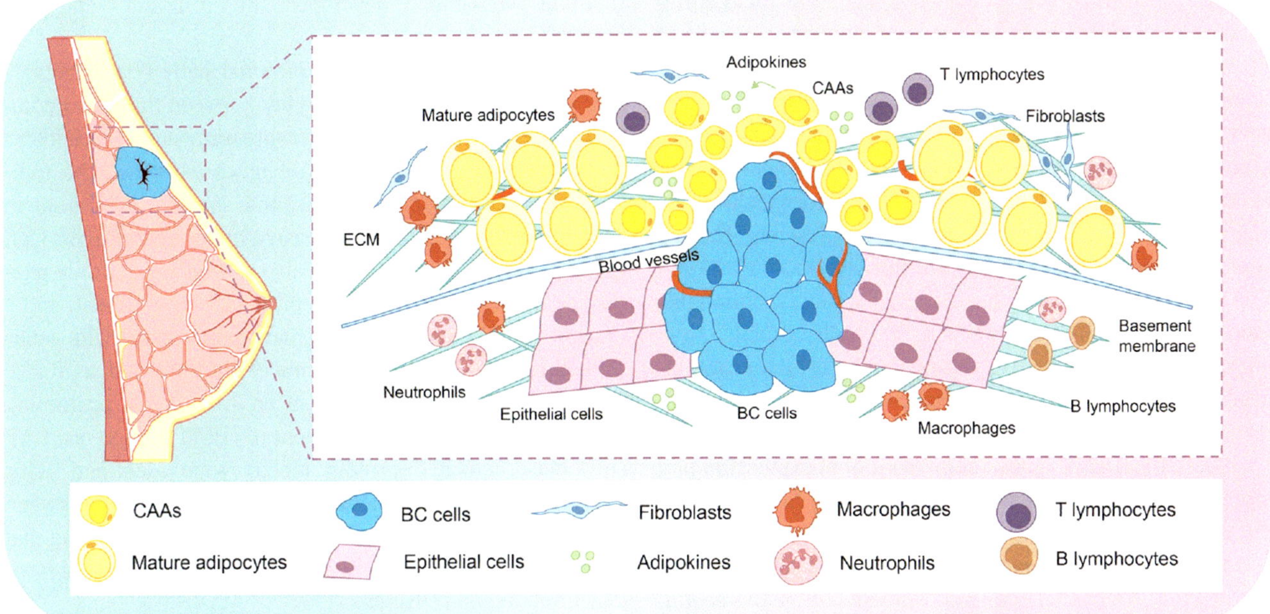

Fig. 23.2 The figure illustrates the components of a breast tumor, including the normal and tumor epithelial cells, structures, and other constituents representing the tumor microenvironment. Their spatial relations stimulate the idea of close interactions between the different cell populations. *BC* breast cancer, *CAA* cancer-associated adipocytes, *ECM* extracellular matrix. *With permission, reprinted from C. Zhao et al. (ref. [38]), J Exp Clin Cancer Res 2020. doi: 10.1186/ s13046-020-01666-z*

Allinen and colleagues were among the first to point to the "bulk tissue approach" as problematic, when exploring stromal tissue features by gene expression analyses [41]. They therefore aimed to elucidate cellular interactions along with paracrine regulatory modules in breast cancer, reporting the transcriptional and genetic alterations in various cell types in invasive breast cancer, ductal carcinoma in situ, and normal breast tissue. All cell types were purified, and the gene expression profiles of the cell types such as the epithelial cells, myoepithelial cells, myofibroblasts, fibroblasts, endothelial cells, and leukocytes were described. The identification of upregulated CXCL14 and CXCL12 specifically in tumor myoepithelial cells and myofibroblasts, causing epithelial cell proliferation and invasion via the binding of these ligands to their cognate receptors on epithelial tumor cells, were among their novel findings [41]. This study uniquely examined cell type-specific gene expression programs and additionally validated the functional consequences of these alterations, proposing novel analysis approaches to study the tumor-stroma interactions.

Gene Expression Signatures Reflecting the Bulk Cancer-Associated Stroma

As the cancer stroma is composed of several cellular components, examination of general stromal gene expression alterations may bring us into challenges of low specificity regarding which cell type the different expression signals originate from. However, the literature on general stromal signatures demonstrates new information as compared to what was derived from the studies on "whole tissue approaches," as elucidated in the following section.

Several gene expression signatures derived from the tumor stroma have been published, some of them investigated in relation to disease progress. Two studies explored the differences in the tumor stroma by assessing pre-invasive ductal carcinoma in situ lesions and invasive breast carcinomas. Ma and colleagues assessed the global expression alterations specifically in the stromal and epithelial compartments [42], and demonstrated comprehensive gene expression changes in the tumor-associated stroma during progression from normal to the pre-invasive and invasive states. A gene expression signature reflecting histologic tumor grade was identified in the stromal compartment. This study embraced the hypothesis that tumor-stromal-related changes contribute to tumor progression, specifically in the step from pre-invasive to invasive disease.

In a similar manner, Roman-Peréz and colleagues compared the expression pattern of tumor-adjacent tissue from invasive carcinomas and ductal carcinoma in situ, identifying breast cancer subtypes defined by extratumoral expression patterns [43]. Two distinct "microenvironmental subtypes" were identified, denoted as "Active" and "Inactive" types. Tumors with "active signature" shared features of claudin-low breast cancer and were associated with TGF-β induced activation score. The "active signature" also correlated with tumor aggressiveness and clinical outcome in ER-positive breast cancer.

In supervised analyses of global gene expression data, gene expression patterns between different pre-defined groups have been examined. What would be the best groups to compare when investigating the microenvironmental alterations that support or drive tumor progression? Normal versus cancer? Normal versus pre-invasive in situ lesions? The pre-invasive cases versus cancer? Or simply, although a more complex analytical approach, the whole sequence from normal through pre-invasive and eventually invasive carcinomas? In the following section, studies approaching this challenge in different ways are summarized.

Troester and colleagues compared global expression patterns of normal breast tissue from reduction mammoplasty resections and normal breast tissue adjacent to tumor tissue. A 155-gene "cancer adjacent normal tissue" signature was derived [44]. Genes reflecting constituents of the extracellular matrix, and remodeling of this, as well as genes of inflammation were enriched in this signature. Further, some of the signature genes were known to be involved in cell adhesion, angiogenesis, and re-epithelialization such as keratins. Interpreting these transcriptional findings in a functional manner, similarities to wound healing were seen, and the signature was regarded to reflect an in vivo "wound response." Further, the signature is strongly associated with breast cancer survival, indicating that tumor-related microenvironmental responses might be of importance in the progression of breast carcinomas.

Finak and colleagues applied laser capture tissue microdissection to assess the gene expression pattern of tumor stroma in primary breast cancer. Several gene expression signatures identified in this series are associated with disease course. The 26-gene signature denoted *"stroma derived prognostic predictor"* pointed to contrasting immune responses and angiogenic and hypoxic responses in different tumors [45]. This signature also predicted prognosis, as validated in multiple breast cancer data sets. Based on clustering of the 26-gene signature, the authors suggested stroma-dependent breast cancer subtypes. Also, the stroma signature by Finak predicted clinical outcome independent of other signatures, which were also associated with prognosis, indicating that their stroma-derived prognosticator mirrors specific biological processes taking part in directing the clinical disease course. In this study, Finak and colleagues demonstrated an independent stromal impact within the tumor, showing that genes of their stroma-derived prognostic marker did not predict prognosis when assessed in the epithelial component. The prediction of metastatic disease improved when combining the stroma signatures by Finak with other signature scores of prognostic value, indicating an improved reflection of the stroma-related processes when

merging signatures developed by different analytical approaches.

How do the stromal and epithelial cells communicate? Are we able to reflect the interplay between these two compartments by the use of gene expression data? To address these questions, Casey and colleagues examined the transcriptomic pattern of epithelial and stromal cells, both in normal breast tissue and in invasive breast cancer [46]. Cell type-specific interactions were also assessed. A "motile phenotype" was identified in the epithelial compartment, and a "reactive phenotype" in the stromal compartment, with genes reflecting remodeling of the extracellular matrix in a proteolytic manner in the invasive cancer. Also, genes promoting epithelial-mesenchymal interaction (EMT), such as FAP (fibroblast activated protein alpha) were identified. This study interestingly supports a molecular crosstalk between the epithelial and stromal cell compartments, suggesting that alterations facilitating invasion are one of the features of cancer-associated stroma.

By examining global gene expression alterations relating to specific tumor microenvironment elements that are microscopically assessable, it might be possible to identify underlying alterations of the histopathologic phenotype. Van den Eynden examined fibrotic tumor foci and associated gene expression patterns [47], and demonstrated Ras signaling and HIF1A-pathway activation along with other hypoxia- and angiogenesis-related genes in the large fibrotic foci. Also, fibrotic foci correlated with an activated wound healing signature and with earlier development of distant metastases.

What would be the model system best fit to capture ongoing microenvironmental processes promoting tumor progression? Marchini and colleagues examined the transcriptomic alterations in A17 mouse mammary carcinoma cells [48]. Three gene expression signatures reflecting stroma-related features and processes were identified: One "stemness signature," one "angiogenesis signature," and one "signal transduction signature." These signatures are associated with mesenchymal stem cell signatures, ER-negative breast cancer, a basal-like phenotype and breast cancer bone metastases. In post-treatment assessment of breast cancer xenograft models, the A17 angiogenesis- and signal transduction signatures were more highly expressed after hormonal therapy. This study indicates a linkage between mesenchymal features, tumor progression and therapy resistance, directing an interpretation of these findings towards EMT, as regarded having critical importance in tumor progression. Recent studies indicate that epithelial-mesenchymal plasticity contributes to stem-like tumor features and generates cancer stem cells [49–51].

Are the tumor microenvironmental changes in cancer progression common or specific across tumor types? Planche and colleagues examined this question by laser microdissecting stromal cells of invasive breast and prostate carcinoma. These two tumor types displayed distinctly different stromal gene expression patterns [52]. Gene expression alterations of the cancer type-specific stromal genes clustered both breast and prostate cancer samples into groups with different disease courses. Of note, genes of extracellular matrix constituents and proteolytic enzymes were upregulated in the invasive breast cancer stroma, in line with the observations done on the tumor histology sections.

In most mRNA expression studies, RNA is extracted from tissue that is snap frozen in the surgical theatre, as the RNA is best preserved for quantitative analyses in this manner, as compared to when extracted from formalin fixed paraffin embedded (FFPE) tissue. However, as of the writing of this chapter, FFPE patient-derived tissue is widely available, as this is stored in pathology archives worldwide. Winslow and colleagues made a critical step forward in this field when they succeeded in studying gene expression alterations from laser dissected tumor epithelial and stromal compartments from FFPE invasive breast cancer samples. This study showed that stroma-specific gene expression signatures were segregated into three major thematic groups; (1) extracellular matrix and fibroblast-related genes; (2) vascular-related genes; and (3) immune cell-related genes. Strikingly, the immune-related signature is associated with basal-like breast cancer subtype [53]. As the results from this study were in line with other similarly designed studies on fresh frozen tissue, the study gave new hope for RNA studies on FFPE tissue.

A few studies have related global gene expression data to specific molecular microenvironmental alterations. Specifically, a relationship between CD10+ stromal cell expression and breast cancer progression was previously reported [41], and Desmedt and colleagues followed up on this by exploring gene expression alterations related to CD10+ stromal cells [54]. A "*CD10+ stroma signature*" of 12 genes was generated by comparing the gene expression patterns of CD10+ cells isolated from breast carcinomas and normal breast tissue. In co-culture experiments, the CD10+ cells were characterized as specific cell populations: fibroblasts, myoepithelial, and mesenchymal stem cells. As seen in many of the stroma- and CAF-derived signatures, the CD10+ signature was composed of genes related to matrix remodeling. Interestingly, genes related to osteoblast differentiation (*e.g.,* osteopontin) were also upregulated in the CD10+ signature. All the different CD10+ cell types contributed to this stroma-related signature, however, the highest CD10+ stroma signature score was found in mesenchymal stem cells. Of clinical value, the signature was able to differentiate in situ and invasive breast cancer lesions. Also, the CD10+ signature demonstrated a potential to predict response to chemotherapy, and high CD10+ stroma score was associated with reduced survival in HER2 positive breast

cancer cases. This study is a good example of how to combine in vivo and in vitro studies, specifically with respect to validating the functionality of a gene expression signature.

In another study describing gene expression alterations reflecting specific molecular alterations, Rajski and colleagues identified a signature associated with IGF-I stimulated stromal cells [55]. Amongst the IGF-I signature genes, there was enrichment of proliferation-associated genes. This signature clustered the cancer samples in two major groups: those with upregulated IGF-1 and those without. Cases in the cluster with genes upregulated by IGF-I experienced shorter survival. An example of a signature related to specific histopathologic tumor features is one necrosis-related signature derived from gene expression alterations between endometrial carcinomas with and without tumor necrosis [56]. In this case, tumor necrosis was found to be associated with gene expression programs of hypoxia, angiogenesis, and inflammatory responses.

The cancer biology underlying phenotypic features of various cancer types may be cancer specific, but also share commonalities with other diseases and non-cancerous conditions. West and colleagues exploited the potential of approaching the research question from a different angle, when postulating that fibroblasts present with different activation states. In their approach to this question, they distinguished fibroblast populations in non-cancerous samples [57], demonstrating that solitary fibrous tumors and desmoid-type fibromatosis exhibited different expression patterns. In particular, the expression of growth factors and extracellular matrix genes were differentially expressed. When assessing the gene signature separating solitary fibrous tumor from desmoid-type fibromatosis in a series of invasive breast cancer, two groups of breast carcinomas were identified and associated with different survival. The cases with an expression pattern similar to the desmoid-type fibromatosis showed more favorable outcome, while the other group was observed with poorer prognosis. These findings supported the hypothesis that tumor stromal response varies among carcinomas of different aggressiveness.

After the first breast cancer subtype classification by Perou et al. [16], further subgroups of the subtypes are identified based on molecular alterations, like the Lehman subgrouping of triple-negative breast cancer into basal-like, immunomodulatory, mesenchymal, mesenchymal-like, and luminal androgen receptor subtypes—some of the subtypes associated with distinct survival patterns [58]. A recent study by Bareche and coworkers aimed to characterize the tumor microenvironment of triple-negative breast cancer subtypes, elucidating how the microenvironment heterogeneity may contribute to the different clinical pictures seen in triple-negative subsets [59]. A broad signature approach was applied, incorporating gene sets reflecting immune activation, angiogenesis, hypoxia, cancer-associated fibroblast, and metabolism (*e.g.,* glycolysis, lipid metabolism) in the analyses. Distinct TME profiles and specific immune cell composition and localization were associated with the different triple-negative subgroups—and associated differently with clinical outcomes. Next, 16 signatures reflecting innate and adaptive immune responses [60] were mapped to the triple-negative subtypes, demonstrating enrichment of adaptive immune response in the immune modulatory subtype, and enriched innate response in the mesenchymal-like subtype. The mesenchymal and basal-like subtypes showed poor immune responses, both innate and adaptive.

Qian and coworkers described in 2020 a *"pan-cancer blueprint of the heterogeneous tumor microenvironment"*—adding substantially to our knowledge about heterogenous microenvironment by analyzing single-cell RNA and proteins [61]. By profiling 233,591 single cells from lung, colorectal, ovary and breast tumors and corresponding tumor-free tissue, profiles of 68 stromal cell populations were identified, 22 unique and 46 shared between cancer types. The stromal cell populations were characterized phenotypically by marker genes, metabolic activities, and tissue-specific expression differences. Applying the analysis approaches to an independent subset of melanoma tumors treated with checkpoint immune inhibitors, a naïve CD4+ T-cell phenotype predictive of response to checkpoint immunotherapy was identified. By applying single cell and signature analyses approaches, this study replies in interesting ways to whether and how the tumor microenvironment heterogeneity is present across cancer types, and generates, as the authors state, *"the first panoramic view on the shared complexity of stromal cells in different cancers"*—with potential for identification of strong prognostic and predictive cancer biomarkers. interactions.

Gene Expression Signatures Reflecting Cancer-Associated Fibroblasts

Most of the studies above have investigated bulk tissue stroma and have thereby potentially reflected expression contribution from the combination of different stromal cell types. Many of the stromal signatures correlate with clinicopathologic features and disease course, potentially reflecting underlying stroma biology. Still, it is tempting to ask: What is the contribution to the signatures from each of the specific stromal cell types?

Chang and colleagues were among the first to generate a pure fibroblast gene expression signature, where the expression alterations were generated by fibroblasts being exposed to serum [62]. The signature was denoted a *"core serum response."* Functional analyses revealed involvement of the signature genes in myofibroblast activation, matrix remodeling, and cell motility. All these processes contribute to wound healing. Based on the expression of this wound healing-related signature, breast cancer samples are segregated into two groups. The group with activated signature pattern was associated with increased risk of metastatic disease and death from breast cancer. Further, the signature pattern was consistent in paired samples of locally advanced breast carcinomas, biopsied before and after chemotherapy, indicating stability of the biological program reflected in this signature. Interestingly, the basal-like molecular breast cancer subtype is significantly associated with the expression pattern of the wound healing-related signature, suggesting that the signature points to intrinsic properties of the basal-like phenotype. The signature was also examined in gene expression data sets of various tumor types, and the findings were striking: The expression pattern of the signature separated the cases into two groups, with significantly increased risk of metastatic disease in the group with the activated signature pattern. Harold F. Dvorak suggested in a review in 1986 that the wound is an analog to the stromal processes observed in tumors [63]. The gene expression signature by Chang might have captured some of the alterations observed by Dvorak.

Tchou and colleagues added information about subtype-specific stromal gene expression patterns in breast cancer [64]. Their analyses demonstrated distinctly different expression profiles in CAFs from breast cancer samples of the HER2 positive subtype, triple-negative cases and ER-positive cases. In particular pathways linked to the cytoskeleton and integrin signaling were differentially enriched in the different CAF groups. The results from this study add to the arguments of specific stroma-related breast cancer subtypes, supporting the hypothesis that fibroblasts participate to the disease biology underlying clinically relevant breast cancer subtypes.

Two projects exploring transcriptional alterations in tumor-associated fibroblasts compared to normal mammary fibroblasts, demonstrated an increased expression of genes involved in tumor progression in the CAFs. Cytokines, genes related to remodeling of the extracellular matrix, and genes reflecting paracrine or intracellular signaling, as well as cell-matrix interactions, were upregulated in the tumor-associated fibroblasts [65, 66]. In the study by Singer, it was noted that these gene expression alterations also take place in the isolated cell culture state, in the absence of adjacent malignant epithelium [66]. In the study by Bauer, the CAF-associated genes were incorporated into a 31-gene signature that was validated by qPCR. Some of the genes upregulated in CAFs were validated at protein levels by immunohistochemistry, with respect to location and quantitation [65]. Taken together, the findings from these two studies indicate fibroblastic subpopulations of the tumor stroma, facilitating tumor progress.

By comparing global gene expression patterns of platelet-derived growth factor (PDGF)-stimulated human fibroblasts and resting fibroblasts, Frings and colleagues identified a 113-gene expression signature reflecting PDGF-activated fibroblasts [67]. This signature had the potential to identify breast cancers with a stroma of PDGF-stimulated fibroblasts. The signature correlated with high expression of the PDGF receptor β (PDGFRB) and its ligands and was enriched for genes related to angiogenesis and regulation of the extracellular matrix. Signature analyses in several breast cancer data sets demonstrated associations between the PDGF signature score and clinicopathologic features reflecting aggressive tumors, such as large tumor size, high histologic grade, HER2 positive, and ER-negative tumors. Moreover, signature activation is correlated with the HER2 positive, basal-like and Luminal B subtypes of breast cancer. In line with these observations, the signature demonstrated a robust association with survival; a high signature score was associated with reduced survival, also in multivariate analyses, when adjusted for other stroma signatures and a proliferation signature.

Sonnenblick et al. developed a stromal gene expression signature based on reactive breast cancer stroma in HER2 positive cases, containing increased amounts of reactive myofibroblasts surrounding the tumor cell nests [68]. This "reactive stroma signature" was associated with trastuzumab resistance in estrogen receptor (ER)-negative tumors, but not in ER-positive tumors, suggesting the reactive stroma and its accompanying signature as a potential predictive marker for Trastuzumab in subsets of breast cancer.

Siletz and colleagues assessed transcription factor signatures and activity specific for mammary CAFs versus normal mammary fibroblasts [69]. A transcription factor activity signature included activation of reporters for ELK1, GATA1, retinoic acid receptor, serum response factor, and vitamin D receptor. An increased activation of reporters for HIF1 and several STAT and proliferation-related transcription factors was seen after induction of fibroblasts by conditioned medium from breast cancer cell lines. These transcription factor activity profiles indicate CAF subtype-specific signaling promoting tumor progression through a pro-invasive stroma.

In recent years, single-cell RNA sequencing has allowed for identification and deep characterization of CAF subpopulations. By defining CAF subpopulations by single-cell RNA sequencing of transcriptomes of mesenchymal cells from a genetically engineered mouse model of breast cancer, Bartoschek and colleagues added knowledge about CAF heterogeneity with functional and clinical implications [70]. Gene signatures reflecting angiogenesis and vascular development, matrix-related genes, cell cycle activation, and development and differentiation were enriched in the CAF groups that accordingly were annotated vascular, matrix, cycling, and developmental CAFs (vCAFs, mCAFs, cCAFs, dCAFs). The vCAFs and mCAFs signatures were validated by RNA sequencing of bulk breast cancer tissue, demonstrating biological and clinical relevance (Fig. 23.3).

Wu and colleagues aimed to elucidate stromal heterogeneity in triple-negative breast cancer [71]. Two CAF and two perivascular-like (PVL) subpopulations were identified in the stroma, with distinct spatial relationships and functional properties. The gene signatures reflecting inflammatory CAFs and differentiated PVL revealed associations with cytotoxic T-cell dysfunction in independent cohorts of triple-negative breast cancer, pointing to potential candidate biomarkers for new therapeutic strategies in the treatment of triple-negative breast cancer.

Woelfle and colleagues derived a signature of 86 genes differentially expressed between primary tumors with and without bone marrow metastases [72]. Although the tumor microenvironment was not the focus of this study, most of the signature genes were related to extracellular matrix remodeling, cytoskeleton plasticity and cell adhesion. Also, RAS- and HIF1A signaling were enriched in tumors with bone marrow metastases. The many similarities between this signature and the stroma- and CAF-related signatures described above lead to an intriguing perspective on this signature. In addition to facilitate invasive growth and tumor progression, perhaps the tumor stroma is heavily involved in directing tumor metastases to different locations? Another interesting perspective of this signature was that 77 of the 86 signature genes were downregulated in primary tumors with bone marrow metastases, indicating transcriptional repression as part of the picture in tumor progressive processes.

A few studies have examined transcriptional alterations related specifically to the extracellular matrix in breast cancer. Bergamaschi and colleagues set out to classify breast carcinomas based on constituents of the extracellular matrix (ECM), selecting 278 ECM-related from the literature [73]. The ECM-related genes segregated the breast cancer samples into four ECM classes with different clinical courses. The ECM group associated with best survival showed upregulation of protease inhibitors of the serpin family. The ECM group associated with poorest survival presented with overexpression of integrins and metallopeptidases, and low expression of laminin chains. In a follow-up study, Triulzi and colleagues demonstrated that one of the ECM groups consistently predicted one cluster in several independent breast cancer data sets [74]. The 58-gene signature of this ECM subset contained 43 genes encoding structural ECM proteins. Investigation of gene expression data sets on separate cancer epithelial and stromal cells demonstrated that genes of this ECM signature were expressed both by the epithelial and stromal compartments. In vitro experiments

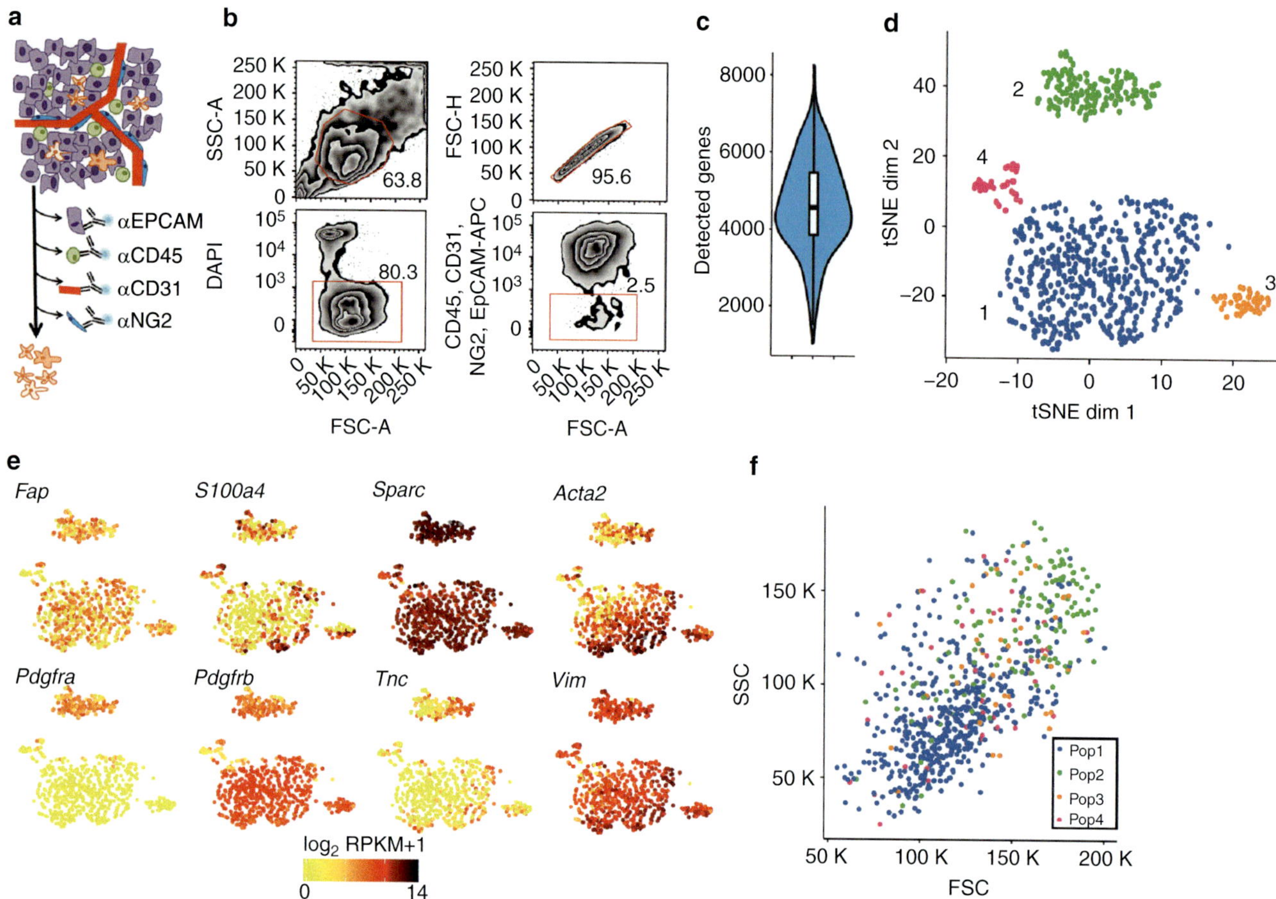

Fig. 23.3 Unbiased clustering of fibroblast single-cell transcriptomic data reveals four populations. (**a**) Schematic representation of negative selection strategy. (**b**) gating strategy and quantification of flow cytometry for single-cell sequencing. *FSC* forward scatter, *SCC* side scatter. (**c**) Violin plot of detected genes in 784 sorted fibroblasts. (**d**) t-SNE layout of CAFs ($n = 716$) by RPKM-normalized transcriptomic data. (**e**) Expression plots on t-SNE layout. Log2(RPKM+1) levels of CAFs marker genes in individual cells. (**f**) Cell size and granularity as determined by forward-scattered light (FSC) and side-scattered light (SSC) of different CAF populations. *With permission, reprinted from M. Bartoschek et al. (ref. [70]), Nat Commun 2018. doi: 10.1038/s41467-018-07582-3*

showed induction of signature genes, in particular in fibroblasts and in ER-negative breast cancer cells. Single genes and gene sets reflecting EMT were significantly associated with this ECM signature. In another study validating the functionality of the identified CAF subsets, Bartoschek and colleagues (see above) characterized transcription of genes encoding ECM proteins included in the matrisome. Each of the CAF populations demonstrated distinct ECM transcriptional signatures, supporting their different biological functions [70].

Gene Expression Signatures Reflecting Vascular Biology

Various measures of histologically verified tumor vasculature (*e.g.,* mean vessel density, vascular proliferation) are related to tumor progress and metastatic disease in solid cancer types. The vasculature is viewed as a target for therapy, as exploited in therapeutic programs in several tumor types. Studies on genomic programs measuring the transcriptional alterations have a potential to reveal novel aspects of vascular biology in malignant tumors. With this in mind, Wallgard and colleagues sought to elucidate the transcriptome and molecular processes specific to endothelial cells [75]. Fifty-eight genes specifically linked to microvascular expression were identified, many of them not previously described in relation to functions of endothelial cells. Wallgard suggested several genes and related proteins to be further explored in relation to drugs targeting the microvasculature, like Eltd1, Gpr116, Ramp2, Rasip1. In a recent study, Cleuren and colleagues further characterized the endothelial cell biology by facilitating isolation of endothelial cell (EC) ribosome-associated transcripts, also known as the translatome [76]. By combined endothelial-specific translating ribosome affinity purification (EC-TRAP) and high-throughput RNA sequencing analyses, known and new pan EC-enriched gene signatures and tissue-specific EC transcripts were identified,

Fig. 23.4 Identification of enriched transcripts after EC-TRAP. (**a**) GO analysis of the 500 top-ranked genes with the highest enrichment scores after EC-TRAP (FDR < 10%) shows overrepresentation of transcripts involved in vascular-related processes. (**b**) Unsupervised hierarchical clustering of EC-enriched genes shows distinct, highly heterogenous vascular bed-specific EC expression patterns. (**c**) Comparison of the 500 most enriched genes per tissue identifies a group of pan-endothelial and subsets of tissue-specific EC-enriched genes. *With permission, reprinted from A.C.A. Cleuren et al. [76], Proc Natl Acad Sci USA 2019. doi: 10.1073/ pnas.1912409116*

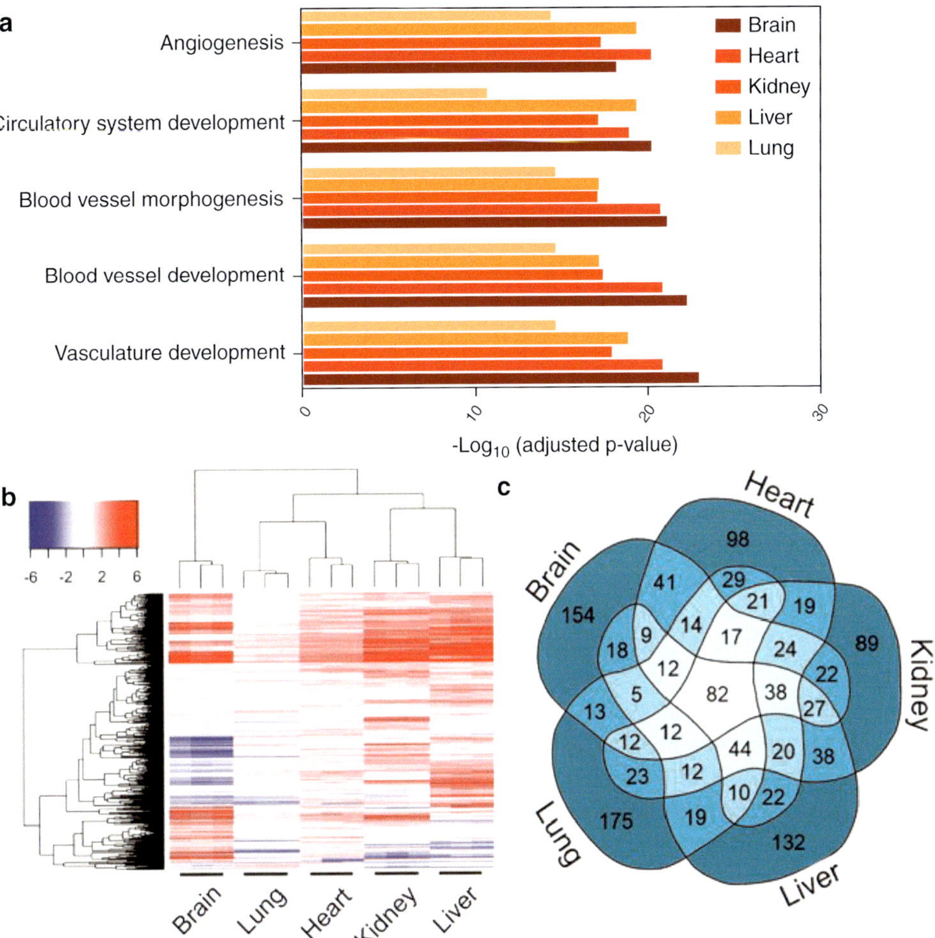

also demonstrating endothelial cell heterogeneity across tissue types and disease states (Fig. 23.4). Results from this study indicated that the transcriptome of a tissue lysate can serve as a proxy for the corresponding tissue translatome, supporting relevance of the mRNA expression analysis approaches applied in previous studies on vascular biology in cancer.

The vasculature is regarded as the main route for breast cancer metastases. Hu and colleagues compared the global transcription pattern of primary tumors and distant metastases, identifying an in vivo hypoxia signature reflecting VEGF activation and predicting poor clinical outcome in breast cancer and other tumor types [77]. This 13-gene signature was composed of several angiogenesis-related genes. Eight of the 13 signature genes contained binding sites for the hypoxia-related transcription factor HIF1α and had been demonstrated to be regulated by HIF1α.

Pepin and colleagues identified two distinct tumor vasculature types by analyzing global transcription patterns across laser capture microdissected tumor-associated and matched normal vasculature [78]. The two tumor vasculature types demonstrated specific gene expression signatures, whereas one related to anti-angiogenic signaling. Samples enriched

for this signature demonstrated lower mean vessel density as compared to the group enriched for the gene signature associated with active vascular remodeling and reduced vascular shear stress. Reduced vascular shear stress is suggested to reflect reduced vessel flow rate and may reflect inappropriate tumor perfusion. Significantly, several therapeutic targets with potential relevance in anti-angiogenic treatment (*e.g.,* MET, PDGFRβ, ITGAV) were differentially expressed between the vasculature subtypes.

When studying alterations in vascular gene expression, different study designs may reveal different layers of the complete picture. Bender and colleagues demonstrated by supervised analyses of angiogenesis-related genes that the gene expression of the VEGF and semaphorin families was altered in pro-angiogenic manners in triple-negative breast cancer [79]. Compiling these genes into a composite biomarker, the gene expression signature is associated with triple-negative breast cancer and reduced survival in non-triple-negative subtypes.

Wallace and colleagues approached angiogenesis-related biology in a more indirect manner. In an analysis of genes and pathways mediating fibroblast contribution in cancer progression [80], the authors studied how Ets2 function varied between mammary stromal fibroblasts and epithelial cells. In HER2 positive breast cancer mouse models, Ets2 inactivation in fibroblasts reduced tumor growth. The same effects were not seen when inhibiting Ets2 in epithelial cells. An Ets2-dependent gene signature was derived, enriched in genes related to remodeling of the extracellular matrix, cell migration, and angiogenesis. Supportive to these functional interpretations, fewer functional blood vessels were found in tumors lacking fibroblast Ets2. The Ets2-dependent gene expression signature was able to segregate human breast cancer stroma and normal stroma and indicated a link between Ets2 and the fibroblast-endothelial crosstalk, pointing to a contribution of Ets2 in the angiogenic process.

Xiao and colleagues [81] developed in vitro models studying breast cancer-specific endothelial cells, identifying multiple subpopulations of tumor-associated endothelial cells, each population with distinct gene expression patterns. A relationship with tumor-associated endothelial cells had not previously been established for several genes. Irx2 and Zfp503 were without previously known relevance to vascular biology, but were found highly upregulated in tumor endothelial cells. These genes are known to regulate neuronal patterning and developmental differentiation [82, 83], and may point to new information on vascular-related mechanisms and co-regulatory circuits in vascular biology.

Mannelqvist and colleagues published an 18-gene expression signature related to vascular invasion in endometrial carcinomas, also relating to features of aggressive disease and disease outcome [84]. In a follow-up study on multiple breast cancer gene expression data sets, the vascular invasion signature was associated with tumor progression and clinical course in breast cancer [85]. Also, a high signature score was associated with the basal-like phenotype and response to neoadjuvant chemotherapy. The signature was composed of genes related to angiogenesis, immune responses, and extracellular matrix biology. Further, the signature was correlated with other gene expression profiles of vascular biology, hypoxia, EMT, immune response, and tumor progression.

The same research group later published a 32-gene signature reflecting tissue-based vascular proliferation. Microvessel proliferation was assessed by dual endothelial immunostaining of Factor-VIII/Ki67, and global gene expression data as well as copy number information were explored in supervised manners [86]. Several genes in the signature had previously been linked to processes such as neovascularization, endothelial cell migration and adhesion, supporting this signature as relevant for tumor angiogenesis. Also, amplification of the region 6p21, potentially harboring VEGF, is associated with high microvessel proliferation.

Tobin et al. elucidated how gene transcripts representative of normal endothelium related to breast cancer progress. A composite microvasculature (MV) score was derived from expression values of 57 mouse microvasculature transcripts [87]. In 993 breast cancer tumors, the MV score did not associate with microvessel density, but indicated decreased risk of metastasis in endocrine-treated patients. Further, the MV score was increased from pre-treatment to post-treatment samples in metastatic breast tumors after treatment with sunitinib and docetaxel, compared to cases with only docetaxel treatment, supporting the concept of vascular normalization following treatment with an angiogenic inhibitor.

Physiological angiogenesis is regarded molecularly different from the pathologic angiogenesis, indicating different mechanisms involved in the two processes. Guarischi-Sousa and colleagues followed up on this idea, identifying a 153-gene signature reflecting pathologic angiogenesis from oxygen-induced retinopathy [88]. Applying a machine learning algorithm, a signature of 11 of the 153 genes was compiled together with information on age and stage into a signature strongly predicting breast cancer survival. The authors propose the signature as a potential marker for pointing to tumors relevant for angiogenesis-targeted therapies.

Harrell and colleagues sought to determine whether tumor-associated vascular properties could identify mechanisms contributing to the different risks of metastatic disease across the intrinsic subtypes of breast cancer [89]. They found that claudin-low and basal-like tumors were enriched for transcriptional programs reflecting vascular quantity, vascular proliferation, and a VEGF/Hypoxia signature. Incorporating several of the vascular gene signatures described above-added information about risk of metastatic disease. Furthermore, experimental studies demonstrated that claudin-low cells exhibited endothelial-like morphology, and claudin-low xenograft tumors were highly perfused through intercellular spaces and non-vascular tumor cell lined channels. This study combined the transcriptional studies with experimental validation in an interesting manner, demonstrating both endothelial-like characteristics of cancer cells, and how the vasculature in conceptually new manners may contribute to breast cancer progression. Also, the gene expression signatures were suggested as predictive markers to anti-angiogenic therapy.

Mendiola and colleagues set out to identify a biomarker predicting response to bevacizumab and paclitaxel in metastatic breast cancer by exploring angiogenesis-related genes and clinical markers [90]. An 11-gene signature predicted improved progression-free and overall survival in patients on bevacizumab–paclitaxel treatment, with added prognostic value when combining the signature with five clinical covariates. The value of these composite biomarkers as predictive markers to bevacizumab in metastatic breast cancer should be tested.

Krüger et al. recently studied predictive markers for combined neoadjuvant bevacizumab and chemotherapy treatment in a randomized trial [91]. Along with tissue-based angiogenesis biomarkers (microvessel density, proliferative microvessel density, glomeruloid microvascular proliferation), the authors explored how an angiogenesis-based mRNA signature previously published from the same group [86], reflected pathologic complete response. High baseline MVD predicted pCR in the bevacizumab-arm, whereas vascular proliferation and a high angiogenesis score were associated with the triple-negative and basal-like phenotypes but did not predict therapy response.

Inflammation is regarded to promote tumor angiogenesis. Pro-inflammatory cytokines work through mediators, enhancing or suppressing angiogenesis. Combinations of these factors may contribute to the tumor's vascular invasive and metastasizing properties. Pitroda and colleagues explored how vascular inflammation influences cancer prognosis [92]. A gene expression signature reflecting inflammation in tumor-associated endothelial cells was developed. The endothelial-derived 6-gene inflammatory signature predicted reduced overall survival in breast cancer and other tumor types. Also, inflammatory pathways activated in endothelial cells are linked to tumor progression in mice, supporting a vasculo-immunogenic link contributing to tumor progression in breast cancer.

Oshi et al. aimed to explore relations between intratumoral angiogenesis, inflammation, and metastasis in breast cancer [93]. They derived an angiogenesis-related signature score that did not correlate with clinicopathologic variables or survival, nor with breast cancer molecular subtypes. However, a high score is associated with a low fraction of immune cell infiltrations, both favorable and unfavorable. Unfavorable inflammation-related gene sets (IL6, TNFα, TGFβ) and metastasis-related gene sets were enriched in high-score tumors. Further, a high angiogenesis score was significantly associated with metastasis to brain and bone.

Gene Expression Signatures Reflecting Immune-Related Alterations

The immune system is considered to play an important role in cancer initiation and progression and is a promising multifaceted target in novel therapeutic strategies [94]. Important interactions between the immune cells and other tumor microenvironmental elements are brought to discussion [95]. How immune system alterations contribute to cancer progress is not yet well understood. Studies on breast cancer have demonstrated survival benefit from immunotherapy, mainly in advanced triple-negative and HER2 subtypes [96–100]. European Medicine Agency approved in 2020 the PD-L1 checkpoint inhibitor atezolizumab in combination with chemotherapy (nab-paclitaxel), to patients with PD-L1 positive, unresectable, locally advanced or metastatic triple-negative breast cancer [99, 101]. PD-L1 immunohistochemistry is

approved as a predictive biomarker test for this treatment regimen, but study results indicate a need for improved predictive biomarkers for checkpoint inhibitors. Although the field of cancer immunology has been extensively explored and exploited for diagnostic and therapeutic purposes, the words of Winston Churchill still seem valid: *"This is not the end. It is not even the beginning of the end. But it is, perhaps, the end of the beginning."*

Perou and colleagues touched upon the transcriptional heterogeneity of ER-negative breast cancer in their early breast cancer classification study [16]. Teschendorff et al. followed up on this, demonstrating transcriptional alterations associated with the clinical course of ER-negative breast cancer [102]. Distinct subclasses among ER-negative tumors were shown based on transcriptional patterns. One of the classes consisted of basal-like tumors with upregulation of genes related to immune response and complement activation. This subset of ER-negative samples demonstrated better survival pattern as compared to the rest of ER-negative tumors. Based on this study, a seven-gene immune response signature was derived. Downregulation of this module is associated with increased risk of advanced disease. In a later study, Rody and colleagues focused on the clinically and prognostically heterogenous triple-negative breast cancer subtype [103]. The basal-like and claudin-low subtypes were described by metagenes reflecting angiogenesis, inflammation, and non-neoplastic cell types like immune cells, adipocytes, and fibroblasts. High immune cell score is associated with improved survival, and high inflammation and angiogenesis scores are correlated with reduced survival. By applying a ratio of the B-cell and IL-8 metagenes, Rody identified a subgroup (32%) of triple-negative cases with high B-cell and low IL-8 scores, experiencing improved outcome. Further, two other breast cancer studies have underpinned the association between an immune response and tumor subsets with milder disease courses [104, 105]. In the study by Alexe and colleagues, a HER2-positive subtype with low recurrence rate was associated with high expression of lymphocyte-associated genes [104]. Also, a prominent lymphocytic infiltration was seen by histologic examination of these tumor cases. In the study by Schmidt and colleagues, a high B-cell metagene score was associated with metastasis-free survival in node-negative cases with high proliferation, as validated both in high-grade cases and in young breast cancer patients [105]. Schmidt and colleagues [106] followed up on this study, aiming to identify one single immune system marker for cancer progression. Immunoglobulin κC (IGKC) demonstrated similarly predictive and prognostic value as the entire B-cell metagene [105]. IGKC gene expression is associated with improved survival across different molecular subtypes in node-negative breast cancer. Also, levels of IGKC measured by immunostaining in a series of FFPE breast cancer tissues correlated with clinical outcomes.

Tumor-infiltrating plasma cells were identified as the source of the protein. These findings suggest relevance of further exploration of the humoral immune response and its relevance in the therapeutic setting.

One study pointing in this direction, specifically examined genes related to TH1-mediated adaptive immunity in breast cancer [107], and demonstrated that inflammation and immune suppression predicted tumor subsets with different clinical outcomes. Data sets on various tumor types were analyzed, and Hsu showed that upregulation of the TH1-mediated adaptive immunity genes correlated with good prognosis in young breast cancer patients (<45 years). Two other studies demonstrated better survival in cases of high immune signature score in breast cancer [108, 109]. Bianchini et al. demonstrated association between high expression of a B-cell/plasma cell signature and improved survival in ER-positive cases with high proliferation, also when adjusting for standard prognostic variables and other transcriptional scores [108]. In the study by Nagalla and coworkers, a cluster of cases without distant metastases was associated with genes related to immunological functions. These genes could be clustered into three major "immune metagenes," one cluster reflecting B-cells and/or plasma cells, another cluster reflecting T-cells and natural killer cells, and a third cluster reflecting monocytes and/or dendritic cells [109]. In tumors of high proliferation, high immune metagene score was associated with reduced risk of metastasis—cases with low immune metagene scores are associated with poorer outcome.

A few studies of immune-related signatures have suggested therapy strategies based on their findings. Ascierto and colleagues elucidated how immune function networks related to tumor-infiltrating immune cells were more highly expressed in cases without recurrent disease [110]. The network genes were related to B-cell development, interferon signaling, autoimmune reactions, and antigen presentation pathways. The results indicated crosstalk between the adaptive and innate immune systems. Five B-cell response genes predicted relapse-free survival (>85% accuracy), also validated by qPCR. The authors thus suggested immunotherapy, in the neoadjuvant setting, to patients with high risk of recurrent disease, potentially by inducing genes of immune function.

Iglesia and colleagues aimed to elucidate transcriptional alterations related to the cancer immune response of breast and ovarian cancers with high lymphocyte infiltration and improved survival [111]. RNAseq data and a microarray dataset were applied to identify signatures reflecting the adaptive immune response. The B-cell signatures predicted improved survival in the basal-like and HER2 subtypes. Further, analyses of B-cell receptor (BCR) sequences were assessed through RNAseq data. It was previously shown that a clonal expansion of the B-cells and somatic hypermuta-

tions in B-cell tumor-infiltrating lymphocytes in breast tissue represent an antigen-directed response [112–114], and the response of antigen-specific B-cell populations actively demonstrate features of clonal expansion. A part of the basal-like and HER2-enriched cases with shorter survival showed upregulation of BCR gene segments with low diversity, indicating lack of B-cell clonal expansion, and were also indicative of an ineffective antigen-directed response in these cases, potentially contributing to their poorer prognosis. More and varied BCR segments with increased expression are associated with improved prognosis. The results indicate a limited B-cell antitumor response in a subset of basal-like breast cancer. Also, immunomodulatory therapies were suggested, and supporting B-cell responses may be one relevant approach in B-cell infiltrated carcinomas.

Perez and coworkers developed a transcriptional signature of immune-related genes predicting clinical benefit in a clinical trial of adjuvant Trastuzumab in combination with chemotherapy in HER2 positive breast cancer [115]. Signature enrichment is associated with increased recurrence-free survival only in the study arms receiving Trastuzumab. Cases in the Trastuzumab study arms without immune signature enrichment did not benefit from Trastuzumab, suggesting interactions between immune-related genes and therapy response. Immune-related signatures associate with improved survival in several studies. However, when it comes to immune responses, the picture is not black and white. Rody and colleagues elucidated how the transcriptional changes of immune metagenes related to clinical outcomes [116]. An IgG metagene, which was found to be a marker for B-cells, did not associate with prognosis. However, high expression of a T-cell/lymphocyte-specific kinase signature is associated with survival in ER-negative cases and cases of concurrently ER and HER2 positivity. This study also suggests inhibition of the IL-8 pathway as a potential therapeutic strategy in breast cancer. Adding to the complexity, a link between the EMT program and immune evasion seen in cancer has been suggested [117–120].

By unsupervised analysis, identifying co-expressed breast cancer transcripts in global gene expression data, Yang and coworkers identified two co-expressed gene clusters with significant enrichment of gene sets reflecting immune responses and cell cycle activity. A condensed 17-gene signature was derived, correlating well with overall levels of tumor-infiltrating lymphocytes in triple-negative breast cancer [121]. The immune cell signature demonstrated prognostic value in subtype- and immunity-adjusted risk of distant metastasis (iRDM) analysis, as validated by independent cohorts.

The immune microenvironment in triple-negative breast cancer has been in the spotlight over the last years. The study by Zhang and colleagues contributes to our understanding of the mechanisms that promote cancer progress in triple-negative breast cancer, exploring the gene expression profiles of tumor-infiltrating CD4⁺T cells, elucidating how they contribute to modulating immune cell functions in triple-negative breast cancer [122]. The contribution of CD4 + T cells to the tumor-promoting biology was examined by assessing differentially expressed genes between tumor and peripheral blood CD4⁺T cells from patients with triple-negative breast cancer. Expression patterns associated with increased levels of T regulatory (Treg) cells and exhausted lymphocytes, and decreased effector/memory and cytotoxic T-cells were demonstrated in tumor samples. Additionally, genes overexpressed in CD4⁺ TILs contributed to exhaustion of lymphocytes and regulation of chemotaxis.

Adding information about spatial gene- and protein relations is recently increasingly focused on translational cancer studies. Considering the risk of losing compartment-specific information by studies on bulk tumor, Gruosso et al. integrated spatial tissue immune response information and gene expression profiling data from matched stromal and epithelial tumor compartments, identifying distinct tumor immune microenvironment (TIME) profiles in the triple-negative subgroup (Fig. 23.5) [123].

Biological processes identified by analyses of gene expression data from laser capture microdissected tissue from matched stromal and epithelial tumor compartments, pointed to distinct TIME subtypes, believed to support the development of TIME-dependent targeted therapeutic approaches to treat triple-negative breast cancer. Based on the high versus low tumor core or margin CD8⁺ T-cell infiltration, with information on stromal and epithelial T-cell infiltration, the triple-negative subset was grouped into "margin-restricted" (MR), "immune desert" (ID), "fully inflamed" (FI), and "stroma-restricted." The tumor characterization based on CD8⁺ T-cell localization identified

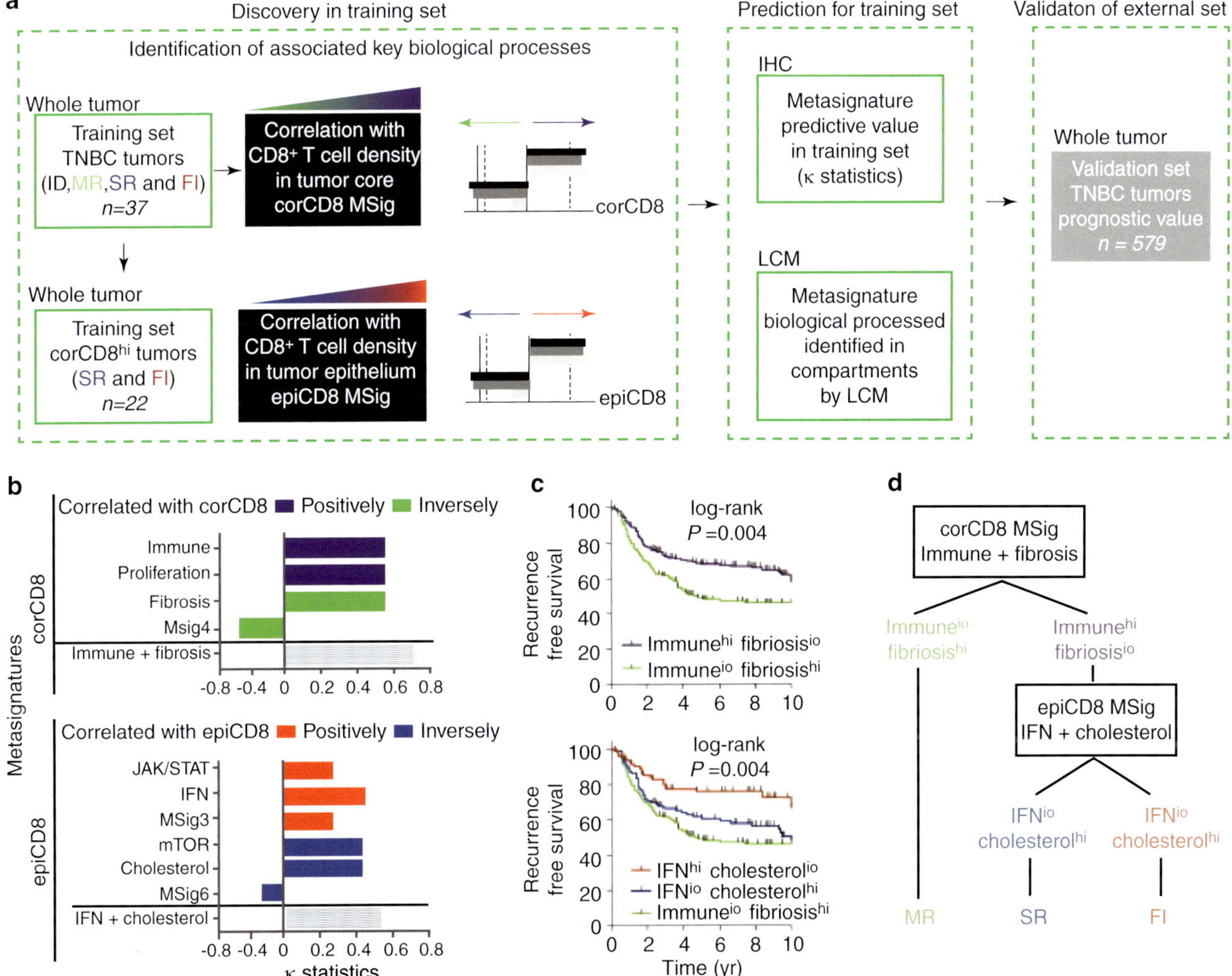

Fig. 23.5 (**a**) The analysis pipeline from Gruosso et al. [123], demonstrating discovery and validation of gene expression signatures identifying spatially context-dependent immune cell profiles. The authors visualize correlations between the immune cell profiles and pathway signaling (**b**), how signature combinations into meta-signatures stratify clinical outcome (**c**), and propose identification of new tumor phenotypes (**d**). *With permission, reprinted from Gruosso et al. [123], J Clin Invest 2019. doi: 10.1172/JCI96313*

mRNA signatures identify distinct biological processes in the different tumor compartments, like enrichment of cholesterol biosynthesis and IL17-related immunosuppression in restricted stromal tumors. The TIME subtype-specific mRNA signatures provided new survival knowledge within the group of triple-negative breast cancer.

Adipocytes and Glycolysis-Related Gene Signatures

At the invasive front of breast cancer, we frequently find the adipocytes, more specifically the breast cancer-associated adipocytes (CAAs). The crosstalk between adipocytes and cancer cells results in phenotypical and functional changes for both cell types [38, 124]. Ultimately, the interplay between CAAs and tumor cells shapes the tumor microenvironment towards an oncogene-driven state favoring proliferation, angiogenesis, invasion, and metastasis.

CAAs are proposed as key players in breast cancer progression, like in the study by Wu and colleagues [124], where the authors investigated the adipocyte-cancer cell crosstalk to gain insight into tumor biology and uncover novel therapeutic targets. Adipocytes are regarded as a giant energy storage upon interaction with BC cells, providing high energy metabolites. With this in mind, theories discuss that tumors may induce reprogramming of metabolic cooperation in adipocytes, adjusting to intracellular metabolic processes supporting proliferation through interplay and interactions between CAAs and breast cancer cells [125, 126]. Importantly, dividing cells demand extreme amounts of energy, and to meet these requirements, alterations in the metabolism of all macromolecules take place in cancer cells. Metabolic changes are well known as a hallmark of cancer [32], and glucose utilization and uptake are heavily increased in order to fuel cell growth and division in multiple cancer types. Interestingly, glycolysis is preferred in malignant tumors rather than oxidative phosphorylation in mitochondria [38, 127].

Targeting tumor metabolism has become a promising therapeutic strategy in cancer treatment. Investigating tumor glycolysis was the main objective for Tang and colleagues [128], who presented a glycolysis-related gene expression signature aiming to predict the prognosis of breast cancer patients. A total of 878 patients were included in the analyses, revealing 129 glycolysis-related genes significantly associated with breast cancer prognosis. From these, a robust four-gene signature was established in a prognostic model, separating breast cancer patients into high- and low-risk groups. Survival analysis demonstrated significantly better prognosis in the low-risk group. Moreover, the glycolysis-related gene signature showed excellent prognostic accuracy, also when stratified by clinicopathological risk factors. To validate the prognostic value of the signature, external validation sets were applied, demonstrating both statistically significant and clinical relevance of the signature.

Accompanying the hunt for glycolysis-related gene signatures in breast cancer, Li and colleagues [129] identified a prognosis-associated signature related to energy metabolism in triple-negative breast cancer (TNBC). Herein, 1097 cases were studied. An 8-gene signature associated with energy metabolism were identified, distinguishing patients' outcome into low-risk and high-risk groups. The 8-gene signature is distinctively associated with the patients' clinical characteristics, representing an independent factor in predicting TNBC patient prognosis. Also, the signature could potentially be used as a prognostic marker and for predicting response to therapy targeting the energy metabolism.

With similar study design, Zhang and colleagues [130] identified a glycolysis-related 11-gene signature for prognostic evaluation of breast cancer patients. In contrast to the common workflow applied in most studies working on gene expression and gene signature identification, this study selected genes mainly by performing gene set enrichment analysis (GSEA). The authors argued that as GSEA does not require significant differences in gene thresholds and screens genes based on overall expression levels, the risk of overlooking genes with important biological functions decreases. This study was the first in line to identify glycolysis-related genes with prognostic information in breast cancer. The 11-gene signature was proposed as a promising prognostic marker in breast cancer, and potentially with value as a screening tool to identify persons at high risk of developing breast cancer.

Regarding the topic of evading risk of overlooking important genes, protein–protein interaction network analysis (PPI) has become a popular tool when screening for prognostic factors in cancer, appearing to be a more effective method due to its ability to compare the relationship between candidate genes through network interactions. Moreover, interaction networks allow for visualization, which invites the human perspective along with computed calculations to inspect candidate genes based on their network relations, thus minimizing the risk of overlooking potential genes that may seem unimportant at first. When mining for key genes, protein–protein interaction analyses can be applied to single out genes with dense connections and central roles either in the network as a whole or in specific sub-clusters.

Studying the gene expression differences in distant and tumor-adjacent adipose tissues may reflect distance to the tumor, rather than the presence of tumor cells. By gene expression analyses on distant and tumor-adjacent adipose tissue related to invasive breast cancers and on adipose tissue from non-malignant breasts from postmenopausal women, Sturtz and colleagues aimed to identify genes supporting tumor development and progression [131]. The authors demonstrated that highly expressed genes in tumor-adjacent compared to distant adipose tissue promote tumor growth and progression, due to increased cellular proliferation, invasion, migration, metastasis, and angiogenesis.

Methodological Aspects of Gene Expression Signatures

When exploring biological characteristics of the tumor microenvironment and the ongoing processes underlying cancer development and progression, we may feel like Mr. Jones in the song of Bob Dylan (1941–): "*... something is happening here, but you don't know what it is. Do you, Mr. Jones?*" How can we best capture the "something happening here" in the microenvironment surrounding the tumor? When using global gene expression data, is there a "perfect" way of picturing the stromal activities? The statistician George E.P. Box (1919–2013) stated that "*All models are wrong, but some are useful,*" indicating that not one single model is able to catch the complete picture, and combining different and complementary approaches is probably one way out.

In dealing with gene expression analyses as one model, we most likely assess relevant information about the processes and pathway signaling taking place in the tumor microenvironment. The results from these studies are dependent on the input and analysis strategies. Gene expression analysis approaches can be divided into *unsupervised* and *supervised* analyses. The former requires no supplementary information to the expression data and provides great exploratory potential. The latter is driven by sample characteristics, typically in two groups, *e.g.,* "positive" versus "negative" molecular phenotype, or high versus low tumor stage.

Unsupervised Analyses and Class Discovery: Unbiased Exploring

By unsupervised analyses, without guidance by additional data except for the gene expression information itself, the aim is to find patterns in the expression profiles where no pre-defined class is presented. *Hierarchical clustering* is one example of unsupervised analysis. This method aims to group together objects based on measures of similarity and dissimilarities between them [132]. Hierarchical clustering requires specification of *similarity metrics* and *linkage*. The *similarity metric* describes how similar two samples are, by reflecting the distance between them. Additional information for the distance between clusters is needed, as reflected by the *linkage method* (single, average, or complete linkage). Complete linkage is demonstrated to be superior for clustering genes, while for clustering of samples, both average and complete linkage is proven useful [133]. Validation of the identified clusters is crucial, including validation of both biological and clinical plausibility, and the level of statistical evidence.

Supervised Analyses: Genes Differentially Expressed Between Groups

Identifying genes with known functions that are differentially expressed between two groups may provide better understanding of biological differences between the pre-defined groups [133]. If the genes identified are of unknown function, the analyses have the potential to provide novel insight into new gene functions. Supervised analyses require supplementary information about the groups, such as clinicopathologic or molecular phenotypic data. An increased risk of false-positive findings due to *multiple testing* occurs as we run, *e.g.,* 20,000 tests simultaneously on the same data, when searching for genes differentially expressed between classes. There are various methods to adjust for multiple testing, all of them with the aim to provide greater certainty that the genes in our analysis output are truly differentially expressed between the groups we examine, and not listed due to chance. Being very strict in the adjustment of the multiple testing might mask true biological effects. The adjustments will thus be a "trade-off" between too few and too many genes correctly identified as differentially expressed between classes. It is generally accepted that applying filters that results in no false-positive genes in the output is a too stringent approach, with a high risk of losing relevant biological findings in the analysis output. When searching for single genes differentially expressed between classes, the genes identified should nevertheless be further validated, and elimination of false-positive candidate genes or biomarkers occurs at these stages. In the search for the optimal cut-off on the output lists, it is important to remember that statistical significance does not imply biological relevance—and that biological relevance will not always provide statistical significance.

The number of genes differentially expressed between classes might be reduced to a limited number of genes with specific biological and/or prognostic information, and may be presented as *gene expression signatures*. Such signatures (*i.e.,* gene sets) might be regarded as *metagenes* with respect to expression value, and a *signature score* is calculated to evaluate the *metagene expression value* [26]. Such signature scores have been derived in various ways. One simple approach is to generate a "sum score" or "average score" (the score value of one sample equals the sum or the average of the expression values of the genes in the signature). One potential way of better preserving the biological information in a signature score is an algorithm where each sample is given a score value by subtracting the sum of downregulated genes from the sum of upregulated signature genes. More complex algorithms for derivation of gene expression signatures exists [134]. Which algorithm to select depends on how the signature gene list is derived, and the question you want to reply to by use of the signature.

Gene Networks Differentially Enriched Between Classes

Gaining further insight into biological mechanisms involved in a given process is a major challenge when working on high-throughput gene expression data. Subramanian et al. pointed to a few of the obstacles in how to interpret the single-gene lists into new and/or relevant biological information [35]: We may miss information about pathway alterations by single-gene analyses, as the interpretation of these is heavily dependent on the researcher's pre-existing knowledge of the field. Pathway signaling may involve large gene networks and thus should not be too focused on "large enough" fold changes of single genes in the search for biological information in our data output. Minor changes in all genes known to be involved in a signaling pathway may be of higher importance than large fold changes of a few genes.

Gene Set Enrichment Analysis (GSEA) is a method that determines whether an *a priori* defined set of genes shows statistically significant differences between two classes (*e.g.,* phenotypes). GSEA is an open access tool (*www.broadinstitute.org/gsea*), incorporating The Molecular Signatures Database (MSigDB), a publicly available collection of seven major classes of annotated gene sets (www.broadinstitute.org/gsea/msigdb). The gene expression signatures applied in GSEA/MSigDB are generated in various ways, and caution needs to be drawn when interpreting the results. To draw conclusions on gene set analyses, it is crucial to understand how the gene sets and signatures in question are generated, evaluating whether the specific gene sets are relevant for the current study. As for all large-scale analyses, considering the adjustment for multiple testing is required before interpreting the analysis output.

Linking gene expression alterations to network patterns of experimentally verified protein–protein interactions (PPI) provides improved understanding of the transcriptional patterns underlying the tumor and microenvironmental phenotypic characteristics [135, 136]. When analyzing the microenvironmental alterations and the interplay between the epithelial and microenvironmental compartments in tumor progression, integrating multiple levels of data will likely add information [137]. Large breast cancer studies have aimed at such integrative analyses, although a similar "all-level approach" not yet has been done with the microenvironment in focus.

Some Future Perspectives

Over the last decade, RNA sequencing has increasingly replaced the gene expression microarray method for global gene expression profiling. Analysis approaches have advanced, although a lot of the same analysis approaches are applied. Assessment of large-scale DNA, RNA, and protein single-cell information is one of the later methodological adds. Adding spatial information on top of the single-cell profiling seems like a promising approach for better elucidating network biology, intratumor heterogeneity, and the accompanying biological and clinical consequences. Imaging mass cytometry (IMC) assesses multiple protein-based markers with high-dimensional spatial resolution at the single-cell level—a promising tool for developing complex models of cellular interactions with particular relevance for the tumor microenvironment [138]. The method provides possibilities for multiplexed detection of up to 40 metal-bound proteins, showing promise regarding improved understanding of cancer biology, with accompanying development of functional biomarkers [139–141]. By applying this method, Jackson et al. recently described novel microenvironment subgroups splitting the classic molecular subtypes, informing clinical outcome [139]. More recent developments of the IMC method have provided a possibility to concurrently detect multiple mRNA and proteins at single-cell level, preserving the spatial information. A recent study describing this technology demonstrated strong correlation between HER2 mRNA and proteins at the cell population level in breast cancer (Fig. 23.6) [142]. Also, other platforms provide the possibility to detect concurrent single-cell co-expression of multiple transcripts and proteins [143, 144]. Combining mRNA and protein information into multi-level signatures, pointing to new subclasses in cancer, will likely be an approach exploited in future biomarker research.

To understand how metastases are initiated and how they progress, Lawson and colleagues aimed to elucidate the properties of metastasis-initiating cells in human breast cancer. By single-cell analyses from early-stage metastatic lesions, Lawson demonstrated that cells from these lesions are characterized by a gene expression signature reflecting stemness [145]. Strikingly, the gene expression signature patterns in metastatic cells from tissues in early and advanced stage metastatic disease (patient-derived xenograft models) were distinctly different. The early-stage metastatic cells demonstrated increased expression of stem cell markers, epithelial-to-mesenchymal transition, as well as pro-survival and dormancy-associated genes. The metastatic cells from the advanced stage were more heterogeneous and displayed an expression pattern like the matched primary tumor. This study adds important information about the role of stem-like cells to the picture of the early stages of the metastasis process.

Fig. 23.6 To build comprehensive models of cellular states and interactions in normal and diseased tissue, genetic and proteomic information must be extracted with single-cell and spatial resolution. Schulz et al. extended imaging mass cytometry to enable multiplexed detection of mRNA and proteins in tissues. Three mRNA target species were detected by RNAscope-based metal in situ hybridization with simultaneous antibody detection of 16 proteins. Analysis of 170 breast cancer samples showed that HER2 and CK19 mRNA and protein levels are moderately correlated on the single-cell level, but only HER2, and not CK19, has strong mRNA-to-protein correlation on the cell population level. The chemoattractant CXCL10 was expressed in stromal cell clusters, and the frequency of CXCL-expressing cells correlated with T-cell presence. *With permission, reprinted from D. Schulz et al. [142], Cell Syst 2018. doi: 10.1016/j.cels.2017.12.001*

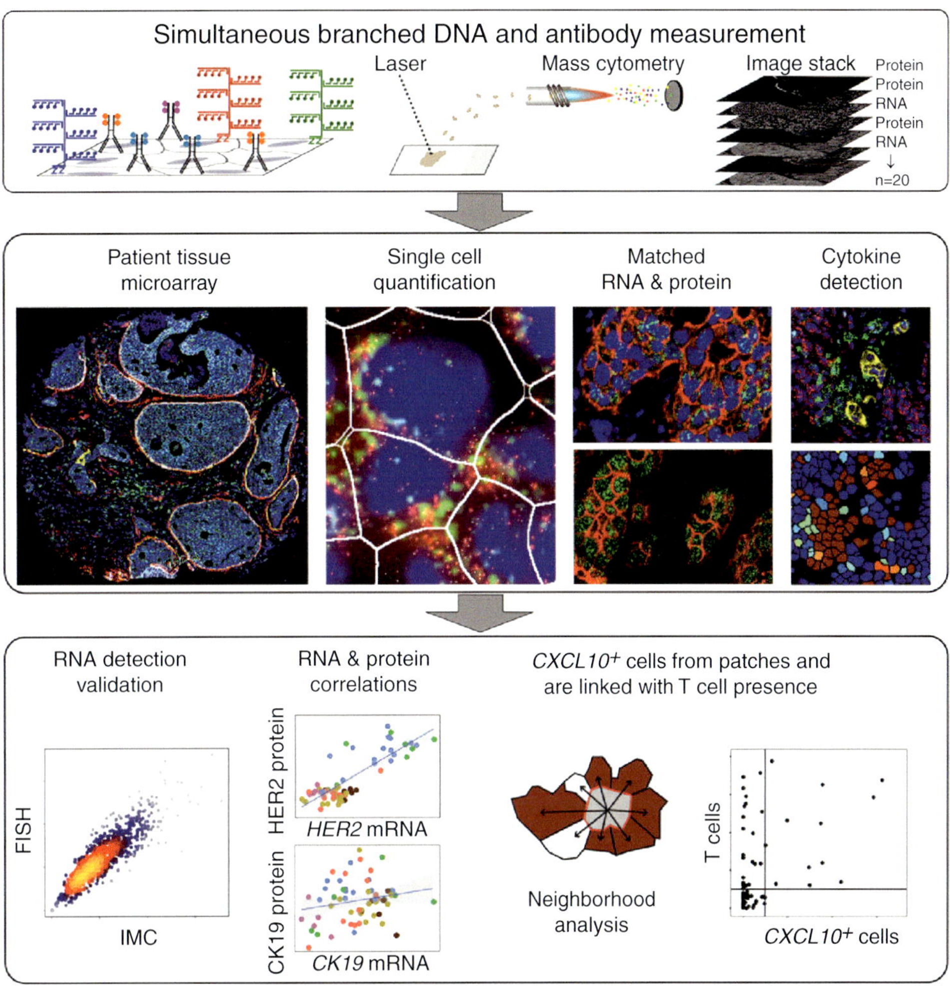

Two elegantly designed studies, linking information about tumor-stroma interactions, pointed at integrin signaling as being of major importance in tumor progression and in the organotropism of the metastatic lesions. Reuter and colleagues profiled gene expression data of both epithelium and stroma at specific time points during tumor progression in an experimental 3D tumor model [146]. A *"core cancer progression signature"* was identified, and data indicated extracellular matrix-interacting network hubs as essential in tumor progression. Blocking the β1-integrin hub, inhibited tumor development. A study on the role of exosomes in the metastatic process demonstrated that tumor-derived exosomes prepare the pre-metastatic niche in organ-specific cells [147]. Lung and liver metastases were associated with specific integrin expression patterns. Targeting these integrins decreased the exosome uptake as well as lung and liver metastases, and Hoshino suggested that exosomal integrins have a potential role in directing metastatic cells in organotropic manners.

Deconvolution methods, a computational dissection of bulk gene expression data, providing cell compartment or cell type-specific counts or expression profiles, is a novel approach, potentially assisting in decoding complex data, with improved understanding of the tumor compartments [40, 148–150]. In a recent study by Zhu et al., gene expression data (by RNAseq) was analyzed from 50 primary breast tumors and their matched metastatic tumors [151]. Based on gene expression data, deconvolution methods demonstrated lower abundance of immune cells in the metastatic lesions, except for M2 macrophages, that occurred with higher levels in the metastatic lesions compared to primary tumors. Validation by immunohistochemistry analyses of tumor tissue confirmed the mRNA results, proposing immune escape as a potential mechanism for the lower infiltration of immune cells in metastases.

Concluding Remarks/Summary

Do signature approaches, as outlined in this chapter, seem promising when searching to understand the microenvironment biology in cancer? The summarized studies indicate that signature analyses are valuable tools in cancer research. Capturing gene expression alterations in multigene signatures may better reflect the complex biological programming both driving and supporting tumor development and progression. Stroma-related alterations are probably exploitable with respect to treatment identification. As underlined from many of the studies on transcriptional alterations of the tumor-associated microenvironment, interplay between extracellular remodeling, vascular biology and immune-related signaling appears to be critically important features of tumor subtypes and their associated patient outcomes. How to best reflect the functional interactions between the compartments is a daunting task. Integrating, interpreting, and validating results from global gene expression analyses are still major challenges, as deRisi stated in the very beginning of the "omics" era [24]. Developing new technology and analysis approaches, and steadily increasing the detection possibilities and the level of molecular complexity outlined, including molecular networks across molecular levels, provide new knowledge potentially impacting how we understand tumor biology and clinical diseases. Adding context-depending spatial information to large-scale single-cell data is proposed as a promising way forward—potentially further improving our understanding of microenvironment heterogeneity, and its biological and clinical consequences. How we embrace this methodology, should likely go along the line suggested by the mathematician Richard W. Hamming (1915–1998): *If you believe too much, you will never notice the flaws; if you doubt too much you won't get started. It requires a lovely balance.*

References

1. Fidler IJ. The pathogenesis of cancer metastasis: the 'seed and soil' hypothesis revisited. Nat Rev Cancer. 2003;3(6):453–8.
2. Talmadge JE, Fidler IJ. AACR centennial series: the biology of cancer metastasis: historical perspective. Cancer Res. 2010;70(14):5649–69.
3. Paget S. The distribution of secondary growths in cancer of the breast. Lancet. 1889;1:571–3.
4. Nguyen DX, Massague J. Genetic determinants of cancer metastasis. Nat Rev Genet. 2007;8(5):341–52.
5. Nguyen DX, Bos PD, Massague J. Metastasis: from dissemination to organ-specific colonization. Nat Rev Cancer. 2009;9(4):274–84.
6. Bhat R, Bissell MJ. Of plasticity and specificity: dialectics of the microenvironment and macroenvironment and the organ phenotype. Wiley Interdiscip Rev Dev Biol. 2014;3(2):147–63.
7. Boudreau A, van't Veer LJ, Bissell MJ. An "elite hacker": breast tumors exploit the normal microenvironment program to instruct their progression and biological diversity. Cell Adhes Migr. 2012;6(3):236–48.
8. Wculek SK, Malanchi I. Neutrophils support lung colonization of metastasis-initiating breast cancer cells. Nature. 2015;528(7582):413–7.
9. Valastyan S, Weinberg RA. Tumor metastasis: molecular insights and evolving paradigms. Cell. 2011;147(2):275–92.
10. Oppenheimer SB. Cellular basis of cancer metastasis: a review of fundamentals and new advances. Acta Histochem. 2006;108(5):327–34.
11. Kaplan RN, Rafii S, Lyden D. Preparing the "soil": the premetastatic niche. Cancer Res. 2006;66(23):11089–93.
12. Kaplan RN, Riba RD, Zacharoulis S, Bramley AH, Vincent L, Costa C, et al. VEGFR1-positive haematopoietic bone marrow progenitors initiate the pre-metastatic niche. Nature. 2005;438(7069):820–7.
13. Alizadeh AA, Eisen MB, Davis RE, Ma C, Lossos IS, Rosenwald A, et al. Distinct types of diffuse large B-cell lymphoma identified by gene expression profiling. Nature. 2000;403(6769):503–11.
14. Golub TR, Slonim DK, Tamayo P, Huard C, Gaasenbeek M, Mesirov JP, et al. Molecular classification of cancer: class discovery and class prediction by gene expression monitoring. Science. 1999;286(5439):531–7.
15. Kim H, Nam SW, Rhee H, Shan Li L, Ju Kang H, Hye Koh K, et al. Different gene expression profiles between microsatellite instability-high and microsatellite stable colorectal carcinomas. Oncogene. 2004;23(37):6218–25.
16. Perou CM, Sorlie T, Eisen MB, van de Rijn M, Jeffrey SS, Rees CA, et al. Molecular portraits of human breast tumours. Nature. 2000;406(6797):747–52.
17. Sorlie T, Perou CM, Tibshirani R, Aas T, Geisler S, Johnsen H, et al. Gene expression patterns of breast carcinomas distinguish tumor subclasses with clinical implications. Proc Natl Acad Sci U S A. 2001;98(19):10869–74.
18. Sotiriou C, Neo SY, McShane LM, Korn EL, Long PM, Jazaeri A, et al. Breast cancer classification and prognosis based on gene expression profiles from a population-based study. Proc Natl Acad Sci U S A. 2003;100(18):10393–8.
19. Li W, Wang R, Yan Z, Bai L, Sun Z. High accordance in prognosis prediction of colorectal cancer across independent data-sets by multi-gene module expression profiles. PLoS One. 2012;7(3):e33653.
20. van 't Veer LJ, Dai H, van de Vijver MJ, He YD, Hart AA, Mao M, et al. Gene expression profiling predicts clinical outcome of breast cancer. Nature. 2002;415(6871):530–6.
21. Wang Y, Klijn JG, Zhang Y, Sieuwerts AM, Look MP, Yang F, et al. Gene-expression profiles to predict distant metastasis of lymph-node-negative primary breast cancer. Lancet. 2005;365(9460):671–9.
22. van de Vijver MJ, He YD, van't Veer LJ, Dai H, Hart AA, Voskuil DW, et al. A gene-expression signature as a predictor of survival in breast cancer. N Engl J Med. 2002;347(25):1999–2009.
23. Rouzier R, Rajan R, Wagner P, Hess KR, Gold DL, Stec J, et al. Microtubule-associated protein tau: a marker of paclitaxel sensitivity in breast cancer. Proc Natl Acad Sci U S A. 2005;102(23):8315–20.
24. DeRisi JL, Iyer VR, Brown PO. Exploring the metabolic and genetic control of gene expression on a genomic scale. Science. 1997;278(5338):680–6.
25. Hughes TR, Marton MJ, Jones AR, Roberts CJ, Stoughton R, Armour CD, et al. Functional discovery via a compendium of expression profiles. Cell. 2000;102(1):109–26.
26. Huang E, Ishida S, Pittman J, Dressman H, Bild A, Kloos M, et al. Gene expression phenotypic models that predict the activity of oncogenic pathways. Nat Genet. 2003;34(2):226–30.
27. Bild AH, Yao G, Chang JT, Wang Q, Potti A, Chasse D, et al. Oncogenic pathway signatures in human cancers as a guide to targeted therapies. Nature. 2006;439(7074):353–7.
28. Black EP, Huang E, Dressman H, Rempel R, Laakso N, Asa SL, et al. Distinct gene expression phenotypes of cells lacking Rb and Rb family members. Cancer Res. 2003;63(13):3716–23.
29. Lamb J, Ramaswamy S, Ford HL, Contreras B, Martinez RV, Kittrell FS, et al. A mechanism of cyclin D1 action encoded in the patterns of gene expression in human cancer. Cell. 2003;114(3):323–34.

30. Biomarkers Definitions Working G. Biomarkers and surrogate endpoints: preferred definitions and conceptual framework. Clin Pharmacol Ther. 2001;69(3):89–95.

31. Hanahan D, Weinberg RA. The hallmarks of cancer. Cell. 2000;100(1):57–70.

32. Hanahan D, Weinberg RA. Hallmarks of cancer: the next generation. Cell. 2011;144(5):646–74.

33. Lamb J, Crawford ED, Peck D, Modell JW, Blat IC, Wrobel MJ, et al. The Connectivity Map: using gene-expression signatures to connect small molecules, genes, and disease. Science. 2006;313(5795):1929–35.

34. Lamb J. The Connectivity Map: a new tool for biomedical research. Nat Rev Cancer. 2007;7(1):54–60.

35. Subramanian A, Tamayo P, Mootha VK, Mukherjee S, Ebert BL, Gillette MA, et al. Gene set enrichment analysis: a knowledge-based approach for interpreting genome-wide expression profiles. Proc Natl Acad Sci U S A. 2005;102(43):15545–50.

36. Sorlie T, Tibshirani R, Parker J, Hastie T, Marron JS, Nobel A, et al. Repeated observation of breast tumor subtypes in independent gene expression data sets. Proc Natl Acad Sci U S A. 2003;100(14):8418–23.

37. Manjili MH, Najarian K, Wang XY. Signatures of tumor-immune interactions as biomarkers for breast cancer prognosis. Future Oncol. 2012;8(6):703–11.

38. Zhao C, Wu M, Zeng N, Xiong M, Hu W, Lv W, et al. Cancer-associated adipocytes: emerging supporters in breast cancer. J Exp Clin Cancer Res. 2020;39(1):156.

39. Newman AM, Liu CL, Green MR, Gentles AJ, Feng W, Xu Y, et al. Robust enumeration of cell subsets from tissue expression profiles. Nat Methods. 2015;12(5):453–7.

40. Peng XL, Moffitt RA, Torphy RJ, Volmar KE, Yeh JJ. De novo compartment deconvolution and weight estimation of tumor samples using DECODER. Nat Commun. 2019;10(1):4729.

41. Allinen M, Beroukhim R, Cai L, Brennan C, Lahti-Domenici J, Huang H, et al. Molecular characterization of the tumor microenvironment in breast cancer. Cancer Cell. 2004;6(1):17–32.

42. Ma XJ, Dahiya S, Richardson E, Erlander M, Sgroi DC. Gene expression profiling of the tumor microenvironment during breast cancer progression. Breast Cancer Res. 2009;11(1):R7.

43. Roman-Perez E, Casbas-Hernandez P, Pirone JR, Rein J, Carey LA, Lubet RA, et al. Gene expression in extratumoral microenvironment predicts clinical outcome in breast cancer patients. Breast Cancer Res. 2012;14(2):R51.

44. Troester MA, Lee MH, Carter M, Fan C, Cowan DW, Perez ER, et al. Activation of host wound responses in breast cancer microenvironment. Clin Cancer Res. 2009;15(22):7020–8.

45. Finak G, Bertos N, Pepin F, Sadekova S, Souleimanova M, Zhao H, et al. Stromal gene expression predicts clinical outcome in breast cancer. Nat Med. 2008;14(5):518–27.

46. Casey T, Bond J, Tighe S, Hunter T, Lintault L, Patel O, et al. Molecular signatures suggest a major role for stromal cells in development of invasive breast cancer. Breast Cancer Res Treat. 2009;114(1):47–62.

47. Van den Eynden GG, Smid M, Van Laere SJ, Colpaert CG, Van der Auwera I, Bich TX, et al. Gene expression profiles associated with the presence of a fibrotic focus and the growth pattern in lymph node-negative breast cancer. Clin Cancer Res. 2008;14(10):2944–52.

48. Marchini C, Montani M, Konstantinidou G, Orru R, Mannucci S, Ramadori G, et al. Mesenchymal/stromal gene expression signature relates to basal-like breast cancers, identifies bone metastasis and predicts resistance to therapies. PLoS One. 2010;5(11):e14131.

49. Guo W, Keckesova Z, Donaher JL, Shibue T, Tischler V, Reinhardt F, et al. Slug and Sox9 cooperatively determine the mammary stem cell state. Cell. 2012;148(5):1015–28.

50. Mani SA, Guo W, Liao MJ, Eaton EN, Ayyanan A, Zhou AY, et al. The epithelial-mesenchymal transition generates cells with properties of stem cells. Cell. 2008;133(4):704–15.

51. Morel AP, Lievre M, Thomas C, Hinkal G, Ansieau S, Puisieux A. Generation of breast cancer stem cells through epithelial-mesenchymal transition. PLoS One. 2008;3(8):e2888.

52. Planche A, Bacac M, Provero P, Fusco C, Delorenzi M, Stehle JC, et al. Identification of prognostic molecular features in the reactive stroma of human breast and prostate cancer. PLoS One. 2011;6(5):e18640.

53. Winslow S, Leandersson K, Edsjo A, Larsson C. Prognostic stromal gene signatures in breast cancer. Breast Cancer Res. 2015;17:23.

54. Desmedt C, Majjaj S, Kheddoumi N, Singhal SK, Haibe-Kains B, El Ouriaghli F, et al. Characterization and clinical evaluation of CD10+ stroma cells in the breast cancer microenvironment. Clin Cancer Res. 2012;18(4):1004–14.

55. Rajski M, Zanetti-Dallenbach R, Vogel B, Herrmann R, Rochlitz C, Buess M. IGF-I induced genes in stromal fibroblasts predict the clinical outcome of breast and lung cancer patients. BMC Med. 2010;8:1.

56. Bredholt G, Mannelqvist M, Stefansson IM, Birkeland E, Bo TH, Oyan AM, et al. Tumor necrosis is an important hallmark of aggressive endometrial cancer and associates with hypoxia, angiogenesis and inflammation responses. Oncotarget. 2015;6(37):39676–91.

57. West RB, Nuyten DS, Subramanian S, Nielsen TO, Corless CL, Rubin BP, et al. Determination of stromal signatures in breast carcinoma. PLoS Biol. 2005;3(6):e187.

58. Lehmann BD, Bauer JA, Chen X, Sanders ME, Chakravarthy AB, Shyr Y, et al. Identification of human triple-negative breast cancer subtypes and preclinical models for selection of targeted therapies. J Clin Invest. 2011;121(7):2750–67.

59. Bareche Y, Buisseret L, Gruosso T, Girard E, Venet D, Dupont F, et al. Unraveling triple-negative breast cancer tumor microenvironment heterogeneity: towards an optimized treatment approach. J Natl Cancer Inst. 2020;112(7):708–19.

60. Tamborero D, Rubio-Perez C, Muinos F, Sabarinathan R, Piulats JM, Muntasell A, et al. A pan-cancer landscape of interactions between solid tumors and infiltrating immune cell populations. Clin Cancer Res. 2018;24(15):3717–28.

61. Qian J, Olbrecht S, Boeckx B, Vos H, Laoui D, Etlioglu E, et al. A pan-cancer blueprint of the heterogeneous tumor microenvironment revealed by single-cell profiling. Cell Res. 2020;30(9):745–62.

62. Chang HY, Sneddon JB, Alizadeh AA, Sood R, West RB, Montgomery K, et al. Gene expression signature of fibroblast serum response predicts human cancer progression: similarities between tumors and wounds. PLoS Biol. 2004;2(2):E7.

63. Dvorak HF. Tumors: wounds that do not heal. Similarities between tumor stroma generation and wound healing. N Engl J Med. 1986;315(26):1650–9.

64. Tchou J, Kossenkov AV, Chang L, Satija C, Herlyn M, Showe LC, et al. Human breast cancer associated fibroblasts exhibit subtype specific gene expression profiles. BMC Med Genet. 2012;5:39.

65. Bauer M, Su G, Casper C, He R, Rehrauer W, Friedl A. Heterogeneity of gene expression in stromal fibroblasts of human breast carcinomas and normal breast. Oncogene. 2010;29(12):1732–40.

66. Singer CF, Gschwantler-Kaulich D, Fink-Retter A, Haas C, Hudelist G, Czerwenka K, et al. Differential gene expression profile in breast cancer-derived stromal fibroblasts. Breast Cancer Res Treat. 2008;110(2):273–81.

67. Frings O, Augsten M, Tobin NP, Carlson J, Paulsson J, Pena C, et al. Prognostic significance in breast cancer of a gene signature capturing stromal PDGF signaling. Am J Pathol. 2013;182(6):2037–47.

68. Sonnenblick A, Salmon-Divon M, Salgado R, Dvash E, Ponde N, Zahavi T, et al. Reactive stroma and trastuzumab resistance in HER2-positive early breast cancer. Int J Cancer. 2020;147(1):266–76.

69. Siletz A, Kniazeva E, Jeruss JS, Shea LD. Transcription factor networks in invasion-promoting breast carcinoma-associated fibroblasts. Cancer Microenviron. 2013;6(1):91–107.

70. Bartoschek M, Oskolkov N, Bocci M, Lovrot J, Larsson C, Sommarin M, et al. Spatially and functionally distinct subclasses of breast cancer-associated fibroblasts revealed by single cell RNA sequencing. Nat Commun. 2018;9(1):5150.

71. Wu SZ, Roden DL, Wang C, Holliday H, Harvey K, Cazet AS, et al. Stromal cell diversity associated with immune evasion in human triple-negative breast cancer. EMBO J. 2020;39(19):e104063.

72. Woelfle U, Cloos J, Sauter G, Riethdorf L, Janicke F, van Diest P, et al. Molecular signature associated with bone marrow micrometastasis in human breast cancer. Cancer Res. 2003;63(18):5679–84.

73. Bergamaschi A, Tagliabue E, Sorlie T, Naume B, Triulzi T, Orlandi R, et al. Extracellular matrix signature identifies breast cancer subgroups with different clinical outcome. J Pathol. 2008;214(3):357–67.

74. Triulzi T, Casalini P, Sandri M, Ratti M, Carcangiu ML, Colombo MP, et al. Neoplastic and stromal cells contribute to an extracellular matrix gene expression profile defining a breast cancer subtype likely to progress. PLoS One. 2013;8(2):e56761.

75. Wallgard E, Larsson E, He L, Hellstrom M, Armulik A, Nisancioglu MH, et al. Identification of a core set of 58 gene transcripts with broad and specific expression in the microvasculature. Arterioscler Thromb Vasc Biol. 2008;28(8):1469–76.

76. Cleuren ACA, van der Ent MA, Jiang H, Hunker KL, Yee A, Siemieniak DR, et al. The in vivo endothelial cell translatome is highly heterogeneous across vascular beds. Proc Natl Acad Sci U S A. 2019;116(47):23618–24.

77. Hu Z, Fan C, Livasy C, He X, Oh DS, Ewend MG, et al. A compact VEGF signature associated with distant metastases and poor outcomes. BMC Med. 2009;7:9.

78. Pepin F, Bertos N, Laferriere J, Sadekova S, Souleimanova M, Zhao H, et al. Gene-expression profiling of microdissected breast cancer microvasculature identifies distinct tumor vascular subtypes. Breast Cancer Res. 2012;14(4):R120.

79. Bender RJ, Mac GF. Expression of VEGF and semaphorin genes define subgroups of triple negative breast cancer. PLoS One. 2013;8(5):e61788.

80. Wallace JA, Li F, Balakrishnan S, Cantemir-Stone CZ, Pecot T, Martin C, et al. Ets2 in tumor fibroblasts promotes angiogenesis in breast cancer. PLoS One. 2013;8(8):e71533.

81. Xiao L, Harrell JC, Perou CM, Dudley AC. Identification of a stable molecular signature in mammary tumor endothelial cells that persists in vitro. Angiogenesis. 2014;17(3):511–8.

82. Chang CW, Tsai CW, Wang HF, Tsai HC, Chen HY, Tsai TF, et al. Identification of a developmentally regulated striatum-enriched zinc-finger gene, Nolz-1, in the mammalian brain. Proc Natl Acad Sci U S A. 2004;101(8):2613–8.

83. Matsumoto K, Nishihara S, Kamimura M, Shiraishi T, Otoguro T, Uehara M, et al. The prepattern transcription factor Irx2, a target of the FGF8/MAP kinase cascade, is involved in cerebellum formation. Nat Neurosci. 2004;7(6):605–12.

84. Mannelqvist M, Stefansson IM, Bredholt G, Hellem Bo T, Oyan AM, Jonassen I, et al. Gene expression patterns related to vascular invasion and aggressive features in endometrial cancer. Am J Pathol. 2011;178(2):861–71.

85. Mannelqvist M, Wik E, Stefansson IM, Akslen LA. An 18-gene signature for vascular invasion is associated with aggressive features and reduced survival in breast cancer. PLoS One. 2014;9(6):e98787.

86. Stefansson IM, Raeder M, Wik E, Mannelqvist M, Kusonmano K, Knutsvik G, et al. Increased angiogenesis is associated with a 32-gene expression signature and 6p21 amplification in aggressive endometrial cancer. Oncotarget. 2015;6(12):10634–45.

87. Tobin NP, Wennmalm K, Lindstrom LS, Foukakis T, He L, Genove G, et al. An endothelial gene signature score predicts poor outcome in patients with endocrine-treated, low genomic grade breast tumors. Clin Cancer Res. 2016;22(10):2417–26.

88. Guarischi-Sousa R, Monteiro JS, Alecrim LC, Michaloski JS, Cardeal LB, Ferreira EN, et al. A transcriptome-based signature of pathological angiogenesis predicts breast cancer patient survival. PLoS Genet. 2019;15(12):e1008482.

89. Harrell JC, Pfefferle AD, Zalles N, Prat A, Fan C, Khramtsov A, et al. Endothelial-like properties of claudin-low breast cancer cells promote tumor vascular permeability and metastasis. Clin Exp Metastasis. 2014;31(1):33–45.

90. Mendiola M, Martinez-Marin V, Herranz J, Heredia V, Yebenes L, Zamora P, et al. Predictive value of angiogenesis-related gene profiling in patients with HER2-negative metastatic breast cancer treated with bevacizumab and weekly paclitaxel. Oncotarget. 2016;7(17):24217–27.

91. Kruger K, Silwal-Pandit L, Wik E, Straume O, Stefansson IM, Borgen E, et al. Baseline microvessel density predicts response to neoadjuvant bevacizumab treatment of locally advanced breast cancer. Sci Rep. 2021;11(1):3388.

92. Pitroda SP, Zhou T, Sweis RF, Filippo M, Labay E, Beckett MA, et al. Tumor endothelial inflammation predicts clinical outcome in diverse human cancers. PLoS One. 2012;7(10):e46104.

93. Oshi M, Newman S, Tokumaru Y, Yan L, Matsuyama R, Endo I, et al. Intra-tumoral angiogenesis is associated with inflammation, immune reaction and metastatic recurrence in breast cancer. Int J Mol Sci. 2020;21(18):6708.

94. Chen DS, Mellman I. Elements of cancer immunity and the cancer-immune set point. Nature. 2017;541(7637):321–30.

95. Joyce JA, Fearon DT. T cell exclusion, immune privilege, and the tumor microenvironment. Science. 2015;348(6230):74–80.

96. Adams S, Diamond JR, Hamilton E, Pohlmann PR, Tolaney SM, Chang CW, et al. Atezolizumab plus nab-paclitaxel in the treatment of metastatic triple-negative breast cancer with 2-year survival follow-up: a phase 1b clinical trial. JAMA Oncol. 2019;5(3):334–42.

97. Loi S, Giobbie-Harder A, Gombos A, Bachelot T, Hui R, Curigliano G, et al. Pembrolizumab plus trastuzumab in trastuzumab-resistant, advanced, HER2-positive breast cancer (PANACEA): a single-arm, multicentre, phase 1b-2 trial. Lancet Oncol. 2019;20(3):371–82.

98. Schmid P, Adams S, Rugo HS, Schneeweiss A, Barrios CH, Iwata H, et al. Atezolizumab and nab-paclitaxel in advanced triple-negative breast cancer. N Engl J Med. 2018;379(22):2108–21.

99. Schmid P, Rugo HS, Adams S, Schneeweiss A, Barrios CH, Iwata H, et al. Atezolizumab plus nab-paclitaxel as first-line treatment for unresectable, locally advanced or metastatic triple-negative breast cancer (IMpassion130): updated efficacy results from a randomised, double-blind, placebo-controlled, phase 3 trial. Lancet Oncol. 2020;21(1):44–59.

100. Solinas C, Gombos A, Latifyan S, Piccart-Gebhart M, Kok M, Buisseret L. Targeting immune checkpoints in breast cancer: an update of early results. ESMO Open. 2017;2(5):e000255.

101. Emens LA. Immunotherapy in triple-negative breast cancer. Cancer J. 2021;27(1):59–66.

102. Teschendorff AE, Miremadi A, Pinder SE, Ellis IO, Caldas C. An immune response gene expression module identifies a good prognosis subtype in estrogen receptor negative breast cancer. Genome Biol. 2007;8(8):R157.

103. Rody A, Karn T, Liedtke C, Pusztai L, Ruckhaeberle E, Hanker L, et al. A clinically relevant gene signature in triple negative and basal-like breast cancer. Breast Cancer Res. 2011;13(5):R97.

104. Alexe G, Dalgin GS, Scanfeld D, Tamayo P, Mesirov JP, DeLisi C, et al. High expression of lymphocyte-associated genes in node-negative HER2+ breast cancers correlates with lower recurrence rates. Cancer Res. 2007;67(22):10669–76.

105. Schmidt M, Bohm D, von Torne C, Steiner E, Puhl A, Pilch H, et al. The humoral immune system has a key prognostic impact in node-negative breast cancer. Cancer Res. 2008;68(13):5405–13.

106. Schmidt M, Hellwig B, Hammad S, Othman A, Lohr M, Chen Z, et al. A comprehensive analysis of human gene expression profiles identifies stromal immunoglobulin kappa C as a compatible prognostic marker in human solid tumors. Clin Cancer Res. 2012;18(9):2695–703.

107. Hsu DS, Kim MK, Balakumaran BS, Acharya CR, Anders CK, Clay T, et al. Immune signatures predict prognosis in localized cancer. Cancer Investig. 2010;28(7):765–73.

108. Bianchini G, Qi Y, Alvarez RH, Iwamoto T, Coutant C, Ibrahim NK, et al. Molecular anatomy of breast cancer stroma and its prognostic value in estrogen receptor-positive and -negative cancers. J Clin Oncol. 2010;28(28):4316–23.

109. Nagalla S, Chou JW, Willingham MC, Ruiz J, Vaughn JP, Dubey P, et al. Interactions between immunity, proliferation and molecular subtype in breast cancer prognosis. Genome Biol. 2013;14(4):R34.

110. Ascierto ML, Kmieciak M, Idowu MO, Manjili R, Zhao Y, Grimes M, et al. A signature of immune function genes associated with recurrence-free survival in breast cancer patients. Breast Cancer Res Treat. 2012;131(3):871–80.

111. Iglesia MD, Vincent BG, Parker JS, Hoadley KA, Carey LA, Perou CM, et al. Prognostic B-cell signatures using mRNA-seq in patients with subtype-specific breast and ovarian cancer. Clin Cancer Res. 2014;20(14):3818–29.

112. Coronella JA, Spier C, Welch M, Trevor KT, Stopeck AT, Villar H, et al. Antigen-driven oligoclonal expansion of tumor-infiltrating B cells in infiltrating ductal carcinoma of the breast. J Immunol. 2002;169(4):1829–36.

113. Hansen MH, Nielsen H, Ditzel HJ. The tumor-infiltrating B cell response in medullary breast cancer is oligoclonal and directed against the autoantigen actin exposed on the surface of apoptotic cancer cells. Proc Natl Acad Sci U S A. 2001;98(22):12659–64.

114. Nzula S, Going JJ, Stott DI. Antigen-driven clonal proliferation, somatic hypermutation, and selection of B lymphocytes infiltrating human ductal breast carcinomas. Cancer Res. 2003;63(12):3275–80.

115. Perez EA, Thompson EA, Ballman KV, Anderson SK, Asmann YW, Kalari KR, et al. Genomic analysis reveals that immune function genes are strongly linked to clinical outcome in the north central cancer treatment group n9831 adjuvant trastuzumab trial. J Clin Oncol. 2015;33(7):701–8.

116. Rody A, Holtrich U, Pusztai L, Liedtke C, Gaetje R, Ruckhaeberle E, et al. T-cell metagene predicts a favorable prognosis in estrogen receptor-negative and HER2-positive breast cancers. Breast Cancer Res. 2009;11(2):R15.

117. Akalay I, Janji B, Hasmim M, Noman MZ, Andre F, De Cremoux P, et al. Epithelial-to-mesenchymal transition and autophagy induction in breast carcinoma promote escape from T-cell-mediated lysis. Cancer Res. 2013;73(8):2418–27.

118. Akalay I, Tan TZ, Kumar P, Janji B, Mami-Chouaib F, Charpy C, et al. Targeting WNT1-inducible signaling pathway protein 2 alters human breast cancer cell susceptibility to specific lysis through regulation of KLF-4 and miR-7 expression. Oncogene. 2015;34(17):2261–71.

119. Kudo-Saito C, Shirako H, Takeuchi T, Kawakami Y. Cancer metastasis is accelerated through immunosuppression during Snail-induced EMT of cancer cells. Cancer Cell. 2009;15(3):195–206.

120. Ye X, Weinberg RA. Epithelial-mesenchymal plasticity: a central regulator of cancer progression. Trends Cell Biol. 2015;25(11):675–86.

121. Yang B, Chou J, Tao Y, Wu D, Wu X, Li X, et al. An assessment of prognostic immunity markers in breast cancer. NPJ Breast Cancer. 2018;4:35.

122. Zhang H, Qin G, Yu H, Han X, Zhu S. Comprehensive genomic and immunophenotypic analysis of CD4 T cell infiltrating human triple-negative breast cancer. Cancer Immunol Immunother. 2021;70(6):1649–65.

123. Gruosso T, Gigoux M, Manem VSK, Bertos N, Zuo D, Perlitch I, et al. Spatially distinct tumor immune microenvironments stratify triple-negative breast cancers. J Clin Invest. 2019;129(4):1785–800.

124. Wu Q, Li B, Li Z, Li J, Sun S, Sun S. Cancer-associated adipocytes: key players in breast cancer progression. J Hematol Oncol. 2019;12(1):95.

125. Nieman KM, Kenny HA, Penicka CV, Ladanyi A, Buell-Gutbrod R, Zillhardt MR, et al. Adipocytes promote ovarian cancer metastasis and provide energy for rapid tumor growth. Nat Med. 2011;17(11):1498–503.

126. Wang YY, Attane C, Milhas D, Dirat B, Dauvillier S, Guerard A, et al. Mammary adipocytes stimulate breast cancer invasion through metabolic remodeling of tumor cells. JCI Insight. 2017;2(4):e87489.

127. Wu Z, Wu J, Zhao Q, Fu S, Jin J. Emerging roles of aerobic glycolysis in breast cancer. Clin Transl Oncol. 2020;22(5):631–46.

128. Tang J, Luo Y, Wu G. A glycolysis-related gene expression signature in predicting recurrence of breast cancer. Aging (Albany NY). 2020;12(24):24983–94.

129. Li C, Li X, Li G, Sun L, Zhang W, Jiang J, et al. Identification of a prognosisassociated signature associated with energy metabolism in triplenegative breast cancer. Oncol Rep. 2020;44(3):819–37.

130. Zhang D, Zheng Y, Yang S, Li Y, Wang M, Yao J, et al. Identification of a novel glycolysis-related gene signature for predicting breast cancer survival. Front Oncol. 2020;10:596087.

131. Sturtz LA, Deyarmin B, van Laar R, Yarina W, Shriver CD, Ellsworth RE. Gene expression differences in adipose tissue associated with breast tumorigenesis. Adipocytes. 2014;3(2):107–14.

132. Eisen MB, Spellman PT, Brown PO, Botstein D. Cluster analysis and display of genome-wide expression patterns. Proc Natl Acad Sci U S A. 1998;95(25):14863–8.

133. Simon RMKE, McShane LM, Radmacher MD, Wright GW, Zhao Y. Statistics for biology and health: design and analysis of DNA microarray investigations. New York, NY: Springer; 2004.

134. Kato K. Algorithm for in vitro diagnostic multivariate index assay. Breast Cancer. 2009;16(4):248–51.

135. Deng JL, Xu YH, Wang G. Identification of potential crucial genes and key pathways in breast cancer using bioinformatic analysis. Front Genet. 2019;10:695.

136. Tang D, Zhao X, Zhang L, Wang Z, Wang C. Identification of hub genes to regulate breast cancer metastasis to brain by bioinformatics analyses. J Cell Biochem. 2019;120(6):9522–31.

137. Petersen K, Rajcevic U, Abdul Rahim SA, Jonassen I, Kalland KH, Jimenez CR, et al. Gene set based integrated data analysis reveals phenotypic differences in a brain cancer model. PLoS One. 2013;8(7):e68288.

138. Giesen C, Wang HA, Schapiro D, Zivanovic N, Jacobs A, Hattendorf B, et al. Highly multiplexed imaging of tumor tissues with subcellular resolution by mass cytometry. Nat Methods. 2014;11(4):417–22.

139. Jackson HW, Fischer JR, Zanotelli VRT, Ali HR, Mechera R, Soysal SD, et al. The single-cell pathology landscape of breast cancer. Nature. 2020;578(7796):615–20.

140. Wagner J, Rapsomaniki MA, Chevrier S, Anzeneder T, Langwieder C, Dykgers A, et al. A single-cell atlas of the tumor and immune

ecosystem of human breast cancer. Cell. 2019;177(5):1330–45 e18.

141. Schapiro D, Jackson HW, Raghuraman S, Fischer JR, Zanotelli VRT, Schulz D, et al. histoCAT: analysis of cell phenotypes and interactions in multiplex image cytometry data. Nat Methods. 2017;14(9):873–6.

142. Schulz D, Zanotelli VRT, Fischer JR, Schapiro D, Engler S, Lun XK, et al. Simultaneous multiplexed imaging of mRNA and proteins with subcellular resolution in breast cancer tissue samples by mass cytometry. Cell Syst. 2018;6(1):25–36 e5.

143. Brady L, Kriner M, Coleman I, Morrissey C, Roudier M, True LD, et al. Inter- and intra-tumor heterogeneity of metastatic prostate cancer determined by digital spatial gene expression profiling. Nat Commun. 2021;12(1):1426.

144. Merritt CR, Ong GT, Church SE, Barker K, Danaher P, Geiss G, et al. Multiplex digital spatial profiling of proteins and RNA in fixed tissue. Nat Biotechnol. 2020;38(5):586–99.

145. Lawson DA, Bhakta NR, Kessenbrock K, Prummel KD, Yu Y, Takai K, et al. Single-cell analysis reveals a stem-cell program in human metastatic breast cancer cells. Nature. 2015;526(7571):131–5.

146. Reuter JA, Ortiz-Urda S, Kretz M, Garcia J, Scholl FA, Pasmooij AM, et al. Modeling inducible human tissue neoplasia identifies an extracellular matrix interaction network involved in cancer progression. Cancer Cell. 2009;15(6):477–88.

147. Hoshino A, Costa-Silva B, Shen TL, Rodrigues G, Hashimoto A, Tesic Mark M, et al. Tumour exosome integrins determine organotropic metastasis. Nature. 2015;527(7578):329–35.

148. Li B, Li T, Liu JS, Liu XS. Computational deconvolution of tumor-infiltrating immune components with bulk tumor gene expression data. Methods Mol Biol. 2020;2120:249–62.

149. Racle J, Gfeller D. EPIC: a tool to estimate the proportions of different cell types from bulk gene expression data. Methods Mol Biol. 2020;2120:233–48.

150. Newman AM, Steen CB, Liu CL, Gentles AJ, Chaudhuri AA, Scherer F, et al. Determining cell type abundance and expression from bulk tissues with digital cytometry. Nat Biotechnol. 2019;37(7):773–82.

151. Zhu L, Narloch JL, Onkar S, Joy M, Broadwater G, Luedke C, et al. Metastatic breast cancers have reduced immune cell recruitment but harbor increased macrophages relative to their matched primary tumors. J Immunother Cancer. 2019;7(1):265.

Eugene Kim, Morteza Esmaeili, Siver A. Moestue,
and Tone F. Bathen

Abstract

Magnetic resonance (MR) can be exploited in various ways to obtain a wide range of anatomical and physiological information in a safe and non-invasive manner. This makes MR imaging (MRI) and spectroscopy (MRS) valuable tools in cancer research and clinical oncology, among other fields. This chapter provides a brief and basic introduction to MR physics and describes how different in vivo MR techniques noninvasively characterize tumors and the tumor microenvironment. Contrast-enhanced MRI methods are used to evaluate tumor vascularization and vascular function by measuring the kinetics and distribution of intravenously administered contrast agents. Diffusion-weighted MRI is sensitive to the diffusion of water molecules in tissue, from which inferences about tumor cellularity and tissue microstructure can be made. Blood oxygen level-dependent MRI can distinguish between oxygenated and deoxygenated blood as a proxy to tumor oxygenation. In addition, efforts have been made to develop targeted contrast agents to directly image hypoxia. MRS can be used to measure the levels of various metabolites such as lactate and choline that are involved in metabolic reprogramming in cancer. Both endogenous and exogenous pH-sensitive indicators enable spectroscopic measurement of tumor pH. While this chapter does not provide an exhaustive overview of the MR methods used for cancer characterization, it discusses both clinical and experimental techniques that highlight the versatility of MR as a tool for exploring some key aspects of the tumor microenvironment.

E. Kim
Department of Neuroimaging, Institute of Psychiatry, Psychology and Neuroscience, King's College London, London, UK
e-mail: eugene.kim@kcl.ac.uk

M. Esmaeili
Department of Diagnostic Imaging, Akershus University Hospital, Lørenskog, Norway
e-mail: moresm@ahus.no

S. A. Moestue
Department of Clinical and Molecular Medicine,
NTNU - Norwegian University of Science and Technology, Trondheim, Norway

Department of Pharmacy, Nord University, Bodø, Norway
e-mail: siver.a.moestue@ntnu.no

T. F. Bathen (✉)
Department of Circulation and Medical Imaging,
NTNU - Norwegian University of Science and Technology, Trondheim, Norway
e-mail: tone.f.bathen@ntnu.no

L. A. Akslen, R. S. Watnick (eds.), *Biomarkers of the Tumor Microenvironment*, https://doi.org/10.1007/978-3-030-98950-7_24

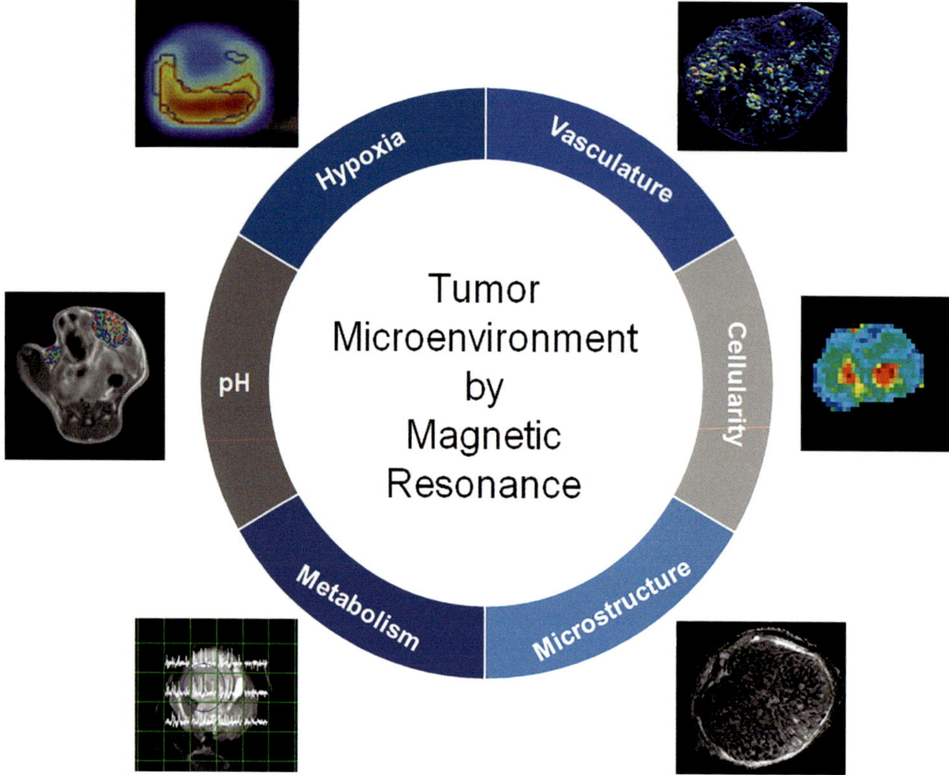

Tumor microenvironment by magnetic resonance.

Take-Home Lessons

- There are several contrast-enhanced MRI methods for characterizing tumor vascularization that can aid cancer diagnosis and treatment evaluation.
- Diffusion-weighted MRI offers promising biomarkers for cancer detection and evaluation of treatment response, and opens a window for in vivo, noninvasive characterization of the tumor microenvironment.
- Experimental techniques, such as blood oxygen level-dependent MRI, can provide information on oxygen levels in tissues. However, several clinically available PET tracers allow direct imaging of hypoxic tissues and may be a more suitable alternative for imaging hypoxia.
- Both MRSI of hyperpolarized ^{13}C bicarbonate and chemical exchange saturation transfer (CEST) MRI can be used to perform in vivo measurements of tumor pH, with both methods showing clear potential for translation to clinical practice.
- Metabolic response measured by ^{13}C hyperpolarized pyruvate and lactate provide assessment of early treatment response in breast cancer.

Magnetic Resonance Basics

Magnetic resonance (MR) signals arise from the intrinsic magnetic moments possessed by certain atomic nuclei in the body. MR imaging (MRI) and MR spectroscopy (MRS) are sensitive to nuclides with an odd number of protons and/or neutrons. The most utilized is the ^1H nuclide (proton) due to its high intrinsic sensitivity and 99.99% natural abundance. Others include ^{31}P phosphorus, ^{13}C carbon, and ^{19}F fluorine.

In an MRI scanner, these nuclear magnetic moments align with each other and precess at a specific resonance frequency, the Larmor frequency, to produce a net magnetization pointing in the direction of the scanner's main magnetic field, B_0. This equilibrium magnetization can be perturbed by applying a radiofrequency (RF) excitation pulse at the Larmor frequency—the nuclei absorb this RF energy, causing the magnetization to tilt away from the B_0 axis. Conceptualizing the magnetization as a vector, this reduces the component parallel to B_0 (longitudinal magnetization) and produces a component perpendicular to B_0 (transverse magnetization). When the RF pulse is turned off, the nuclei re-emit the energy they absorbed as the magnetization returns, i.e., relaxes, to its equilibrium state. This emitted RF energy is detected by an RF receiver coil tuned to the Larmor frequency of the excited nuclei.

The rate at which excited nuclei return to their equilibrium state is characterized by the longitudinal relaxation rate R_1, which can be measured with MRI. There is a concomitant decay (relaxation) in the transverse magnetization caused by two distinct phenomena—R_2 refers to the transverse relaxation rate due to microscopic magnetic field fluctuations created by random molecular motion, and R_2' is the transverse relaxation rate due to static magnetic field inhomogeneities. R_2^* is the sum of R_2 and R_2' and can be measured with a gradient echo sequence. The effect of static field inhomogeneities can be reversed by a spin echo sequence, allowing the measurement of R_2. The reciprocals of the relaxation rates are called the relaxation times T_1, T_2, and T_2^*. Intrinsic MR image contrast can be manipulated by exploiting the different relaxation properties of different tissues; e.g., in T_1-weighted (T_1w) images, tissues with shorter T_1 appear brighter.

There are many intrinsic MR contrast mechanisms that can be exploited to investigate a wide range of anatomical and functional characteristics. Also, exogenous contrast agents can be administered to increase tissue relaxation rates and enhance image contrast. This inherent versatility allows investigation of various aspects of the tumor microenvironment using MR. This chapter will discuss MR techniques for characterizing tumor vasculature, cellularity and tissue microstructure, metabolism, hypoxia, and pH.

Imaging Tumor Vasculature

For tumors to grow and metastasize, a vascular network is required to deliver oxygen and nutrients, remove waste products, and disseminate cancer cells. In many cancers, hypoxia and genetic alterations induce increased expression of vascular endothelial growth factor (VEGF), which is the primary mediator of tumor angiogenesis [1]. VEGF-driven angiogenesis produces structurally and functionally abnormal vessels that are characteristically hyperpermeable [2]. Increased vascularization and vessel leakiness can result in increased delivery of an intravenously (i.v.) injected contrast agent to tumors, making contrast-enhanced imaging methods like dynamic contrast-enhanced (DCE)-MRI a potential method for in vivo characterization of tumor angiogenesis.

DCE-MRI is a commonly used technique in clinical oncology for cancer detection, diagnosis, and characterization. It involves the serial acquisition of T_1w images before, during, and after i.v. administration of a gadolinium-based contrast agent (GBCA) in order to capture the dynamic signal enhancement caused by the T_1-shortening effect of the GBCA as it extravasates from the blood vessels to the extravascular extracellular space (EES). Calculating contrast agent concentration from the signal enhancement is possible with an additional scan to measure pre-contrast T_1 values.

DCE-MRI data can be analyzed by: (1) qualitative inspection of signal intensity-time curves, (2) semi-quantitative characterization of signal intensity or concentration-time curves, or (3) pharmacokinetic (PK) modeling of concentration-time curves.

PK modeling allows quantification of physiological parameters, e.g. the widely used Tofts model provides estimates of v_e (the EES volume fraction) and K^{trans} (the volume transfer constant between the intravascular space and the EES), which depends on blood flow, vessel permeability, and vessel surface area [3]. However, PK modeling requires high temporal resolution and the additional measurement of an arterial input function (AIF), which is the time-dependent contrast agent concentration in the blood plasma of the vessel that supplies the tissue of interest. This is not a trivial task, and population-averaged AIFs are often used instead of measuring individual AIFs.

DCE-MRI gives indirect measures of tumor angiogenesis, and the interpretation of these measurements is not straightforward. Studies have reported correlations between DCE-MRI parameters and microvessel density (MVD) [4, 5]. However, other studies have reported that DCE-MRI does not correlate with MVD or VEGF expression [6, 7]. MVD measures the number of blood vessels, whereas DCE-MRI measures vascular function and perfusion. It is not surprising that the two do not always correlated, especially in tumors, which have characteristically abnormal and dysfunctional vessels. Still, DCE-MRI has been demonstrated to provide useful diagnostic and prognostic indicators.

DCE-MRI signal enhancement depends on perfusion, vessel surface area, and vessel permeability; these in turn reflect angiogenic activity, which is associated with tumor aggressiveness and metastatic potential [8]. Studies have shown that pre-treatment DCE-MRI examinations can predict breast cancer patient survival. For example, several semi-quantitative parameters such as relative signal enhancement and area under the enhancement curve (AUC) correlated with disease free survival and overall survival (OS) of breast cancer patients who received neoadjuvant chemotherapy [9]. Another study reported significantly faster enhancement kinetics (measured by the maximum enhancement in the first minute and the steepest slope of the enhancement curve) in breast cancer patients who developed local recurrence or distant metastases after surgery compared to those without recurrence or metastases [10].

The shape of DCE-MRI signal intensity-time curves has been shown to have diagnostic value in breast cancer [11]. Enhancement curves are typically classified as one of three types—persistent (continuous enhancement over time), plateau (enhancement reaches a plateau), or washout (initial enhancement followed by signal decrease). Most benign breast tumors (83.0%) displayed persistent enhancement, whereas malignant lesions were characterized by plateau

(33.6%) or washout (57.4%) type curves [11]. Such qualitative classification of enhancement curves may still be the most common form of DCE-MRI analysis, but efforts have been made to automate this classification to eliminate intra- and inter-observer variability [12, 13].

Quantitative parameters are desirable in the context of treatment monitoring and drug trials as they enable better assessment of longitudinal changes and comparison between different centers and studies. It has been recommended that K^{trans} or IAUC, the initial area under the contrast agent concentration-time curve, should be used as primary endpoints in early phase cancer drug trials [14]. Anti-angiogenic therapies are expected to decrease vascularization, perfusion, and/or vessel permeability, which would lead to decreases in K^{trans} and IAUC. Many clinical and preclinical studies have utilized DCE-MRI for monitoring response to various anti-angiogenic and vascular disrupting agents, with most reporting significant reductions in K^{trans} and IAUC (Fig. 24.1A) [15, 16]. However, some studies showed no sig-

nificant change, which may simply indicate drug resistance, or point to the complexity of the therapeutic mechanisms of action and of the physiological meanings of the DCE-MRI readouts. It is still not fully clear how antivascular agents work, and this uncertainty is also present in the interpretation of K^{trans} and IAUC, which are dependent on several factors (perfusion, vessel permeability, and surface area) that may change and affect these parameters in different ways after treatment. There are other, more generalized PK models that provide separate estimates of blood flow and the vessel permeability-surface area product, which are reviewed by Sourbron and Buckley [17]. But they are also more complex, computationally expensive, require higher temporal resolution, and have not been widely adopted in clinical practice.

Susceptibility contrast MRI utilizes (super)paramagnetic contrast agents to measure vascular function and morphology. The difference in the magnetic susceptibilities of the i.v.-administered contrast agent and biological tissue locally enhance transverse relaxation rates ($R_2^{(*)}$) in and around

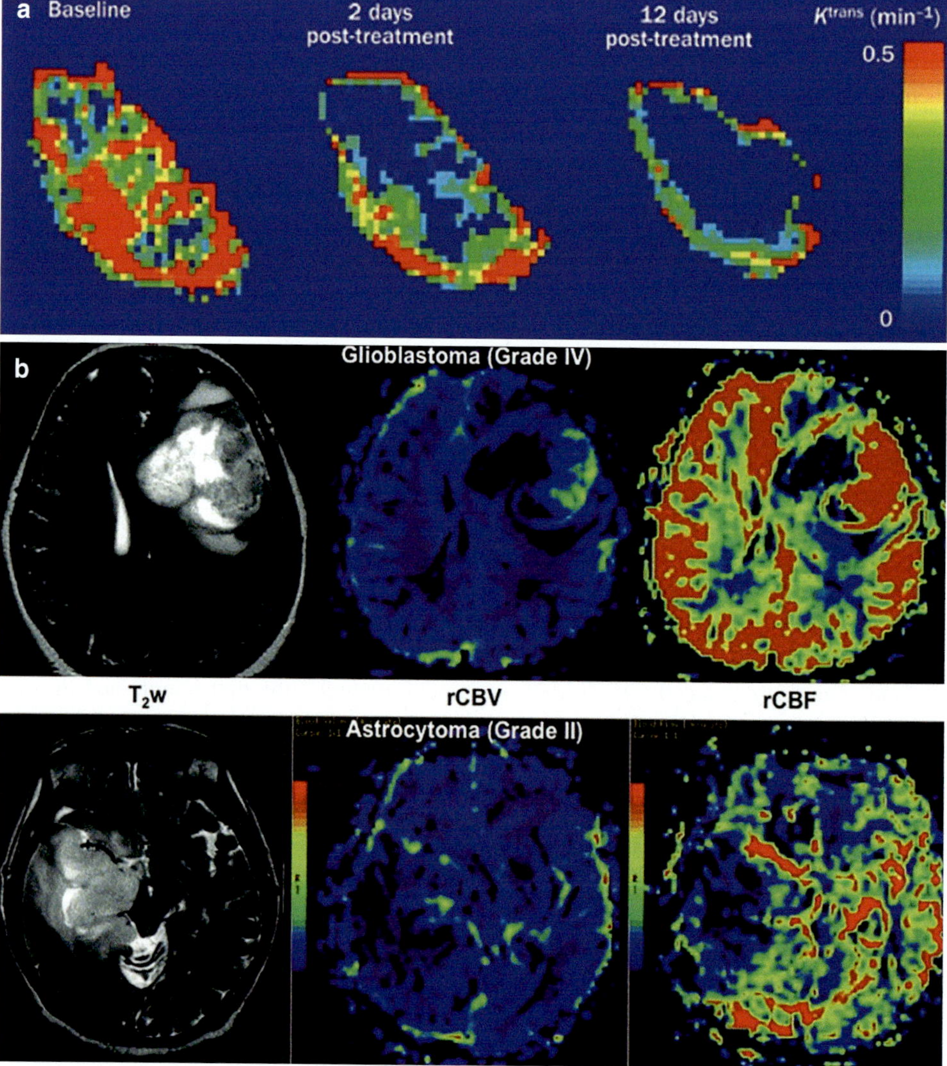

Fig. 24.1 (**a**) K^{trans} maps from a patient with a colorectal liver metastasis showing decreased perfusion, vascularization, and/or vessel permeability after bevacizumab treatment. Reprinted by permission from Macmillan Publishers Ltd.: Nature Reviews Clinical Oncology [15], copyright 2012. (**b**) Conventional T_2-weighted (T_2w) images (left), and DSC-MRI-derived rCBV (center) and rCBF maps (right) from a patient with grade IV glioblastoma (top) and a patient with grade II astrocytoma (bottom). The differences in rCBV and rCBF between the high- and low-grade gliomas are readily apparent. Reprinted from [20], Copyright 2005, with permission from Elsevier

blood vessels. Pre- and post-contrast images are acquired to measure the increase in relaxation ($\Delta R_2^{(*)}$), which is dependent on contrast agent concentration and distribution.

In the clinic, dynamic susceptibility contrast (DSC)-MRI is used to measure perfusion, primarily in the brain. A series of pre- and post-contrast T_2w or T_2*w images are acquired with high temporal resolution to capture the first pass of a GBCA bolus through the vasculature. Relative cerebral blood volume (rCBV) can be estimated from the signal intensity-time curve [18]; an AIF in addition to complex mathematics are required for quantification of absolute CBV and cerebral blood flow (CBF) [19]. DSC-MRI has been shown to be able to distinguish between high- and low-grade gliomas, with the high-grade lesions having significantly higher rCBV and rCBF (Fig. 24.1B) [20]. Similarly, Schmainda et al. showed that rCBV is predictive of OS in patients with recurrent high-grade glioma who received bevacizumab treatment, with OS being significantly longer if the rCBV of the lesion was below a certain threshold [21]. DSC-MRI is also sensitive to therapeutic response, but differentiating tumor progression from pseudoprogression and, in the case of anti-angiogenic therapy, response from pseudo-response can be challenging [22, 23].

The safety of GBCAs has come into question in recent years, sparked by a 2014 study by Kanda et al. that residual amounts of GBCAs were deposited and retained in the brain in a dose-dependent manner [24]. This and subsequent corroborative studies led the US Food and Drug Administration to require new warning labels and safety measures for all GBCAs [25], while the European Medicines Agency suspended approval of certain linear GBCAs [26], which are less stable than macrocyclic variants [27]. In response, recent studies have investigated the feasibility of DCE-MRI using lower GBCA doses (10–15% of the standard 0.1 mmol/kg dose). Low-dose DCE-MRI was shown to be comparable to standard dose in detecting breast [28] and prostate cancer [29]. These studies also found moderate to strong correlations between kinetic parameters calculated from low-dose and standard-dose data.

The ongoing uncertainty surrounding GBCAs has also helped regalvanize the development of a different class of contrast agents—superparamagnetic iron oxide (SPIO) nanoparticles. Currently, there are no commercially available SPIOs approved for use as MRI contrast agents, but ferumoxytol, an ultrasmall SPIO (USPIO) indicated for the treatment of iron deficiency anemia, is increasingly being used "off-label" as a contrast agent for various MRI applications [30]. In addition, other SPIO contrast agents continue to be developed [31–35].

While GBCAs leak relatively quickly from the blood pool into the extravascular space, USPIO nanoparticles like ferumoxytol have long circulation times, making them better suited for vascular imaging techniques like angiography [36] and DSC-MRI [37]. For example, a study comparing DSC-MRI using ferumoxytol and the GBCA gadoteridol showed that rCBV calculated using ferumoxytol could differentiate between tumor progression and pseudoprogression after chemo- and radiotherapy in glioblastoma multiforme patients; in comparison, additional contrast agent leakage correction was necessary for gadoteridol rCBV to be significantly associated with survival [38].

Intravascular contrast agents USPIOs are also used for steady-state susceptibility contrast (SSC)-MRI (i.e. vessel size imaging). Instead of acquiring images at high temporal resolution to capture the contrast agent kinetics, pre- and post-contrast spin and gradient echo images are acquired to measure steady-state ΔR_2 and ΔR_2*, respectively. These can be used to calculate various parameters that estimate mean vessel density [39], fractional blood volume, and mean vessel diameter [40]. SSC-MRI parameters have been shown to correlate with vascular measurements from histology [41] and high-resolution micro-CT [42, 43]. A review by Emblem et al. discusses the potential use of vessel size imaging parameters as clinical biomarkers of treatment response [44].

To summarize, there are multiple MRI techniques that are widely used preclinically and in clinical oncology for the characterization of the vascular phenotype, diagnosis, and treatment evaluation. The development of new contrast agents is an active area of research that could improve existing techniques and enable new vascular imaging applications. Still, a better understanding of the underlying biophysics that effect the MRI measurements and of the mechanisms of action of anti-angiogenic drugs and other therapies are needed for the development of clinically validated MRI-based biomarkers of tumor angiogenesis.

Imaging Tissue Cellularity and Microstructure

Diffusion-weighted MRI (DWI) is currently one of the fastest developing MRI-based techniques in oncology. DWI allows the mapping of water diffusion due to the Brownian motion of water molecules in vivo. The water diffusion is measured indirectly as a signal loss induced by diffusion sensitizing magnetic field gradients applied during the MRI pulse sequence. The diffusion can be quantitatively assessed by calculating the apparent diffusion coefficient (ADC) value. This assessment is done by acquiring several (at least two) images with different diffusion sensitization, from which the ADC value can be derived by exponential fitting. High ADC values indicate relatively free diffusion while low indicate restricted diffusion. The distribution of ADC values is commonly illustrated in parametric maps (Fig. 24.2).

The contrast in DWI arises from the different compositions of biological tissue, such as cell membranes, macro-

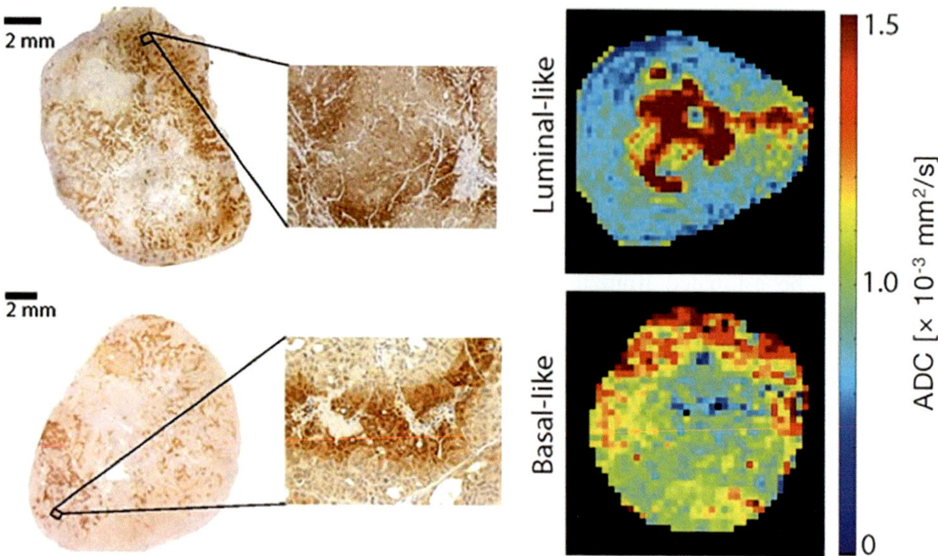

Fig. 24.2 Pimonidazole staining of luminal-like breast cancer xenografts (top left) demonstrates that these tumors are more hypoxic than basal-like breast cancer xenografts (bottom left). ADC values (shown in parametric maps) were significantly lower in the luminal-like (top right) compared to the basal-like tumors (bottom right), which demonstrates the inverse correlation between hypoxia and ADC and also reflects the higher content of collagen and fibronectin in the stroma of the luminal-like tumors [155, 156]. Reprinted with permission from [120], Copyright 2011 Wiley Periodicals, Inc

molecules, fibers, or other tissue components, all of which restrict water diffusion. Diffusion is also affected by water exchange between intracellular and extracellular compartments, the shape of the extracellular space, and tissue cellularity. Diffusion patterns can therefore reveal microscopic details about the tissue architecture. Due to this complex mixture of contributions to the measured DWI signal, the complete biophysical interpretation is still not fully clear.

Several studies have been performed to better understand the association between the microenvironment and the obtained diffusion properties. Importantly, tumor tissue is usually characterized by low water diffusivity, which is most likely related to higher cellular density [45] and proliferation [46]. Low ADC values have also been associated with high hypoxic fraction (Fig. 24.2), interstitial hypertension, and elevated metastatic propensity in melanoma xenografts [45].

Epithelial to mesenchymal transition (EMT) is important for tumor metastasis. It has been proposed that an increasing ADC value can be detected in tumor cells undergoing EMT [47]. Water diffusion is altered during the transition between epithelial and mesenchymal phenotypes due to changes in cell-cell contact and the volume of extracellular space. Subcutaneous xenograft tumors with epithelial-like phenotypes showed significantly lower ADC values compared to those with mesenchymal-like phenotypes.

Exploiting the diffusion properties by histogram analysis of ADC values across a tumor volume enables a better description of intratumoral heterogeneity compared to using mean or median ADC. Such analyses have for example been utilized to differentiate gliomas [48] and predict progression free survival [49]. Moreover, histogram analysis of ADC values of glioma contributed to distinguish between isocitrate dehydrogenase gene mutation-positive and—negative high-grade gliomas, which could be relevant for clinical patient management since the mutation-positive patients have a favorable prognosis [50].

Restriction spectrum imaging (RSI) is a new extension of the DWI methodology [51]. Restricted diffusion is a term used to describe the trapping of water molecules within an enclosed compartment, for example as defined by the cell plasma membrane. RSI requires the use of high diffusion sensitization in addition to directionality, and enables quantitative estimates of tissue microstructure based on modeling of tissue properties such as cell size, density, and orientation as a function of diffusion sensitization. The calculated cellularity index, an in vivo measure of spherically restricted water, has shown promising clinical results in improving the tumor conspicuity of high-grade brain tumors [52], capturing the treatment response of anti-angiogenic treatment [53], and improving visualization of white matter pathways through regions of peritumoral edema [54]. More recently, the RSI-derived cellularity index was found to be associated with the aggressiveness of prostate cancer (Gleason score) [55] and significantly contributed to prostate cancer staging based on accurate detection of extraprostatic extension of the tumor [56]. Recently, it was also shown that RSI had better specificity than ADC in the detection of transition sone prostate tumors [57].

Anti-cancer treatment changes the structural features of the tumor tissue and cells. Treatment-induced cell death is usually reflected by increased ADC values, due to loss of cell membrane integrity and decreased cell density caused by both necrosis and apoptosis, and this may be observed prior to any significant reduction of the tumor volume [58]. Increased diffusion due to treatment response has been shown after standard cytotoxic treatment [59–61], targeted treatment [60–62], anti-angiogenic treatment [63, 64], and radiation therapy [65, 66]. A comprehensive review of DWI in oncologic applications can be found in [67].

Increased deposition and reorientation of stromal collagen fibers are associated with breast cancer progression and invasiveness [68], and DWI can potentially provide noninvasive biomarkers to characterize this. The relationship between diffusion and the tumor stroma has been investigated in breast cancer [69], where ADC values were negatively correlated with tumor:stroma ratio, most likely because stroma-poor tumors have greater cellularity. However, diffusion was observed to be lower in collagen-dominant stroma types compared to fibroblast or lymphocyte-dominant types [69]. This is further confirmed in a study where area fractions of cellular and collagen content in histologic sections were quantified and compared with the corresponding in vivo DWI information [70]. Stromal collagen content increased the diffusivity and was associated with higher ADC. In prostate cancer, ADC correlates with the tumor tissue composition, and a positive association between ADC and the volume of the luminal space has been identified [71].

An interesting extension of DWI is diffusion tensor imaging (DTI), which adds information about tissue microstructure by addressing diffusion direction. In DTI, diffusion sensitizing gradients are applied in many (at least six) different directions, and the diffusion profile is fitted to a tensor model. The tensor model assumes that one dominant direction of diffusion is present and that the diffusion anisotropy can be described by an ellipsoidal symmetry [72]. DTI has been suggested as a new approach for the detection of breast cancer based on tracking the mammary architectural elements [73]. The breast's fibroglandular tissue is orientated along tubular ducts and ligaments, and the diffusion properties of the mammary fibroglandular tissue change during malignant transformation. The sensitivity of DTI to detect breast cancer was found to be high, particularly in dense breasts. However, other studies report that ADC is still the most important parameter for distinguishing benign and malignant breast lesions, while the anisotropy measures derived from DTI help to further characterize tumor microstructure and microenvironment [74]. A challenge in the management of breast cancer is the detection of early response to therapy. DTI could potentially aid in this, as changes in diffusion anisotropy reflect changes in tissue structure induced by neoadjuvant therapy [75]. Fractional anisotropy (FA) describes the degree of anisotropy of the diffusion process. FA and ADC were found to correlate with collagen fiber density in breast cancer xenografts [76]. The hypoxic regions of the same xenografts contained lower density of collagen fibers and simultaneously exhibited lower FA and ADC, suggesting that ADC and FA could serve as clinically relevant, noninvasive markers of fiber density as well as hypoxia.

Intravoxel incoherent motion (IVIM) imaging is another advanced DWI approach that was first described nearly three decades ago but is now gaining huge interest in oncology [77]. This technique considers the fact that the motion of water molecules contributing to the diffusion signal not only arises from extra- and intracellular diffusion, but also from intravascular blood flow (perfusion). This is especially apparent for images acquired with low diffusion sensitization [78]. IVIM allows for the separation of motion of water molecules due to microcirculation from motion due to diffusion, which is promising for response measurement in treatment studies targeting both vasculature and cell proliferation [79]. Recently, the applicability to detect early treatment changes exploiting IVIM has been highlighted in several cancers such as esophageal squamous cell carcinoma [80], liver metastases [81], osteosarcoma [82], and breast cancer [83, 84]. Importantly, this reflection of tissue diffusivity and microcapillary perfusion is obtained without contrast agent injection. However, most studies investigating IVIM for assessment of treatment response are small, and the added value compared to the simple and robust ADC measurement needs further examination.

Recently, radiomics approaches and machine learning techniques have made their entrance in the utilization of DWI data. This high-throughput extraction and analysis of features from medical images, is a promising field for characterizing tumor phenotype and assessing treatment response [85]. A number of studies have proven this approach to be useful in the differentiation of subtypes, e.g. in breast cancer [86] and ovarian cancer [87]. The ability to quantify image features in a standardized way and further exploit this information in modelling of relevant target characteristics has promising prospects in DWI.

In summary, DWI is now frequently used as one of the sequences in multiparametric MRI for preclinical and clinical oncological applications. The DWI signal, and the derived ADC value, largely depends on the tissue cellularity. To establish ADC as a robust biomarker, standardization of the DWI acquisition (how to apply the diffusion sensitization) and subsequent post-processing and analysis is necessary [88]. Importantly, preclinical studies have shown that absolute ADC values are comparable between sites and equipment, provided standardized protocols are employed [89]. Advanced extensions of DWI, such as DTI, RSI, and IVIM broaden the applicability of the methodology. DWI offers promising biomarkers for both cancer detection and evaluation of treatment response, and opens a window for in vivo, noninvasive characterization of the tumor microenvironment.

Investigating Cancer Metabolism

During cancer progression, molecular changes are associated with metabolic reprogramming [90, 91], which is a hallmark of cancer [92]. Cancer metabolism is regulated by intrinsic cellular responses for emerging needs or external forces from the tumor microenvironment. Several studies have developed quantification and imaging methods to investigate cancer metabolism's unusual alterations [93–95]. Clinical molecular imaging modalities, such as MRS and positron emission tomography (PET), can quantify metabolite concentrations in vivo. Also, metabolic changes can be measured within cell/or tissue extracts and intact tissue samples in laboratory settings using high-resolution MRS [96, 97].

MRS exploits the fact that the Larmor frequency is different for every nuclide and also depends on the magnetic field strength. Different nuclei experience slightly different magnetic fields depending on their molecular environment and chemical shielding and therefore precess at slightly different frequencies. These resonance offsets can be described on a field-independent dimensionless scale called chemical shift (δ), which is expressed in parts per million (ppm). Individual molecular properties can be characterized by a single or multiple resonance in MR frequency spectra, thereby allowing detection and quantification of the relative concentrations of different metabolites and other molecules by MRS.

One of the most common metabolic anomalies observed in cancer is the Warburg effect. Partly due to hypoxia, and partly due to direct metabolic regulation through oncogenic signaling, most cancer cells exhibit high glycolytic activity and convert a substantial fraction of their glucose to lactate even in the presence of adequate oxygen levels [98]. The lactate dehydrogenase (LDH) enzyme catalyzes the reversible conversion of pyruvate to lactate. LDH expression and high tumor lactate are required for the progression of many tumors. MRS-measured lactate concentration can be a sensitive indicator of the metabolic adaptation in cancer cells, and many studies have revealed its correlation with prognosis, treatment efficacy, and clinical outcome in a variety of human cancers [99]. Some other commonly measured metabolites in ^{1}H MRS include choline-containing compounds, lipids, N-acetyl aspartate, creatine, glutamate, glutamine, GABA, myo-inositol, citrate, and 2-hydroxyglutarate.

Altered membrane choline phospholipid metabolism is associated with malignancies, oncogenesis, and tumor progression [100]. Changes in choline-containing metabolite concentrations have been shown to be potential early biomarkers of targeted anti-tumor therapies. Increased levels of choline-containing metabolites, referred to as total choline (tCho), in cancer cells has been interpreted to be associated with cancer cells' demands for increased proliferation, upregulation of choline kinase activity, and oncogenic cell signaling such as overactivity of PI3K signaling [100]. ^{1}H MRS can detect tCho noninvasively on clinically available MR scanners. ^{31}P MRS is another useful tool for noninvasive investigation of phospholipid metabolism in vivo. Compared to ^{1}H MRS, this technique is less prone to water and lipid contamination; however, it is less sensitive and requires an additional dedicated phosphorus coil. Several key metabolites involved in phospholipid metabolism are detected by ^{31}P MRS, such as phosphocholine (PCho), phosphoethanolamine (PE), glycerophosphocholine (GPC), and glycerophosphoethanolamine (GPE). Other potential applications of ^{31}P MRS include the evaluation of high-energy phosphates: phosphocreatine (PCr), adenosine-triphosphate (ATP) and adenosine diphosphate (ADP) and the intracellular redox state estimation by quantifying NAD+ over NADH [101].

With 1.1% natural abundance of the ^{13}C isotope, ^{13}C MRS of endogenous metabolites is less sensitive than ^{1}H MRS. However, exogenous ^{13}C MRS is feasible following administration of a ^{13}C-labeled substrate, including ^{13}C-labeled glucose, and subsequent incorporation of the ^{13}C-label from the exogenous substrate into other molecules. For instance, glycolytic rates can be measured by investigating the uptake and metabolism of [^{13}C]-glucose in vivo. However, the utility of ^{13}C MRS is limited due to its relatively low sensitivity and that most commercial MR systems are only capable of ^{1}H MRS. One of the most important innovations in recent years has been the development of dynamic nuclear polarization (DNP, or "hyperpolarization") of ^{13}C-labeled metabolic substrates, enhancing the sensitivity of the ^{13}C MRS experiment dramatically (>10,000-fold higher than non-hyperpolarized ^{13}C) [102]. This improvement allows the analysis of several metabolic pathways and metabolic fluxes through select enzyme-catalyzed steps. Due to its excellent polarization properties, rapid transport into important metabolic pathways, and longer relaxation time, [1-^{13}C]pyruvate has been the most widely studied substrate to date. In addition to indicating the presence of the Warburg effect in tumors, [1-^{13}C]pyruvate has been employed to investigate the response to anti-cancer therapies by noninvasively evaluating real-time flux of pyruvate to lactate and LDH activity in preclinical [103, 104] and more recently, clinical studies [95, 105]. A recent clinical study [105] has successfully demonstrated the feasibility of ^{13}C hyperpolarized imaging on breast cancer patients. The authors showed a significant correlation between [1-^{13}C]pyruvate metabolism and the tumor's molecular characteristics. They observed a considerable accumulation of ^{13}C-lactate in a more aggressive TNBCs grade 3 than TNBCs grade 2. When com-

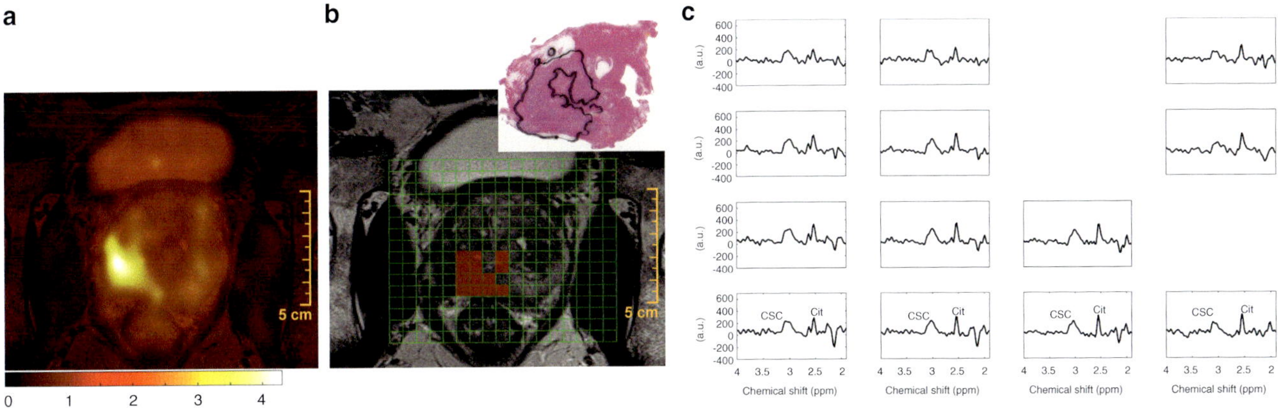

Fig. 24.3 Representative PET, MRI, and MRSI images acquired from a 66-year-old patient with prostate cancer by an integrated 3.0 T PET/MRI system. (**a**) ^{18}F-fluciclovine image shows a focal uptake in the right lobe of the peripheral zone of the prostate. (**b**) Axial T2-weighted MR image and overlaid MRSI-derived (Choline + Spermine + Creatine)/Citrate (CSC/Cit) metabolic map. Corresponding whole-mount histopathology slide indicates the lesion margin. (**c**) MR spectra from the red color voxels in **b**. PET, positron emission tomography; MRSI, Magnetic resonance spectroscopic imaging. Adapted from [112], under CC-BY license

pared to DCE-derived parameters, K^{trans} and washout (k_{ep}), the metabolic response Lactate/Pyruvate ratio and pyruvate-lactate exchange rate (k_{PL}) measured by ^{13}C hyperpolarized showed more reliable early assessment of neoadjuvant chemotherapy in a TNBC patient [95]. A decrease in the K^{trans} and k_{ep} followed by neoadjuvant chemotherapy is frequently associated with response [95], however, the authors unexpectedly observed increased levels of these DCE-derived parameters. Contrarily, the authors demonstrated that Lactate/Pyruvate ratio and k_{PL} decreased significantly (-34% and -37%, respectively), providing early assessment biomarkers to TNBC neoadjuvant chemotherapy. [1,4-^{13}C$_2$]fumarate has been used to investigate cell necrosis and treatment response in tumors [106]. Hyperpolarized [1-^{13}C]pyruvate and [1,4-^{13}C$_2$]fumarate have also been used to detect early changes in tumor metabolism following administration of a vascular disrupting agent [107].

PET is a sensitive and quantitative method for measuring the uptake and trapping of different radio-labeled PET substrates, such as ^{18}F-fluorodeoxyglucose (^{18}F-FDG), a radioactive form of glucose. This technique allows noninvasive molecular imaging of cancer cell metabolism, heterogeneity, and metastases in systems ranging from advanced tumor models to patients in the clinical setting. When combined with computed tomography (CT), PET/CT provides both anatomical localization and functional information. There is a wide range of novel and established PET radiotracers, which can be used to investigate various aspects of cancer, including carbohydrate, amino acid, and fatty acid metabolism. ^{18}F-FDG-PET by far is the most successful tracer in in vivo cancer studies. The reduction in ^{18}F-FDG uptake has been used to detect treatment response in some cancer subtypes [108].

Integration of ^{18}F-FDG-PET and MRS may potentially increase the sensitivity and accuracy in tumor localization [109] and specificity of tumor detection [110–112] (Fig. 24.3). The increased availability of clinical PET/MR scanners has recently raised the interest in simultaneous DNP-MRS and PET imaging [111, 113]. PET provides relatively higher sensitivity than DNP-MRS, detecting in the range of nano- to picomolar compared to the millimolar range sensitivity of MRS. Due to low sensitivity, the concentrations of DNP substrates that have to be administered may exceed that of physiologic levels, which may perturb normal metabolism. The short half-life (in tens of seconds) is another notable limitation of DNP-MRS, which calls for improvement in fast-MRS data acquisition. But unlike PET, DNP-MRS does not employ ionizing radiation and can detect injected substrate and its metabolic products simultaneously. The latter enables the observation of both the uptake of the targeted molecule and its downstream metabolic products.

Multimodal imaging techniques have provided novel opportunities for cancer treatment by providing comprehensive cancer metabolomics information. In clinical cancer management, there has been a great tendency towards personalized therapies—including targeting specific metabolic pathways, enzymes, and/or oncogenes—and away from aggressive or cytotoxic treatments. Integration of anatomical information of MRI and metabolic information provided by multivoxel MRS imaging (MRSI) or PET can significantly improve the assessment of cancer location, extent, aggressiveness, and response to treatment.

Imaging Tumor Hypoxia

Hypoxia can be defined as subnormal levels of oxygen in tissue, and is a frequent phenomenon in solid tumors. A functional mismatch between cell proliferation and vascularization often leads to poor oxygenation of tumor regions—either because the cancer cells are located so far from the nearest blood vessel that oxygen supply through diffusion is insufficient, or because the tumor vasculature is dysfunctional and cannot provide oxygen to meet the demands of the surrounding tumor tissue.

During the lifespan of a tumor, there will be both temporal and spatial variation in the degree of hypoxia. This will in turn induce adaptive changes in the biology of the cancer cells. These changes are predominantly mediated through the hypoxia-inducible factors (HIFs) and hypoxia response elements, which transcriptionally regulate genes that are relevant for cancer cell growth and disease development [114].

A well-documented clinical consequence of low partial oxygen pressure in tumors is resistance to radiotherapy caused by insufficient production of free oxygen radicals [115]. However, it has also been shown that hypoxia, measured with electrodes inserted directly into tumor tissue, is associated with poor prognosis in several cancers [116]. Furthermore, it has been demonstrated that hypoxia promotes local invasion and metastatic dissemination of cancer cells [117, 118].

Since hypoxia is a driving force for cancer progression, and since the outcome of radiotherapy is strongly associated with oxygenation of the target tissue, measuring the level of hypoxia in solid tumors has potential clinical implications, such as a more precise prognosis and facilitation of personalized treatment. There is therefore significant interest in the development of noninvasive imaging methods that can report on the degree of hypoxia in solid tumors, preferably with high spatial resolution. This can be achieved either through direct approaches using oxygen level-sensitive contrast agents, or through indirect approaches using functional proxy markers of hypoxia.

MRI cannot directly measure the partial pressure of oxygen in tissue. Therefore, hypoxia has traditionally been imaged using indirect markers of oxygen concentration. Oxygen delivery and consumption depend on vascular perfusion and cellular density, which can be imaged using DCE-MRI and DW-MRI, respectively. While these methods do not provide information on actual tissue oxygenation, several reports describe relationships between standard DCE-MRI and DW-MRI readouts and hypoxia in preclinical model systems. For example, an inverse correlation between K^{trans} and ADC and the fraction of hypoxic cells has been demonstrated in several experimental model systems (Fig. 24.2) [45, 119–121]. However, this may represent an indirect association because hypoxia can arise from the imbalance between oxygen supply and demand created by high cellular density. Interestingly, these studies have also demonstrated associations between these functional MRI parameters, hypoxia, and metastatic potential, emphasizing the potential clinical value of imaging the hypoxic tumor microenvironment.

Using blood oxygen level-dependent (BOLD) MRI, the ratio of oxygenated to deoxygenated blood can be measured through differences in intrinsic magnetic susceptibility between oxy- and deoxy-hemoglobin—the presence of paramagnetic deoxy-hemoglobin will increase the $R_2{*}$ relaxation rate of water protons. In cancer, it has been suggested that changes in $R_2{*}$ in response to inhalation of hyperoxic gas can be used to identify hypoxic tumor fractions [122]. However, changes in $R_2{*}$ are not directly proportional to changes in tissue oxygenation levels, and this technique has therefore not yet found clinical use [123, 124]. The same problem applies to R_1 relaxivity-based tissue oxygen level-dependent (TOLD) MRI, which recently has been suggested as a tool for mapping regional oxygenation in tumors [125]. Before these methods can be introduced in the clinic, there is a need for both technical validation, improved understanding of the relationship between imaging biomarkers and underlying biology, and identification of clinical application where these imaging biomarkers provide diagnostic or prognostic value [126].

The direct approach to imaging hypoxia through oxygen-sensitive contrast agents is predominantly based on 2-nitroimidazole derivatives, a group of compounds that form covalent bonds with cellular macromolecules at oxygen levels below 10 mmHg pO2 [127]. Nitroimidazole adducts can be detected ex vivo using immunohistochemistry [128], but contrast agents for in vivo labeling and imaging have also been developed. Several fluorinated nitroimidazole derivatives have been tested clinically, using ^{19}F MRS to detect accumulation of contrast agent in hypoxic tumor regions [129]. Recently, a gadolinium-labeled nitroimidazole contrast agent (GdDO$_3$NI), was found to accumulate in poorly perfused regions of xenografted tumors, suggesting that T_1-based MRI of hypoxia may be a possibility [130]. However, efforts to develop hypoxia-targeted MRI contrast agents are hampered by the inherent low sensitivity of this imaging modality.

In contrast, PET imaging is highly suitable for quantitative imaging of contrast agents present in low concentrations in tissue. Several PET probes, such as ^{18}F-fluoromisonidazole [^{18}F-MISO] and ^{18}F-flortanidazole [^{18}F-HX4] bind to viable hypoxic cells in vivo, thereby allowing direct imaging of hypoxia in cancer. Using quantitative readouts such as tumor:blood or tumor:muscle signal intensity ratios, it has been shown that ^{18}F-MISO can accurately and reproducibly image regional insufficiencies in pO2 across a wide range of cancers [131, 132]. In several trials, pre-treatment ^{18}F-MISO uptake predicted the outcome of radiation therapy, demonstrating the value of noninvasive hypoxia assessment [133,

134]. The technique has been cross-validated against DCE-MRI, demonstrating that high ^{18}F-MISO uptake correlates with low K^{trans}. Based on the current clinical evidence, the FDA has granted an Investigational New Drug (IND) status for ^{18}F-MISO. However, due to the pharmacokinetic properties of ^{18}F-MISO, the image contrast is frequently insufficient for the assessment of intratumor heterogeneity. Second-generation tracers, such as ^{18}F-HX4 and FAZA are less lipophilic and have faster clearance, which enables imaging of small, poorly vascularized, hypoxic regions in tumor tissue [135]. Clinical trials which describe the prognostic and predictive performance of these tracers in specific patient contexts will be crucial for clinical implementation of hypoxia-sensitive PET imaging [136, 137].

In summary, the clinical implications of noninvasive assessment of tumor tissue oxygen levels are significant, predominantly due to its predictive value in radiotherapy. Currently, PET imaging with ^{18}F-MISO is the most widely used imaging approach, but second-generation tracers may display higher diagnostic performance in clinical trials. As the BOLD and TOLD MRI techniques do not require the use of exogenous contrast, further understanding of how they reflect tumor tissue oxygenation would make them attractive for clinical use.

Probing Intratumoral pH

As mentioned above, most cancer cells have high glycolytic rates and the resulting pyruvate is converted to lactate instead of being oxidized in the mitochondria, even under normoxic conditions. To maintain a sustainable intracellular pH (pH_i), excess lactate is transported out of the cells via the monocarboxylate transporter system. This contributes to the acidification of the extracellular compartment, which has been associated with tumorigenic transformation, decreased genetic stability, induction of growth factors and proteases and, ultimately, increased migration and invasion leading to increased metastatic potential [138, 139]. The extracellular pH (pH_e) in solid tumors can be as low as 6.0, in contrast to normal tissues where pH_i (7.2–7.4) normally is slightly lower than pH_e [140].

Noninvasive pH measurement is therefore of clinical interest—both since pH may provide independent prognostic/predictive information, and since pH measurements may be relevant for early response monitoring as well as guiding treatment with pH-sensitive drugs or drug delivery systems [141, 142].

Imaging pH in vivo has been a challenge for the scientific communities for several decades, partly because it requires an exogenous or endogenous pH indicator that has a pKA in the relevant range, as well as the ability to provide sufficient signal at non-toxic/endogenous concentrations. One approach has been to develop self-quenching fluorescent probes that are activated at low pH [143]. This approach, however, is only semi-quantitative by nature. Using quantitative MRS for simultaneous measurement of the protonated and ionic fractions of weak acids through differences in chemical shift is therefore a more accurate method for non-invasive determination of pH.

The chemical shift of inorganic phosphate (Pi) is pH-dependent, and ^{31}P MRS can therefore estimate pH based on the resonance frequency of Pi within 0.05 pH units [144]. However, it has been confirmed that Pi primarily represents the intracellular pH, which is neutral/slightly alkaline even in highly acidic tumors [145, 146]. This led to the development of membrane impermeant phosphonate-based probes, such as 3-aminopropylphosphonate (3-APP), which can be used to measure pH_e. Despite the limited sensitivity of ^{31}P MRS, these compounds unequivocally demonstrated that the acidic pH in tumors is due to the low extracellular pH.

Attempts to develop more clinically relevant extracellular NMR-detectable agents also include several imidazole-based pH indicators for ^{1}H MRS [147, 148]. Preclinical experiments have demonstrated that MRSI of these agents can describe pH heterogeneity in tumors with differences as large as 0.5 pH units within less than a centimeter in distance. Co-registration studies suggest that the extracellular pH correlates to regional lactate concentration, but also that low pH is associated with poor perfusion.

In recent years, it has also been demonstrated that Chemical Exchange Saturation Transfer (CEST) MRI can be used to determine pH in tumors. This technique is based on the pH-dependent transfer of magnetization to water molecules from protons in endogenous or exogenous molecules. As the average chemical exchange rates of some labile protons are pH-dependent, and because CEST effects from two labile protons can be selectively detected, a ratio of two CEST effects from the same agent can be used to measure pH in a manner that is independent of concentration [149]. This has led to the development of the acidoCEST protocol, which uses the clinically accepted contrast agent iopromide as a CEST agent [150]. AcidoCEST has been extensively validated in various preclinical models, and a recent proof-of-concept study has demonstrated the clinical translatability of the method [151–153].

An intriguing new approach to in vivo pH measurements is the use of hyperpolarized ^{13}C bicarbonate, allowing real-time assessment of HCO3- and dissolved CO2 concentrations with ^{13}C MRS, from which pH can be calculated using the Henderson-Hasselbalch equation [154]. Preclinical studies with this tracer have confirmed the presence of a pH gradient across cell membranes ($pH_i > pH_e$), and that the method reports on pH across the physiologically relevant range.

In summary, MRI/MRS offers several approaches for measurement of tissue pH. Depending on the need for accuracy and spatial resolution, as well as access to specialized equipment, several methods may be of value in clinical cancer management.

Concluding Remarks/Summary

Magnetic resonance is a versatile method to obtain a wide range of anatomical and physiological information, relevant for cancer characterization. The methodology is non-invasive and has the potential to provide biomarkers for tumor vascularization, cellularity, tissue microstructure, oxygenation, and pH, as well as metabolic reprogramming. Biomarkers derived from preclinical research can easily be translated to the clinical setting.

References

1. Kerbel RS. Tumor angiogenesis. N Engl J Med. 2008;358(19):2039–49.
2. Weis SM, Cheresh DA. Pathophysiological consequences of VEGF-induced vascular permeability. Nature. 2005;437(7058):497–504.
3. Tofts PS, Brix G, Buckley DL, Evelhoch JL, Henderson E, Knopp MV, et al. Estimating kinetic parameters from dynamic contrast-enhanced T(1)-weighted MRI of a diffusable tracer: standardized quantities and symbols. J Magn Reson Imaging. 1999;10(3):223–32.
4. Buckley DL, Drew PJ, Mussurakis S, Monson JR, Horsman A. Microvessel density of invasive breast cancer assessed by dynamic Gd-DTPA enhanced MRI. J Magn Reson Imaging. 1997;7(3):461–4.
5. Gaustad JV, Brurberg KG, Simonsen TG, Mollatt CS, Rofstad EK. Tumor vascularity assessed by magnetic resonance imaging and intravital microscopy imaging. Neoplasia. 2008;10(4):354–62.
6. Atkin G, Taylor NJ, Daley FM, Stirling JJ, Richman P, Glynne-Jones R, et al. Dynamic contrast-enhanced magnetic resonance imaging is a poor measure of rectal cancer angiogenesis. Br J Surg. 2006;93(8):992–1000.
7. Su MY, Cheung YC, Fruehauf JP, Yu H, Nalcioglu O, Mechetner E, et al. Correlation of dynamic contrast enhancement MRI parameters with microvessel density and VEGF for assessment of angiogenesis in breast cancer. J Magn Reson Imaging. 2003;18(4):467–77.
8. Weidner N, Semple JP, Welch WR, Folkman J. Tumor angiogenesis and metastasis--correlation in invasive breast carcinoma. N Engl J Med. 1991;324(1):1–8.
9. Pickles MD, Manton DJ, Lowry M, Turnbull LW. Prognostic value of pre-treatment DCE-MRI parameters in predicting disease free and overall survival for breast cancer patients undergoing neoadjuvant chemotherapy. Eur J Radiol. 2009;71(3):498–505.
10. Tuncbilek N, Tokatli F, Altaner S, Sezer A, Ture M, Omurlu IK, et al. Prognostic value DCE-MRI parameters in predicting factor disease free survival and overall survival for breast cancer patients. Eur J Radiol. 2012;81(5):863–7.
11. Kuhl CK, Mielcareck P, Klaschik S, Leutner C, Wardelmann E, Gieseke J, et al. Dynamic breast MR imaging: are signal intensity time course data useful for differential diagnosis of enhancing lesions? Radiology. 1999;211(1):101–10.
12. Chen W, Giger ML, Bick U, Newstead GM. Automatic identification and classification of characteristic kinetic curves of breast lesions on DCE-MRI. Med Phys. 2006;33(8):2878–87.
13. El Khouli RH, Macura KJ, Jacobs MA, Khalil TH, Kamel IR, Dwyer A, et al. Dynamic contrast-enhanced MRI of the breast: quantitative method for kinetic curve type assessment. AJR Am J Roentgenol. 2009;193(4):W295–300.
14. Leach MO, Brindle KM, Evelhoch JL, Griffiths JR, Horsman MR, Jackson A, et al. The assessment of antiangiogenic and anti-vascular therapies in early-stage clinical trials using magnetic resonance imaging: issues and recommendations. Br J Cancer. 2005;92(9):1599–610.
15. O'Connor JP, Jackson A, Parker GJ, Roberts C, Jayson GC. Dynamic contrast-enhanced MRI in clinical trials of antivascular therapies. Nat Rev Clin Oncol. 2012;9(3):167–77.
16. Nielsen T, Wittenborn T, Horsman MR. Dynamic contrast-enhanced magnetic resonance imaging (DCE-MRI) in preclinical studies of antivascular treatments. Pharmaceutics. 2012;4(4):563–89.
17. Sourbron SP, Buckley DL. Tracer kinetic modelling in MRI: estimating perfusion and capillary permeability. Phys Med Biol. 2012;57(2):R1–33.
18. Knopp EA, Cha S, Johnson G, Mazumdar A, Golfinos JG, Zagzag D, et al. Glial neoplasms: dynamic contrast-enhanced T2*-weighted MR imaging. Radiology. 1999;211(3):791–8.
19. Shiroishi MS, Castellazzi G, Boxerman JL, D'Amore F, Essig M, Nguyen TB, et al. Principles of T2 *-weighted dynamic susceptibility contrast MRI technique in brain tumor imaging. J Magn Reson Imaging. 2015;41(2):296–313.
20. Hakyemez B, Erdogan C, Ercan I, Ergin N, Uysal S, Atahan S. High-grade and low-grade gliomas: differentiation by using perfusion MR imaging. Clin Radiol. 2005;60(4):493–502.
21. Schmainda KM, Prah M, Connelly J, Rand SD, Hoffman RG, Mueller W, et al. Dynamic-susceptibility contrast agent MRI measures of relative cerebral blood volume predict response to bevacizumab in recurrent high-grade glioma. Neuro-Oncology. 2014;16(6):880–8.
22. Huang RY, Neagu MR, Reardon DA, Wen PY. Pitfalls in the neuroimaging of glioblastoma in the era of antiangiogenic and immuno/targeted therapy - detecting illusive disease, defining response. Front Neurol. 2015;6:33.
23. Hygino da Cruz LC Jr, Rodriguez I, Domingues RC, Gasparetto EL, Sorensen AG. Pseudoprogression and pseudoresponse: imaging challenges in the assessment of posttreatment glioma. AJNR Am J Neuroradiol. 2011;32(11):1978–85.
24. Kanda T, Ishii K, Kawaguchi H, Kitajima K, Takenaka D. High signal intensity in the dentate nucleus and globus pallidus on unenhanced T1-weighted MR images: relationship with increasing cumulative dose of a gadolinium-based contrast material. Radiology. 2014;270(3):834–41.
25. FDA. FDA Drug Safety Communication: FDA warns that gadolinium-based contrast agents (GBCAs) are retained in the body; requires new class warnings. https://www.fda.gov/Drugs/DrugSafety/ucm589213.htm: FDA Communication; 2017.
26. Editor EM. EMA's final opinion confirms restrictions on use of linear gadolinium agents in body scans https://www.ema.europa.eu/en/medicines/human/referrals/gadolinium-containing-contrast-agents2017 [updated 19/12/2017].
27. Runge VM. Critical questions regarding gadolinium deposition in the brain and body after injections of the gadolinium-based contrast agents, safety, and clinical recommendations in consideration of the EMA's pharmacovigilance and risk assessment committee recommendation for suspension of the marketing authorizations for 4 linear agents. Investig Radiol. 2017;52(6):317–23.
28. Wang N, Xie Y, Fan Z, Ma S, Saouaf R, Guo Y, et al. Five-dimensional quantitative low-dose multitasking dynamic contrast-enhanced MRI: preliminary study on breast cancer. Magn Reson Med 2021.
29. He D, Chatterjee A, Fan X, Wang S, Eggener S, Yousuf A, et al. Feasibility of dynamic contrast-enhanced magnetic resonance imaging using low-dose gadolinium: comparative performance

with standard dose in prostate cancer diagnosis. Investig Radiol. 2018;53(10):609–15.

30. Daldrup-Link HE. Ten things you might not know about iron oxide nanoparticles. Radiology. 2017;284(3):616–29.

31. Wei H, Bruns OT, Kaul MG, Hansen EC, Barch M, Wisniowska A, et al. Exceedingly small iron oxide nanoparticles as positive MRI contrast agents. Proc Natl Acad Sci U S A. 2017;114(9):2325–30.

32. Zhang H, Li L, Liu XL, Jiao J, Ng CT, Yi JB, et al. Ultrasmall ferrite nanoparticles synthesized via dynamic simultaneous thermal decomposition for High-performance and multifunctional T1 magnetic resonance imaging contrast agent. ACS Nano. 2017;11(4):3614–31.

33. Wang L, Huang J, Chen H, Wu H, Xu Y, Li Y, et al. Exerting enhanced permeability and retention effect driven delivery by ultrafine iron oxide nanoparticles with T1-T2 switchable magnetic resonance imaging contrast. ACS Nano. 2017;11(5):4582–92.

34. Xiao WL, Chevallier P, Lagueux J, Oh KW, Fortin MA. Superparamagnetic iron oxide nanoparticles stabilized with multidentate block copolymers for optimal vascular contrast in T1-weighted magnetic resonance imaging. ACS Appl Nano Mater 2018;1(2):14.

35. Bao YS, Sherwood JA, Sun Z Magnetic iron oxide nanoparticles as T1 contrast agents for magnetic resonance imaging. J Mater Chem C 2018(6):10.

36. Hope MD, Hope TA, Zhu C, Faraji F, Haraldsson H, Ordovas KG, et al. Vascular imaging with Ferumoxytol as a contrast agent. AJR Am J Roentgenol. 2015;205(3):W366–73.

37. Varallyay CG, Nesbit E, Horvath A, Varallyay P, Fu R, Gahramanov S, et al. Cerebral blood volume mapping with ferumoxytol in dynamic susceptibility contrast perfusion MRI: comparison to standard of care. J Magn Reson Imaging. 2018;48(2):441–8.

38. Gahramanov S, Muldoon LL, Varallyay CG, Li X, Kraemer DF, Fu R, et al. Pseudoprogression of glioblastoma after chemo- and radiation therapy: diagnosis by using dynamic susceptibility-weighted contrast-enhanced perfusion MR imaging with ferumoxytol versus gadoteridol and correlation with survival. Radiology. 2013;266(3):842–52.

39. Jensen JH, Chandra R. MR imaging of microvasculature. Magn Reson Med. 2000;44(2):224–30.

40. Tropres I, Grimault S, Vaeth A, Grillon E, Julien C, Payen JF, et al. Vessel size imaging. Magn Reson Med. 2001;45(3):397–408.

41. Tropres I, Lamalle L, Peoc'h M, Farion R, Usson Y, Decorps M, et al. In vivo assessment of tumoral angiogenesis. Magn Reson Med. 2004;51(3):533–41.

42. Kim E, Cebulla J, Ward BD, Rhie K, Zhang J, Pathak AP. Assessing breast cancer angiogenesis in vivo: which susceptibility contrast MRI biomarkers are relevant? Magn Reson Med. 2013;70(4):1106–16.

43. Ungersma SE, Pacheco G, Ho C, Yee SF, Ross J, van Bruggen N, et al. Vessel imaging with viable tumor analysis for quantification of tumor angiogenesis. Magn Reson Med. 2010;63(6):1637–47.

44. Emblem KE, Farrar CT, Gerstner ER, Batchelor TT, Borra RJ, Rosen BR, et al. Vessel caliber--a potential MRI biomarker of tumour response in clinical trials. Nat Rev Clin Oncol. 2014;11(10):566–84.

45. Hompland T, Ellingsen C, Galappathi K, Rofstad EK. DW-MRI in assessment of the hypoxic fraction, interstitial fluid pressure, and metastatic propensity of melanoma xenografts. BMC Cancer. 2014;14:92.

46. Karavaeva E, Harris RJ, Leu K, Shabihkhani M, Yong WH, Pope WB, et al. Relationship between [18F]FDOPA PET uptake, apparent diffusion coefficient (ADC), and proliferation rate in recurrent malignant gliomas. Mol Imaging Biol. 2015;17(3):434–42.

47. Chen YW, Pan HB, Tseng HH, Chu HC, Hung YT, Yen YC, et al. Differentiated epithelial- and mesenchymal-like phenotypes in subcutaneous mouse xenografts using diffusion weighted-magnetic resonance imaging. Int J Mol Sci. 2013;14(11):21943–59.

48. Kang Y, Choi SH, Kim YJ, Kim KG, Sohn CH, Kim JH, et al. Gliomas: histogram analysis of apparent diffusion coefficient maps with standard- or high-b-value diffusion-weighted MR imaging--correlation with tumor grade. Radiology. 2011;261(3):882–90.

49. Kondo M, Uchiyama Y. Apparent diffusion coefficient histogram analysis for prediction of prognosis in glioblastoma. J Neuroradiol. 2018;45(4):236–41.

50. Lee S, Choi SH, Ryoo I, Yoon TJ, Kim TM, Lee SH, et al. Evaluation of the microenvironmental heterogeneity in high-grade gliomas with IDH1/2 gene mutation using histogram analysis of diffusion-weighted imaging and dynamic-susceptibility contrast perfusion imaging. J Neuro-Oncol. 2015;121(1):141–50.

51. White NS, McDonald C, Farid N, Kuperman J, Karow D, Schenker-Ahmed NM, et al. Diffusion-weighted imaging in cancer: physical foundations and applications of restriction spectrum imaging. Cancer Res. 2014;74(17):4638–52.

52. White NS, McDonald CR, Farid N, Kuperman JM, Kesari S, Dale AM. Improved conspicuity and delineation of high-grade primary and metastatic brain tumors using "restriction spectrum imaging": quantitative comparison with high B-value DWI and ADC. AJNR Am J Neuroradiol 2013;34(5):958–64, S1.

53. Kothari PD, White NS, Farid N, Chung R, Kuperman JM, Girard HM, et al. Longitudinal restriction spectrum imaging is resistant to pseudoresponse in patients with high-grade gliomas treated with bevacizumab. AJNR Am J Neuroradiol. 2013;34(9):1752–7.

54. McDonald CR, White NS, Farid N, Lai G, Kuperman JM, Bartsch H, et al. Recovery of white matter tracts in regions of peritumoral FLAIR hyperintensity with use of restriction spectrum imaging. AJNR Am J Neuroradiol. 2013;34(6):1157–63.

55. Liss MA, White NS, Parsons JK, Schenker-Ahmed NM, Rakow-Penner R, Kuperman JM, et al. MRI-derived restriction spectrum imaging cellularity index is associated with high grade prostate cancer on radical prostatectomy specimens. Front Oncol. 2015;5:30.

56. Rakow-Penner RA, White NS, Parsons JK, Choi HW, Liss MA, Kuperman JM, et al. Novel technique for characterizing prostate cancer utilizing MRI restriction spectrum imaging: proof of principle and initial clinical experience with extraprostatic extension. Prostate Cancer Prostatic Dis. 2015;18(1):81–5.

57. Felker ER, Raman SS, Shakeri S, Mirak SA, Bajgiran AM, Kwan L, et al. Utility of restriction spectrum imaging among men undergoing first-time biopsy for suspected prostate cancer. AJR Am J Roentgenol. 2019;213(2):365–70.

58. Hamstra DA, Rehemtulla A, Ross BD. Diffusion magnetic resonance imaging: a biomarker for treatment response in oncology. J Clin Oncol. 2007;25(26):4104–9.

59. Papaevangelou E, Almeida GS, Jamin Y, Robinson SP, deSouza NM. Diffusion-weighted MRI for imaging cell death after cytotoxic or apoptosis-inducing therapy. Br J Cancer. 2015;112(9):1471–9.

60. Cebulla J, Huuse EM, Pettersen K, van der Veen A, Kim E, Andersen S, et al. MRI reveals the in vivo cellular and vascular response to BEZ235 in ovarian cancer xenografts with different PI3-kinase pathway activity. Br J Cancer. 2015;112(3):504–13.

61. Pereira NP, Curi C, Osorio C, Marques EF, Makdissi FB, Pinker K, et al. Diffusion-weighted magnetic resonance imaging of patients with breast cancer following neoadjuvant chemotherapy provides early prediction of pathological response - a prospective study. Sci Rep. 2019;9(1):16372.

62. Tang L, Li J, Li ZY, Li XT, Gong JF, Ji JF, et al. MRI in predicting the response of gastrointestinal stromal tumor to targeted therapy: a patient-based multi-parameter study. BMC Cancer. 2018;18(1):811.

63. Moestue SA, Huuse EM, Lindholm EM, Bofin A, Engebraaten O, Maelandsmo GM, et al. Low-molecular contrast agent dynamic contrast-enhanced (DCE)-MRI and diffusion-weighted (DW)-MRI in early assessment of bevacizumab treatment in breast cancer xenografts. J Magn Reson Imaging. 2013;38(5):1043–53.

64. Matikas A, Souglakos J, Katsaounis P, Kotsakis A, Kouroupakis P, Pantazopoulos N, et al. MINOAS: a single-arm translational phase II trial of FOLFIRI plus Aflibercept as first-line therapy in unresectable, metastatic colorectal cancer. Target Oncol. 2019;14(3):285–93.

65. Liu L, Wu N, Ouyang H, Dai JR, Wang WH. Diffusion-weighted MRI in early assessment of tumour response to radiotherapy in high-risk prostate cancer. Br J Radiol. 2014;87(1043):20140359.

66. Philippe J, Jochen F, Mathias S, Gunther S, Christian R, Arno B, et al. Diffusion-weighted MRI improves response assessment after definitive radiotherapy in patients with NSCLC. Cancer Imaging. 2021;21(1):15.

67. Bonekamp S, Corona-Villalobos CP, Kamel IR. Oncologic applications of diffusion-weighted MRI in the body. J Magn Reson Imaging. 2012;35(2):257–79.

68. Provenzano PP, Inman DR, Eliceiri KW, Knittel JG, Yan L, Rueden CT, et al. Collagen density promotes mammary tumor initiation and progression. BMC Med. 2008;6:11.

69. Ko ES, Han BK, Kim RB, Cho EY, Ahn S, Nam SJ, et al. Apparent diffusion coefficient in estrogen receptor-positive invasive ductal breast carcinoma: correlations with tumor-stroma ratio. Radiology. 2014;271(1):30–7.

70. Egnell L, Vidic I, Jerome NP, Bofin AM, Bathen TF, Goa PE. Stromal collagen content in breast tumors correlates with in vivo diffusion-weighted imaging: a comparison of multi b-value DWI with histologic specimen from benign and malignant breast lesions. J Magn Reson Imaging. 2020;51(6):1868–78.

71. Kobus T, van der Laak JA, Maas MC, Hambrock T, Bruggink CC, Hulsbergen-van de Kaa CA, et al. Contribution of histopathologic tissue composition to quantitative MR spectroscopy and diffusion-weighted imaging of the prostate. Radiology. 2015;142889

72. Basser PJ, Mattiello J, LeBihan D. MR diffusion tensor spectroscopy and imaging. Biophys J. 1994;66(1):259–67.

73. Nissan N, Furman-Haran E, Feinberg-Shapiro M, Grobgeld D, Eyal E, Zehavi T, et al. Tracking the mammary architectural features and detecting breast cancer with magnetic resonance diffusion tensor imaging. J Vis Exp. 2014;94

74. Luo J, Hippe DS, Rahbar H, Parsian S, Rendi MH, Partridge SC. Diffusion tensor imaging for characterizing tumor microstructure and improving diagnostic performance on breast MRI: a prospective observational study. Breast Cancer Res. 2019;21(1):102.

75. Furman-Haran E, Nissan N, Ricart-Selma V, Martinez-Rubio C, Degani H, Camps-Herrero J. Quantitative evaluation of breast cancer response to neoadjuvant chemotherapy by diffusion tensor imaging: initial results. J Magn Reson Imaging. 2018;47(4):1080–90.

76. Kakkad SM, Zhang J, Akhbardeh A, Jacob D, Solaiyappan M, Jacobs MA, et al., editors. In vivo and ex vivo diffusion tensor imaging parameters follow Collagen 1 fiber distribution in breast cancer xenograft model. Proc Intl Soc Magn Reson Med; 2015; Toronto, Ontario, Canada.

77. Le Bihan D. Intravoxel incoherent motion imaging using steady-state free precession. Magn Reson Med. 1988;7(3):346–51.

78. Mannelli L, Nougaret S, Vargas HA, Do RK. Advances in diffusion-weighted imaging. Radiol Clin N Am. 2015;53(3):569–81.

79. Gaeta M, Benedetto C, Minutoli F, D'Angelo T, Amato E, Mazziotti S, et al. Use of diffusion-weighted, intravoxel incoherent motion, and dynamic contrast-enhanced MR imaging in the assessment of response to radiotherapy of lytic bone metastases from breast cancer. Acad Radiol. 2014;21(10):1286–93.

80. Song T, Yao Q, Qu J, Zhang H, Zhao Y, Qin J, et al. The value of intravoxel incoherent motion diffusion-weighted imaging in predicting the pathologic response to neoadjuvant chemotherapy in locally advanced esophageal squamous cell carcinoma. Eur Radiol 2020.

81. Zhang H, Li W, Fu C, Grimm R, Chen Z, Zhang W, et al. Comparison of intravoxel incoherent motion imaging, diffusion kurtosis imaging, and conventional DWI in predicting the chemotherapeutic response of colorectal liver metastases. Eur J Radiol. 2020;130:109149.

82. Baidya Kayal E, Kandasamy D, Khare K, Bakhshi S, Sharma R, Mehndiratta A. Intravoxel incoherent motion (IVIM) for response assessment in patients with osteosarcoma undergoing neoadjuvant chemotherapy. Eur J Radiol. 2019;119:108635.

83. Cho GY, Gennaro L, Sutton EJ, Zabor EC, Zhang Z, Giri D, et al. Intravoxel incoherent motion (IVIM) histogram biomarkers for prediction of neoadjuvant treatment response in breast cancer patients. Eur J Radiol Open. 2017;4:101–7.

84. Kim Y, Kim SH, Lee HW, Song BJ, Kang BJ, Lee A, et al. Intravoxel incoherent motion diffusion-weighted MRI for predicting response to neoadjuvant chemotherapy in breast cancer. Magn Reson Imaging. 2018;48:27–33.

85. Li H, El Naqa I, Rong Y. Current status of Radiomics for cancer management: challenges versus opportunities for clinical practice. J Appl Clin Med Phys. 2020;21(7):7–10.

86. Vidic I, Egnell L, Jerome NP, Teruel JR, Sjobakk TE, Ostlie A, et al. Support vector machine for breast cancer classification using diffusion-weighted MRI histogram features: preliminary study. J Magn Reson Imaging. 2018;47(5):1205–16.

87. Jian J, Li Y, Pickhardt PJ, Xia W, He Z, Zhang R, et al. MR image-based radiomics to differentiate type iota and type IotaIota epithelial ovarian cancers. Eur Radiol. 2021;31(1):403–10.

88. Padhani AR, Liu G, Koh DM, Chenevert TL, Thoeny HC, Takahara T, et al. Diffusion-weighted magnetic resonance imaging as a cancer biomarker: consensus and recommendations. Neoplasia. 2009;11(2):102–25.

89. Doblas S, Almeida GS, Ble FX, Garteiser P, Hoff BA, McIntyre DJ, et al. Apparent diffusion coefficient is highly reproducible on preclinical imaging systems: evidence from a seven-center multivendor study. J Magn Reson Imaging 2015;42(6):1759–64.

90. Dang CV, Semenza GL. Oncogenic alterations of metabolism. Trends Biochem Sci. 1999;24(2):68–72.

91. Phan LM, Yeung SC, Lee MH. Cancer metabolic reprogramming: importance, main features, and potentials for precise targeted anticancer therapies. Cancer Biol Med. 2014;11(1):1–19.

92. Hanahan D, Weinberg RA. Hallmarks of cancer: the next generation. Cell. 2011;144(5):646–74.

93. Mankoff DA, Farwell MD, Clark AS, Pryma DA. Making molecular imaging a clinical tool for precision oncology: a review. JAMA Oncol. 2017;3(5):695–701.

94. Sun C, Li T, Song X, Huang L, Zang Q, Xu J, et al. Spatially resolved metabolomics to discover tumor-associated metabolic alterations. Proc Natl Acad Sci U S A. 2019;116(1):52–7.

95. Woitek R, McLean MA, Gill AB, Grist JT, Provenzano E, Patterson AJ, et al. Hyperpolarized (13)C MRI of tumor metabolism demonstrates early metabolic response to neoadjuvant chemotherapy in breast cancer. Radiol Imaging Cancer. 2020;2(4):e200017.

96. Griffin JL, Shockcor JP. Metabolic profiles of cancer cells. Nat Rev Cancer. 2004;4(7):551–61.

97. Bathen TF, Sitter B, Sjobakk TE, Tessem MB, Gribbestad IS. Magnetic resonance metabolomics of intact tissue: a biotechnological tool in cancer diagnostics and treatment evaluation. Cancer Res. 2010;70(17):6692–6.

98. Warburg O. On respiratory impairment in cancer cells. Science. 1956;124(3215):269–70.

99. Le A, Cooper CR, Gouw AM, Dinavahi R, Maitra A, Deck LM, et al. Inhibition of lactate dehydrogenase a induces oxidative stress and inhibits tumor progression. Proc Natl Acad Sci U S A. 2010;107(5):2037–42.

100. Glunde K, Bhujwalla ZM, Ronen SM. Choline metabolism in malignant transformation. Nat Rev Cancer. 2011;11(12):835–48.

101. Ren J, Malloy CR, Sherry AD. Quantitative measurement of redox state in human brain by (31) P MRS at 7T with spectral simplification and inclusion of multiple nucleotide sugar components in data analysis. Magn Reson Med. 2020;84(5):2338–51.

102. Ardenkjaer-Larsen JH, Fridlund B, Gram A, Hansson G, Hansson L, Lerche MH, et al. Increase in signal-to-noise ratio of > 10,000 times in liquid-state NMR. Proc Natl Acad Sci U S A. 2003;100(18):10158–63.

103. Day SE, Kettunen MI, Gallagher FA, Hu DE, Lerche M, Wolber J, et al. Detecting tumor response to treatment using hyperpolarized 13C magnetic resonance imaging and spectroscopy. Nat Med. 2007;13(11):1382–7.

104. Ward CS, Venkatesh HS, Chaumeil MM, Brandes AH, Vancriekinge M, Dafni H, et al. Noninvasive detection of target modulation following phosphatidylinositol 3-kinase inhibition using hyperpolarized 13C magnetic resonance spectroscopy. Cancer Res. 2010;70(4):1296–305.

105. Gallagher FA, Woitek R, McLean MA, Gill AB, Manzano Garcia R, Provenzano E, et al. Imaging breast cancer using hyperpolarized carbon-13 MRI. Proc Natl Acad Sci U S A. 2020;117(4):2092–8.

106. Gallagher FA, Kettunen MI, Hu DE, Jensen PR, Zandt RI, Karlsson M, et al. Production of hyperpolarized [1,4-13C2] malate from [1,4-13C2]fumarate is a marker of cell necrosis and treatment response in tumors. Proc Natl Acad Sci U S A. 2009;106(47):19801–6.

107. Bohndiek SE, Kettunen MI, Hu DE, Witney TH, Kennedy BW, Gallagher FA, et al. Detection of tumor response to a vascular disrupting agent by hyperpolarized 13C magnetic resonance spectroscopy. Mol Cancer Ther. 2010;9(12):3278–88.

108. Plathow C, Weber WA. Tumor cell metabolism imaging. J Nucl Med. 2008;49(Suppl 2):43S–63S.

109. Testa C, Schiavina R, Lodi R, Salizzoni E, Corti B, Farsad M, et al. Prostate cancer: sextant localization with MR imaging, MR spectroscopy, and 11C-choline PET/CT. Radiology. 2007;244(3):797–806.

110. Tozaki M, Hoshi K. 1H MR spectroscopy of invasive ductal carcinoma: correlations with FDG PET and histologic prognostic factors. AJR Am J Roentgenol. 2010;194(5):1384–90.

111. Gutte H, Hansen AE, Henriksen ST, Johannesen HH, Ardenkjaer-Larsen J, Vignaud A, et al. Simultaneous hyperpolarized (13) C-pyruvate MRI and (18)F-FDG-PET in cancer (hyperPET): feasibility of a new imaging concept using a clinical PET/MRI scanner. Am J Nucl Med Mol Imaging. 2015;5(1):38–45.

112. Esmaeili M, Tayari N, Scheenen T, Elschot M, Sandsmark E, Bertilsson H, et al. Simultaneous (18)F-fluciclovine positron emission tomography and magnetic resonance spectroscopic imaging of prostate cancer. Front Oncol. 2018;8:516.

113. Gutte H, Hansen AE, Larsen M, Rahbek S, Henriksen S, Johannesen H, et al. Simultaneous hyperpolarized 13C-pyruvate MRI and 18F-FDG-PET (hyperPET) in 10 canine cancer patients. J Nucl Med 2015;56(11):1786–92

114. Semenza GL. Defining the role of hypoxia-inducible factor 1 in cancer biology and therapeutics. Oncogene. 2010;29(5):625–34.

115. Thomlinson RH, Gray LH. The histological structure of some human lung cancers and the possible implications for radiotherapy. Br J Cancer. 1955;9(4):539–49.

116. Ragnum HB, Vlatkovic L, Lie AK, Axcrona K, Julin CH, Frikstad KM, et al. The tumour hypoxia marker pimonidazole reflects a transcriptional programme associated with aggressive prostate cancer. Br J Cancer. 2015;112(2):382–90.

117. Rofstad EK, Galappathi K, Mathiesen B, Ruud EB. Fluctuating and diffusion-limited hypoxia in hypoxia-induced metastasis. Clin Cancer Res. 2007;13(7):1971–8.

118. Semenza GL. The hypoxic tumor microenvironment: a driving force for breast cancer progression. Biochim Biophys Acta 2015.

119. Ellingsen C, Hompland T, Galappathi K, Mathiesen B, Rofstad EK. DCE-MRI of the hypoxic fraction, radioresponsiveness, and metastatic propensity of cervical carcinoma xenografts. Radiother Oncol. 2014;110(2):335–41.

120. Huuse EM, Moestue SA, Lindholm EM, Bathen TF, Nalwoga H, Kruger K, et al. In vivo MRI and histopathological assessment of tumor microenvironment in luminal-like and basal-like breast cancer xenografts. J Magn Reson Imaging. 2012;35(5):1098–107.

121. Ovrebo KM, Hompland T, Mathiesen B, Rofstad EK. Assessment of hypoxia and radiation response in intramuscular experimental tumors by dynamic contrast-enhanced magnetic resonance imaging. Radiother Oncol. 2012;102(3):429–35.

122. Stubbs M, Robinson SP, Rodrigues LM, Parkins CS, Collingridge DR, Griffiths JR. The effects of host carbogen (95% oxygen/5% carbon dioxide) breathing on metabolic characteristics of Morris hepatoma 9618a. Br J Cancer. 1998;78(11):1449–56.

123. Baudelet C, Gallez B. How does blood oxygen level-dependent (BOLD) contrast correlate with oxygen partial pressure (pO2) inside tumors? Magn Reson Med. 2002;48(6):980–6.

124. McPhail LD, Robinson SP. Intrinsic susceptibility MR imaging of chemically induced rat mammary tumors: relationship to histologic assessment of hypoxia and fibrosis. Radiology. 2010;254(1):110–8.

125. Burrell JS, Walker-Samuel S, Baker LC, Boult JK, Jamin Y, Halliday J, et al. Exploring DeltaR(2) * and DeltaR(1) as imaging biomarkers of tumor oxygenation. J Magn Reson Imaging. 2013;38(2):429–34.

126. O'Connor JPB, Robinson SP, Waterton JC. Imaging tumour hypoxia with oxygen-enhanced MRI and BOLD MRI. Br J Radiol. 2019;92(1095):20180642.

127. Gross MW, Karbach U, Groebe K, Franko AJ, Mueller-Klieser W. Calibration of misonidazole labeling by simultaneous measurement of oxygen tension and labeling density in multicellular spheroids. Int J Cancer. 1995;61(4):567–73.

128. Raleigh JA, Chou SC, Bono EL, Thrall DE, Varia MA. Semiquantitative immunohistochemical analysis for hypoxia in human tumors. Int J Radiat Oncol Biol Phys. 2001;49(2):569–74.

129. Lee CP, Payne GS, Oregioni A, Ruddle R, Tan S, Raynaud FI, et al. A phase I study of the nitroimidazole hypoxia marker SR4554 using 19F magnetic resonance spectroscopy. Br J Cancer. 2009;101(11):1860–8.

130. Gulaka PK, Rojas-Quijano F, Kovacs Z, Mason RP, Sherry AD, Kodibagkar VD. GdDO3NI, a nitroimidazole-based T1 MRI contrast agent for imaging tumor hypoxia in vivo. J Biol Inorg Chem. 2014;19(2):271–9.

131. Okamoto S, Shiga T, Yasuda K, Ito YM, Magota K, Kasai K, et al. High reproducibility of tumor hypoxia evaluated by 18F-fluoromisonidazole PET for head and neck cancer. J Nucl Med. 2013;54(2):201–7.

132. Rasey JS, Koh WJ, Evans ML, Peterson LM, Lewellen TK, Graham MM, et al. Quantifying regional hypoxia in human tumors with positron emission tomography of [18F]fluoromisonidazole: a pretherapy study of 37 patients. Int J Radiat Oncol Biol Phys. 1996;36(2):417–28.

133. Kikuchi M, Yamane T, Shinohara S, Fujiwara K, Hori SY, Tona Y, et al. 18F-fluoromisonidazole positron emission tomography before treatment is a predictor of radiotherapy outcome and survival prognosis in patients with head and neck squamous cell carcinoma. Ann Nucl Med. 2011;25(9):625–33.

134. Rischin D, Hicks RJ, Fisher R, Binns D, Corry J, Porceddu S, et al. Prognostic significance of [18F]-misonidazole positron emission tomography-detected tumor hypoxia in patients with advanced head and neck cancer randomly assigned to chemoradiation with

or without tirapazamine: a substudy of trans-Tasman radiation oncology group study 98.02. J Clin Oncol. 2006;24(13):2098–104.

135. Souvatzoglou M, Grosu AL, Roper B, Krause BJ, Beck R, Reischl G, et al. Tumour hypoxia imaging with [18F]FAZA PET in head and neck cancer patients: a pilot study. Eur J Nucl Med Mol Imaging. 2007;34(10):1566–75.

136. Sakso M, Mortensen LS, Primdahl H, Johansen J, Kallehauge J, Hansen CR, et al. Influence of FAZA PET hypoxia and HPV-status for the outcome of head and neck squamous cell carcinoma (HNSCC) treated with radiotherapy: long-term results from the DAHANCA 24 trial (NCT01017224). Radiother Oncol. 2020;151:126–33.

137. Capitanio U, Pepe G, Incerti E, Larcher A, Trevisani F, Luciano R, et al. The role of 18F-FAZA PET/CT in detecting lymph node metastases in renal cell carcinoma patients: a prospective pilot trial. Eur J Nucl Med Mol Imaging 2020.

138. Estrella V, Chen T, Lloyd M, Wojtkowiak J, Cornnell HH, Ibrahim-Hashim A, et al. Acidity generated by the tumor microenvironment drives local invasion. Cancer Res. 2013;73(5):1524–35.

139. Stubbs M, McSheehy PM, Griffiths JR, Bashford CL. Causes and consequences of tumour acidity and implications for treatment. Mol Med Today. 2000;6(1):15–9.

140. Fukumura D, Jain RK. Tumor microenvironment abnormalities: causes, consequences, and strategies to normalize. J Cell Biochem. 2007;101(4):937–49.

141. Gillies RJ, Robey I, Gatenby RA. Causes and consequences of increased glucose metabolism of cancers. J Nucl Med. 2008;49(Suppl 2):24S–42S.

142. Liu J, Huang Y, Kumar A, Tan A, Jin S, Mozhi A, et al. pH-sensitive nano-systems for drug delivery in cancer therapy. Biotechnol Adv. 2014;32(4):693–710.

143. Wang L, Zhu X, Xie C, Ding N, Weng X, Lu W, et al. Imaging acidosis in tumors using a pH-activated near-infrared fluorescence probe. Chem Commun (Camb). 2012;48(95):11677–9.

144. Hashim AI, Zhang X, Wojtkowiak JW, Martinez GV, Gillies RJ. Imaging pH and metastasis. NMR Biomed. 2011;24(6):582–91.

145. Gillies RJ, Raghunand N, Garcia-Martin ML, Gatenby RA. pH imaging. A review of pH measurement methods and applications in cancers. IEEE Eng Med Biol Mag. 2004;23(5):57–64.

146. Soto GE, Zhu Z, Evelhoch JL, Ackerman JJ. Tumor 31P NMR pH measurements in vivo: a comparison of inorganic phosphate and intracellular 2-deoxyglucose-6-phosphate as pHnmr indicators in murine radiation-induced fibrosarcoma-1. Magn Reson Med. 1996;36(5):698–704.

147. Garcia-Martin ML, Herigault G, Remy C, Farion R, Ballesteros P, Coles JA, et al. Mapping extracellular pH in rat brain gliomas in vivo by 1H magnetic resonance spectroscopic imaging: comparison with maps of metabolites. Cancer Res. 2001;61(17):6524–31.

148. Provent P, Benito M, Hiba B, Farion R, Lopez-Larrubia P, Ballesteros P, et al. Serial in vivo spectroscopic nuclear magnetic resonance imaging of lactate and extracellular pH in rat gliomas shows redistribution of protons away from sites of glycolysis. Cancer Res. 2007;67(16):7638–45.

149. Liu G, Li Y, Sheth VR, Pagel MD. Imaging in vivo extracellular pH with a single paramagnetic chemical exchange saturation transfer magnetic resonance imaging contrast agent. Mol Imaging. 2012;11(1):47–57.

150. Chen LQ, Howison CM, Jeffery JJ, Robey IF, Kuo PH, Pagel MD. Evaluations of extracellular pH within in vivo tumors using acidoCEST MRI. Magn Reson Med. 2014;72(5):1408–17.

151. Jones KM, Randtke EA, Yoshimaru ES, Howison CM, Chalasani P, Klein RR, et al. Clinical translation of tumor acidosis measurements with AcidoCEST MRI. Mol Imaging Biol. 2017;19(4):617–25.

152. High RA, Randtke EA, Jones KM, Lindeman LR, Ma JC, Zhang S, et al. Extracellular acidosis differentiates pancreatitis and pancreatic cancer in mouse models using acidoCEST MRI. Neoplasia. 2019;21(11):1085–90.

153. Akhenblit PJ, Hanke NT, Gill A, Persky DO, Howison CM, Pagel MD, et al. Assessing metabolic changes in response to mTOR inhibition in a mantle cell lymphoma xenograft model using AcidoCEST MRI. Mol Imaging 2016;15.

154. Gallagher FA, Kettunen MI, Day SE, Hu DE, Ardenkjaer-Larsen JH, Zandt R, et al. Magnetic resonance imaging of pH in vivo using hyperpolarized 13C-labelled bicarbonate. Nature. 2008;453(7197):940–3.

155. Bergamaschi A, Hjortland GO, Triulzi T, Sorlie T, Johnsen H, Ree AH, et al. Molecular profiling and characterization of luminal-like and basal-like in vivo breast cancer xenograft models. Mol Oncol. 2009;3(5–6):469–82.

156. Bergamaschi A, Tagliabue E, Sorlie T, Naume B, Triulzi T, Orlandi R, et al. Extracellular matrix signature identifies breast cancer subgroups with different clinical outcome. J Pathol. 2008;214(3):357–67.

The Influence of Tissue Architecture on Drug Response: Anticancer Drug Development in High-Dimensional Combinatorial Microenvironment Platforms

Tiina A. Jokela, Eric G. Carlson, and Mark A. LaBarge

Abstract

Predicting how anticancer therapeutics will function in people based on preclinical studies remains a significant challenge. High rates of phase II clinical trial failures indicate that many candidate therapeutics that pass preclinical studies lack efficacy in patients. The discovery of oncogenes and tumor suppressors has led to vast investments into developing technologies that enable exploration of the total complexity of genomes and proteomes intrinsic to cells. These technologies seek to define how mutations contribute to cancer development and progression. An important and unexpected outcome of those massive investments to understand cancer as a cell-intrinsic problem is the undeniable conclusion that mutations do not explain everything. Indeed, the fact that frankly malignant cells can be phenotypically normal, when exposed to a normal tissue microenvironment (ME), suggests that there is a dominant role of the ME. Tumor microenvironments modulate the malignant phenotypes of cells and impact drug responses. In most drug screens, conventional two-dimensional plastic dishes are the substrate of choice for cell culture and rodents are used as the primary in vivo model, but these modalities lack context in a way that is relevant to predicting drug activity. Alternatively, combinatorial microenvironment microarray platforms provide a high-throughput means of exploring cell-based functional responses in diverse microenvironmental milieus. Data from these techniques are single-cell resolution and encapsulate cell–cell heterogeneity, which provides direct linkages between cellular phenotypes, such as drug responses, and MEs. This chapter focuses on the applications and analytic approaches used for functional cell-based exploration of combinatorial MEs using microarray technology.

T. A. Jokela
Department of Population Sciences, Beckman Research Institute, Duarte, CA, USA

The Faculty of Sport and Health Sciences, University of Jyväskylä, Finland, Jyväskylä, Finland
e-mail: Tiina.a.jokela@jyu.fi

E. G. Carlson
Department of Population Sciences, Beckman Research Institute, Duarte, CA, USA

Irell and Manella Graduate School of Biological Sciences, Duarte, CA, USA
e-mail: ecarlson@coh.org

M. A. LaBarge (✉)
Department of Population Sciences, Beckman Research Institute, Duarte, CA, USA

Center for Cancer and Aging Research, City of Hope, Duarte, CA, USA

Center for Cancer Biomarkers Research (CCBIO), University of Norway, Bergen, Norway
e-mail: mlabarge@coh.org

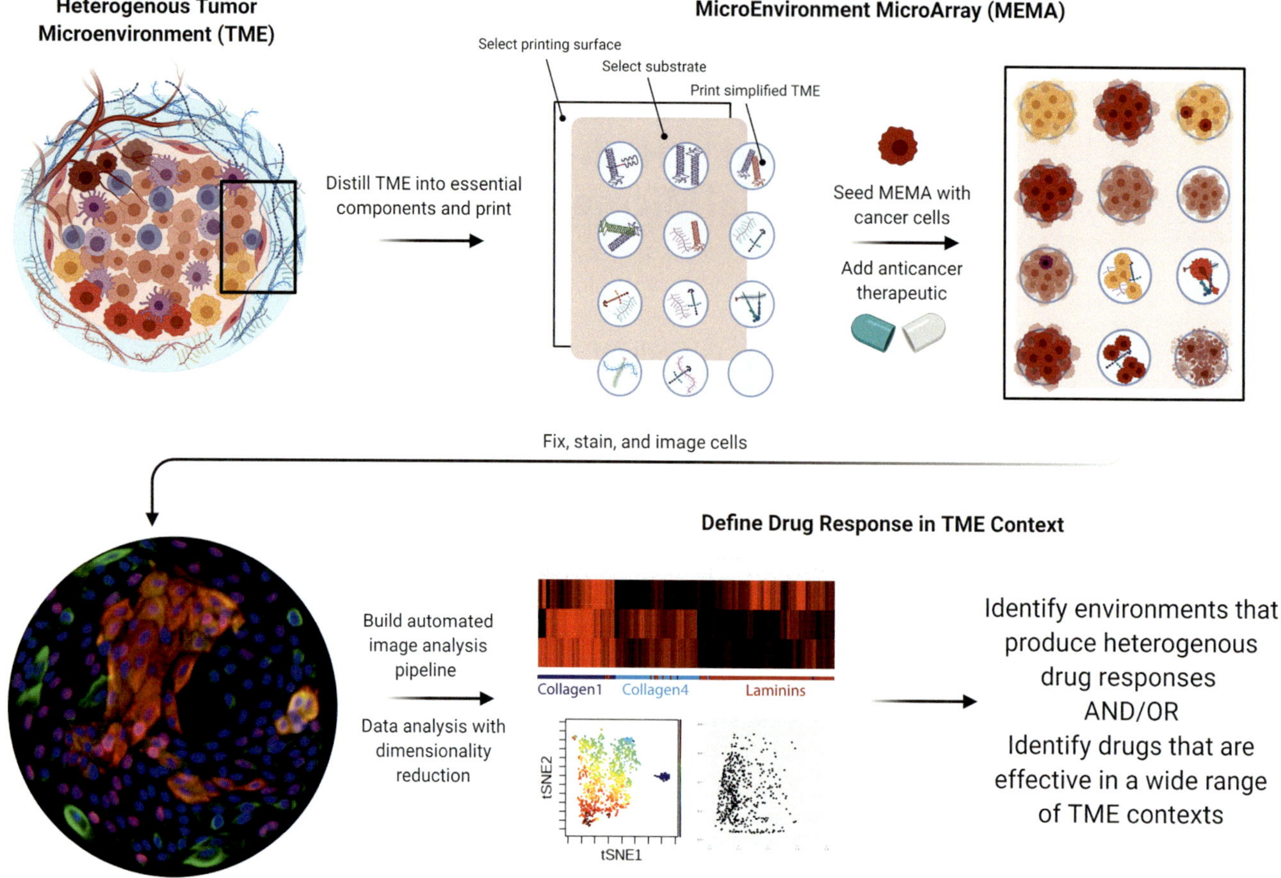

Functional dissection of a tumor microenvironment. A microarray printer deposits combinations of TME-relevant components on a printing substrate that best mimics the in vivo microenvironment being studied. After relevant cancer cells are seeded on the simplified, printed TMEs, anticancer therapeutics are added to culture. Following culture, cells are fixed, stained, and imaged leading to the acquisition of high-dimensional, single-cell data.

Take-Home Lessons

- Tumor microenvironments have dominant effects on cellular phenotypes and can impact anticancer drug responses but are often ignored during drug development.
- MicroEnvironment MicroArrays (MEMAs) are functional, cell-based, high-throughput platforms to study cancer cell phenotypes and functions in combinatorial microenvironments.
- MEMAs provide a fast and cost-effective in vitro platform to predict microenvironment components that will modify anticancer drug performance.
- MEMA experiments produce high-dimensional, single-cell datasets that necessitate optimized automated workflows for ease of analysis.
- Quality control and data analysis may benefit greatly from the application of both traditional machine learning and convolutional neural network algorithms.

The Challenge of Predicting Efficacy

In anticancer drug development, a suboptimal ability to predict how therapeutics will perform in humans based on preclinical drug screening often delays the progress of drug discovery. In the last few decades, tremendous resources have been invested into translating preclinical anticancer therapeutics to drugs used clinically. From 2000 to 2015, the probability of success for a new anticancer therapeutic to gain FDA approval was 3.4% [1], which has allowed manufacturers to justify skyrocketing drug prices [2].

Advancements in cell and molecular biology, as well as engineering, have ushered in the modern era of pharmacology. In this era, new therapeutics with potentially selective activity against tumors are identified by using cell-based high-throughput screenings, and then the efficacy of the selected therapeutics is further validated in animal model systems, with rodents being the most popular mammalian system. Increased knowledge about the molecular underpinnings of tumor biology has accelerated the development of novel therapeutics over the past two decades. For instance, the Cancer Genome Atlas program has identified a broad range of recurrent gene mutations and structural rearrangements that putatively drive tumorigenesis. A number of drugs have been selected to target protein changes resulting from those specific genetic mutations, but while a number of candidates show promising effects in small animals, they have had much less success in patients [3]. Almost 70% of new cancer drugs exhibit no efficacy in phase II despite meeting safety standards established in phase I trials [1]. Several potential explanations for why anticancer therapeutics fail at such high rates are the significant differences in expressed genomes of mice and men [4], as well as the significant differences that arise at the level of physiology and tissue architecture that can impact drug responses [5, 6].

The tumor microenvironment (TME), i.e., the sum of cell–cell, cell-extracellular matrix (ECM), cell-soluble factor interactions, and the physical properties and geometry of the tumor, has been shown to impact cancer progression, drug responses, and many other tumor properties [7, 8]. Thus, it is important to identify preclinical screening modalities that take microenvironment (ME) into account. Implementation of techniques that are more reflective of the relevant biology in human tissues may provide more predictable outcomes in cancer drug development.

Tumors Are Heterogenous "Organs" and Tumor Microenvironments Are Important Determinants in Therapeutic Responses

Innate inter- and intra-tumor heterogeneity is thought to be a major contributor to acquisition of drug resistance. Tumors rarely are homogenous expansions of neoplastic cells and may be better framed as abnormal "organs" with multiple cell types and dynamic microenvironmental ecologies [9]. These organs interact with the body via unique vascular systems and changes to immune homeostasis that together contribute to hampered immunosurveillance as well as dampened efficacy of cancer treatments [10]. ECM, growth factors, cytokines, mechanical stress, and oxygen tension construct combinatorial and dynamic TMEs, which contribute to control the malignant progression, metastasis, and drug responses of cancer [8, 11–15].

The cancer stem cell (CSC) hypothesis offers attractive explanations for generation of heterogeneity within tumors, metastatic dissemination, and resistance to therapy. The underlying logic is modeled on normal developmental hierarchies that are delineated for several adult tissues. Undifferentiated stem cells give rise to less potent progenitors, which produce the most specialized cells of a given tissue. Analogously, only CSCs are thought capable of

self-renewal, of initiating tumors at primary and distant locations, and of giving rise to more differentiated daughters that are less capable of reestablishing the tumor. Normal stem cell activity is maintained in niches; therefore, employing the same logic used for developmental hierarchies, niches that maintain CSCs, should also exist [16–18]. Niches are specialized MEs wherein stem cells reside (reviewed in [19, 20]), which exert control over cell function. Niches are immensely instructive, as progenitors in both skin and skeletal muscle can adopt residency in vacated stem cell niches, where they reacquire stem cell traits [21–23]. Impressively, testicular and neural stem cells from male mice were shown to give rise to lactating mammary glands when transplanted into the mammary fat pads of female mice [24, 25]. And in true reductionist models that used defined ME components, embryonic and adult stem and progenitor cell fate decisions were shown to be quantifiably flexible in response to combinatorial MEs [26–29].

The ability of the niche to determine the functional spectrum of stem cell activities led us to hypothesize that stem cell niches beget stem cell functions [30, 31]. Due to their role in maintaining stem cell activity, disrupting CSC-niche interactions may be crucial for overcoming barriers to therapeutic resistance [32]. In fact, putative components of the CSC niche that increase drug tolerance in malignant breast cancer cells have been identified using combinatorial microenvironment microarrays (MEMAs, formerly known as MEarrays) [33]. Thus, understanding the interactions between TMEs and cancer cells is important for the identification of druggable mechanisms (e.g., proliferation, differentiation, and quiescence) that may improve drug efficacy in humans.

Deconstructing Tumor Microenvironments into Experimentally Tractable Combinations

Tissues are collections of cells and ECM knit together into unique spatial configurations that cooperatively carry out specialized functions. Remarkably, tissue with an intact architecture can maintain many basic functions despite the presence of gene mutations that cause dysfunctions when introduced into cells cultured on tissue culture plastic (TCP) [34]. Disrupted MEs can unleash the malignant potential of transformed cells, which further demonstrates the principle that tissue architecture and composition confers normal function in the face of cell-intrinsic perturbations [35]. Organized asymmetry is therefore an important basic feature of metazoan tissues; there must be distinctive topologies on which receptors assemble to correctly integrate the signaling patterns associated with tissue-specific functions. TMEs should as well possess combinatorial signaling asymmetries, though the MEs may be less obviously organized. One hypothesis is that the normal and tumor MEs integrate the signaling apparatuses differently. Accordingly, therapeutic targets could be identified to selectively harm the tumor cells, with ME composition functioning as a determinant of drug efficacy. Those potential differences in signal integration can be revealed by technologies that recapitulate aspects of in vivo MEs, using defined physical, geometric, and molecular elements. This allows one to assess the contribution of each attribute of the ME to emergent properties of tissues.

The complexity of MEs is a major impediment to understanding their impact on cells. A majority of our understanding of biological mechanisms in human cells has been built upon studies using two-dimensional (2D) plastic plates or dishes. Since the first human cell line, HeLa, was established on cell culture dishes, 2D cell culture has been a mainstay of biological research. However, as the dominant nature of the ME over physiological processes has become increasingly appreciated, engineered 2D and three-dimensional (3D) culture platforms that better recapitulate the molecular and physical nuances of tissues in vivo are being developed.

It is an oversimplification to distinguish 2D and 3D culture platforms based on dimensionality. The details of the culture MEs need to be considered with care to understand how each definable property affects cell physiology. Although 2D TCP has been used extensively for biological research, it does not offer an accurate physiological representation of tissues. In addition to the synthetic polymer composition of the plastic, cells in conventional 2D culture systems adhere to surfaces that are nonphysiologically rigid (elastic modulus of >2 Gigapascals (GPa)) as opposed to the rigidity of normal tissue (hundreds of Pa in soft tissue to tens of thousands of Pa for stiffer tissues like cartilage and bone) [36, 37]. As the importance of ME in therapeutic response has become better understood, and more widely accepted, the urgency to identify tractable organotypic culture systems for studying human tissues in vitro has manifested. Matrigel, HuBiogel, and other commercially available laminin-rich ECM are widely used to provide 3D cell growth environments. These gels are used increasingly to study the impact of drugs on cells grown in 3D and have allowed for adoption of 3D culture to high-throughput systems where the rate-limiting steps are quality imaging and analysis [38]. Biopolymers used for 3D culture systems better mimic tissue than plastic as Matrigel has an elastic modulus between 400 Pa and 1 kPa and collagen gels can range from 500 Pa to >12 kPa depending on collagen concentration and attachment to the culture vessel. Matrigel, which is harvested from a rodent sarcoma cell line, is comprised of hundreds of proteins that can vary significantly in their exact composition and properties between production lots [39–41]. While Matrigel has made 3D high-throughput systems less daunting, placing human cells in an undefined rodent sarcoma 3D context may not mimic the intended in vivo ME, and variability in the molecular components may confound interpretations and reproducibility of the results. Synthetic 3D culture hydrogels, such as polyethylene glycol-based systems, offer precision tunability of the elastic modulus, which covers a range similar to collagen gels while allowing for greater control over molecular composition [42].

Every in vitro system for studying tissue ME sacrifices important aspects of the in vivo situation, but there is merit in studying microenvironmental properties in isolation. Although engineered and biopolymer-derived systems necessarily oversimplify TMEs, they can reveal important mechanistic elements of cellular responses by winnowing down the possible candidate pathways involved in a given functional response. The ME can be dissected into biophysical (e.g., rigidity, shear force), biochemical (e.g., ECM, growth factors, cytokines), and architectural (e.g., dimension and geometry) properties, and each property plays a role in regulating various cellular functions. For instance, by examining normal mammary epithelial cells in the context of matrix rigidity, in isolation from many other ME properties, we discovered age-dependent regulation of the mechano-transducing YAP and TAZ transcription factors [43]. Similarly, by using engineered polymer surfaces, we showed that substrate rigidity is a determinant for HER2-targeted therapeutic efficacy via YAP and TAZ signaling, both in vitro and in vivo [44]. In vitro screens of thousands of MEs comprised of unique combinations of ECM, growth factors, and cytokines revealed combinations that induced expression of CSC markers in malignant breast cancer cells that in turn led to increased resistance to chemotherapeutics [33]. In addition to rigidity and composition of the MEs being major determinants of cell fate, it has been found that shape and geometry contribute to producing diverse cellular responses [45, 46]. Kilian et al. found that similar shapes with pentagonal symmetry, but slightly different subcellular curvature, could bias differentiation of human mesenchymal stem cells toward either osteoblasts or adipocytes [45]. As MEs are deconstructed and different properties are studied individually or in defined combinations, the knowledge that we accrue over time allows us to form a portrait that models, and possibly explains, ME effects on cellular functions.

Combinatorial Microenvironment Platforms Mimic Diverse and Defined Milieus and Allow for High-Throughput Experimentation

Established human cell lines and primary cells propagated in 2D culture are amenable to high-throughput experimentation. Potentially powerful tools for performing cancer drug design in TME contexts are being developed by merging the flexibility of functional cell-based screening with the highly parallel nature of microarray-type experiments. A microarray is a tool that contains thousands of functionalized probes immobilized on a substrate. These tools provide both complexity and scalability and are used to explore diversity in various biological systems. Broadly speaking, the microarray technology can be classified into protein arrays, gene chips, or carbohydrate microarrays, depending upon what probes are immobilized on the substrate [47–49]. An interesting innovation in this technology space has been to fabricate microarrays in 2D and 3D contexts, printing substratum that supports adhesion of cultured cells. These types of combinatorial MEMAs facilitate highly parallel cell-based functional screening. Indeed, using different ECM, soluble ligands, and pathway-blocking or pathway-activating antibodies in various combinations as printed probes enables molecular dissection of complicated MEs and TMEs [26–29, 33, 42, 50–58].

While these array platforms create caricatures of in vivo MEs, they enable researchers to functionally define molecular components that maintain cell fate, thus revealing molecular regulators and pathways of cell states. We predict that this type of functional cell-based dissection of combinatorial MEs will have particular high impact in understanding normal and malignant human stem cells, because human in vivo experiments are essentially impossible. For instance, putative niche molecules and other tissue-specific ligands have been identified using MEMA, and validated in vivo in some cases, that were relevant to human embryonic [51], neural [28] and mammary stem cells [27, 29, 33]. MEMAs were also used to profile cell-ECM adhesion biases [59] and to optimize growth conditions of cultured cells [53, 60]. Taking a combinatorial approach, relative to a candidate-based approach, allows screening combinations of multiple tissue-specific ME molecules to identify extracellular cues that are the basis for emergent cell behaviors. Figure 25.1 summarizes several MEMA experiments that highlight the importance of including components of the TME when studying anticancer drug activity. TME context was found to produce dramatically different responses in various cancer cell lines even when using standard of care therapeutics.

The successful application of MEMA requires managing many technical details that are, in many cases, on the edge of discovery themselves. The remainder of this chapter will elaborate on some of the issues that arise most often when producing MEMA on 2D substrates and provide some discussion of how we are managing them. There are relatively fewer examples of MEMA-type platforms in 3D, perhaps because some of the high-throughput liquid handling and 3D imaging requirements raise the barrier to entry; however, there are successful examples of 3D MEMAs [42, 61].

Selecting the Printing Substrate: It Depends on the Biological Questions Being Asked

There are numerous materials used to immobilize ME molecules. But the primary objectives remain the same where MEMA fabrication is concerned: a suitable surface coating for printing molecules upon should provide high adsorption capacity, low cell attachment in areas not printed with molecules (i.e., non-fouling), and low spot-to-spot variation. Other important considerations include the capacity of the material to retain the structure, functionality, and binding sites of any given ME component.

The most commonly used substrata for immobilizing ME components are untreated polystyrene plastic surfaces, chemically modified surfaces of glass slides (with aldehydes or epoxies), or polymer (e.g., polydimethylsiloxane (PDMS))-coated glass slides. Slides with these surfaces adsorb proteins through hydrophobic interactions, covalent bonds, or strong electrostatic interactions, respectively. Covalent modifications provide irreversible attachment; however, protein 3D structures may not be well maintained. Unintended cell attachment can also occur on all substrata. The addition of non-fouling coatings, like synthetic blocking copolymers or bovine serum albumin, can lessen the extent of nonspecific cell adherence. Another option is to coat glass surfaces with polyacrylamide (PA) or poly (ethylene glycol) (PEG) hydrogels. These hydrogels physically absorb proteins through relatively weak electrostatic interactions, which retain most of the native protein conformation at the cost of higher variation in protein-binding capacity [62]. One of the most convenient properties of PA and PEG gels is their native non-fouling character, which reduces nonspecific cell attachment.

Rigidity of the substrate is another important property to consider. Untreated polystyrene and modified glass surfaces provide extremely stiff substratum (>2 GPa), which is not representative of the physical range of human tissues. PDMS is inexpensive, and its elastic modulus is easy to manipulate by altering the cure:polymer ratio, covering a range of elastic moduli similar to cartilage, skin, and tendon (0.6 to 3.5 MPa). PEG represents a range of elastic moduli from 0.5 to 1600 MPa. PA is another inexpensive substrate, which can be tuned from 150 Pa to 0.4 MPa, which is closer to the biological ME for soft tissues like brain and breast, and a reasonable range of elastic moduli to simulate normal and malignant breast, 100 to 4000 Pa [37, 63]. The substrate used for protein immobilization ultimately depends upon the characteristics of the cells used, the tissue being mimicked, and the outcomes being measured.

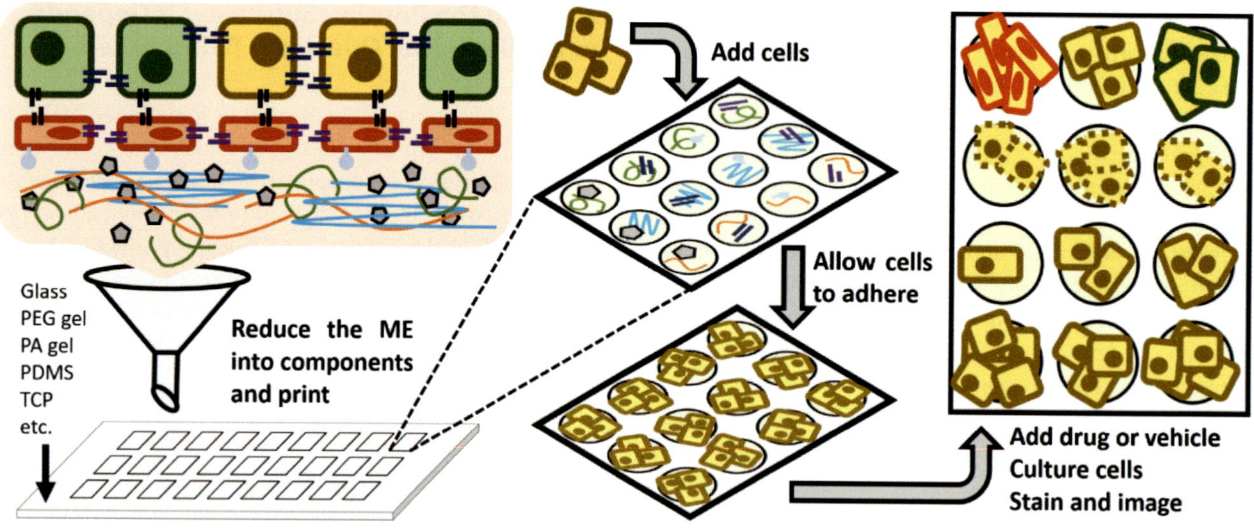

Cell type	Substrate and MEs	Drugs	Measured outcomes	Highlights	Reference
A549 lung adenocarcinoma cells	Polyacrylamide hydrogel 55 ME comprised of single and two-factor combinations of 10 ECM proteins	Alkylating agent and 5 tyrosine kinase inhibitors: cisplatin, cabozantinib, nilotinib, gefitinib, sunitinib, vandetanib	Cell number, BrdU, and cleaved caspase-3	Lung adenocarcinoma cells with known genetic drivers responded differently to therapeutics depending on ME context	(52)
HER2-amplified HCC1569 breast cancer cell line, HER2-negative BT549 breast cancer cell line, A549 non-small cell lung cancer (NSCLC) cell line, PC3 prostate cancer cell line	Polyacrylamide hydrogel tuned to stiffness of 2.5 and 40 kPa 70 ME comprised of two-factor combinations of 7 ligands and 5 ECM proteins	Lapatinib and Lapatinib + Verteporfin (YAP inhibitor)	Cellular morphology, HER2/pHER2 protein expression, and cell proliferation	Standard of care therapeutics in combination with drugs that target ME-imposed phenotypes can improve therapeutic response	(54)
AU565 breast cancer cell line (L-HER2+ subtype) and HCC1954 breast cancer cell line (HER2E subtype)	TCP >2,500 ME comprised of combinations of 56 ligands and 46 ECM proteins	Lapatinib	Cell proliferation	ME-induced resistance is potent even in the face of combination therapy if the combination does not consider ME Drug delivered in the wrong context can stimulate cancer cell growth	(55)
Isogenic human mammary epithelial cell malignant progression series: 184, 184A1, 184AA3	Polyacrylamide hydrogel tuned to stiffness of 4.5 kPa 228 ME comprised of combinations 16 ligands, 4 cell surface and 13 ECM proteins	Paclitaxel (drug was added to specific ME and not to array screen)	Cellular morphology, AXL and c-KIT expression	Defined components of the CSC niche that produce drug resistant phenotypes and understand how a breakdown in the architecture of the tissue can contribute to the production of more potent cells capable of resisting chemotherapeutics	(33)

Fig. 25.1 Examples of MEMA platforms used to analyze anticancer drug response in various cancer cell lines

MEMA Data Analysis: Seeing the Forest for the Trees

The main goal of MEMA-type experiments is to provide causal links between cellular responses and specific MEs. Both inter- and intra-ME heterogeneity of cellular responses are to be expected and can be instructive about the continuum of phenotypic plasticity within the experimental system. Measuring heterogeneity of drug responses in a diversity of contexts may result in more realistic expectations of drug responses in vivo. By incorporating sufficient numbers of replicate features into the design of a MEMA, significant associations between MEs and cell phenotypes can be identified. Still, the high dimensionality of the data is a hindrance to the extraction of meaningful information. Most MEMA platforms use fluorescent probes to visualize biochemical and functional phenotypes and fluorescent and phase microscopy to capture colorimetric and morphological phenotypes. There are no specialized high-throughput imaging systems for this type of work currently available; however, microarray scanners and programmable, motorized epifluorescence or laser scanning confocal microscopes have been successfully used to acquire the necessary images [27, 42, 64].

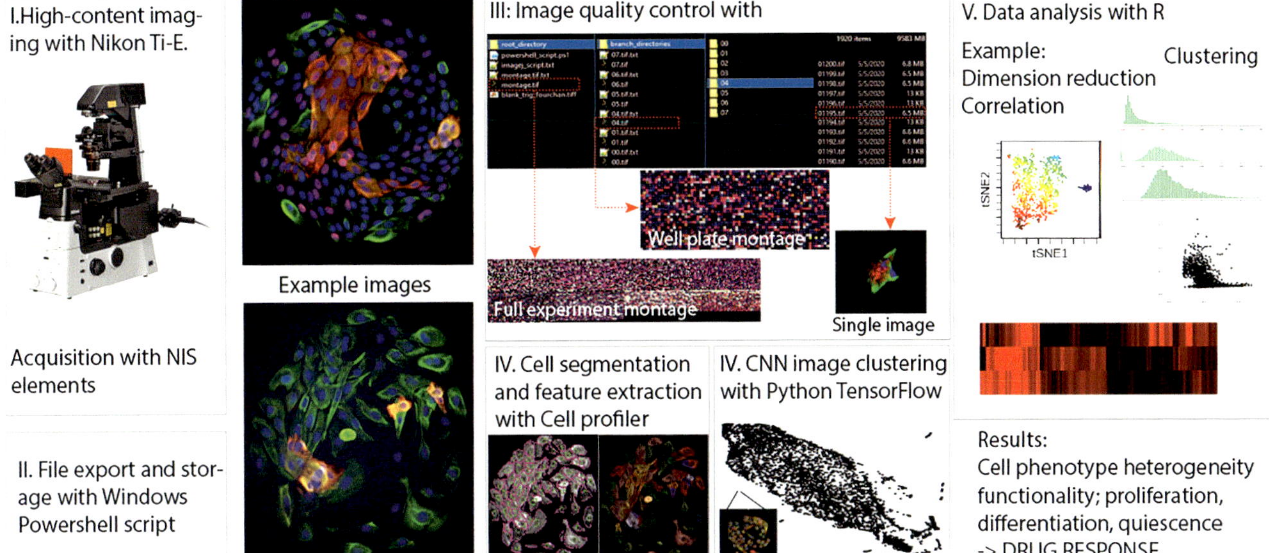

Fig. 25.2 Example of MEMA imaging and data analysis workflow

Imaging Quality Control

When implementing automated high-throughput imaging, there is a need for practical quality control steps. The variability of substratum that is inherent to the MEMA platform demands an autofocusing step for each individual spot and therefore increases acquisition time and poses a challenge for high-content imaging. Failed autofocusing generates blurry images, which cause distortion in downstream analyses. Background artifacts and image saturation cause similar problems. Manual and automated approaches can be applied to exclude these poor quality images from the dataset [65]. For manual quality control inspection, we have developed a "montage"-image navigating tool, which allows quick browsing of the entire dataset using Fiji open-source software (Fig. 25.2) [64]. For an automated quality control system, machine learning algorithms work very efficiently because they can be trained to recognize images with artifacts and automatically exclude them from the dataset (Fig. 25.2) (described here [65]).

Cell Segmentation and Feature Extraction

Flow cytometry and single-cell transcriptome sequencing analyses have shown that tissues and tumors contain substantially heterogeneous cell subpopulations [66], the significance of which is evident when identifying tumor cell subpopulations that play a significant role in initiating tumor metastasis, drug resistance, or relapse [66]. Likewise, tissue homeostasis and repair are driven by rare stem cell popula-

tions [67]. To achieve cellular resolution of cell-ME analyses, MEMA images must be analyzed with cell segmentation algorithms found in image analysis software, such as Fiji and CellProfiler (Fig. 25.2) [68–70]. Cell segmentation provides information about the morphological features of cells and provides further insight about ME-imposed changes to cellular phenotypes. In summary, cell segmentation and multiparametric feature extraction in MEMA data analysis need to be part of an automated workflow that demands optimization and rigorous quality control to provide informative single-cell resolution, high-dimensional datasets.

Data Analysis

Even in cases where a MEMA experiment is designed to have reasonably low complexity, e.g., 100 or fewer unique ME combinations, the analytical challenges are significant. The complexity of the information space generated by MEMA experiments increases rapidly when taking into consideration multiple ME properties such as rigidity, geometry, and molecular composition. And in addition to this, multiparametric data collected at single-cell resolution provides many dependent variables that can make meaningful interpretations difficult. In practice, the statistical analysis of MEMA experiments is a rate-limiting step for this technology, and there are multiple solutions for addressing this challenge. The data processing workflow for MEMA experiments includes signal normalization, identification of functionally similar MEs by clustering, dimension reduction, data visualization, and pathway analysis (Fig. 25.2).

Data Normalization

All microarray-like data contain some useful information and a significant degree of noise; thus, proper normalization is crucial. The data analysis begins with measuring fluorescence intensity or colorimetric density of each target protein in cells on each array feature. In this context, intensity typically reflects the relative abundance of the target protein. Intensities are impacted by factors such as the characteristics of the dye (antibody), spatial location, cell morphology, and uneven surfaces of the slides that cause inconsistent background [71]. Unlike DNA microarrays, which load the same amount of cDNA onto the array and then use total intensity as an internal reference, the number of cells attached to MEMA features varies by ME. Thus, we may use the average of the entire signal from all cells on all or spatially defined array features as a reference for normalization of arrays of the same treatment condition. A signal emanating from cells on a control ME, which is known a priori to reproducibly bias toward a given phenotype, can be used as a reference [27, 57]. An alternative is to use whole cell staining dyes such as CellMask that fluorescently labels the entire cell, which can be used as an internal control to normalize fluorescent signal between cells.

Statistical Considerations

The primary purpose of MEMA experiments is to identify the specific MEs that modulate certain cellular states by comparing cellular phenotypes between treatment and control groups. Compared to using a Student's t-test, a Dunnett's test is a better option for correcting false p-values due to multiple comparisons and identifying MEs that impose phenotypes that are significantly different from the control [27]. The Z-score standardization is a simple method used to identify meaningful groups that are distinct from the global mean. Z-scores have been used successfully to identify and optimize culture conditions for rare cell populations [72]. However, the Z-score has several limitations, like skewing of values due to outliers within a dataset as well as decreased accuracy when cell numbers are reduced. Moreover, the Z-score assumes that the data fit a Gaussian distribution, which is not the case in many biological systems. Thus, Guyon et al. proposed the Φ-score as a cell-to-cell phenotypic scoring method for selecting the hit discovery in cell-based assays (Table 25.1). The Φ-score ranks cells instead of averaging them and performs better than the Z-score despite the limitations previously mentioned. Indeed, the Φ-score can be more sensitive (more true hits) and more specific (fewer false positives) compared to other conventional methods [73].

Along with a large number of dependent variables, MEMA data often have many independent variables to contend with as well. It is biologically relevant to study the synergistic effects of ME factors and this is a greater challenge than studying the

Table 25.1 Examples of data analysis and visualization techniques used with MEMA-type data

Methods	Type	Advantages	Limitations
Φ-score	Normalization	Overcomes the limitation of Z-score	
PCA	Dimension reduction	A simple, deterministic method to identify patterns due to variance	Only reflects linear relationships
tSNE, UMAP	Visualization	Nonlinear methods to identify patterns due to variance	Stochastic. Global trends are not accurately represented in mapping. Cannot handle incomplete data
Multiple linear regression model, General Linear Model (GLM)	Statistical test	Can analyze multiple independent variables	Data need to be linear and normally distributed
Chi-Square	Statistical test	Suitable for categorical variables	Sensitive to sample size

effect of each individual ME factor on cellular phenotypes. Multiple linear regression is a regression model capable of estimating the relationship between the dependent variable and two or more independent variables (Table 25.1). It expands upon the linear regression model and therefore makes many of the same assumptions as the linear regression model, so data need to be normally distributed and linear. With the multiple linear regression model, it is possible to estimate how specific ME components (independent variables) change cell phenotype variables (dependent variable) [33, 42, 54, 74]. When some independent variables are categorical variables, such as specific ME components, the appropriate regression model to employ is called the General Linear Model (GLM) (Table 25.1). If all variables are categorical, a Chi-squared test provides an effective way to evaluate whether there is a significant association between the variables (Table 25.1). The Chi-squared test has been used to evaluate the co-occurrence of immune cell populations in patients with triple-negative breast cancer (TNBC) to define the coordinated immune response that occurs within the TNBC TME [75].

Clustering, Dimension Reduction, and Data Visualization

Clustering methods commonly used for DNA microarray datasets, such as hierarchical or *k*-means clustering, also are used with MEMA data to identify meaningful groups. Konagaya et al. interrogated a relatively small number of growth factor combinations to optimize neural progenitor cell culture MEs and then used hierarchical cluster analysis to reveal three major clusters of ME combinations that facilitated growth versus astrocyte or neuron differentiation [60]. Although these analyses can reveal the meaningful groups within simple datasets, like traditional two-color DNA microarray data, they become ineffective as the complexity of the data increases which has been described as the "curse of dimensionality" [76]. To overcome the challenges of working with high-dimensional datasets, dimension reduction techniques have been developed.

Improvements in computational processing power better facilitate analysis of high-dimensional data because they have enabled researchers to use algorithms that do not make painful compromises in the name of efficiency. Dimension reduction essentially distills vast amounts of information into snapshots that are emblematic of the underlying biology. Principal component analysis (PCA) is used for dimension reduction and can reveal the most variable factors that contribute to certain phenotypes (Table 25.1) [77]. However, not all biological questions are related to the variables with the highest variance in the dataset, and in such cases, PCA is less well-equiped to identify the contributing factors. Linear techniques such as PCA focus on separating dissimilar data points far away in low-dimensional representations after data transformation. However, biological data are often nonlinear, and for high-dimensional data, it is usually more important to keep similar data points close together in low-dimensional representations, which is typically not feasible with linear mapping techniques. t-Distributed Stochastic Neighbor Embedding (t-SNE) and Uniform Manifold Approximation and Projection (UMAP) provide nonlinear approaches for high-dimensional data visualization (Table 25.1) [78, 79]. These two approaches consider the major and minor sources of variance within a dataset and represent them on a lower dimensional surface. Once the meaningful information has been extracted, the data collected from MEMA need to be connected to the existing body of knowledge to perform further biological validation.

Machine Learning

In addition to feature extraction analysis, high content MEMA image sets provide excellent material for machine learning-based classification and clustering analysis. Deep learning algorithms, like convolution neural network (CNN), are useful and efficient ways to analyze MEMA image sets [80]. When supervised, the CNN model can be utilized during the image quality control step, where the algorithm can be trained to recognize and discard low-quality images. Another supervised approach is to use machine learning to classify MEMA images based on a provided training set that could include example images of cell morphology (differen-tiated versus non differentiated) or by cell proliferation rate. Following training, the algorithms are able to classify the remaining images in the dataset automatically with varying levels of accuracy, specificity, and sensitivity. Unsupervised deep learning can be used to optimize single-cell segmentation and improve the accuracy of single-cell level analysis [81]. Unsupervised clustering of MEMA images provides the potential to compare how different MEs affect not only the morphology of a single cell, but also how specific MEs influence cell–cell contact and self-organization. Currently, most of the deep learning image analysis algorithms are trained on 2D images, but promising deep learning 3D image analysis algorithms have been published recently [82, 83], and in the future, these algorithms may be excellent tools used to study 3D-MEMA data.

Open Access MEMA Data

MEMA is a core technology of the Microenvironment Perturbagen (MEP)—LINCS center (https://lincsproject. org/LINCS/centers/data-and-signature-generating-centers/ mep-lincs), which is one of six Data and Signature Generating Centers of the NIH Library of Integrated Network-Based Cellular Signatures (LINCS) program [84]. The broad aim of the LINCS program is to advance the understanding of health and disease by identifying how a broad range of perturbations to different tissues and cells generate patterns of common networks and cellular responses. MEP-LINCS complements the LINCS program by elucidating how ME signals affect molecular networks to generate experimentally observable cellular phenotypes. To this end, MEP-LINCS employs MEMA experiments to measure how close to 3000 pairwise MEs impact the proliferation, differentiation status, and cell cycle of 22 cell lines. Using rigorous data analysis workflows, researchers addressed how ME-induced cellular phenotypes were regulated by specific molecular networks, whether certain ME subsets that produce similar phenotypic responses were due to modulation of common molecular networks, and if specific molecular networks were capable of producing multiple cellular phenotypes. Integration of MEP-LINCS generated datasets with other datasets from the LINCS program will allow researchers to determine whether ME-induced network changes bear similarity to genetic or chemically induced network changes in the same cell lines. MEP-LINCS generated data are freely available online (https://www.synapse.org/#!Synapse:syn2862345/wiki/), as are details of the data processing steps necessary to generate meaningful conclusions from MEMA experiments (data processing pipelines available at https://github.com/MEP-LINCS). Two of the several tools available on the website are the Virtual Lab and MEMA Board. The Virtual Lab tool allows user to interact with MEMA experiments by selecting cell lines, ECM proteins, and ligands and then observing images for the selections along with selected data. The MEMA Board app allows for exploration of the datasets using dimension reduction methods and interactive heatmaps. The webpage is routinely updated with the most recent datasets which can be downloaded to a local device for further analysis.

Concluding Remarks/Summary

One important, and wholly unexpected, outcome of the massive efforts to understand cancer as an entirely cell-intrinsic problem is the undeniable conclusion that mutations do not explain everything. Indeed, the fact that frankly malignant cells can be phenotypically normal, when held in check by a normal microenvironment, suggests that there is a dominant role of the microenvironment. New investments need to be made in technologies that facilitate the dissection and exploration of tissue MEs. MEMA-type platforms, and their successors, will provide opportunities to gain a comprehensive understanding of how the ME modulates drug responses in human cells and will provide functional cell-based data for preclinical drug screening that is ultimately more predictive of in vivo biology.

These platforms are amenable to high-throughput scale-up using several imaging modalities for quantification. The main challenges of this approach are access to purified extracellular proteins, managing the combinatorial complexity to minimize cost and maximize the combinatorial space that is evaluated, data visualization, and statistical analysis to identify microenvironment components that contribute to a given outcome. An important component that is still in its infancy is robust network analysis that can provide a systematic understanding of how microenvironments are linked to activity in specific signaling pathways, which underlie cell phenotypes, and reveal candidates for further investigation. Tapping into the accumulated knowledge, represented in public databases and tools for pathway mapping like GO (Gene Ontology) enrichment analysis and KEGG (*Kyoto Encyclopedia of Genes and Genomes*), will increase the possibility that we can connect ME-imposed phenotypes to known signaling pathways and, hence, to cellular functions. Different ME components, such as ECM or substrate rigidity, are the input, and the measurements, such as morphometrics and other protein markers, are the output. The major object of pathway analysis is to delineate the relationship between input and output.

There is an obvious need to improve preclinical drug discovery and evaluation. Overall, MEMAs are meant to address the shortcomings of experimentation that uses standard human cell culture models (i.e., the nonphysiological contexts), rodent models (i.e., the nonhuman context), and human beings (i.e., the intractable model). One of the approaches is to consider the microenvironmental impact on drug responses during the earliest design stages of therapeutics. The combinatorial nature of MEMAs provides the advantages of exquisitely controlling microenvironmental properties and enabling high throughput. MEMA data are high-content, single-cell resolution and can capture cell-to-cell heterogeneity; hence, it may provide a more realistic picture of drug performance. However, it remains to be seen whether data from MEMA-type experiments can build in vivo response models. Improved knowledge of microenvironmental impact on drug responses will economize and hasten drug development by making the preclinical stage more predictive and aid in the deployment of more precision therapeutics.

References

1. Wong CH, Siah KW, Lo AW. Estimation of clinical trial success rates and related parameters. Biostatistics. 2018;20:273–86.
2. Light DW, Kantarjian H. Market spiral pricing of cancer drugs. Cancer. 2013;119:3900–2.
3. Talmadge JE, Singh RK, Fidler IJ, Raz A. Murine models to evaluate novel and conventional therapeutic strategies for cancer. Am J Pathol. 2007;170:793–804.
4. Yue F, Cheng Y, Breschi A, Vierstra J, Wu W, Ryba T, Sandstrom R, Ma Z, Davis C, Pope BD, Shen Y, Pervouchine DD, Djebali S, Thurman RE, Kaul R, Rynes E, Kirilusha A, Marinov GK, Williams BA, Trout D, Amrhein H, Fisher-Aylor K, Antoshechkin I, DeSalvo G, See L-H, Fastuca M, Drenkow J, Zaleski C, Dobin A, Prieto P, Lagarde J, Bussotti G, Tanzer A, Denas O, Li K, Bender MA, Zhang M, Byron R, Groudine MT, McCleary D, Pham L, Ye Z, Kuan S, Edsall L, Wu Y-C, Rasmussen MD, Bansal MS, Kellis M, Keller CA, Morrissey CS, Mishra T, Jain D, Dogan N, Harris RS, Cayting P, Kawli T, Boyle AP, Euskirchen G, Kundaje A, Lin S, Lin Y, Jansen C, Malladi VS, Cline MS, Erickson DT, Kirkup VM, Learned K, Sloan CA, Rosenbloom KR, Lacerda de Sousa B, Beal K, Pignatelli M, Flicek P, Lian J, Kahveci T, Lee D, James Kent W, Ramalho Santos M, Herrero J, Notredame C, Johnson A, Vong S, Lee K, Bates D, Neri F, Diegel M, Canfield T, Sabo PJ, Wilken MS, Reh TA, Giste E, Shafer A, Kutyavin T, Haugen E, Dunn D, Reynolds AP, Neph S, Humbert R, Scott Hansen R, De Bruijn M, Selleri L, Rudensky A, Josefowicz S, Samstein R, Eichler EE, Orkin SH, Levasseur D, Papayannopoulou T, Chang K-H, Skoultchi A, Gosh S, Disteche C, Treuting P, Wang Y, Weiss MJ, Blobel GA, Cao X, Zhong S, Wang T, Good PJ, Lowdon RF, Adams LB, Zhou X-Q, Pazin MJ, Feingold EA, Wold B, Taylor J, Mortazavi A, Weissman SM, Stamatoyannopoulos JA, Snyder MP, Guigo R, Gingeras TR, Gilbert DM, Hardison RC, Beer MA, Ren B, The Mouse EC. A comparative encyclopedia of DNA elements in the mouse genome. Nature. 2014;515:355–64.
5. Uhl EW, Warner NJ. Mouse models as predictors of human responses: evolutionary medicine. Curr Pathobiol Rep. 2015;3:219–23.
6. Weigelt B, Lo AT, Park CC, Gray JW, Bissell MJ. HER2 signaling pathway activation and response of breast cancer cells to HER2-targeting agents is dependent strongly on the 3D microenvironment. Breast Cancer Res Treat. 2010;122:35–43.
7. Baghban R, Roshangar L, Jahanban-Esfahlan R, Seidi K, Ebrahimi-Kalan A, Jaymand M, Kolahian S, Javaheri T, Zare P. Tumor microenvironment complexity and therapeutic implications at a glance. Cell Commun Signal. 2020;18:59.
8. Bissell MJ, Hines WC. Why don't we get more cancer? A proposed role of the microenvironment in restraining cancer progression. Nat Med. 2011;17:320.

9. Egeblad M, Nakasone ES, Werb Z. Tumors as organs: complex tissues that interface with the entire organism. Dev Cell. 2010;18:884–901.

10. Junttila MR, de Sauvage FJ. Influence of tumour microenvironment heterogeneity on therapeutic response. Nature. 2013;501:346–54.

11. Mlecnik B, Bindea G, Kirilovsky A, Angell HK, Obenauf AC, Tosolini M, Church SE, Maby P, Vasaturo A, Angelova M. The tumor microenvironment and Immunoscore are critical determinants of dissemination to distant metastasis. Sci Transl Med. 2016;8:327ra26.

12. Northcott JM, Dean IS, Mouw JK, Weaver VM. Feeling stress: the mechanics of cancer progression and aggression. Front Cell Dev Biol. 2018;6:17.

13. Mpekris F, Angeli S, Pirentis AP, Stylianopoulos T. Stress-mediated progression of solid tumors: effect of mechanical stress on tissue oxygenation, cancer cell proliferation, and drug delivery. Biomech Model Mechanobiol. 2015;14:1391–402.

14. Correia AL, Bissell MJ. The tumor microenvironment is a dominant force in multidrug resistance. Drug Resist Updat. 2012;15:39–49.

15. Son B, Lee S, Youn H, Kim E, Kim W, Youn B. The role of tumor microenvironment in therapeutic resistance. Oncotarget. 2017;8:3933–45.

16. Flynn CM, Kaufman DS. Donor cell leukemia: insight into cancer stem cells and the stem cell niche. Blood. 2007;109:2688–92.

17. Ingangi V, Minopoli M, Ragone C, Motti ML, Carriero MV. Role of microenvironment on the fate of disseminating cancer stem cells. Front Oncol. 2019;9

18. Plaks V, Kong N, Werb Z. The cancer stem cell niche: how essential is the niche in regulating stemness of tumor cells? Cell Stem Cell. 2015;16:225–38.

19. Fuchs E, Tumbar T, Guasch G. Socializing with the neighbors: stem cells and their niche. Cell. 2004;116:769–78.

20. Scadden DT. The stem-cell niche as an entity of action. Nature. 2006;441:1075–9.

21. Collins CA, Olsen I, Zammit PS, Heslop L, Petrie A, Partridge TA, Morgan JE. Stem cell function, self-renewal, and behavioral heterogeneity of cells from the adult muscle satellite cell niche. Cell. 2005;122:289–301.

22. Nishimura EK, Jordan SA, Oshima H, Yoshida H, Osawa M, Moriyama M, Jackson IJ, Barrandon Y, Miyachi Y, Nishikawa S-I. Dominant role of the niche in melanocyte stem-cell fate determination. Nature. 2002;416:854–60.

23. Sacco A, Doyonnas R, Kraft P, Vitorovic S, Blau HM. Self-renewal and expansion of single transplanted muscle stem cells. Nature. 2008;456:502–6.

24. Bruno RD, Fleming JM, George AL, Boulanger CA, Schedin P, Smith GH. Mammary extracellular matrix directs differentiation of testicular and embryonic stem cells to form functional mammary glands in vivo. Sci Rep. 2017;7:40196.

25. Booth BW, Mack DL, Androutsellis-Theotokis A, McKay RD, Boulanger CA, Smith GH. The mammary microenvironment alters the differentiation repertoire of neural stem cells. Proc Natl Acad Sci U S A. 2008;105:14891–6.

26. Flaim CJ, Chien S, Bhatia SN. An extracellular matrix microarray for probing cellular differentiation. Nat Methods. 2005;2:119–25.

27. LaBarge MA, Nelson CM, Villadsen R, Fridriksdottir A, Ruth JR, Stampfer MR, Petersen OW, Bissell MJ. Human mammary progenitor cell fate decisions are products of interactions with combinatorial microenvironments. Integr Biol (Camb). 2009;1:70–9.

28. Soen Y, Mori A, Palmer TD, Brown PO. Exploring the regulation of human neural precursor cell differentiation using arrays of signaling microenvironments. Mol Syst Biol. 2006;2:37.

29. Au-Lin C-H, Au-Lee JK, Au-LaBarge MA (2012) Fabrication and use of microenvironment microarrays (MEArrays). JoVE. e4152.

30. LaBarge MA, Petersen OW, Bissell MJ. Of microenvironments and mammary stem cells. Stem Cell Rev. 2007;3:137–46.

31. Jokela TA, LaBarge MA. Integration of mechanical and ECM microenvironment signals in the determination of cancer stem cell states. Curr Stem Cell Rep. 2020.

32. LaBarge MA. The difficulty of targeting cancer stem cell niches. Clin Cancer Res. 2010;16:3121–9.

33. Jokela TA, Engelsen AST, Rybicka A, Pelissier Vatter FA, Garbe JC, Miyano M, Tiron C, Ferariu D, Akslen LA, Stampfer MR, Lorens JB, LaBarge MA. Microenvironment-induced non-sporadic expression of the AXL and cKIT receptors are related to epithelial plasticity and drug resistance. Front Cell Dev Biol. 2018;6:41.

34. Bissell MJ, LaBarge MA. Context, tissue plasticity, and cancer: Are tumor stem cells also regulated by the microenvironment? Cancer Cell. 2005;7:17–23.

35. Kenny PA, Bissell MJ. Tumor reversion: correction of malignant behavior by microenvironmental cues. Int J Cancer. 2003;107:688–95.

36. Engler AJ, Sen S, Sweeney HL, Discher DE. Matrix elasticity directs stem cell lineage specification. Cell. 2006;126:677–89.

37. Paszek MJ, Zahir N, Johnson KR, Lakins JN, Rozenberg GI, Gefen A, Reinhart-King CA, Margulies SS, Dembo M, Boettiger D, Hammer DA, Weaver VM. Tensional homeostasis and the malignant phenotype. Cancer Cell. 2005;8:241–54.

38. Booij TH, Price LS, Danen EHJ. 3D cell-based assays for drug screens: challenges in imaging, image analysis, and high-content analysis. SLAS Discov. 2019;24:615–27.

39. Hansen KC, Kiemele L, Maller O, O'Brien J, Shankar A, Fornetti J, Schedin P. An in-solution ultrasonication-assisted digestion method for improved extracellular matrix proteome coverage. Mol Cell Proteomics. 2009;8:1648–57.

40. Soofi SS, Last JA, Liliensiek SJ, Nealey PF, Murphy CJ. The elastic modulus of Matrigel™ as determined by atomic force microscopy. J Struct Biol. 2009;167:216–9.

41. Hughes CS, Postovit LM, Lajoie GA. Matrigel: a complex protein mixture required for optimal growth of cell culture. Proteomics. 2010;10:1886–90.

42. Ranga A, Gobaa S, Okawa Y, Mosiewicz K, Negro A, Lutolf M. 3D niche microarrays for systems-level analyses of cell fate. Nat Commun. 2014;5:1–10.

43. Pelissier FA, Garbe JC, Ananthanarayanan B, Miyano M, Lin C, Jokela T, Kumar S, Stampfer MR, Lorens JB, LaBarge MA. Age-related dysfunction in mechanotransduction impairs differentiation of human mammary epithelial progenitors. Cell Rep. 2014;7:1926–39.

44. Lin C-H, Pelissier FA, Zhang H, Lakins J, Weaver VM, Park C, LaBarge MA. Microenvironment rigidity modulates responses to the HER2 receptor tyrosine kinase inhibitor lapatinib via YAP and TAZ transcription factors. Mol Biol Cell. 2015;26:3946–53.

45. Kilian KA, Bugarija B, Lahn BT, Mrksich M. Geometric cues for directing the differentiation of mesenchymal stem cells. Proc Natl Acad Sci U S A. 2010;107:4872–7.

46. Yu S-M, Li B, Granick S, Cho Y-K. Mechanical adaptations of epithelial cells on various protruded convex geometries. Cell. 2020;9:1434.

47. Sealfon SC, Chu TT. RNA and DNA microarrays. Methods Mol Biol. 2011;671:3–34.

48. Sutandy FXR, Qian J, Chen C-S, Zhu H (2013) Overview of protein microarrays. Curr Protoc Protein Sci. Chapter 27: 2711–27.1.

49. Shin I, Park S, Mr L. Carbohydrate microarrays: an advanced technology for functional studies of glycans. Chemistry. 2005;11:2894–901.

50. Flaim CJ, Teng D, Chien S, Bhatia SN. Combinatorial signaling microenvironments for studying stem cell fate. Stem Cells Dev. 2008;17:29–39.

51. Brafman DA, Shah KD, Fellner T, Chien S, Willert K. Defining long-term maintenance conditions of human embryonic stem cells with arrayed cellular microenvironment technology. Stem Cells Dev. 2009;18:1141–54.

52. Kaylan KB, Gentile SD, Milling LE, Bhinge KN, Kosari F, Underhill GH. Mapping lung tumor cell drug responses as a function of matrix context and genotype using cell microarrays. Integr Biol (Camb). 2016;8:1221–31.

53. Hou L, Kim JJ, Wanjare M, Patlolla B, Coller J, Natu V, Hastie TJ, Huang NF. Combinatorial extracellular matrix microenvironments for probing endothelial differentiation of human pluripotent stem cells. Sci Rep. 2017;7:6551.

54. Lin CH, Jokela T, Gray J, LaBarge MA. Combinatorial microenvironments impose a continuum of cellular responses to a single pathway-targeted anti-cancer compound. Cell Rep. 2017;21:533–45.

55. Watson SS, Dane M, Chin K, Tatarova Z, Liu M, Liby T, Thompson W, Smith R, Nederlof M, Bucher E, Kilburn D, Whitman M, Sudar D, Mills GB, Heiser LM, Jonas O, Gray JW, Korkola JE. Microenvironment-mediated mechanisms of resistance to HER2 inhibitors differ between HER2+ breast cancer subtypes. Cell Syst. 2018;6:329–42.e6.

56. Kaylan KB, Berg IC, Biehl MJ, Brougham-Cook A, Jain I, Jamil SM, Sargeant LH, Cornell NJ, Raetzman LT, Underhill GH. Spatial patterning of liver progenitor cell differentiation mediated by cellular contractility and Notch signaling. eLife. 2018;7:e38536.

57. Smith R, Devlin K, Kilburn D, Gross S, Sudar D, Bucher E, Nederlof M, Dane M, Gray JW, Heiser L, Korkola JE. Using microarrays to interrogate microenvironmental impact on cellular phenotypes in cancer. J Vis Exp. 2019. https://doi.org/10.3791/58957

58. Gaharwar AK, Arpanaei A, Andresen TL, Dolatshahi-Pirouz A. 3D biomaterial microarrays for regenerative medicine: current state-of-the-art, emerging directions and future trends. Adv Mater. 2016;28:771–81.

59. Kuschel C, Steuer H, Maurer AN, Kanzok B, Stoop R, Angres B. Cell adhesion profiling using extracellular matrix protein microarrays. BioTechniques. 2006;40:523–31.

60. Konagaya S, Kato K, Nakaji-Hirabayashi T, Arima Y, Iwata H. Array-based functional screening of growth factors toward optimizing neural stem cell microenvironments. Biomaterials. 2011;32:5015–22.

61. Floren M, Tan W. Three-dimensional, soft neotissue arrays as high throughput platforms for the interrogation of engineered tissue environments. Biomaterials. 2015;59:39–52.

62. Angenendt P. Progress in protein and antibody microarray technology. Drug Discov Today. 2005;10:503–11.

63. Kim HN, Kang D-H, Kim MS, Jiao A, Kim D-H, Suh K-Y. Patterning methods for polymers in cell and tissue engineering. Ann Biomed Eng. 2012;40:1339–55.

64. Jokela T, Todhunter ME, LaBarge MA. High-throughput microenvironment microarray (MEMA) high resolution imaging. Biosens Biodetect. 2021;

65. Bray M-A, Carpenter AE. Quality control for high-throughput imaging experiments using machine learning in CellProfiler. In: High content screening. Springer; 2018. p. 89–112.

66. Lawson DA, Kessenbrock K, Davis RT, Pervolarakis N, Werb Z. Tumour heterogeneity and metastasis at single-cell resolution. Nat Cell Biol. 2018;20:1349–60.

67. Rué P, Martinez AA. Cell dynamics and gene expression control in tissue homeostasis and development. Mol Syst Biol. 2015;11:792.

68. Abramoff M, Magalhães P, Ram SJ. Image processing with ImageJ. Biophoton Int. 2004;11:36–42.

69. Schindelin J, Arganda-Carreras I, Frise E, Kaynig V, Longair M, Pietzsch T, Preibisch S, Rueden C, Saalfeld S, Schmid B, Tinevez J-Y, White DJ, Hartenstein V, Eliceiri K, Tomancak P, Cardona A. Fiji: an open-source platform for biological-image analysis. Nat Methods. 2012;9:676–82.

70. Kamentsky L, Jones TR, Fraser A, Bray MA, Logan DJ, Madden KL, Ljosa V, Rueden C, Eliceiri KW, Carpenter AE. Improved structure, function and compatibility for CellProfiler: modular high-throughput image analysis software. Bioinformatics. 2011;27:1179–80.

71. Yang YH, Dudoit S, Luu P, Lin DM, Peng V, Ngai J, Speed TP. Normalization for cDNA microarray data: a robust composite method addressing single and multiple slide systematic variation. Nucleic Acids Res. 2002;30:e15.

72. Brafman DA, Chien S, Willert K. Arrayed cellular microenvironments for identifying culture and differentiation conditions for stem, primary and rare cell populations. Nat Protoc. 2012;7:703.

73. Guyon L, Lajaunie C, Fer F, Bhajun R, Sulpice E, Pinna G, Campalans A, Radicella JP, Rouillier P, Mary M. Φ-score: a cell-to-cell phenotypic scoring method for sensitive and selective hit discovery in cell-based assays. Sci Rep. 2015;5:14221.

74. Edwards AL (1985) Multiple regression and the analysis of variance and covariance (WH Freeman/Times Books/Henry Holt & Co).

75. Keren L, Bosse M, Marquez D, Angoshtari R, Jain S, Varma S, Yang S-R, Kurian A, Van Valen D, West R, Bendall SC, Angelo M. A structured tumor-immune microenvironment in triple negative breast cancer revealed by multiplexed ion beam imaging. Cell. 2018;174:1373–87.e19.

76. Bellman RE. Adaptive control processes: a guided tour. Princeton University Press; 1961.

77. Hilsenbeck SG, Friedrichs WE, Schiff R, O'Connell P, Hansen RK, Osborne CK, Fuqua SA. Statistical analysis of array expression data as applied to the problem of tamoxifen resistance. J Natl Cancer Inst. 1999;91:453–9.

78. McInnes L, Healy J, Melville J (2018) Umap: Uniform manifold approximation and projection for dimension reduction. arXiv preprint arXiv:1802.03426.

79. Lvd M, Hinton G. Visualizing data using t-SNE. J Mach Learn Res. 2008;9:2579–605.

80. Moen E, Bannon D, Kudo T, Graf W, Covert M, Van Valen D. Deep learning for cellular image analysis. Nat Methods. 2019;16:1233–46.

81. Yao K, Rochman ND, Sun SX. Cell type classification and unsupervised morphological phenotyping from low-resolution images using deep learning. Sci Rep. 2019;9:13467.

82. Haberl MG, Churas C, Tindall L, Boassa D, Phan S, Bushong EA, Madany M, Akay R, Deerinck TJ, Peltier ST, Ellisman MH. CDeep3M—Plug-and-Play cloud-based deep learning for image segmentation. Nat Methods. 2018;15:677–80.

83. Tokuoka Y, Yamada TG, Hiroi NF, Kobayashi TJ, Yamagata K, Funahashi A. Convolutional neural network-based instance segmentation algorithm to acquire quantitative criteria of early mouse development. bioRxiv. 2018. 324186.

84. Keenan AB, Jenkins SL, Jagodnik KM, Koplev S, He E, Torre D, Wang Z, Dohlman AB, Silverstein MC, Lachmann A, Kuleshov MV, Ma'ayan A, Stathias V, Terryn R, Cooper D, Forlin M, Koleti A, Vidovic D, Chung C, Schürer SC, Vasiliauskas J, Pilarczyk M, Shamsaei B, Fazel M, Ren Y, Niu W, Clark NA, White S, Mahi N, Zhang L, Kouril M, Reichard JF, Sivaganesan S, Medvedovic M, Meller J, Koch RJ, Birtwistle MR, Iyengar R, Sobie EA, Azeloglu EU, Kaye J, Osterloh J, Haston K, Kalra J, Finkbiener S, Li J, Milani P, Adam M, Escalante-Chong R, Sachs K, Lenail A, Ramamoorthy D, Fraenkel E, Daigle G, Hussain U, Coye A, Rothstein J, Sareen D, Ornelas L, Banuelos M, Mandefro B, Ho R, Svendsen CN, Lim RG, Stocksdale J, Casale MS, Thompson TG, Wu J, Thompson LM, Dardov V, Venkatraman V, Matlock A, Van Eyk JE, Jaffe JD, Papanastasiou M, Subramanian A, Golub TR, Erickson SD, Fallahi-Sichani M, Hafner M, Gray NS, Lin JR, Mills CE, Muhlich JL, Niepel M, Shamu CE, Williams EH, Wrobel D, Sorger PK, Heiser LM, Gray JW, Korkola JE, Mills GB, LaBarge M, Feiler HS, Dane MA, Bucher E, Nederlof M, Sudar D, Gross S, Kilburn DF, Smith R, Devlin K, Margolis R, Derr L, Lee A, Pillai A. The library of integrated network-based cellular signatures NIH Program: system-level cataloging of human cells response to perturbations. Cell Syst. 2018;6:13–24.

Models of Tumor Progression in Prostate Cancer

Waqas Azeem, Yaping Hua, Karl-Henning Kalland, Xisong Ke, Jan Roger Olsen, Anne Margrete Oyan, and Yi Qu

Abstract

Human prostate cancer is initiated in a benign prostate epithelial cell which gains the potential to progress to invasive and metastatic disease. The exact cell of origin of prostate cancer has not been finally determined. The plasticity of cell differentiation, the evolutionary potential of cancer cells, and differences between human and mouse prostate glands may underlie differences in the results from different experimental models. Numerous experimental models are available for the study of prostate cancer progression and include benign and transformed cells in monolayer or three-dimensional cultures, patient-derived explant and organoid cultures, xenografted and genetically modified animals, and animal models with spontaneous prostate cancer development. Technological developments, such as lab-on-a-chip and three-dimensional tissue printing, are ongoing with the aim to achieve standardized, miniaturized, and high-capacity models that capture essential features of cancer development in vivo. Recently, the development of high-resolution assays has opened new avenues to the understanding of the complexity of prostate carcinogenesis, including such techniques as single-cell sequencing and mass cytometry. The choice of model will depend on the exact question that will be investigated. Here we review different types of experimental models that are available for increasing insight into prostate carcinogenesis.

W. Azeem
Department of Clinical Science, University of Bergen, Bergen, Norway

Centre for Cancer Biomarkers CCBIO, University of Bergen, Bergen, Norway

Y. Hua · J. R. Olsen
Department of Clinical Science, University of Bergen, Bergen, Norway

K.-H. Kalland (✉)
Department of Clinical Science, University of Bergen, Bergen, Norway

Centre for Cancer Biomarkers CCBIO, University of Bergen, Bergen, Norway

Department of Microbiology, Haukeland University Hospital, Bergen, Norway
e-mail: Kalland@uib.no

X. Ke · Y. Qu
Center for Chemical Biology, Institute of Interdisciplinary Integrative Medicine Research, Shanghai University of Traditional Chinese Medicine, Shanghai, People's Republic of China

A. M. Oyan
Department of Clinical Science, University of Bergen, Bergen, Norway

Department of Immunology and Transfusion Medicine, Haukeland University Hospital, Bergen, Norway

© The Author(s), under exclusive license to Springer Nature Switzerland AG 2022
L. A. Akslen, R. S. Watnick (eds.), *Biomarkers of the Tumor Microenvironment*, https://doi.org/10.1007/978-3-030-98950-7_26

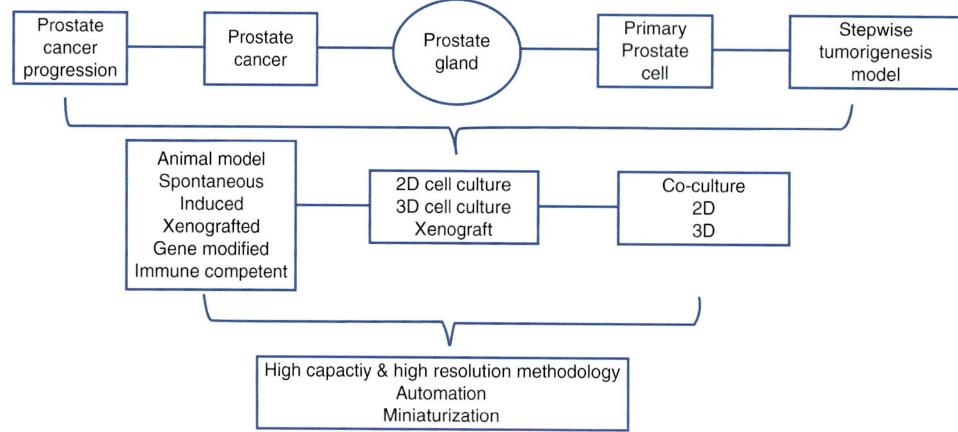

Heterogeneity and context dependency represent complicated challenges in prostate cancer research and therapy. Choice of appropriate experimental models is critical in experimental design and for therapeutic relevance. Single cell resolution, automation and bioinformatic analyses and an increasing number of available models promise advances ahead.

> **Take-Home Lessons**
> - Large number of experimental models are available.
> - Choice of model depends upon scientific question.
> - Technological development is ongoing.
> - High-resolution methods improve detailed insight.

Origin of the Prostate Cancer Cell

The prostate gland consists of multiple small glandular elements embedded in a vascularized connective tissue stroma (Fig. 26.1). Each small glandular element is defined by an outer basement membrane on which a layer of basal epithelial cells is situated (Fig. 26.1). The master transcription factor, the androgen receptor (AR), is silenced in basal cells and expressed in luminal cells. One prevailing view regarding normal prostate epithelial differentiation is that when AR is induced by unknown mechanisms in the presence of androgen, basal cells differentiate into luminal (secretory) cells and a minor population of neuroendocrine cells. Early passages of primary prostate cells can recapitulate such differentiation, e.g. with androgen and fibroblast growth factor 7 (FG7) added to the growth medium [1]. Immortalized basal cells can be propagated indefinitely as transit amplifying (TA) cells in culture media with low calcium concentration [2], but we have found that such long-term cultures are very resistant to luminal differentiation [3]. The explanation could be that normal luminal cells become terminally differentiated, and consequently the selection pressure favors TA cells that do not differentiate. The lineage relationships between basal, luminal and neuroendocrine prostate cells, and in particular which one is the cell of origin of prostate cancer, and

of putative prostate cancer stem cells (CSCs), have been vigorously debated [4, 5]. The bulk of prostate adenocarcinoma cells express mostly luminal cell expression patterns, but recently evidence has been provided to support all the different lineages of benign epithelial prostate cells as the cell of origin of prostate cancer [6–12]. These cumulative results underscore considerable plasticity of prostate cell differentiation, but also that there are differences between the human and mouse prostate and the experimental models used. There are, however, strong clues that the key regulatory mechanisms in normal prostate epithelial differentiation are retained in a perverted form in advanced prostate cancer. This notion is exemplified by the importance of the AR transcription factor during prostate cancer progression, including in castration resistant prostate cancer (CRPC) [10, 13], and by the neuroendocrine differentiation [14, 15] in end-stage prostate cancer. The unknown activation status of AR in putative prostate CSCs remains an important unresolved question with significant therapeutic consequences [10, 16].

Cell Culture Modeling of Prostate Carcinogenesis

Primary prostate epithelial cells (PrECs) can be obtained from biopsies and surgical material, as well as commercially, and can be propagated for a limited number of passages in monolayers until senescence ensues. PrECs have been immortalized using either hTERT (human telomerase reverse transcriptase) or the transforming elements of DNA viruses [17–19]. The 957E/hTERT cells [20, 21] and EP156T cells [22] were immortalized by exogenous expression of hTERT. PZ-HPV7, CA-HPV10, and RWPE-1 cells were immortalized by human papilloma virus (HPV) transforming elements [23]. Immortalization of PrECs has been achieved without exogenous gene expression [5, 24–26], but there is no model available of PrECs that spontaneously have transformed into malignant cell lines in vitro.

Many attempts have been made to study the malignant transformation of benign prostate cells in culture, but the use of strong carcinogens or oncogenic viral elements was necessary to achieve transformation [27]. Forced transformation may be useful for many purposes, but is suboptimal when physiological mechanisms of transcriptional reprogramming during prostate carcinogenesis are investigated. Physiological selection pressure was applied to EP156T cells by keeping the cells in a confluent monolayer with regular replacement

of fresh growth medium. After several months, progeny EPT1 cells with reduced cell-to-cell contact inhibition dominated the culture. EPT1 cells had undergone EMT but were not tumorigenic [27]. EMT turned out to be the first step in the accumulation of malignant traits in a succession of progeny cells, eventually resulting in tumorigenic EPT3 cells (Fig. 26.2) [28, 29]. This model encompasses benign transit amplifying epithelial cells (EP156T), benign (EPT1) and pre-malignant (EPT2) mesenchymal type cells, tumorigenic (EPT3-N04/EPT3-PT1) and metastatic (EPT3-M1) cells in mice (Fig. 26.2). The very different phenotypes share a common genotype. Forensic-grade DNA microsatellite, karyotype and copy number break point analyses verified progeny

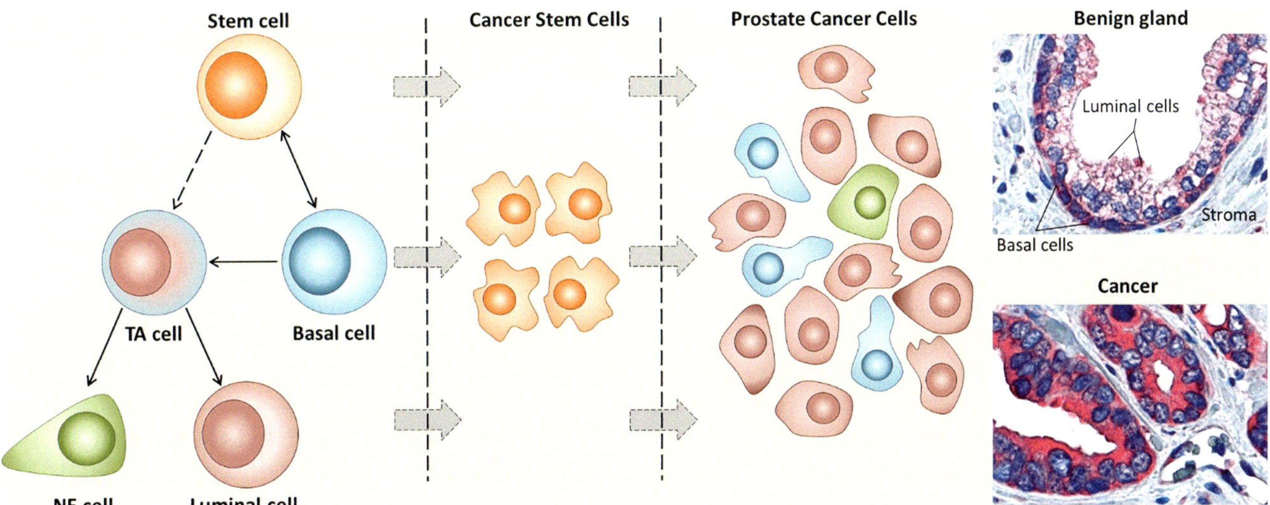

Fig. 26.1 Possible normal differentiation pathways from prostate stem cells to epithelial basal cells, luminal cells and neuroendocrine (NE) cells and possible transformation pathways to prostate cancer stem cells and cancer cells (TA = Transit Amplifying cell). Stained histological sections of prostate benign (upper) and cancer (lower) tissue are from reference [142]

	Epithelial	Mesenchymal	Soft agar colonies	Prostaspheres	Tumor
Phenotype	EP156T	EPT1	EPT2	EPT2-D5-HS	EPT3
Loss of contact inhibition	−	+	+	+	+
EMT	−	+	+	+	+
Postconfluent proliferation	−	+	++	NA	NA
Apoptosis resistance	−	−	+	+	+
Anchorage indep. growth	−	−	+	+	NA
Growth factor indep. growth	−	−	+	+	NA
Tumor formation in mouse	−	−	−	+	++
Tumor metastases	−	−	−	−	++

Fig. 26.2 Overview of the EPT prostate stepwise tumorigenesis model. EPT1 cells were selected for loss of cell contact inhibition. EPT2 cells were selected from foci of confluent EPT1 cells and cloned in soft agar. EPT2-D5-HS were selected in protein-free medium. EPT3 cells were selected following subcutaneous injection. Cells were recovered from the EPT3 tumor. The progressive accumulation of malignant hallmarks is summarized [29]

authenticity [29]. Each of the different cell types can be passaged indefinitely and to high cell numbers in sub-confluent monolayers. Subpopulations of tumor initiating EPT3 cells (TICs) show activation of an autocrine IL6/STAT3 loop and show increased resistance to apoptosis and anoikis [29]. Genome-wide analyses revealed that epigenetic promoter patterns at different steps of the model corresponded strongly with coordinated expression changes of regulatory gene modules, such as HOX and microRNA genes, and structural gene modules, such as desmosome and adherens junction genes [27, 28, 30]. The model demonstrates, however, an absence of gene expression patterns characteristic of the bulk cellular population of prostate adenocarcinomas. Prostate luminal gene expression is strikingly absent, and the model is more likely to represent features of mesenchymal type cells in prostate cancer progression. In fact, evidence of EMT in the progression of primary prostate cancer has been shown in patient tissue [31]. However, the role of EMT, and its significance, in early prostate carcinogenesis, in metastasis and in the development of resistance to androgen deprivation treatment (ADT) and other prostate cancer therapy requires further investigation in available cell cultures, preclinical models and patient samples [32]. A particular pressing issue is the mounting evidence that ADT and highly potent inhibitors of AR function, such as enzalutamide, might induce EMT and more aggressive cancer, possibly involving prostate CSCs [3, 33, 34]. Alternative hypotheses have been discussed, such as the existence of a common progenitor prostate cancer stem cell that gives rise to both the neuroendocrine like and adenocarcinoma components and both these components continue to evolve and respond to selective pressures in parallel [34]. A very interesting feature of this EPT stepwise prostate tumorigenesis model is that exogenous expression of the AR in EP156T cells strongly induced the androgen-responsive AR target genes typical of prostate luminal cells, such as *KLK3* (PSA), *TMPRSS2*, *FKBP5*, in EP156T epithelial cells, but endogenous AR was not induced [3]. One possible explanation of the very restricted expression of AR could be that its expression is selected against because of its ability to induce terminal luminal cell differentiation in the presence of androgen in this context. It is additionally noteworthy that in the mesenchymal context of EPT3 cells in this model, exogenous AR expression and androgen are unable to induce the AR target genes that are readily induced by this treatment in epithelial EP156T cells [3].

Prostate Cancer Cell Lines

LNCaP, PC3, and DU145 and their metastatic derivatives are still the most widely used human prostate cancer cell lines despite the length of time these "classical" cell lines have been in culture since isolated from human metastases [10, 19, 35–39]. It has proven to be difficult to establish stable cell lines from primary prostate cancer. LNCaP cells are androgen responsive in contrast to the AR negative PC3 and DU145 cell lines, but are less effective in forming tumors and metastatic colonies in mouse xenografts. Reviews summarize in vitro models of AR signaling in prostate cancer [35] and useful cell lines for mouse xenografting [38]. Among additional prostate cancer cell lines, the VCaP and DuCaP cell lines express AR and the androgen-responsive TMPRSS-ERG fusion, and the 22Rv1 cell line is considered an in vitro model of CRPC [35]. 22Rv1 cells express the androgen-independent AR splice variant denoted AR-V7 [40]. These and additional prostate cancer cell lines have provided important information on prostate cancer, but also have many limitations. With their origin in metastatic tissue and lack of exact passage history they cannot be used to recapitulate prostate carcinogenesis, and it is difficult to estimate which genetic changes are due to in vitro culture selection [10]. Thus, in one genome-wide ChIP-seq study only 3% overlap in AR binding sites were found between prostate cancer cell lines and prostate cancer tissue prior to treatment [41]. Since most cell lines were isolated from patients who had undergone treatment this could also be a factor in the differential gene expression.

In Vitro Modeling of the Prostate Cancer Microenvironment and 3-Dimensional (3D) Growth Conditions

Cancer cells develop, proliferate, and invade in crosstalk with a microenvironment consisting of fibroblasts, immune cells, vessels, and nerves embedded in a connective tissue matrix (Fig. 26.1). Both gene expression and functional properties have been shown to differ between the same cells cultured in 3-dimensional (3D) compared to 2D cultures, and with 3D conditions corresponding better to the in vivo features and with the advantage when models are sought for drug discovery and development. Many models recapitulate selected aspects of cancer growth in 3D or microenvironment conditions [42–45]. One simple experimental approximation to the in vivo situation is to co-culture prostate cancer cells and stromal cells in monolayer or double layers. Primary and stable cell lines can be embedded in a variety of matrix materials, e.g., collagen, fibronectin, vitronectin, or commercially available gels, such as Matrigel or Geltrex or alternatively synthetically bioengineered scaffolds that may support 3D growth of both benign and malignant prostate cells [46, 47].

Several techniques are available to support the 3D spheroid growth of prostate cells with or without extracellular matrices. When grown on surfaces with ultralow attachment, prostate cells tend to form spheroids or prostaspheres resulting in the enrichment of cells with stem cell features [29]. Spheroids grown either in the extracellular matrix or in ultralow attachment plates or as hanging drops may all reproduce the nutrition, oxygen, and pH gradients that are found in cancer tissues that outgrow their blood supply [48–52].

Nanotechnology applied on bioreactors and lab-on-a-chip solutions is a developing field [43]. The potential advantages are to standardize experimental conditions, such as stiffness, shear stress, hydrostatic pressure, and concentration gradients, and by miniaturization to save on patient samples and reagents. Inbuilt sensor mechanisms could increase sensitivity and reduce analyses time [53, 54]. So far microfluidics, lab- or organ-on-a-chip and bioreactors have nevertheless not been widely applied in prostate cancer experimental models. Disadvantages include the cost and labor to establish such systems. A prostate-on-a-chip system to mimic the functional epithelial-stromal interface lining the ductal systems of a human prostate gland was recently reported [55]. 3D and even 4D bioprinting aiming to establish physiologically relevant tissue models promise future potential [56–58]. 4D bioprinting infers that printed biomaterials are able to relevant change of their shape or function over time as a response to developmental or external stimuli [59, 60].

Organoid Cultures Versus Tissue Explants

Both tissue culture explants and organoids are highly useful 3D experimental models whenever patient tissues are available. Ex vivo tissue explants are thin slices or sections of surgical cancer tissue in short-term cultures [48, 61–63]. It is possible to cut slices manually using a razor blade or scalpel, but commercial microslicers and microchoppers can prepare more standardized and thinner slices down to the micrometer scale [62]. Neighboring slices may then be processed for histology or immunohistochemistry to validate representative tissue. The advantage of tissue explants is that they preserve most of the features of the tissue architecture as well as its heterogeneity, although it is difficult to maintain and propagate the cultures for more than a few weeks. Ex vivo explants can be useful for hormone and drug testing. This model has potential usefulness in designing personalized medicine and in experiments that assay morphological or signal pathway changes in a tissue context.

The basis of organoid cultures is the availability of a matrix that supports 3D growth in vitro and an essential cocktail of compounds that modulate defined signal transduction pathways. In this way, adult stem cells have been able to differentiate and self-organize into organoids that retain many features of the organ of origin [64, 65]. Organoid culture technology has significantly improved the success rate of establishing in vitro cultures of cancer cells [66]. Organoid

technology has successfully generated benign epithelial prostate cultures [25, 67] and cultures that represent different subtypes of prostate cancer [68]. Prostate organoids have been established from metastatic cells, though the establishment of in vitro cultures of primary prostate cancer cells remains a challenge [26, 68]. Organoid cultures have the additional advantage of being able to be propagated indefinitely and can be stored in liquid nitrogen as a living biobank. Compared to monolayer cultures of stable cancer cell lines, organoid cultures may recapitulate more features of original cancer although more experience needs to be gathered regarding the extent and for how many passages essential aspects of the original tumor can be preserved. The outcome will be very important for the use of organoids in personalized medicine in order to test drug sensitivity in vitro and to have an expandable antigen source that may be exploited in individualized immunoassays and dendritic cell-based vaccine development in the immunotherapy field. In prostate cancer experimental research the availability of organoids established from distinct cancer subtypes should facilitate investigation of critical molecular signaling pathways. Tissue explants and organoids may find their place between traditional cell cultures and animal models [66, 69] (Fig. 26.3).

In the design of animal experiments, it should be considered whether organoids could replace traditional cell lines for ethical, cost, and capacity reasons. The CRISPR-Cas9 genome editing system has transformed genome editing by its efficiency to knock out or knock in genes in cells and animals [70–72]. When used in combination with organoid technology, CRISPR-Cas9, and additionally induced pluripotent stem cell technology, may generate attractive experimental systems with systematic manipulation of single cancer-relevant genes or combinations of genes [25, 73–75].

The main disadvantage with organoids is their limited take rate. In particular for prostate cancer, the take rate may be very low and establishment may fail in most cases. Additionally, one should be aware that critical elements of the in vivo tissue microenvironment could be missing [44, 69].

Animal Models

Animal models are useful for better understanding of how cancer cells interact with the tumor microenvironment and with the entire organism during metastasis. Spontaneous development of prostate cancer is relatively common in dogs and some rat strains, but less common in mouse strains. Mouse models can be broadly divided into xenograft models and genetically engineered models [76]. While immunodeficient mouse strains are critical for xenograft models, the current interest in immunotherapy has increased the demand for immunocompetent (syngeneic) and humanized mouse models [49, 77].

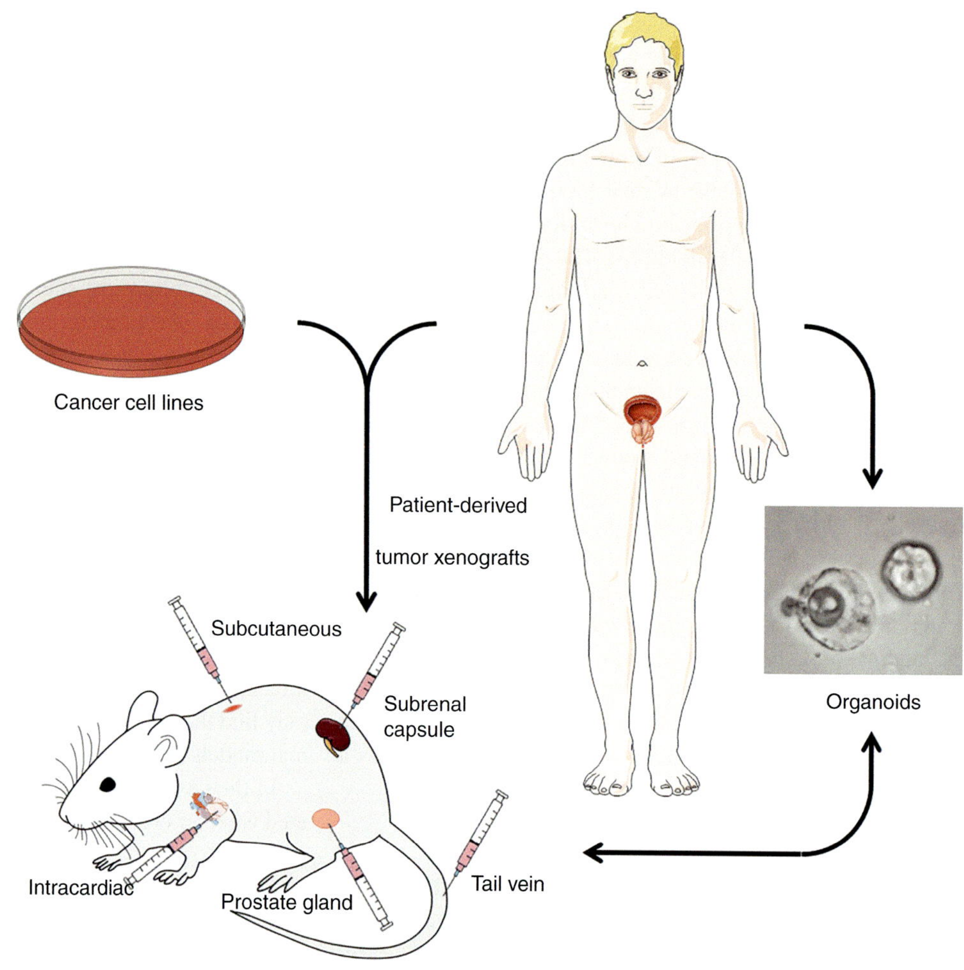

Fig. 26.3 Prostate cancer cell lines have most commonly been used for mouse xenograft models. Patient-derived xenografts (PDXs) have several advantages in retaining heterogeneity and features of original cancer tissue. Organoids can be established directly from prostate cancer tissues or via PDXs and vice versa. Patient derived organoids (PDOs) have advantages when it comes to capacity and biobanking and several experimental types. In the panel to the right are shown short-term organoids grown from a primary prostate cancer core biopsy obtained at our Haukeland University Hospital from a patient in a Phase I Clinical Trial of cryoimmunotherapy against metastatic castration resistant prostate cancer

Mouse Xenograft Models

Xenografts can be grown from any tumorigenic prostate cell culture or pieces of tissue. LNCaP, PC3, and DU145 are the three most commonly used prostate cancer cell lines in xenograft models and have provided insight into disease biology, but with limitations [10, 78]. Technically, the simplest approach is to inject tumorigenic cells subcutaneously with or without an intercellular matrix support, such as Matrigel. Tail vein injection or technically more demanding orthotopic injection into the prostate gland may be advantageous to answer questions related to metastasis and stromal invasion. Sub-renal capsular injection of cells that are otherwise difficult to graft may be successful in part due to the high vascularization at this site. Tissue recombination models in which dissociated adult prostate cells are combined with embryonic urogenital sinus mesenchymal cells and implanted under the renal capsule have been useful for cell differentiation studies and epithelial-stroma interactions [44, 79].

The choice of mouse strain, and in particular the extent of immunodeficiency, may also affect the efficiency of xenograft formation. The "nude" mouse was first established more than 40 years ago, and the advancement of immunodeficient mice to model human tumor growth has been reviewed [44, 80].

Patient Derived Xenografts

Although cell culture-based xenografts may provide useful information on cancer biology, these models have important limitations. In recent years the cancer research field has become highly aware of the importance of cancer cell heterogeneity which cannot be recapitulated by available cell culture-based xenografts. Patient-derived tumor xenografts (PDX) have emerged as a powerful technology: capable of retaining the molecular heterogeneity of their originating sample and have been shown to exhibit genomic clonal dynamics reminiscent of their originating tumor sample [81–83]. In contrast to cell-based xenografts, PDXs have original tumor morphology. PDXs have the potential to improve basic research on cancer subtypes with specific genomic lesions and could provide mouse avatars in personalized medicine drug evaluation and co-clinical trials [44, 83–85]. The establishment of prostate cancer PDXs is still challenging, with a take rate of 10–40% and prolonged latency time, although immunodeficient mice have proved very helpful to establish serially transplantable PDXs [49, 74]. Relevant stromal or immune drivers of malignant progression could, however, be missing when immunodeficient mice are used as recipients [82].

Genetically Engineered Mouse Models (GEMMS)

In genetically engineered mouse models (GEMMs) selected genes are introduced or deleted in order to study the effect of defined pathways on carcinogenesis and tumor progression [39, 76, 86–91]. Advantages compared to xenografted mouse models are that GEMMs are compatible with intact immune systems and stromal microenvironments of the same species as the tumor. The limitation of GEMMs is related to differences between mouse and men, regarding prostate architecture, cancer propensity in rodents and the small size of mice compared to humans. The TRAMP model is one of the most commonly used early transgenic models [39, 92]. The model was generated by the introduction of a gene construct with the minimal rat probasin promoter driving expression of the SV40 virus early region. Androgen-responsive expression of the SV40 large T antigen inhibits p53 and Rb and the small t antigen inhibits protein phosphatase 2A [88]. C57BL/6 TRAMP mice develop prostatic intraepithelial neoplasia (PIN) by 3 months of age. PIN typically progresses to neuroendocrine carcinoma within half a year with lymph nodes and lungs as metastatic predilection sites. The model has been extensively used in preclinical testing and studies on carcinogenesis and tumor progression, but several limitations exist [39, 88, 89]. DNA virus oncoproteins, such as SV40 large T antigen or Human papilloma virus E6 or E7, have a special power to force cancer development, but these viruses have not been shown to induce prostate cancer. Furthermore, neuroendocrine differentiation is a feature of end-stage human prostate cancer and is seen in less than 2% of primary human cancers [14]. Furthermore, TRAMP mice rarely develop bone metastases, a common event in human patients.

The LADY model provides a modification compared to the TRAMP model by using a larger region of the rat probasin promoter to drive the SV40 large T antigen expression without small t antigen. Thereby a panel of less aggressive tumor lines, collectively referred to as LADY, was generated to study cancer-preventing factors and the synergistic effects of different oncogenes [39, 76, 86–88, 90].

Transgenic mouse models have since been generated to study signal transduction pathways involved in prostate carcinogenesis and progression in humans. Overexpression of the transcription factor MYC is prevalent in early prostate cancer [93], overexpression of which immortalizes primary prostate cells, induces PIN in normal prostate tissue, and stimulates the growth of both early-stage and CRPC [94, 95]. Mouse models of prostate cancer based on c-Myc have been reviewed [39, 76, 86–89, 96].

The most frequently mutated single genes in primary prostate cancers are *SPOP, TP53, FOXA1* and *PTEN* [97]. In one analysis of 333 primary prostate carcinomas, 15% harbored homozygous deletions spanning the *PTEN* locus [98]. The homozygotic knockout of *Pten* is lethal in mouse embryos, while heterozygotic knockout results in a spectrum of prostate phenotypes that, combined with other genetic lesions, such as p27$^{Kip1-/-}$ or Nkx3.1$^{-/-}$ mice, result in the progression to PIN and invasive prostate cancer [86]. The health problems associated with *Pten* knockout mice and the value of this genetic background in the study of additional genes and pathways in prostate cancer have encouraged the development of several conditional *Pten* knockout mouse models [39, 76, 86–90, 96].

A system that introduces genes directly into the prostate glands of mice using tissue electroporation was used to study WNT signaling in prostate cancer metastasis [99].

Genomic Editing of Mouse Models

Traditional GEMMs have exploited genetic engineering and homologous recombination of embryonic stem cells followed by injection of the manipulated stem cells into wild-type blastocysts. Selected chimeric mice are then crossed to generate single-gene knockout or double-mutant mice [100]. Genetic elements that allow inducible gene expression [101], such as tetracycline inducible element, or conditional knockout [102], such as the Cre-Lox system, or knock-in [103], have further expanded the utility of GEMMs [104]. The generation of these useful models has, however, been costly and time-consuming. The CRISPR-Cas9 genome editing system may lead to a breakthrough in easy, fast and effective generation of precision mouse cancer models [75, 100, 105].

Prostate Neuroendocrine Tumor Models

Small-cell neuroendocrine carcinoma is a rare form of primary prostate cancer [14]. When the common acinar adenocarcinoma has reached the stage of CRPC it can often still be efficiently targeted by AR inhibiting compounds, such as enzalutamide and darolutamide, and androgen synthesis inhibitor abiraterone. Tumor relapse is, however, the eventual outcome and often in the form of aggressive neuroendocrine cancer. Neuroendocrine trans-differentiation may provide important clues to the nature of putative prostate CSCs. Recently, high-resolution single-cell RNA sequencing has uncovered mechanisms of neuroendocrine differentiation [6, 11, 106]. Models of neuroendocrine prostate cancer, such as xenograft and genetically engineered mouse models, are of increasing importance [14, 15, 34, 107]. The TRAMP model described above generates neuroendocrine mouse tumors [39].

Bone Metastasis Models

The bone is a predilection site for metastases of prostate cancer resulting in high morbidity associated with late stages of this disease [108–110]. Dogs spontaneously may develop benign prostate hyperplasia and prostate cancer with osteoblastic bone metastases similar to the natural course of prostate cancer in men [111]. DPC-1, Ace-1, Leo and Probasco represent four dog cell lines available for research on bone metastases, including xenograft models. The human prostate cancer cell line PC3 also forms bone metastases in xenograft models. A mouse model of bone metastasis was generated by grafting human lung and bone tissue followed by tail vein injection of LNCaP cells. The LNCaP cells preferentially metastasized to the human bone tissue [112]. A 3D in-vitro model to examine bone metastatic prostate cancer under dynamic conditions has been reported [113]. Available prostate cell lines and xenograft models of prostate bone metastases have been reviewed [42, 110, 114].

Spontaneous Cancer Development

In general, mice do not develop spontaneous prostate cancer with an incidence that makes them useful prostate cancer models. ApcMin/+ mice, which were originally selected from randomly mutagenized mice, develop multiple intestinal neoplasia (min), presumably due to *Apc* gene inactivation and consequently β-catenin activation [115]. It has been shown that up to 40% of male ApcMin/+ mice developed histological features of both PIN and prostate carcinoma at 5 to 6 months of age, thus mimicking the early stages of prostate cancer in aging men [116] making this an interesting model not only for intestinal tumors, but also for prostate cancer [117].

Several rat models are prone to spontaneous or chemically induced prostate cancer [76, 114]. Almost one-third of Lobund-Wistar rats develop spontaneous androgen-sensitive metastatic prostate adenocarcinomas at a mean age of 26 months. These tumors subsequently become androgen independent and metastasize primarily to the lung. The model has been useful in studies of chemical and dietary effects on carcinogenesis [118].

Dog Models

Many breeds of domestic dogs are prone to develop spontaneous age-dependent benign prostatic hyperplasia (BPH, high-grade prostatic intraepithelial neoplasia, and invasive prostate cancer [114, 119–121]. Development of bone metastases with mixed osteoblastic and osteolytic lesions, and the emergence of new woven bone in the later stages of prostate cancer are similarities shared between dogs and humans [122]. The use of next-generation sequencing and a greater level, and depth, of information generated by large-scale sequencing of human prostate cancers [98] could increase the utility of dog models in studies of the relevance of selected genes in cancer development and progression. Dog breeding records would facilitate association analysis and family-based linkage studies [119].

Pet dogs could be valuable in preparing for Phase I Clinical Trials of novel targeted therapies, immunotherapies, and personalized innovative combination therapies. When considering the dog model, potential advantages, such as animal size and the propensity of skeletal metastases, should be balanced against potential limitations. Specifically, in contrast to what has been observed in castrated humans, castration of dogs does not seem to protect against development of prostate cancer. Additionally, the effect of androgen deprivation therapy may differ between human and dog prostate cancers [114].

Model Organisms

The zebrafish and fruit fly models have become useful in cancer research [123, 124]. These model organisms are particularly useful in the study of defined oncogenes and signal transduction pathways. The zebrafish has become a widely used model organism for prostate cancer research with several advantages regarding optical clarity, fecundity, rapid embryo development, and absence of immune system development until 14 days post-fertilization. Genomic tools have made possible disease modeling and large phenotype-based screens in zebrafish models [124]. The zebrafish model offers a rapid and inexpensive means of evaluating the metastatic potential of prostate cancer cells. By injection into the perivitelline space of 2 day old embryos, DU145 prostate cancer cells can be found throughout the body after only 24–48 h, and knockdown of WASF3 led to suppression of metastasis in zebrafish [125]. In addition, the zebrafish model can be used for identification of prostate tumor initiating cells from cultured cells and primary prostate cancer cells and shows advantages over mouse models in prediction of therapy response, because its translucent nature allows non-invasive observation of tumor progression in real time [126].

Zebrafish might also provide an excellent vertebrate tool to accelerate cancer drug discovery and development, including high-throughput screening, toxicology, and target identification. In our group, we have evaluated compounds that inhibit Wnt/β-catenin signaling in vivo using a transgenic zebrafish harboring the Tcf/Lef-miniP:dGFP reporter [127]. Imaging of the fluorescent protein reporter allows real-time determination of drug potency, targeting specificity and body toxicity in vivo.

Cancer Immunotherapy and Co-Culture Models

Cancer immunotherapy represents a most encouraging breakthrough during the last decade. Prostate cancer is, however, not among the solid tumors that has responded best to immune checkpoint inhibitors or other immunotherapy and has been considered an immunologically "cold" cancer type. Experimental in vitro models to investigate interactions between immune cells and cancers are improving [128]. Several published models could potentially be applied on prostate cancer. Co-cultures of autologous tumor organoids and peripheral blood lymphocytes were used to study invasion and attack of cytotoxic lymphocytes on cancer cells [129, 130]. Additional examples are provided by the effect on cancer stem cells in co-cultures with dendritic cells and immune cells [131] and assays of co-cultures between dendritic cells and keratinocytes [132]. Co-culture systems for exploring cancer immunology has been reviewed [133–135].

Animal models for experimental cancer immunotherapy pose challenges due to differences between human and mouse immune systems and because immunodeficient mice have been extensively used to establish xenografts, but relevant immune competent and humanized animal models are improving [136–139].

Future Perspectives

Multiple experimental and preclinical models are available and under development for future prostate cancer research. Presently, no single experimental model can capture all features of the complicated biology and evolution that is ongoing in patient with prostate cancer. Mice represent the most common animal model in drug discovery and preclinical development [140], but the small size of the mouse may have its disadvantages as a tumor model. Even large tumor masses in mice could have a volume one thousand-fold smaller than a human tumor of the same stage. Consequently, the cancer cell number would be proportionately lower in mice tumors and the cancer cell heterogeneity problem could be underes-

timated. This could be one reason why mouse tumors often have a higher cure rate than what is found in subsequent clinical testing in patients. The trend nevertheless is that the repertoire and sophistication of experimental models are advancing, and so are high-resolution methods, such as single-cell sequencing and mass cytometry, that may offer fresh looks if previously established models are revisited. In silico modeling is another developing field [135, 141].

Ultimately, the choice of model should be carefully evaluated during experimental design to secure optimal scientific results with due attention given to statistics, ethics, capacity, and costs.

References[1]

1. Lamb LE, Knudsen BS, Miranti CK. E-cadherin-mediated survival of androgen-receptor-expressing secretory prostate epithelial cells derived from a stratified in vitro differentiation model. J Cell Sci. 2010;123(Pt 2):266–76.
2. Antony L, van der Schoor F, Dalrymple SL, Isaacs JT. Androgen receptor (AR) suppresses normal human prostate epithelial cell proliferation via AR/beta-catenin/TCF-4 complex inhibition of c-MYC transcription. Prostate. 2014;74(11):1118–31.
3. Olsen JR, Azeem W, Hellem MR, Marvyin K, Hua Y, Qu Y, et al. Context dependent regulatory patterns of the androgen receptor and androgen receptor target genes. BMC Cancer. 2016;16:377.
4. Lee SH, Shen MM. Cell types of origin for prostate cancer. Curr Opin Cell Biol. 2015;37:35–41.
5. Strand DW, Goldstein AS. The many ways to make a luminal cell and a prostate cancer cell. Endocr Relat Cancer. 2015;22(6):T187–97.
6. Dong B, Miao J, Wang Y, Luo W, Ji Z, Lai H, et al. Single-cell analysis supports a luminal-neuroendocrine transdifferentiation in human prostate cancer. Commun Biol. 2020;3(1):778.
7. Karthaus WR, Hofree M, Choi D, Linton EL, Turkekul M, Bejnood A, et al. Regenerative potential of prostate luminal cells revealed by single-cell analysis. Science. 2020;368(6490):497–505.
8. Kwon OJ, Zhang L, Jia D, Zhou Z, Li Z, Haffner M, et al. De novo induction of lineage plasticity from human prostate luminal epithelial cells by activated AKT1 and c-Myc. Oncogene. 2020;39(48):7142–51.
9. Li JJ, Shen MM. Prostate stem cells and cancer stem cells. Cold Spring Harb Perspect Med 2019;9(6).
10. Maitland NJ. Resistance to antiandrogens in prostate cancer: is it inevitable, intrinsic or induced? Cancers. 2021;13(2)
11. Park JW, Lee JK, Sheu KM, Wang L, Balanis NG, Nguyen K, et al. Reprogramming normal human epithelial tissues to a common, lethal neuroendocrine cancer lineage. Science. 2018;362(6410):91–5.
12. Guo W, Li L, He J, Liu Z, Han M, Li F, et al. Single-cell transcriptomics identifies a distinct luminal progenitor cell type in distal prostate invagination tips. Nat Genet. 2020;52(9):908–18.
13. Watson PA, Arora VK, Sawyers CL. Emerging mechanisms of resistance to androgen receptor inhibitors in prostate cancer. Nat Rev Cancer 2015.
14. Berman-Booty LD, Knudsen KE. Models of neuroendocrine prostate cancer. Endocr Relat Cancer. 2015;22(1):R33–49.

[1]Space constraints allow only for selected references.

15. Terry S, Beltran H. The many faces of neuroendocrine differentiation in prostate cancer progression. Front Oncol. 2014;4:60.

16. Rane JK, Pellacani D, Maitland NJ. Advanced prostate cancer--a case for adjuvant differentiation therapy. Nat Rev Urol. 2012;9(10):595–602.

17. Rhim JS, Li H, Furusato B. Novel human prostate epithelial cell culture models for the study of carcinogenesis and of normal stem cells and cancer stem cells. Adv Exp Med Biol. 2011;720:71–80.

18. Sobel RE, Wang Y, Sadar MD. Molecular analysis and characterization of PrEC, commercially available prostate epithelial cells. In Vitro Cell Dev Biol Anim. 2006;42(1–2):33–9.

19. van Bokhoven A, Varella-Garcia M, Korch C, Johannes WU, Smith EE, Miller HL, et al. Molecular characterization of human prostate carcinoma cell lines. Prostate. 2003;57(3):205–25.

20. Litvinov IV, Vander Griend DJ, Xu Y, Antony L, Dalrymple SL, Isaacs JT. Low-calcium serum-free defined medium selects for growth of normal prostatic epithelial stem cells. Cancer Res. 2006;66(17):8598–607.

21. Yasunaga Y, Nakamura K, Ewing CM, Isaacs WB, Hukku B, Rhim JS. A novel human cell culture model for the study of familial prostate cancer. Cancer Res. 2001;61(16):5969–73.

22. Kogan I, Goldfinger N, Milyavsky M, Cohen M, Shats I, Dobler G, et al. hTERT-immortalized prostate epithelial and stromal-derived cells: an authentic in vitro model for differentiation and carcinogenesis. Cancer Res. 2006;66(7):3531–40.

23. Bello D, Webber MM, Kleinman HK, Wartinger DD, Rhim JS. Androgen responsive adult human prostatic epithelial cell lines immortalized by human papillomavirus 18. Carcinogenesis. 1997;18(6):1215–23.

24. Jiang M, Strand DW, Fernandez S, He Y, Yi Y, Birbach A, et al. Functional remodeling of benign human prostatic tissues in vivo by spontaneously immortalized progenitor and intermediate cells. Stem Cells. 2010;28(2):344–56.

25. Karthaus WR, Iaquinta PJ, Drost J, Gracanin A, van Boxtel R, Wongvipat J, et al. Identification of multipotent luminal progenitor cells in human prostate organoid cultures. Cell. 2014;159(1):163–75.

26. Palechor-Ceron N, Suprynowicz FA, Upadhyay G, Dakic A, Minas T, Simic V, et al. Radiation induces diffusible feeder cell factor(s) that cooperate with ROCK inhibitor to conditionally reprogram and immortalize epithelial cells. Am J Pathol. 2013;183(6):1862–70.

27. Ke XS, Qu Y, Goldfinger N, Rostad K, Hovland R, Akslen LA, et al. Epithelial to mesenchymal transition of a primary prostate cell line with switches of cell adhesion modules but without malignant transformation. PLoS One. 2008;3(10):e3368.

28. Ke XS, Li WC, Hovland R, Qu Y, Liu RH, McCormack E, et al. Reprogramming of cell junction modules during stepwise epithelial to mesenchymal transition and accumulation of malignant features in vitro in a prostate cell model. Exp Cell Res. 2011;317(2):234–47.

29. Qu Y, Oyan AM, Liu R, Hua Y, Zhang J, Hovland R, et al. Generation of prostate tumor-initiating cells is associated with elevation of reactive oxygen species and IL-6/STAT3 signaling. Cancer Res. 2013;73(23):7090–100.

30. Ke XS, Qu Y, Cheng Y, Li WC, Rotter V, Oyan AM, et al. Global profiling of histone and DNA methylation reveals epigenetic-based regulation of gene expression during epithelial to mesenchymal transition in prostate cells. BMC Genomics. 2010;11:669.

31. Gravdal K, Halvorsen OJ, Haukaas SA, Akslen LA. A switch from E-cadherin to N-cadherin expression indicates epithelial to mesenchymal transition and is of strong and independent importance for the progress of prostate cancer. Clin Cancer Res. 2007;13(23):7003–11.

32. Xie D, Gore C, Liu J, Pong RC, Mason R, Hao G, et al. Role of DAB2IP in modulating epithelial-to-mesenchymal transition and prostate cancer metastasis. Proc Natl Acad Sci U S A. 2010;107(6):2485–90.

33. Jadaan DY, Jadaan MM, McCabe JP. Cellular plasticity in prostate cancer bone metastasis. Prostate Cancer. 2015;2015:651580.

34. Nouri M, Ratther E, Stylianou N, Nelson CC, Hollier BG, Williams ED. Androgen-targeted therapy-induced epithelial mesenchymal plasticity and neuroendocrine transdifferentiation in prostate cancer: an opportunity for intervention. Front Oncol. 2014;4:370.

35. Sampson N, Neuwirt H, Puhr M, Klocker H, Eder IE. In vitro model systems to study androgen receptor signaling in prostate cancer. Endocr Relat Cancer. 2013;20(2):R49–64.

36. Sobel RE, Sadar MD. Cell lines used in prostate cancer research: a compendium of old and new lines--part 2. J Urol. 2005;173(2):360–72.

37. Sobel RE, Sadar MD. Cell lines used in prostate cancer research: a compendium of old and new lines--part 1. J Urol. 2005;173(2):342–59.

38. Wu X, Gong S, Roy-Burman P, Lee P, Culig Z. Current mouse and cell models in prostate cancer research. Endocr Relat Cancer. 2013;20(4):R155–70.

39. Saranyutanon S, Deshmukh SK, Dasgupta S, Pai S, Singh S, Singh AP. Cellular and molecular progression of prostate cancer: models for basic and preclinical research. Cancers. 2020;12(9).

40. Lu J, Van der Steen T, Tindall DJ. Are androgen receptor variants a substitute for the full-length receptor? Nat Rev Urol. 2015;12(3):137–44.

41. Sharma NL, Massie CE, Ramos-Montoya A, Zecchini V, Scott HE, Lamb AD, et al. The androgen receptor induces a distinct transcriptional program in castration-resistant prostate cancer in man. Cancer Cell. 2013;23(1):35–47.

42. Costard LS, Hosn RR, Ramanayake H, O'Briena BCF, Curtin CM. Influences of the 3D microenvironment on cancer cell behaviour and treatment responsiveness: a recent update on lung, breast and prostate cancer models. Acta Biomater 2021.

43. Fernandes DC, Canadas RF, Reis RL, Oliveira JM. Dynamic culture systems and 3D interfaces models for cancer drugs testing. Adv Exp Med Biol. 2020;1230:137–59.

44. Kato M, Sasaki T, Inoue T. Current experimental human tissue-derived models for prostate cancer research. Int J Urol. 2021;28(2):150–62.

45. Linxweiler J, Hammer M, Muhs S, Kohn M, Pryalukhin A, Veith C, et al. Patient-derived, three-dimensional spheroid cultures provide a versatile translational model for the study of organ-confined prostate cancer. J Cancer Res Clin Oncol. 2019;145(3):551–9.

46. Lopes D, Fernandes C, Nobrega JM, Patricio SG, Oliveira MB, Mano JF. Screening of perfused combinatorial 3D microenvironments for cell culture. Acta Biomater. 2019;96:222–36.

47. Unal AZ, West JL. Synthetic ECM: bioactive synthetic hydrogels for 3D tissue engineering. Bioconjug Chem. 2020;31(10):2253–71.

48. Ellem SJ, De-Juan-Pardo EM, Risbridger GP. In vitro modeling of the prostate cancer microenvironment. Adv Drug Deliv Rev. 2014;79-80:214–21.

49. Namekawa T, Ikeda K, Horie-Inoue K, Inoue S. Application of prostate cancer models for preclinical study: advantages and limitations of cell lines, patient-derived xenografts, and three-dimensional culture of patient-derived cells. Cell 2019;8(1).

50. Kim SJ, Kim EM, Yamamoto M, Park H, Shin H. Engineering multi-cellular spheroids for tissue engineering and regenerative medicine. Adv Healthc Mater. 2020:e2000608.

51. Fontana F, Raimondi M, Marzagalli M, Sommariva M, Gagliano N, Limonta P. Three-dimensional cell cultures as an in vitro tool for prostate cancer modeling and drug discovery. Int J Mol Sci. 2020;21(18).

52. Rodriguez-Dorantes M, Cruz-Hernandez CD, Cortes-Ramirez SA, Cruz-Burgos JM, Reyes-Grajeda JP, Peralta-Zaragoza O, et al.

Prostate cancer spheroids: a three-dimensional model for studying tumor heterogeneity. Methods Mol Biol. 2021;2174:13–7.

53. Han SJ, Park HK, Kim KS. Applications of microfluidic devices for urology. Int Neurourol J. 2017;21(Suppl 1):S4–9.

54. Egger D, Fischer M, Clementi A, Ribitsch V, Hansmann J, Kasper C. Development and characterization of a parallelizable perfusion bioreactor for 3D cell culture. Bioengineering (Basel) 2017;4(2).

55. Jiang L, Ivich F, Tahsin S, Tran M, Frank SB, Miranti CK, et al. Human stroma and epithelium co-culture in a microfluidic model of a human prostate gland. Biomicrofluidics. 2019;13(6):064116.

56. Pavlovich MJ, Hunsberger J, Atala A. Biofabrication: a secret weapon to advance manufacturing, economies, and healthcare. Trends Biotechnol. 2016;34(9):679–80.

57. Dey M, Ozbolat IT. 3D bioprinting of cells, tissues and organs. Sci Rep. 2020;10(1):14023.

58. Gebeyehu A, Surapaneni SK, Huang J, Mondal A, Wang VZ, Haruna NF, et al. Polysaccharide hydrogel based 3D printed tumor models for chemotherapeutic drug screening. Sci Rep. 2021;11(1):372.

59. Peng W, Unutmaz D, Ozbolat IT. Bioprinting towards physiologically relevant tissue models for pharmaceutics. Trends Biotechnol. 2016;34(9):722–32.

60. Shah Mohammadi M, Buchen JT, Pasquina PF, Niklason L, Alvarez LM, Jariwala SH. Critical considerations for regeneration of vascularized composite tissues. Tissue Eng Part B Rev 2020.

61. Centenera MM, Raj GV, Knudsen KE, Tilley WD, Butler LM. Ex vivo culture of human prostate tissue and drug development. Nat Rev Urol. 2013;10(8):483–7.

62. Rosales Gerpe MC, van Vloten JP, Santry LA, de Jong J, Mould RC, Pelin A, et al. Use of precision-cut lung slices as an ex vivo tool for evaluating viruses and viral vectors for gene and oncolytic therapy. Mol Ther Methods Clin Dev. 2018;10:245–56.

63. Tieu T, Irani S, Bremert KL, Ryan NK, Wojnilowicz M, Helm M, et al. Patient-derived prostate cancer explants: a clinically relevant model to assess siRNA-based nanomedicines. Adv Healthc Mater 2020:e2001594.

64. Jung P, Sato T, Merlos-Suarez A, Barriga FM, Iglesias M, Rossell D, et al. Isolation and in vitro expansion of human colonic stem cells. Nat Med. 2011;17(10):1225–7.

65. Sato T, Vries RG, Snippert HJ, van de Wetering M, Barker N, Stange DE, et al. Single Lgr5 stem cells build crypt-villus structures in vitro without a mesenchymal niche. Nature. 2009;459(7244):262–5.

66. Sachs N, Clevers H. Organoid cultures for the analysis of cancer phenotypes. Curr Opin Genet Dev. 2014;24:68–73.

67. Chua CW, Shibata M, Lei M, Toivanen R, Barlow LJ, Bergren SK, et al. Single luminal epithelial progenitors can generate prostate organoids in culture. Nat Cell Biol 2014;16(10):951–61, 1–4.

68. Gao D, Vela I, Sboner A, Iaquinta PJ, Karthaus WR, Gopalan A, et al. Organoid cultures derived from patients with advanced prostate cancer. Cell. 2014;159(1):176–87.

69. Gleave AM, Ci X, Lin D, Wang Y. A synopsis of prostate organoid methodologies, applications, and limitations. Prostate. 2020;80(6):518–26.

70. Cho SW, Kim S, Kim JM, Kim JS. Targeted genome engineering in human cells with the Cas9 RNA-guided endonuclease. Nat Biotechnol. 2013;31(3):230–2.

71. Cong L, Ran FA, Cox D, Lin S, Barretto R, Habib N, et al. Multiplex genome engineering using CRISPR/Cas systems. Science. 2013;339(6121):819–23.

72. Mali P, Yang L, Esvelt KM, Aach J, Guell M, DiCarlo JE, et al. RNA-guided human genome engineering via Cas9. Science. 2013;339(6121):823–6.

73. Drost J, van Jaarsveld RH, Ponsioen B, Zimberlin C, van Boxtel R, Buijs A, et al. Sequential cancer mutations in cultured human intestinal stem cells. Nature. 2015;521(7550):43–7.

74. Hepburn AC, Sims CHC, Buskin A, Heer R. Engineering prostate cancer from induced pluripotent stem cells-new opportunities to develop preclinical tools in prostate and prostate cancer studies. Int J Mol Sci 2020;21(3).

75. Hazafa A, Mumtaz M, Farooq MF, Bilal S, Chaudhry SN, Firdous M, et al. CRISPR/Cas9: a powerful genome editing technique for the treatment of cancer cells with present challenges and future directions. Life Sci. 2020;263:118525.

76. Ittmann M, Huang J, Radaelli E, Martin P, Signoretti S, Sullivan R, et al. Animal models of human prostate cancer: the consensus report of the New York meeting of the mouse models of human cancers consortium prostate pathology committee. Cancer Res. 2013;73(9):2718–36.

77. Wang M, Yao LC, Cheng M, Cai D, Martinek J, Pan CX, et al. Humanized mice in studying efficacy and mechanisms of PD-1-targeted cancer immunotherapy. FASEB J. 2018;32(3):1537–49.

78. Toivanen R, Taylor RA, Pook DW, Ellem SJ, Risbridger GP. Breaking through a roadblock in prostate cancer research: an update on human model systems. J Steroid Biochem. 2012;131(3–5):122–31.

79. Zong Y, Goldstein AS, Witte ON. Dissociated prostate regeneration under the renal capsule. Cold Spring Harb Protoc 2015;2015(11):pdb prot078063.

80. Shultz LD, Goodwin N, Ishikawa F, Hosur V, Lyons BL, Greiner DL. Human cancer growth and therapy in immunodeficient mouse models. Cold Spring Harb Protoc. 2014;2014(7):694–708.

81. Eirew P, Steif A, Khattra J, Ha G, Yap D, Farahani H, et al. Dynamics of genomic clones in breast cancer patient xenografts at single-cell resolution. Nature. 2015;518(7539):422–6.

82. Cassidy JW, Caldas C, Bruna A. Maintaining tumor heterogeneity in patient-derived tumor xenografts. Cancer Res. 2015;75(15):2963–8.

83. Palanisamy N, Yang J, Shepherd PDA, Li-Ning-Tapia EM, Labanca E, Manyam GC, et al. The MD Anderson prostate cancer patient-derived xenograft series (MDA PCa PDX) captures the molecular landscape of prostate cancer and facilitates marker-driven therapy development. Clin Cancer Res. 2020;26(18):4933–46.

84. Malaney P, Nicosia SV, Dave V. One mouse, one patient paradigm: new avatars of personalized cancer therapy. Cancer Lett. 2014;344(1):1–12.

85. Navone NM, van Weerden WM, Vessella RL, Williams ED, Wang Y, Isaacs JT, et al. Movember GAP1 PDX project: an international collection of serially transplantable prostate cancer patient-derived xenograft (PDX) models. Prostate. 2018;78(16):1262–82.

86. Grabowska MM, DeGraff DJ, Yu X, Jin RJ, Chen Z, Borowsky AD, et al. Mouse models of prostate cancer: picking the best model for the question. Cancer Metastasis Rev. 2014;33(2–3):377–97.

87. Irshad S, Abate-Shen C. Modeling prostate cancer in mice: something old, something new, something premalignant, something metastatic. Cancer Metast Rev. 2013;32(1–2):109–22.

88. Jeet V, Russell PJ, Khatri A. Modeling prostate cancer: a perspective on transgenic mouse models. Cancer Metastasis Rev. 2010;29(1):123–42.

89. Parisotto M, Metzger D. Genetically engineered mouse models of prostate cancer. Mol Oncol. 2013;7(2):190–205.

90. Saxena M, Christofori G. Rebuilding cancer metastasis in the mouse. Mol Oncol. 2013;7(2):283–96.

91. van Marion DM, Domanska UM, Timmer-Bosscha H, Walenkamp AM. Studying cancer metastasis: Existing models, challenges and future perspectives. Crit Rev Oncol Hematol. 2015.

92. Greenberg NM, DeMayo F, Finegold MJ, Medina D, Tilley WD, Aspinall JO, et al. Prostate cancer in a transgenic mouse. Proc Natl Acad Sci U S A. 1995;92(8):3439–43.

93. Hawksworth D, Ravindranath L, Chen Y, Furusato B, Sesterhenn IA, McLeod DG, et al. Overexpression of C-MYC oncogene in

prostate cancer predicts biochemical recurrence. Prostate Cancer Prostatic Dis. 2010;13(4):311–5.

94. Gil J, Kerai P, Lleonart M, Bernard D, Cigudosa JC, Peters G, et al. Immortalization of primary human prostate epithelial cells by c-Myc. Cancer Res. 2005;65(6):2179–85.

95. Iwata T, Schultz D, Hicks J, Hubbard GK, Mutton LN, Lotan TL, et al. MYC overexpression induces prostatic intraepithelial neoplasia and loss of Nkx3.1 in mouse luminal epithelial cells. PLoS One 2010;5(2):e9427.

96. Mimeault M, Batra SK. Animal models relevant to human prostate carcinogenesis underlining the critical implication of prostatic stem/progenitor cells. Biochim Biophys Acta. 2011;1816(1):25–37.

97. Barbieri CE, Rubin MA. Molecular characterization of prostate cancer following androgen deprivation: the devil in the details. Eur Urol. 2014;66(1):40–1.

98. Cancer Genome Atlas Research Network. Electronic address scmo, Cancer Genome Atlas Research N. The Molecular Taxonomy of Primary Prostate Cancer. Cell 2015;163(4):1011–1025.

99. Leibold J, Ruscetti M, Cao Z, Ho YJ, Baslan T, Zou M, et al. Somatic tissue engineering in mouse models reveals an actionable role for WNT pathway alterations in prostate cancer metastasis. Cancer Discov. 2020;10(7):1038–57.

100. Mou HW, Kennedy Z, Anderson DG, Yin H, Xue W. Precision cancer mouse models through genome editing with CRISPR-Cas9. Genome Med 2015;7.

101. Saunders TL. Inducible transgenic mouse models. Methods Mol Biol. 2011;693:103–15.

102. Friedel RH, Wurst W, Wefers B, Kuhn R. Generating conditional knockout mice. Methods Mol Biol. 2011;693:205–31.

103. Roebroek AJ, Gordts PL, Reekmans S. Knock-in approaches. Methods Mol Biol. 2011;693:257–75.

104. Kasper S. Survey of genetically engineered mouse models for prostate cancer: analyzing the molecular basis of prostate cancer development, progression, and metastasis. J Cell Biochem. 2005;94(2):279–97.

105. Huijbers IJ. Generating genetically modified mice: a decision guide. Methods Mol Biol. 2017;1642:1–19.

106. Yamada Y, Beltran H. Clinical and biological features of neuroendocrine prostate cancer. Curr Oncol Rep. 2021;23(2):15.

107. Yu C, Hu K, Nguyen D, Wang ZA. From genomics to functions: preclinical mouse models for understanding oncogenic pathways in prostate cancer. Am J Cancer Res. 2019;9(10):2079–102.

108. Coleman RE. Clinical features of metastatic bone disease and risk of skeletal morbidity. Clin Cancer Res. 2006;12(20 Pt 2):6243s–9s.

109. Mehra R, Kumar-Sinha C, Shankar S, Lonigro RJ, Jing X, Philips NE, et al. Characterization of bone metastases from rapid autopsies of prostate cancer patients. Clin Cancer Res. 2011;17(12):3924–32.

110. Simmons JK, Hildreth BE 3rd, Supsavhad W, Elshafae SM, Hassan BB, Dirksen WP, et al. Animal models of bone metastasis. Vet Pathol. 2015;52(5):827–41.

111. LeRoy BE, Thudi NK, Nadella MV, Toribio RE, Tannehill-Gregg SH, van Bokhoven A, et al. New bone formation and osteolysis by a metastatic, highly invasive canine prostate carcinoma xenograft. Prostate. 2006;66(11):1213–22.

112. Yonou H, Yokose T, Kamijo T, Kanomata N, Hasebe T, Nagai K, et al. Establishment of a novel species- and tissue-specific metastasis model of human prostate cancer in humanized non-obese diabetic/severe combined immunodeficient mice engrafted with human adult lung and bone. Cancer Res. 2001;61(5):2177–82.

113. Jasuja H, Kar S, Katti DR, Katti K. Perfusion bioreactor enabled fluid-derived shear stress conditions for novel bone metastatic prostate cancer testbed. Biofabrication 2021.

114. Winter SF, Cooper AB, Greenberg NM. Models of metastatic prostate cancer: a transgenic perspective. Prostate Cancer Prostatic Dis. 2003;6(3):204–11.

115. Bruxvoort KJ, Charbonneau HM, Giambernardi TA, Goolsby JC, Qian CN, Zylstra CR, et al. Inactivation of Apc in the mouse prostate causes prostate carcinoma. Cancer Res. 2007;67(6):2490–6.

116. Poutahidis T, Rao VP, Olipitz W, Taylor CL, Jackson EA, Levkovich T, et al. CD4+ lymphocytes modulate prostate cancer progression in mice. Int J Cancer. 2009;125(4):868–78.

117. Valkenburg KC, Hostetter G, Williams BO. Concurrent Hepsin overexpression and adenomatous polyposis coli deletion causes invasive prostate carcinoma in mice. Prostate. 2015;75(14):1579–85.

118. Pollard M, Suckow MA. Dietary prevention of hormone refractory prostate cancer in Lobund-Wistar rats: a review of studies in a relevant animal model. Comp Med. 2006;56(6):461–7.

119. Davis BW, Ostrander EA. Domestic dogs and cancer research: a breed-based genomics approach. ILAR J. 2014;55(1):59–68.

120. Leroy BE, Northrup N. Prostate cancer in dogs: comparative and clinical aspects. Vet J. 2009;180(2):149–62.

121. Waters DJ, Bostwick DG. The canine prostate is a spontaneous model of intraepithelial neoplasia and prostate cancer progression. Anticancer Res. 1997;17(3A):1467–70.

122. Rosol TJ, Tannehill-Gregg SH, LeRoy BE, Mandl S, Contag CH. Animal models of bone metastasis. Cancer. 2003;97(3 Suppl):748–57.

123. White RM. Cross-species oncogenomics using zebrafish models of cancer. Curr Opin Genet Dev. 2015;30:73–9.

124. Amawi H, Aljabali AAA, Boddu SHS, Amawi S, Obeid MA, Ashby CR, Jr., et al. The use of zebrafish model in prostate cancer therapeutic development and discovery. Cancer Chemother Pharmacol 2021.

125. Teng Y, Xie X, Walker S, White DT, Mumm JS, Cowell JK. Evaluating human cancer cell metastasis in zebrafish. BMC Cancer. 2013;13:453.

126. Bansal N, Davis S, Tereshchenko I, Budak-Alpdogan T, Zhong H, Stein MN, et al. Enrichment of human prostate cancer cells with tumor initiating properties in mouse and zebrafish xenografts by differential adhesion. Prostate. 2014;74(2):187–200.

127. Shimizu N, Kawakami K, Ishitani T. Visualization and exploration of Tcf/Lef function using a highly responsive Wnt/beta-catenin signaling-reporter transgenic zebrafish. Dev Biol. 2012;370(1):71–85.

128. Yunger S, Bar El A, Zeltzer LA, Fridman E, Raviv G, Laufer M, et al. Tumor-infiltrating lymphocytes from human prostate tumors reveal anti-tumor reactivity and potential for adoptive cell therapy. Onco Targets Ther. 2019;8(12):e1672494.

129. Cattaneo CM, Dijkstra KK, Fanchi LF, Kelderman S, Kaing S, van Rooij N, et al. Tumor organoid-T-cell coculture systems. Nat Protoc. 2020;15(1):15–39.

130. Dijkstra KK, Cattaneo CM, Weeber F, Chalabi M, van de Haar J, Fanchi LF, et al. Generation of tumor-reactive T cells by co-culture of peripheral blood lymphocytes and tumor organoids. Cell. 2018;174(6):1586–98 e12.

131. Yang T, Zhang W, Wang L, Xiao C, Wang L, Gong Y, et al. Co-culture of dendritic cells and cytokine-induced killer cells effectively suppresses liver cancer stem cell growth by inhibiting pathways in the immune system. BMC Cancer. 2018;18(1):984.

132. Thelu A, Catoire S, Kerdine-Romer S. Immune-competent in vitro co-culture models as an approach for skin sensitisation assessment. Toxicology In Vitro. 2020;62:104691.

133. Fitzgerald AA, Li E, Weiner LM. 3D culture systems for exploring cancer immunology. Cancers 2020;13(1).

134. Ye W, Luo C, Li C, Huang J, Liu F. Organoids to study immune functions, immunological diseases and immunotherapy. Cancer Lett. 2020;477:31–40.

135. Lee MW, Miljanic M, Triplett T, Ramirez C, Aung KL, Eckhardt SG, et al. Current methods in translational cancer research. Cancer Metastasis Rev 2020.
136. Chulpanova DS, Kitaeva KV, Rutland CS, Rizvanov AA, Solovyeva VV. Mouse tumor models for advanced cancer immunotherapy. Int J Mol Sci 2020;21(11).
137. Schachtschneider KM, Schwind RM, Newson J, Kinachtchouk N, Rizko M, Mendoza-Elias N, et al. The oncopig cancer model: an innovative large animal translational oncology platform. Front Oncol. 2017;7:190.
138. Yin L, Wang XJ, Chen DX, Liu XN, Wang XJ. Humanized mouse model: a review on preclinical applications for cancer immunotherapy. Am J Cancer Res. 2020;10(12):4568–84.
139. Morillon YM 2nd, Sabzevari A, Schlom J, Greiner JW. The development of next-generation PBMC humanized mice for preclinical investigation of cancer immunotherapeutic agents. Anticancer Res. 2020;40(10):5329–41.
140. Valkenburg KC, Pienta KJ. Drug discovery in prostate cancer mouse models. Expert Opin Drug Discov. 2015;10(9):1011–24.
141. Wang Y, Xing J, Xu Y, Zhou N, Peng J, Xiong Z, et al. In silico ADME/T modelling for rational drug design. Q Rev Biophys. 2015;48(4):488–515.
142. Rostad K, Mannelqvist M, Halvorsen OJ, Oyan AM, Bo TH, Stordrange L, et al. ERG upregulation and related ETS transcription factors in prostate cancer. Int J Oncol. 2007;30(1):19–32.

Prostate Cancer Biomarkers: The Old and the New

Anette L. Magnussen and Ian G. Mills

Abstract

Triggered by the urgent need for greater accuracy in predicting the biological behaviour of diseases, foremost cancer, the search for the ideal biomarker—a molecule, gene or any other characteristic that can be objectively measured and evaluated—is relentless. The search for exemplary candidates has been encouraged by the rapid progress in profiling and detection technologies which have enhanced throughput and accuracy of protein, transcript and mutation detection. These advances are reflected in the sheer number of publications reporting discoveries and clinical evaluation of new genes or proteins of biomarker potential.

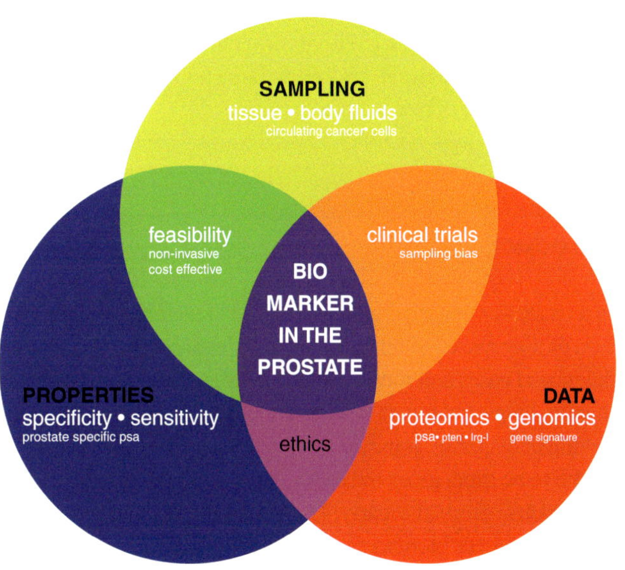

The pictured Venn—diagram suggests, in a non-mathematical sense, the relation between the three major pre-sets that determine the potential of a biological feature to become a prognostic signpost for prostate cancer. In the centre where the circles overlap in the most favourable way, we can find the perfect biomarker.

Take-Home Lessons

- Prostate cancer biomarkers can in principle have an impact in stratifying patients based on progression risk at diagnosis or to predict the risk of treatment relapse.
- Very few biomarkers have progressed into routine clinical practice and kallikreins remain, so far, the prime examples.
- Biomarker adoption and routine use requires independent validation and careful cost–benefit assessments. The latter should be a continuous process as detection technologies and data accumulate and this process therefore is costly in time and resources. This process is exemplified for PSA.

A. L. Magnussen (✉)
Nuffield Department of Surgical Sciences, University of Oxford, Oxford, UK
e-mail: anette.magnussen@nds.ox.ac.uk

I. G. Mills
Nuffield Department of Surgical Sciences, University of Oxford, Oxford, UK

Patrick G Johnston Centre for Cancer Research, Queen's University of Belfast, Belfast, UK

Centre for Cancer Biomarkers, University of Bergen, Bergen, Norway

Department of Clinical Science, University of Bergen, Bergen, Norway
e-mail: ian.mills@nds.ox.ac.uk

L. A. Akslen, R. S. Watnick (eds.), *Biomarkers of the Tumor Microenvironment*, https://doi.org/10.1007/978-3-030-98950-7_27

- By contrast the discovery of candidate biomarkers occurs with much shorter timelines and the costs of discovery research fall as profiling and detection technologies evolve.
- Transcript gene signatures detectable in tissue; mutation detection in circulating cell-free tumour DNA and the detection of circulation tumour cells exemplify biomarkers on the cusp of adoption in selected clinical contexts.
- In considering secreted protein biomarkers we exemplify their challenges and potential by describing leucine-rich glycoprotein-1, LRG-1, and its role in prostate cancer and other cancer types.
- We conclude by discussing the importance of informed patient and clinician choice in bringing biomarkers into clinical practice.

Introduction

In a cancer setting, biomarkers are needed to enhance the precision of diagnosis and disease staging as well as to prognosticate diagnosed cases and monitor disease progression. A potent biomarker helps treatment selection for patients and to monitor treatment response. It may even function as a therapeutic target. At the same time, given the nearly 40,000 references for 'cancer biomarkers' from the early 1940s to present, the number of approved cancer biomarkers is relatively small (Fig. 27.1). The disparity is, on reflection, not very surprising as the ideal biomarker has to comply with a number of high demands such as:

- originates only from tumour tissue
- highly sensitive and highly specific
- able to detect cancer at an early stage
- discriminatory between indolent and clinically significant tumours
- easily detectable by non-invasive test
- inexpensive

In reality no single biomarker will fulfil all of these criteria. Instead, the predictive value is determined by combining a series of biomarkers with other biological parameters and clinical risk factors.

Biomarkers for Prostate Cancer

Prostate cancer is the second most commonly diagnosed cancer amongst men worldwide. Statistically, one in eight men will develop prostate cancer at some time in their lives. The rate is even higher, six in ten, for men above 65 and in men of colour [1]. At the same time the overall rate of men dying from prostate cancer in the European Union, for example, is on the decline [2]. This apparent paradox is due to the wide spectrum of clinical behaviour with men surviving long enough to die of other causes and the high frequency with which relatively indolent cases are diagnosed. Such heterogeneity of clinical behaviour poses challenges for early detection of the disease. When a man is concerned about prostate cancer and seeks medical advice, two major questions arise that frame a particularly important context in which to add complementary prostate cancer biomarkers to existing detection strategies:

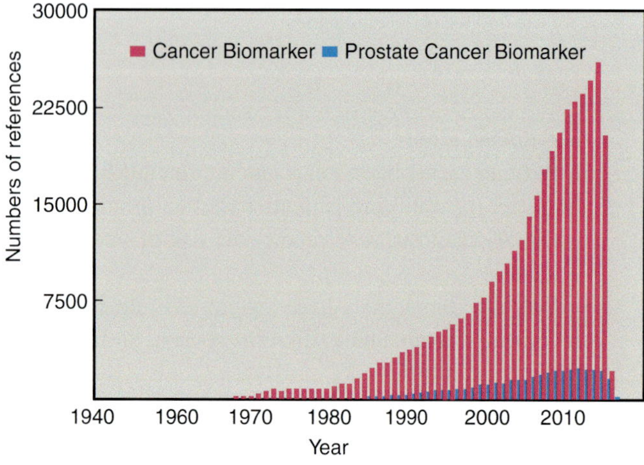

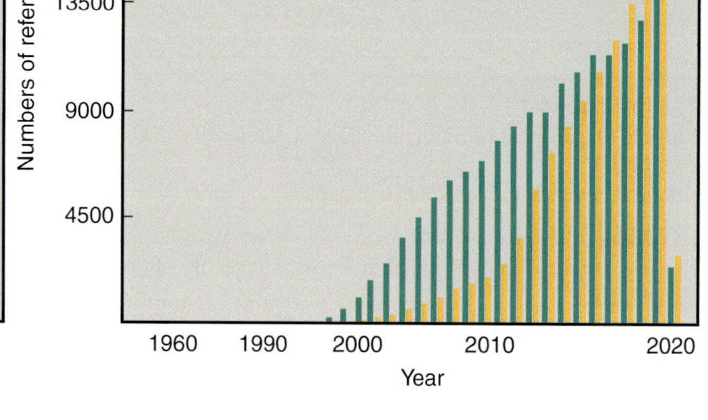

Fig. 27.1 The number of references has risen continuously from the first two publications on fetuin as a potential biomarker in the early 1940s to the present. A keyword query of 'cancer biomarkers' yields nearly 350'000 hits. Especially in the last 15 years, a particular steep increase in publications addressing biomarkers in cancer is recorded simultaneously with the advances made in proteomic and transcriptomic pattern recognition and the ability of analysing very large data sets. Despite those efforts, however, the number of reliable biomarkers for cancer remains low. [Source https://pubmed.ncbi.nlm.nih.gov February 2021]

Table 27.1 Table is a digest of FDA approved biomarkers for prostate cancer to be applied in combination with classic means of diagnosis

Name of marker	Type of marker	Source	Target	Application
BRCA1/BRCA1	Gene mutation	Blood and bone marrow	Breast cancer Ovarian cancer Prostate cancer	Treatment specification for breast and ovarian cancer; Risk assessment
Circulating cancer cells cell search	Protein detection on circulating cancer cells	Blood	Breast cancer Prostate cancer	Assist with clinical decision making
PAP	Protein (Prostatic acid phosphatase)	Blood	Metastatic prostate cancer	Diagnosis of poorly differentiated tumours
PSA	Protein (Prostate specific antigen)	Blood	Prostate cancer	Diagnosis and monitoring of treatment response and/or recurrence
Pca3 mRNA	RNA (Transcriptome)	Urine	Prostate cancer	Assessment if second biopsy is needed
17-Gene signature oncotype DX	RNA (Transcriptome)	Tumour tissue	Prostate cancer	Stratification
46-Gene signature prolaris	RNA (Transcriptome)	Tumour tissue	Prostate cancer	Monitor tumour progression and assist disease management

Those markers mainly serve clinicians in monitoring treatment response and disease management. Source: NCI.org April 2021 [3]

1. Should an individual be tested for prostate cancer and by what means?
2. If he is diagnosed with prostate cancer, what is the risk of potentially lethal versus clinically insignificant disease?

The classification of high-risk prostate cancer is based on any one of the following: evidence of metastasis; a Gleason score of 8 to 10 representing poorly differentiated or undifferentiated (immature) cells which often grow and spread quickly; a clinical stage where the tumour is large or spread beyond the prostate; or a very high PSA level. Each of these factors indicate real potential for the cancer to develop into a fatal type and definitive treatment of high-risk prostate cancer is paramount. However, it is among patients with low- or intermediate-risk prostate cancer that the concern about choosing the most befitting treatment is greatest. All approved prostate cancer biomarkers are intended to assist with this choice as an addition to conventional diagnosis methods. They are either detected as circulating biomarkers in blood or urine or isolated from tumour tissues [Table 27.1].

Circulating Biomarkers

One of the earliest discovered markers for prostate cancer is the increased blood level of prostatic acid phosphatase (PAP), an enzyme produced in the prostate gland. The clinical testing for PAP proved to be impractical, marred by the relative instability of the enzyme and the low sensitivity in early-stage disease. PAP, however, is surprisingly accurate in identifying high-risk patients and raised levels point to poorly differentiated tumours [4, 5]. In clinic PAP made way in favour for the most widely implemented diagnostic reference point: the change of prostate-specific antigen levels (PSA) in the blood.

Prostate-Specific Antigen Measurements in the Blood Are the Standard Molecular Diagnostic and Prognostic Tools

PSA Testing

PSA testing to aid diagnosis has been used in clinic since the early 1980s. The approval as diagnostic maker by the FDA followed in 1994. Its diagnostic and disease monitoring properties have been decidedly beneficial for many patients, but it comes with a critical limitation: PSA is not a cancer-specific marker, it is an organ-specific marker. Measuring PSA levels can be deceptive as the concentrations in the blood also rise during infection/inflammation and through benign prostatic hyperplasia. If a malignancy is indeed present, the PSA level does not provide information about the stage of the disease nor its aggressiveness [6].

PSA, also known as kallikrein 3 or hK3, is a serine protease and a member of a family of glandular kallikrein-related peptidases. The genes for glandular kallikreins are clustered on chromosome 19 (Chr19q13-4) and the transcription of PSA is regulated by androgens. The function of PSA is to liquefy seminal fluid through its action on the gel-forming proteins semenogelin and fibronectin. A healthy prostate is surrounded by a continuous layer of basal cells and a basement membrane. Both act as a barrier and prevent PSA leaking from in the prostate into the circulation, hence the low normal PSA baseline. During abnormal processes accompanied by inflammation this barrier becomes weaker and blood vessels more permeable for PSA. Despite extensive research and testing it is very difficult to define the optimal threshold (or cut-off value) for PSA in a patient. Traditionally, it was set at the range between 4–10 ngml^{-1} providing a sensitive test, with a positive predictive value of 37% and a negative predictive value of 91%. In other words, three quarters of men with blood PSA within that range and who undergo biopsy are not diagnosed with a malignancy. Still, even with a threshold as low as 4 ng/ml, the risk that a cancerous growth might exist cannot be ignored. The Prostate Cancer Prevention Trial (PCPT), for example, reported that 27% of men whose digital rectal examination (DRE) had been normal and the serum PSA value just below the 4 ng/ml mark did have prostate cancer at the time of examination. On the other hand, lowering the PSA cut-off below 4 ng/ml had no preventative effect in the long term and would only lead to more unnecessary biopsies of clinical insignificant prostate cancer.

Differentiation Between Benign and Malignant Prostatic Hyperplasia by the Prostate Health Index

Honing PSA testing is built on protein-complexation and isomeric variants of PSA and their ratio to each other. PSA can circulate in the blood in its native form aka 'free PSA' (fPSA) or in complex of PSA (cPSA) binding to α1-antichymotrypsin (ACT), α2-macroglobulin (A2M) and α1-protease inhibitor (API)). The relative amount of fPSA was found to be a decisive factor between prostate cancer and benign conditions and the percentage, PSA/(fPSA + cPSA) × 100, is in clinical use as a stratification guide for patients whose PSA lies within the critical range. The lower the percentage the higher becomes the probability for a malignancy to be present. Native fPSA exists in multiple isoforms, including inactive precursor PSA (pro-PSA), benign prostatic hyperplasia associated PSA (BPSA) and intact PSA (iPSA), the un-cleaved enzymatically inactive form of PSA [7]. Several studies provided evidence that levels of pro-PSA are significantly higher in patients with prostate cancer, whereas the levels of BPSA and iPSA are decreased [8, 9]. Tests of blood samples for the 'two amino acid' truncated variant of pro-PSA (p2PSA) demonstratively out-perform the percentage-fPSA guide and classic PSA screening in both sensitivity and specificity. The presence of relatively elevated p2PSA is especially dominant in men with metastatic prostate [10]. By reference to this information the Prostate Health Index (PHI) is assessed. PHI combines the ratio of fPSA to p2PSA with the total PSA into a single score which is calculated by the mathematical formula :p2PSA/fPSA × $\sqrt{\text{total PSA}}$. As mentioned above, patients with moderately high PSA and negative DRE results still may be at risk and the PHI was introduced by the FDA in 2012 to aid in the distinction between benign and malignant condition. The PHI is also helpful in monitoring men after interventions. The probability that cancer is present or has recurred rises proportional to the increase of the index, but impact of the PHI on the clinical decision making remained below expectations.

4 Kallikrein Predictive Score Model

The 4Kscore® is a statistical test that has shown to accurately diagnose prostate cancer of Gleason grade >2 before biopsy and to prognose distant metastases [11]. The statistical power of 4Kscore® rests on the measurement of four prostate-specific kallikreins: tPSA, fPSA, iPSA and human kallikrein-related peptidase2 (hK2). A data-based analysis from 2015 pooled 10 independent studies into one cohort of 14,580 patients, whose levels of all four kallikreins were measured before biopsy. The results of an assessment of the discrimination potential assessed showed that iPSA and hK2 were key factors to the success of accurate prognosis of biopsies and the 4Kscore® consequentially outperformed the conventional age-related tPSA approach [12].

Circulating Tumour Cells

A less commonly applied biomarker is the standardised assay CellSearch®, which captures circulating (epithelial) tumour cells (CTC) with an antibody against the epithelial adhesion molecule (anti-epCAM antibody) in the patient's blood [13, 14]. The cells are further classified as cytokeratin+/CD45-/DAPI+ to exclude immune cells or erythrocytes. CTCs are considered a 'liquid biopsy' and are invaluable material to study tumour cell behaviour without taking tissues, especially after recurrence of a growth when yet another biopsy is considered unethical for a patient. The CellSearch® assay has a high prognostic power, meaning number of CTCs in the blood helps to forecast a patient's outcome without treatment. CellSearch® seems to fare less well in its predictive power, meaning the number of CTCs is less helpful in the estimate of a likely benefit a patient would receive from treatment [15]. Extending the verification markers of the commercial CellSearch® by additional specific molecular markers that are also easy therapeutic targets enhances the predictive power of the assay [16]. For prostate cancer a suitable target is the androgen receptor, and more specifically the splice variant AR-V7, which could become a marker directing either to hormone or chemotherapy [17]. The detection of AR-V7 on CTCs is in general a sign for the presence of metastatic castration-resistant prostate cancer and the majority of those patients would not benefit from further androgen deprivation therapy. This group of prostate cancer patients are more likely to respond to chemotherapy or to the emerging category of novel small molecule inhibitors that directly bind to the intrinsically disordered N-terminus of the androgen receptors and its splice variants [18, 19].

Other Circulating Biomarkers

In addition to the search for protein biomarkers, germline genetic variants have been identified through genome-wide association studies. Genetic variation accounts for up to one-third of the cumulative lifetime risk of being diagnosed with prostate cancer and this has been based on genome-wide association studies (GWAS) focussing predominantly on common single nucleotide polymorphisms (SNPs). Usefully SNPs can be detected in germline DNA extracted from either saliva or blood samples fulfilling the criterion of a minimally invasive test. The focus of many of these GWAS studies has been on European Caucasian cases and controls. More recent multi-ethnic studies suggest that distinct genetic risk landscapes underpin heritable risk aligned to differing ethnicities. Genetic testing can provide a cost-effective approach to focussed diagnostic testing using PSA, multi-parametric magnetic resonance imaging and other modalities. Whereas the germline genetic landscape associated with prostate cancer risk is rich enough to lend itself to the development of polygenic risk scores (PRS) [20], more work is needed to offer risk stratification tools for people from all ethnic backgrounds [21]. As the costs of genetic testing fall further and capacity increases it will be possible to identify rare genetic variants associated with poor prognosis, metastatic disease risk rather than the lifetime risk of developing prostate cancer [22]. Some of this work indicates that such variants will associate with biological mechanisms that are known to be dysregulated in tumours, including DNA repair pathways [23]. Clinically that will provide the possibility of selecting bespoke imaging and biomarker panels aligned to these genetic features and also to actionable molecular targets and improved treatment outcomes.

The prostate cancer gene 3 (Pca3 mRNA) is upregulated in all cancerous tissues of the prostate, in comparison with benign prostatic hyperplasia, and hence a better discriminating factor than PSA. Pca3 mRNA can be detected in the urine after DRE (prostate massage). For patients with raised PSA levels and negative biopsy the Pca3 mRNA score helps to decide whether a second biopsy is advisable or not [24, 25].

Prostate cancer is by nature a 'male' disease, but a hereditary link between men and women exists: the BRCA1 and BRCA2 gene. BRCA1 and BRCA2 are co-regulators of the androgen/oestrogen receptor and a germline mutation in those genes increases the risk for breast cancer in women. Their presence is usually detected in blood and bone marrow samples. Inherited BRCA2 mutations via the female line also cause an increase in risk for men to develop prostate cancer [26]. The results from the IMPACT study, a collaboration between 65 centres in 20 countries, showed that carriers of BRCA2 mutations had higher incidences in developing prostate cancer. Within the carrier cohort prostate cancer was also diagnosed at younger age and number of clinically significant tumours was elevated compared to the cohort of non-carriers [27]. The genetic screening of BRCA2 mutations has been extended to men with suspected prostate cancer to guide treatment specification.

Tissue-Based Biomarkers

Biopsy or surgical removal of the prostate gland provides tissue samples for classic pathological evaluation, specific immunohistochemistry, or used for molecular profiling. Grade scoring of tissue samples by proliferative markers, cell adhesion molecules protein expressed by tumour-suppressor gene are no official prostate biomarkers but are useful co-indicators.

Proliferation Index: Ki67

The Ki67 protein is found in the nuclei of proliferating cells and can be detected by immunohistochemistry. Ki67 is particularly attractive due to its ease of interpretation of stained tissues and high reproducibility of observational results. For prostate cancer samples the proportion of tumour cells staining positive for Ki-67 was higher in malignant than in benign phenotype and strongly related to the Gleason Scoring [28, 29].

E-Cadherin

Cell adhesion molecules preserve the structure integrity in a tissue, for example, 'calcium dependent adhesion' molecules called cadherins. E-cadherin is the epithelial cell–cell adhesion molecule that ensures cell polarity and epithelial integrity. The loss of E-cadherin and/or the switch to N-Cadherin signals the transition to a less differentiated and more aggressive tumour cell type in prostate cancer and could therefore pass as a disease progression marker [30, 31].

PTEN

Phosphatase and tensin homologue (PTEN) is the protein of the tumour-suppressor gene *pten* on chromosome 10q23. PTEN antagonises the PI-3 K/Akt signalling pathway which regulates cell cycle and cell motility and the loss of the protein in (prostate) cancer cells leads to their increased proliferation and cell survival [32]. The loss of PTEN is generally suggestive of adverse oncological outcome and resistance to a number of conventional therapies, which may be accountable for the high probability of recurrence in patients that show a low expression of PTEN [33]. The features of PTEN loss could be instrumental for prognosis, especially for distinction between indolent and malignant tumours, and predictive for the course of treatment.

As mentioned earlier, it is unlikely that one single biomolecule will combine all mandatory criteria that make an ideal biomarker and compromises must be made. At the same time, even the most hopeful candidate must be abandoned in the face of conflicting data. Gene fusion genes are known to be driver of carcinogenesis. For prostate cancer, recurrent fusion of the 5′ untranslated region of androgen-regulated trans-membrane protease serine (TMPRSS2) and Oncogene ERG of the ETS transcription factor family was first reported in 2005 [34]. The true value of fusion gene TMPRSS2-ERG as diagnostic, prognostic and predictive biomarker, however, could not be established but the specificity to prostate cancer could make it a strong therapeutic target [35, 36]. Although the enhancer of zeste homologue 2 (EZH2) gene is upregulated in prostate and other cancer types, its credentials as a biomarker have not been shown to date [37]. EZH2 mediates trimethylation of histone H3 lysine 27 (H3K27), which leads to repression of transcription and silencing of gene expression including the E-cadherin gene, which is vital for maintaining the epithelial integrity [38, 39]. On its own EHZ2 remains a meaningful therapeutic target rather than a convincing tissue biomarker, but as part of a 14 gene panel the diagnostic and prognostic results are promising [40].

Approved Tissue Markers for Prostate Cancer

The 17 gene signature is a qRT-PCR assay to measure the expression levels of 12 cancer related genes and five house-keeping genes (control) in needle biopsy tissue samples. A total of three clinical studies were conducted to validate the gene panel. The first two studies consisted of a discovery cohort of 441 samples and another cohort of 167 samples from patients that were at intermediate to low risk but subject to active surveillance. From the genetic data of those two studies a multigene-based signature, the genomic prostate score (GPS) on a scale from 0–100 was developed. A third study was designed to validate the GPS. A logistic regression of 395 samples tested the GPS in correlation to pathological stage and grade at the time of prostatectomy. The results showed that the GPS accurately discriminated the aggressiveness of prostate cancer, despite tumour heterogeneity and multifocal occurrences and may aid in clinic to separate patients for active surveillance from those that need immediate treatment [41–43].

The 46 gene signature is an extension to the aforementioned 17 gene signature and is also based on tissue qRT-PCR. The 46 gene panel includes 31 cell cycle genes and 15 house-keeping genes and is also known as cell cycle progression (CCP) test. The CCP scale is an empirical score system of arbitrary units on a dynamic range normalised to the expression levels of the 15 house-keeping genes [44, 45]. In 16 independent studies the CCP score reliably paired the prediction of biochemical recurrence and disease-specific progression and mortality with conventional means of diagnosis and prognosis [46].

Both 17 and 46 gene signatures are prognostic tests and tools for an individualised risk assessment. The two molecular assays are commercially available and traded under the product name of Oncotype DX Genomic Prostate Score (17 gene signature; Genomic Health, Inc.) and Prolaris CCP (46 gene signature; Myriad Genetics, Inc.). Both are approved by the FDA for patient stratification, treatment monitoring and disease management.

Leucine-Rich Alpha2 Glycoprotein: A Biomarker in Many Contexts

Biopsies and tissue samples will never totally be avoidable and a tissue section provides invaluable information about stage, grade and general pathology of a tumour. Paraffin embedded tissue samples are well preserved and easy to archive. However, collecting tissue samples comes at a price. Prostate cancer, for example, is an inter and intra-heterogeneic tumour, a feature that adds to the difficulty of biopsy stratification. A needle biopsy can, involuntarily, introduce sampling bias by simply not piercing the 'right part'. Prostate cancer is also multifocal: several small islands of cancerous tissue appear within the organ and might be missed by needle biopsy. If a patient is under active surveillance and monitored for treatment response and/or recurrence, it is ethically untenable to submit them repeatedly to a biopsy. One top breakthrough in cancer detection is the 'liquid biopsy': a circulating biomarker in blood or other bodily fluids, independent of tumour location. Samples can be easily and frequently collected by minimal invasive or even non-invasive procedures. As discussed in the previous chapter, the standard biomarker for prostate cancer still is PSA which has the great benefit of being detectable in the blood but falls short in other ways.

Over the last decades, elevated levels of leucine-rich alpha2 glycoprotein (LRG-1) were detected in multiple studies scrutinising the transcriptome and proteome of cancer cells and in tissues of other proliferative diseases [47–51] (Fig. 27.2). In cancer elevated LRG-1 levels are present in tumour tissues but appealingly, also in blood and other bodily fluids of the patients. The consistency of

Fig. 27.2 Graphic that summarises the clinical studies conducted to explore LRG-1 as a marker for tumour progression, prognosis and risk stratification. *Figure designed with BioRender*

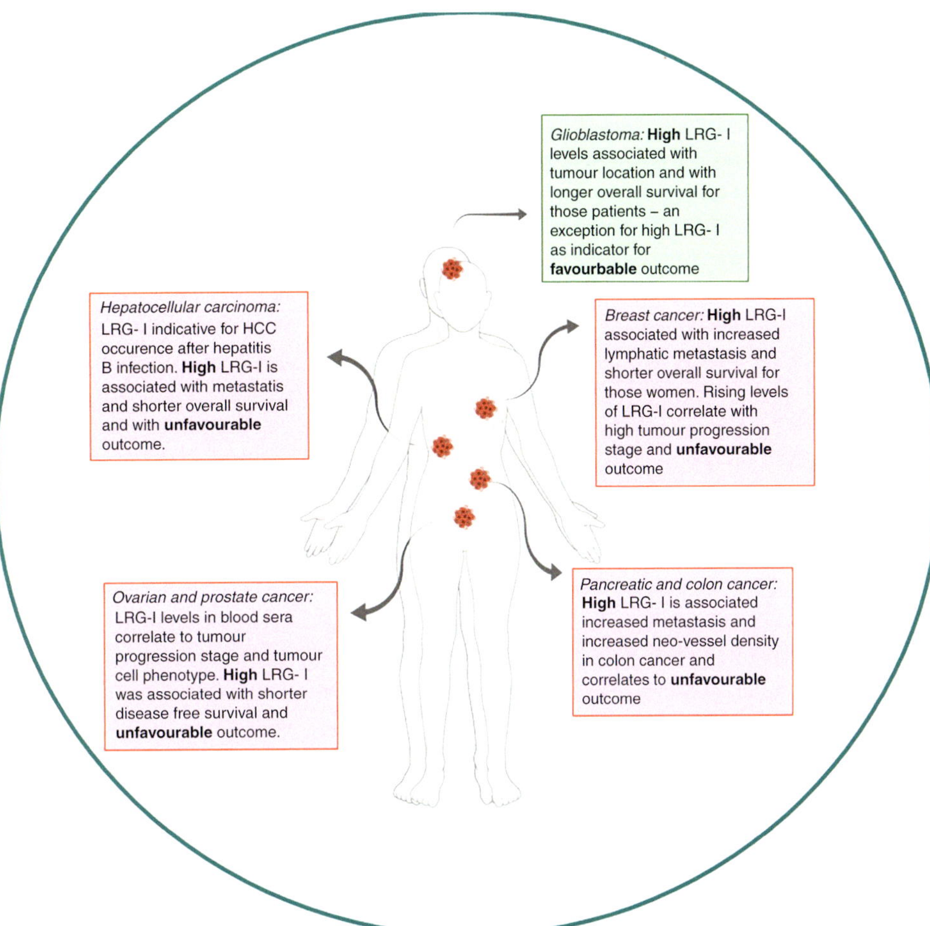

finding LRG-1 enrichment as a sign for abnormal processes makes a strong case for LRG-1 becoming a powerful and versatile biomarker facilitating diagnosis and prognosis in the future.

LRG-1 is found in a number of normal cell types in a number of organs: in the alveolar cells of the lung, duct cells of the pancreas and the glandular cells of the prostate but it is particularly enriched in the hepatocytes of the liver. In the eye, heart muscle, skin, placenta and prostate, LRG-1 is also enriched in endothelial cells of the blood vessels and it is found in neutrophils and monocytes of the blood. LRG-1 is packaged into the granules of the neutrophiles and released upon activation [52, 53]. In cultured hepatocytes LRG-1 is enclosed in vesicles in the cytoplasm and believed to be excreted [54]. LRG-1 can therefore be detected in blood serum and to some extent in other bodily fluids such as urine.

LRG-1 a Diagnostic Biomarker for Cancers That Are Hard-to-Detect

Early detection is a problem for any cancer; however, some cancers are harder to discover than others. Liver, pancreatic and kidney cancer diagnosis is made more difficult by the location of the organs that are either sheltered by the ribcage or hidden deep in the torso. Ovarian cancer is notoriously overlooked and early symptoms are mundane and attributed to 'indigestion' rather than to a deadly growth [55]. The same is true for brain tumours: protected by the skull tumours in the brain are not palpable and headaches are common without a serious condition and slight changes in personality can be explained by external factors [56]. By the time the symptoms are so severe to raise concern, it is often too late.

Hepatocellular Carcinoma

Unsurprisingly, upregulation of LRG-1 was first detected on hepatocellular carcinoma (HCC) tissue, as the cells in the liver are naturally expressing the protein. One of the earliest publications reported a mass spectroscopy analysis of glycolproteins isolated by lectin-based chromatography from the cancerous tissue, which could otherwise be masked when screening the proteome in whole. In the sub-selection, LRG-1 was one of the most prominent proteins in the tumour tissue [57]. A later study of sera from patients with HCC came to similar results. In this study the aim had been to see if the distribution of bio markers in the serum, including LRG-1, could be used to identify the origin of the cancer, here after infection with Hepatis B virus (HBV). The result was that patients whose liver tumour correlated with earlier HBV infection showed significant higher levels of LRG-1 in the serum samples, than the patients that carried no virus [58]. Those results were picked up and expanded with a large cohort of 777 HCC patient samples (both tumour and adjacent non-tumour liver samples). In 51.4% of the 777 samples LRG-1 (based on mRNA and protein) levels were significantly raised and correlated with the pathological data of consistently larger late-stage tumours, poor tumour differentiation and higher rate of vascular invasion. For the individuals in that particular group the overall survival rate and disease-free time period were shortened, the recurrence probability and the tendency to develop metastases were increased (Fig. 27.3). The statistical difference was significant for all criteria and the diagnostic power of the screening found to be as high as 95% [59]. Almost simultaneously a second, very similar study was published which came to the exact opposite results, reporting that LRG-1 was downregulated in HCC tissue samples. Alas, no clinical patient data had been available. The study also showed that LRG-1 had no effect on HCC cell proliferation but could inhibit HCC cell migration and invasion concluding LRG-1 as a potential anti-metastatic factor [60].

Glioblastoma

LRG-1 was found in patients diagnosed with glioma. A clinical study that had been conducted and results published in 2020. A cohort of 155 glioma tissue samples, in which 114 were identified as glioblastoma, 27 as astrocytoma and 14 as oligodendroglioma was analysed for LRG-1 [61]. All samples showed increase of LRG-1 levels compared to control tissues from normal brain cortex samples. The assessment of the samples followed a scoring system from 0 (negative) to 4 (positive liver control). Within the glioma group the level of LRG-1 expression varied. The occurrences of high LRG-1 in the non-glioblastoma samples were significantly fewer than in the major group of glioblastomas. In the astrocytoma and oligodendroglioma subgroups only 3 (21%) and 1 (4%) case, respectively, had high levels of LRG-1. In the major group of glioblastomas, 47 (41%) cases showed high LRG-1 levels. As for clinical outcome: after surgery, patients that had tumours with high levels of LRG-1 had an advantage in their 'overall survival' but not in 'progression free survival' over patients whose samples showed lower LRG-1 levels (Fig. 27.3). Case samples for this study were matched in their 'extension of resection' (EOR) index. Yet, the tumours that showed high levels of LRG-levels had been located further away from the subventricular zone (SVZ) and were predominantly removed from the periphery of the brain, those with lower LRG-levels were closer to the SVZ.

Ovarian Cancer

LRG-1 was found to be a novel protein marker after deep depletion of abundant proteins from ovarian cancer tissue samples and blood serum of women with ovarian cancer [62, 63]. In a cohort of 114 women, 58 diagnosed with ovarian cancer and 56 healthy women, LRG-1 concentrations were indicative to the stage the cancer had been at the time of sampling. In blood serum (and tissue samples) the mean LRG-1 level was consistently raised and significantly (2-fold) higher

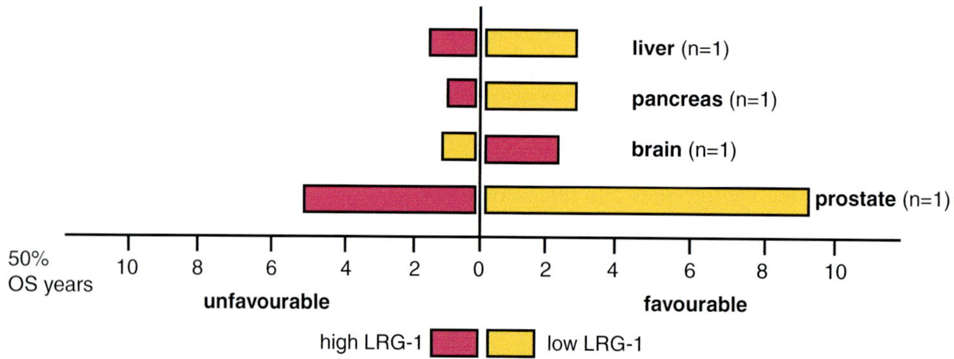

Fig. 27.3 Graph that shows qualitatively LRG-1 levels relating to overall survival. The bar-graph matches LRG-1 levels to the patient's clinical outcome and is based on 50% death rate in the highest risks groups in each study. All patients had received maximum treatment depending on their diagnosis and circumstances. The term 'high' and 'low' LRG-1 in this graphic is a general term to describe the empirical threshold concentrations that vary for each study. Other variables are the source of LRG-1 (circulating protein in blood vs tissue samples) and the methods with which LRG-1 was detected in the clinical samples. Liver: IHC and scoring system of patient samples [59]; Pancreas: LRG-1 plasma levels by ELISA [90]; Brain: IHC and scoring system of patient samples [61]; Prostate: LRG-1 plasma levels by ELISA [105]. n = number of clinical studies. *Figure designed in BioRender*

in cancer patients than in the healthy cohort. The highest concentrations were measured in women diagnosed with late-stage (III/IV) ovarian cancer. Compelling data, however, was obtained from pre-operative blood samples taken from a separate cohort of 193 women that underwent surgery for suspicious adnexal growth. In this study the mean LRG-levels in those patients that actually had a malignant growth (serous and clear ovarian cancer) were 1.7 fold higher than in the women whose tissue pathology report returned as 'benign', manifesting the hypothesis that LRG-1 could be a distinction marker between malignant and benign phenotypes [64, 65]. In a later (but much smaller study) the concentrations of LRG-1 in the urine of women diagnosed with early-stage ovarian were compared to an age-matched cohort of heathy volunteers. The women with early-stage ovarian cancer had a mean LRG-1 content in their urine that was significantly higher than in the control group [66, 67]. This result is insofar worth noting as many women with early-stage ovarian cancer show normal levels of cancer antigen 125 (CA125), one of the FDA approved marker of ovarian cancer to assist diagnoses and to monitor treatment response.

Breast Cancer

High LRG-1 in tissues of breast cancer linked the patients to the malignant progression of the disease. In 2020, a tissue study of 330 breast cancer samples showed that the elevated LRG-1 levels went along with climbing numbers of lymph metastases and raised scores in the TNM pathological staging system. Those women went through shorter disease-free survival and shorter overall survival than the women whose tissue samples showed significantly lower LRG-1 concentrations [68].

Other Harder to Diagnose Cancer Types

LRG-1 upregulation has also been observed in plasma samples from patients with pancreatic cancer and in patients with colon cancer [69, 70]. A different study on colon cancer patients made the case that not only the raised levels of LRG-1 in the tumour tissue are indicative for disease progression but also showed that the micro-vessel density in those tissues had been greater. Greater micro-vessel density is a nod to the angiogenic properties of LRG-1 and suggestive for increased risk that tumour cell invades the blood vessels [71]. LRG-1 protein was also upregulated in tissue samples, glycoprotein-enriched serum samples and urine samples from lung cancer patients. For this study no correlation between LRG-1 levels in those samples and the clinical outcome of the patients was drawn [72–74]. A study on patients diagnosed with non-small cell lung cancer (NSCLC) however, showed that high levels of LRG-1 in biopsies were associated with the tendency for metastasis and shorter overall survival [75]. Similar results derived from clinical studies on patients with thyroid cancer [76].

The History of LRG-1 Protein

In 1977, an unknown human serum protein was isolated from the by-product of the large-scale preparation of albumin and g-globulin: the 347 amino acids long leucine-rich alpha2 glycoprotein (LRG-1). The amino acid content is unusual in that the leucine content is almost 17%, which means that one fifth of the amino acid content is a leucine [77]. Crystal structure analysis shows the protein as a single polypeptide chain with one galactosamine and four glucosamine attached. Of the 312 amino acids, 66 are leucine. The peptide can be divided into 13 segments with 24 residues each. Eight residues present a periodic pattern of leucine, proline and asparagine. The protein contains domains capable of bipolar surface orientation and shows homology to segments of mitochondrial proteins, viral envelope proteins and oncogene proteins [78, 79]. The 3D protein model, based on NetrinG2 template, reveals a coiling amino acid ß-chain that forms a barrel or tube-like tertiary structure and features a short amino acid α-helix towards the C-terminus. The structure is stabilised by four cysteines that form di-sulphide bonds, one bond at either end [80, 81].

LRG-1: The Transforming Growth Factor Connection

For the longest time LRG-1 was classified as 'a serum protein with unknown function' and its true biological role is still not very well understood [77, 82]. First hints about role of LRG-1 in the cell cycle came from a report in 1995. A study of differentially expressed genes in human hepatoma cells was laid out to search for novel factors involved in the transforming growth factor b (TGF-ß) signalling pathway and identified mRNA for a gene, SB31, that was 100% homologous with LRG-1. This gene was co-ordinately expressed with mRNA of the TGF-ßR2 gene, which suggested an interaction between the both [83].

TGF-ß Signalling in a Nutshell

What makes the function of LRG-1 hard to discern in its relation to TGF-ß, is the fact that TGF-ß itself has several roles with often opposite consequences in the grand scheme of cell signalling. In order to interpret the effect LRG-1 has on TGF-ß signalling we need to understand the role of TGF-ß first. TGF-ß is a multifunctional growth factor of, and name-giver to, the *transforming growth factor superfamily* (which in fact comprises a large number of proteins). Their downstream signalling pathways regulate the cell cycle, and can either suppress or stimulate cell proliferation and differentiation. Although downstream *effects* of TGF-ß pathways are heavily dependent on cellular context, the downstream *signalling* is, at least partially, conserved in many cell types. There are three known and highly homologues isomers of TGF-ß, numbered 1–3. All three act via the same receptors, which are single strand serine/threonine kinase receptors R1, R2 and R3. R3 possesses no kinase activity and is not directly involved in the TGF-ß signal transduction pathway but works as a reservoir for the growth factor. TGF-ß is a ligand to R2 and the TGF-ß/R2 complex recruits and phosphorylates R1. Depending on R1/R2 phosphorylation pattern a canonical (also called 'SMAD') signalling pathway or a non-canonical signalling pathway is triggered. In the SMAD signalling pathway, activated R1 in return phosphorylates receptor-regulated transcription factors SMAD (R-SMAD), that is then able to bind to coSMAD. The R-SMAD/coSMAD complex translocates to the nucleus and modulates gene expression depending on the cellular context. In the non-canonical signalling pathway TGF-ß–R1/R2 complex carries an additional phosphate and activates several other signalling pathways including Rho/Rock that regulates the tight junctions, MAPK and Erk pathways, both transcriptional regulators, and P13K/Akt pathway that controls protein synthesis. Both TGF-ß signalling pathways contribute to the regulation of proliferation, differentiation, apoptosis and epithelial–mesenchymal transition—key events in cell biology [84]. Upon secretion by various cell types, including macrophages, TGF-ß is present in its latent form bound mainly by two TGF-ß binding proteins (LTBP and LAP). Proteinases, for example, plasmin, can cleave the complex binding and release activated TGF-ß into the extracellular space. Other TGF-ß activating factors are integrins, reactive oxygen species (ROS) and thrombospondin. On the surface of macrophages, for example, the latent TGF-ß complex is bound to CD36 via thrombospondin-1 (TSB-1). In response to inflammatory stimuli plasmin levels rise and the release of activated TGF-ß1 is turned on, hence the regulatory role of TGF-ß in inflammation [85, 86].

TGF-ß: Cancers Double Agent

In normal cells TGF-ß signalling arrests the cells in G1 phase of the cell cycle. In the early stages of tumour growth TGF-ß indeed exerts an anti-proliferative influence on the cells but in the later stages of tumour progression this effect wears off. There it is replaced by loss of control over proliferation and apoptotic response while sustaining angiogenesis. The dual effect could be explained by significant downregulation of receptor expression on cancer cells as the disease moves ahead and with mutations of the growth and other downstream factors involved in cell cycle regulation [87, 88]. At the same time, many types of tumour cells and cells of the tumour microenvironment start to overexpress the growth factor, which skews the ligand/receptor balance. TGF-ß is also a potent immunosuppressor adding to the formidable ability of the cancer cells to evade attack by the immune system of their host [89].

LRG-1 and TGF-ß: Brothers in Arms

LRG-1 and TGF-ß and TGF-ß receptor enrichment is often simultaneously observed in human tissues and fluids of various proliferate diseases. It was, for example, discovered in patients with idiopathic normal pressure hydrocephalus (INPH), a neuro-degenerative disease with excess cerebrospinal fluid (CSF) build-up in the brain ventricles. Analysis of the INPH-CFS showed a markedly higher concentration of LRG-1 and TGF-ß1 and TGF-ßR2 than in the CFS of healthy controls [49]. How the upregulation of two but not the third mandatory factor, TGF-ßR1, in the conserved three-factor activation pathway effects TGF-ß1 downstream signalling was not clear. In cultured NSCLC, LRG-1 affects TGF-ß1 dependent cell proliferation, migration and invasion and promotes TGF-ß1 dependent angiogenesis. A549 (lung cancer) cells were manipulated to either lose or to overexpress LRG-1. In the knockout variant proliferation and cell motility were significantly reduced and enhanced in LRG-1 overexpressing cells. LRG-1 rich exosomes isolated [75]. NSCLC patient blood samples and cells lines encouraged an angiogenic response in HUVECs and the effect could be negated by selective TGF-ß1 receptor blocker SM-16. The analysis of HUVECs for TGF-ß1 expression (on mRNA and protein level) before and after exosome exposure on mRNA revealed a significant increase of the growth factor, which the authors concluded, was due to the presence of LRG-1. In LRG-1 expressing clones of human pancreatic ductal adenocarcinoma (PDAC) cell line Panc1/LRG, TGF-ß1 induced transition from epithelial phenotype to mesenchymal phenotype took place and was observed in the change of the shape in the majority of cells [90]. Those cells showed a drop of phosphorylated Smad2, part of the Smad-transcription factor complex that control expression of cell–cell adhesions molecules such as E-cadherin, occludins and claudins (tight junction molecules) and tissue specific cytokeratins. The loss of E-cadherin in general and here in Panc1/LRG clones, is a distinctive (but not exclusive) sign that EMT commences.

LRG-1 Regulates Angiogenesis

In 2013 a study was published, presenting data that linked LRG-1 upregulation tightly to TGF-ß induced angiogenesis in the mouse retina and for the first time reported a distinct function of LRG-1 [91]. Prominent *Lrg1* gene upregulation in the transcriptome of three mouse models simulating retinal vessel architecture and retinal degeneration was observed in the first instance. LRG-1 protein in all three models was almost exclusively found in the blood vessels of the retina and to some lesser extent the choroid, which is the vascularised layer of tissue that separates the retina from the sclera. Upregulation of *Lrg1* gene in the retina was also observed in angiogenic phase in mouse models of oxygen induced retinopathy (OIR) and choroidal neovascularisation (CNV) days after laser injury. The retinas of LRG-1 knockout mice are only slightly less developed than those of their wild-type littermates, but LRG-1−/− did not display active angiogenesis in the OIR model or CNV after injury. Cultured endothelial cells (HUVEC) were responsive both after LRG-1 activation and LRG-1 inhibitions in angiogenesis assays. Immunoprecipitation of LRG-1 with TGF-ßR2 and endoglin (auxiliary receptor to TGF-ßR2 on endothelial cells), this time in primary mouse brain endothelial cells, suggested the direct interaction of LRG-1 with those receptors. Endoglin is not a direct receptor for the growth factor, but the interaction with LRG-1 promotes TGF-ß receptor configuration and that flips the angiogenic switch via the canonical signalling pathway.

LRG-1 also promotes angiogenesis in normal wound healing. LRG-1 is a necessary angiogenic factor in the proliferative stage of the healing process, when fibroblasts are recruited to form the primary granulation tissue. The healing process is significantly delayed in LRG-1−/− mice. At the same time, it does not promote wound healing in diabetic mice, although the sites of wounding were infused with LRG-1 [50]. In kidneys of diabetic mice, LRG-1 is predominantly localised to the capillaries in glomeruli and contributed to adverse events such as glomerular angiogenesis, diabetic glomerulopathy and podocyte loss [92, 93]. Although the supportive role of LRG-1 in angiogenesis is amply cited, little is known about the role LRG-1 actually plays in tumour angiogenesis. A niche in vitro study that makes a link to angiogenic, long non-coding RNA, specifically taurine-upregulated 1 (TUC1) by way of LRG-1 expressing ovarian cancer cells, was published in 2019 [94]. In this study the authors report the various angiogenic effects of conditioned media taken from TUC1 knockdown ovarian cancer cells. They established a negative correlation between low LRG-1 and angiogenic factors (reduction in VEGF and Ang1 but not in TGF-ß) in the supernatant of TUC knockdown cells and the limited activation of HUVECs, observed by absence of typical vascular structure elements and immobilisation of endothelial cells assessed in classic angiogenesis and migration assays. HUVEC activation could be rescued by the addition of recombinant LRG-1 to the experimental mix, hence the conclusion that LRG-1 coming from the cancer cells regulates the angiogenic response of HUVECs.

The Cytochrome c Connection

Alerted by the diminished sensitivity to cytochrome c (Cyt c) in ELISA assays in the presence of serum, a mass spectroscopy study was conducted in 2006 to find that in both human and bovine foetal serum the inhibitory factor was LRG-1 [95].

Cytochrome c in Apoptosis

In response to stress (or developmental signals) the intrinsic, or mitochondrial, pathway of apoptosis can be triggered from within the cells. Cty c is a protein that normally resides in the mitochondria where it is part of the mitochondrial electron-transport chain. Upon release into the cytosol the role of Cyt c changes and it binds to an adaptor protein called apoptosis-protease activation factor (Apaf1). The binding causes Apaf1 to oligomerise into a hexamer called the apotosome. Apotosomes recruit initiator caspase-9 protein that sets off the caspase cascade leading to apoptosis [96, 97].

LRG-1 Is a Competitive Ligand to Cyt c

The region on LRG-1 and Apaf1 that binds to Cyt c is very similar in the amino acid sequence and both proteins home to the same binding region on Cyt c. In controlled cytotoxicity experiments however, the apoptotic effect of Cyt c on lymphocytes was blocked by LRG-1, suggesting that despite LRG-1 being in competition with Apaf1 as a ligand to Cyt c, only Apaf1 is able to activate the caspase pathway of apoptosis [98]. Blocking the mitochondrial pathway of apoptosis could have critical consequences on the natural suppression of cancer cell proliferation. A study that investigated this hypothesis was published in 2021 [99]. A three-way cytotoxicity experiment was designed, taking breast cancer cells MCF-7 and additionally transfecting them: a) with the lrg1 gene to generate an LRG-1 overexpressing genotype and b) transfecting them with interfering hairpin RNA to generate an LRG-1 knock down genotype. In the parental MCF-7 cells LRG-1 was confined to the cytosol and was not secreted in detectable amounts. Apoptosis assays revealed a significant resistance of the transfected cells to enter the apoptotic cycle. The LRG-1 seems to instantly trap Cyt c that was released from the mitochondria before Apaf1 binding could occur. The affinity with which LRG-1 bound to Cyt c is extremely high, which, on the other hand, makes Cyt c an extremely sensitive substate for LRG-1 detection [100].

LRG-1: Prognosticator Prostate Cancer Progression

In 2007 and 2008, LRG-1 was identified in the proteome of PC3, LNCaP and 22Rv1 prostate cancer cell lines (supernatant and cell membrane), but at the time the researchers had focussed on different proteins and the potential of LRG-1 as a biomarker in patient samples had not been investigated [101, 102]. LRG-1 makes several appearances in supplemental data in publications analysing human serum proteins and mouse *pten* knock out prostate cancer models [103, 104]. It was in a comprehensive study published in 2020 where LRG-1 first took centre stage in its role as biomarker and with convincing results. Data had been generated suggesting LRG-1 measurements could be a new standard for improved risk stratification for patients with prostate cancer [105]. For this project, archival blood samples spanning three decades were analysed and classified into four independent cohorts of prostate cancer patients: discovery cohort, confirmation cohort (with follow-up data ≥ 10 years), and exploration cohort. The final validation cohort covered 451 blood samples. The study confirmed that LRG-1 levels were consistently elevated in cancer patients over those in healthy control volunteers (discovery cohort). The variations within cancer patients correlated with the progressions of the tumours, being highest in the group of patients that were diagnosed with metastases and those whose outcome was fatal, approximately two-fold increase in serum LRG-1 over the second highest group, that of indolent prostate cancer. The LRG-1 serum concentration in the group of men that were cancer free at the time of blood draw, but developed the disease later on however, were baseline (confirmation cohort), meaning that there was no evidence that serum LRG-1 could predict a pre-cancer status. A clear relation between rising LRG-1 concentration in the blood serum and increasing risk factor in those patients to emerge with metastasis and unfavourable outcome was found (Fig. 27.3). Few deaths were registered in the group of men with low LRG-1 levels, whereas men with high LRG-1 levels were more likely subject to disease progression, metastasis and ultimately, death (exploration cohort).

The Challenges in Translating Novel Biomarkers into Clinical Practice: An Epilogue

The Natural Function of LRG-1 Remains a Mystery

Good efforts—and progress—have been made to shed light on the function of LRG-1 in cell biology. In all the published clinical studies, LRG-1 levels are pronounced in tumours (of various sources), in blood sera and sometimes also urine of cancer patients or patients with other proliferative diseases. Apart from very few exceptions, high-rise LRG-1 seems associated to an unfavourable outcome. Biologically, LRG-1 interferes with the TGF-ß signalling cascade and the effect is noticeable in both epithelial and endothelial cells. LRG-1 actively causes an angiogenic switch via the canonical TGF-ß signalling pathway and furthers endothelial cell activation in vitro and in vivo (mouse). Even so, many questions are waiting for an answer. Why is LRG-1 elevated in the first place? Do baseline levels of LRG-1 in healthy tissues in any way impact the upregulation of the protein under pathological conditions? Does LRG-1 inhibit TGF-ß *anti-proliferative* or support TGF-ß *proliferative* function in tumour cells? How important is LRG-1 in tumour angiogenesis? In the healthy prostate, for example, LRG-1 is expressed in basal glandular cells and urothelial cells but is highest in the endothelium. Would that mean, LRG-1 effect on tumour angiogenesis would be dominant and would prostate cancer tissue with high LRG-1 also be more vascularised? Does LRG-1 wield an inhibitory effect on mitochondrial programmed cell death in cancer [106]? Ideally, the biological function of LRG-1 should be completely understood to maximise the extent for LRG-1 as a clinical marker. Regardless of the perforated knowledge about LRG-1, sound circumstantial evidence that LRG-1 is a high-performing biomarker might be sufficient for clinicians, in unison with their patients, to make informed decisions in treatment. Unravelling the biological function of LRG-1 in all its particulars may not be strictly necessary. Testing for LRG-1 in blood or even urine samples is comparably simple and could work together with other markers, such as PSA.

In the meantime, PSA stays as the most widely used biomarker for prostate cancer diagnosis, prognosis and prediction. Much research and efforts went and still go into the refinement of PSA testing. A protein produced only in the prostate exerts a strong attraction and the high specificity reconciles scientists and clinicians alike with the lack in sensitivity. Although various biomarkers for prostate cancer have been implemented in discrete clinical settings, none of them rivals the convenience of PSA. For progressive scientists and clinicians, the search for novel candidates continues and funding for clinical studies to do so has surged in the last decade, not the least due to the enormous societal impact a success promises. Alas, poor reproducibility taints the results from many of those studies. The more we ask of a biomarker, for example, as a prognosticator when the gap between diagnosis and outcome can be 10 years or more, the more biomarkers succumb to variables that may still validate their biological significance but may invalidate their clinical translation. We have moved into the era of precision technology and image-guided biopsy and as a result a much higher proportion of tumour biopsies taken presently are of intermediate to advanced stage (according to the Gleason score) than in the past. In other words, a substantial proportion of archival tissue samples are non-malignant. This sampling bias creates difficulties for direct performance comparison between tissue biomarkers assessed in samples from one era versus the other and some biomarkers will need re-evaluation. Vital data about progression free survival, overall survival and quality of life are often missing from the documentation collected the past and the lesson has been taken no longer to neglect those aspects when building a tissue archive and planning future studies.

Fundamentally the question of whether medical testing will improve patient outcome endures. Desirable and beneficial advances in screening and prognosis are overshadowed by the inherently ethical dilemma between the right of patients to full and accurate information about their own medical condition and the psychological impact this information, above all in the absence of symptoms, may have on the individual. This challenge is most acute when considering the use of germline genetics but applies for many other types of biomarker. Applications of testing and treatments must still be aligned to the needs of a patient and not to indulge scientific curiosity nor for corporate financial gain. It is hard to establish whether a particular test/biomarker actually influences the clinical decision making, since planning a route of treatment does not follow an algorithm but is influenced by many factors. Nor can the economic benefit be assessed objectively. Statistically, any healthcare system might save money otherwise spent on over-treatment but in reality, the human factor might offset this benefit. In 2017, the independent organisation Health Quality Ontario, Canada published a systematic review that addresses the questions of cost efficiency of genomic profiling of prostate cancer and whether such an approach should be funded under the existing health care plan. Based on a possible offer of a Prolaris CCP test evidence for clinical and economic benefit for patients with low-and intermediate-risk localised prostate cancer was sought [107]. Although the analysis was admittedly flawed by gaps in crucial data, the investigation found no evidence that additional Prolaris CCP testing has an impact on the patient-important outcome. Neither would a routine CCP test pay-off in the short term, rather it would load significant costs onto the local health care system. In interviews with prostate cancer patients, it transpired that many of the men were initially overwhelmed with the diagnosis and most of them put great value on the recommendations from their physicians. For all patients the emotional impact of the diagnosis took hold over their decision making and the fear of metastasis weighed heavily on most patients' minds. The anxiety that the cancer may spread beyond the prostate led some men decide against active surveillance and opt for more drastic interventions. Some men had doubts that a CCP test result, which they feared may only further com-

plicate the decision-making process, had let them change the course of treatment, others would not exclude a change of mind if the CCP results were unambiguous. An evaluation of the Prolaris® CCP test from 2016 by the National Institute for Health and Care Excellence (NICE), UK came to similar results as to cost efficiency, although their conclusions were based on the questionnaires given to clinicians only and did not involve actual patients [108]. More recently in 2019, a clinical trial by the Leeds Centre for Personalised Medicine and Health was launched to collect data if a precise genetic profiling (Prolaris®) would help to avoid unnecessary surgery and radiotherapy in men that developed prostate cancer [109]. The design of the study, which is in partnership with Myriad, has placed an emphasis on how the test had influenced the participants in their decision making about treatment and their quality of life. The trial results are expected in 2022.

Routinely consulting novel and intricate biomarkers, and complex tests such as gene profiling, are in its infancy, and the temptation to stick to time-proven methods like PSA testing and Gleason scoring is strong. In a matter of time, however, what is new and intimidating will become familiar and chances are that novel or complex biomarkers will be a habitual part of any anti-cancer regime in the near future.

Concluding Remarks/Summary

With technological advances it has become possible to sensitively profile tissue, blood and urine samples from prostate cancer patients to identify candidate biomarkers reflecting metabolic, protein, RNA, DNA and epigenetic changes. Aligning those measurements, often arising from diagnostic or pre-diagnostic samples, to the ultimate outcome of the disease for a given patient remains a huge challenge. This is because a significant time-lag may exist between diagnosis and progression, but also because the disease is highly heterogenous and a given patient may present with an array of histopathologically, molecularly and spatially different alterations in the prostate gland. Furthermore, some informative biomarkers may reflect changes in the tumour micro-environment in response to these alterations. In this chapter, we have chosen to highlight some of this complexity for one biomarker, LRG1. The next phase in the translation of this and many other markers will need to focus on understanding their spatial expression and biological function, their relationship to imaging modalities now being incorporated into diagnostic pathways and their contribution alongside other markers in predicting treatment responses and outcome. To achieve this, new clinical and research environments will need to emerge to enhance data sharing, technology adoption and the development and application of data type-agnostic analytical workflows.

References

1. Rawla P. Epidemiology of prostate cancer. World J Oncol. 2019;10(2):63–89.

2. Carioli G, et al. European cancer mortality predictions for the year 2020 with a focus on prostate cancer. Ann Oncol. 2020;31(5):650–8.

3. https://www.cancer.gov/about-cancer/diagnosis-staging/diagnosis/tumor-markers-list.

4. Taira A, et al. Reviving the acid phosphatase test for prostate cancer. Oncology (Williston Park). 2007;21(8):1003–10.

5. Xu H, et al. Prostatic acid phosphatase (PAP) predicts prostate cancer Progress in a population-based study: the renewal of PAP? Dis Markers. 2019;2019:7090545.

6. Farshchi F, Hasanzadeh M. Nanomaterial based aptasensing of prostate specific antigen (PSA): recent progress and challenges in efficient diagnosis of prostate cancer using biomedicine. Biomed Pharmacother. 2020;132:110878.

7. Slawin KM, Shariat S, Canto E. BPSA: a novel serum marker for benign prostatic hyperplasia. Rev Urol. 2005;7(Suppl 8):S52–6.

8. Mikolajczyk SD, Rittenhouse HG. Pro PSA: a more cancer specific form of prostate specific antigen for the early detection of prostate cancer. Keio J Med. 2003;52(2):86–91.

9. Mikolajczyk SD, et al. A truncated precursor form of prostate-specific antigen is a more specific serum marker of prostate cancer. Cancer Res. 2001;61(18):6958–63.

10. Sottile A, et al. A pilot study evaluating serum pro-prostate-specific antigen in patients with rising PSA following radical prostatectomy. Oncol Lett. 2012;3(4):819–24.

11. Punnen S, Pavan N, Parekh DJ. Finding the wolf in sheep's clothing: the 4Kscore is a novel blood test that can accurately identify the risk of aggressive prostate cancer. Rev Urol. 2015;17(1):3–13.

12. Vickers A, et al. Value of intact prostate specific antigen and human Kallikrein 2 in the 4 Kallikrein predictive model: an individual patient data meta-analysis. J Urol. 2018;199(6):1470–4.

13. Andree KC, van Dalum G, Terstappen LWMM. Challenges in circulating tumor cell detection by the CellSearch system. Mol Oncol. 2016;10(3):395–407.

14. Galletti G, et al. Circulating tumor cells in prostate cancer diagnosis and monitoring: an appraisal of clinical potential. Mol Diagn Ther. 2014;18(4):389–402.

15. Wang L, et al. Promise and limits of the CellSearch platform for evaluating pharmacodynamics in circulating tumor cells. Semin Oncol. 2016;43(4):464–75.

16. Sharp A, et al. Clinical utility of circulating tumour cell androgen receptor splice Variant-7 status in metastatic castration-resistant prostate cancer. Eur Urol. 2019;76(5):676–85.

17. Tagawa ST, et al. Expression of AR-V7 and ARv567es in circulating tumor cells correlates with outcomes to Taxane therapy in men with metastatic prostate cancer treated in TAXYNERGY. Clin Cancer Res. 2019;25(6):1880.

18. Antonarakis ES, et al. Androgen receptor variant-driven prostate cancer: clinical implications and therapeutic targeting. Prostate Cancer Prostatic Dis. 2016;19(3):231–41.

19. Sadar MD. Discovery of drugs that directly target the intrinsically disordered region of the androgen receptor. Expert Opin Drug Discovery. 2020;15(5):551–60.

20. Lambert SA, Abraham G, Inouye M. Towards clinical utility of polygenic risk scores. Hum Mol Genet. 2019;28(R2):R133–42.

21. Huynh-Le MP, et al. Polygenic hazard score is associated with prostate cancer in multi-ethnic populations. Nat Commun. 2021;12(1):1236.

22. Saunders EJ, Kote-Jarai Z, Eeles RA. Identification of germline genetic variants that increase prostate cancer risk and influence development of aggressive disease. Cancers (Basel). 2021;13(4)

23. Darst BF, et al. Germline sequencing DNA repair genes in 5,545 men with aggressive and non-aggressive prostate cancer. J Natl Cancer Inst. 2020;

24. Li M, et al. Urine PCA3 mRNA level in diagnostic of prostate cancer. J Cancer Res Ther. 2018;14(4):864–6.

25. Shappell SB, et al. PCA3 urine mRNA testing for prostate carcinoma: patterns of use by community urologists and assay performance in reference laboratory setting. Urology. 2009;73(2):363–8.

26. López-Abente G, Mispireta S, Pollán M. Breast and prostate cancer: an analysis of common epidemiological features in mortality trends in Spain. BMC Cancer. 2014;14(1):874.

27. Page EC, et al. Interim results from the IMPACT study: evidence for prostate-specific antigen screening in BRCA2 mutation carriers. Eur Urol. 2019;76(6):831–42.

28. Tretiakova MS, et al. Prognostic value of Ki67 in localized prostate carcinoma: a multi-institutional study of >1000 prostatectomies. Prostate Cancer Prostatic Dis. 2016;19(3):264–70.

29. Verma R, et al. Significance of p53 and ki-67 expression in prostate cancer. Urol Ann. 2015;7(4):488–93.

30. Olson A, et al. The comprehensive role of E-cadherin in maintaining prostatic epithelial integrity during oncogenic transformation and tumor progression. PLoS Genet. 2019;15(10):e1008451.

31. Tomita K, et al. Cadherin switching in human prostate cancer progression. Cancer Res. 2000;60(13):3650.

32. Jamaspishvili T, et al. Clinical implications of PTEN loss in prostate cancer. Nat Rev Urol. 2018;15(4):222–34.

33. Geybels MS, et al. PTEN loss is associated with prostate cancer recurrence and alterations in tumor DNA methylation profiles. Oncotarget. 2017;8(48):84338–48.

34. Petrovics G, et al. Frequent overexpression of ETS-related gene-1 (ERG1) in prostate cancer transcriptome. Oncogene. 2005;24:3847–52.

35. Gasi Tandefelt D, et al. ETS fusion genes in prostate cancer. Endocr Relat Cancer. 2014;21(3):R143–52.

36. Kumar-Sinha C, Tomlins SA, Chinnaiyan AM. Recurrent gene fusions in prostate cancer. Nat Rev Cancer. 2008;8(7):497–511.

37. Varambally S, et al. The polycomb group protein EZH2 is involved in progression of prostate cancer. Nature. 2002;419(6907):624–9.

38. Duan R, Du W, Guo W. EZH2: a novel target for cancer treatment. J Hematol Oncol. 2020;13(1):104.

39. Yang YA, Yu J. EZH2, an epigenetic driver of prostate cancer. Protein Cell. 2013;4(5):331–41.

40. Guo J, et al. Establishing a urine-based biomarker assay for prostate cancer risk stratification. Front Cell Dev Biol. 2020;8:597961.

41. Klein EA, et al. A 17-gene assay to predict prostate cancer aggressiveness in the context of Gleason grade heterogeneity, tumor multifocality, and biopsy undersampling. Eur Urol. 2014;66(3):550–60.

42. Eggener S, et al. A 17-gene panel for prediction of adverse prostate cancer pathologic features: prospective clinical validation and utility. Urology. 2019;126:76–82.

43. Cullen J, et al. The 17-gene genomic prostate score test as a predictor of outcomes in men with unfavorable intermediate risk prostate cancer. Urology. 2020;143:103–11.

44. Crawford ED, et al. CCP score and risk stratification for prostate cancer patients at biopsy. J Clin Oncol. 2014;32(4_suppl):47.

45. Cuzick J, et al. Validation of an RNA cell cycle progression score for predicting death from prostate cancer in a conservatively managed needle biopsy cohort. Br J Cancer. 2015;113(3):382–9.

46. Sommariva S, et al. Prognostic value of the cell cycle progression score in patients with prostate cancer: a systematic review and meta-analysis. Eur Urol. 2016;69(1):107–15.

47. Gillott DJ, et al. Specific isoforms of leucine-rich alpha2-glycoprotein detected in the proliferative endometrium of women undergoing assisted reproduction are associated with spontaneous pregnancy. Fertil Steril. 2008;90(3):761–8.

48. Kentsis A, et al. Detection and diagnostic value of urine leucine-rich α-2-glycoprotein in children with suspected acute appendicitis. Ann Emerg Med. 2012;60(1):78–83.e1.

49. Li X, et al. Expression of TGF-betas and TGF-beta type II receptor in cerebrospinal fluid of patients with idiopathic normal pressure hydrocephalus. Neurosci Lett. 2007;413(2):141–4.

50. Liu C, et al. A multifunctional role of leucine-rich α-2-glycoprotein 1 in cutaneous wound healing under Normal and diabetic conditions. Diabetes. 2020;69(11):2467–80.

51. Wang Y, et al. TNF-α-induced LRG1 promotes angiogenesis and mesenchymal stem cell migration in the subchondral bone during osteoarthritis. Cell Death Dis. 2017;8(3):e2715.

52. Ai J, et al. LRG-accelerated differentiation defines unique G-CSFR signaling pathways downstream of PU.1 and C/EBPepsilon that modulate neutrophil activation. J Leukoc Biol. 2008;83(5):1277–85.

53. Druhan LJ, et al. Leucine rich α-2 glycoprotein: a novel neutrophil granule protein and modulator of myelopoiesis. PLoS One. 2017;12(1):e0170261.

54. proteinatlas.org.

55. Lengyel E. Ovarian cancer development and metastasis. Am J Pathol. 2010;177(3):1053–64.

56. Perkins A, Liu G. Primary brain tumors in adults: diagnosis and treatment. Am Fam Physician. 2016;93(3):211–7.

57. Chaerkady R, et al. O labeling for a quantitative proteomic analysis of glycoproteins in hepatocellular carcinoma. Clin Proteomics. 2008;4(3–4):137–55.

58. Sarvari J, et al. Comparative proteomics of sera from HCC patients with different origins. Hepat Mon. 2014;14(1):e13103.

59. Wang CH, et al. LRG1 expression indicates unfavorable clinical outcome in hepatocellular carcinoma. Oncotarget. 2015;6(39):42118–29.

60. Zhang Y, et al. LRG1 suppresses the migration and invasion of hepatocellular carcinoma cells. Med Oncol. 2015;32(5):146.

61. Furuta T, et al. The multipotential of leucine-rich α-2 glycoprotein 1 as a clinicopathological biomarker of glioblastoma. J Neuropathol Exp Neurol. 2020;79(8):873–9.

62. Lin B, et al. Deep depletion of abundant serum proteins reveals low-abundant proteins as potential biomarkers for human ovarian cancer. Proteomics Clin Appl. 2009;3(7):853–61.

63. Boylan KL, et al. Quantitative proteomic analysis by iTRAQ(R) for the identification of candidate biomarkers in ovarian cancer serum. Proteome Sci. 2010;8:31.

64. Andersen JD, et al. Leucine-rich alpha-2-glycoprotein-1 is upregulated in sera and tumors of ovarian cancer patients. J Ovarian Res. 2010;3:21.

65. Wu J, et al. Altered expression of sialylated glycoproteins in ovarian cancer sera using lectin-based ELISA assay and quantitative glycoproteomics analysis. J Proteome Res. 2013;12(7):3342–52.

66. Mu AK, et al. Identification of O-glycosylated proteins that are aberrantly excreted in the urine of patients with early stage ovarian cancer. Int J Mol Sci. 2013;14(4):7923–31.

67. Smith CR, et al. Deciphering the peptidome of urine from ovarian cancer patients and healthy controls. Clin Proteomics. 2014;11(1):23.

68. Zhang YS, et al. Prognostic value of LRG1 in breast cancer: a retrospective study. Oncol Res Treat. 2020:1–6.

69. Kakisaka T, et al. Plasma proteomics of pancreatic cancer patients by multi-dimensional liquid chromatography and two-dimensional difference gel electrophoresis (2D-DIGE): up-regulation of leucine-rich alpha-2-glycoprotein in pancreatic cancer. J Chromatogr B Analyt Technol Biomed Life Sci. 2007;852(1–2):257–67.

70. Choi JW, et al. Proteomic and cytokine plasma biomarkers for predicting progression from colorectal adenoma to carcinoma in human patients. Proteomics. 2013;13(15):2361–74.

71. Sun DC, et al. Leucine-rich alpha-2-glycoprotein-1, relevant with microvessel density, is an independent survival prognostic factor for stage III colorectal cancer patients: a retrospective analysis. Oncotarget. 2017;8(39):66550–8.

72. Heo SH, et al. Identification of putative serum glycoprotein biomarkers for human lung adenocarcinoma by multi-lectin affinity chromatography and LC-MS/MS. Proteomics. 2007;7(23):4292–302.

73. Li Y, et al. Proteomic identification of exosomal LRG1: a potential urinary biomarker for detecting NSCLC. Electrophoresis. 2011;32(15):1976–83.

74. Liu Y, et al. Integrative proteomics and tissue microarray profiling indicate the association between overexpressed serum proteins and non-small cell lung cancer. PLoS One. 2012;7(12):e51748.

75. Li Z, et al. Exosomal leucine-rich-Alpha2-glycoprotein 1 derived from non-small-cell lung cancer cells promotes angiogenesis via TGF-β signal pathway. Mol Ther Oncolytics. 2019;14:313–22.

76. Ban Z, et al. LRG-1 enhances the migration of thyroid carcinoma cells through promotion of the epithelial-mesenchymal transition by activating MAPK/p38 signaling. Oncol Rep. 2019;41(6):3270–80.

77. Haupt H, Baudner S. Isolation and characterization of an unknown, leucine-rich 3.1-S-alpha2-glycoprotein from human serum (author's transl). Hoppe Seylers Z Physiol Chem. 1977;358(6):639–46.

78. uniprot.org.

79. Takahashi N, Takahashi Y, Putnam FW. Periodicity of leucine and tandem repetition of a 24-amino acid segment in the primary structure of leucine-rich alpha 2-glycoprotein of human serum. Proc Natl Acad Sci. 1985;82(7):1906.

80. swissmodel.expasy.org.

81. Brasch J, et al. Crystal structure of the ligand binding domain of netrin G2. J Mol Biol. 2011;414(5):723–34.

82. Schwick HG, Haupt H. Purified human plasma proteins of unknown function. Jpn J Med Sci Biol. 1981;34(5):299–327.

83. Sun D, Kar S, Carr BI. Differentially expressed genes in TGF-beta 1 sensitive and resistant human hepatoma cells. Cancer Lett. 1995;89(1):73–9.

84. Xu J, Lamouille S, Derynck R. TGF-beta-induced epithelial to mesenchymal transition. Cell Res. 2009;19(2):156–72.

85. Vander Ark A, Cao J, Li X. TGF-β receptors: in and beyond TGF-β signaling. Cell Signal. 2018;52:112–20.

86. Morikawa M, Derynck R, Miyazono K. TGF-β and the TGF-β family: context-dependent roles in cell and tissue physiology. Cold Spring Harb Perspect Biol. 2016;8(5)

87. Haque S, Morris JC. Transforming growth factor-β: a therapeutic target for cancer. Hum Vaccin Immunother. 2017;13(8):1741–50.

88. Principe DR, et al. TGF-β: duality of function between tumor prevention and carcinogenesis. JNCI: J Natl Cancer Inst. 2014;106(2)

89. Wojtowicz-Praga S. Reversal of tumor-induced immunosuppression by TGF-β inhibitors. Investig New Drugs. 2003;21(1):21–32.

90. Otsuru T, et al. Epithelial-mesenchymal transition via transforming growth factor beta in pancreatic cancer is potentiated by the inflammatory glycoprotein leucine-rich alpha-2 glycoprotein. Cancer Sci. 2019;110(3):985–96.

91. Wang X, et al. LRG1 promotes angiogenesis by modulating endothelial TGF-β signalling. Nature. 2013;499(7458):306–11.

92. Hong Q, et al. LRG1 promotes diabetic kidney disease progression by enhancing TGF-β-induced angiogenesis. J Am Soc Nephrol. 2019;30(4):546–62.

93. Zhang A, et al. Role of VEGF-A and LRG1 in abnormal angiogenesis associated with diabetic nephropathy. Front Physiol. 2020;11:1064.

94. Fan M, et al. Knockdown of long noncoding RNA-taurine-upregulated gene 1 inhibits tumor angiogenesis in ovarian cancer by regulating leucine-rich α-2-glycoprotein-1. Anti-Cancer Drugs. 2019;30(6):562–70.

95. Cummings C, et al. Serum leucine-rich alpha-2-glycoprotein-1 binds cytochrome c and inhibits antibody detection of this apoptotic marker in enzyme-linked immunosorbent assay. Apoptosis. 2006;11(7):1121–9.

96. Alberts B, et al. The molecular biology of the cell. 2014;1025.

97. Garrido C, et al. Mechanisms of cytochrome c release from mitochondria. Cell Death Differ. 2006;13(9):1423–33.

98. Codina R, et al. Cytochrome c-induced lymphocyte death from the outside in: inhibition by serum leucine-rich alpha-2-glycoprotein-1. Apoptosis. 2010;15(2):139–52.

99. Jemmerson R, et al. Intracellular leucine-rich alpha-2-glycoprotein-1 competes with Apaf-1 for binding cytochrome c in protecting MCF-7 breast cancer cells from apoptosis. Apoptosis. 2021;

100. Shirai R, et al. Autologous extracellular cytochrome c is an endogenous ligand for leucine-rich alpha2-glycoprotein and beta-type phospholipase A2 inhibitor. J Biol Chem. 2010;285(28):21607–14.

101. Sardana G, et al. Proteomic analysis of conditioned media from the PC3, LNCaP, and 22Rv1 prostate cancer cell lines: discovery and validation of candidate prostate cancer biomarkers. J Proteome Res. 2008;7(8):3329–38.

102. Sardana G, Marshall J, Diamandis EP. Discovery of candidate tumor markers for prostate cancer via proteomic analysis of cell culture-conditioned medium. Clin Chem. 2007;53(3):429–37.

103. Cima I, et al. Cancer genetics-guided discovery of serum biomarker signatures for diagnosis and prognosis of prostate cancer. Proc Natl Acad Sci. 2011;108(8):3342.

104. Murphy K, et al. Integrating biomarkers across omic platforms: an approach to improve stratification of patients with indolent and aggressive prostate cancer. Mol Oncol. 2018;12(9):1513–25.

105. Guldvik IJ, et al. Identification and validation of leucine-rich α-2-glycoprotein 1 as a noninvasive biomarker for improved precision in prostate cancer risk stratification. Eur Urol Open Sci. 2020;21:51–60.

106. Lopez J, Tait SW. Mitochondrial apoptosis: killing cancer using the enemy within. Br J Cancer. 2015;112(6):957–62.

107. Health Quality O. Prolaris cell cycle progression test for localized prostate cancer: a Health technology assessment. Ontario Health Technol Assess Ser. 2017;17(6):1–75.

108. https://www.nice.org.uk/advice/mib65/chapter/Technology-overview.

109. https://personalisedhealthleeds.com/news-events/new-hope-for-prostate-cancer-care-as-leeds-launches-uk-first-study/.

Michael S. Rogers

Abstract

Phenotypes viewed as distinctive to cancer are often recapitulated in benign disease and consideration of these diseases can inform our understanding of the cancer microenvironment. Endometriosis is an estrogen-dependent inflammatory disease characterized by the presence of "metastatic" endometrium-like glands and stroma, together with hemosiderin and (often) fibrosis outside the uterine lumen. It is most often diagnosed as a result of pain and/or infertility and results in substantial economic and personal costs. However, in contrast to cancer it is typically not dysplastic and rarely causes death, though it increases the risk of several ovarian cancer subtypes. Like cancers, the disease is angiogenesis-dependent and genetic studies demonstrate that the VEGFR2 signaling axis plays a key role in the disease. In addition, molecular studies demonstrate that the immune/inflammatory milieu of endometriosis lesions is more similar to that of endometriosis-associated ovarian cancers (EAOCs) than it is to eutopic endometrium. This is consistent with the dysregulation of a host of immune/inflammatory cells and cytokines in disease tissue in ways that often resemble dysregulation observed in ovarian cancer. However, in contrast to EAOC, pain is often a key early symptom of endometriosis and can accompany even very small lesions. Another key contrast with cancers is the very limited range of medical treatments available. This is partially driven by the much more limited range of side effects that is acceptable for treatment of a non-life-threatening illness in women of childbearing age, but is also a function of the limited study of endometriosis pathophysiology that has occurred thus far.

M. S. Rogers (✉)
Vascular Biology Program, Boston Children's Hospital, Harvard Medical School, Boston, MA, USA
e-mail: michael.rogers@childrens.harvard.edu

Take-Home Lessons

- Endometriosis is an estrogen-dependent inflammatory disease that affects ~10% of women of childbearing age.
- Like cancer, endometriosis is proliferative, invasive, and metastatic.
- Endometriosis predisposes to "endometriosis associated ovarian cancers."
- Endometriosis shares key microenvironmental features with gynecologic malignancies, including activated angiogenesis and an altered immune/inflammatory milieu.
- Available treatments for endometriosis (NSAIDs, hormonal therapy, surgery) are frequently ineffective; new treatments are urgently needed.

Endometriosis is an estrogen-dependent gynecological disease characterized by the presence of endometrium-like glands, stroma, and hemosiderin in locations other than the lumen of the uterus. While endometriosis prevalence has not been clearly determined, the condition is estimated to affect ~10% of the general female population [1, 2], and is present in >50% of women and teenage girls with chronic pelvic pain and up to 50% of infertile women [3]. The annual costs of endometriosis in the USA have been estimated at $69.4 billion during the peridiagnostic period; however, this number is likely substantially higher once the ten years surrounding diagnosis are considered [4]. The disease incurs similar per-capita costs in Europe as well, emphasizing the high economic burden of the disease [5]. Current endometriosis therapies include medical and surgical options, but the success of these treatments is often limited and recurrence of symptoms is common [6]. Pain scores frequently return toward baseline levels after discontinuation of medication [7–9] and about half of patients report recurrence of pain by 12 months postoperatively [10].

L. A. Akslen, R. S. Watnick (eds.), *Biomarkers of the Tumor Microenvironment*, https://doi.org/10.1007/978-3-030-98950-7_28

Endometrium as a Model of Cancer-Like Microenvironment

There are several microenvironmental alterations that are often described as key hallmarks of cancer. These include angiogenesis, immune dysregulation, inflammation, invasion, and metastasis [11]. Cancers are also often characterized by rapid cell growth. The intense study of malignancy over the last half century has sometimes obscured the extent to which non-cell-autonomous features of cancer are also exhibited by both normal physiology and benign pathologies. In this context a useful comparison can be made between cancer and the endometrium and the most common endometrial pathology, endometriosis (Fig. 28.1).

Endometriosis is most commonly characterized by infertility and/or chronic pain, especially in the pelvic or abdominal region [3]. The disease is associated with the growth of proliferative, invasive, endometrium-like tissue, often located on sites such as the ovaries, posterior cul-de-sac, or

bladder. The best supported hypothesis for the origin of these lesions is Sampson's theory of retrograde menstruation [12]. It posits that endometriosis results when menstrual fluid flows through the Fallopian tubes into the abdominal and/or pelvic spaces where it seeds lesions. Endometriosis can lead to several cancers, but is not itself usually considered a precursor lesion. The fraction of endometriosis cases that lead to malignancy is relatively small (~1%). And though there are several "endometriosis-associated ovarian carcinomas" (EAOCs), the odds ratios for women with endometriosis being later diagnosed with these cancers is substantially smaller than with typical precursor lesions; for clear cell ovarian cancer (OR, 3.73), endometrioid ovarian cancer (OR, 2.32), and low-grade serous ovarian cancer (OR, 2.02) [13, 14]. Endometriosis is not usually dysplastic (though nuclear atypia is sometimes observed, especially in conjunction with EAOC).

Importantly, although endometriosis is associated with individual cancer-associated mutations (in, e.g., KRAS, ARID1A, PIK3CA [15]), most lesions have no cancer-associated mutations and those that do have only a single cancer gene mutated. In addition, disease symptoms commonly manifest themselves in young women shortly after menarche, suggesting that the local microenvironment, rather than mutational processes (that take time) predominates in disease susceptibility. Thus, comparing endometriosis pathophysiology with that of EAOC can help differentiate mutation-driven processes from those that result from maladaptive results of normal biology.

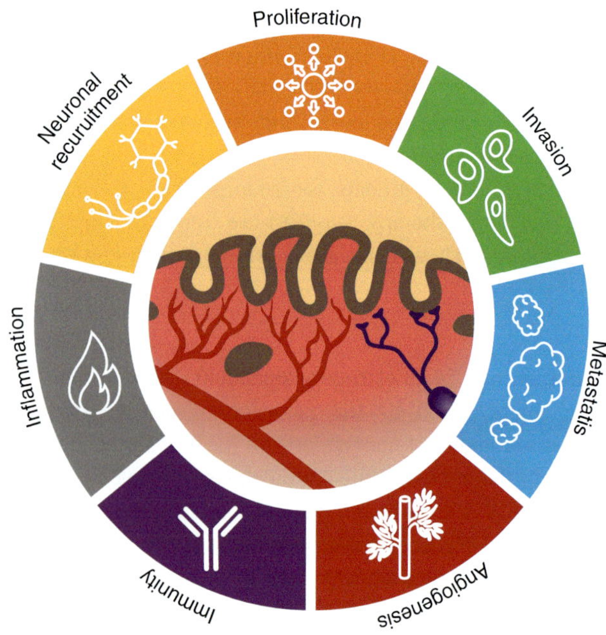

Fig. 28.1 Key Hallmarks of Endometriosis. Endometriosis shares multiple microenvironmental hallmarks of cancer, including: *Proliferation*; eutopic endometrium is highly proliferative and endometriosis tissue reflects this. Some normal differentiation is lost as endometriosis only rarely decidualizes. Importantly, the disease is highly responsive to steroid hormone manipulation. *Invasion*; essentially all lesions invade the mesothelium, with deep invasion into organ structures in a significant subset of women. *Metastasis*; metastatic tissue implants are produced without oncogenic transformation. Distal metastases are observed. *Angiogenesis*; robust angiogenesis defines lesion color. *Immunity*; dysfunctional innate immunity that fails to clear shed tissue and no longer reflects cyclic recruitment of immune cell types to lesions. *Inflammation*; lesions and surrounding tissue are characterized by ongoing sterile inflammation. *Neuronal recruitment* is dramatically increased in a subset of individuals, potentially contributing to lesion growth via neuroimmune communication

The Endometrium Is an Extraordinarily Proliferative Tissue

The endometrium is the lining of the uterus and its major function is to enable embryo implantation, placenta formation, and gestation. It is composed of two layers, the basalis, a ~ 0.5 mm thick [16] layer of compact stromal tissue with "rhizome-like" horizontal glands [17, 18] that is not shed during menstruation. Overlying and arising from the basalis is the functionalis, an often spongy layer containing a characteristic stroma with vertical glands and an overlying luminal epithelium. This layer ranges in thickness from 0 to >8 mm in thickness, depending on the menstrual phase.

Menstruation is induced when a drop in progesterone causes the dense network of spiral arteries feeding the functionalist to constrict, resulting in tissue hypoxia/ischemia, apoptosis, and shedding of the vast majority, if not all, of the functionalis. The shedding process is followed by an extraordinarily rapid proliferation of endometrial epithelial and stromal cells, that rivals the fastest tumor growth rates. Within a few days of the onset of menstruation, epithelial cells from glands in the basalis and any residual functionalis proliferate and cover the newly denuded lumen of the endometrium, forming a new luminal epithelium by the end of the menstrual phase. Then, during the proliferative phase, the endometrium rapidly expands, more than doubling in size in a week [19]. The proliferative phase ends with ovulation. The next phase is called the secretory phase and is named for the secretion by the endometrial glands of histotroph, which nourishes the developing embryo prior to establishment of the placenta. During this phase, modest continued glandular proliferation is accompanied by decidualization of the stroma and continued vascular proliferation in preparation for embryo implantation. If these steps do not occur, progesterone drops and the cycle repeats. In modern humans this can occur >400 times in a lifetime.

Dissemination/Colonization: Endometriosis as "Metastatic" Endometrium

Because the Fallopian tubes are open to the pelvic space, retrograde menstruation (flow of menstrual fluid through the Fallopian tubes, in addition to through the cervix) is common, being observed in ~90% of women. About 10% of women experience endometriosis, the presence of endometrium-like tissue in a location other than the uterine lumen [20]. The most widely accepted hypothesis for the origin of endometriosis is that it represents metastatic dissemination of eutopic endometrium via retrograde menstruation [12]. The retrograde menstruation hypothesis is supported by the observation that risk of endometriosis is increased by anything that is likely to increase the amount of menstrual tissue deposited in the pelvic space (earlier menarche, decreased cycle length, heavier flow, obstructed flow) [20, 21]. In bilateral endometrioma, lesions in a given patient typically do not share mutations [22], suggesting that the capacity for dissemination and implantation is not rate limiting in lesion generation. Importantly, endometriosis is not limited to the pelvic and abdominal spaces. Lesions have been reported throughout the body, including lungs, brain, etc. It is commonly assumed that lesions arrive at these locations via lymphatic or hematogenous spread, but this has not been clearly demonstrated. Thus, in addition to very rapid proliferation, endometrium exhibits the ability to metastasize. In the context of EAOC, and especially cancers that arise from endometriosis lesions, this means that the tissue has metastasized to a new location *before* oncogenic transformation.

Invasion in Endometriosis

In addition to high proliferative rates, endometriosis can also be invasive. (Adenomyosis, which consists of endometrium invading into the myometrium is typically considered a separate disease and will not be discussed here.) Endometriosis lesions are commonly divided into 3 types according to location and invasivity. Most endometriosis lesions are of the superficial peritoneal type and invade the mesothelium, but only exhibit shallow (<5 mm) invasion into surrounding tissue. Deep infiltrating endometriosis is most commonly found in the cul-de-sac, but can be found anywhere. Lesions of this type can invade deep into surrounding organs (bladder, bowel, etc.) complicating surgical removal and causing organ dysfunction. Finally, endometriomas consist of cysts of endometriosis tissue on the ovary. While not typically considered invasive, these lesions can grow to large sizes that compromise ovarian function.

Thus, endometrial tissue and endometriosis exhibit many of the hallmarks typically associated with cancer. However, there are also important differences with EAOC. Among these is a lack of dysplasia and maintenance of apparently normal histology. And although stroma typically does not decidualize, differentiation in lesion glands is otherwise normal, in marked contrast to EAOC. Based on the appearance of a greater proportion of fibrotic lesions in older women, it is also likely that glandular cells are not immortal and can exhaust their proliferative potential in some cases.

The Microenvironment in Endometriosis

Notwithstanding these differences, it is clear that endometriosis and EAOC (and cancer, more broadly) share several key microenvironmental characteristics (Fig. 28.2). Lesions in both diseases are strongly angiogenic, with disease driven by VEGF and other angiogenic regulators. In the case of endometriosis, the angiogenic nature of the disease is emphasized by the strong genetic evidence that polymorphisms in angiogenic regulators affect disease susceptibility. Both diseases are also characterized by an ongoing sterile inflammatory response that is responsible for a significant fraction of disease pathophysiology and progression. It is likely that the inflammatory response is driven by release of damage-associated molecular patterns (DAMPs), including apoptotic and/or necrotic cell debris, as well as heme and other iron species. Differences in inflammatory state among diseases may reflect differences in the profile of DAMPs released by disease tissue (e.g., apoptotic, necrotic, and hematogenous debris), but co-clustering experiments show that there is considerable overlap among diseases. One important characteristic of endometriosis is the increased participation of sensory neurons, especially nociceptors, in the disease. These clearly contribute to the intense pain that can be an important feature of the disease. However, it is also likely that they participate in neuroimmune communication [23] that may support lesion growth. In the case of cancer, inflammatory effectors may also increase the mutational burden, thereby contributing to lesion progression. Each of these features of the endometriosis microenvironment is described in more detail below.

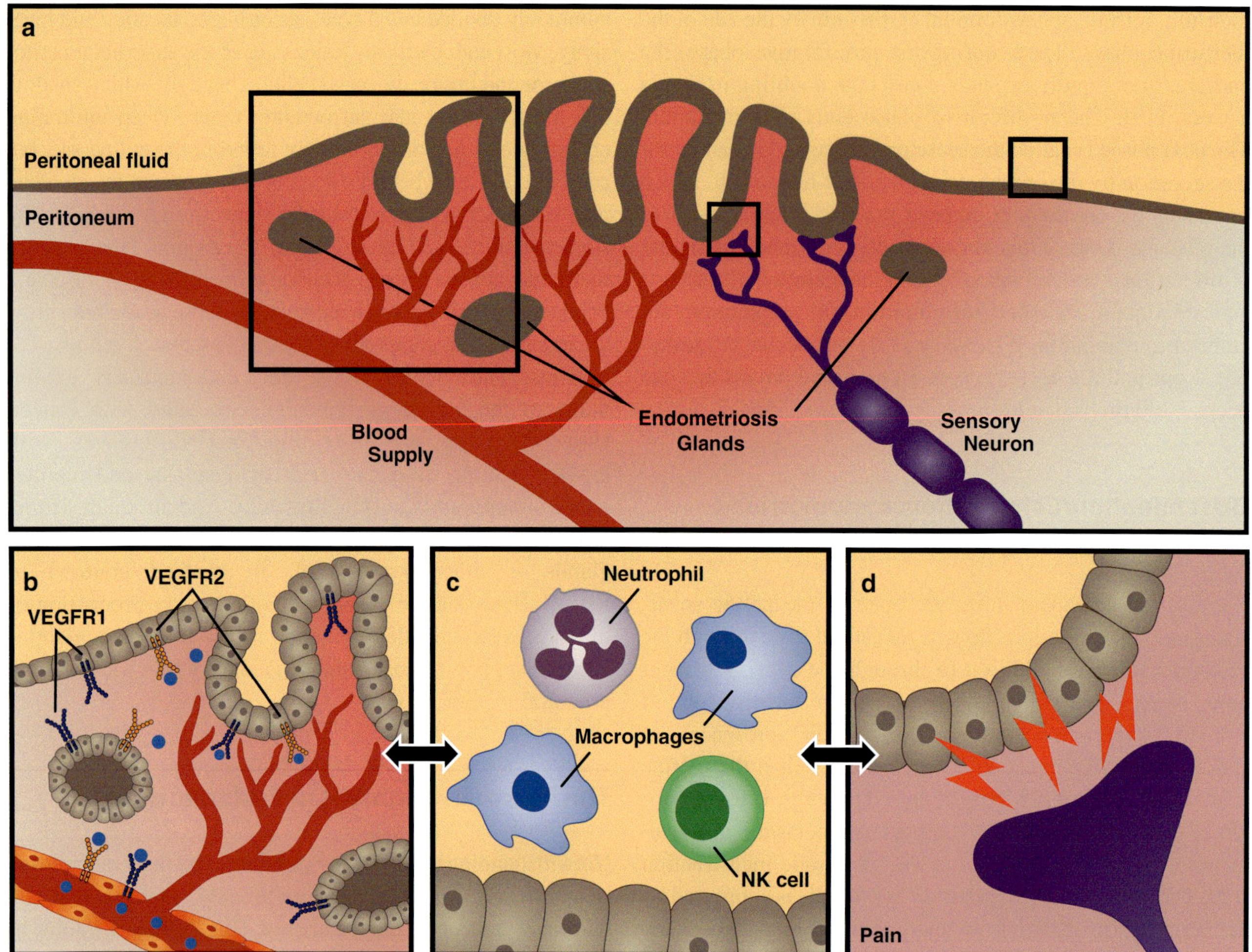

Fig. 28.2 Key pathalogical features of the endometriosis microenvironment. (**a**) Lesions consist of endometrium-like glands and stroma in an inflammatory milieu that is innervated and often highly angiogenic. (**b**) Angiogenesis is stimulated by a variety of growth factors, including VEGF, which is induced by local tissue hypoxia. VEGF signals not only through VEGF receptors on the endothelial surface, but VEGFR1 and VEGFR2 are also found on the surface of lesion tissue, suggesting direct support of lesion cells. (**c**) An altered immune and inflammatory milieu may contribute both to local inflammation and to angiogenic and neurogenic signaling without clearing lesion tissue. (**d**) Recruitment of neurites, especially from nociceptors is a common feature of endometriosis. It contributes to pain and may also be involved in neural immune communication that supports ongoing pathology

Angiogenesis and Endometriosis

The angiogenic response in cancers is described in detail in other chapters and will not be detailed here, except for a few comparisons. Rather, we will focus on the pro-angiogenic microenvironment in endometriosis. Ever since Dr. Judah Folkman proposed that tumors are angiogenesis-dependent and could be treated by antiangiogenic agents [24], the notion that this might apply to other pathologies was evident. The highly vascular nature of most endometriosis lesions, their irregular behavior, and their heterogeneous presentation made endometriosis a natural candidate for such a hypothesis.

VEGF and Angiogenesis

Vascular endothelial growth factor A (VEGF-A, also known as VEGF) is a member of the VEGF family of growth factors and is an important inducer of angiogenesis. VEGF-A signaling through VEGF receptor 2 (VEGFR2) plays an essential role during many important physiological processes such as embryonic development, organ remodeling, and wound healing [25–28]. VEGF-mediated angiogenesis also plays a key role in numerous pathologies where the formation of new blood vessels is required [29], including cancer tumor angiogenesis [30, 31]. VEGF is also implicated in the etiology of endometriosis. Importantly, polymorphisms in VEGFR2 are strongly associated with endometriosis risk

[32], underlining the importance of this pathway in disease establishment and progression.

Angiogenesis is the generation of new blood vessels from existing vessels. It is required for the generation or growth of new tissue beyond the oxygen diffusion distance, which is typically <1 mm in living tissue. Angiogenesis regulators include a long list of stimulators, such as VEGFs, basic fibroblast growth factor (bFGF), platelet-derived growth factor (PDGF), hepatocyte growth factor (HGF), bone morphogenetic proteins BMP-9 and BMP-10, interleukins IL-6 and IL-8, angiopoietin-2, and lysophosphatidic acid. Normally, angiogenesis is inhibited by molecules including thrombospondin, angiopoietin-1, tissue inhibitors of metalloproteinases (TIMPs), and collagen fragments (e.g., endostatin, arresten, canstatin, etc.). Most research over the last two decades has focused on the VEGF-VEGFR2 axis, partially because in contrast with other angiogenesis stimulators, VEGF-A had few recognized non-angiogenic activities other than to increase the permeability of endothelial cells. VEGF-A is also dramatically upregulated upon hypoxia (via HIF1α) [33, 34], and thus consistently upregulated during tissue remodeling [35].

In mammals, the VEGF family of growth factors includes VEGF-A, VEGF-B, VEGF-C, VEGF-D, and placental growth factor (PlGF). The best characterized is VEGF-A; its role in angiogenesis is well defined [25, 36]. VEGF family receptors include the tyrosine kinases VEGFR1, VEGFR2, VEGFR3, and the co-receptors NRP1 and NRP2 [37]. VEGF-A induces angiogenesis via VEGFR2 (either as a homodimer or as a heterodimer with other VEGF ligands), inducing complex intracellular signaling cascades resulting in endothelial cell responses such as proliferation, migration, survival, and permeability [38].
Aberrant expression of soluble VEGFR1 and VEGFR2 is associated with several pathologies [39–42]. Given the existence of multiple ligands and both membrane-bound and soluble receptors, measurement of a single factor can result in incomplete understanding as results can be confounded by other pathway members. Rather than a single factor controlling disease state, the net sum of all pro- and anti-angiogenic effectors is more likely to determine whether a given microenvironment supports lesion growth.

Genetic Associations Between Angiogenesis and Endometriosis

Genetic studies clearly link the VEGF-VEGFR2 pathway to endometriosis susceptibility. In GWAS, polymorphisms in VEGFR2 are associated with a ~10% difference in risk of disease [32], an effect that is stronger with increasing disease stage (and therefore, generally increased lesion burden). Candidate gene studies replicate this association [43, 44], and the absence

of a cis-eQTL for VEGFR2 expression in whole uterine and other tissues [44] is consistent with altered expression of VEGFR2 in a minor cell population, such as endothelial cells.

Other angiogenesis regulators implicated in endometriosis susceptibility by GWAS include IL1A, CDKN2B-AS1, FN1, and ID4 [32]. Interleukin (IL)-1α promotes tumor growth, invasion, migration, and angiogenesis *in vitro* [45], and it also likely influences the immune/inflammatory microenvironment of lesions. The antisense RNA encoded by CDKN2B-AS1 is involved in the epigenetic silencing of the CDKN2B-CDKN2A cluster on chromosome 9 [46], which includes of tumor suppressors genes [47, 48] linked to multiple angiogenesis-dependent pathologies [49–51]. FN1 encodes fibronectin, an extracellular matrix protein that plays a key role in vessel growth by regulating cell adhesion, migration, and differentiation [52]. ID4 is a transcriptional regulator that affects multiple processes including angiogenesis [53–55].

The GWAS locus at 1p36.12 near the WNT gene may also be angiogenesis-linked. The Wnt4/β-catenin pathway regulates angiogenesis. But eQTL analyses does not support changes in WNT4 expression as mediating the effect [56] at this locus. While this may be another example of the insensitivity of eQTL analysis to differential gene expression in minor cell types such as endothelial cells, an eQTL for CDC42 (a Rho GTPase) was identified. CDC42 regulates multiple angiogenic cells processes, including cell migration [57]. It also increases VEGF-expression and promotes endothelial cell proliferation [58]. Strikingly, a significant fraction of genes identified by GWAS in both the 2017 study discussed here [32] and a more recent study currently available as only a preprint can play a role (either directly or indirectly) in regulating the local microenvironment.

Finally, candidate gene studies, including large meta-analysis associate VEGF-A polymorphisms with endometriosis [59–62]. The absence of signal in GWAS studies might be explained by stochastic effects; however, the nature of GWAS study design may also hamper detection. In GWAS, individual polymorphisms stand in for more complex haplotypes. As long as simple haplotype–phenotype associations are observed, this is effective; however, the VEGF gene exhibits a complex haplotype structure with no single polymorphism predicting changes in gene expression [60], violating key GWAS assumptions. Thus, when viewed together, the findings of candidate gene studies, combined with appropriate interpretation of GWAS results support the idea that genetically-mediated changes in the regulation of the VEGF signaling cause some individuals to generate a microenvironment more supportive of ectopic growth of endometrial tissue than others.

VEGF-A Expression in Endometriosis

Measurements of VEGF-A in tissues from endometriosis support a role for the protein in the disease; however, important caveats must be considered for all such studies [63, 64]. Key among these is the nature of controls. In contrast with genetic studies, identification and collection of appropriate control samples can be as challenging as disease tissue collection. Controls are most often collected from patients who need surgery for other indications (e.g., fibroids, infertility not related to endometriosis, etc.), which could result in false positives if VEGF-A were dysregulated in control samples. Best practice is to include controls from multiple indications, allowing Occam's razor to be applied to infer that the outlier is the disease where dysregulation occurs. However, since controls often have angiogenesis-dependent diseases, as well (e.g., fibroids), the studies outlined below may underestimate the role of VEGF-A in endometriosis.

A few studies report that VEGF-C is upregulated in endometriosis tissue [65–67], but many more studies have looked at VEGF-A. VEGF-A is upregulated in both epithelial and stromal cells [68–80] and peritoneal fluid (PF) [49, 50, 62–74] in endometriosis. In endometriosis patients, peritoneal fluid VEGF-A concentration varies with cycle phase [81], potentially as a result of regulation by 17β-estradiol [80, 82]. VEGF-A levels in PF also correlate with disease stage [83], though the direction of causality is not clear. Increased expression may enable lesion implantation and growth or increased lesion burden, but it may also be that VEGF release is caused by increased disease burden and associated inflammatory signals (e.g., VEGF-A release from neutrophils induced by IL-8 or TNFα [84]). Indeed, treatment of endometrial and endometriotic cell cultures with PF from endometriosis PF upregulates VEGF-A expression to a greater extent than treatment with control PF does [85]. Importantly, VEGF-A may not only act on the vasculature because endometriosis epithelial and stromal cells both express VEGFR1 and VEGFR2 [86].

There is striking visual heterogeneity in endometriosis lesion color, which is driven by the presence of blood vessels and blood breakdown products (e.g., hemosiderin) [87]. As might be anticipated, histology demonstrates that peritoneal red lesions are the most highly vascularized and the most mitotic [88], a result consistent with the fact that VEGF-A concentrations in the peritoneal fluid of women with endometriotic lesions are also the highest [89], demonstrating that this growth factor is angiogenically active [89].

In addition to ectopic tissue, the eutopic endometrium of women with endometriosis exhibits higher overall VEGF-A [90, 91] and greater VEGFR2 expression on blood vessels [75] when compared to eutopic endometrium in disease-free controls. However, in cultured endometrium there are no detectable differences between these two groups in either

VEGF-A secretion or endothelial cell stimulation [92]. Thus, differences in the local microenvironment (e.g., menstruation-associated ischemia [93]) likely account for these differences.

Plasma VEGF-A concentrations are also correlated with endometriosis [94, 95], though it is important to take menstrual phase into account in such measurements; VEGF-A is highest during the menstruation phase [94, 95], likely as a result of tissue hypoxia. In contrast to plasma and peritoneal fluid, evidence that serum VEGF-A levels rise in endometriosis is less compelling [96–102]. The lack of consensus on the use of serum VEGF-A as a biomarker may be the result of the large number of underpowered studies on the hypothesis, the frequent use of comparators who themselves have angiogenesis-dependent diseases, dilution into the circulation, or the high variation in VEGF-A released when platelets degranulate. However, some studies do suggest a positive correlation [75, 103–107]. Overall, to the extent that it exists, the contribution of endometriosis to the overall variation in serum VEGF is small, while more substantial changes are observed locally and in plasma.

Other Angiogenesis Regulators

VEGF-A is only one of dozens of angiogenesis regulators that may affect endometriosis lesion implantation and growth, but others have received much less attention. Among those that have been studied, both HGF and its receptor (cMet) are upregulated in eutopic endometrium of patients vs. controls [108]. The observation that expression is highest in red peritoneal lesions [108] indicates that an important function of this overexpression is regulation of angiogenesis, but their involvement in cell migration suggests that they may also enable lesion establishment. RNA studies have also found that many other angiogenesis regulators are differentially expressed in the eutopic endometrium of advanced patients vs. unaffected controls, including VEGF-A, TNFRSF12A, RGCC, NR4A1, EREG, CYR61, and S100A7 [91].

As is true of VEGF-A measurements, the comparator tissue chosen can affect outcomes. Among the most common are other benign disease tissue and eutopic endometrium. For example, compared to benign cysts, VEGF and IL-8 are increased in the cyst fluid of both EAOC and endometrioma [109]. When ectopic and eutopic tissues are compared, additional regulators are differentially expressed, including inflammatory lipids such as prostaglandins. Prostaglandin F2α (PGF2α) is an angiogenesis stimulator and both the enzymes that synthesize it as well as its receptor are upregulated in peritoneal lesions [110]. Importantly, NSAIDs target this pathway. Since NSAIDs are known to be effective in treating endometriosis-associated pain in some women, this suggests that similar comparisons may identify additional drug targets. Thus, the observation that VEGFR2, HIF1A,

PDGFB, NRP1, EPH4B, and HGF are all upregulated in ectopic vs. eutopic tissue [111] may point toward additional therapeutic targets. Based on similar observations and in an effort to identify additional druggable targets, Lin et al. compared cell surface proteins expressed in endometriosis tissue vs. eutopic endometrium [112]. Overexpression of ANTXR2, an angiogenesis regulator [113], in endometriosis tissue vs. matched eutopic endometrium, was confirmed by qRT-PCR, western blot, and immunohistochemistry (n = 43, 42) [112]. Then, the antiangiogenic ANTXR2 inhibitor PGG [114] was found to inhibit lesion implantation and growth in a mouse model [112].

Immune/Inflammatory Microenvironment

Dysregulation of the immune/inflammatory system is an important driver of malignant transformation [13, 14]. Key cell types in this system are dynamically regulated in the eutopic endometrium throughout the menstrual cycle. During the secretory phase, macrophages, neutrophils, natural killer, and dendritic cells are increased and all but NK cells remain high during the menstrual phase. In contrast, increased T-cells are recruited during the proliferative phase. In lesion tissue, many of these cyclic fluctuations are lost or damped, indicating a (partial) loss of normal differentiation cues [115]. In addition, the sterile inflammation that contributes to both diseases is characterized by molecular changes, including upregulation of multiple immune and/or inflammatory mediators that themselves contribute to disease pathophysiology.

Immune/Inflammatory Cell Changes

In the endometrium, M1 macrophage polarization may decrease shedding thereby increasing lesion formation, but once in the ectopic location, the predominance of M2 macrophages likely contributes to lesion formation [115]. In the endometrium, (anti-inflammatory) M2 macrophages predominate in healthy women, while in endometriosis, M1 macrophages are more common. However, in ectopic lesions, M2 macrophages are commonly found to predominate and may play a role in lesion growth and/or maintenance [115, 116]. Also, in contrast to eutopic tissue, macrophages do not rise in the secretory phase in endometriosis, potentially contributing to the decrease in shedding in disease tissue [116, 117].

In lesions, a pro-inflammatory environment is generating by increased TNFα, IL-Iβ, and IL-6 [115–117], but notwithstanding their high activation state, macrophage phagocytic ability is decreased as a result of PGE2-mediated downregulation of CD36. Reversal of this effect may account for some of the effect of NSAIDs on disease pathology [116, 117].

NK cells normally protect the endometrium from infection. They also participate in blood vessel remodeling, increasing in the secretory phase in preparation for shedding at the end of that phase [115]. In endometriosis, the cytolytic activity of these cells decreases, both locally and, to a lesser extent, in the periphery [115–117]. Binding of NKG2D and c-type lectin-like NK cell receptor by MICA and MICB may decrease NK cell activity [116, 117]. NKG2D function may be further modulated by proteolysis as evidenced by increases in soluble NKG2D ligands in the peritoneal fluid of endometriosis patients allowing lesions to evade NK cell recognition [118]. This decrease may also be a consequence of high levels of IL-6, IL-10, IL-15, and TGF-β, as well as increased NKB1 and EB6 expression [116, 117].

In endometriosis patients, neutrophil numbers are increased in both the eutopic endometrium and the peritoneal cavity. Inasmuch as neutrophil depletion in a mouse model results in decreased lesion size, it is likely that these cells promote lesion growth. This may occur as a result of production of VEGF and IFN-γ [115, 117].

In endometriosis, dendritic cell maturation decreases and increased immature dendritic cells may contribute to neurogenesis and angiogenesis. The absence of mature dendritic cells may also decrease the efficacy of phagocytic clearing during menstruation, increasing the odds that any cells deposited in the pelvic space will survive long enough to implant [115].

In endometriosis, CD8+ T-cells increase vs. eutopic endometrium and the cyclic changes in T-cell number (increased in proliferative vs. secretory phases) are lost [115]. CD4+ cells increase to a greater extent resulting in an increased CD4+/CD8+ ratio. Importantly, the increased CD4+ cells are mostly Tregs and other anti-inflammatory subtypes [115, 116]. For example, in endometriosis Th17 cells are increased in ectopic lesions, peritoneal fluid, and peripheral blood, and their number correlates positively with disease stage [115, 117]. These changes may be a result of changes in cytokine patterns (see below). In the peritoneal fluid and peripheral blood of endometriosis patients, both Th1 (pro-inflammatory) and Th2 (anti-inflammatory) cytokines are increased with Th2 cytokines (e.g., IL-4 and IL-10) increased slightly more [115, 117].

Another potential modulator of T-cell function is B-cells. B lymphocyte stimulator (BLyS) is increased in endometriosis, suggests an induced state [115, 116], which may change CD4+ T-cell maturation via both ligand–receptor interaction and cytokine release [115, 117, 119]. Auto-antibodies are also a common feature of endometriosis [120].

Molecular Changes

At the molecular level, a macrophage-driven signature of peritoneal inflammation describes the peritoneal fluid of a significant subset of long-term endometriosis patients [121]. The core of this signature is defined by upregulation of IL-1β, IL1ra, IL-6 IL-8, IL-10, G-CSF, MCP-1, and RANTES; with HGF, IL-16, GROα, MIF, and MIG also contributing [121]. In patients with severe (stage III/IV) disease, IL-9, IL-4, IFN-γ, and TNFα are also increased [121]. The cytokine signature is associated with deep infiltrating disease [121], suggesting that inflammatory cells contribute to invasion.

Similar inflammatory processes likely contribute to EAOC, as well. In unsupervised clustering of immune transcriptome genes, most endometriosis tissue clusters with EAOC, demonstrating that the diseases often share a closely related immune microenvironment [13]. This environment is characterized, in part, by upregulation of elements of the complement cascade (C5, C7, CFD, CFB, CFH, and MASP1) [13, 122]. Likewise, IL-6 is increased in both endometriosis and EAOC [123, 124], and similarly, TNFα is increased in both diseases, both locally and systemically [123]. In the case of IL-10, there is a gradient of increased expression from endometriosis up to frank ovarian carcinoma [125]. This may be relevant to immune evasion in both diseases because IL-10 can increase HLA-G transcription [126]. HLA-G, in turn, can allow downregulation of HLA genes without inducing NK-mediated killing [127]. This may enable lesions to evade clearing by immune/inflammatory cells notwithstanding the presence of substantial DAMPs (in the case of endometriosis) as well as neoantigens (in case of EAOC). Increased HLA-G is, in fact observed in endometriosis [126], as well as in healthy eutopic endometrium during menstruation, suggesting that this is another example of disease hijacking normal processes.

CXCR3 is upregulated in both EAOC and endometriosis, while the fraction of (pro-inflammatory) CXCR3-expressing lymphocytes decreases modestly [128]. CXCR3 receptor and cognate CXC chemokines recruit a subset of T-cells and NK cells, thereby contributing to Th1-dependent T-cell responses [128]. This combination likely contributes to a response that is pro-inflammatory, but insufficient to clear disease tissue and thus prolonged, contributing to overall disease pathology. However, the extent of these changes can differ between malignant and benign disease, contributing to the former. For example, CXCR3B and its ligand CXCL4 are reduced in CCC compared to endometriosis [129]. The decrease in CXCR3B signaling decrease may reduce the effectiveness of any anti-tumor responses, thereby contributing to malignant transformation [109]. CXCR3 and CXC chemokines also inhibit angiogenesis [128]; for example, the CXCR3B ligand CXCL4 inhibits both VEGF and fibroblast growth factor, thereby reducing angiogenesis. In endometriosis, CD68 + macrophages express CXCL4 and CXCL4L1, but this gradually decreases in the transition zone to EAOC [130] likely contributing to a further increase in angiogenesis concomitant with oncogenic transformation and demonstrating another key distinction between the endometriosis and cancer microenvironments.

The Role of the Microenvironment in Endometriosis-Associated Pain

Pain is a key presenting symptom of endometriosis. Pain (dysmenorrhea, chronic pelvic and/or abdominal pain, dyspareunia, and dyschezia) correlates poorly with lesion type, size, anatomic location, or stage of disease [131, 132]. Women with endometriosis exhibit greater overall sensitivity to painful stimuli than women without disease [133–136], suggesting that systemic changes predispose to or result from the disease. In addition, several features of the local microenvironment correlate with pain. In rat models, increased NGF correlates with hyperalgesia [137] and both human endometriosis tissue and ectopic rat uterine tissue cause sensory nerve invasion [138]. In humans, TRPV1 staining in and around lesions is positively correlated with chronic pelvic pain, vs pain-free controls [139] and in painful endometriosis vs. pain-free woman having surgery for adnexal masses [140]. More generally, women with endometriosis-associated pain have nerve fiber densities 6 times higher than pain-free and disease-free controls, and there are functional differences in the types of neurons innervating both the eutopic endometrium and myometrium [141, 142].

Finally, it has long been known that there is correlation between angiogenic stimulation and innervation and endometriosis is no exception. In endometriosis, lesion microvessel density is correlated with pain [143, 144], and VEGF-A, acting through VEGFR1 has been shown to modulate pain in the context of cancer [30]. Thus, variation in the expression of angiogenesis stimulators has been suggested to explain variation in pelvic pain symptoms, including cyclicity and intensity [135]. However, in endometriosis expression of VEGF-A (tissue or plasma) is not correlated with pain [143, 144], suggesting that other angiogenesis drivers (e.g., NGF) play a larger role in driving pain.

Therapies Targeting the Microenvironment in Endometriosis Therapy

Endometriosis is an estrogen-dependent inflammatory disease and existing therapies leverage those characteristics. Early disease management strategies typically focus on

NSAIDs, which damp production of inflammatory lipids, such as prostaglandins. This strategy can reduce the initiating drive toward inflammation, but is less effective at resolving existing inflammation [145]. For the significant fraction of women for whom NSAIDs are insufficient to resolve symptoms, hormonal manipulations targeting the estrogen receptors are next pursued. However, such approaches are often unsuccessful and new approaches to medical therapy of endometriosis are urgently needed [146].

Antiangiogenic agents are effect treatments for cancer [147, 148] and neovascular eye disease [149] and several lines of evidence indicate that direct targeting of the VEGF pathway can be successful in treating endometriosis. First, increased serum soluble VEGFR1 (sVEGFR1, a natural VEGF antagonist) was associated with lower rASRM stage of disease in a study comparing serum and urinary angiogenic factors among endometriosis patients [150]. Second, VEGF-A inhibitors (sVEGFR1 and anti-VEGF antibody) reduce lesion burden and microvessel density in mouse models of endometriosis [151]. Third, some drugs that have been used to treat endometriosis affect VEGF-A and angiogenesis. Danazol decreases serum VEGF-A levels to normal [152]; and gonadotropin-releasing hormone (GnRH) analog activity is partially mediated by VEGF-A-regulation. VEGF-A is a survival factor for endometrial epithelial cells [86] treated with leuprolide [153], which reduces VEGF-A production in culture [154–156]. *In vivo*, in a rat model as leuprolide reduces VEGF-A production concomitant with reduction in lesion size [157]. In humans, GnRH analog treatment reduces peritoneal fluid VEGF-A [83]. Thus, a portion of the effects of hormonal agents may be mediated by regulation of VEGF-A and angiogenesis in the lesion microenvironment.

In animal models, agents that target the VEGF-VEGFR2 axis reduce cell growth, microvessel density, and lesion size and number [158–171]. However, both anti-VEGF agents and small molecule antagonists of VEGFR2 kinase activity are classified as pregnancy category D agents, and thus not suitable for fertile women during their reproductive years. Nevertheless, regression of endometriosis lesions has been observed in patients treated for malignancy with small molecule inhibitors of VEGFR2 [172]. In addition, VEGFR2 may be targetable via non-teratogenic means. Dopamine-signaling through DRD2 inhibits angiogenesis by downregulating VEGFR2 protein via endocytosis [173]. DRD2 is expressed in human endometriosis lesions, as well as eutopic endometrium [174], and the DRD2 agonists cabergoline and quinagolide inhibit angiogenesis in mice [175]. Cabergoline inhibits the growth of human endometrial tissue xenografts in mice [174] by reducing VEGFR2 activation and angiogenesis [176]. In humans, a small number of women with both hyperprolactinemia (which can be treated with quinagolide) and endometriosis were treated with quinagolide, which reduced the size of endometriosis lesions [177]. Since DRD2 agonists are generally considered to have no known risks during pregnancy, they may prove to be an effective means of disrupting VEGF-induced angiogenesis thereby treating endometriosis and clinical trials are currently underway to test this hypothesis.

Finally, agents targeting non-VEGF aspects of angiogenesis regulation should be considered. For example, in a mouse xenograft model, ABT-898 (an analog of the endogenous angiogenesis inhibitor thrombospondin-1) reduced endometriosis lesion vascularization and growth without affecting fertility or embryonic development [178, 179]. However, this agent is no longer in development, so alternative means of activating the Tsp-1 pathway would be needed to pursue this therapeutic avenue. In summary, existing therapeutics clearly target the abnormal microenvironment of endometriosis lesions and it is likely that identification and exploitation of new targets in this milieu will result in new therapeutics for this debilitating disease.

Concluding Remarks/Summary

Many phenotypes currently viewed as distinctive to cancer are recapitulated in benign disease, emphasizing the extent to which the normal milieu regulates the phenotype of both genotypically normal and malignant tissue. In the case of endometriosis, both eutopic tissue and disease lesions are characterized by rapid proliferation. Lesions exhibit a generally normal histology, with a modest decrease in cyclic differentiation. Lesions are less sensitive to progestin signals and do not typically decidualize. Cyclic recruitment of immune/inflammatory cell types is also absent. These differences suggest that a least some loss of differentiation that is evident in cancers may not result from genetic abnormalities; rather, loss of environmental signals may decrease tissue specialization.

Invasion and metastasis are often considered key hallmarks of cancer. However, endometriosis lesions exhibit both characteristics. By definition, endometriosis is metastatic, meaning that cancers that arise from metastatic lesions have metastasized *before* oncogenic transformation. Lesions also invade other structures, at least the mesothelium, but often deep into other organs. These observations demonstrate that neither invasion nor metastatic dissemination is unique to cancer. They also show that both processes proceed more readily than is sometimes imagined and do not require mutation. Nevertheless, the relative rarity of distal dissemination in endometriosis shows that there is some barrier to distal metastasis.

Blood and blood-derived hemosiderin play a key role in the wide variety of colors observed by surgeons in endometriosis. Angiogenesis is the key determinant of the vascularization of endometriosis lesions, and cancers as well. Both diseases release a variety of angiogenesis stimulators, including VEGF. In the case of endometriosis, genetically regulated angiogenic responsiveness plays a key role in disease susceptibility. Multiple cancers are effectively treated by angiogenesis inhibitors, and there is emerging evidence that these drugs can effectively treat endometriosis. Importantly, such treatment is contraindicated with currently available direct VEGF and VEGFR2 antagonists because they are teratogenic. However, non-teratogenic antiangiogenic therapeutics can be expected to be highly effective.

Finally, it is clear that EAOC and endometriosis share important components of a sterile inflammatory microenvironment. Endometriosis is pro-inflammatory, but the innate immune system cannot clear disease tissue in much the same way that cancer has been described as a wound that does not heal. In endometriosis, there is growing evidence that this is supplemented by neuroimmune communication that further supports disease growth.

In summary, endometriosis and cancer share many microenvironmental changes and these changes support key hallmarks of both diseases. In the case of EAOC, these changes precede oncogenic transformation. A better understanding of pathophysiology of non-malignant disease may help understand mutation-driven processes and distinguish those from physiological responses to DAMPs, reactive iron, and hypoxia, thereby enabling improved targeting of the microenvironment in both cancer and endometriosis.

References

1. Eskenazi B, Warner ML. Epidemiology of endometriosis. Obstet Gynecol Clin N Am. 1997;24(2):235–58.
2. Missmer SA, Hankinson SE, et al. Incidence of laparoscopically confirmed endometriosis by demographic, anthropometric, and lifestyle factors. Am J Epidemiol. 2004;160(8):784–96.
3. Giudice LC. Clinical practice. Endometriosis. N Engl J Med. 2010;362(25):2389–98.
4. Fuldeore M, Yang H, et al. Healthcare utilization and costs in women diagnosed with endometriosis before and after diagnosis: a longitudinal analysis of claims databases. Fertil Steril. 2015;103(1):163–71.
5. Simoens S, Dunselman G, et al. The burden of endometriosis: costs and quality of life of women with endometriosis and treated in referral centres. Hum Reprod. 2012;27(5):1292–9.
6. Ozkan S, Arici A. Advances in treatment options of endometriosis. Gynecol Obstet Investig. 2009;67(2):81–91.
7. Hornstein MD, Hemmings R, et al. Use of nafarelin versus placebo after reductive laparoscopic surgery for endometriosis. Fertil Steril. 1997;68(5):860–4.
8. Parazzini F, Fedele L, et al. Postsurgical medical treatment of advanced endometriosis: results of a randomized clinical trial. Am J Obstet Gynecol. 1994;171(5):1205–7.
9. Telimaa S, Puolakka J, et al. Placebo-controlled comparison of danazol and high-dose medroxyprogesterone acetate in the treatment of endometriosis. Gynecol Endocrinol. 1987;1(1):13–23.
10. Candiani GB, Fedele L, et al. Presacral neurectomy for the treatment of pelvic pain associated with endometriosis: a controlled study. Am J Obstet Gynecol. 1992;167(1):100–3.
11. Hanahan D, Robert A (2011) Hallmarks of cancer: the next generation. Cell 144.
12. Sampson JA, Albany NY (1927) Peritoneal endometriosis due to the menstrual dissemination of endometrial tissue into the peritoneal cavity. Am J Obstet Gynecol 14.
13. Suryawanshi S, Huang X, et al. (2014) Complement pathway is frequently altered in endometriosis and endometriosis-associated ovarian cancer. Clin Cancer Res 20.
14. Wendel JRH, Wang X, et al. (2018) The Endometriotic tumor microenvironment in ovarian cancer. Cancers (Basel) 10.
15. Anglesio MS, Papadopoulos N, et al. Cancer-associated mutations in endometriosis without cancer. N Engl J Med. 2017;376(19):1835–48.
16. McLennan CE, Rydell AH. Extent of endometrial shedding during normal menstruation. Obstet Gynecol. 1965;26(5):605–21.
17. Yamaguchi M, Yoshihara K, et al. Three-dimensional understanding of the morphological complexity of the human uterine endometrium. iScience. 2021;24(4):102258.
18. Tempest N, Jansen M, et al. Histological 3D reconstruction and in vivo lineage tracing of the human endometrium. J Pathol. 2020;251(4):440–51.
19. Baerwald AR, Pierson RA. Endometrial development in association with ovarian follicular waves during the menstrual cycle. Ultrasound Obstet Gynecol. 2004;24(4):453–60.
20. Shafrir AL, Farland LV, et al. Risk for and consequences of endometriosis: a critical epidemiologic review. Best Pract Res Clin Obstet Gynaecol. 2018;51:1–15.
21. Zondervan KT, Becker CM, et al. Endometriosis. Nat Rev Dis Primers. 2018;4(1):9.
22. Suda K, Nakaoka H, et al. Clonal expansion and diversification of cancer-associated mutations in endometriosis and normal endometrium. Cell Rep. 2018;24(7):1777–89.
23. Fattori V, Ferraz CR, et al. Neuroimmune communication in infection and pain: friends or foes? Immunol Lett. 2021;229:32–43.
24. Folkman J. Tumor angiogenesis: therapeutic implications. N Engl J Med. 1971;285(21):1182–6.
25. Ferrara N, Gerber HP, et al. The biology of VEGF and its receptors. Nat Med. 2003;9(6):669–76.
26. Carmeliet P, Ferreira V, et al. Abnormal blood vessel development and lethality in embryos lacking a single VEGF allele. Nature. 1996;380(6573):435–9.
27. Azar DT. Corneal angiogenic privilege: angiogenic and antiangiogenic factors in corneal avascularity, vasculogenesis, and wound healing (an American Ophthalmological Society thesis). Trans Am Ophthalmol Soc. 2006;104:264–302.
28. Johnson KE, Wilgus TA. Vascular endothelial growth factor and angiogenesis in the regulation of cutaneous wound repair. Adv Wound Care (New Rochelle). 2014;3(10):647–61.
29. Carmeliet P, Jain RK. Angiogenesis in cancer and other diseases. Nature. 2000;407(6801):249–57.
30. Selvaraj D, Gangadharan V, et al. A functional role for VEGFR1 expressed in peripheral sensory neurons in cancer pain. Cancer Cell. 2015;27(6):780–96.
31. Marcoval J, Moreno A, et al. Angiogenesis and malignant melanoma. Angiogenesis is related to the development of vertical (tumorigenic) growth phase. J Cutan Pathol. 1997;24(4):212–8.
32. Sapkota Y, Steinthorsdottir V, et al. Meta-analysis identifies five novel loci associated with endometriosis highlighting key genes involved in hormone metabolism. Nat Commun. 2017;8:15539.
33. Forsythe JA, Jiang BH, et al. Activation of vascular endothelial growth factor gene transcription by hypoxia-inducible factor 1. Mol Cell Biol. 1996;16(9):4604–13.
34. Shweiki D, Itin A, et al. Vascular endothelial growth factor induced by hypoxia may mediate hypoxia-initiated angiogenesis. Nature. 1992;359(6398):843–5.

35. Pugh CW, Ratcliffe PJ. Regulation of angiogenesis by hypoxia: role of the HIF system. Nat Med. 2003;9(6):677–84.

36. Lohela M, Bry M, et al. VEGFs and receptors involved in angiogenesis versus lymphangiogenesis. Curr Opin Cell Biol. 2009;21(2):154–65.

37. Roskoski R Jr. VEGF receptor protein-tyrosine kinases: structure and regulation. Biochem Biophys Res Commun. 2008;375(3):287–91.

38. Koch S, Claesson-Welsh L. Signal transduction by vascular endothelial growth factor receptors. Cold Spring Harb Perspect Med. 2012;2(7):a006502.

39. Artini PG, Ruggiero M, et al. Vascular endothelial growth factor and its soluble receptor in benign and malignant ovarian tumors. Biomed Pharmacother. 2008;62(6):373–7.

40. Pavlakovic H, Becker J, et al. Soluble VEGFR-2: an anti-lymphangiogenic variant of VEGF receptors. Ann N Y Acad Sci. 2010;1207(Suppl 1):E7–15.

41. Wu FT, Stefanini MO, et al. A systems biology perspective on sVEGFR1: its biological function, pathogenic role and therapeutic use. J Cell Mol Med. 2010;14(3):528–52.

42. Kumasawa K, Ikawa M, et al. Pravastatin induces placental growth factor (PGF) and ameliorates preeclampsia in a mouse model. Proc Natl Acad Sci USA. 2011;108(4):1451–5.

43. Albertsen HMCR, Ward K. Endometriosis GWAS Replicate Association Near the Kinase Insert Domain Receptor Gene (KDR); 2017 18 May 2017; Vancouver, CA.

44. Steinthorsdottir V, Thorleifsson G, et al. Common variants upstream of KDR encoding VEGFR2 and in TTC39B associate with endometriosis. Nat Commun. 2016;7:12350.

45. Salmeron K, Aihara T, et al. IL-1alpha induces angiogenesis in brain endothelial cells in vitro: implications for brain angiogenesis after acute injury. J Neurochem. 2016;136(3):573–80.

46. Aguilo F, Zhou MM, et al. Long noncoding RNA, polycomb, and the ghosts haunting INK4b-ARF-INK4a expression. Cancer Res. 2011;71(16):5365–9.

47. Traves PG, Luque A, et al. Macrophages, inflammation, and tumor suppressors: ARF, a new player in the game. Mediat Inflamm. 2012;2012:568783.

48. Zerrouqi A, Pyrzynska B, et al. P14ARF inhibits human glioblastoma-induced angiogenesis by upregulating the expression of TIMP3. J Clin Invest. 2012;122(4):1283–95.

49. Burd CE, Jeck WR, et al. Expression of linear and novel circular forms of an INK4/ARF-associated non-coding RNA correlates with atherosclerosis risk. PLoS Genet. 2010;6(12):e1001233.

50. Yoshino S, Cilluffo R, et al. Single nucleotide polymorphisms associated with abnormal coronary microvascular function. Coron Artery Dis. 2014;25(4):281–9.

51. Nanda V, Downing KP, et al. CDKN2B regulates TGFbeta signaling and smooth muscle cell investment of hypoxic neovessels. Circ Res. 2016;118(2):230–40.

52. Pankov R, Yamada KM. Fibronectin at a glance. J Cell Sci. 2002;115(Pt 20):3861–3.

53. Kuzontkoski PM, Mulligan-Kehoe MJ, et al. Inhibitor of DNA binding-4 promotes angiogenesis and growth of glioblastoma multiforme by elevating matrix GLA levels. Oncogene. 2010;29(26):3793–802.

54. Martini M, Cenci T, et al. Epigenetic silencing of Id4 identifies a glioblastoma subgroup with a better prognosis as a consequence of an inhibition of angiogenesis. Cancer. 2013;119(5):1004–12.

55. Nio-Kobayashi J, Narayanan R, et al. Expression and localization of inhibitor of differentiation (ID) proteins during tissue and vascular remodelling in the human corpus luteum. Mol Hum Reprod. 2013;19(2):82–92.

56. Powell JE, Fung JN, et al. Endometriosis risk alleles at 1p36.12 act through inverse regulation of CDC42 and LINC00339. Hum Mol Genet. 2016;25(22):5046–58.

57. Qadir MI, Parveen A, et al. Cdc42: role in cancer management. Chem Biol Drug Des. 2015;86(4):432–9.

58. Ma J, Xue Y, et al. Role of activated rac1/cdc42 in mediating endothelial cell proliferation and tumor angiogenesis in breast cancer. PLoS One. 2013;8(6):e66275.

59. Rogers MS, D'Amato RJ. The effect of genetic diversity on angiogenesis. Exp Cell Res. 2006;312(5):561–74.

60. Rogers MS, D'Amato RJ (2012) Common polymorphisms in angiogenesis. Cold Spring Harb Perspect Med 2(11).

61. Li YZ, Wang LJ, et al. Vascular endothelial growth factor gene polymorphisms contribute to the risk of endometriosis: an updated systematic review and meta-analysis of 14 case-control studies. Genet Mol Res. 2013;12(2):1035–44.

62. Cardoso JV, Abrao MS, et al. Combined effect of vascular endothelial growth factor and its receptor polymorphisms in endometriosis: a case-control study. Eur J Obstet Gynecol Reprod Biol. 2017;209:25–33.

63. Holt VL, Weiss NS. Recommendations for the design of epidemiologic studies of endometriosis. Epidemiology. 2000;11(6):654–9.

64. Zondervan KT, Cardon LR, et al. What makes a good case-control study? Design issues for complex traits such as endometriosis. Hum Reprod. 2002;17(6):1415–23.

65. Takehara M, Ueda M, et al. Vascular endothelial growth factor A and C gene expression in endometriosis. Hum Pathol. 2004;35(11):1369–75.

66. Song WW, Lu H, et al. Expression of vascular endothelial growth factor C and anti-angiogenesis therapy in endometriosis. Int J Clin Exp Pathol. 2014;7(11):7752–9.

67. Xu H, Zhang T, et al. Vascular endothelial growth factor C is increased in endometrium and promotes endothelial functions, vascular permeability and angiogenesis and growth of endometriosis. Angiogenesis. 2013;16(3):541–51.

68. Tan CW, Lee YH, et al. (2014) CD26/DPPIV down-regulation in endometrial stromal cell migration in endometriosis. Fertil Steril 102(1): 167–177 e169.

69. Braza-Boils A, Mari-Alexandre J, et al. MicroRNA expression profile in endometriosis: its relation to angiogenesis and fibrinolytic factors. Hum Reprod. 2014;29(5):978–88.

70. Meng Q, Sun W, et al. Identification of common mechanisms between endometriosis and ovarian cancer. J Assist Reprod Genet. 2011;28(10):917–23.

71. van den Berg LL, Crane LM, et al. Analysis of biomarker expression in severe endometriosis and determination of possibilities for targeted intraoperative imaging. Int J Gynaecol Obstet. 2013;121(1):35–40.

72. Di Carlo C, Bonifacio M, et al. Metalloproteinases, vascular endothelial growth factor, and angiopoietin 1 and 2 in eutopic and ectopic endometrium. Fertil Steril. 2009;91(6):2315–23.

73. Machado DE, Abrao MS, et al. Vascular density and distribution of vascular endothelial growth factor (VEGF) and its receptor VEGFR-2 (Flk-1) are significantly higher in patients with deeply infiltrating endometriosis affecting the rectum. Fertil Steril. 2008;90(1):148–55.

74. Ramon LA, Braza-Boils A, et al. microRNAs expression in endometriosis and their relation to angiogenic factors. Hum Reprod. 2011;26(5):1082–90.

75. Bourlev V, Volkov N, et al. The relationship between microvessel density, proliferative activity and expression of vascular endothelial growth factor-A and its receptors in eutopic endometrium and endometriotic lesions. Reproduction. 2006;132(3):501–9.

76. Gilabert-Estelles J, Ramon LA, et al. Expression of angiogenic factors in endometriosis: relationship to fibrinolytic and metalloproteinase systems. Hum Reprod. 2007;22(8):2120–7.

77. Oliveira VA, Abreu LG, et al. Vascular endothelial growth factor in the plasma, follicular fluid and granulosa cells of women with

endometriosis submitted to in vitro fertilization – a pilot study. Gynecol Endocrinol. 2005;20(5):284–8.

78. Takehara M, Ueda M, et al. Vascular endothelial growth factor A and C gene expression in endometriosis. Hum Pathol. 2004;35(11):1369–75..

79. Tan XJ, Lang JH, et al. Expression of vascular endothelial growth factor and thrombospondin-1 mRNA in patients with endometriosis. Fertil Steril. 2002;78(1):148–53.

80. Zhang L, Xiong W, et al. 17 β-Estradiol promotes vascular endothelial growth factor expression via the Wnt/β-catenin pathway during the pathogenesis of endometriosis. Mol Hum Reprod. 2016;22(7):526–35.

81. Fujishita A, Hasuo A, et al. Immunohistochemical study of angiogenic factors in endometrium and endometriosis. Gynecol Obstet Investig. 1999;48(Suppl 1):36–44.

82. Mueller MD, Vigne JL, et al. Regulation of vascular endothelial growth factor (VEGF) gene transcription by estrogen receptors alpha and beta. Proc Natl Acad Sci USA. 2000;97(20):10972–7.

83. Kupker W. Paracrine changes in the peritoneal environment of women with endometriosis. Hum Reprod Update. 1998;4(5):719–23.

84. Na YJ, Yang SH, et al. Effects of peritoneal fluid from endometriosis patients on the release of vascular endothelial growth factor by neutrophils and monocytes. Hum Reprod. 2006;21(7):1846–55.

85. Braza-Boils A, Gilabert-Estelles J, et al. Peritoneal fluid reduces angiogenesis-related microRNA expression in cell cultures of endometrial and endometriotic tissues from women with endometriosis. PLoS One. 2013;8(4):e62370.

86. Wang HB, Lang JH, et al. Expression of vascular endothelial growth factor receptors in the ectopic and eutopic endometrium of women with endometriosis. Zhonghua Yi Xue Za Zhi. 2005;85(22):1555–9.

87. Martin DC. Laparoscopic appearance of endometriosis. 2nd ed. Resurge Press; 2017.

88. Nisolle M, Casanas-Roux F, et al. Morphometric study of the stromal vascularization in peritoneal endometriosis. Fertil Steril. 1993;59(3):681–4.

89. Khan KN, Masuzaki H, et al. Higher activity by opaque endometriotic lesions than nonopaque lesions. Acta Obstet Gynecol Scand. 2004;83(4):375–82.

90. Donnez J, Smoes P, et al. Vascular endothelial growth factor (VEGF) in endometriosis. Hum Reprod. 1998;13(6):1686–90.

91. Zhao L, Gu C, et al. Identification of global transcriptome abnormalities and potential biomarkers in eutopic endometria of women with endometriosis: A preliminary study. Biomed Rep. 2017;6(6):654–62.

92. Print C, Valtola R, et al. Soluble factors from human endometrium promote angiogenesis and regulate the endothelial cell transcriptome. Hum Reprod. 2004;19(10):2356–66.

93. Sharkey AM, Day K, et al. Vascular endothelial growth factor expression in human endometrium is regulated by hypoxia. J Clin Endocrinol Metab. 2000;85(1):402–9.

94. Vodolazkaia A, El-Aalamat Y, et al. Evaluation of a panel of 28 biomarkers for the non-invasive diagnosis of endometriosis. Hum Reprod. 2012;27(9):2698–711.

95. Vodolazkaia A, Yesilyurt BT, et al. Vascular endothelial growth factor pathway in endometriosis: genetic variants and plasma biomarkers. Fertil Steril. 2016;105(4):988–96.

96. Kalu E, Sumar N, et al. Cytokine profiles in serum and peritoneal fluid from infertile women with and without endometriosis. J Obstet Gynaecol Res. 2007;33(4):490–5.

97. Kianpour M, Nematbakhsh M, et al. Serum and peritoneal fluid levels of vascular endothelial growth factor in women with endometriosis. Int J Fertil Steril. 2013;7(2):96–9.

98. Pupo-Nogueira A, de Oliveira RM, et al. Vascular endothelial growth factor concentrations in the serum and peritoneal fluid of women with endometriosis. Int J Gynaecol Obstet. 2007;99(1):33–7.

99. Gagne D, Page M, et al. Levels of vascular endothelial growth factor (VEGF) in serum of patients with endometriosis. Hum Reprod. 2003;18(8):1674–80.

100. Kim JG, Kim JY, et al. Association between endometriosis and polymorphisms in endostatin and vascular endothelial growth factor and their serum levels in Korean women. Fertil Steril. 2008;89(1):243–5.

101. Othman Eel D, Hornung D, et al. Serum cytokines as biomarkers for nonsurgical prediction of endometriosis. Eur J Obstet Gynecol Reprod Biol. 2008;137(2):240–6.

102. Gogacz M, Gałczyński K, et al. Concentration of selected angiogenic factors in serum and peritoneal fluid of women with endometriosis. Polish Gynaecol. 2015;86(3):188–92.

103. Bourlev V, Iljasova N, et al. Signs of reduced angiogenic activity after surgical removal of deeply infiltrating endometriosis. Fertil Steril. 2010;94(1):52–7.

104. Wang H, Gorpudolo N, et al. Elevated vascular endothelia growth factor-A in the serum and peritoneal fluid of patients with endometriosis. J Huazhong Univ Sci Technolog Med Sci. 2009;29(5):637–41.

105. Xavier P, Belo L, et al. Serum levels of VEGF and TNF-alpha and their association with C-reactive protein in patients with endometriosis. Arch Gynecol Obstet. 2006;273(4):227–31.

106. Kopuz A, Kurt S, et al. Relation of peritoneal fluid and serum vascular endothelial growth factor levels to endometriosis stage. Clin Exp Obstet Gynecol. 2014;41(5):547–50.

107. Mohamed ML, El Behery MM, et al. Comparative study between VEGF-A and CA-125 in diagnosis and follow-up of advanced endometriosis after conservative laparoscopic surgery. Arch Gynecol Obstet. 2013;287(1):77–82.

108. Khan KN, Masuzaki H, et al. Immunoexpression of hepatocyte growth factor and c-Met receptor in the eutopic endometrium predicts the activity of ectopic endometrium. Fertil Steril. 2003;79(1):173–81.

109. Fasciani A, D'Ambrogio G, et al. (2001) Vascular endothelial growth factor and interleukin-8 in ovarian cystic pathology. Fertil Steril 75.

110. Rakhila H, Al-Akoum M, et al. Augmented angiogenic factors expression via FP signaling pathways in peritoneal endometriosis. J Clin Endocrinol Metabol. 2016;101(12):4752–63.

111. Yerlikaya G, Balendran S, et al. Comprehensive study of angiogenic factors in women with endometriosis compared to women without endometriosis. Eur J Obst Gynecol Reprod Biol. 2016;204:88–98.

112. Lin SC, Lee HC, et al. Targeting anthrax toxin receptor 2 ameliorates endometriosis progression. Theranostics. 2019;9(3):620–32.

113. Rogers MS, Christensen KA, et al. Mutant anthrax toxin B moiety (protective antigen) inhibits angiogenesis and tumor growth. Cancer Res. 2007;67(20):9980–5.

114. Cryan LM, Bazinet L, et al. 1,2,3,4,6-Penta-O-galloyl-beta-d-glucopyranose inhibits angiogenesis via inhibition of capillary morphogenesis gene 2. J Med Chem. 2013;56(5):1940–5.

115. Vallve-Juanico J, Houshdaran S, et al. (2019) The endometrial immune environment of women with endometriosis. Hum Reprod Update 25.

116. Riccio LDGC, Santulli P, et al. (2018) Immunology of endometriosis. Best Pract Res Clin Obstet Gynaecol 50.

117. Symons LK, Miller JE, et al. (2018) The immunopathophysiology of endometriosis. Trends Mol Med 24.

118. González-Foruria I, Santulli P, et al. (2015) Soluble ligands for the NKG2D receptor are released during endometriosis and correlate with disease severity. PLoS One 10.

119. Shen P, Fillatreau S (2015) Antibody-independent functions of B cells: a focus on cytokines. Nat Rev Immunol 15.

120. Lang GA, Yeaman GR. Autoantibodies in endometriosis sera recognize a Thomsen-Friedenreich-like carbohydrate antigen. J Autoimmun. 2001;16(2):151–61.

121. Beste MT, Pfaffle-Doyle N, et al. Molecular network analysis of endometriosis reveals a role for c-Jun-regulated macrophage activation. Sci Transl Med. 2014;6(222):222ra216.

122. Aslan C, Ak H, et al. Overexpression of complement C5 in endometriosis. Clin Biochem. 2014;47(6):496–8.

123. Darai E, Detchev R, et al. (2003) Serum and cyst fluid levels of interleukin (IL) -6, IL-8 and tumour necrosis factor-alpha in women with endometriomas and benign and malignant cystic ovarian tumours. Hum Reprod 18.

124. Schroder W, Ruppert C, et al. (1994) Concomitant measurements of interleukin-6 (IL-6) in serum and peritoneal fluid of patients with benign and malignant ovarian tumors. Eur J Obstet Gynecol Reprod Biol 56.

125. Sipak-Szmigiel O, Wlodarski P, et al. (2017) Serum and peritoneal fluid concentrations of soluble human leukocyte antigen, tumor necrosis factor alpha and interleukin 10 in patients with selected ovarian pathologies. J Ovarian Res 10.

126. Mach P, Blecharz P, et al. (2010) Differences in the soluble HLA-G blood serum concentration levels in patients with ovarian cancer and ovarian and deep endometriosis. Am J Reprod Immunol 63.

127. Liu L, Wang L, et al. The role of HLA-G in tumor escape: manipulating the phenotype and function of immune cells. Front Oncol. 2020;10:597468.

128. Furuya M, Suyama T, et al. (2007) Up-regulation of CXC chemokines and their receptors: implications for proinflammatory microenvironments of ovarian carcinomas and endometriosis. Hum Pathol 38.

129. Furuya M, Yoneyama T, et al. (2011) Differential expression patterns of CXCR3 variants and corresponding CXC chemokines in clear cell ovarian cancers and endometriosis. Gynecol Oncol 122.

130. Furuya M, Tanaka R, et al. (2012) Impaired CXCL4 expression in tumor-associated macrophages (TAMs) of ovarian cancers arising in endometriosis. Cancer Biol Ther 13.

131. Fedele L, Parazzini F, et al. Stage and localization of pelvic endometriosis and pain. Fertil Steril. 1990;53(1):155–8.

132. Adamson GD. Diagnosis and clinical presentation of endometriosis. Am J Obstet Gynecol. 1990;162(2):568–9.

133. He W, Liu X, et al. Generalized hyperalgesia in women with endometriosis and its resolution following a successful surgery. Reprod Sci. 2010;17(12):1099–111.

134. Bajaj P, Bajaj P, et al. Endometriosis is associated with central sensitization: a psychophysical controlled study. J Pain. 2003;4(7):372–80.

135. Morotti M, Vincent K, et al. Mechanisms of pain in endometriosis. Eur J Obstet Gynecol Reprod Biol. 2017;209:8–13.

136. Mowers EL, Lim CS, et al. Prevalence of endometriosis during abdominal or laparoscopic hysterectomy for chronic pelvic pain. Obstet Gynecol. 2016;127(6):1045–53.

137. Zhang G, Dmitrieva N, et al. Endometriosis as a neurovascular condition: estrous variations in innervation, vascularization, and growth factor content of ectopic endometrial cysts in the rat. Am J Physiol Regul Integr Comp Physiol. 2008;294(1):R162–71.

138. Berkley KJ, Dmitrieva N, et al. Innervation of ectopic endometrium in a rat model of endometriosis. Proc Natl Acad Sci. 2004;101(30):11094–8.

139. Rocha MG, e Silva JC, et al. TRPV1 expression on peritoneal endometriosis foci is associated with chronic pelvic pain. Reprod Sci. 2011;18(6):511–5.

140. Poli-Neto OB, Filho AA, et al. Increased capsaicin receptor TRPV1 in the peritoneum of women with chronic pelvic pain. Clin J Pain. 2009;25(3):218–22.

141. Tokushige N, Markham R, et al. Nerve fibres in peritoneal endometriosis. Hum Reprod. 2006;21(11):3001–7.

142. Tokushige N, Markham R, et al. High density of small nerve fibres in the functional layer of the endometrium in women with endometriosis. Hum Reprod. 2006;21(3):782–7.

143. García-Manero M, Alcazar JL, et al. Vascular endothelial growth factor (VEGF) and ovarian endometriosis: correlation between VEGF serum levels, VEGF cellular expression, and pelvic pain. Fertil Steril. 2007;88(2):513–5.

144. Garcia-Manero M, Santana GT, et al. Relationship between microvascular density and expression of vascular endothelial growth factor in patients with ovarian endometriosis. J Womens Health (Larchmt). 2008;17(5):777–82.

145. Serhan CN, Levy BD. Resolvins in inflammation: emergence of the pro-resolving superfamily of mediators. J Clin Invest. 2018;128(7):2657–69.

146. Zondervan KT, Becker CM, et al. Endometriosis. N Engl J Med. 2020;382(13):1244–56.

147. Shih T, Lindley C. Bevacizumab: an angiogenesis inhibitor for the treatment of solid malignancies. Clin Ther. 2006;28(11):1779–802.

148. Cook KM, Figg WD. Angiogenesis inhibitors: current strategies and future prospects. CA Cancer J Clin. 2010;60(4):222–43.

149. Chang J-H, Garg NK, et al. Corneal neovascularization: an anti-VEGF therapy review. Surv Ophthalmol. 2012;57(5):415–29.

150. Cho SH, Oh YJ, et al. Evaluation of serum and urinary angiogenic factors in patients with endometriosis. Am J Reprod Immunol. 2007;58(6):497–504.

151. Hull ML, Charnock-Jones DS, et al. Antiangiogenic agents are effective inhibitors of endometriosis. J Clin Endocrinol Metab. 2003;88(6):2889–99.

152. Matalliotakis IM, Goumenou AG, et al. Serum concentrations of growth factors in women with and without endometriosis: the action of anti-endometriosis medicines. Int Immunopharmacol. 2003;3(1):81–9.

153. Bilotas M, Meresman G, et al. Effect of vascular endothelial growth factor and interleukin-1beta on apoptosis in endometrial cell cultures from patients with endometriosis and controls. J Reprod Immunol. 2010;84(2):193–8.

154. Tesone M, Bilotas M, et al. The role of GnRH analogues in endometriosis-associated apoptosis and angiogenesis. Gynecol Obstet Investig. 2008;66(Suppl 1):10–8.

155. Huang F, Wang H, et al. Effect of GnRH-II on the ESC proliferation, apoptosis and VEGF secretion in patients with endometriosis in vitro. Int J Clin Exp Pathol. 2013;6(11):2487–96.

156. Meresman GF, Bilotas MA, et al. Effect of GnRH analogues on apoptosis and release of interleukin-1beta and vascular endothelial growth factor in endometrial cell cultures from patients with endometriosis. Hum Reprod. 2003;18(9):1767–71.

157. Dogan E, Saygili U, et al. Regression of endometrial explants in rats treated with the cyclooxygenase-2 inhibitor rofecoxib. Fertil Steril. 2004;82(Suppl 3):1115–20.

158. Liu S, Xin X, et al. Efficacy of anti-VEGF/VEGFR agents on animal models of endometriosis: a systematic review and meta-analysis. PLoS One. 2016;11(11):e0166658.

159. Ozer H, Boztosun A, et al. The efficacy of bevacizumab, sorafenib, and retinoic acid on rat endometriosis model. Reprod Sci. 2013;20(1):26–32.

160. Soysal D, Kızıldağ S, et al. (2014) A novel angiogenesis inhibitor bevacizumab induces apoptosis in the rat endometriosis model. Balkan J Med Genet 17(2).

161. Ricci AG, Olivares CN, et al. Effect of vascular endothelial growth factor inhibition on endometrial implant development in a murine model of endometriosis. Reprod Sci. 2011;18(7):614–22.

162. Sevket O, Sevket A, et al. The effects of ranibizumab on surgically induced endometriosis in a rat model: a preliminary study. Reprod Sci. 2013;20(10):1224–9.

163. Laschke MW, Elitzsch A, et al. Combined inhibition of vascular endothelial growth factor (VEGF), fibroblast growth factor and

platelet-derived growth factor, but not inhibition of VEGF alone, effectively suppresses angiogenesis and vessel maturation in endometriotic lesions. Hum Reprod. 2006;21(1):262–8.

164. Yildiz C, Kacan T, et al. Effects of pazopanib, sunitinib, and sorafenib, anti-VEGF agents, on the growth of experimental endometriosis in rats. Reprod Sci. 2015;22(11):1445–51.

165. Abbas MA, Disi AM, et al. Sunitinib as an anti-endometriotic agent. Eur J Pharm Sci. 2013;49(4):732–6.

166. Pala HG, Erbas O, et al. The effects of sunitinib on endometriosis. J Obstet Gynaecol. 2015;35(2):183–7.

167. Fallon EM, Nehra D, et al. Sunitinib reduces recurrent pelvic adhesions in a rabbit model. J Surg Res. 2012;178(2):860–5.

168. Meisel JA, Fallon EM, et al. Sunitinib inhibits postoperative adhesions in a rabbit model. Surgery. 2011;150(1):32–8.

169. Kim S, Lee S, et al. Inhibition of intra-abdominal adhesion formation with the angiogenesis inhibitor sunitinib. J Surg Res. 2008;149(1):115–9.

170. Moggio A, Pittatore G, et al. Sorafenib inhibits growth, migration, and angiogenic potential of ectopic endometrial mesenchymal stem cells derived from patients with endometriosis. Fertil Steril. 2012;98(6):1521–1530 e1522.

171. Leconte M, Santulli P, et al. Inhibition of MAPK and VEGFR by sorafenib controls the progression of endometriosis. Reprod Sci. 2015;22(9):1171–80.

172. Mir O, Ropert S, et al. Clinical activity of sunitinib and regorafenib in endometriosis. Mayo Clin Proc. 2019;94(12):2591–3.

173. Basu S, Nagy JA, et al. The neurotransmitter dopamine inhibits angiogenesis induced by vascular permeability factor/vascular endothelial growth factor. Nat Med. 2001;7(5):569–74.

174. Novella-Maestre E, Carda C, et al. Identification and quantification of dopamine receptor 2 in human eutopic and ectopic endometrium: a novel molecular target for endometriosis therapy. Biol Reprod. 2010;83(5):866–73.

175. Delgado-Rosas F, Gomez R, et al. The effects of ergot and non-ergot-derived dopamine agonists in an experimental mouse model of endometriosis. Reproduction. 2011;142(5):745–55.

176. Novella-Maestre E, Carda C, et al. Dopamine agonist administration causes a reduction in endometrial implants through modulation of angiogenesis in experimentally induced endometriosis. Hum Reprod. 2009;24(5):1025–35.

177. Gomez R, Abad A, et al. Effects of hyperprolactinemia treatment with the dopamine agonist quinagolide on endometriotic lesions in patients with endometriosis-associated hyperprolactinemia. Fertil Steril. 2011;95(3):882–888 e881.

178. Nakamura DS, Edwards AK, et al. Thrombospondin-1 mimetic peptide ABT-898 affects neovascularization and survival of human endometriotic lesions in a mouse model. Am J Pathol. 2012;181(2):570–82.

179. Nakamura DS, Edwards AK, et al. Compatibility of a novel thrombospondin-1 analog with fertility and pregnancy in a xenograft mouse model of endometriosis. PLoS One. 2015;10(3):e0121545.

Tumor-Vascular Interactions in Non-Small Cell Lung Cancer

Maria Ramnefjell and Lars A. Akslen

Abstract

Despite improved diagnostics leading to early discovery and potentially curable disease, and with new promising treatment options, lung cancer remains the leading cause of cancer-related deaths worldwide.

As will be shown in this chapter, tumor cell interaction with lung vasculature in NSCLC is complicated. Angiogenesis, defined as the sprouting of new capillaries from pre-existing vessels, has been found as an important prognostic factor in lung cancer. There are several new potential treatments aiming to inhibit angiogenesis, either alone or in combination with other chemotherapeutic substances or lately also with immunotherapy. The major problem seems to be the increased risk of adverse events, and possibly not a long-lasting effect on survival. Also, there is a constant and yet unmet need for reliable biomarkers for selecting patients who will benefit from such advanced treatment.

Meanwhile, as researchers try to find new treatments with increasingly complicated methods, vascular invasion represents a tumor feature that is currently included in pathology reports in our environment, and that in numerous publications is reported to have a clear impact on survival. We believe that this important and easily accessible prognostic factor should be taken more into consideration, not only concerning primary staging, but also to select a group of patients that need close follow-up.

Take-Home Lessons
- Vascular invasion in lung cancer can be evaluated by routine staining methods, and is a strong and independent prognostic factor.
- Angiogenesis is an important factor in tumor progression, also in lung cancer.
- There is still an unmet need for validated predictive biomarkers for anti-angiogenic therapy in lung cancer.

Background

Lung cancer is the most common cause of cancer-related deaths in the world today, with an estimated 1.8 million deaths in 2020 [1]. Non-small cell lung cancer (NSCLC) comprises around 80% of the cases [2]. Although the five-year relative survival rate has increased over the past ten years [3], lung cancer is still the leading cause of cancer-related deaths, only surpassed by breast cancer for women worldwide [1].

This implies a constant need for more efficient and targeted treatment regimes. Several new potential therapies are in the pipeline, and we realize that a constant focus on the basic biological characteristics of non-small cell lung cancers is important in the treatment and follow-up of these patients.

Lung cancer is divided broadly into small cell carcinoma, non-small cell carcinoma (NSCLC), and other main types like sarcomas [4]. NSCLC is further divided into subtypes according to histopathological features as described in the 2015 WHO Classification of Lung Tumors [5, 6], adenocarcinoma and squamous cell carcinoma being the two most common. These cancers frequently metastasize to other organs, with contralateral lung, regional and distant lymph nodes, the nervous system, liver, adrenals, skin, and the skeletal system as the most common sites for NSCLC [7, 8].

M. Ramnefjell (✉)
Department of Clinical Medicine, Centre for Cancer Biomarkers CCBIO, University of Bergen, Bergen, Norway
e-mail: maria.ramnefjell@uib.no

L. A. Akslen
Centre for Cancer Biomarkers CCBIO, Department of Clinical Medicine, University of Bergen, Bergen, Norway
e-mail: lars.akslen@uib.no

© The Author(s), under exclusive license to Springer Nature Switzerland AG 2022
L. A. Akslen, R. S. Watnick (eds.), *Biomarkers of the Tumor Microenvironment*, https://doi.org/10.1007/978-3-030-98950-7_29

Lung cancers are staged using the TNM Classification of Malignant Tumors (eighth edition from 2017, [9]), which takes into account tumor size, node involvement, pleural involvement, and distant metastasis. The T denominator describes mainly the tumor size, but also whether the tumor infiltrates the pleura, or adjacent structures such as the diaphragm, the mediastinum, or the heart. The N denominator describes lymph nodes affected by tumor metastasis and is subdivided depending on their localization. The M denominator describes whether distant metastases are present or not. These three denominators are then combined to give stages I–IV.

Traditionally, the treatment of NSCLC is primarily based on the stage category [10]. For early-stage NSCLC (stages I–II), surgery is the primary choice for curative therapy. Whether surgery is performed will also depend on the localization of the tumor and the patient's general health. Alternatively, patients in stages I–III who are technically or medically inoperable, stereotactic ablative radiotherapy is an option for curative treatment. To date, no randomized controlled studies comparing surgery and radiotherapy are published, but smaller studies indicate comparable results [11, 12].

For stage IIIA tumors, treatment options depend on prognostic factors such as tumor size, weight loss, and the ECOG status (daily functioning level). Stages IIIB and IV are considered inoperable, but patients in stage IIIB can be offered chemotherapy with curative intent depending on prognostic factors as described above. For patients in which palliative care is the remaining option, the choice of treatment is often discussed in multidisciplinary teams. Choice of chemotherapy regimen depends on tumor subtype and stage with platinum doublets as the standard of care.

Recently, there has been an exciting development in targeted treatment options, mostly linked to epidermal growth factor receptor (*EGFR*) mutations and anaplastic lymphoma kinase (*ALK*) rearrangements. These genetic alterations occur most often in female non-smokers of Asian descent with adenocarcinoma [13]. Current recommendations indicate that all new cases of non-squamous NSCLC will be tested for *EGFR* mutations, *ALK* rearrangements, and *ROS1* mutations [14, 15]. Given a positive result, the patient will be treated with tyrosine kinase inhibitors (TKI). Also, as part of a broader molecular profiling, it is now recommended to test for METex14 skipping mutations, NTRK1/2/3 gene fusions, and RET rearrangements [15].

The latest and most promising development is immunotherapy, where immune checkpoint inhibitors like ipilimumab first showed improved survival in patients with advanced stages of metastatic melanoma [16]. This monoclonal antibody blocks the cytotoxic T-lymphocyte-associated protein-4 (CTLA-4), thus enabling T-cells to recognize tumor cells as foreign and initiate an immunogenic response. Ipilimumab has not shown the same effect in non-small cell lung cancer, but it has proven effective in combination with standard chemotherapy, especially for the subgroup of squamous cell carcinomas [17].

Another mechanism of targeting the immune system is by blocking the interaction between programmed cell death 1 (PD-1) and its ligand PD-L1, an interaction which inactivates cytotoxic T-cells that normally would attack tumor cells [18–20]. For lung cancer, the first monoclonal antibody presented was pembrolizumab, a humanized monoclonal IgG4 kappa antibody against PD-1 [21], followed by nivolumab [22]. Both drugs are now approved by the FDA for the treatment of advanced non-small cell carcinoma [23].

The Tumor Microenvironment

The tumor microenvironment (TME), or supporting tumor stroma, consists of fibroblasts, vascular cells, inflammatory cells, fat cells, and the extracellular matrix including various growth factors and inhibitors [24, 25]. The microenvironment in lung tissue is characterized by high vascularity, and the normal lung has anatomical and cellular characteristics to protect against foreign particles and pathogens [24, 26]. However, it is known that patients with increased inflammatory activity, such has those with chronic interstitial lung disease, have an increased risk of developing lung cancer [27], and that this comorbidity is related to reduced survival [28].

The interplay between tumor cells and the TME has been known since the mid-1800's when Virchow found tumors growing at sites of chronic inflammation [29]. However, it is only recently that this relationship has gathered increased attention among researchers, emerging as a new area for targeted therapies and combination treatments [30, 31].

Of specific interest was the immune system, where increasing evidence throughout the late 1990s pointed to immune cells not only being able to suppress tumor growth, but also facilitate and sustain the development of malignant tumors [32]. The concept of tumor immunoediting emerged, consisting of the three E's: *elimination, equilibrium, and escape* [33]. This theory has later been revisited [18, 34], and integrated into the *hallmarks of cancer* [35]. In lung cancer, it served as a basis for the development of immunotherapy mentioned above.

Tumor cells interact with their microenvironment not only at the primary site, but importantly also at metastatic sites. As mentioned, Paget introduced the concept of "seed and soil" in 1889 [36], whereby the tumor cells (*seed*) prefer certain secondary sites (*soil*) that are the most suitable in terms of potential growth, and this theory was consolidated further by Fidler et al. in the 1970s [37]. At the metastatic site, circulating or disseminated tumor cells are faced with a different microenvironment than at the primary site. In 2005,

Kaplan et al. published their seminal paper describing the *"pre-metastatic niche"* [38], reporting that hematopoietic progenitor cells that expressed VEGFR-1 were present at the metastatic site before detectable tumor cells. Further studies have shown that these pre-metastatic niches are diverse and include both fibronectin, cytokines, growth factors, and matrix metalloproteinases, all contributing to attracting tumor cells and facilitating not only extravasation of tumor cells, but also the shift from a micrometastasis to a detectable macrometastasis [39]. The latter shift occurs among other mechanisms through the initiation of angiogenesis.

Tumor Angiogenesis in Lung Cancer

As defined by Hanahan and Folkman, angiogenesis represents the sprouting of new capillaries from pre-existing vessels, and this process is regarded as one of the hallmarks of cancer development and progression [35, 40, 41]. Malignant tumors require angiogenesis to grow beyond 1–2 mm³ in size and to be able to metastasize as proposed by Judah Folkman [42]. Angiogenesis is initiated physiologically during embryogenesis [43] and also in wound healing [44–46], being carefully balanced by positive and negative angiogenic regulators. In tumors, the induction of angiogenesis is thought to commence through the "angiogenic switch," whereby proangiogenic signals (such as VEGF) overcome the antiangiogenic signals (such as thrombospondin-1) [40].

The newly formed vessels are often small, branched, leaky, and distorted [47], and they represent a promising target for tumor treatment, also in lung cancer [48]. The vessels are subject to mechanical compression by surrounding cancer cells, fibroblasts, and extracellular matrix, which affects vessel formation and function [49]. In addition, they have abnormal function as a result of overexpression of proangiogenic molecules such as VEGF described below.

As a main driver of angiogenesis, VEGF was first reported as a stimulator of the vasculature (the vascular permeability factor, VPF) by Senger and Dvorak in 1983 [50], and later specified as a vascular endothelial growth factor (VEGF) in 1989 by Ferrara and Henzel [51]. The VEGF family consists of five members, given the letters A through E. They bind to transmembrane tyrosine kinase receptors (VEGFR-1, 2, and 3) on endothelial cells, thereby initiating intracellular signaling (such as RAS/RAF and PI3K) and eventually endothelial proliferation, migration, and survival, along with increased vascular permeability [52–54]. The VEGF family of proteins (VEGF-A, VEGF-C, and VEGF-D) and their receptors (VEGFR-1, VEGFR-2, and VEGFR-3) are considered one of the most important angiogenic pathways, and the expression of these proteins might be studied on endothelial cells, stromal cells, and tumor cells by immunohistochemistry using paraffin-embedded tissues [55–58].

Two other major proangiogenic factors are platelet-derived growth factors (PDGF) and fibroblast growth factors (FGF). Both of these bind to transmembrane receptors (PDGFR-α, PDGFR-β, FGFR-1, and FGFR-2), and this leads to initiation of downstream signaling mainly through the PI3K pathway, inducing angiogenesis [59, 60]. Other proangiogenic factors include TGF-β, ANG, TIE, NOTCH, and WNT as described in a review by Carmeliet and Jain [61].

VEGF upregulation has been associated with poor prognosis in several tumors [62], such as breast, melanoma, gastric adenocarcinoma, and synovial sarcoma [63–66]. Upregulation of VEGF has also been related to reduced survival in NSCLC [67, 68]. Studies have shown that high tumor cell expression of VEGF-A and VEGFR-2 was associated with poor prognosis in NSCLC [69]. In contrast, high stromal expression of angiogenic markers favors a good prognosis with VEGF-C as an independent prognostic factor [56]. Others found that tumor cell expression of PDGF-A correlated with lymph node metastasis and that high levels of PDGFR- β, VEGF-A, and VEGFR-3 in tumor cells were associated with lymph node metastasis and subsequent poor prognosis [57, 58, 70].

The many complex networks of ligands, receptors, and signaling pathways underline the difficulties in targeting a single factor in order to prohibit angiogenesis. Adding to this picture are other described mechanisms whereby a tumor can form functioning vascular structures; vasculogenesis, intussusception, vessel co-option, vascular mimicry, and endothelial cells formed from cancer stem-like cells by reprogramming [61, 71]. Vessel co-option is a process of vascularization where tumor cells grow toward and along already existing vessels and where tumor cells infiltrate between these vessels and incorporate them into the tumor itself [72]; this process was first described for brain tumors [73]. Vessel co-option is regarded as a possible mechanism for resistance to anti-angiogenic therapy, which is directed toward newly formed vessels such as by angiogenesis [72–74]. This demonstrates the complexity by which tumors ensure sufficient perfusion and delivery of nutrients and oxygen.

Biomarkers of Angiogenesis

Microvessel Density

Counting microvessel density (MVD) has been considered an appropriate estimate for tumor-associated angiogenesis [75], but there have been discussions on how to measure and report MVD in a standardized way [76, 77]. Actively proliferating vessels (pMVD), vascular proliferation index (VPI), and glomeruloid microvascular proliferation (GMP) are more closely correlated to disease progression and prognosis than MVD [78–80] in some tumor types. Such comparative studies have so far mainly focused on melanomas, endometrial cancer, prostate cancer, and breast cancer.

Regarding the prognostic value of MVD in lung cancer, previous studies have given somewhat conflicting results, as pointed out in a meta-analysis by Meert et al. where 23 studies from 1992 through 2001 were included [81]. The first study to report negative prognostic impact of MVD in lung cancer was published in 1992 relating high MVD to increased metastatic rate [82]. Since the review by Meert, there are reports on MVD in NSCLC, but only a few where the prognostic value was evaluated. Medetoglu et al. found that a high MVD, evaluated by staining for CD105, was an independent adverse prognostic factor in 114 stage I adenocarcinomas and squamous cell carcinomas [83]. Pomme et al. recently presented results from a study of MVD evaluated by CD34 and CD105 in TMAs of 371 NSCLC, where they found a decreased MVD in the tumor center to be independently associated with reduced survival [84]. Although no survival analysis was performed, Mlika et al. in their study from 2015 pointed out that MVD was significantly different among growth patterns in lung adenocarcinoma, with acinar and papillary patterns having the highest MVD, compared to the solid growth pattern with a proposed worse prognosis [85]. However, this study was rather small with only 46 patients included.

Vascular Proliferation

Although microvascular density can be used as an indicator of overall tumor vascularity, it only captures the presence of these vessels. In 2000, Eberhard et al. proposed that ongoing angiogenesis measured by studying endothelial cell proliferation would give a more realistic picture of the angiogenic status in tumors [86]. Stefansson et al. used this metric in their 2006 paper, showing for the first time that increased vascular proliferation, measured by the vascular proliferation index (VPI) and using Factor VIII/Ki67 for dual immunohistochemical detection, was associated with reduced survival in endometrial carcinoma [79]. The prognostic sensitivity of VPI was supported in 2009 by Gravdal et al. using a novel marker for neo-angiogenesis, by combining Nestin for immature endothelial cells with Ki67 expression for dividing endothelial cells (Nestin/Ki67) [78]. In these studies, vascular proliferation had stronger prognostic impact than standard MVD.

As mentioned, angiogenesis in non-small cell lung cancer has previously been reported using microvascular density as such. In the study by Yazdani et al. [87], a dual staining for CD31 and Ki67 was applied, but any prognostic impact of this ratio was not found. In contrast, our recent study using vascular proliferation index [88] presents a novel marker (Nestin/Ki67) for angiogenesis in NSCLC, and our findings are in line with those reported for endometrial carcinoma [79], prostatic adenocarcinoma [78], breast carcinoma [89–91], pancreatic adenocarcinoma [92], and melanoma [93] using this marker for ongoing tumor associated angiogenesis.

Glomeruloid Microvascular Proliferation (GMP)

GMP is the formation of focal proliferative buddings of endothelial cells resembling a renal glomerulus. First described as a feature of glioblastoma, GMP was later reported as a prognostic factor in other solid tumors by Straume et al. [80]. Subsequently, Tanaka et al. reported in 2003 that GMP was an independent adverse prognostic factor for overall survival in NSCLC [94]. However, in the same study the authors found that for adenocarcinomas, GMP negative patients had worse prognosis. This difference was not discussed in the paper.

Nestin Expression

Nestin was identified in the early 1990s as an intermediate filament protein, and was initially thought to be related to neuroepithelial stem cells alone [95–97]. Since then, Nestin has been found to be expressed in cells harboring characteristics like multipotency, limited self-renewal, and regenerative capacity [98], both in healthy tissues, tissue undergoing repair after injury [99], and in tumor cells [98, 99]. Nestin expression in tumor cells has been related to poor prognosis [100–105].

In lung carcinoma, the first publication on Nestin expression in tumor cells and vasculature occurred in 2010, where it was associated with another stem cell marker, CD133 [106], but no association with patient survival was found. High Nestin expression in tumor cells has been associated with lymphangiogenesis, lymph node metastasis, and reduced patient survival [107–111]. In contrast, Skarda et al. did not find any prognostic effect of Nestin expression in tumor cells, either for overall survival or for disease-free survival [112].

The results concerning a prognostic value of Nestin positivity in lung cancer cells might be conflicting. Could Nestin expression in the tumor microenvironment give better and more promising results? In the aforementioned work by Skarda et al., the authors also looked at Nestin expression in intratumoral microvessels in TMAs from 114 patients with surgically resected NSCLC, both in primary tumors and in 35 matched brain metastases [112]. The authors found that Nestin positive vessels were more frequent in higher tumor stages, but relations to patient prognosis by survival analyses were not presented.

As reported, tumor angiogenesis has been evaluated by many different methods. The use of Nestin in this setting has received attention since the early 2000s when it was found to be a marker of immature endothelial cells [113]. In 2009,

Gravdal et al. published a paper showing that neo-angiogenesis evaluated by the vascular proliferation index (VPI) had a greater impact on patient prognosis than counting microvessels alone [78]. A double staining of Nestin for immature endothelial cells, combined with the proliferation marker Ki67, was used, and the authors counted both the MVD and the density of proliferating vessels. This is the same method that Stefansson et al. previously used with FactorVIII-Ki67 [79]. Later, Krüger et al. and Kraby et al. found that VPI evaluated by Nestin-Ki67 was associated with aggressive tumor features and a basal-like phenotype in breast carcinomas [91, 114].

Whereas in lung cancer the focus has mainly been on Nestin expression in tumor cells, as described above, Onisim et al. in their review from 2015 [115] found that Nestin expression in vessels has been related to angiogenesis in cancers from multiple organs, like CNS, skin (melanoma), the gastrointestinal tract, pancreas, liver, prostate, and ovaries, including non-small cell lung cancer. However, the combination of Nestin and Ki67 in the vessels of lung carcinomas was first published by our group in 2017 [88] (Fig. 29.1). We have not been able to find other studies reporting a prognostic effect on patient survival for microvessel density evaluated by Nestin positive vessels in NSCLC. In our study, we found that Nestin demarcated endothelial cells nicely with homogenous cytoplasmic staining and that expression in small vessels and single endothelial cells was more intense than in established larger vessels [88]. We observed some staining in scattered stromal cells resembling fibroblasts, but these were distinguishable from endothelial cells by their morphology and distribution. Therefore, we found Nestin to be a valuable marker for assessment of endothelial cells.

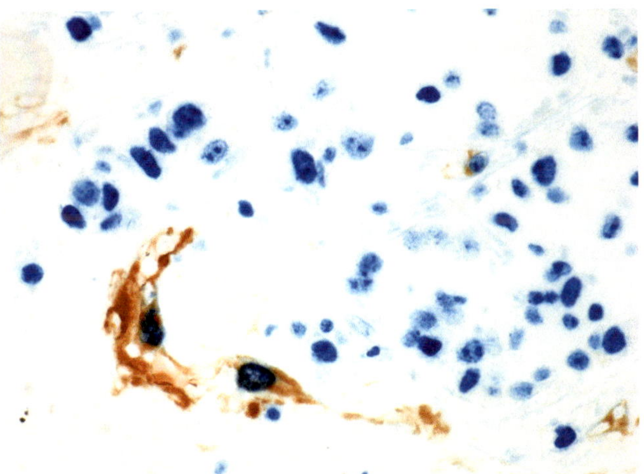

Fig. 29.1 Dual immunohistochemical staining of endothelial cells (in red) and cellular proliferation by Ki67 expression (in blue). The vascular structure (lower part) shows evidence of endothelial cell proliferation (blue nuclear staining), whereas groups of tumor cells above show a high proportion of proliferating cells. (×400) (Photo by L.A.A.)

Vascular Invasion in Lung Cancer

The newly formed vessels not only supply tumors with the necessary nutrients for growth, but also serve as possible routes for tumor cells to spread and metastasize. Invasion by tumor cells into vascular structures such as blood vessels and lymphatic vasculature has been described as an adverse prognostic factor in several tumor types, including NSCLC, since the 1950s [116].

Lymphatic invasion has been reported as a prognostic factor for reduced survival in non-small cell lung cancer [117], relating to both local recurrence and survival as described in a recent paper by Matsuura et al. [118].

How to report vascular invasion in the routine work-up of lung cancer cases has been subject to much debate, and may be a contributing factor as to why this feature is not yet implemented as a factor in the TNM staging. In the following section, we argue that this prognostic biomarker can be evaluated by standard HE staining on surgical specimens and should be taken into account with regard to a closer follow-up of this patient group after surgery.

In a study done by our group, vascular invasion was recorded in accordance with previously published studies [119], and evaluated without additional staining [120]. We interpreted blood vessel invasion as groups of tumor cells in a space covered by endothelial lining with at least in part a preserved elastic layer. Invasion into lymphatic vessels had to be seen around central airways, in the subpleural area, or along interlobular septa. No muscular outer layer should be present, and the vessels should not contain red blood cells. For vascular invasion, uncertain cases were grouped together with negative tumors for further analysis. This was done to show that by routine preparation as in daily practice, we were able to identify invasion into both blood and lymphatic vessels. Other studies have argued that elastin staining and IHC are necessary in order to accurately identify and separate all blood and lymphatic vessels with tumor invasion [121, 122].

In a subset of these cases, we then added a marker for blood vessels, CD31, and a marker for lymphatic channels, D2–40 (Fig. 29.2), to explore if we were able to detect more vessels than on conventional slides, but also to evaluate if we incorrectly recorded vessel invasion in spaces not covered by endothelial cells (false negative and false positive cases) [121]. Additionally, we wanted to examine how well we were able to distinguish between blood and lymphatic vessels, as this is a well-known challenge on HE staining, especially for smaller vessels. We randomly selected 50 adenocarcinoma cases from our cohort that on first review were negative for vessel invasion, 25 cases positive for BVI alone, and 25 cases positive for LVI alone, by examination of HE slides. The results indicated that by IHC, 5 additional cases with BVI and 7 additional cases with LVI were detected

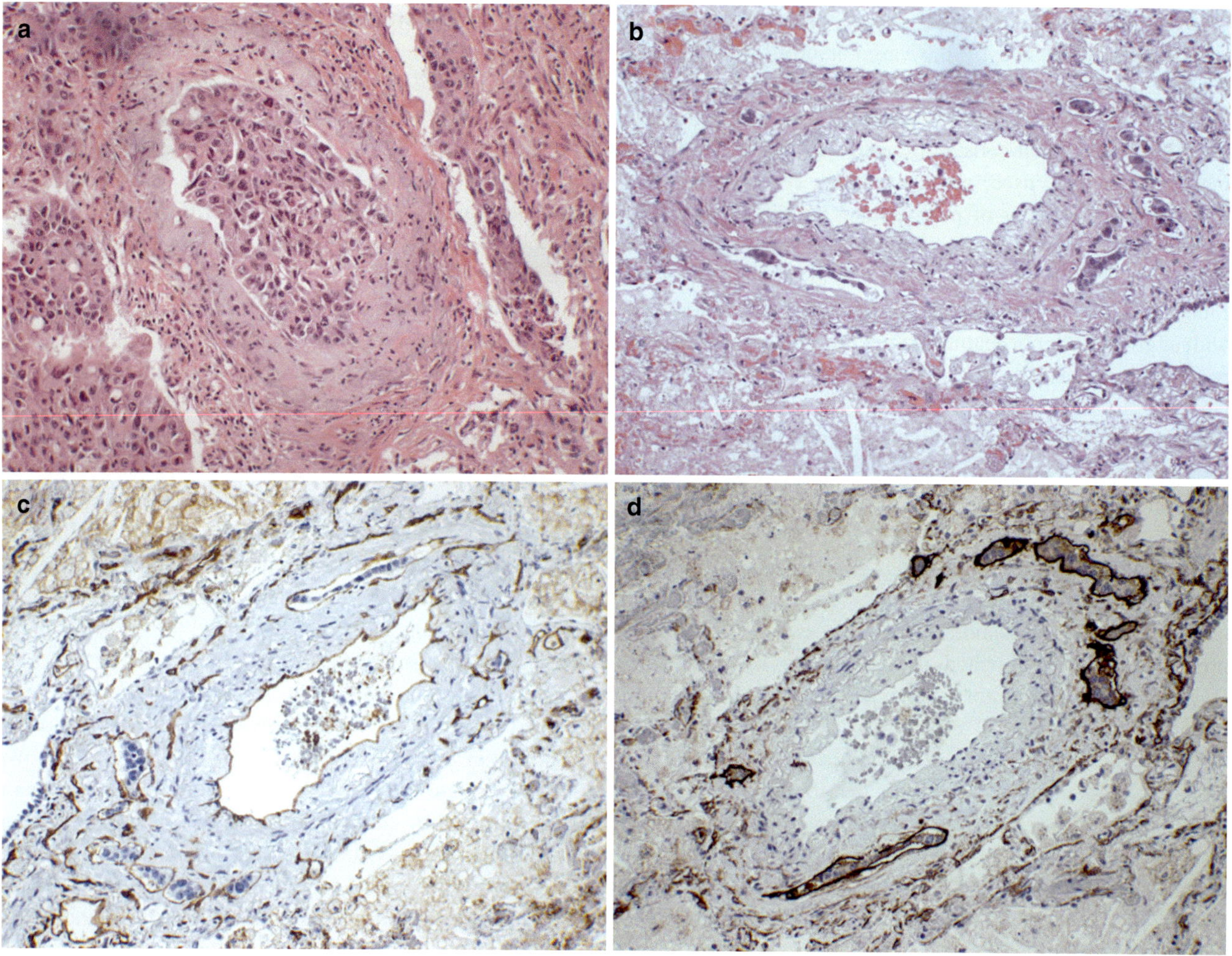

Fig. 29.2 Blood vessel invasion (**a**). Invasion into lymphatic vessels around a central blood vessel (**b**), supported by endothelial markers CD31 (**c**) and D2–40 (**d**) (×400) (Photo by M.R.)

among the negative cases. These vessels represented for the most part smaller vascular channels embedded between tumor islands. This discrepancy could in part be explained by the use of deeper tissue levels for IHC than the original HE slides. In this sub-study, only the master blocks were examined, whereas on first evaluation of the tumors (by HE slides), all available tumor slides were used, and thus, we were able to find vessels with tumor invasion in slides other than from the master blocks. Overall, we found by our criteria that there was a good correlation for distinguishing between blood and lymphatic vessels. Previous studies point to this distinction as a major shortcoming if only using HE slides [121]. We did, however, show that by standard methods, we were able to differentiate between BVI and LVI, and moreover, both were found to have independent prognostic value.

The prognostic implication of invasion into vascular structures for lung cancer was first described in the 1950s by researchers such as Aylwin et al. and Collier et al. [123–125],

who found reduced survival for patients harboring vessel invasion. The impact of vascular invasion has since been studied along with other clinicopathologic factors in various publications through the past few decades [116, 126–128]. In 2018, Sung et al. found that lymphovascular invasion (defined here as combined BVI and LVI) was significantly associated with reduced disease-free survival related to nodal metastases and distant metastases in stage I–IIa patients with complete surgical excision [129]. The most recent publication regarding vascular invasion in NSCLC found that these, alongside tumor size and advanced stage, were independent factors of early recurrence among patients with metastatic cancers [130]. Here, Shimizu et al. stated that patients with vascular invasion need more careful follow-up even after recurrence, as they showed shorter post-recurrence survival.

In the TNM Classification (eighth edition), tumor size, nodal status, and invasion into adjacent structures like pleura, mediastinum, and the diaphragm are all factors to be taken into consideration. Meanwhile, several studies have reported the negative prognostic value of invasion into lymphovascular spaces, that is blood vessels, lymphatic vessels, or both [119, 131–139]. It was proposed that infiltration into blood vessels should be included in the TNM Classification [122]. However, vascular invasion is mentioned as an important prognostic factor, but not a prerequisite for staging [140].

In our studies, we found that vascular invasion was related to decreased survival rates in non-small cell lung carcinomas. This was not a new finding, but multivariate analysis with separate models for adenocarcinomas and squamous cell carcinomas was performed in a large population-based cohort, and this was a novel aspect. Also, we showed in our study that regular HE staining is sufficient to reach a confident diagnosis of vascular invasion if thorough slide evaluation is performed, and that this provided independent prognostic information. Further, the prognostic effect of BVI and LVI was best when the two were combined, with the worst prognosis for patients with the presence of both LVI and BVI [120].

The results were equally significant for lung cancer-specific survival and time to recurrence, supporting the timely discussion of vascular invasion as another factor to be taken into account on pathological examination of surgically resected non-small cell lung cancer specimens, but not yet included in the TNM staging system.

Anti-angiogenic Therapy in Lung Cancer

In recent years, the development of anti-angiogenic treatments has emerged, targeting proangiogenic factors such as the vascular endothelial growth factor (VEGF), platelet-derived growth factor (PDGF), and fibroblast growth factor (FGF). These have all been found to be upregulated in tumor-associated angiogenesis [141–143], and their upregulation in tumors has been related to reduced survival in NSCLC [67, 144, 145].

There are two main classes of anti-angiogenic drugs developed. The first are monoclonal antibodies targeting VEGF or its receptor (VEGFR), and the second are small molecule oral TKIs [146]. Among the first is bevacizumab (Avastin®), which was approved by the FDA in 2007, and is now standard of care for advanced non-squamous lung carcinomas in the USA and some European countries [147]. Although showing a modest effect on disease-free and overall survival, there are concerns about toxicity, especially an increased risk of fatal hemorrhage [148–150]. In Norway, bevacizumab is recommended only in patients with EGFR or ALK mutations as second-line treatment [151, 152].

Other monoclonal antibodies against VEGF (aflibercept) and VEGFR (ramucirumab) have been tested in clinical trials (phase II–III) without convincing effects on survival to date [153, 154]. However, ramucirumab was approved by the FDA in 2014 for the treatment of metastatic NSCLC patients who had progressed on chemotherapy [155]. The approval was based on the REVEL trial (phase III) where the authors found a modest increase in median progression-free survival (4.5 months compared to 3.0 months) [156]. Notably, the National Institute for Health and Care Excellence (NICE) declined the approval of ramucirumab in 2016 based on the same study [157].

The second mode of treatment consists of oral TKIs targeting different combinations of VEGFR, EGFR, PDGFR, c-Kit, and RET. Examples include nintedanib, sorafenib, sunitinib, cediranib, motesanib, and vandetanib. They have all been tested in combination with standard chemotherapy for advanced NSCLC (phase II and III), and despite some effect on progression free survival, none have given improved overall survival rates [158]. Nintedanib is to date the only one approved by the FDA and in the EU for use in second-line treatment of advanced adenocarcinoma combined with docetaxel based on results from the LUME-1 study [159, 160].

However, a common denominator for all available anti-angiogenic drugs is that there is currently no validated biomarkers for selecting which patients will have the best effect of this treatment. A limited number of studies have addressed the use of predictive biomarkers. Mok et al. published results from a phase II clinical trial called ABIGAIL in 2014, where correlations between biomarkers including VEGF-A and VEGFR-1/VEGFR-2 were studied with regard to response to bevacizumab combined with platinum-doublet chemotherapy [161, 162]. The only significant finding was that patients with higher plasma levels of VEGF-A at baseline had shorter progression-free survival than those with low VEGF-A levels. In contrast, tumor expression of VEGF had no impact on survival. Also, MVD has been suggested as a possible predictive biomarker for the effect of bevacizumab in NSCLC, as Zhao et al. showed in a small study published in 2012. Here, they found that high percentage of so-called undifferentiated intratumoral vessels labeled by CD31/CD34 correlated with better response to treatment [163]. No larger studies on the predictive value of MVD have been published to our knowledge.

As described above, anti-angiogenic drugs target the tumor microenvironment and aim to normalize the tumor vasculature. This normalization can improve the delivery of traditional chemotherapeutic agents to reach tumor cells by increasing permeability and blood supply to the tumor, thereby increasing sensitivity to treatment, as described in a recent review by Qiang et al. [164].

Anti-angiogenic drugs may also have synergistic effects with tyrosine kinase inhibitors, as VEGF upregulation has been shown to contribute to TKI resistance [165] due to partially shared downstream pathways. For example, inhibiting both VEGF and EGFR pathways in combination could improve the effect of treatment [166].

Further, anti-angiogenic drugs have the ability to not only normalize the tumor vasculature, but also to enhance infiltration of immune cells, thus making the TME more susceptible to immune-checkpoint inhibitors [167, 168].

Finding reliable biomarkers in order to identify patients who will benefit from these combined treatments is essential. As described earlier in this chapter, angiogenesis biomarkers do exist, and there have been several studies on biomarkers like VEGF and MVD related to the efficacy of anti-angiogenic agents such as bevacizumab in NSCLC [161, 163]. However, none of these markers are in current use due to limited predictive value. Although biomarkers for immunotherapy are in clinical use, e.g., PD-L1, the complex interactions of combination therapies represent a significant challenge. Therefore, additional studies are called for in the field of predictive biomarkers in NSCLC, with particular attention to the vascular systems.

References

1. Sung H, Ferlay J, Siegel RL, Laversanne M, Soerjomataram I, Jemal A, et al. Global cancer statistics 2020: GLOBOCAN estimates of incidence and mortality worldwide for 36 cancers in 185 countries. CA Cancer J Clin. 2021;71(3):209–49.
2. Stewart BW, Wild C. International Agency for Research on Cancer, World Health Organization, World cancer report 2014. Lyon, France, Geneva, Switzerland: International Agency for Research on Cancer,WHO Press; 2014. xiv, 630 pages p.
3. Lu T, Yang X, Huang Y, Zhao M, Li M, Ma K, et al. Trends in the incidence, treatment, and survival of patients with lung cancer in the last four decades. Cancer Manag Res. 2019;11:943–53.
4. Travis WD, Brambilla E, Muller-Hermelink HK, Harris CC, editors. World health organization classification of tumours. Pathology and genetics of tumours of the lung, pleura, thymus and heart. Lyon: IARC Press; 2004.
5. Travis WD, Brambilla E, Nicholson AG, Yatabe Y, Austin JH, Beasley MB, et al. The 2015 world health organization classification of lung tumors: impact of genetic, clinical and radiologic advances since the 2004 classification. J Thorac Oncol. 2015;10(9):1243–60.
6. Travis WD, Brambilla E, Burke AP, Marx A, Niholson AG, editors. WHO classification of tumours of the lung, pleura, thymus and heart. 4th ed. Lyon: IARC; 2015.
7. Quint LE, Tummala S, Brisson LJ, Francis IR, Krupnick AS, Kazerooni EA, et al. Distribution of distant metastases from newly diagnosed non-small cell lung cancer. Ann Thorac Surg. 1996;62(1):246–50.
8. Stenbygaard LE, Sorensen JB, Larsen H, Dombernowsky P. Metastatic pattern in non-resectable non-small cell lung cancer. Acta Oncol. 1999;38(8):993–8.
9. Brierley J, Gospodarowicz MK, Wittekind C. TNM classification of malignant tumours. 8th ed. Chichester, West Sussex: Wiley; 2017.
10. Postmus PE, Kerr KM, Oudkerk M, Senan S, Waller DA, Vansteenkiste J, et al. Early and locally advanced non-small-cell lung cancer (NSCLC): ESMO Clinical Practice Guidelines for diagnosis, treatment and follow-up. Ann Oncol. 2017;28(suppl_4):iv1–iv21.
11. Chang JY, Senan S, Paul MA, Mehran RJ, Louie AV, Balter P, et al. Stereotactic ablative radiotherapy versus lobectomy for oper-
able stage I non-small-cell lung cancer: a pooled analysis of two randomised trials. Lancet Oncol. 2015;16(6):630–7.
12. Hamaji M. Surgery and stereotactic body radiotherapy for early-stage non-small cell lung cancer: prospective clinical trials of the past, the present, and the future. Gen Thorac Cardiovasc Surg. 2020;68(7):692–6.
13. Rosell R, Moran T, Queralt C, Porta R, Cardenal F, Camps C, et al. Screening for epidermal growth factor receptor mutations in lung cancer. N Engl J Med. 2009;361(10):958–67.
14. Helsedirektoratet. Nasjonalt handlingsprogram med retningslinjer for diagnostikk, behandling og oppfølging av lungekreft. 01/2014 ed2014.
15. Ettinger DS, Wood DE, Aisner DL, Akerley W, Bauman JR, Bharat A, et al. NCCN guidelines insights: non-small cell lung cancer, version 2.2021. J Natl Compr Cancer Netw. 2021;19(3):254–66.
16. Hodi FS, O'Day SJ, McDermott DF, Weber RW, Sosman JA, Haanen JB, et al. Improved survival with ipilimumab in patients with metastatic melanoma. N Engl J Med. 2010;363(8):711–23.
17. Lynch TJ, Bondarenko I, Luft A, Serwatowski P, Barlesi F, Chacko R, et al. Ipilimumab in combination with paclitaxel and carboplatin as first-line treatment in stage IIIB/IV non-small-cell lung cancer: results from a randomized, double-blind, multicenter phase II study. J Clin Oncol. 2012;30(17):2046–54.
18. Mittal D, Gubin MM, Schreiber RD, Smyth MJ. New insights into cancer immunoediting and its three component phases – elimination, equilibrium and escape. Curr Opin Immunol. 2014;27:16–25.
19. Topalian SL, Drake CG, Pardoll DM. Immune checkpoint blockade: a common denominator approach to cancer therapy. Cancer Cell. 2015;27(4):450–61.
20. Vesely MD, Schreiber RD. Cancer immunoediting: antigens, mechanisms, and implications to cancer immunotherapy. Ann N Y Acad Sci. 2013;1284:1–5.
21. Garon EB, Rizvi NA, Hui R, Leighl N, Balmanoukian AS, Eder JP, et al. Pembrolizumab for the treatment of non-small-cell lung cancer. N Engl J Med. 2015;372(21):2018–28.
22. Borghaei H, Paz-Ares L, Horn L, Spigel DR, Steins M, Ready NE, et al. Nivolumab versus docetaxel in advanced nonsquamous non-small-cell lung cancer. N Engl J Med. 2015;373(17):1627–39.
23. Morgensztern D, Herbst RS. Nivolumab and pembrolizumab for non-small cell lung cancer. Clin Cancer Res. 2016;22(15):3713–7.
24. Mittal V, El Rayes T, Narula N, McGraw TE, Altorki NK, Barcellos-Hoff MH. The microenvironment of lung cancer and therapeutic implications. Adv Exp Med Biol. 2016;890:75–110.
25. Pattabiraman DR, Weinberg RA. Tackling the cancer stem cells – what challenges do they pose? Nat Rev Drug Discov. 2014;13(7):497–512.
26. Altorki NK, Markowitz GJ, Gao D, Port JL, Saxena A, Stiles B, et al. The lung microenvironment: an important regulator of tumour growth and metastasis. Nat Rev Cancer. 2019;19(1):9–31.
27. Young RP, Hopkins RJ, Gamble GD, Etzel C, El-Zein R, Crapo JD. Genetic evidence linking lung cancer and COPD: a new perspective. Appl Clin Genet. 2011;4:99–111.
28. Zhai R, Yu X, Shafer A, Wain JC, Christiani DC. The impact of coexisting COPD on survival of patients with early-stage non-small cell lung cancer undergoing surgical resection. Chest. 2014;145(2):346–53.
29. Balkwill F, Mantovani A. Inflammation and cancer: back to Virchow? Lancet. 2001;357(9255):539–45.
30. Pitt JM, Marabelle A, Eggermont A, Soria JC, Kroemer G, Zitvogel L. Targeting the tumor microenvironment: removing obstruction to anticancer immune responses and immunotherapy. Ann Oncol. 2016;27(8):1482–92.
31. Wood SL, Pernemalm M, Crosbie PA, Whetton AD. The role of the tumor-microenvironment in lung cancer-metastasis and its relationship to potential therapeutic targets. Cancer Treat Rev. 2014;40(4):558–66.

32. Coussens LM, Werb Z. Inflammation and cancer. Nature. 2002;420(6917):860–7.
33. Dunn GP, Old LJ, Schreiber RD. The three Es of cancer immunoediting. Annu Rev Immunol. 2004;22:329–60.
34. Schreiber RD, Old LJ, Smyth MJ. Cancer immunoediting: integrating immunity's roles in cancer suppression and promotion. Science. 2011;331(6024):1565–70.
35. Hanahan D, Weinberg RA. Hallmarks of cancer: the next generation. Cell. 2011;144(5):646–74.
36. Paget S. The distribution of secondary growths in cancer of the breast. 1889. Cancer Metastasis Rev. 1989;8(2):98–101.
37. Fidler IJ, Kripke ML. Metastasis results from preexisting variant cells within a malignant tumor. Science. 1977;197(4306):893–5.
38. Kaplan RN, Riba RD, Zacharoulis S, Bramley AH, Vincent L, Costa C, et al. VEGFR1-positive haematopoietic bone marrow progenitors initiate the pre-metastatic niche. Nature. 2005;438(7069):820–7.
39. Psaila B, Lyden D. The metastatic niche: adapting the foreign soil. Nat Rev Cancer. 2009;9(4):285–93.
40. Hanahan D, Folkman J. Patterns and emerging mechanisms of the angiogenic switch during tumorigenesis. Cell. 1996;86(3):353–64.
41. Hanahan D, Weinberg RA. The hallmarks of cancer. Cell. 2000;100(1):57–70.
42. Folkman J. What is the evidence that tumors are angiogenesis dependent? J Natl Cancer Inst. 1990;82(1):4–6.
43. Risau W, Flamme I. Vasculogenesis. Annu Rev Cell Dev Biol. 1995;11:73–91.
44. Demidova-Rice TN, Durham JT, Herman IM. Wound healing angiogenesis: innovations and challenges in acute and chronic wound healing. Adv Wound Care (New Rochelle). 2012;1(1):17–22.
45. Eming SA, Brachvogel B, Odorisio T, Koch M. Regulation of angiogenesis: wound healing as a model. Prog Histochem Cytochem. 2007;42(3):115–70.
46. Tonnesen MG, Feng X, Clark RA. Angiogenesis in wound healing. J Investig Dermatol Symp Proc. 2000;5(1):40–6.
47. Nagy JA, Chang SH, Shih SC, Dvorak AM, Dvorak HF. Heterogeneity of the tumor vasculature. Semin Thromb Hemost. 2010;36(3):321–31.
48. Hong S, Tan M, Wang S, Luo S, Chen Y, Zhang L. Efficacy and safety of angiogenesis inhibitors in advanced non-small cell lung cancer: a systematic review and meta-analysis. J Cancer Res Clin Oncol. 2015;141(5):909–21.
49. Jain RK. Antiangiogenesis strategies revisited: from starving tumors to alleviating hypoxia. Cancer Cell. 2014;26(5):605–22.
50. Senger DR, Galli SJ, Dvorak AM, Perruzzi CA, Harvey VS, Dvorak HF. Tumor cells secrete a vascular permeability factor that promotes accumulation of ascites fluid. Science. 1983;219(4587):983–5.
51. Ferrara N, Henzel WJ. Pituitary follicular cells secrete a novel heparin-binding growth factor specific for vascular endothelial cells. Biochem Biophys Res Commun. 1989;161(2):851–8.
52. Ballas MS, Chachoua A. Rationale for targeting VEGF, FGF, and PDGF for the treatment of NSCLC. Onco Targets Ther. 2011;4:43–58.
53. Ferrara N. Vascular endothelial growth factor. Trends Cardiovasc Med. 1993;3(6):244–50.
54. Ferrara N, Gerber HP, LeCouter J. The biology of VEGF and its receptors. Nat Med. 2003;9(6):669–76.
55. Donnem T, Al-Saad S, Al-Shibli K, Busund LT, Bremnes RM. Co-expression of PDGF-B and VEGFR-3 strongly correlates with lymph node metastasis and poor survival in non-small-cell lung cancer. Ann Oncol. 2010;21(2):223–31.
56. Donnem T, Al-Saad S, Al-Shibli K, Delghandi MP, Persson M, Nilsen MN, et al. Inverse prognostic impact of angiogenic marker expression in tumor cells versus stromal cells in non small cell lung cancer. Clin Cancer Res. 2007;13(22 Pt 1):6649–57.
57. Donnem T, Al-Shibli K, Al-Saad S, Busund LT, Bremnes RM. Prognostic impact of fibroblast growth factor 2 in non-small cell lung cancer: coexpression with VEGFR-3 and PDGF-B predicts poor survival. J Thorac Oncol. 2009;4(5):578–85.
58. Donnem T, Al-Shibli K, Al-Saad S, Delghandi MP, Busund LT, Bremnes RM. VEGF-A and VEGFR-3 correlate with nodal status in operable non-small cell lung cancer: inverse correlation between expression in tumor and stromal cells. Lung Cancer. 2009;63(2):277–83.
59. Rusnati M, Presta M. Fibroblast growth factors/fibroblast growth factor receptors as targets for the development of anti-angiogenesis strategies. Curr Pharm Des. 2007;13(20):2025–44.
60. Wu E, Palmer N, Tian Z, Moseman AP, Galdzicki M, Wang X, et al. Comprehensive dissection of PDGF-PDGFR signaling pathways in PDGFR genetically defined cells. PLoS One. 2008;3(11):e3794.
61. Carmeliet P, Jain RK. Molecular mechanisms and clinical applications of angiogenesis. Nature. 2011;473(7347):298–307.
62. Toi M, Matsumoto T, Bando H. Vascular endothelial growth factor: its prognostic, predictive, and therapeutic implications. Lancet Oncol. 2001;2(11):667–73.
63. Boone B, Brochez L. Clinical markers and driving mechanisms in melanoma progression: VEGF-C, RhoC, c-Ski/SnoN and EGFR. Verh K Acad Geneeskd Belg. 2009;71(5):251–94.
64. Feng Q, Guo P, Wang J, Zhang X, Yang HC, Feng JG. High expression of SDF-1 and VEGF is associated with poor prognosis in patients with synovial sarcomas. Exp Ther Med. 2018;15(3):2597–603.
65. Gasparini G. Clinical significance of determination of surrogate markers of angiogenesis in breast cancer. Crit Rev Oncol Hematol. 2001;37(2):97–114.
66. Ozdemir F, Akdogan R, Aydin F, Reis A, Kavgaci H, Gul S, et al. The effects of VEGF and VEGFR-2 on survival in patients with gastric cancer. J Exp Clin Cancer Res. 2006;25(1):83–8.
67. Fontanini G, Vignati S, Boldrini L, Chine S, Silvestri V, Lucchi M, et al. Vascular endothelial growth factor is associated with neovascularization and influences progression of non-small cell lung carcinoma. Clin Cancer Res. 1997;3(6):861–5.
68. Mattern J, Koomagi R, Volm M. Vascular endothelial growth-factor expression and angiogenesis in nonsmall cell lung carcinomas. Int J Oncol. 1995;6(5):1059–62.
69. O'Byrne KJ, Koukourakis MI, Giatromanolaki A, Cox G, Turley H, Steward WP, et al. Vascular endothelial growth factor, platelet-derived endothelial cell growth factor and angiogenesis in non-small-cell lung cancer. Br J Cancer. 2000;82(8):1427–32.
70. Donnem T, Al-Shibli K, Andersen S, Al-Saad S, Busund LT, Bremnes RM. Combination of low vascular endothelial growth factor A (VEGF-A)/VEGF receptor 2 expression and high lymphocyte infiltration is a strong and independent favorable prognostic factor in patients with nonsmall cell lung cancer. Cancer. 2010;116(18):4318–25.
71. Jain RK, Carmeliet P. SnapShot: tumor angiogenesis. Cell. 2012;149(6):1408-e1.
72. Kuczynski EA, Reynolds AR. Vessel co-option and resistance to anti-angiogenic therapy. Angiogenesis. 2020;23(1):55–74.
73. Donnem T, Hu J, Ferguson M, Adighibe O, Snell C, Harris AL, et al. Vessel co-option in primary human tumors and metastases: an obstacle to effective anti-angiogenic treatment? Cancer Med. 2013;2(4):427–36.
74. Bridgeman VL, Vermeulen PB, Foo S, Bilecz A, Daley F, Kostaras E, et al. Vessel co-option is common in human lung metastases and mediates resistance to anti-angiogenic therapy in preclinical lung metastasis models. J Pathol. 2017;241(3):362–74.

75. Weidner N, Semple JP, Welch WR, Folkman J. Tumor angiogenesis and metastasis – correlation in invasive breast carcinoma. N Engl J Med. 1991;324(1):1–8.

76. Vermeulen PB, Gasparini G, Fox SB, Colpaert C, Marson LP, Gion M, et al. Second international consensus on the methodology and criteria of evaluation of angiogenesis quantification in solid human tumours. Eur J Cancer. 2002;38(12):1564–79.

77. Vermeulen PB, Gasparini G, Fox SB, Toi M, Martin L, McCulloch P, et al. Quantification of angiogenesis in solid human tumours: an international consensus on the methodology and criteria of evaluation. Eur J Cancer. 1996;32A(14):2474–84.

78. Gravdal K, Halvorsen OJ, Haukaas SA, Akslen LA. Proliferation of immature tumor vessels is a novel marker of clinical progression in prostate cancer. Cancer Res. 2009;69(11):4708–15.

79. Stefansson IM, Salvesen HB, Akslen LA. Vascular proliferation is important for clinical progress of endometrial cancer. Cancer Res. 2006;66(6):3303–9.

80. Straume O, Chappuis PO, Salvesen HB, Halvorsen OJ, Haukaas SA, Goffin JR, et al. Prognostic importance of glomeruloid microvascular proliferation indicates an aggressive angiogenic phenotype in human cancers. Cancer Res. 2002;62(23):6808–11.

81. Meert AP, Paesmans M, Martin B, Delmotte P, Berghmans T, Verdebout JM, et al. The role of microvessel density on the survival of patients with lung cancer: a systematic review of the literature with meta-analysis. Br J Cancer. 2002;87(7):694–701.

82. Macchiarini P, Fontanini G, Hardin MJ, Squartini F, Angeletti CA. Relation of neovascularisation to metastasis of non-small-cell lung cancer. Lancet. 1992;340(8812):145–6.

83. Medetoglu B, Gunluoglu MZ, Demir A, Melek H, Buyukpinarbasili N, Fener N, et al. Tumor angiogenesis in predicting the survival of patients with stage I lung cancer. J Thorac Cardiovasc Surg. 2010;140(5):996–1000.

84. Pomme G, Augustin F, Fiegl M, Droeser RA, Sterlacci W, Tzankov A. Detailed assessment of microvasculature markers in non-small cell lung cancer reveals potentially clinically relevant characteristics. Virchows Arch. 2015;467(1):55–66.

85. Mlika M, Makhlouf C, Boudaya MS, Haddouchi C, Tritar F, Mezni F. Evaluation of the microvessel density and the expression of metalloproteases 2 and 9 and ttf1 in the different subtypes of lung adenocarcinoma in Tunisia: a retrospective study of 46 cases. J Immunoassay Immunochem. 2015;36(2):111–8.

86. Eberhard A, Kahlert S, Goede V, Hemmerlein B, Plate KH, Augustin HG. Heterogeneity of angiogenesis and blood vessel maturation in human tumors: implications for antiangiogenic tumor therapies. Cancer Res. 2000;60(5):1388–93.

87. Yazdani S, Miki Y, Tamaki K, Ono K, Iwabuchi E, Abe K, et al. Proliferation and maturation of intratumoral blood vessels in non-small cell lung cancer. Hum Pathol. 2013;44(8):1586–96.

88. Ramnefjell M, Aamelfot C, Aziz S, Helgeland L, Akslen LA. Microvascular proliferation is associated with aggressive tumour features and reduced survival in lung adenocarcinoma. J Pathol Clin Res. 2017;3(4):249–57.

89. Arnes JB, Stefansson IM, Straume O, Baak JP, Lonning PE, Foulkes WD, et al. Vascular proliferation is a prognostic factor in breast cancer. Breast Cancer Res Treat. 2012;133(2):501–10.

90. Nalwoga H, Arnes JB, Stefansson IM, Wabinga H, Foulkes WD, Akslen LA. Vascular proliferation is increased in basal-like breast cancer. Breast Cancer Res Treat. 2011;130(3):1063–71.

91. Kruger K, Stefansson IM, Collett K, Arnes JB, Aas T, Akslen LA. Microvessel proliferation by co-expression of endothelial nestin and Ki-67 is associated with a basal-like phenotype and aggressive features in breast cancer. Breast. 2013;22(3):282–8.

92. Hoem D, Straume O, Immervoll H, Akslen LA, Molven A. Vascular proliferation is associated with survival in pancreatic ductal adenocarcinoma. APMIS. 2013;121(11):1037–46.

93. Hugdahl E, Bachmann IM, Schuster C, Ladstein RG, Akslen LA. Prognostic value of uPAR expression and angiogenesis in primary and metastatic melanoma. PLoS One. 2019;14(1):e0210399.

94. Tanaka F, Oyanagi H, Takenaka K, Ishikawa S, Yanagihara K, Miyahara R, et al. Glomeruloid microvascular proliferation is superior to intratumoral microvessel density as a prognostic marker in non-small cell lung cancer. Cancer Res. 2003;63(20):6791–4.

95. Dahlstrand J, Collins VP, Lendahl U. Expression of the class VI intermediate filament nestin in human central nervous system tumors. Cancer Res. 1992;52(19):5334–41.

96. Dahlstrand J, Zimmerman LB, McKay RD, Lendahl U. Characterization of the human nestin gene reveals a close evolutionary relationship to neurofilaments. J Cell Sci. 1992;103(Pt 2):589–97.

97. Lendahl U, Zimmerman LB, McKay RD. CNS stem cells express a new class of intermediate filament protein. Cell. 1990;60(4):585–95.

98. Wiese C, Rolletschek A, Kania G, Blyszczuk P, Tarasov KV, Tarasova Y, et al. Nestin expression – a property of multi-lineage progenitor cells? Cell Mol Life Sci. 2004;61(19–20):2510–22.

99. Krupkova O Jr, Loja T, Zambo I, Veselska R. Nestin expression in human tumors and tumor cell lines. Neoplasma. 2010;57(4):291–8.

100. Bae HS, Chung YW, Lee JK, Lee NW, Yeom BW, Lee KW, et al. Nestin expression as an indicator of cervical cancer initiation. Eur J Gynaecol Oncol. 2013;34(3):238–42.

101. He QZ, Luo XZ, Zhou Q, Wang K, Li SX, Li Y, et al. Expression of nestin in ovarian serous cancer and its clinicopathologic significance. Eur Rev Med Pharmacol Sci. 2013;17(21):2896–901.

102. Kleeberger W, Bova GS, Nielsen ME, Herawi M, Chuang AY, Epstein JI, et al. Roles for the stem cell associated intermediate filament Nestin in prostate cancer migration and metastasis. Cancer Res. 2007;67(19):9199–206.

103. Liu C, Chen B, Zhu J, Zhang R, Yao F, Jin F, et al. Clinical implications for nestin protein expression in breast cancer. Cancer Sci. 2010;101(3):815–9.

104. Qin Q, Sun Y, Fei M, Zhang J, Jia Y, Gu M, et al. Expression of putative stem marker nestin and CD133 in advanced serous ovarian cancer. Neoplasma. 2012;59(3):310–5.

105. Zhong B, Wang T, Lun X, Zhang J, Zheng S, Yang W, et al. Contribution of nestin positive esophageal squamous cancer cells on malignant proliferation, apoptosis, and poor prognosis. Cancer Cell Int. 2014;14:57.

106. Janikova M, Skarda J, Dziechciarkova M, Radova L, Chmelova J, Krejci V, et al. Identification of CD133+/nestin+ putative cancer stem cells in non-small cell lung cancer. Biomed Pap Med Fac Univ Palacky Olomouc Czech Repub. 2010;154(4):321–6.

107. Chen Z, Wang J, Cai L, Zhong B, Luo H, Hao Y, et al. Role of the stem cell-associated intermediate filament nestin in malignant proliferation of non-small cell lung cancer. PLoS One. 2014;9(2):e85584.

108. Chen Z, Wang T, Luo H, Lai Y, Yang X, Li F, et al. Expression of nestin in lymph node metastasis and lymphangiogenesis in non-small cell lung cancer patients. Hum Pathol. 2010;41(5):737–44.

109. Narita K, Matsuda Y, Seike M, Naito Z, Gemma A, Ishiwata T. Nestin regulates proliferation, migration, invasion and stemness of lung adenocarcinoma. Int J Oncol. 2014;44(4):1118–30.

110. Ryuge S, Sato Y, Jiang SX, Wang G, Matsumoto T, Katono K, et al. Prognostic impact of nestin expression in resected large cell neuroendocrine carcinoma of the lung. Lung Cancer. 2012;77(2):415–20.

111. Ryuge S, Sato Y, Wang GQ, Matsumoto T, Jiang SX, Katono K, et al. Prognostic significance of nestin expression in resected non-small cell lung cancer. Chest. 2011;139(4):862–9.

112. Skarda J, Kolar Z, Janikova M, Radova L, Kolek V, Fridman E, et al. Analysis of the prognostic impact of nestin expression in

non-small cell lung cancer. Biomed Pap Med Fac Univ Palacky Olomouc Czech Repub. 2012;156(2):135–42.

113. Mokry J, Cizkova D, Filip S, Ehrmann J, Osterreicher J, Kolar Z, et al. Nestin expression by newly formed human blood vessels. Stem Cells Dev. 2004;13(6):658–64.

114. Kraby MR, Kruger K, Opdahl S, Vatten LJ, Akslen LA, Bofin AM. Microvascular proliferation in luminal A and basal-like breast cancer subtypes. J Clin Pathol. 2015;68(11):891–7.

115. Onisim A, Achimas-Cadariu A, Vlad C, Kubelac P, Achimas-Cadariu P. Current insights into the association of Nestin with tumor angiogenesis. J BUON. 2015;20(3):699–706.

116. Mosely JM, Dickson DR. Vascular invasion in lung cancer. Clinical-pathologic significance. Am Rev Respir Dis. 1960;82:807–9.

117. Harada M, Hato T, Horio H. Intratumoral lymphatic vessel involvement is an invasive indicator of completely resected pathologic stage I non-small cell lung cancer. J Thorac Oncol. 2011;6(1):48–54.

118. Matsuura N, Go T, Fujiwara A, Nakano T, Nakashima N, Tarumi S, et al. Lymphatic invasion is a cause of local recurrence after wedge resection of primary lung cancer. Gen Thorac Cardiovasc Surg. 2019;67(10):861–6.

119. Neri S, Yoshida J, Ishii G, Matsumura Y, Aokage K, Hishida T, et al. Prognostic impact of microscopic vessel invasion and visceral pleural invasion in non-small cell lung cancer: a retrospective analysis of 2657 patients. Ann Surg. 2014;260(2):383–8.

120. Ramnefjell M, Aamelfot C, Helgeland L, Akslen LA. Vascular invasion is an adverse prognostic factor in resected non-small-cell lung cancer. APMIS. 2017;125(3):197–206.

121. Hamanaka R, Yokose T, Sakuma Y, Tsuboi M, Ito H, Nakayama H, et al. Prognostic impact of vascular invasion and standardization of its evaluation in stage I non-small cell lung cancer. Diagn Pathol. 2015;10:17.

122. Kudo Y, Saji H, Shimada Y, Matsubayashi J, Nagao T, Kakihana M, et al. Proposal on incorporating blood vessel invasion into the T classification parts as a practical staging system for stage I non-small cell lung cancer. Lung Cancer. 2013;81(2):187–93.

123. Aylwin JA. Avoidable vascular spread in resection for bronchial carcinoma. Thorax. 1951;6(3):250–67.

124. Collier FC, Blakemore WS, Kyle RH, Enterline HT, Kirby CK, Johnson J. Carcinoma of the lung: factors which influence five year survival with special reference to blood vessel invasion. Ann Surg. 1957;146(3):417–23.

125. Collier FC, Enterline HT, Kyle RH, Tristan TT, Greening R. The prognostic implications of vascular invasion in primary carcinomas of the lung; a clinicopathologic correlation of two hundred twenty-five cases with one hundred per cent follow-up. AMA Arch Pathol. 1958;66(4):594–603.

126. Elson CE, Roggli VL, Vollmer RT, Greenberg SD, Fraire AE, Spjut HJ, et al. Prognostic indicators for survival in stage I carcinoma of the lung: a histologic study of 47 surgically resected cases. Mod Pathol. 1988;1(4):288–91.

127. Macchiarini P, Dulmet E, De Montpreville V, Chapelier A, Cerrina J, Le Roy LF, et al. Prognostic significance of peritumoural blood and lymphatic vessel invasion by tumour cells in T4 non-small cell lung cancer following induction therapy. Surg Oncol. 1995;4(2):91–9.

128. Rigau V, Molina TJ, Chaffaud C, Huchon G, Audouin J, Chevret S, et al. Blood vessel invasion in resected non small cell lung carcinomas is predictive of metastatic occurrence. Lung Cancer. 2002;38(2):169–76.

129. Sung SY, Kwak YK, Lee SW, Jo IY, Park JK, Kim KS, et al. Lymphovascular invasion increases the risk of nodal and distant recurrence in node-negative stage I-IIA non-small-cell lung cancer. Oncology. 2018;95(3):156–62.

130. Shimizu R, Kinoshita T, Sasaki N, Uematsu M, Sugita Y, Shima T, et al. Clinicopathological factors related to recurrence patterns of resected non-small cell lung cancer. J Clin Med. 2020;9(8)

131. Al-Alao BS, Gately K, Nicholson S, McGovern E, Young VK, O'Byrne KJ. Prognostic impact of vascular and lymphovascular invasion in early lung cancer. Asian Cardiovasc Thorac Ann. 2014;22(1):55–64.

132. Higgins KA, Chino JP, Ready N, D'Amico TA, Berry MF, Sporn T, et al. Lymphovascular invasion in non-small-cell lung cancer: implications for staging and adjuvant therapy. J Thorac Oncol. 2012;7(7):1141–7.

133. Hishida T, Yoshida J, Maeda R, Ishii G, Aokage K, Nishimura M, et al. Prognostic impact of intratumoural microvascular invasion and microlymphatic permeation on node-negative non-small-cell lung cancer: which indicator is the stronger prognostic factor? Eur J Cardiothorac Surg. 2013;43(4):772–7.

134. Kato T, Ishikawa K, Aragaki M, Sato M, Okamoto K, Ishibashi T, et al. Angiolymphatic invasion exerts a strong impact on surgical outcomes for stage I lung adenocarcinoma, but not non-adenocarcinoma. Lung Cancer. 2012;77(2):394–400.

135. Kessler R, Gasser B, Massard G, Roeslin N, Meyer P, Wihlm JM, et al. Blood vessel invasion is a major prognostic factor in resected non-small cell lung cancer. Ann Thorac Surg. 1996;62(5):1489–93.

136. Ma KF, Chu XY, Liu Y. Clinical significance of lymphatic vessel invasion in stage I non-small cell lung cancer patients. Genet Mol Res. 2015;14(1):1819–27.

137. Usui S, Minami Y, Shiozawa T, Iyama S, Satomi K, Sakashita S, et al. Differences in the prognostic implications of vascular invasion between lung adenocarcinoma and squamous cell carcinoma. Lung Cancer. 2013;82(3):407–12.

138. Wang J, Chen J, Chen X, Wang B, Li K, Bi J. Blood vessel invasion as a strong independent prognostic indicator in non-small cell lung cancer: a systematic review and meta-analysis. PLoS One. 2011;6(12):e28844.

139. Wang J, Wang B, Zhao W, Guo Y, Chen H, Chu H, et al. Clinical significance and role of lymphatic vessel invasion as a major prognostic implication in non-small cell lung cancer: a meta-analysis. PLoS One. 2012;7(12):e52704.

140. Brierley JD, Gospodarowicz MK, Wittekind C. TNM classification of malignant tumours. 8th ed.

141. Alvarez RH, Kantarjian HM, Cortes JE. Biology of platelet-derived growth factor and its involvement in disease. Mayo Clin Proc. 2006;81(9):1241–57.

142. Ferrara N. Role of vascular endothelial growth factor in regulation of physiological angiogenesis. Am J Physiol Cell Physiol. 2001;280(6):C1358–66.

143. Presta M, Dell'Era P, Mitola S, Moroni E, Ronca R, Rusnati M. Fibroblast growth factor/fibroblast growth factor receptor system in angiogenesis. Cytokine Growth Factor Rev. 2005;16(2):159–78.

144. Andersen S, Donnem T, Al-Saad S, Al-Shibli K, Busund LT, Bremnes RM. Angiogenic markers show high prognostic impact on survival in marginally operable non-small cell lung cancer patients treated with adjuvant radiotherapy. J Thorac Oncol. 2009;4(4):463–71.

145. Donnem T, Andersen S, Al-Saad S, Al-Shibli K, Busund LT, Bremnes RM. Prognostic impact of angiogenic markers in non-small-cell lung cancer is related to tumor size. Clin Lung Cancer. 2011;12(2):106–15.

146. Li BT, Barnes TA, Chan DL, Naidoo J, Lee A, Khasraw M, et al. The addition of anti-angiogenic tyrosine kinase inhibitors to chemotherapy for patients with advanced non-small-cell lung cancers: A meta-analysis of randomized trials. Lung Cancer. 2016;102:21–7.

147. Cohen MH, Gootenberg J, Keegan P, Pazdur R. FDA drug approval summary: bevacizumab (Avastin) plus Carboplatin

and Paclitaxel as first-line treatment of advanced/metastatic recurrent nonsquamous non-small cell lung cancer. Oncologist. 2007;12(6):713–8.

148. Reck M, von Pawel J, Zatloukal P, Ramlau R, Gorbounova V, Hirsh V, et al. Phase III trial of cisplatin plus gemcitabine with either placebo or bevacizumab as first-line therapy for non-squamous non-small-cell lung cancer: AVAil. J Clin Oncol. 2009;27(8):1227–34.

149. Reck M, von Pawel J, Zatloukal P, Ramlau R, Gorbounova V, Hirsh V, et al. Overall survival with cisplatin-gemcitabine and bevacizumab or placebo as first-line therapy for nonsquamous non-small-cell lung cancer: results from a randomised phase III trial (AVAiL). Ann Oncol. 2010;21(9):1804–9.

150. Sandler A, Gray R, Perry MC, Brahmer J, Schiller JH, Dowlati A, et al. Paclitaxel-carboplatin alone or with bevacizumab for non-small-cell lung cancer. N Engl J Med. 2006;355(24):2542–50.

151. Helsedirektoratet. Nasjonalt handlingsprogram med retningslinjer for diagnostikk, behandling og oppfølging av lungekreft, mesoteliom og thymom. 2021.

152. Reck M, Mok TSK, Nishio M, Jotte RM, Cappuzzo F, Orlandi F, et al. Atezolizumab plus bevacizumab and chemotherapy in non-small-cell lung cancer (IMpower150): key subgroup analyses of patients with EGFR mutations or baseline liver metastases in a randomised, open-label phase 3 trial. Lancet Respir Med. 2019;7(5):387–401.

153. Doebele RC, Spigel D, Tehfe M, Thomas S, Reck M, Verma S, et al. Phase 2, randomized, open-label study of ramucirumab in combination with first-line pemetrexed and platinum chemotherapy in patients with nonsquamous, advanced/metastatic non-small cell lung cancer. Cancer. 2015;121(6):883–92.

154. Ramlau R, Gorbunova V, Ciuleanu TE, Novello S, Ozguroglu M, Goksel T, et al. Aflibercept and Docetaxel versus Docetaxel alone after platinum failure in patients with advanced or metastatic non-small-cell lung cancer: a randomized, controlled phase III trial. J Clin Oncol. 2012;30(29):3640–7.

155. Fala L. Cyramza (ramucirumab) approved for the treatment of advanced gastric cancer and metastatic non-small-cell lung cancer. Am Health Drug Benefits 2015;8(Spec Feature):49–53.

156. Garon EB, Ciuleanu TE, Arrieta O, Prabhash K, Syrigos KN, Goksel T, et al. Ramucirumab plus docetaxel versus placebo plus docetaxel for second-line treatment of stage IV non-small-cell lung cancer after disease progression on platinum-based therapy (REVEL): a multicentre, double-blind, randomised phase 3 trial. Lancet. 2014;384(9944):665–73.

157. Hall CJ, Umeweni N, Knight H, Smith L. NICE guidance on ramucirumab for previously treated locally advanced or metastatic non-small-cell lung cancer. Lancet Oncol. 2016;17(10):1357–8.

158. Chu BF, Otterson GA. Incorporation of Antiangiogenic Therapy Into the Non-Small-Cell Lung Cancer Paradigm. Clin Lung Cancer. 2016;17(6):493–506.

159. Reck M, Kaiser R, Mellemgaard A, Douillard JY, Orlov S, Krzakowski M, et al. Docetaxel plus nintedanib versus docetaxel plus placebo in patients with previously treated non-small-cell lung cancer (LUME-Lung 1): a phase 3, double-blind, randomised controlled trial. Lancet Oncol. 2014;15(2):143–55.

160. Hall CJ, Hay N, George E, Adler AI. NICE guidance on nint-edanib for previously treated locally advanced, metastatic, or locally recurrent non-small-cell lung cancer. Lancet Oncol. 2015;16(9):1019–20.

161. Mok T, Gorbunova V, Juhasz E, Szima B, Burdaeva O, Orlov S, et al. A correlative biomarker analysis of the combination of bevacizumab and carboplatin-based chemotherapy for advanced nonsquamous non-small-cell lung cancer: results of the phase II randomized ABIGAIL study (BO21015). J Thorac Oncol. 2014;9(6):848–55.

162. Mok TS, Hsia TC, Tsai CM, Tsang K, Chang GC, Chang JW, et al. Efficacy of bevacizumab with cisplatin and gemcitabine in Asian patients with advanced or recurrent non-squamous non-small cell lung cancer who have not received prior chemotherapy: a substudy of the Avastin in Lung trial. Asia Pac J Clin Oncol. 2011;7(Suppl 2):4–12.

163. Zhao YY, Xue C, Jiang W, Zhao HY, Huang Y, Feenstra K, et al. Predictive value of intratumoral microvascular density in patients with advanced non-small cell lung cancer receiving chemotherapy plus bevacizumab. J Thorac Oncol. 2012;7(1):71–5.

164. Qiang H, Chang Q, Xu J, Qian J, Zhang Y, Lei Y, et al. New advances in antiangiogenic combination therapeutic strategies for advanced non-small cell lung cancer. J Cancer Res Clin Oncol. 2020;146(3):631–45.

165. De Luca A, Carotenuto A, Rachiglio A, Gallo M, Maiello MR, Aldinucci D, et al. The role of the EGFR signaling in tumor microenvironment. J Cell Physiol. 2008;214(3):559–67.

166. Masuda C, Yanagisawa M, Yorozu K, Kurasawa M, Furugaki K, Ishikura N, et al. Bevacizumab counteracts VEGF-dependent resistance to erlotinib in an EGFR-mutated NSCLC xenograft model. Int J Oncol. 2017;51(2):425–34.

167. Manegold C, Dingemans AC, Gray JE, Nakagawa K, Nicolson M, Peters S, et al. The potential of combined immunotherapy and antiangiogenesis for the synergistic treatment of advanced NSCLC. J Thorac Oncol. 2017;12(2):194–207.

168. Datta M, Coussens LM, Nishikawa H, Hodi FS, Jain RK. Reprogramming the tumor microenvironment to improve immunotherapy: emerging strategies and combination therapies. Am Soc Clin Oncol Educ Book. 2019;39:165–74.

Tumor–Host Interactions in Malignant Gliomas

30

Lina Leiss, Ercan Mutlu, Mohummad Aminur Rahman, Mette Hartmark Nilsen, and Per Øyvind Enger

Abstract

Malignant gliomas are infiltrative tumors arising in the brain, characterized by neurodegeneration, degradation of the extracellular matrix, and tumor cell migration along white matter tracts. The most aggressive form displays angiogenesis and recruitment of host vessels, whereas host-derived cells are re-programmed to mediate pro-tumorigenic effects and counteract immune recognition of the tumor. Thus, tumor–stroma interactions regulate critical aspects of brain tumor progression. These interactions are shaped by the structural organization of the central nervous system (CNS) and involve various cell types, extracellular matrix (ECM) components, and host cell-derived soluble factors that are unique to the CNS. Here, we will first provide an overview of the CNS microenvironment, followed by a review of how these elements engage in the brain tumor–host interplay.

Take-Home Messages

- Malignant gliomas are incurable and almost invariably fatal.
- Tumor–stroma interactions are an essential and integral part of tumor progression:
  - Tumor cells migrate along ECM components and myelinated nerve fibers into the surrounding brain parenchyma.
  - Cystine uptake from the brain tumor microenvironment via the xCT antiport is essential for glutathione synthesis that protects glioma cells against oxidative stress.
  - Glutamate release via the xCT antiport to the extracellular space mediates neurodegeneration and may trigger epilepsy.
  - Hypoxia induced release of angiogenic factors from glioma cells and tumor-associated glial cells triggers vessel sprouting from the host vasculature, coinciding with a marked shortening of survival.
  - Tumor-associated macrophages, microglia, and regulatory T cells have critical roles in maintaining an immunosuppressive brain tumor microenvironment.
- In contrast to other cancer types, no anti-angiogenic or immune-based therapy have yet been documented to provide a survival benefit for glioma patients.

L. Leiss
Department of Oncology-Pathology, Karolinska Institutet, Stockholm, Sweden
e-mail: lina.wik.leiss@ki.se

E. Mutlu
Karolinska Sjukhuset, Stockholm, Sweden

M. A. Rahman · M. H. Nilsen · P. Ø. Enger (✉)
Department of Biomedicine, University of Bergen, Bergen, Norway
e-mail: Aminur.Rahman@uib.no; mni020@student.uib.no; per.enger@uib.no

Constituents of the Central Nervous System

Tumor–stroma interactions are heavily influenced by the histoarchitecture of the host tissue. The main cell types found in the CNS are neurons, astrocytes, oligodendrocytes, ependymal cells, neural stem cells, progenitor cells, microglia, immune cells, endothelial cells, and pericytes. The extracellular matrix comprises hyaluronic acid, proteoglycans, and glycoproteins and accounts for 10–20% of the volume of the CNS tissue [1].

L. A. Akslen, R. S. Watnick (eds.), *Biomarkers of the Tumor Microenvironment*, https://doi.org/10.1007/978-3-030-98950-7_30

Neurons

These cells exert the core function of the central nervous system by propagating information coded as electric impulses, action potentials [2]. Through cellular extensions, neurons establish contacts, synapses, with other neurons. Across these synapses, information is transmitted in the form of chemical substances called neurotransmitters. Thus, neurons are interconnected via synapses in a functional network that allows flow of information between different CNS regions. The brains' neuronal cell bodies are mostly located underneath the brains' surface where they form the gray matter or cerebral cortex. Action potentials are generated near the cell body and transmitted to other neurons along the nerve fibers, axons. These axons may be covered by a lipid-rich sheet called myelin that serves to insulate the axons and increase the transmission velocity of the electric pulses. The myelin is formed from the cell membrane of a glial cell type called oligodendrocytes and is wrapped as concentric lamellas around the axons. The brain parenchyma underneath the cerebral cortex contains bundles of these myelinated fibers that appear white, referred to as white matter tracts. Moreover, neurons also communicate with astrocytes located in the immediate vicinity of the neuronal pre- and post-synaptic membranes. Collectively, these elements constitute the tripartite synapses that mediate reciprocal interactions impacting both on neuronal activity and astrocyte function [3].

Glial Cells

These cells are the most numerous in the CNS and are classified into subtypes based on morphology and function which comprise astrocytes, oligodendrocytes, ependymal cells, and microglia [4, 5]. They do not generate action potentials but have multiple roles linked to homeostatic functions and maintaining structural support and integrity of the brain parenchyma. Astrocytes represent a major subgroup of glial cells that are present in both gray matter and white matter. They control ion concentration and osmotic pressure in the extracellular space, and they express transporters for uptake of neurotransmitters. Astrocytes express intermediate filaments, including glial fibrillary acidic protein (GFAP), which provide a robust cytoskeleton, consistent with their role in structural support [6]. Importantly, astrocytes are coupled via gap junctions [7] and also form cellular protrusions with enlargements at the distal end that lie in close contact with neurons. Through these gap junctions, astrocytes form a functional networks that regulate synaptic transmission and neuronal activity by providing neurons with glucose and lactate for energy production and through glutamate clearance and removal of K^+ from the extracellular space [8]. Astrocytes

also form the so-called foot processes or end-feet, which establish contacts with cerebral capillaries and contribute to the structural and functional integrity of the blood-brain barrier [9, 10].

Oligodendrocytes are glial cells whose primary function is to produce the myelin sheets that insulate nerve axons in the CNS, enabling faster propagation of action potentials [11]. The myelin sheets comprise multiple layers of cell membranes concentrically wrapped around the nerve axons. Oligodendrocytes produce myelin basic protein (MBP) which are part of the myelin sheet and essential for its function and structure [12]. Due to their role in nerve fiber myelination, oligodendrocytes are abundantly present in areas containing nerve fibers, such as the white matter of the brain. However, they also exist in the gray matter where myelin lamellae surround fibers traversing the cerebral cortex.

Immune Cells

The paradigm of the brain as an immune-privileged organ has been dispelled by studies that have established the presence of extensive immune regulatory networks within the CNS which both conduct a monitoring function and activate immune responses in response to specific cues. As such, both the afferent and efferent elements of the immune system access the brain and operate in a coordinated manner. Due to several factors however, immune suppression is a prominent feature of CNS immunity and differs markedly from other organs. Firstly, the blood-brain barrier limits access to the central nervous system of cells, blood-borne pathogens and molecules. In a similar manner, exchange between the cerebrospinal fluid (CSF) and the blood is restricted by the blood–CSF barrier. Moreover, apart from some neuronal subsets, MHC class I antigens are not expressed at detectable levels in the normal state in neurons or glial cells, although they can be induced [13, 14]. From a developmental perspective, these unique features likely represent a necessary adaption to the non-compliant skull that encloses the brain. Thus, a massive immune response with increased local perfusion, tissue necrosis, and vasogenic edema would cause a life-threatening elevation of the intracranial pressure.

Microglia are smaller than astrocytes and oligodendrocytes, they account for 5–20% of all glial cells and mediate the CNS' innate immunity toward harmful events. They are derived from myeloid progenitors of the yolk sac and populate the CNS during fetal development [15, 16]. Throughout adult life, microglia reside in the brain parenchyma and renew through replication. While they represent the primary, local, and innate immune defense they may also trigger the adaptive immune system [17]. Furthermore, they maintain CNS homeostasis through phagocytosis of debris from dead cells and provision of trophic factors to surrounding neurons and other glial cell types. In the healthy state, microglia adapt a resting state in which they sample the CNS microenvironment through cellular extensions that contact neurons, astrocytes, and oligodendrocytes. Upon detection of pathological changes they undergo activation accompanied by proliferation, phagocytosis, and migration to the area of pathology. This is accompanied by upregulation of MHC class I antigens and the release of inflammatory mediators and chemo-attractants that recruit immune cells from the peripheral circulation including dendritic cells, monocytes, macrophages, NK cells, and various T-cell subtypes [18, 19]. These cells enter the CNS via the (1) Blood–CSF barrier through the vascular stroma of the choroid plexus, (2) Postcapillary venules of the brain parenchyma, and (3) The perivascular space that surrounds arteries entering the brain parenchyma and that communicates with CSF in the subarachnoid space. Prior to activation however, peripheral immune cells cluster at various anatomical locations in close vicinity to the CNS where they serve a sentinel function. As such, bone marrow-derived cells populate the perivascular space and dendritic cells are present in proximity to the meninges and in the choroid plexus [17]. These cells as well as microglia in the brain parenchyma may detect and phagocytose foreign antigens and present these to T cells, either locally at the site or possibly in peripheral lymph nodes by dendritic cells that have returned from the CNS. T cells may also enter the CNS by directly traversing the BBB, a process that is facilitated by cell surface molecules that bind vascular adhesion molecules on the membrane of endothelial cells.

Importantly, several afferent routes are available for trafficking substances and immune cells out of the CNS and back to the systemic circulation and lymph nodes. As such, the glymphatic system is a key regulator of solute exchange between the brain interstitium and the lymphatic system, as CSF flowing from the subarachnoid to the perivascular space subsequently enters the CNS interstitium via aquaporin 4 water channels [20]. From this compartment fluid can exit and return to CSF in the perivascular space around veins. Recently, studies have also established the presence of a functional lymphatic network in the meninges providing a direct drainage pathway from the CNS to the peripheral immune system and cervical lymph nodes [21]. Moreover, antigens and T cells can traverse the arachnoid coverings of olfactory nerves to reach cervical lymph nodes via the nasal mucosa.

The Blood-Brain Barrier

The CNS is highly vascularized, reflecting the neurons' high consumption of oxygen and vulnerability to oxygen deprivation. The cerebral capillaries in the CNS have unique structural features that markedly restrict the exchange of hydrophilic compounds between blood and nervous tissue and is referred to as the blood-brain barrier (BBB). This affects the transport of glucose, various nutrients, macromolecules as well as polar or charged molecules. Many of these substances gain entry to the CNS by means of selective transporters and channels. Hence, the BBB prevents interstitial levels of ions and neuroactive substances from being affected by fluctuating concentrations of these compounds in the blood stream. Conversely, O_2, CO_2, and lipophilic molecules up to a certain size diffuse freely through the BBB. Notably, endothelial cells in the CNS are not fenestrated like in other organs, but sealed closely together with the so-called tight junctions that effectively block transport between the cells. These junctions are formed by various transmembrane proteins, including claudins, junctional adhesion molecules (JAMs), and occludins [22]. The endothelial cells are further surrounded by a continuous basal lamina that again is covered by pericytes. Astrocytic end-feet form an outer layer that insulates the capillaries. Collectively these structural elements are referred to as the blood-brain barrier and serve to maintain a stable concentration of ions and other solutes which is critical for normal neuronal functioning [10].

Extracellular Matrix (ECM): Apart from its cellular constituents, the CNS comprises an extracellular matrix that accounts for 10–20% of the brain volume. In the adult CNS, this matrix provides structural support and regulates synaptic plasticity and function. The ECM is organized into a looser neural interstitial matrix of ECM molecules occupying the extracellular space between the cells, the basement membrane which supports and separates endothelial cells from the brain parenchyma, and perineuronal nets which are a mesh-like structure that surrounds the neuronal cell bodies and dendrites [23]. The interstitial matrix consists of proteoglycans, glycoproteins with one or more side-chains of unbranched glycosaminoglycans covalently bound to a core protein [24]. In addition, it has a high content of hyaluronan, a glycosaminoglycan without binding to a core protein, tenascin, and linker proteins. Glycosaminoglycans are negatively charged and thus bind water molecules and cations. The basal lamina is a specialized ECM structure built from fibrous proteins including collagen, fibronectin, and laminin. These molecules have other physical properties than the glycosaminoglycans and create a firmer structure than the neural interstitial matrix. The basal lamina contributes to the integrity of the blood-brain barrier, and it also forms the glia limitans together with astrocytic end-feet at the outer surface of the CNS, underneath the pia covering. The perineuronal nets are condensed matrix structures lying around the neuronal cell bodies in areas such as the cerebral cortex and the hippocampus. Its chemical composition includes elements such as the chondroitin sulfate proteoglycans, hyaluronan,

Tenascin R, and link proteins. The perineuronal nets regulate synaptic function and stabilize the microenvironment around the neuronal cell bodies.

Gliomas: A Brief Overview

Gliomas are the most common malignant primary brain tumors. They are classified according to WHO based on their resemblance with glial cell types, and the most common classes are astrocytomas, oligodendrogliomas, and tumors with mixed histology. Furthermore, tumors are graded based on their degree of malignancy according to histopathological criteria, including nuclear atypia, the presence of mitotic figures, microvascular proliferation, and necrosis [25] (Fig. 30.1). Grade II–IV gliomas are highly infiltrative and invasive, characterized by enzymatic degradation of the extracellular matrix (ECM) and glioma cell migration along ECM components and white matter tracts. Gliomas are almost invariably fatal, but virtually never metastasize outside the CNS. Survival is generally shorter for patients with astrocytic than oligodendroglial tumors, and is inversely correlated with tumor grade. However, even for gliomas of identical classification and grade, survival varies considerably between patients. Reported survival outcomes also vary between cohorts of glioma patients but are generally shorter in population based studies than patient trials that evaluate specific treatment regimens. According to the Central Brain Tumor Registry of The United States (CBTRUS) that report incidence and mortality data related to primary brain tumors for the entire US population [26], median survival is: 36 months for diffuse astrocytoma (grade II), 119 months for oligodendroglioma (grade II), 18 months for anaplastic astrocytoma (grade III), 60 months for anaplastic oligodendroglioma (grade III), and 8–9 months for glioblastoma (GBM, grade IV). Lower grade tumors have a tendency to become more malignant over time and usually occur in younger individuals in the third or fourth decade. GBMs mostly occur in patients over 50 years, and are highly vascular, necrotic, and infiltrative tumors. The varying survival time observed between patients with identical tumor histologies has remained a challenge, but molecular markers have emerged which link survival outcome to subclasses based on genetic changes, methylation status as well as gene expression patterns [27, 28]. A classification system that integrates genetic and epigenetic subtypes with transcriptional profiles has not yet been implemented. However, whereas genetic aberrations in the *EGFR* gene is typical of glioblastomas arising *de novo*, mutation in the *IDH* gene is associated with longer survival in glioblastomas that arise from grade II and III astrocytomas that also carry the IDH mutation [29]. Moreover, methylation of the DNA repair gene *MGMT* predicts response to temozolomide and a survival benefit [30]. Although survival is short in epidemiological studies, median survival for GBMs is around 14–16 months if standard multimodal therapy is administered. This involves surgery followed by fractionated radiotherapy and temozolomide administered concomitantly and then adjuvantly in repeated cycles [31, 32]. Tumor-treating field involves delivery of intermittent electric fields using transducers attached to the scalp, and reportedly prolongs overall survival in glioblastoma patients with 5 months [33]. Since this is a patented technology however, the significant treatment costs have precluded its implementation into the standard therapy regimen in many countries.

Brain Tumor Angiogenesis

The onset of angiogenesis is a key event in the malignant progression of gliomas and marks the transition from anaplastic gliomas to glioblastomas, coinciding with a drasti-

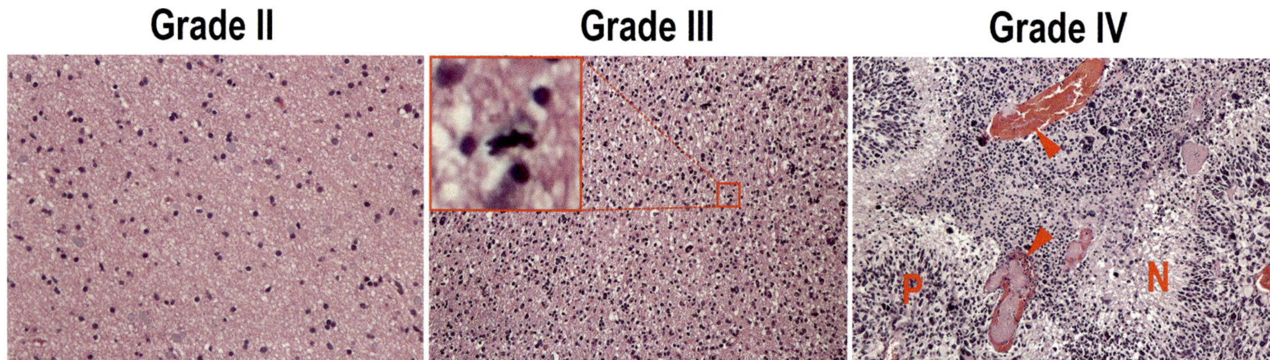

Fig. 30.1 Histological characteristics of WHO grade II–IV gliomas. Shown are H/E staining of formalin fixed 5 μm thick glioma section, grades as indicated. Grade II astrocytoma displays slight hypercellularity and moderate cellular pleomorphism. Grade III, or anaplastic astrocytoma, shows pronounced hypercellularity, nuclear atypia, and occasional mitotic figures (insert). Grade IV tumors or glioblastoma exhibits hypercellularity, striking nuclear atypia, as well as necrotic regions (N) surrounded by pseudopalisading cells (P) with microvascular proliferations and enlarged vessels (red arrowheads). H hematoxylin, E eosin, magnification: x 100

cally shortened survival [34]. Similar to other cancer types, brain tumor angiogenesis is triggered by hypoxia resulting from the tumor outgrowing its vascular supply and increasing oxygen demands. This subsequently elevates the levels of the HIF-1α transcription factor which again increases glioma cells' expression of the angiogenic vascular endothelial growth factor (VEGF), the most important factor driving brain tumor angiogenesis. Importantly, hypoxia as well as oncogene activation and matrix degradation also trigger the release of other angiogenic factors including fibroblast growth factors (FGF), platelet growth factors (PDGF), angiopoietins, matrix metalloproteases (MMPs), and transforming growth factor-β (TGF-β) [35]. Many of these are released by glioma cells, and high expression levels of FGF2 and TGF-β have been reported to correlate with shorter overall survival in glioma patients [36, 37]. Through binding of their receptors these factors coordinate the different steps leading to formation of new tumor vessels by sprouting from existing vessels. Initially, disintegration of the vessel wall and proliferation of endothelial cells are accompanied by enzymatic degradation of the basement membrane and ECM. Synthesis of ECM components then serve as a migratory substrate for endothelial cells and formation of capillary tubes. This sprouting from existing vessels is assumed to be the main mechanism of brain tumor angiogenesis, although various other cellular processes and biological mechanisms have been implicated, including co-option of the host vasculature by invading cells, vascular mimicry, vessel intussusception, recruitment of bone marrow-derived endothelial precursors, and transdifferentiation of cancer stem-like cells into endothelial cells [38].

Histopathologically, necrotic regions in glioblastomas are surrounded by dilated vessels and microvascular proliferations with endothelial hyperplasia, forming non-laminated structures referred to as glomeruloid bodies or vascular tufts, due to their resemblance with glomeruli in the kidneys. The proliferation index of tumor endothelial cell has been estimated to be 22–29% in GBMs, higher than in lower grade gliomas, whereas proliferation of endothelial cells in normal brain tissue is largely absent [39]. Furthermore, VEGF expression is particularly upregulated in palisading tumor cells around necrotic regions [40]. In addition, the VEGF receptor is abundantly expressed in these endothelial cells but hardly detectable in the normal brain vasculature. These findings also explain the striking presence of endothelial cell proliferations surrounding necrotic areas.

Animal studies also suggest that GBM cells with a stem-like phenotype had the ability to integrate into the vessel wall and transdifferentiate into endothelial cells [41]. Others have reported that endothelial cells carrying mutations found in the GBM cells occur at a very low rate mostly outside the endothelial lining of the vessel wall [41]. Thus, the experimental findings regarding this phenomenon are conflicting,

and no clinical data has established a role for cancer stem cell transdifferentiation in human glioma angiogenesis.

Several studies implicate bone marrow-derived cells in brain tumor angiogenesis. In particular, macrophages may acquire an M1-, tumor-inhibitory phenotype or an M2-, tumor-promoting phenotype. These cells exert their effects in vivo by releasing cytokines that promote tumor cell growth and angiogenesis. In experimental studies, integration of bone marrow-derived cells into the vessel wall seems to occur at a low rate and has not been demonstrated in human gliomas [38].

Brain Tumor Angiogenesis from a Therapeutic Perspective

Glioblastomas have been considered attractive candidates for anti-angiogenic therapy, due to their highly vascular nature. However, two prospective multi-center trials randomizing more than 1500 patients with newly diagnosed GBMs to treatment with the humanized monoclonal anti-VEGF antibody, Bevacizumab, or placebo failed to demonstrate a survival benefit in patients receiving Bevacizumab [42, 43]. The escape mechanisms mediating brain tumor progression during Bevacizumab treatment are incompletely characterized. However, both experimental studies and analyses of autopsied tumors from GBM patients receiving Bevacizumab suggest that other angiogenic factors are upregulated, and that tumors undergoing anti-angiogenic treatment acquire a more invasive growth pattern, possibly by coopting the host vasculature [44, 45]. Hence, subsequent efforts have explored targeting other and multiple angiogenic factors. However, this has not been successful in patients so far. Notably, the angiopoietin inhibitor Trebananib did not provide a survival benefit when administered to GBM patients in the recurrent setting, either as monotherapy or in combination with Bevacizumab [46].

Brain Tumor Immunity

Already several decades ago, histopathological studies demonstrated immune cell tumor infiltration in glioma patients. Whereas a high degree of lymphocyte infiltration in the perivascular space was reported to be associated with up to 4 months longer survival in one study [47], others found that lymphocytes infiltrating the tumor correlated with a poor prognosis [48]. With the introduction of antibodies allowing for identification of lymphocyte subtypes however, it became clear that these conflicting findings were consistent with the presence of functionally distinct classes of lymphocytes. Furthermore, studies also reported that glioma patients displayed reduced peripheral cellular and humoral immunity

[49]. Since then, numerous experimental and clinical studies have shown that glioma cells interact extensively with the immune system. These interactions involve both the innate and adaptive arm of the immune system, as well as local and peripheral immune cells. Despite the presence of the blood-brain barrier, peripheral immune cells may enter the brain parenchyma and the tumor bed via postcapillary venules, across the CSF–blood barrier in the choroid plexus, and via the perivascular space around arteries that enter the CNS. Moreover, the BBB is typically disrupted in malignant gliomas due to reduced pericyte coverage, gaps between the endothelial cells, and basement membrane defects in the brain tumor vasculature [50, 51], allowing peripheral immune cells to enter the CNS. In the opposite direction, interstitial fluid drains to the perivascular space, enabling tumor antigens in the brain parenchyma to reach antigen-presenting cells present around the meninges and in the subarachnoid space [52]. It has also been demonstrated that CSF communicates with deep cervical lymphatic drainage, and that antigens in the ventricles may induce antibody-producing cells in cervical lymph nodes [53]. Despite the multiple routes by which CNS communicates with the peripheral immune system, the brain tumor microenvironment is held in an immune-suppressive state by various mechanisms. The most prevalent cells in the brain tumor microenvironment are tumor-associated macrophages (TAMs) [54] that are derived both from peripheral monocytes recruited to the tumor bed and microglia. The recruitment and transformation of monocytes into TAMs is mediated by the chemokine CCL2 and colony-stimulating factor 1 (CSF1). However, whereas T-cell lymphocytes are the main cell type mediating adaptive antitumor immunity in the CNS, tumor-infiltrating lymphocytes (TILs) are far fewer than TAMs, and a less striking feature in gliomas than in many other tumor types [19, 55]. In addition, there is a shift toward a higher presence of T-cell subclasses with immunosuppressive functions in TILs compared to T cells in peripheral blood from patients [18]. Notably, regulatory T cells, T_{regs}, with an immunosuppressive phenotype not present in the peripheral blood are induced in the brain tumor microenvironment. Conversely, the proportion of CD3+CD4+ helper T cells in GBM biopsies is reduced compared to peripheral blood from the patient. Moreover, CD3+CD8+ cytotoxic lymphocytes (CTLs) are present among TILs, but their expressions of the costimulatory molecule CD28 and the adhesion molecule CD56 are reduced [18]. Thus, whereas several studies show that the glioma-infiltrating effector cells correlate positively with tumor grade as well as survival in glioblastomas [56, 57], this immune response is counteracted to varying degree by Tregs, astrocytes, TAMs, and tumor-derived factors, which impair the function of CTLs and helper T cells [58]. Notably, astrocytes, TAMs, and Tregs release IL-10 and TGF-β that inhibit activation of CTLs [59]. TAMs also mediate its immunosuppressive effect through arginase expression which deplete L-arginine from the brain tumor microenvironment where it is critical for T-cell function [60]. In addition, glioma cells metabolize tryptophan through their release of indoleamine-2,3-dioxygenase (IDO) into kynurenine. Apart from the effect of tryptophan starvation in itself, which induce T-cell anergy and cell death, kynurenine inhibits T-cell activation and skew T-cell differentiation toward suppressive phenotypes [61, 62]. The cellular participants and factors with critical roles in the tumor–host interplay are outlined in Fig. 30.2.

Immunotherapy for Gliomas

The immune-suppressive brain tumor environment has proven difficult to target and primary brain tumors have so far not been included on the growing list of malignancies for which immunotherapeutic drugs have been approved. The strategies to overcome glioma-related immunosuppression have largely involved inhibitors of immune suppressors, cancer vaccines, cellular therapies, and immune check point therapies or combinations of these. Cellular therapy has involved adoptive T-cell transfer with T cells immunized against tumor antigens, including genetically modified T cells with chimeric antigen receptors, CAR T cells, that activate T cells upon antigen binding [63]. Patient trials have demonstrated bioactivity and acceptable safety [64], although no survival benefit has been shown so far. Both obtaining robust delivery to the tumor site, gliomas' relatively low number of coding mutations and gliomas' heterogeneity in antigen expression are likely factors that can explain the lack of success whereas compelling effects have been observed for some other tumor types [65]. Tumor vaccines involve tumor-associated antigens that are preferentially expressed by tumor cells but also expressed by normal cells, or tumor-specific antigens that are confined to the malignant cell pool. Tumor-specific vaccines have been developed against the epidermal growth factor receptor variant III (EGFRvIII), a mutation occurring in 30% of GBMs, and cytomegalovirus (CMV), since CMV encoded proteins are present in most GBMs. Although both vaccines have triggered responses, a randomized phase III trial validating the EGFRvIII vaccine Rindopepimut enrolled 745 patients, but reported no survival benefit compared to standard treatment [66]. Immune checkpoints serve to ensure an appropriate T cells response toward foreign antigens while maintaining self-tolerance. Inhibitory checkpoints suppress T-cell function. Blockage of two of these, the cytotoxic T-lymphocyte-associated antigen-4 (CTLA-4) and programmed cell death protein 1(PD-1) or its ligands PD-L1 and PD-L2, has successfully prolonged overall and progression-free survival in patients with metastatic cancers [63, 67]. Notably, combinatorial blockage of

Fig. 30.2 Summary of the brain tumor–host interplay in the tumor core and the invasion zone. Hypoxia in the tumor core triggers angiogenesis, whereas immune cells and tumor-associated glial cells maintain an immunosuppressive microenvironment. Growth factors and a connexin-dependent astrocyte–glioma network facilitate glioma cell proliferation and invasion. The xCT antiport has a crucial role in providing precursors for glioma cell synthesis of glutathione that protects against oxidative stress, whereas glutamate released via the same antiport to the extracellular fluid causes neuronal cell death. The infiltrative zone is characterized by tumor cell migration along ECM components, white matter tracts, and smaller vessels (Created with BioRender.com)

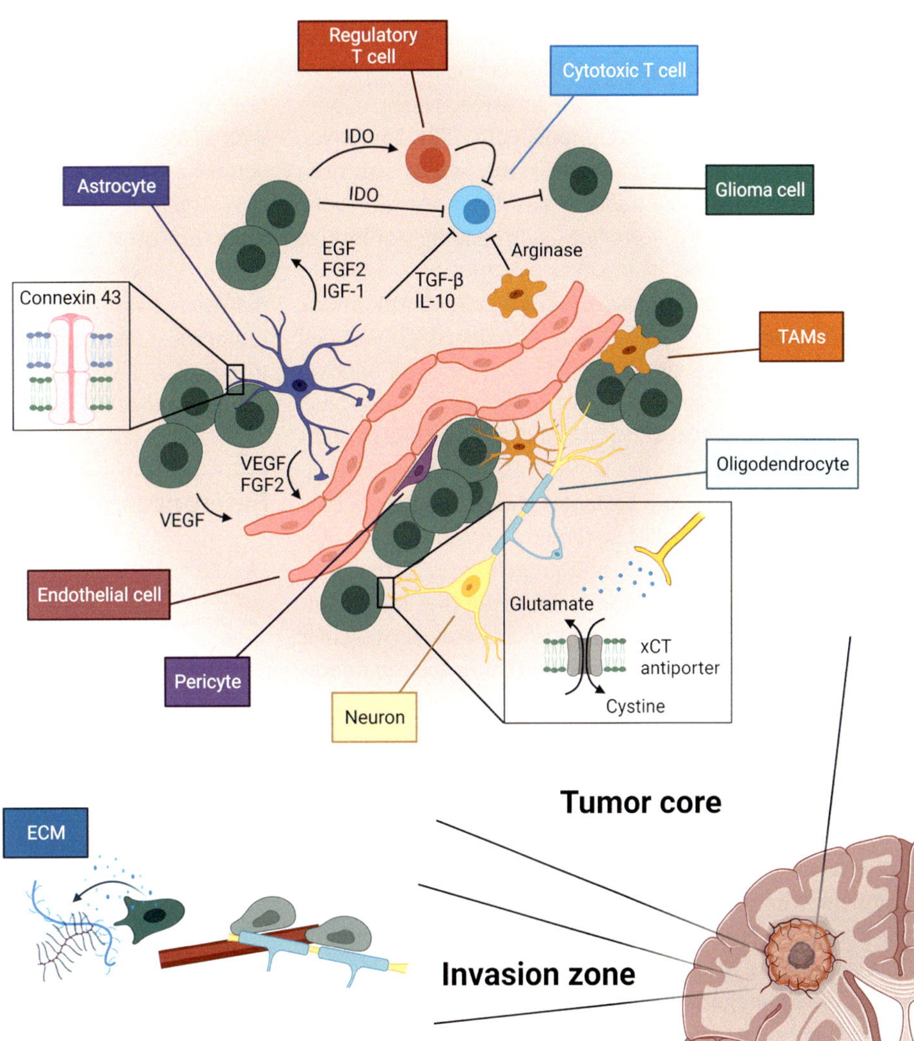

CTLA-4 and PD-L1 has demonstrated anti-tumor activity in animal glioma models [68]. Currently a phase II randomized trial compares ipilimumab that targets CTLA-4 and temozolomide to temozolomide alone after surgery and adjuvant chemotherapy in patients with newly diagnosed glioblastoma [69]. However, the PD-1 inhibitor Nivolumab failed to demonstrate a survival benefit when validated against Bevacizumab in a randomized phase 3 trial enrolling patients with GBM recurrences [70].

Tumor-Associated Glial Cells and Neurons

Glial cell types including astrocytes and oligodendrocytes represent the most abundant cell types in the CNS. These cells provide structural support and maintain homeostasis in the normal brain, but are also present in the brain tumor microenvironment (Fig. 30.2), where they can influence multiple aspects of glioma growth and sensitivity to treatment.

Reactive astrocytes are abundantly present in the tumor bed among infiltrating glioma cells, and brain tumor growth is accompanied by astrogliosis [71]. This process represents an activated state of astrocytes accompanied by secretion of factors that also promote the proliferation of glioma cells and/or angiogenesis, including EGF, IGF-1, GDF-15, IL-10, TGF-β, VEGF, and FGF2 [72–75]. Recently, it has also been shown that tumor-associated glial cells and astrocytes promote tumor growth in animal models [75, 76]. Gene expression analysis of astrocytes isolated from human GBM xenografts in immunodeficient mice revealed an upregulation of fetal transcription factors suggesting that tumor-associated glial cells adapted a stem-like phenotype [75]. In human GBM samples, the presence of peritumoral astrocytes expressing PDGFr-α and GFAP was associated with shorter survival, suggesting a prognostic relevance to astrocytes residing in the tumor bed [77].

Similarly, several studies have clearly demonstrated a pro-invasive effect of tumor-associated astrocytes on glioma cells both in *vitro* [74, 78] and in *vivo* [79, 80], involving multiple mechanisms: Astrocytes have been shown to secrete an inactive preform of matrix metalloproteinase-2, a proteolytic enzyme linked to cancer cell invasion, which is converted into an active form by glioma cells [78]. Moreover, connective tissue growth factor (CTGF), which has been implicated in cancer metastasis, has been shown to be secreted from reactive astrocytes surrounding infiltrative gliomas and bind to tyrosine kinase receptor type a (TrkA) present on the cell membrane of glioma cells. Furthermore, targeting either CTGF or TrkA both reduced glioma cell infiltration [80]. Whereas the Gap junction protein Connexin 43 (CX43) is overexpressed by astrocytes in the tumor bed [79], gliomas in CX43 knockout mice have more circumscribed margins. This implies a role for CX43 in tumor invasion, suggesting that CX43 promotes glioma cell detachment from the tumor core. A role in tumor angiogenesis has also been ascribed to oligodendrocyte progenitor cells that may enhance angiogenesis in gliomas by disrupting the blood-brain barrier, thereby abrogating the effect of perivascular pericytes, and by promoting vessel sprouting and tubule formation [81].

Gliomas are characterized by chemoresistance, and several studies show that astrocytes can modulate the response of the tumor cell compartment to chemotherapy. Co-cultures of astrocytes and a panel of glioma cell lines showed that the presence of astrocytes increased glioma cell survival after treatment with Temozolomide and Doxorubicin in several cell lines [82]. However, the gap junction channel inhibitor CBX as well as CX43 siRNA knockdown abolished this protective effect suggesting that the presence of gap junction channels between glioma cells and astrocytes is essential for mediating chemoresistance [83].

Gliomas are also associated with intra- and peritumoral neurodegeneration that is mediated by glutamate release from glioma cells via the xCT antiport in exchange for cystine uptake from the microenvironment. Cystine is essential for synthesis of glutathione that protects glioma cells against increased ROS levels resulting from elevated metabolic rates and biosynthesis. Glutamate is an excitatory neurotransmitter but excessive extracellular concentrations are neurotoxic and may cause epilepsy and neuronal cell deaths. Whereas physiological levels of extracellular glutamate typically range from 1–4 μM [84], concentrations up to 250 μM, which is known to be neurotoxic, have been measured in extracellular fluid derived from tumors [85]. Thus xCT appears to have a dual role in brain tumor progression: Apart from its role in protecting glioma cells against oxidative stress it also mediates neurodegeneration thereby vacating space for tumor growth. Notably, xCT expression is associated with tumor-associated epilepsy and a poorer survival outcome in glioma patients [86].

Concluding Remarks/Summary

Malignant gliomas are characterized by dynamic interactions with the immune system, glial cells in the tumor bed as well as recruitment of the host vasculature. Since these interactions are critical to tumor progression, they may be attractive targets for glioma therapy. Unlike some other cancer types however, neither anti-angiogenic nor immune-based therapies have demonstrated any survival benefit in glioma patients, suggesting that the mechanisms that regulate tumor–host interactions in the CNS are in many ways unique to gliomas. Thus, therapeutic progress in this field requires that those mechanisms are explored in further detail.

References

1. Cragg B. Brain extracellular space fixed for electron microscopy. Neurosci Lett. 1979;15(2–3):301–6.
2. Brodal P. The central nervous system. 4th ed. Oxford University Press; 2010.
3. Charveriat M, Naus CC, Leybaert L, Saez JC, Giaume C. Connexin-dependent neuroglial networking as a new therapeutic target. Front Cell Neurosci. 2017;11:174.
4. Andriezen WL. The neuroglia elements in the human brain. Br Med J. 1893;2(1700):227–30.
5. Freeman MR, Rowitch DH. Evolving concepts of gliogenesis: a look way back and ahead to the next 25 years. Neuron. 2013;80(3):613–23.
6. Maunoury R, Delpech A, Delpech B, Vidard MN, Vedrenne C, Constans JP, Hillereau J. Immunocytochemical localization of gliofibrillary proteins (GDAP) in human cerebral tumors. Histological and in vitro studies. Neuro-Chirurgie. 1977;23(3):173–85.
7. Orthmann-Murphy JL, Freidin M, Fischer E, Scherer SS, Abrams CK. Two distinct heterotypic channels mediate gap junction coupling between astrocyte and oligodendrocyte connexins. J Neurosci. 2007;27(51):13949–57.
8. Wallraff A, Kohling R, Heinemann U, Theis M, Willecke K, Steinhauser C. The impact of astrocytic gap junctional coupling on potassium buffering in the hippocampus. J Neurosci. 2006;26(20):5438–47.
9. Aird RB. The role of tissue permeability with particular reference to the blood-brain barrier in diseases of the central nervous system. Calif Med. 1948;69(5):360–3.
10. Brightman MW. Morphology of blood-brain interfaces. Exp Eye Res. 1977;25(Suppl):1–25.
11. Luse SA. Formation of myelin in the central nervous system of mice and rats, as studied with the electron microscope. J Biophys Biochem Cytol. 1956;2(6):777–84.
12. Kornguth SE, Anderson JW. Localization of a basic protein in the myelin of various species with the aid of fluorescence and electron microscopy. J Cell Biol. 1965;26(1):157–66.
13. Owens T, Bechmann I, Engelhardt B. Perivascular spaces and the two steps to neuroinflammation. J Neuropathol Exp Neurol. 2008;67(12):1113–21.
14. Lampson LA, Hickey WF. Monoclonal antibody analysis of MHC expression in human brain biopsies: tissue ranging from "histologically normal" to that showing different levels of glial tumor involvement. J Immunol. 1986;136(11):4054–62.
15. Li Q, Barres BA. Microglia and macrophages in brain homeostasis and disease. Nat Rev Immunol. 2018;18(4):225–42.

16. Ginhoux F, Greter M, Leboeuf M, Nandi S, See P, Gokhan S, Mehler MF, Conway SJ, Ng LG, Stanley ER, et al. Fate mapping analysis reveals that adult microglia derive from primitive macrophages. Science. 2010;330(6005):841–5.

17. Ousman SS, Kubes P. Immune surveillance in the central nervous system. Nat Neurosci. 2012;15(8):1096–101.

18. Kmiecik J, Poli A, Brons NH, Waha A, Eide GE, Enger PO, Zimmer J, Chekenya M. Elevated CD3+ and CD8+ tumor-infiltrating immune cells correlate with prolonged survival in glioblastoma patients despite integrated immunosuppressive mechanisms in the tumor microenvironment and at the systemic level. J Neuroimmunol. 2013;264(1–2):71–83.

19. Sampson JH, Gunn MD, Fecci PE, Ashley DM. Brain immunology and immunotherapy in brain tumours. Nat Rev Cancer. 2020;20(1):12–25.

20. Gallina P, Nicoletti C, Scollato A, Lolli F. The "glymphatic-lymphatic system pathology" and a new categorization of neurodegenerative disorders. Front Neurosci. 2021;15:669681.

21. Louveau A, Herz J, Alme MN, Salvador AF, Dong MQ, Viar KE, Herod SG, Knopp J, Setliff JC, Lupi AL, et al. CNS lymphatic drainage and neuroinflammation are regulated by meningeal lymphatic vasculature. Nat Neurosci. 2018;21(10):1380–91.

22. Bodnar CN, Watson JB, Higgins EK, Quan N, Bachstetter AD. Inflammatory regulation of cns barriers after traumatic brain injury: a tale directed by interleukin-1. Front Immunol. 2021;12:688254.

23. Lau LW, Cua R, Keough MB, Haylock-Jacobs S, Yong VW. Pathophysiology of the brain extracellular matrix: a new target for remyelination. Nat Rev Neurosci. 2013;14(10):722–9.

24. Zimmermann DR, Dours-Zimmermann MT. Extracellular matrix of the central nervous system: from neglect to challenge. Histochem Cell Biol. 2008;130(4):635–53.

25. Louis DN, Ohgaki H, Wiestler OD, Cavenee WK, Burger PC, Jouvet A, Scheithauer BW, Kleihues P. The 2007 WHO classification of tumours of the central nervous system. Acta Neuropathol. 2007;114(2):97–109.

26. Ostrom QT, Patil N, Cioffi G, Waite K, Kruchko C, Barnholtz-Sloan JS. CBTRUS statistical report: primary brain and other central nervous system tumors diagnosed in the United States in 2013–2017. Neuro-Oncology 2020, 22(12 Suppl 2):iv1–iv96.

27. Wen PY, Weller M, Lee EQ, Alexander BM, Barnholtz-Sloan JS, Barthel FP, Batchelor TT, Bindra RS, Chang SM, Chiocca EA, et al. Glioblastoma in adults: a Society for Neuro-Oncology (SNO) and European Society of Neuro-Oncology (EANO) consensus review on current management and future directions. Neuro-Oncology. 2020;22(8):1073–113.

28. Verhaak RG, Hoadley KA, Purdom E, Wang V, Qi Y, Wilkerson MD, Miller CR, Ding L, Golub T, Mesirov JP, et al. Integrated genomic analysis identifies clinically relevant subtypes of glioblastoma characterized by abnormalities in PDGFRA, IDH1, EGFR, and NF1. Cancer Cell. 2010;17(1):98–110.

29. Cancer Genome Atlas Research N: Comprehensive genomic characterization defines human glioblastoma genes and core pathways. Nature 2008;455(7216):1061–1068.

30. McAleenan A, Kelly C, Spiga F, Kernohan A, Cheng HY, Dawson S, Schmidt L, Robinson T, Brandner S, Faulkner CL, et al. Prognostic value of test(s) for O6-methylguanine-DNA methyltransferase (MGMT) promoter methylation for predicting overall survival in people with glioblastoma treated with temozolomide. Cochrane Database Syst Rev. 2021;3:CD013316.

31. Vigneswaran K, Neill S, Hadjipanayis CG. Beyond the World Health Organization grading of infiltrating gliomas: advances in the molecular genetics of glioma classification. Ann Transl Med. 2015;3(7):95.

32. Stupp R, Mason WP, van den Bent MJ, Weller M, Fisher B, Taphoorn MJ, Belanger K, Brandes AA, Marosi C, Bogdahn U, et al. Radiotherapy plus concomitant and adjuvant temozolomide for glioblastoma. N Engl J Med. 2005;352(10):987–96.

33. Stupp R, Taillibert S, Kanner AA, Kesari S, Steinberg DM, Toms SA, Taylor LP, Lieberman F, Silvani A, Fink KL, et al. Maintenance therapy with tumor-treating fields plus temozolomide vs temozolomide alone for glioblastoma: a randomized clinical trial. JAMA. 2015;314(23):2535–43.

34. Cancer TiAfRo: WHO classification of tumours of the central nervous system, 4th edn; 2007.

35. Ahir BK, Engelhard HH, Lakka SS. Tumor development and angiogenesis in adult brain tumor: glioblastoma. Mol Neurobiol. 2020;57(5):2461–78.

36. Sooman L, Freyhult E, Jaiswal A, Navani S, Edqvist PH, Ponten F, Tchougounova E, Smits A, Elsir T, Gullbo J, et al. FGF2 as a potential prognostic biomarker for proneural glioma patients. Acta Oncol. 2015;54(3):385–94.

37. Bruna A, Darken RS, Rojo F, Ocana A, Penuelas S, Arias A, Paris R, Tortosa A, Mora J, Baselga J, et al. High TGFbeta-Smad activity confers poor prognosis in glioma patients and promotes cell proliferation depending on the methylation of the PDGF-B gene. Cancer Cell. 2007;11(2):147–60.

38. Plate KH, Scholz A, Dumont DJ. Tumor angiogenesis and anti-angiogenic therapy in malignant gliomas revisited. Acta Neuropathol. 2012;124(6):763–75.

39. Lebelt A, Dzieciol J, Guzinska-Ustymowicz K, Lemancewicz D, Zimnoch L, Czykier E. Angiogenesis in gliomas. Folia histochemica et cytobiologica/Polish Academy of Sciences, Polish Histochemical and Cytochemical Society 2008;46(1):69–72.

40. Plate KH, Breier G, Weich HA, Risau W. Vascular endothelial growth factor is a potential tumour angiogenesis factor in human gliomas in vivo. Nature. 1992;359(6398):845–8.

41. Ricci-Vitiani L, Pallini R, Biffoni M, Todaro M, Invernici G, Cenci T, Maira G, Parati EA, Stassi G, Larocca LM, et al. Tumour vascularization via endothelial differentiation of glioblastoma stem-like cells. Nature. 2010;468(7325):824–8.

42. Gilbert MR, Dignam JJ, Armstrong TS, Wefel JS, Blumenthal DT, Vogelbaum MA, Colman H, Chakravarti A, Pugh S, Won M, et al. A randomized trial of bevacizumab for newly diagnosed glioblastoma. N Engl J Med. 2014;370(8):699–708.

43. Chinot OL, Wick W, Mason W, Henriksson R, Saran F, Nishikawa R, Carpentier AF, Hoang-Xuan K, Kavan P, Cernea D, et al. Bevacizumab plus radiotherapy-temozolomide for newly diagnosed glioblastoma. N Engl J Med. 2014;370(8):709–22.

44. Lucio-Eterovic AK, Piao Y, de Groot JF. Mediators of glioblastoma resistance and invasion during antivascular endothelial growth factor therapy. Clin Cancer Res. 2009;15(14):4589–99.

45. Okamoto S, Nitta M, Maruyama T, Sawada T, Komori T, Okada Y, Muragaki Y. Bevacizumab changes vascular structure and modulates the expression of angiogenic factors in recurrent malignant gliomas. Brain Tumor Pathol 2016.

46. Reardon DA, Lassman AB, Schiff D, Yunus SA, Gerstner ER, Cloughesy TF, Lee EQ, Gaffey SC, Barrs J, Bruno J, et al. Phase 2 and biomarker study of trebananib, an angiopoietin-blocking peptibody, with and without bevacizumab for patients with recurrent glioblastoma. Cancer. 2018;124(7):1438–48.

47. Brooks WH, Markesbery WR, Gupta GD, Roszman TL. Relationship of lymphocyte invasion and survival of brain tumor patients. Ann Neurol. 1978;4(3):219–24.

48. Safdari H, Hochberg FH, Richardson EP Jr. Prognostic value of round cell (lymphocyte) infiltration in malignant gliomas. Surg Neurol. 1985;23(3):221–6.

49. Mahaley MS Jr, Brooks WH, Roszman TL, Bigner DD, Dudka L, Richardson S. Immunobiology of primary intracranial tumors. Part 1: studies of the cellular and humoral general immune competence of brain-tumor patients. J Neurosurg. 1977;46(4):467–76.

50. Long DM. Capillary ultrastructure and the blood-brain barrier in human malignant brain tumors. J Neurosurg. 1970;32(2):127–44.

51. Nystrom SH. Electron microscopical structure of the wall of small blood vessels in human multiform glioblastoma. Nature. 1959;184:65.

52. Ransohoff RM, Engelhardt B. The anatomical and cellular basis of immune surveillance in the central nervous system. Nat Rev Immunol. 2012;12(9):623–35.

53. Walter BA, Valera VA, Takahashi S, Matsuno K, Ushiki T. Evidence of antibody production in the rat cervical lymph nodes after antigen administration into the cerebrospinal fluid. Arch Histol Cytol. 2006;69(1):37–47.

54. Graeber MB, Scheithauer BW, Kreutzberg GW. Microglia in brain tumors. Glia. 2002;40(2):252–9.

55. Mohme M, Neidert MC. Tumor-specific T cell activation in malignant brain tumors. Front Immunol. 2020;11:205.

56. Lohr J, Ratliff T, Huppertz A, Ge Y, Dictus C, Ahmadi R, Grau S, Hiraoka N, Eckstein V, Ecker RC, et al. Effector T-cell infiltration positively impacts survival of glioblastoma patients and is impaired by tumor-derived TGF-beta. Clin Cancer Res. 2011;17(13):4296–308.

57. Han S, Zhang C, Li Q, Dong J, Liu Y, Huang Y, Jiang T, Wu A. Tumour-infiltrating CD4(+) and CD8(+) lymphocytes as predictors of clinical outcome in glioma. Br J Cancer. 2014;110(10):2560–8.

58. Rolle CE, Sengupta S, Lesniak MS. Mechanisms of immune evasion by gliomas. Adv Exp Med Biol. 2012;746:53–76.

59. Vitkovic L, Maeda S, Sternberg E. Anti-inflammatory cytokines: expression and action in the brain. Neuroimmunomodulation. 2001;9(6):295–312.

60. Zhang I, Alizadeh D, Liang J, Zhang L, Gao H, Song Y, Ren H, Ouyang M, Wu X, D'Apuzzo M, et al. Characterization of arginase expression in glioma-associated microglia and macrophages. PLoS One. 2016;11(12):e0165118.

61. Zhai L, Bell A, Ladomersky E, Lauing KL, Bollu L, Sosman JA, Zhang B, Wu JD, Miller SD, Meeks JJ, et al. Immunosuppressive IDO in cancer: mechanisms of action, animal models, and targeting strategies. Front Immunol. 2020;11:1185.

62. Platten M, Weller M, Wick W. Shaping the glioma immune microenvironment through tryptophan metabolism. CNS Oncol. 2012;1(1):99–106.

63. Reardon DA, Freeman G, Wu C, Chiocca EA, Wucherpfennig KW, Wen PY, Fritsch EF, Curry WT Jr, Sampson JH, Dranoff G. Immunotherapy advances for glioblastoma. Neuro-Oncology. 2014;16(11):1441–58.

64. Brown CE, Badie B, Barish ME, Weng L, Ostberg JR, Chang WC, Naranjo A, Starr R, Wagner J, Wright C, et al. Bioactivity and safety of IL13Ralpha2-redirected chimeric antigen receptor CD8+ T cells in patients with recurrent glioblastoma. Clin Cancer Res. 2015;21(18):4062–72.

65. Petersen CT, Krenciute G. Next generation CAR T cells for the immunotherapy of high-grade glioma. Front Oncol. 2019;9:69.

66. Weller M, Butowski N, Tran DD, Recht LD, Lim M, Hirte H, Ashby L, Mechtler L, Goldlust SA, Iwamoto F, et al. Rindopepimut with temozolomide for patients with newly diagnosed, EGFRvIII-expressing glioblastoma (ACT IV): a randomised, double-blind, international phase 3 trial. Lancet Oncol. 2017;18(10):1373–85.

67. Larkin J, Chiarion-Sileni V, Gonzalez R, Grob JJ, Cowey CL, Lao CD, Schadendorf D, Dummer R, Smylie M, Rutkowski P, et al. Combined nivolumab and ipilimumab or monotherapy in untreated melanoma. N Engl J Med. 2015;373(1):23–34.

68. Wainwright DA, Chang AL, Dey M, Balyasnikova IV, Kim CK, Tobias A, Cheng Y, Kim JW, Qiao J, Zhang L, et al. Durable therapeutic efficacy utilizing combinatorial blockade against IDO, CTLA-4, and PD-L1 in mice with brain tumors. Clin Cancer Res. 2014;20(20):5290–301.

69. Brown NF, Ng SM, Brooks C, Coutts T, Holmes J, Roberts C, Elhussein L, Hoskin P, Maughan T, Blagden S, et al. A phase II open label, randomised study of ipilimumab with temozolomide versus temozolomide alone after surgery and chemoradiotherapy in patients with recently diagnosed glioblastoma: the Ipi-Glio trial protocol. BMC Cancer. 2020;20(1):198.

70. Reardon DA, Brandes AA, Omuro A, Mulholland P, Lim M, Wick A, Baehring J, Ahluwalia MS, Roth P, Bahr O, et al. Effect of nivolumab vs bevacizumab in patients with recurrent glioblastoma: the CheckMate 143 phase 3 randomized clinical trial. JAMA Oncol. 2020;6(7):1003–10.

71. Lee J, Borboa AK, Baird A, Eliceiri BP. Non-invasive quantification of brain tumor-induced astrogliosis. BMC Neurosci. 2011;12:9.

72. Sierra A, Price JE, Garcia-Ramirez M, Mendez O, Lopez L, Fabra A. Astrocyte-derived cytokines contribute to the metastatic brain specificity of breast cancer cells. Laboratory investigation; a journal of technical methods and pathology 1997;77(4):357–368.

73. Roth P, Junker M, Tritschler I, Mittelbronn M, Dombrowski Y, Breit SN, Tabatabai G, Wick W, Weller M, Wischhusen J. GDF-15 contributes to proliferation and immune escape of malignant gliomas. Clin Cancer Res. 2010;16(15):3851–9.

74. Rath BH, Fair JM, Jamal M, Camphausen K, Tofilon PJ. Astrocytes enhance the invasion potential of glioblastoma stem-like cells. PLoS One. 2013;8(1):e54752.

75. Leiss L, Mutlu E, Oyan A, Yan T, Tsinkalovsky O, Sleire L, Petersen K, Rahman MA, Johannessen M, Mitra SS, et al. Tumour-associated glial host cells display a stem-like phenotype with a distinct gene expression profile and promote growth of GBM xenografts. BMC Cancer. 2017;17(1):108.

76. Mega A, Hartmark Nilsen M, Leiss LW, Tobin NP, Miletic H, Sleire L, Strell C, Nelander S, Krona C, Hagerstrand D, et al. Astrocytes enhance glioblastoma growth. Glia. 2020;68(2):316–27.

77. Leiss L, Mega A, Olsson Bontell T, Nister M, Smits A, Corvigno S, Rahman MA, Enger PO, Miletic H, Ostman A. Platelet-derived growth factor receptor alpha/glial fibrillary acidic protein expressing peritumoral astrocytes associate with shorter median overall survival in glioblastoma patients. Glia. 2020;68(5):979–88.

78. Le DM, Besson A, Fogg DK, Choi KS, Waisman DM, Goodyer CG, Rewcastle B, Yong VW. Exploitation of astrocytes by glioma cells to facilitate invasiveness: a mechanism involving matrix metalloproteinase-2 and the urokinase-type plasminogen activator-plasmin cascade. J Neurosci Off J Soc Neurosci. 2003;23(10):4034–43.

79. Sin WC, Aftab Q, Bechberger JF, Leung JH, Chen H, Naus CC. Astrocytes promote glioma invasion via the gap junction protein connexin43. Oncogene 2015.

80. Edwards LA, Woolard K, Son MJ, Li A, Lee J, Ene C, Mantey SA, Maric D, Song H, Belova G, et al. Effect of brain- and tumor-derived connective tissue growth factor on glioma invasion. J Natl Cancer Inst. 2011;103(15):1162–78.

81. Huang Y, Hoffman C, Rajappa P, Kim JH, Hu W, Huse J, Tang Z, Li X, Weksler B, Bromberg J, et al. Oligodendrocyte progenitor cells promote neovascularization in glioma by disrupting the blood-brain barrier. Cancer Res. 2014;74(4):1011–21.

82. Yang N, Yan T, Zhu H, Liang X, Leiss L, Sakariassen PO, Skaftnesmo KO, Huang B, Costea DE, Enger PO, et al. A co-culture model with brain tumor-specific bioluminescence demonstrates astrocyte-induced drug resistance in glioblastoma. J Transl Med. 2014;12:278.

83. Chen W, Wang D, Du X, He Y, Chen S, Shao Q, Ma C, Huang B, Chen A, Zhao P, et al. Glioma cells escaped from cytotoxicity of temozolomide and vincristine by communicating with human astrocytes. Med Oncol. 2015;32(3):43.

84. Lerma J, Herranz AS, Herreras O, Abraira V, Martin del Rio R. In vivo determination of extracellular concentration of amino acids in the rat hippocampus. A method based on brain dialysis and computerized analysis. Brain Res. 1986;384(1):145–55.

85. Savaskan NE, Fan Z, Broggini T, Buchfelder M, Eyupoglu IY. Neurodegeneration and the Brain Tumor Microenvironment [corrected]. Curr Neuropharmacol. 2015;13(2):258–65.

86. Robel S, Buckingham SC, Boni JL, Campbell SL, Danbolt NC, Riedemann T, Sutor B, Sontheimer H. Reactive astrogliosis causes the development of spontaneous seizures. J Neurosci. 2015;35(8):3330–45.

The Role of the Microenvironment in Tumor Promoting Stress Responses

Hanna Dillekås, Cornelia Schuster, Kjersti T. Davidsen, and Oddbjørn Straume

Abstract

All cells need to be able to respond rapidly to changes in their surroundings to be able to survive and multiply. In nature, cells and multicellular organisms are frequently faced with acute changes such as heat and cold, as well as more chronic challenges such as starvation, forcing the cells to come up with responses to be able to grow and thrive. In this chapter, we will discuss how normal cell extrinsic and intrinsic stress responses, emerging in the tumor microenvironment (TME), can promote cancer development under certain circumstances. The scene will be set by showing how systemic responses following tissue trauma and wound healing can ignite the growth of dormant, occult micrometastases. In addition, the role of the adrenergic stress response machinery during development of malignancy will be discussed. Furthermore, the importance of epithelial to mesenchymal transition (EMT) and one of its regulators, the Axl receptor, will be introduced as a fundamental cellular stress response in cancer. Finally, we will discuss how an unfavorable, stressful, and abnormal TME can bring on intrinsic instigators of DNA damage as oncogenic drivers of the mutator phenotype.

Take-Home Lessons

- Cancers follow the laws of nature; species produce mutants and variants to cope with hostile environmental changes; mutations are necessary for evolution.
- Cells respond to changing environments and stress by increased adaptive mutability, which might cause acquired therapy resistance in cancers.
- Instigators of endogenous DNA damage represent an important stress response in *E. coli*, and human homologues have been described.
- The heat-shock response is a powerful adaptive mechanism.
- A phenotypic switch is necessary for cancer cells to establish distant metastases.
- Cancer–host interactions are targetable.
- β-adrenergic signaling can impact multiple hallmarks of cancer; β2-adrenergic receptor blocking drugs can inhibit tumor-promoting processes.
- Interactions with the innate and adaptive immune systems support a pro-tumorigenic environment.
- The receptor tyrosine kinase AXL enables phenotypic plasticity related to epithelial to mesenchymal transition, immune evasion, invasiveness, metastasis, and therapy resistance.
- AXL is induced by stress such as hypoxia, starvation, oxidative stress, and acidosis.

H. Dillekås · K. T. Davidsen
Department of Oncology, Haukeland University Hospital, Bergen, Norway
e-mail: hanna.elisabet.dillekas@helse-bergen.no; kjersti.davidsen@helse-bergen.no

C. Schuster · O. Straume (✉)
Centre of Cancer Biomarkers, University of Bergen, Bergen, Norway
e-mail: cornelia.schuster@uib.no; oddbjorn.straume@helse-bergen.no

Introduction

Cancer is now the leading cause of premature death in developed countries, and the majority of these deaths are caused by metastasis [1]. We have learned that "cancer is, in essence, a genetic disease" [2]. Mutations in the DNA represent the

L. A. Akslen, R. S. Watnick (eds.), *Biomarkers of the Tumor Microenvironment*, https://doi.org/10.1007/978-3-030-98950-7_31

major cause of all cancerous diseases leading to uncontrolled cell proliferation, disrupted tissue homeostasis, metastatic spread, and death. Thus, for cells and organisms, mutations are undesirable and must be prevented, with a few exceptions.

On his round-the-world survey voyage on the HMS Beagle (1831–36) (Fig. 31.1), Charles Darwin observed animals, birds, insects, and plants and their interactions with their macro- and microenvironments. These observations lay the foundation for his evolution theories [3]. Even today, we can use his revolutionary way of thinking when we are trying to understand tumor biology. If a given plant, let us say wheat, grows under favorable conditions, the plant population will thrive and abound. There will be homogeneity and very little individual variation. However, when domesticated and grown under optimal conditions, breeders frequently observe sterility; these plants do not prioritize to spread. Darwin noted that if he traveled from the fertile river valley and up into the cold and barren mountains, the same plants exhibited more variation with crippled, heterogeneous miniature individuals. Darwin called these plants variants and mutants. And interestingly, these plants prioritize seed production and spread over growth. Three billion years of evolution have benefitted the survival of those cells and organisms capable of coping with environmental stress with increased variation encouraged by mutation, a *genotype switch*. The very same stress response mechanisms are in play during the rapid progression of malignant cells and metastasis.

One unexplained phenomenon observed in melanoma patients is that ulcerated primary melanomas (Fig. 31.2a and b) have a poorer prognosis in comparison to non-ulcerated primaries. The question then emerges as to whether the ulcer on the surface of the tumor reflects an underlying aggressive tumor biology *per se*? Or, is it the ulcer itself, and the persistent wound healing events in the environment enclosing the tumor, that drives the cancer cells into a more aggressive and more lethal phenotype? These questions give rise to a larger, more central question as to whether stressful conditions, such as hypoxia, frequently found in rapidly growing and ulcerated tumors, initiate a *phenotype switch* enabling escape of tumor cells from the primary focus to distant sites. These clinically relevant questions may not be so simple at all, and might define how we perceive and interpret cancer with respect to its interactions with the host. Realizing that cancer in general is a distorted and corrupted reflection of our own body tissue, and that the nature of the malignancies basically is a coopted normal,

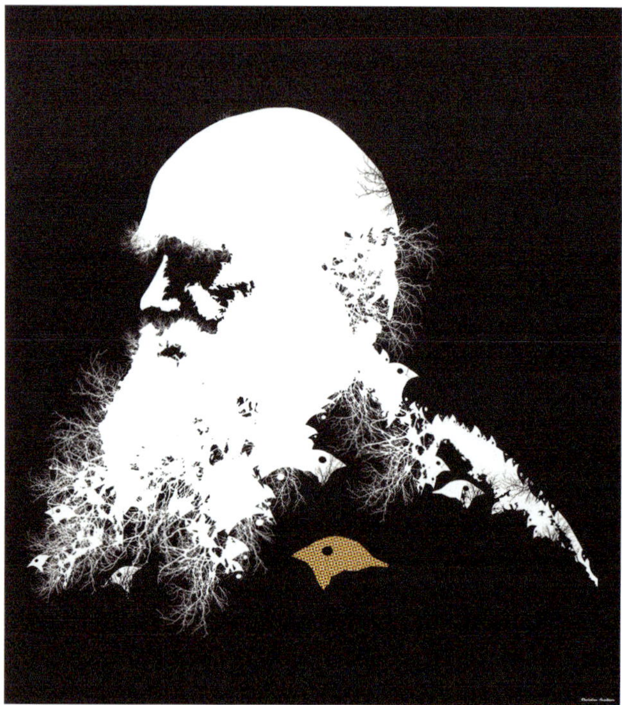

Fig. 31.1 Charles Darwing by Christine Sandtorv

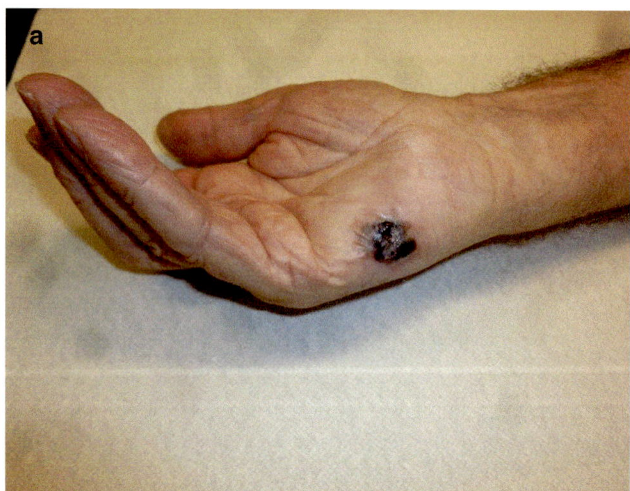

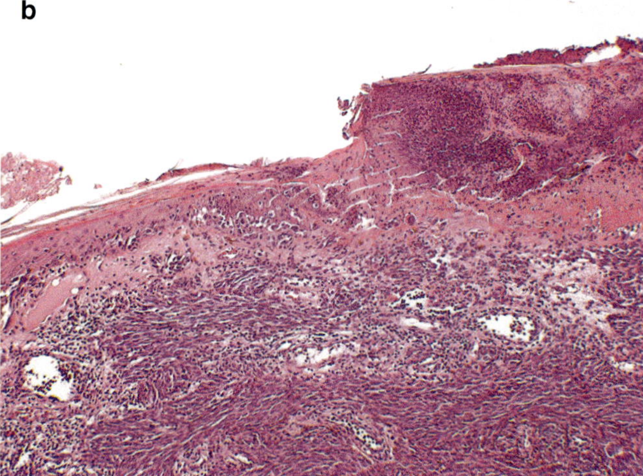

Fig. 31.2 Ulcerated malignant melanoma

out of control, physiologic process, makes it easier to grasp the core of the challenges clinicians and researchers are up against.

A mutated cell is on its own not sufficient to generate a lethal tumor let alone metastatic dissemination to kill the host. Growth and spread do not happen without the contribution from a supportive microenvironment. Clearly, the tumor cell is not an island. Only by taking control over the interactions with normal cells and the extracellular matrix, cancer cells can multiply, grow, and spread. These interactions are essential in tumor biology, *and* they can be targeted therapeutically [4–6].

The Escape from Tumor Dormancy

The Biology of Tumor Dormancy

This section is a brief description of the delicate balance and complex interactions of the tumor microenvironment, as well as those between the tumor and the entire biologic system of the host, regarding escape from dormancy and tumor progression. To begin with, what is tumor dormancy and how is it initiated and maintained?

Tumor dormancy was first described in 1954 [7] and refers to a reversible state of little to no growth of cancer cells with maintained malignant potential. It can further be divided along several different axes. Primary tumor dormancy, where people harbor microscopic tumors without ever having been diagnosed with cancer, has been demonstrated in autopsy studies to be very frequent [8]. Metastatic dormancy on the other hand is characterized by a latency to manifest metastatic disease after apparently successful primary tumor treatment, thus resulting from early dissemination and a period of dormancy at the metastatic site. This has been ascribed to a maladaptation to the new microenvironment of the metastatic site. The metastatic niche may be quite different from the organ of origin, not permitting growth of the cancer cell until it has acquired new characteristics, better suited to this new milieu, or until the microenvironment changes [9]. Cancer treatment with chemotherapy can also induce dormancy, as has been demonstrated in vivo to be mediated by type I interferon (IFN) signaling. An association between serum IFN-β during neoadjuvant chemotherapy and longer time to recurrence suggested a clinical correlate in humans [10].

Withdrawal of hormonal stimulation can maintain cancer in the dormant state, as can be deduced from both the benefit of extended endocrine therapy, even beyond 5 years [11, 12], and the synchronization of metastasis growth at the end of adjuvant endocrine treatment [13]. Animal models support this finding. In an ovariectomized immunocompromised mouse model, ER+ breast cancer micrometastases remained dormant until hormone stimulation was initiated [14].

A distinction can also be made between intrinsic dormancy, caused by genetic or epigenetic mechanisms within the cancer cell [15], and extrinsic dormancy, where micrometastases are kept dormant by immune control [16], lack of angiogenesis [17], growth factor deprivation [18], or other restraints in the microenvironment. Partly overlapping with the classification of intrinsic and extrinsic dormancy is the concept of cellular dormancy, cell cycle arrest in the G0 phase of individual cells, and cell population-based dormancy where there is a balance between proliferation and apoptosis [19] resulting in a stable population of cancer cells. These classifications or variants of tumor dormancy are not mutually exclusive and can thus coexist in the same patient at the same time. The extrinsic pressure from a hostile microenvironment will lead to cell death in some cells, but may activate cell-intrinsic survival mechanisms in others, like upregulation of cell cycle inhibitors p21 and p27 [20], reduced PI3K/Akt signaling, or epigenetic modifications [21]. These stress-response transcriptional programs are expanded on in a later section of this chapter.

Tumor Dormancy as a Clinical Problem

To a patient treated for cancer, learning that physicians cannot guarantee that all cancer cells are eradicated and never will cause a relapse is a grim notion, leading to significant anxiety in some patients. The fact that some cancer forms, breast cancer being perhaps the most widely recognized, can give rise to metastatic disease years or decades after primary treatment is considered indirect evidence of a period of dormancy as this cannot be convincingly explained by other models of tumor growth [22].

A marker for the presence or absence of disseminated dormant cancer cells would be important information for follow-up of cancer patients. As of now, there is no clinically validated biomarker of dormant cancer. In breast cancer, the presence of disseminated tumor cells in the bone marrow after primary treatment is an independent prognostic marker [23], but we are not yet capable of distinguishing if these cells are truly dormant and harbor the potential of awakening. From preclinical models, the nuclear receptor NR2F1 displays potential as a marker of dormancy, and is currently being explored in clinical samples in breast cancer as well as other tumor forms [24, 25]. Liquid biopsies are significantly easier and less invasive than bone marrow aspiration to obtain and have demonstrated usefulness as a prognostic biomarker of late recurrence. In a series of ER positive, HER2 negative breast cancer patients, without evidence of recurrence five years after primary treatment, detection of circulating tumor cells at five years was significantly associated with relapse [26]. In a small group of late relapsing breast cancer patients, significantly differential expression of miRNA-21 and miRNA-200c was discovered in plasma at primary treatment compared to non-relapsing patients [27]. TGF-β2 [28], bone morphogenic protein 30 (BMP) [29], retinoic acid, and IFN-β [10] are other systemic markers explored for potential clinical utility as biomarkers for tumor dormancy. An interesting potential biomarker is growth arrest-specific ligand (GAS6) of the TAM family of receptor tyrosine kinase receptors (TYRO3, AXL, and MER) [30]; details of AXL signaling are outlined in Sect. 4 of this chapter.

What Causes the Awakening?

Even if the mechanisms of dormancy initiation and maintenance are different, as discussed above, the stimulus inducing escape from dormancy may be the same. When the cancer relapse occurs decades after primary treatment, the escape from dormancy may be explained by advanced age in the patient with accompanying increase in inflammation ("inflammaging") or disturbed homeostasis from other systemic diseases that may arise as we age [31]. The escape from dormancy has also been suggested to be predetermined by an internal clock in the cancer cells [32], or elicited by some random event. Systemic signaling promoting cell proliferation and migration, angiogenesis, and immune modulation are all present in tissue trauma and wound healing [33]. Thus, such a process may awaken the dormant micrometastases regardless of the mechanism by which dormancy was first established [34].

Stimulated growth of cancer lesions after tissue trauma and wound healing has been demonstrated repeatedly, both in clinical and experimental settings [35–37]. As mechanisms of dormancy are not yet fully understood, the evidence for how tissue trauma and wound healing can facilitate escape from dormancy is less clear. Coherent with the concepts of extrinsic and population-based dormancy is the theory of an angiogenic switch being capable of inducing escape from dormancy. Dr. Judah Folkman first proposed this in the 1970s. According to his work, tumors of 1–2 mm in size are restricted from further growth by a lack of sufficient blood supply [38]. At some time point, the chronic hypoxic stress resulting from this hypoperfusion stimulates production of angiogenic factors such as VEGF, FGF, angiopoietins, and others, causing blood vessels to sprout and supply the tumor with oxygen and nutrients to support further tumor growth [39]. This switch, from a non-angiogenic to angiogenic phenotype mediating escape from dormancy, has been demonstrated in animal models, but as of yet lacks a convincing clinical correlate [40, 41]. Another angle of the vascular-dormancy interaction is the proposal that the perivascular niche of stable vessel induces and maintains dormancy via enrichment of thrombospondin-1. Tip cells of sprouting neovasculature, on the contrary, produce various factors capable of promoting metastatic growth [42]. Further, the primary tumor is suggested to be capable of maintaining microscopic metastases at a distant site in a dormant state. In models, this effect was demonstrated to be mediated by production of angiogenesis inhibitors [43] or immune modulators [44]. Accordingly, removal of the primary tumor may have a dual stimulating effect on metastasis development. Removing the primary tumor would free the dormant metastases from their homeostatic restraint. At the same time, growth would be stimulated by physiological wound healing signaling.

Inflammation has also been demonstrated to stimulate escape from dormancy. Different studies point to different cells responsible of this effect, like tumor-associated macrophages [45] and neutrophils [46]. The inflammatory stimuli in these studies have come from tobacco smoke [47], LPS (lipopolysaccaride) injection [46], and surgical trauma [45]. In another study, active inflammation was not necessary to induce escape from dormancy, but rather the fibrotic remodeling of the stroma after inflammation [48].

What actually happens in the cell, at the molecular level, that switches it from dormancy to malignant growth is also an area of dedicated research. In cell experiments, a shift in the balance of phosphorylation of the intracellular signaling molecule ERK, central in cell division, in relation to phosphorylation of p38, involved in cell death and growth restriction, has been suggested to be a key event [32]. Adding to the complexity, mechanisms of escape from dormancy may be organ specific; in a mouse model, when dormant breast cancer cells were exposed to the same signaling molecule escape from dormancy was observed in the lung, but not in other organs [9]. To summarize, escape from dormancy can be understood from the molecular level, the cellular level, the microenvironment level, or the systemic level. In order to fully comprehend this ominous event, all of these levels of understanding need to be integrated.

Duality of Immune System Dormancy Effects

The immune system is a powerful weapon that the body can use to attack cancer; in other circumstances, the immune system may stimulate escape from tumor dormancy and fuel cancer growth [49]. A causal correlation between chronic inflammation and cancer was hypothesized already by Virchow, and has been robustly demonstrated in hepatitis and hepatocellular carcinoma as well as inflammatory bowel diseases like ulcerative colitis and Crohn's disease and colon cancer [50].

Indirect evidence for immune mediated dormancy stems from the occurrence of donor-derived cancer, where organ recipients, under immune suppressive treatment, develop cancer originating from donors considered cured from cancer, or that were never diagnosed with cancer. Most reports are on melanoma, but also other cancer forms, including breast carcinomas and renal cancer, have been described [51, 52]. The other side of this coin is the impressive responses seen in some patients treated with immune checkpoint inhibitors [53]. This relatively new form of cancer treatment releases the breaks of the immune system, allowing immune cells to attack cancer cells, leading to long-term responses or perhaps even cures. The cancer-immune system interaction is considered to span a scale of escape, equilibrium, and elimination [54]. Most cells undergoing malignant transformation are recognized and eliminated by the immune system. This is evident from the high proportions of people harboring microscopic cancers seen in autopsy studies, far outnumbering cases of clinical disease. Considering how many cell divisions are happening every day in our bodies, and how many opportunities there are for things to go wrong at some step, leading to uncontrolled growth, it is no wonder control systems are in place to eliminate such cells. Still, some cells, with mechanisms regulating cell growth or dissemination out of control, are able to escape the immune killing and cause clinical cancer [55]. Micrometastatic dormancy is proposed to exist in a state of equilibrium with the immune system, where the micrometastatic deposit is prevented from expanding but still able to survive. Put simply, inflammation and cells of the innate immune system seem to be mainly driving proliferation and re-awakening of cancer cells, while the adaptive immune system preferably conveys either cancer cell killing or dormancy-promoting signals.

Targeting Dormancy

With the mechanisms of dormancy maintenance and evasion still incompletely understood, how to best therapeutically target this problem is not yet determined. Non-dividing, metabolically inactive cells are not considered susceptible to conventional cancer treatment [56]. Still, there are a number of trials targeting residual disease in breast cancer with additional systemic therapy after standard of care adjuvant treatment (NCT00248703, NCT03032406, NCT03400254, NCT01545648). In these studies, residual disease is defined by persistent tumor cells in the bone marrow after chemotherapy, and it may be argued that these cells were resistant to standard therapy rather than truly dormant.

It has been proposed that one feasible approach to target dormant tumor cells would be to stimulate escape from dormancy, as the cells would, once awakened, be susceptible to conventional cancer treatment such as chemotherapy and targeted therapy [57, 58]. The obvious argument against this is that since no cancer treatment today guarantees complete eradication of all malignant cells, one might risk inducing

clinically manifest metastatic disease in a patient who without this intervention never would have suffered from a relapse. Still, it has been attempted in a phase I trial in prostate cancer that was terminated due to low accrual. The strategy in this study was to mobilize dormant prostate cancer cells from the bone marrow to the bloodstream by an anti-CXCR4 agent and then to target these cells with docetaxel (NCT02478125). Another suggestion is to develop therapeutics capable of maintaining dormancy. One phase II trial, investigating the capacity of 5-AZA and ATRA to induce and maintain dormancy in prostate cancer treated patients with a biochemical relapse, is currently recruiting patients (NCT03572387). This seems attractive, as dormant cells cause no problem to the host as long as they remain in the dormant state. However, experience from long-term adjuvant treatment, such as endocrine treatment in breast cancer, informs us that adherence to long-term preventive treatment is low [59]. It is difficult to motivate patients' adherence to therapy over time, where they may experience side effects, but no immediate benefit, and where for a majority, the treatment makes no difference, as they would never have had a relapse even without therapy. Perhaps, the most feasible approach today, with our limited understanding of tumor dormancy mechanisms, would be short-term prevention of escape from dormancy at times when risk is augmented, such as perioperatively. Retrospective studies of short-term anti-inflammatory treatment with NSAIDs during breast cancer surgery demonstrated a significant reduction in metastatic relapse [60]; this was, however, not reproduced in the subsequent prospective trial [61]. Optimal selection of patients, anti-inflammatory agents, and timing is under investigation and may change this. Similar studies with perioperative beta blockers have also given promising results [62].

As we have seen throughout this section, we are beginning to unravel the biology of tumor dormancy and the mechanisms of escape from dormancy. Still, there is a desperate need for a deeper understanding of this intricate feature in order to successfully target it and prevent metastatic relapse.

The Importance of Beta-Adrenergic Signaling in Tumor Progression

Exposure to stressful conditions is part of human life. Physical challenging situations, exposure to extreme environmental circumstances, trauma, or psychosocial factors including emotional loss and isolation can cause stressful surroundings. Activation of "fight or flight" mechanism is a well-conserved stress response to adapt quickly to stressful situations and ensures survival. The idea of a "sympathico-adrenal" communication in response to external or internal stimuli that impact homeostasis, the internal steady state of living beings, was already postulated in the beginning of the twentieth century [63]. Homeostasis is maintained by central coordination of afferent information and response to those signals via peripheral effectors [64, 65]. Stimulation of the hypothalamic–pituitary–adrenal axis increases secretion of the hormones epinephrine (EP) from the adrenal medulla and cortisol from the adrenal cortex. Activation of the autonomic sympathetic nervous system (SNS) increases release of the neurotransmitter norephedrine (NE) at the postganglionic sympathetic nerve endings innervating a wide range of organs and vasculature. NE increases vasoconstriction and heart rate; EP increases metabolic rate, blood glucose levels, and bronchodilatation [65]; consequently, the body is prepared to cope acute stress by "fight or flight" reaction. Thus, the brain as regulator of homeostasis uses NE and EP as effectors to quickly adjust peripheral reactions in stress response [66]. This system works highly efficient in the short term, but chronic activation results in pathophysiological conditions.

NE and EP act through binding to α- or ß-adrenergic receptors (AR) expressed among others in heart, lung, vasculature, and immune cells [65, 67]. ß1, ß2, and ß3 receptors are characterized [68]. Here, we focus on ß2-adrenergic signaling. Stimulation of ß2-AR promotes intracellular signaling either in a classical or non-classical manner (Fig. 31.3). The former induces the second messenger cyclic adenosine monophosphate (cAMP) by Gα$_s$-protein-coupled receptor kinases and activates protein kinase A signaling [68, 69]. ß-arrestin regulates desensitization of the activated receptor [69]. Additionally, ß-arrestins play a role in non-classical signaling through interaction with G-protein-coupled receptor kinases resulting in activation of MAP kinase (mitogen-activated protein kinase) pathway [68–70].

Acute stress responses are indispensable for survival. On the contrary, chronic stress sustains inflammation and impairs immune response as observed in vaccine studies, autoimmune disorders, and chronic disease [71, 72]. The interplay between the adrenergic system and cancer progression gained increased attention during recent years based on epidemiologic, preclinical, and clinical observations. In this context, beta blockers attracted special attention. Both selective ß1-inhibitors or unselective pan-beta blockers bind to ß-AR receptors and inhibit adrenergic signaling [68]. They are commonly used to treat hypertension, cardiac disease, or essential tremor. Patients using beta blockers incidentally showed lower tumor stage at the time of diagnosis and had favorable outcome and improved response to cancer treatment [73–80]. Overexpression of ß-adrenergic receptors in

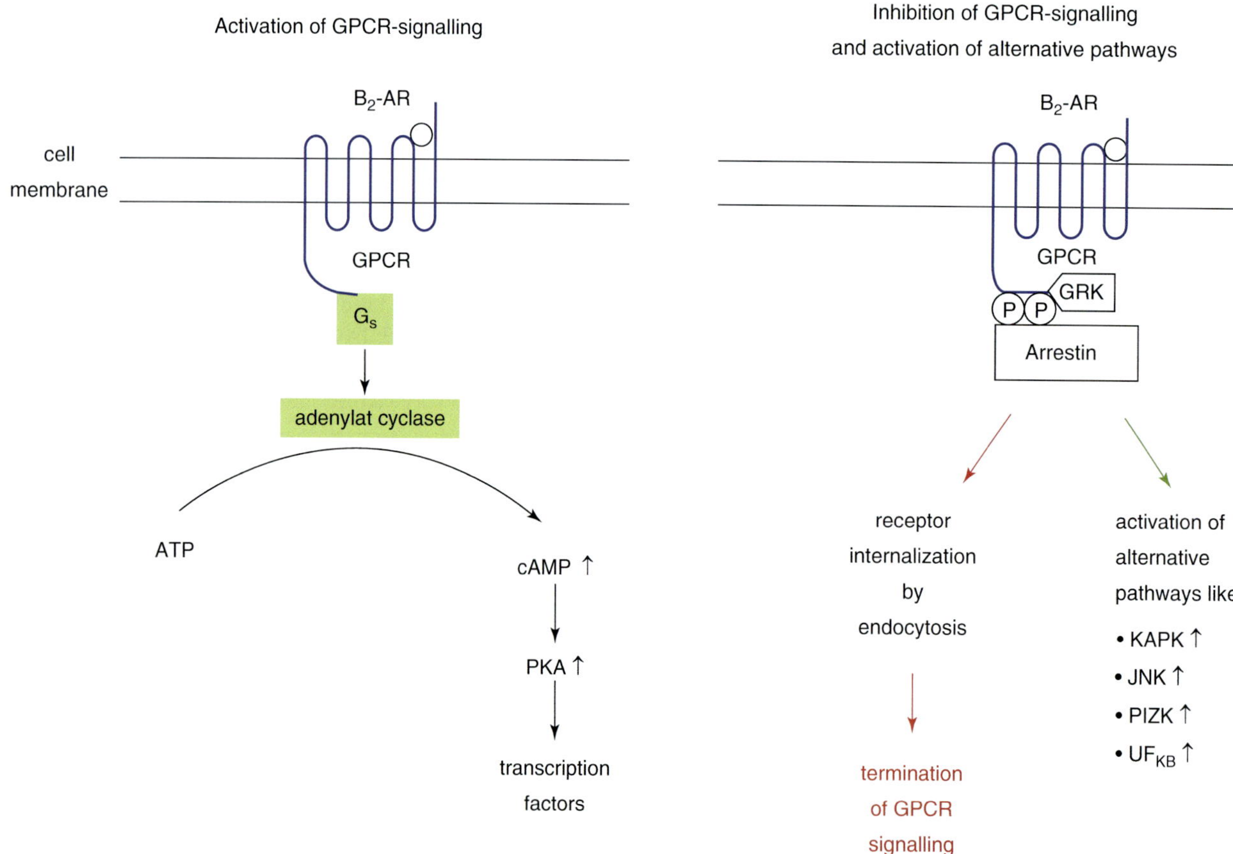

Fig. 31.3 ß2-AR promotes intracellular signaling either in a classical or non-classical manner

tumors correlates with worse prognosis [81–83]. Additionally, multiple in vitro and in vivo models demonstrated the importance of ß-adrenergic signaling in tumor progression, angiogenesis, and immune response. Notably, these unfavorable mechanisms could only be abolished by non-selective ß-adrenergic inhibition but not by ß1-selective inhibition. Thus, selectivity of adrenergic inhibition is crucial. The impact of ß-adrenergic signaling on tumor progression with emphasis on immune response, metastasis, and angiogenesis will be elucidated in the following section.

Immune Response

Immune response is a complex reaction of the body to defeat proteins characterized as foreign and involves the innate and the adaptive immune system. Immune function can be impaired by physical and psychological stressors [84]. With regard to stress response, there is a complex interaction between the central nervous system and peripheral processes controlled by the hypothalamic–pituitary–adrenal axis and the sympathetic–adrenal–medullary system [84]. In the following, we focus on the role of ß-adrenergic signaling in the communication between the sympathetic nervous system (SNS) and the immune response.

The innervation of lymphoid organs by sympathetic nerve fibers [85] and the expression of adrenergic receptors on immune cells [67] are crucial in the cross talk between the brain and the immune system. Communication between SNS and the immune system is predominantly mediated by ß2-adrenergic signaling [67]. Sympathetic innervation of the bone marrow maintains homeostasis in hematopoietic stem cell niches and contributes to mobilization of blood cells into periphery [86]. Adrenergic signaling controls circulation of lymphocytes between periphery and lymph nodes ensuring their availability during daytime [87]. Furthermore, adrenergic signaling influences adaptive and innate immune response. The former can result in impaired CD4+ T-cell proliferation, Th1 cell maturation, and CD8+ T-cell response as well as reduced production of IL-2 and INF-y [88, 89].

Innate immune cells derive from myeloid progenitor cells and include dendritic cells (DCs), myeloid-derived suppressor cells (MDSCs), macrophages, granulocytes, and natural killer cells. ß2-adrenergic signaling supports an immunosuppressive M2-like macrophage phenotype [90, 91] and impairs DC maturation and the ability for antigen presentation [92, 93]. In sum, lasting adrenergic signaling can promote an immunosuppressive condition. On the contrary, acute short-term stress response (minutes to hours) can enhance leukocyte mobilization and activate innate and adaptive immune response. This acute response is beneficial by promoting wound healing and infection which might occur after a "fight or flight" reaction [94]. However, it is not surprising that long-term activation of adrenergic signaling can disrupt the balance of immune response resulting in chronic disease and cancer. "Avoiding immune destruction" is one important hallmark of cancer [95].

Impact of Adrenergic Signaling on Immune Response in Cancer

Preclinical models suggest an impact of ß-adrenergic signaling on tumor development (Fig. 31.4). Physical stress was induced by different housing temperatures in a mouse model.

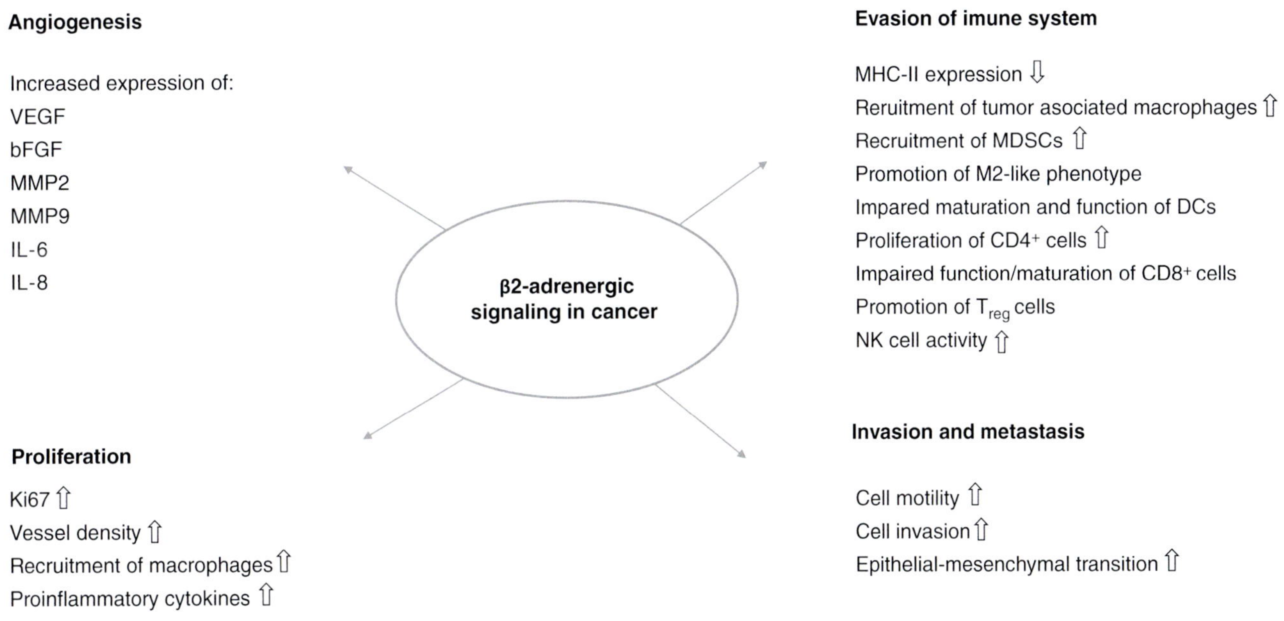

Angiogenesis

Increased expression of:
VEGF
bFGF
MMP2
MMP9
IL-6
IL-8

Evasion of imune system

MHC-II expression ⇓
Reruitment of tumor asociated macrophages ⇑
Recruitment of MDSCs ⇑
Promotion of M2-like phenotype
Impared maturation and function of DCs
Proliferation of CD4+ cells ⇑
Impaired function/maturation of CD8+ cells
Promotion of T_{reg} cells
NK cell activity ⇑

β2-adrenergic signaling in cancer

Proliferation

Ki67 ⇑
Vessel density ⇑
Recruitment of macrophages ⇑
Proinflammatory cytokines ⇑

Invasion and metastasis

Cell motility ⇑
Cell invasion ⇑
Epithelial-mesenchymal transition ⇑

Fig. 31.4 Impact of ß-adrenergic signaling on tumor development

In mice housed at colder conditions compared to mice kept at thermoneutral temperature tumor growth was increased, the number of CD8+ T-cells was decreased, and the number of T$_{reg}$ was enhanced [96]. These observations were reversed in stressed mice treated with propranolol, a non-selective beta blocker [97]. In line with this, another group reported an elevation of activated GranzymB positive CD8+ T-cells as well as increased number of NK-cells and B-cells in a melanoma mouse model treated with propranolol [98]. The same group showed activated T-cell response in human melanoma samples of patients treated with non-selective beta blockers [74]. ß2-adrenergic signaling also mediates innate immune responses. Wrobel et al. described reduced number of tumor infiltrating myeloid cells in primary tumors of mice treated with propranolol compared to untreated animals [98]. In line with this, chemical sympathectomy increased the number of M1-polarized macrophages in the tumor, lowered the number of intratumoral MDSCs, and increased the number of DCs in a lung cancer model in vivo [99].

Tumors can effectively escape the control of the immune system by increased expression of checkpoint molecules that suppress antitumor immune response. One of these proteins is programmed death ligand-1 (PD-L1) expressed by tumor cells. PD-L1 on tumor cells can bind to PD-1 on T-cells and other immune cells to escape immune responses. Immune checkpoint blockade with anti-PD1 is the standard of care in various cancer types. In stressed mice, it did not alter tumor growth significantly. However, anti-PD1 in combination with propranolol reduced tumor growth significantly and enhanced the number of IFNy+ CD8+ T-cells [97]. These observations are underlined by results of another in vivo model that confirmed improved tumor control when propranolol was added to PD1 blockade and data from a retrospective study showing better response to immunotherapy in patients using non-selective betablockers [73]. Altogether, these data suggest that adrenergic signaling promotes an immunosuppressive pro-tumorigenic environment and may result in reduced efficacy of anti-cancer treatment. Preclinical data support that inhibition of adrenergic signaling may promote a more immunogen environment resulting in better tumor control and improved response to treatment. Up to date, there is a lack of prospective clinical data.

Adrenergic Signaling in Tumor Growth and Metastasis

Uncontrolled growth, invasiveness, and metastasis are other hallmarks of cancer. Various in vitro and in vivo models demonstrated tumor growth depending on ß-adrenergic signaling. Qiao et al. give a nice overview of preclinical models for stress-induced tumor progression [100]. During the last few decades, the influence of adrenergic signaling on tumor progression was investigated in melanoma [101], ovarian cancer [82], lung cancer [102], pancreatic cancer [103], breast cancer [104, 105], and prostate cancer [106] but is not limited to these examples. Tumor proliferation can be stimulated pharmacologically by ß-receptor agonists or by creating stressful conditions in vivo. On the contrary, inhibition of ß-adrenergic signaling by a pan-beta blocker, ß2-specific blockade, chemical sympathectomy, or ß2-receptor knockout mice limits tumor growth. Overall, results from in vitro and in vivo models confirm consistently a crucial role of ß-adrenergic signaling in stress-related tumor growth and metastasis. Selected examples will be described in the following passage.

In vitro models described increased tumor cell proliferation and cell migration after stimulation with NE. Inhibition of ß-adrenergic signaling diminished NE promoted cancer cell proliferation and invasion [82, 101, 106, 107]. Furthermore, knockdown and overexpression of ß2-AR in breast cancer cell lines significantly affected invadopodia formation supporting its role in invasiveness [108].

Stress-induced in vivo models demonstrated enhanced tumor growth and metastasis in various tumor types. Inhibition of adrenergic signaling by adding propranolol, injecting cancer cells lacking ß-AR, or silencing ß2-AR by siRNA diminished these effects in ovarian cancer [82, 107]. A lung cancer model could delay tumor development after chemical sympathectomy and observed reduced NE concentration in tumor tissue [99]. In line with these findings, growth of primary melanoma and metastasis was slowed down in mice treated with propranolol compared to untreated animals both in immunodeficient and immunocompetent models [98, 101]. Additionally, the proliferation rate, assessed by Ki67, was significantly reduced in treated mice. Cold stress increased tumor growth compared to mice in neutral housing conditions [73, 97, 109], and propranolol abolished this effect in the stressed group [97]. Furthermore, metastatic spread from breast cancer in stressed mice was significantly attenuated in animals bearing ß2-AR knockdown tumors compared to the control group [108] or by administration of propranolol [104]. In line with this, treatment with a ß-adrenergic agonist provoked metastasis in the control group [104]. Altogether, these in vitro and in vivo models clearly underline the essential role of beta-adrenergic signaling in tumor progression and metastasis. Based on these exciting findings, the role of beta-adrenergic inhibition should be further investigated in cancer patients.

Epithelial mesenchymal transition (EMT) plays a crucial role in metastasis and is characterized by increased expression of vimentin, downregulation of E-cadherin, and a shift toward a mesenchymal like phenotype [110]. Promotion of EMT by ß-adrenergic signaling is described in non-small cell lung cancer (NSLC), colorectal (CRC), ovarian, and breast cancer models [108, 111, 112]. Common findings in these models were stress-induced expression of EMT characteristics, increased cell motility, and invasiveness. In the NSCL and CRC model, the addition of propranolol or TGF b1 inhibitor decreased migration and invasion and diminished expression of HIF-1α, p-Smad3, and Snail [111]. The ovarian cell cancer model investigated the association between NE and telomerase reverse transcriptase (hTERT) [112]. hTERT is related to cancer progression and unfavorable outcome. The model demonstrates NE-induced hTERT expression which in turn promotes the acquirement of an EMT-like phenotype through upregulation of Slug. In line with this, chronic stressed mice developed higher incidence of lung metastasis in a breast cancer model. Here, NE induced downregulation of miRNA 337-3p resulted in STAT3-dependend promotion of EMT [105]. These models illustrate the influence of adrenergic signaling in EMT through various pathways.

In conclusion, ß2-adrenergic signaling is a crucial upstream regulator modifying tumor progression and invasiveness through a plethora of downstream pathways.

Angiogenesis

Angiogenesis, the formation of new vessels from preexisting vasculature, takes place in wound healing, reproduction, and development. Physiologically, the process is localized, time-limited, and controlled by the interplay of pro- and anti-angiogenic factors [113]. Domination of pro-angiogenic mediators topples this balance resulting in enhanced angiogenesis which is another well-established hallmark of cancer [114]. A lack of nutrition or oxygen can trigger this angiogenic switch in the TME promoting tumor growth and dissemination [115, 116]. Neoplastic angiogenesis is orchestrated by vascular endothelial growth factor A (VEGF-A), fibroblast growth factor, cytokines, metalloproteases, and others [113]. In the following, we will concentrate on the mediation of tumor angiogenesis involving ß-adrenergic signaling.

Stimulation with NE or other beta-adrenergic agonists increased the level of well-characterized pro-angiogenic proteins like VEGF-A, MMP-2, MMP-9, IL-6, and IL-8 in ovarian cancer, nasopharyngeal carcinoma, and melanoma cells in preclinical models [81, 82, 107, 117–119]. Induced overexpression of VEGF-A and other factors could be abolished by adding the non-selective beta blocker propranolol [82, 117, 119].

In vivo models confirmed ß2-AR as key mediator in stress-induced angiogenesis. Enhanced vessel density and elevated expression of VEGF-A and other pro-angiogenic mediators were observed in an ovarian cell carcinoma model [82]. Characteristics of immature vasculature were more distinct in stressed animals. It was nicely demonstrated that

VEGF expression is regulated by ß-adrenergic signaling via the PKA pathway. Inhibiting either the ß2-AR or PKA suppressed expression of VEGFA after stimulation with NE [82]. Treatment with propranolol reduced vessel density in primary melanomas and metastasis and attenuated RNA expression of Hif1α [98, 101].

Reduced density of tumor vessels was also observed in a prostate cancer model in mice deficient for ß2- and ß3-AR. Decreased vascularization was elegantly confirmed through orthotopic implantation of a collagen matrix in the prostate of chemically sympathectomized mice compared to the control group [120]. Further investigation in a spontaneous prostate cancer model identified increased vessel and nerve density in high-grade neoplasia along with an increased level of NE and ß2-ARs. The latter was distinctly overexpressed on endothelial cells and is essential to initiate the angiogenic switch in this model [120]. The role of endothelial cells in NE promoted angiogenesis was also emphasized in a model co-culturing breast cancer cells and endothelial cells [121]. Results from this study suggest NE-dependent activation of β2-AR–PKA–mTOR signaling that increases Jagged 1 expression on breast cancer cells and Notch signaling in endothelial cells [121].

An increased number of tumor-associated macrophages (TAMs) are described in tumors with enhanced angiogenesis. TAMs are an important source for VEGF and other pro-angiogenic cytokines [122]. The contribution of M2-polarized macrophages to angiogenesis was demonstrated in a lung cancer model [99]. Catecholamine-treated macrophages increased VEGF secretion and promoted tube formation when co-cultured with HUVECs. Accordingly, the number of M2-polarized macrophages was increased in close relation to neovasculature in vivo. After chemical sympathectomy, vessel and macrophage density declined, and VEGF concentration dropped to lower level [99].

Potential Clinical Implications

Enhanced adrenergic signaling is a stress response mechanism and orchestrates multiple pathways associated with several hallmarks of cancer-immune evasion, invasiveness, proliferation, and angiogenesis. Recent research demonstrated that non-selective beta blockers can abolish essential unfavorable pathways and increase response to treatment. These mechanisms are also crucial in the perioperative period [123]. To date, there is a lack of prospective clinical trials investigating the additional benefit and possible risks of pan-beta blockers in oncological treatment including excision of primary tumors. Two randomized trials investigating perioperative propranolol in breast cancer patients reported promising results [62, 124]. Adding a non-selective beta blocker might promote more epithelial tumor characteristics and a less anti-immunogenic, anti-angiogenic TME, thus increasing response to already established treatment. In line with this, perioperative inflammatory, angiogenic, and immunosuppressive mechanisms might be attenuated and reduce the incidence of metastatic disease.

Axl Signaling and Epithelial to Mesenchymal Transition

Cancer cells are surrounded by stressful conditions. In a normal, healthy tissue, homeostasis is maintained in a strictly regulated process that protects the hierarchy and integrity of the tissue to preserve its function [125]. In a sense, each cell contributes to the greater good and even dies quietly through apoptosis if prompted to do so [126]. In a tumor, anarchy ensues as homeostasis is lost and the cancer cells ignore cues from their environment and resists and overcomes the obstacles a normal tissue represents to achieve their goal of perpetual growth and survival [95]. However, the loss of a well-regulated environment poses a challenge to the individual cancer cell.

The receptor tyrosine kinase AXL has a well-established role in cancer progression, as detailed in Chap. 5. It is upregulated across human cancers, where it enables invasiveness, metastasis, phenotypic plasticity related to epithelial to mesenchymal transition (EMT), therapy resistance, and immune evasion (Fig. 31.5). The following section covers the role of AXL in response to stress in the tumor microenvironment.

In homeostatic tissues, the phospholipid phosphatidyl serine (PS) is scarce, as it is mostly confined to the inner leaflet of the plasma membrane [127]. PS is exposed to the microenvironment during apoptosis [128] on enveloped viruses [129], activated platelets [130], and several immune cells [131–133]. In a well-regulated tissue, apoptotic cells are cleared quickly and quietly, where exposed PS functions as a strong "eat me" signal sensed by the TAM (TYRO 3, AXL, MERTK) family receptors on phagocytic immune cells [134, 135]. However, in the chaotic, hypoxic, nutrient-deprived, inflamed, and therapeutically assaulted tumor microenvironment, PS is readily available [136]. In addition to PS exposed on an abundance of apoptotic cells, the malignant cells themselves expose PS on their membranes [137] and PS can be

Fig. 31.5 Role of AXL in cancer progression

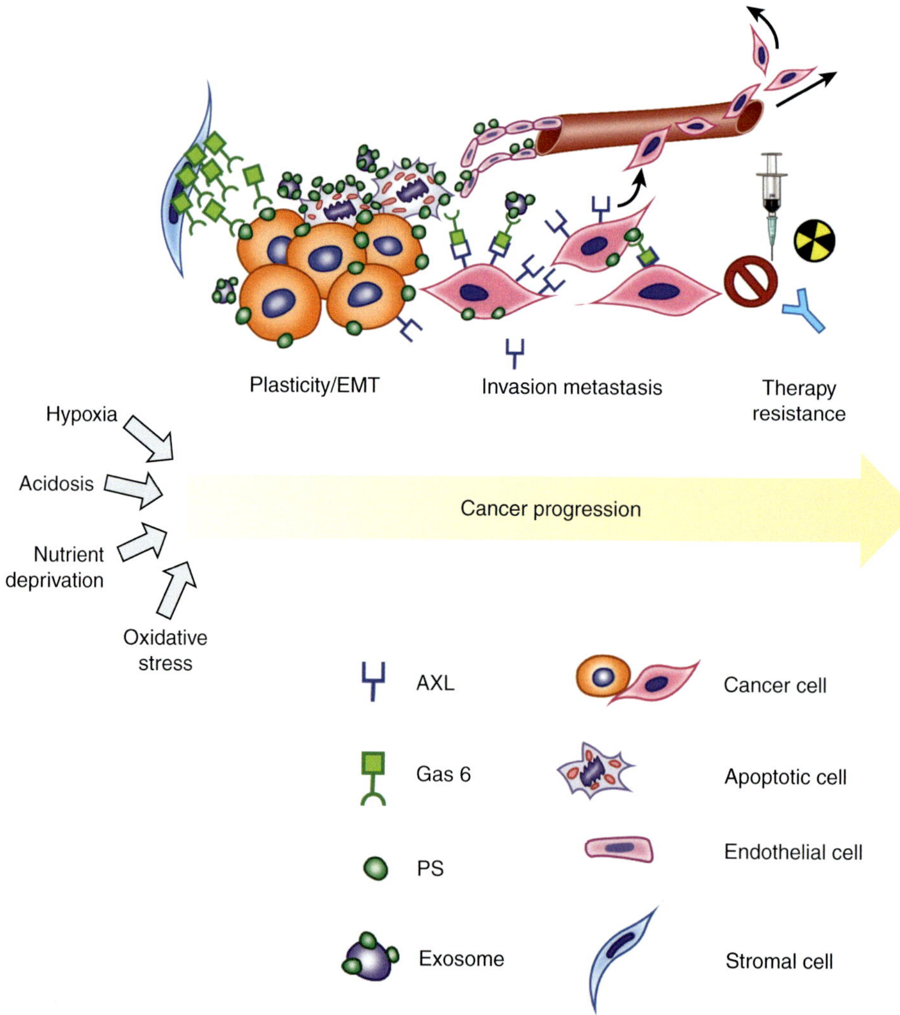

found on exosomes and endothelial cells within tumors [138]. In addition, the AXL ligand GAS6 is produced both by cancer cells [139–142] and by stromal cells in the tumor microenvironment [143]. Together this sets the stage for optimal AXL signaling (as detailed in Chap. 5) during stressful conditions where a proportion of the tumor cells die.

Hypoxia is a dominating feature of the tumor microenvironment [144, 145]. Even though tumors depend on inducing neovascularization for continued growth [146], the tumor vasculature is often dysfunctional with variable success in delivering oxygen [147]. Lack of oxygen is a major threat to survival and hypoxia induces changes in the expression of a large number of genes [148]. Hypoxia-inducible factors (HIFs) are master regulators of the hypoxic stress response and regulate genes that drive cancer progression. A hypoxic tumor microenvironment is linked to cellular phenotypic plasticity, stemness, therapy resistance, metastasis, and poor prognosis [149]. AXL is induced by hypoxia [150–152], and hypoxia-inducible factor 1a (HIF1a) directly regulates AXL expression by binding of HIF-1 and HIF-2 to hypoxia response elements (HRE) in the AXL promoter in response to hypoxia [150]. Strong co-expression of AXL and HIF1a has been reported in prostate and breast cancer [152, 153]. In non-cancerous tissues, it has recently been reported that AXL/GAS6 signaling protects mesenchymal stem cells (MSCs) during hypoxic conditions in myocardial infarction [154].

The dysregulated tumor microenvironment also loses its grip on the normally tightly regulated pH level, as a consequence of altered metabolism with increased output of acidic metabolites like lactate and carbon dioxide [155, 156]. The adaptation to an acidic microenvironment has been reported to drive increased invasiveness and neoangiogenesis as well as EMT and stemness linked to therapy resistance and has been implicated in tumor dormancy [157–160]. In endothelial cells, acidosis upregulates AXL and protects endothelial cells from apoptosis during serum starvation [161]. In melanoma cell lines, acidosis has recently been shown to induce a senescence-like and microphthalmia-associated transcription factor (MITF)^{low}-AXL^{high} phenotype [162], which is linked with therapy resistance in melanoma [163, 164]. AXL upregulation was linked with upregulation and activation of activating transcription factor (ATF)4 and inhibition of eukaryotic translation initiation factor (eIF)2B indicating activation of the integrated stress response (IRS), a pro-survival translational reprogramming response aimed at restoring homeostasis [165]. This has been observed both in response to acidosis, glutamine deprivation, and inflammation [162, 166] and conferred increased invasiveness and metastatic potential. A glutamine starvation gene expression signature furthermore correlated strongly both with the AXL^{high} gene expression pattern of melanomas intrinsically resistant to PD1-targeting immunotherapy and the gene

expression profiles of murine tumors with acquired resistance to T-cell-based immunotherapy [166–168].

Malignant cells also often lack the ability to produce the amino acid arginine, and arginine-depleting agents are being explored as cancer treatment [169]. Arginine starvation stress induced by the arginine-depleting recombinant enzymes leads to rapid AXL activation in melanoma [170, 171] and breast cancer cell lines [171]. Endogenous GAS6 was externalized in response to arginine depletion and was shown to accumulate in the cell membrane, which is important for optimal receptor activation [171].

Oxidative stress in the tumor microenvironment can promote tumorigenesis and has been shown to induce DNA damage and genomic instability, induce EMT, and increase invasiveness of tumors [172, 173]. In lung cancer cells, oxidative stress activates AXL and increases cancer cell migration [174]. In vascular smooth muscle cells, AXL is activated in response to oxidative stress and apoptosis increases in response to concomitant AXL inhibition [175, 176].

The uncontrolled behavior of the malignant cells of the tumor often results in an inhospitable and deprived environment, characterized by the abovementioned conditions of hypoxia, acidification, oxidative stress, and nutrient deprivation. In addition, the aim of cancer therapeutic strategies is to kill cancer cells; however, this will also leave a trail of exposed PS in its wake. This enables one possible road to more aggressive cancer cells through AXL activation, where the demise of some opens the door for optimal AXL signaling in the prevailing cancer cells. The ability of cancer cells to adapt to both the deranged microenvironment of their own making and cancer therapeutics through mechanisms that ultimately fuel cancer progression is a major obstacle to successful treatments for patients with advanced cancers.

Stress Response and Adaptive Mutability

For our cells, mutations are undesirable and must be prevented, with a few exceptions. For a given species to survive changing and stressful life conditions, mutations are welcome and allowed by the cells to drive evolution. Intrinsic instigators of DNA damage are particularly well studied in prokaryotes, such as *E. coli* [177]. Although not well studied in cancer yet, there is emerging evidence that the ever-present stressful conditions that malignant tumors must endure also cause a relaxation of the DNA repair machinery, including homologous recombination [178]. This mutator phenotype (MP) [179] contributes to the heterogeneity in the mutational burden (MB) between primary tumors and subsequent metastases. Moreover, added stress, such as ROS, hypoxia, inflammation, chemotherapy, and radiation, drives cancers cells into evolving therapy resistance through adaptive mutability. This general resistance mechanism was recently demonstrated in CRC [180, 181]. In contrast, with immunotherapy, tumor types with high MB seem to respond better.

More than a century ago, after studying 735 cases of fatal breast cancer, the surgeon Stephen Paget formulated his famous *"seed and soil"* hypothesis. He observed that some environments were more receptive for metastatic growth than others and concluded that secondary tumor growth at distant sites is dependent *both* on properties of the "seed" (cancer cell) *and* of the "soil" (microenvironment) [182]. So, what happens in a cell, whose survival is constantly challenged by changing hostile microenvironments? Let us picture a breast cancer cell, arisen in a primary breast tumor. The cell has a heritage set of driver mutations leading to uncontrolled growth and all the other hallmarks of cancer [95], which includes the capability to metastasize. After arriving in the liver, the cell encounters foreign, stressful, and unforgiving life conditions and must endure a constant attack from hostile host immune cells as well. Most of these refugee cells die, but some are able to cling to life and form small enclaves of cancer cells that can endure as dormant occult cancer for many years after the primary tumor was surgically removed. Just like Darwin observed in the crippled wheat plant, over time, these cells change their genotype and become variants and mutants. Finally, the evolutionary pressure on the cells bring about new generations of cancer cells, well adapted to growth in the liver, and finally, stage IV disease becomes evident on a CT scan. When analyzing biopsies from metastases, pathologists can have a hard time identifying these cells as the same as those in the primary breast tumor, and genomic heterogeneity is frequent [183]. This phenomenon becomes interesting when we discuss whether these cell-intrinsic genomic adaptations happen solely due to the large pool of mutations in cancer cells or if this is actually a controlled biologically conserved stress response, misemployed by cancer cells, meant to facilitate the survival of species during environmental changes. Tumor mutational heterogeneity drives cancer progression and therapy resistance [184, 185]. Therefore, it is of critical importance to learn more about how cellular stress regulates adaptive mutability. To learn more about this we will seek knowledge from microbiologists, who have studied this in relation to microbial pathogenesis and antibiotic resistance [178, 186].

The ability of cells and organisms to detect and respond to fluctuating environmental changes is an essential and ancient trait. Cells must modify proteins, metabolism, cell structure, and RNA levels to maintain homeostasis under stress. Transcriptional control is a key mediator. Global transcriptional programs, such as the environmental stress response (ESR) in eukaryotes [187] and SOS response in *E. coli* [178], are rapidly and transiently induced by a battery of different stresses, indicating a core transcriptional response. We often think of direct DNA damaging effect of external carcinogens, such as ultraviolet light and tobacco smoke, as the main source of mutations. Still, most mutations are actually created endogenously in the cells [188]. In *E. Coli*, a set of proteins were identified as intrinsic instigators of endogenous DNA damage [177], the DNA "damage-up" proteins (DDPs). These can induce reactive oxygen increase, chromosome loss, and reversed replication forks. Human homologues have been discovered [177] and are over-represented among established cancer drivers and associated with reduced prognosis and tumor heterogeneity. As in *E. coli*, evidence shows that these networks of DDPs provoke endogenous DNA damage in humans under stress and represent known and novel cancer-associated proteins such as MSH2, MSH6, MLH1, MITF, and RB1.

As mentioned above, tumor heterogeneity is a major roadblock for treating cancer. Acquired genetic variability during tumor progression together with selection pressure results in more aggressive tumor cells [189]. This concept of *clonal origin of metastases* has been verified and may explain heterogeneity in response to chemotherapy [190]. Artificially induced stress, such as chemotherapy, radiation, and targeted therapies, might also drive evolution and survival of the fittest cancer cells. In an elegant study of colorectal cancers treated with targeted therapy, Russo and coworkers provided evidence that cancer, just like *E. Coli* under antibiotic pressure, exploits adaptive mutability to avoid therapy. EGFR/ BRAF inhibition downregulated mismatch repair (MMR) and homologous recombination (HR) repair genes and upregulated error-prone polymerases in drug-tolerant cells [180].

The heat-shock response is a powerful adaptive mechanism conserved from yeast to humans, fine-tuned to protect cells residing in stressful microenvironments. Upon stress, the heat-shock factor 1 (HSF-1) translocates to the nucleus and induces a chaperone gene expression program of heat-shock elements [191, 192] to protect cells, including cancer cells. Moreover, in cancer, HSF-1 also directly coordinates a network of transcripts that are central in oncogenic processes. A distinct genome-wide transcriptional program, coordinated by HSF-1, was detected in a variety of human cancer types [193], and is significantly related with metastasis and death. HSF-1 is regarded as one of the most potent metastasis promoting genes, and regulates metabolism, cell cycle signaling, apoptosis, cell adhesion, etc., and, importantly, DNA repair [194, 195]. Again, this shows that stress might induce the mutator phenotype as a normal physiologic adaptation in nature.

We have seen that stressful environments lead to transcriptional changes and increased mutation rates within the cells. However, stressed cells will also react by trying to modify their environments to thrive. Micrometastases can only grow up to 1–2 mm in diameter when relying only on passive diffusion of nutrients and oxygen. These tumors will suffer from stress, such as hypoxia and starvation. In addition, if no improvement in the soil occurs, they are kept dormant for years. As discussed above in this chapter, systemic or local events can end this dormant state, by for example an angiogenic switch [196, 197], induced by a set of cytokines and growth factors leading to sustainable and advantageous conditions for metastases to grow. Breast cancer is notorious for late relapses after a seemingly curative primary treatment. Whereas tumor dormancy is desirable, the escape from tumor dormancy is lethal. There is evidence to suggest that stressful events, such as tissue trauma (i.e. surgery) and inflammation, leading to a systemic burst of cytokines and growth factors, might synchronize an escape of multiple occult micrometastases from dormancy resulting in overt metastatic disease [45, 198–201]. HSP27 is a small heat-shock protein with functions not limited to thermotolerance. Evidence shows that HSP27 is a key regulator of tumor dormancy and that suppression of HSP27 induces long-term dormancy in a model of human breast cancer. Further, it was demonstrated that the angiogenic switch is influenced by HSP27-dependent changes in VEGF-A, VEGF-C, and bFGF secretion from tumor cells [202]. This again illustrates that the interactions between cancer cells and the microenvironment, induced as a response to stressful conditions, go both ways.

To conclude, biology has taught us that adaptive mutability under stressful life conditions is a prerequisite for evolution and the survival of species. In tumor evolution, it seems to be a mutation-selection balance and an order in which genomic aberrations occur to lead to robust tumor fitness [203]. Fate mutations and driver mutations can arise randomly or as a result of carcinogens. Then, further gene aberrations are driven *and* selected by microenvironmental conditions. Understanding of the nature of cellular stress responses and insights into the mechanistic interactions driving cancer cell fate might open up for the identification of therapeutic targets for preventing cancer progression and the escape from tumor dormancy.

Concluding Remarks/Summary

In this chapter, we have discussed roles of the tumor microenvironment during development from a malignant cell cluster into lethal disease. We have covered some important effects that microenvironmental changes have on the course of the disease. This knowledge is particularly important as it opens up for the identification of novel candidate targets for therapy. Mutations and other genomic aberrations represent the very foundation of what defines a cancer. To restore the malignant genome is, in essence, impossible. As discussed, recent breakthroughs have revealed that microenvironmental changes causing cellular stress play an important role in the escape from tumor dormancy as well as in ß2-adrenergic signaling, cell plasticity, and phenotypic switching. Finally, even the malignant genome is under influence by cellular stress through adaptive mutability. Further research in the field of normal and malignant cellular stress responses will open up for new strategies to prevent and treat cancer.

References

1. Dillekas H, Rogers MS, Straume O. Are 90% of deaths from cancer caused by metastases? Cancer Med. 2019;8(12):5574–6.
2. Vogelstein B, Kinzler KW. Cancer genes and the pathways they control. Nat Med. 2004;10(8):789–99.
3. Darwin C. On the origin of species. London: John Murray; 1859.
4. Robert C, Schachter J, Long GV, Arance A, Grob JJ, Mortier L, et al. Pembrolizumab versus Ipilimumab in advanced melanoma. N Engl J Med. 2015;372(26):2521–32.
5. Schuster C, Eikesdal HP, Puntervoll H, Geisler J, Geisler S, Heinrich D, et al. Clinical efficacy and safety of bevacizumab monotherapy in patients with metastatic melanoma: predictive importance of induced early hypertension. PLoS One 2012; 7(6).
6. Lotsberg ML, Wnuk-Lipinska K, Terry S, Tan TZ, Lu N, Trachsel-Moncho L, et al. AXL targeting abrogates autophagic flux and induces immunogenic cell death in drug-resistant cancer cells. J Thorac Oncol. 2020;15(6):973–99.
7. Hadfield G. The dormant cancer cell. Br Med J. 1954;2(4888):607–10.
8. Harach HR, Franssila KO, Wasenius VM. Occult papillary carcinoma of the thyroid. A "normal" finding in Finland. A systematic autopsy study. Cancer. 1985;56(3):531–8.
9. Gao HCG, Lee-Lim AP, Mo Q, Decker M, Vonica A, Shen R, Brogi E, Brivanlou AH, Giancotti FG. The BMP inhibitor Coco reactivates breast cancer cells at lung metastatic sites. Cell. 2012;150(4):764–79.
10. Lan Q, Peyvandi S, Duffey N, Huang YT, Barras D, Held W, et al. Type I interferon/IRF7 axis instigates chemotherapy-induced immunological dormancy in breast cancer. Oncogene 2018.
11. Davies C, Pan H, Godwin J, Gray R, Arriagada R, Raina V, et al. Long-term effects of continuing adjuvant tamoxifen to 10 years versus stopping at 5 years after diagnosis of oestrogen receptor-positive breast cancer: ATLAS, a randomised trial. Lancet (London, England). 2013;381(9869):805–16.
12. Pan HGR, Braybrooke J, Davies C, Taylor C, McGale P, Peto R, Pritchard KI, Bergh J, Dowsett M, Hayes DF, EBCTCG. 20-Year risks of breast-cancer recurrence after stopping endocrine therapy at 5 years. N Engl J Med. 2017;377(19):1836–46.
13. Dillekas HTM, Pilskog M, Assmus J, Straume O. Differences in metastatic patterns in relation to time between primary surgery and first relapse from breast cancer suggest synchronized growth of dormant micrometastases. Breast Cancer Res Treat. 2014;146(3):627–36.
14. Ogba N, Manning NG, Bliesner BS, Ambler SK, Haughian JM, Pinto MP, et al. Luminal breast cancer metastases and tumor arousal from dormancy are promoted by direct actions of estradiol and progesterone on the malignant cells. Breast Cancer Res. 2014;16(6):489.
15. Malladi SMD, Jin X, He L, Basnet H, Zou Y, de Stanchina E, Massagué J. Metastatic latency and immune evasion through autocrine inhibition of WNT. Cell. 2016;165(1):45–60.
16. Koebel CMVW, Swann JB, Zerafa N, Rodig SJ, Old LJ, Smyth MJ, Schreiber RD. Adaptive immunity maintains occult cancer in an equilibrium state. Nature. 2007;450(7171):903–7.
17. Naumov GNFJ, Straume O. Tumor dormancy due to failure of angiogenesis: role of the microenvironment. Clin Exp Metastasis. 2009;26(1):51–60.
18. Sosa MSBP, Aguirre-Ghiso JA. Mechanisms of disseminated cancer cell dormancy: an awakening field. Nat Rev Cancer. 2014;14(9):611–22.
19. Aguirre-Ghiso JA. Models, mechansims and clinical evidence for cancer dormancy. Nat Rev Cancer. 2007;7(11):834–46.
20. Fluegen G, Avivar-Valderas A, Wang Y, Padgen MR, Williams JK, Nobre AR, et al. Phenotypic heterogeneity of disseminated tumour cells is preset by primary tumour hypoxic microenvironments. Nat Cell Biol. 2017;19(2):120–32.

21. Crea F, Nur Saidy NR, Collins CC, Wang Y. The epigenetic/noncoding origin of tumor dormancy. Trends Mol Med. 2015;21(4):206–11.

22. Hanin L. Seeing the invisible: how mathematical models uncover tumor dormancy, reconstruct the natural history of cancer, and assess the effects of treatment. Adv Exp Med Biol. 2013;734:261–82.

23. Naume B, Synnestvedt M, Falk RS, Wiedswang G, Weyde K, Risberg T, et al. Clinical outcome with correlation to disseminated tumor cell (DTC) status after DTC-guided secondary adjuvant treatment with docetaxel in early breast cancer. J Clin Oncol Off J Am Soc Clin Oncol. 2014;32(34):3848–57.

24. Borgen E, Rypdal MC, Sosa MS, Renolen A, Schlichting E, Lønning PE, et al. NR2F1 stratifies dormant disseminated tumor cells in breast cancer patients. Breast Cancer Res. 2018;20(1):120.

25. Gao XL, Zheng M, Wang HF, Dai LL, Yu XH, Yang X, et al. NR2F1 contributes to cancer cell dormancy, invasion and metastasis of salivary adenoid cystic carcinoma by activating CXCL12/CXCR4 pathway. BMC Cancer. 2019;19(1):743.

26. Sparano J, O'Neill A, Alpaugh K, Wolff AC, Northfelt DW, Dang CT, et al. Association of circulating tumor cells with late recurrence of estrogen receptor-positive breast cancer: a secondary analysis of a randomized clinical trial. JAMA Oncol. 2018;4(12):1700–6.

27. Papadaki C, Stratigos M, Markakis G, Spiliotaki M, Mastrostamatis G, Nikolaou C, et al. Circulating microRNAs in the early prediction of disease recurrence in primary breast cancer. Breast Cancer Res. 2018;20(1):72.

28. Yumoto K EM, Wang J, Cackowski FC, Decker AM, Lee E, Nobre AR, Aguirre-Ghiso JA, Jung Y, Taichman RS. Axl is required for TGF-β2-induced dormancy of prostate cancer cells in the bone marrow. Sci Rep 2016;7(6).

29. Owens PPM, Novitskiy SV, Giltnane JM, Gorska AE, Hopkins CR, Hong CC, Moses HL. Inhibition of BMP signaling suppresses metastasis in mammary cancer. Oncogene. 2015;34(19):2437–49.

30. Taichman RS, Patel LR, Bedenis R, Wang J, Weidner S, Schumann T, et al. GAS6 receptor status is associated with dormancy and bone metastatic tumor formation. PLoS One. 2013;8(4):e61873.

31. Rodrigues LP, Teixeira VR, Alencar-Silva T, Simonassi-Paiva B, Pereira RW, Pogue R, et al. Hallmarks of aging and immunosenescence: connecteactor Rev 2021.

32. Aguirre-Ghiso JA, Liu D, Mignatti A, Kovalski K, Ossowski L. Urokinase receptor and fibronectin regulate the ERK(MAPK) to p38(MAPK) activity ratios that determine carcinoma cell proliferation or dormancy in vivo. Mol Biol Cell. 2001;12(4):863–79.

33. Martin P, Nunan R. Cellular and molecular mechanisms of repair in acute and chronic wound healing. Br J Dermatol. 2015;173(2):370–8.

34. Antonio N B-BM, Ward L, Collin J, Christensen IJ, Steiniche T, Schmidt H, Feng Y, Martin P. The wound inflammatory response exacerbates growth of pre-neoplastic cells and progression to cancer. EMBO J 2015.

35. Abramovitch RMM, Meir G, Neeman M. Stimulation of tumour growth by wound-derived growth factors. Br J Cancer. 1999;79:1392–8.

36. Hobson J, Gummadidala P, Silverstrim B, Grier D, Bunn J, James T, et al. Acute inflammation induced by the biopsy of mouse mammary tumors promotes the development of metastasis. Breast Cancer Res Treat. 2013;139(2):391–401.

37. Peeters CF, de Waal R, Wobbes T, Westphal JR, Ruers TJ. Outgrowth of human liver metastases after resection of the primary colorectal tumor: a shift in the balance between apoptosis and proliferation. Int J Cancer. 2006;119(6):1249–53.

38. Folkman J, Merler E, Abernathy C, Williams G. Isolation of a tumor factor responsible for angiogenesis. J Exp Med. 1971;133(2):275–88.

39. Naumov GAL, Folkman J. Role of angiogenesis in human tumor dormancy – animal models of the angiogenic switch. Cell Cycle. 2006;5(16):1779–87.

40. Straume OST, Lampa MJ, Carretero J, Øyan AM, Jia D, Borgman CL, Soucheray M, Downing SR, Short SM, Kang SY, Wang S, Chen L, Collett K, Bachmann I, Wong KK, Shapiro GI, Kalland KH, Folkman J, Watnick RS, Akslen LA, Naumov GN. Suppression of heat shock protein 27 induces long-term dormancy in human breast cancer. Proc Natl Acad Sci. 2012;109(22):8699–704.

41. Rogers MS, Novak K, Zurakowski D, Cryan LM, Blois A, Lifshits E, et al. Spontaneous reversion of the angiogenic phenotype to a nonangiogenic and dormant state in human tumors. Mol Cancer Res. 2014;12(5):754–64.

42. Ghajar CM PH, Mori H, Matei IR, Evason KJ, Brazier H, Almeida D, Koller A, Hajjar KA, Stainier DYR, Chen EI, Lyden D, Bissell MJ. The perivascular niche regulates breast tumour dormancy. Nature Cell Biol 2013;15(7).

43. O'Reilly MS, Holmgren L, Shing Y, Chen C, Rosenthal RA, Moses M, et al. Angiostatin: a novel angiogenesis inhibitor that mediates the suppression of metastases by a Lewis lung carcinoma. Cell. 1994;79(2):315–28.

44. Castano Z, San Juan BP, Spiegel A, Pant A, DeCristo MJ, Laszewski T, et al. IL-1beta inflammatory response driven by primary breast cancer prevents metastasis-initiating cell colonization. Nat Cell Biol. 2018;20(9):1084–97.

45. Krall JA, Reinhardt F, Mercury OA, Pattabiraman DR, Brooks MW, Dougan M, et al. The systemic response to surgery triggers the outgrowth of distant immune-controlled tumors in mouse models of dormancy. Sci Transl Med 2018;10(436).

46. De Cock JM, Shibue T, DA, Keckesova Z, Reinhardt F, Weinberg RA. Inflammation triggers Zeb1-dependent escape from tumor latency. Cancer Res. 2016;76(23):6778–84.

47. Albrengues J, Shields MA, Ng D, Park CG, Ambrico A, Poindexter ME, et al. Neutrophil extracellular traps produced during inflammation awaken dormant cancer cells in mice. Science (New York, NY). 2018;361(6409).

48. Barkan DETL, Michalowski AM, Smith JA, Chu I, Davis AS, Webster JD, Hoover S, Simpson RM, Gauldie J, Green JE. Metastatic growth from dormant cells induced by a col-1-enriched fibrotic environment. Cancer Res. 2010;70(14):5706–16.

49. Medler TRCL. Duality of the immune response in cancer: lessons learned from skin. J Invest Dermatol. 2014;134:E23–E8.

50. Coussens LM, Werb Z. Inflammation and cancer. Nature. 2002;420(6917):860–7.

51. Matser YAH, Terpstra ML, Nadalin S, Nossent GD, de Boer J, van Bemmel BC, et al. Transmission of breast cancer by a single multiorgan donor to 4 transplant recipients. Am J Transpl. 2018;18(7):1810–4.

52. Morris-Stiff G, Steel A, Savage P, Devlin J, Griffiths D, Portman B, et al. Transmission of donor melanoma to multiple organ transplant recipients. Am J Transpl. 2004;4(3):444–6.

53. Wolchok JD, Chiarion-Sileni V, Gonzalez R, Rutkowski P, Grob JJ, Cowey CL, et al. Overall survival with combined nivolumab and ipilimumab in advanced melanoma. N Engl J Med. 2017;377(14):1345–56.

54. Koebel CM, Vermi W, Swann JB, Zerafa N, Rodig SJ, Old LJ, et al. Adaptive immunity maintains occult cancer in an equilibrium state. Nature. 2007;450(7171):903–7.

55. Schreiber RD, Old LJ, Smyth MJ. Cancer immunoediting: integrating immunity's roles in cancer suppression and promotion. Science (New York, NY). 2011;331(6024):1565–70.

56. Naumov GNTJ, MacDonald IC, Wilson SM, Bramwell VH, Groom AC, Chambers AF. Ineffectiveness of doxorubicin treatment on solitary dormant mammary carcinoma cells or late-developing metastases. Breast Cancer Res Treat. 2003;82(3):199–206.

57. Bliss SA, Greco SJ, Rameshwar P. Hierarchy of breast cancer cells: key to reverse dormancy for therapeutic intervention. Stem Cells Transl Med. 2014;3(7):782–6.

58. Bliss SASG, Sandiford OA, Williams LM, Engelberth DJ, Guiro K, Isenalumhe LL, Greco SJ, Ayer S, Bryan M, Kumar R, Ponzio NM, Rameshwar P. Mesenchymal stem cell-derived exosomes stimulate cycling quiescence and early breast cancer dormancy in bone marrow. Cancer Res. 2016;76(19):5832–44.

59. Hershman DL, Kushi LH, Shao T, Buono D, Kershenbaum A, Tsai WY, et al. Early discontinuation and nonadherence to adjuvant hormonal therapy in a cohort of 8,769 early-stage breast cancer patients. J Clin Oncol Off J Am Soc Clin Oncol. 2010;28(27):4120–8.

60. Forget P, Bentin C, Machiels JP, Berliere M, Coulie PG, De Kock M. Intraoperative use of ketorolac or diclofenac is associated with improved disease-free survival and overall survival in conservative breast cancer surgery. Br J Anaesth. 2014;113(Suppl 1):i82–7.

61. Forget P, Bouche G, Duhoux FP, Coulie PG, Decloedt J, Dekleermaker A, et al. Intraoperative ketorolac in high-risk breast cancer patients. A prospective, randomized, placebo-controlled clinical trial. PLoS One. 2019;14(12):e0225748.

62. Hiller JG, Cole SW, Crone EM, Byrne DJ, Shackleford DM, Pang JB, et al. Preoperative beta-Blockade with propranolol reduces biomarkers of metastasis in breast cancer: a phase II randomized trial. Clin Cancer Res. 2020;26(8):1803–11.

63. Cannon WB. Organization for physiological homeostasis. Physiol Rev. 1929;9(3):399–431.

64. Goldstein DS, McEwen B. Allostasis, homeostats, and the nature of stress. Stress. 2002;5(1):55–8.

65. Goldstein DS. Sympathetic Nervous System. 2007 7 September 2007. In: Encyclopedia of Stress (Second Edition) [Internet]. Elsevier; [697–703]. Available from: https://doi.org/10.1016/B978-012373947-6.00370-6.

66. Goldstein DS. Concepts of scientific integrative medicine applied to the physiology and pathophysiology of catecholamine systems. Compr Physiol. 2013;3(4):1569–610.

67. Nance DM, Sanders VM. Autonomic innervation and regulation of the immune system (1987–2007). Brain Behav Immun. 2007;21(6):736–45.

68. Wachter SB, Gilbert EM. Beta-adrenergic receptors, from their discovery and characterization through their manipulation to beneficial clinical application. Cardiology. 2012;122(2):104–12.

69. Lorton D, Bellinger DL. Molecular mechanisms underlying beta-adrenergic receptor-mediated cross-talk between sympathetic neurons and immune cells. Int J Mol Sci. 2015;16(3):5635–65.

70. Lefkowitz RJ, Shenoy SK. Transduction of receptor signals by beta-arrestins. Science. 2005;308(5721):512–7.

71. Burns VE, Carroll D, Ring C, Drayson M. Antibody response to vaccination and psychosocial stress in humans: relationships and mechanisms. Vaccine. 2003;21(19–20):2523–34.

72. Marsland AL, Cohen S, Rabin BS, Manuck SB. Associations between stress, trait negative affect, acute immune reactivity, and antibody response to hepatitis B injection in healthy young adults. Health Psychol. 2001;20(1):4–11.

73. Kokolus KM, Zhang Y, Sivik JM, Schmeck C, Zhu J, Repasky EA, et al. Beta blocker use correlates with better overall survival in metastatic melanoma patients and improves the efficacy of immunotherapies in mice. Onco Targets Ther. 2018;7(3):e1405205.

74. Wrobel LJ, Gayet-Ageron A, Le Gal FA. Effects of beta-blockers on melanoma microenvironment and disease survival in human. Cancers (Basel) 2020;12(5).

75. De Giorgi V, Grazzini M, Benemei S, Marchionni N, Botteri E, Pennacchioli E, et al. Propranolol for off-label treatment of patients with melanoma: results from a cohort study. JAMA Oncol. 2018;4(2):e172908.

76. De Giorgi V, Grazzini M, Benemei S, Marchionni N, Geppetti P, Gandini S. beta-Blocker use and reduced disease progression in patients with thick melanoma: 8 years of follow-up. Melanoma Res. 2017;27(3):268–70.

77. Chaudhary KR, Yan SX, Heilbroner SP, Sonett JR, Stoopler MB, Shu C, et al. Effects of beta-adrenergic antagonists on chemoradiation therapy for locally advanced non-small cell lung cancer. J Clin Med 2019;8(5).

78. Lemeshow S, Sorensen HT, Phillips G, Yang EV, Antonsen S, Riis AH, et al. Beta blockers and survival among danish patients with malignant melanoma: a population-based cohort study. Cancer Epidemiol Biomark Prev 2011.

79. Barron TI, Connolly RM, Sharp L, Bennett K, Visvanathan K. Beta blockers and breast cancer mortality: a population-based study. J Clin Oncol. 2011;29(19):2635–44.

80. Melhem-Bertrandt A, Chavez-Macgregor M, Lei X, Brown EN, Lee RT, Meric-Bernstam F, et al. Beta-blocker use is associated with improved relapse-free survival in patients with triple-negative breast cancer. J Clin Oncol. 2011;29(19):2645–52.

81. Moretti S, Massi D, Farini V, Baroni G, Parri M, Innocenti S, et al. beta-adrenoceptors are upregulated in human melanoma and their activation releases pro-tumorigenic cytokines and metalloproteases in melanoma cell lines. Lab Investig. 2013;93(3):279–90.

82. Thaker PH, Han LY, Kamat AA, Arevalo JM, Takahashi R, Lu C, et al. Chronic stress promotes tumor growth and angiogenesis in a mouse model of ovarian carcinoma. Nat Med. 2006;12(8):939–44.

83. Powe DG, Voss MJ, Habashy HO, Zanker KS, Green AR, Ellis IO, et al. Alpha- and beta-adrenergic receptor (AR) protein expression is associated with poor clinical outcome in breast cancer: an immunohistochemical study. Breast Cancer Res Tr. 2011;130(2):457–63.

84. Padgett DA, Glaser R. How stress influences the immune response. Trends Immunol. 2003;24(8):444–8.

85. Felten DL, Felten SY, Carlson SL, Olschowka JA, Livnat S. Noradrenergic and peptidergic innervation of lymphoid tissue. J Immunol. 1985;135(2 Suppl):755s–65s.

86. Katayama Y, Battista M, Kao WM, Hidalgo A, Peired AJ, Thomas SA, et al. Signals from the sympathetic nervous system regulate hematopoietic stem cell egress from bone marrow. Cell. 2006;124(2):407–21.

87. Suzuki K, Hayano Y, Nakai A, Furuta F, Noda M. Adrenergic control of the adaptive immune response by diurnal lymphocyte recirculation through lymph nodes. J Exp Med. 2016;213(12):2567–74.

88. Riether C, Kavelaars A, Wirth T, Pacheco-Lopez G, Doenlen R, Willemen H, et al. Stimulation of beta(2)-adrenergic receptors inhibits calcineurin activity in CD4(+) T cells via PKA-AKAP interaction. Brain Behav Immun. 2011;25(1):59–66.

89. Grebe KM, Hickman HD, Irvine KR, Takeda K, Bennink JR, Yewdell JW. Sympathetic nervous system control of anti-influenza CD8+ T cell responses. Proc Natl Acad Sci USA. 2009;106(13):5300–5.

90. Lamkin DM, Ho HY, Ong TH, Kawanishi CK, Stoffers VL, Ahlawat N, et al. beta-Adrenergic-stimulated macrophages: Comprehensive localization in the M1-M2 spectrum. Brain Behav Immun. 2016;57:338–46.

91. Lamkin DM, Srivastava S, Bradshaw KP, Betz JE, Muy KB, Wiese AM, et al. C/EBPbeta regulates the M2 transcriptome in beta-adrenergic-stimulated macrophages. Brain Behav Immun. 2019;80:839–48.

92. Giordani L, Cuzziol N, Del Pinto T, Sanchez M, Maccari S, Massimi A, et al. beta(2)-Agonist clenbuterol hinders human monocyte differentiation into dendritic cells. Exp Cell Res. 2015;339(2):163–73.

93. Herve J, Dubreil L, Tardif V, Terme M, Pogu S, Anegon I, et al. beta2-Adrenoreceptor agonist inhibits antigen cross-presentation by dendritic cells. J Immunol. 2013;190(7):3163–71.

94. Dhabhar FS. Enhancing versus suppressive effects of stress on immune function: implications for immunoprotection and immunopathology. Neuroimmunomodulation. 2009;16(5):300–17.

95. Hanahan D, Weinberg RA. Hallmarks of cancer: the next generation. Cell. 2011;144(5):646–74.

96. Kokolus KM, Capitano ML, Lee CT, Eng JW, Waight JD, Hylander BL, et al. Baseline tumor growth and immune control in laboratory mice are significantly influenced by sub-thermoneutral housing temperature. Proc Natl Acad Sci USA. 2013;110(50):20176–81.

97. Bucsek MJ, Qiao G, MacDonald CR, Giridharan T, Evans L, Niedzwecki B, et al. beta-Adrenergic signaling in mice housed at standard temperatures suppresses an effector phenotype in CD8(+) T cells and undermines checkpoint inhibitor therapy. Cancer Res. 2017;77(20):5639–51.

98. Jean Wrobel L, Bod L, Lengagne R, Kato M, Prevost-Blondel A, Le Gal FA. Propranolol induces a favourable shift of anti-tumor immunity in a murine spontaneous model of melanoma. Oncotarget. 2016;7(47):77825–37.

99. Xia Y, Wei Y, Li ZY, Cai XY, Zhang LL, Dong XR, et al. Catecholamines contribute to the neovascularization of lung cancer via tumor-associated macrophages. Brain Behavior Immunity. 2019;81:111–21.

100. Qiao GX, Chen MH, Bucsek MJ, Repasky EA, Hylander BL. Adrenergic signaling: a targetable checkpoint limiting development of the antitumor immune response. Front Immunol 2018;9.

101. Wrobel LJ, Le Gal FA. Inhibition of human melanoma growth by a non-cardioselective beta-blocker. J Invest Dermatol. 2015;135(2):525–31.

102. Al-Wadei HA, Ullah MF, Al-Wadei MH. Intercepting neoplastic progression in lung malignancies via the beta adrenergic (beta-AR) pathway: implications for anti-cancer drug targets. Pharmacol Res 2012.

103. Schuller HM, Al-Wadei HA, Ullah MF, Plummer HK 3rd. Regulation of pancreatic cancer by neuropsychological stress responses: a novel target for intervention. Carcinogenesis. 2012;33(1):191–6.

104. Sloan EK, Priceman SJ, Cox BF, Yu S, Pimentel MA, Tangkanangnukul V, et al. The sympathetic nervous system induces a metastatic switch in primary breast cancer. Cancer Res. 2010;70(18):7042–52.

105. Du PX, Zeng H, Xiao YN, Zhao YN, Zheng B, Deng YT, et al. Chronic stress promotes EMT-mediated metastasis through activation of STAT3 signaling pathway by miR-337-3p in breast cancer. Cell Death Dis. 2020;11(9)

106. Barbieri A, Bimonte S, Palma G, Luciano A, Rea D, Giudice A, et al. The stress hormone norepinephrine increases migration of prostate cancer cells in vitro and in vivo. Int J Oncol. 2015;47(2):527–34.

107. Sood AK, Bhatty R, Kamat AA, Landen CN, Han L, Thaker PH, et al. Stress hormone-mediated invasion of ovarian cancer cells. Clin Cancer Res. 2006;12(2):369–75.

108. Chang A, Le CP, Walker AK, Creed SJ, Pon CK, Albold S, et al. beta2-Adrenoceptors on tumor cells play a critical role in stress-enhanced metastasis in a mouse model of breast cancer. Brain Behav Immun. 2016;57:106–15.

109. Eng JW, Reed CB, Kokolus KM, Pitoniak R, Utley A, Bucsek MJ, et al. Housing temperature-induced stress drives therapeutic resistance in murine tumour models through beta2-adrenergic receptor activation. Nat Commun. 2015;6:6426.

110. Thiery JP, Acloque H, Huang RY, Nieto MA. Epithelial-mesenchymal transitions in development and disease. Cell. 2009;139(5):871–90.

111. Zhang J, Deng YT, Liu J, Wang YQ, Yi TW, Huang BY, et al. Norepinephrine induced epithelial-mesenchymal transition in HT-29 and A549 cells in vitro. J Cancer Res Clin Oncol. 2016;142(2):423–35.

112. Choi MJ, Cho KH, Lee S, Bae YJ, Jeong KJ, Rha SY, et al. hTERT mediates norepinephrine-induced Slug expression and ovarian cancer aggressiveness. Oncogene. 2015;34(26):3402–12.

113. Folkman J. Angiogenesis: an organizing principle for drug discovery? Nat Rev Drug Discov. 2007;6(4):273–86.

114. Hanahan D, Weinberg RA. The hallmarks of cancer. Cell. 2000;100(1):57–70.

115. Folkman J. Angiogenesis in cancer, vascular, rheumatoid and other disease. Nat Med. 1995;1(1):27–31.

116. Zetter BR. Angiogenesis and tumor metastasis. Annu Rev Med. 1998;49:407–24.

117. Lutgendorf SK, Cole S, Costanzo E, Bradley S, Coffin J, Jabbari S, et al. Stress-related mediators stimulate vascular endothelial growth factor secretion by two ovarian cancer cell lines. Clin Cancer Res. 2003;9(12):4514–21.

118. Yang EV, Sood AK, Chen M, Li Y, Eubank TD, Marsh CB, et al. Norepinephrine up-regulates the expression of vascular endothelial growth factor, matrix metalloproteinase (MMP)-2, and MMP-9 in nasopharyngeal carcinoma tumor cells. Cancer Res. 2006;66(21):10357–64.

119. Yang EV, Kim SJ, Donovan EL, Chen M, Gross AC, Webster Marketon JI, et al. Norepinephrine upregulates VEGF, IL-8, and IL-6 expression in human melanoma tumor cell lines: implications for stress-related enhancement of tumor progression. Brain Behav Immun. 2009;23(2):267–75.

120. Zahalka AH, Arnal-Estape A, Maryanovich M, Nakahara F, Cruz CD, Finley LWS, et al. Adrenergic nerves activate an angio-metabolic switch in prostate cancer. Science. 2017;358(6361):321–6.

121. Chen HY, Liu D, Yang ZY, Sun LM, Deng Q, Yang S, et al. Adrenergic signaling promotes angiogenesis through endothelial cell-tumor cell crosstalk. Endocr Relat Cancer. 2014;21(5):783–95.

122. De Palma M, Biziato D, Petrova TV. Microenvironmental regulation of tumour angiogenesis. Nat Rev Cancer. 2017;17(8):457–74.

123. Hiller JG, Perry NJ, Poulogiannis G, Riedel B, Sloan EK. Perioperative events influence cancer recurrence risk after surgery. Nat Rev Clin Oncol. 2018;15(4):205–18.

124. Shaashua L, Shabat-Simon M, Haldar R, Matzner P, Zmora O, Shabtai M, et al. Perioperative COX-2 and beta-Adrenergic blockade improves metastatic biomarkers in breast cancer patients in a phase-II randomized trial. Clin Cancer Res. 2017;23(16):4651–61.

125. Biteau B, Hochmuth CE, Jasper H. Maintaining tissue homeostasis: dynamic control of somatic stem cell activity. Cell Stem Cell. 2011;9(5):402–11.

126. Kerr JF, Wyllie AH, Currie AR. Apoptosis: a basic biological phenomenon with wide-ranging implications in tissue kinetics. Br J Cancer. 1972;26(4):239–57.

127. Gordesky SE, Marinetti GV. The asymetric arrangement of phospholipids in the human erythrocyte membrane. Biochem Biophys Res Commun. 1973;50(4):1027–31.

128. Martin SJ, Reutelingsperger CP, McGahon AJ, Rader JA, van Schie RC, LaFace DM, et al. Early redistribution of plasma membrane phosphatidylserine is a general feature of apoptosis regardless of the initiating stimulus: inhibition by overexpression of Bcl-2 and Abl. J Exp Med. 1995;182(5):1545–56.

129. Amara A, Mercer J. Viral apoptotic mimicry. Nat Rev Microbiol. 2015;13(8):461–9.

130. Bevers EM, Comfurius P, van Rijn JL, Hemker HC, Zwaal RF. Generation of prothrombin-converting activity and the exposure of phosphatidylserine at the outer surface of platelets. Eur J Biochem/FEBS. 1982;122(2):429–36.

131. Sen J, Rosenberg N, Burakoff SJ. Expression and ontogeny of CD2 on murine B cells. J Immunol. 1990;144(8):2925–30.

132. Martin S, Pombo I, Poncet P, David B, Arock M, Blank U. Immunologic stimulation of mast cells leads to the reversible exposure of phosphatidylserine in the absence of apoptosis. Int Arch Allergy Immunol. 2000;123(3):249–58.

133. Frasch SC, Henson PM, Nagaosa K, Fessler MB, Borregaard N, Bratton DL. Phospholipid flip-flop and phospholipid scramblase 1 (PLSCR1) co-localize to uropod rafts in formylated Met-Leu-Phe-stimulated neutrophils. J Biol Chem. 2004;279(17):17625–33.

134. Fadok VA, Voelker DR, Campbell PA, Cohen JJ, Bratton DL, Henson PM. Exposure of phosphatidylserine on the surface of apoptotic lymphocytes triggers specific recognition and removal by macrophages. J Immunol. 1992;148(7):2207–16.

135. Lemke G, Burstyn-Cohen T. TAM receptors and the clearance of apoptotic cells. Ann N Y Acad Sci. 2010;1209:23–9.

136. Burstyn-Cohen T, Maimon A. TAM receptors, Phosphatidylserine, inflammation, and Cancer. Cell Commun Signal. 2019;17(1):156.

137. Utsugi T, Schroit AJ, Connor J, Bucana CD, Fidler IJ. Elevated expression of phosphatidylserine in the outer membrane leaflet of human tumor cells and recognition by activated human blood monocytes. Cancer Res. 1991;51(11):3062–6.

138. Ran S, Downes A, Thorpe PE. Increased exposure of anionic phospholipids on the surface of tumor blood vessels. Cancer Res. 2002;62(21):6132–40.

139. Hutterer M, Knyazev P, Abate A, Reschke M, Maier H, Stefanova N, et al. Axl and growth arrest-specific gene 6 are frequently overexpressed in human gliomas and predict poor prognosis in patients with glioblastoma multiforme. Clin Cancer Res. 2008;14(1):130–8.

140. Dirks W, Rome D, Ringel F, Jager K, MacLeod RA, Drexler HG. Expression of the growth arrest-specific gene 6 (GAS6) in leukemia and lymphoma cell lines. Leuk Res. 1999;23(7):643–51.

141. Sun W, Fujimoto J, Tamaya T. Coexpression of Gas6/Axl in human ovarian cancers. Oncology. 2004;66(6):450–7.

142. Sun WS, Fujimoto J, Tamaya T. Coexpression of growth arrest-specific gene 6 and receptor tyrosine kinases Axl and Sky in human uterine endometrial cancers. Ann Oncol. 2003;14(6):898–906.

143. Loges S, Schmidt T, Tjwa M, van Geyte K, Lievens D, Lutgens E, et al. Malignant cells fuel tumor growth by educating infiltrating leukocytes to produce the mitogen Gas6. Blood. 2010;115(11):2264–73.

144. Vaupel P, Mayer A. Hypoxia in cancer: significance and impact on clinical outcome. Cancer Metastasis Rev. 2007;26(2):225–39.

145. Milosevic M, Fyles A, Hedley D, Hill R. The human tumor microenvironment: invasive (needle) measurement of oxygen and interstitial fluid pressure. Semin Radiat Oncol. 2004;14(3):249–58.

146. Gimbrone MA Jr, Leapman SB, Cotran RS, Folkman J. Tumor dormancy in vivo by prevention of neovascularization. J Exp Med. 1972;136(2):261–76.

147. Helmlinger G, Yuan F, Dellian M, Jain RK. Interstitial pH and pO2 gradients in solid tumors in vivo: high-resolution measurements reveal a lack of correlation. Nat Med. 1997;3(2):177–82.

148. Denko NC, Fontana LA, Hudson KM, Sutphin PD, Raychaudhuri S, Altman R, et al. Investigating hypoxic tumor physiology through gene expression patterns. Oncogene. 2003;22(37):5907–14.

149. Bao B, Azmi AS, Ali S, Ahmad A, Li Y, Banerjee S, et al. The biological kinship of hypoxia with CSC and EMT and their relationship with deregulated expression of miRNAs and tumor aggressiveness. Biochim Biophys Acta. 2012;1826(2):272–96.

150. Rankin EB, Fuh KC, Castellini L, Viswanathan K, Finger EC, Diep AN, et al. Direct regulation of GAS6/AXL signaling by HIF promotes renal metastasis through SRC and MET. Proc Natl Acad Sci USA. 2014;111(37):13373–8.

151. Dumas PY, Naudin C, Martin-Lanneree S, Izac B, Casetti L, Mansier O, et al. Hematopoietic niche drives FLT3-ITD acute myeloid leukemia resistance to quizartinib via STAT5-and hypoxia-dependent upregulation of AXL. Haematologica. 2019;104(10):2017–27.

152. Mishra A, Wang J, Shiozawa Y, McGee S, Kim J, Jung Y, et al. Hypoxia stabilizes GAS6/Axl signaling in metastatic prostate cancer. Mol Cancer Res. 2012;10(6):703–12.

153. Nalwoga H, Ahmed L, Arnes JB, Wabinga H, Akslen LA. Strong expression of Hypoxia-Inducible Factor-1alpha (HIF-1alpha) is associated with Axl expression and features of aggressive tumors in African breast cancer. PLoS One. 2016;11(1):e0146823.

154. Shan S, Liu Z, Guo T, Wang M, Tian S, Zhang Y, et al. Growth arrest-specific gene 6 transfer promotes mesenchymal stem cell survival and cardiac repair under hypoxia and ischemia via enhanced autocrine signaling and paracrine action. Arch Biochem Biophys. 2018;660:108–20.

155. Tannock IF, Rotin D. Acid pH in tumors and its potential for therapeutic exploitation. Cancer Res. 1989;49(16):4373–84.

156. Wike-Hooley JL, Haveman J, Reinhold HS. The relevance of tumour pH to the treatment of malignant disease. Radiother Oncol. 1984;2(4):343–66.

157. Martinez-Zaguilan R, Seftor EA, Seftor RE, Chu YW, Gillies RJ, Hendrix MJ. Acidic pH enhances the invasive behavior of human melanoma cells. Clin Exp Metastasis. 1996;14(2):176–86.

158. Rofstad EK, Mathiesen B, Kindem K, Galappathi K. Acidic extracellular pH promotes experimental metastasis of human melanoma cells in athymic nude mice. Cancer Res. 2006;66(13):6699–707.

159. Peppicelli S, Bianchini F, Torre E, Calorini L. Contribution of acidic melanoma cells undergoing epithelial-to-mesenchymal transition to aggressiveness of non-acidic melanoma cells. Clin Exp Metastasis. 2014;31(4):423–33.

160. Peppicelli S, Andreucci E, Ruzzolini J, Laurenzana A, Margheri F, Fibbi G, et al. The acidic microenvironment as a possible niche of dormant tumor cells. Cell Mol Life Sci. 2017;74(15):2761–71.

161. D'Arcangelo D, Gaetano C, Capogrossi MC. Acidification prevents endothelial cell apoptosis by Axl activation. Circ Res. 2002;91(7):e4–12.

162. Bohme I, Bosserhoff A. Extracellular acidosis triggers a senescence-like phenotype in human melanoma cells. Pigment Cell Melanoma Res. 2020;33(1):41–51.

163. Sensi M, Catani M, Castellano G, Nicolini G, Alciato F, Tragni G, et al. Human cutaneous melanomas lacking MITF and melanocyte differentiation antigens express a functional Axl receptor kinase. J Invest Dermatol. 2011;131(12):2448–57.

164. Muller J, Krijgsman O, Tsoi J, Robert L, Hugo W, Song C, et al. Low MITF/AXL ratio predicts early resistance to multiple targeted drugs in melanoma. Nat Commun. 2014;5:5712.

165. Pakos-Zebrucka K, Koryga I, Mnich K, Ljujic M, Samali A, Gorman AM. The integrated stress response. EMBO Rep. 2016;17(10):1374–95.

166. Falletta P, Sanchez-Del-Campo L, Chauhan J, Effern M, Kenyon A, Kershaw CJ, et al. Translation reprogramming is an evolutionarily conserved driver of phenotypic plasticity and therapeutic resistance in melanoma. Genes Dev. 2017;31(1):18–33.

167. Hugo W, Zaretsky JM, Sun L, Song C, Moreno BH, Hu-Lieskovan S, et al. Genomic and transcriptomic features of response to anti-PD-1 therapy in metastatic melanoma. Cell. 2016;165(1):35–44.

168. Landsberg J, Kohlmeyer J, Renn M, Bald T, Rogava M, Cron M, et al. Melanomas resist T-cell therapy through inflammation-induced reversible dedifferentiation. Nature. 2012;490(7420):412–6.

169. Dillon BJ, Prieto VG, Curley SA, Ensor CM, Holtsberg FW, Bomalaski JS, et al. Incidence and distribution of argininosuccinate synthetase deficiency in human cancers: a method for identifying cancers sensitive to arginine deprivation. Cancer. 2004;100(4):826–33.

170. Kuo MT, Long Y, Tsai WB, Li YY, Chen HHW, Feun LG, et al. Collaboration between RSK-EphA2 and Gas6-Axl RTK signaling in arginine starvation response that confers resistance to EGFR inhibitors. Transl Oncol. 2020;13(2):355–64.

171. Tsai WB, Long Y, Park JR, Chang JT, Liu H, Rodriguez-Canales J, et al. Gas6/Axl is the sensor of arginine-auxotrophic response in targeted chemotherapy with arginine-depleting agents. Oncogene. 2016;35(13):1632–42.

172. Radisky DC, Levy DD, Littlepage LE, Liu H, Nelson CM, Fata JE, et al. Rac1b and reactive oxygen species mediate MMP-3-induced EMT and genomic instability. Nature. 2005;436(7047):123–7.

173. Canli O, Nicolas AM, Gupta J, Finkelmeier F, Goncharova O, Pesic M, et al. Myeloid cell-derived reactive oxygen species induce epithelial mutagenesis. Cancer Cell. 2017;32(6):869–83 e5.

174. Huang JS, Cho CY, Hong CC, Yan MD, Hsieh MC, Lay JD, et al. Oxidative stress enhances Axl-mediated cell migration through an Akt1/Rac1-dependent mechanism. Free Radic Biol Med. 2013;65:1246–56.

175. Konishi A, Aizawa T, Mohan A, Korshunov VA, Berk BC. Hydrogen peroxide activates the Gas6-Axl pathway in vascular smooth muscle cells. J Biol Chem. 2004;279(27):28766–70.

176. Smolock EM, Korshunov VA. Pharmacological inhibition of Axl affects smooth muscle cell functions under oxidative stress. Vasc Pharmacol. 2010;53(3–4):185–92.

177. Xia J, Chiu LY, Nehring RB, Bravo Nunez MA, Mei Q, Perez M, et al. Bacteria-to-human protein networks reveal origins of endogenous DNA damage. Cell. 2019;176(1–2):127–43 e24.

178. Galhardo RS, Hastings PJ, Rosenberg SM. Mutation as a stress response and the regulation of evolvability. Crit Rev Biochem Mol Biol. 2007;42(5):399–435.

179. Loeb LA. Human cancers express a mutator phenotype: hypothesis, origin, and consequences. Cancer Res. 2016;76(8):2057–9.

180. Russo M, Crisafulli G, Sogari A, Reilly NM, Arena S, Lamba S, et al. Adaptive mutability of colorectal cancers in response to targeted therapies. Science. 2019;366(6472):1473–80.

181. Fahrer J. Switching off DNA repair-how colorectal cancer evades targeted therapies through adaptive mutability. Signal Transduct Target Ther. 2020;5(1):19.

182. Paget S. The distribution of secondary growths in cancer of the breast. Lancet. 1889;133(3421):571–3.

183. Heppner GH. Tumor heterogeneity. Cancer Res. 1984;44(6):2259–65.

184. Vogelstein B, Papadopoulos N, Velculescu VE, Zhou S, Diaz LA Jr, Kinzler KW. Cancer genome landscapes. Science. 2013;339(6127):1546–58.

185. Mirzayans R, Murray D. Intratumor heterogeneity and therapy resistance: contributions of dormancy, apoptosis reversal (anastasis) and cell fusion to disease recurrence. Int J Mol Sci 2020;21(4).

186. Wright BE. Does selective gene activation direct evolution? FEBS Lett. 1997;402(1):4–8.

187. Hackley RK, Schmid AK. Global transcriptional programs in archaea share features with the eukaryotic environmental stress response. J Mol Biol. 2019;431(20):4147–66.

188. Tubbs A, Nussenzweig A. Endogenous DNA damage as a source of genomic instability in cancer. Cell. 2017;168(4):644–56.

189. Nowell PC. The clonal evolution of tumor cell populations. Science. 1976;194(4260):23–8.

190. Talmadge JE, Fidler IJ. AACR centennial series: the biology of cancer metastasis: historical perspective. Cancer Res. 2010;70(14):5649–69.

191. Pelham HR. A regulatory upstream promoter element in the Drosophila hsp 70 heat-shock gene. Cell. 1982;30(2):517–28.

192. Sakurai H, Enoki Y. Novel aspects of heat shock factors: DNA recognition, chromatin modulation and gene expression. FEBS J. 2010;277(20):4140–9.

193. Mendillo ML, Santagata S, Koeva M, Bell GW, Hu R, Tamimi RM, et al. HSF1 drives a transcriptional program distinct from heat shock to support highly malignant human cancers. Cell. 2012;150(3):549–62.

194. Kang GY, Kim EH, Lee HJ, Gil NY, Cha HJ, Lee YS. Heat shock factor 1, an inhibitor of non-homologous end joining repair. Oncotarget. 2015;6(30):29712–24.

195. Dayalan Naidu S, Dinkova-Kostova AT. Regulation of the mammalian heat shock factor 1. FEBS J. 2017;284(11):1606–27.

196. Hanahan D, Folkman J. Patterns and emerging mechanisms of the angiogenic switch during tumorigenesis. Cell. 1996;86(3):353–64.

197. Naumov GN, Folkman J, Straume O. Tumor dormancy due to failure of angiogenesis: role of the microenvironment. Clin Exp Metastas. 2009;26(1):51–60.

198. Dillekas H, Transeth M, Pilskog M, Assmus J, Straume O. Differences in metastatic patterns in relation to time between primary surgery and first relapse from breast cancer suggest synchronized growth of dormant micrometastases. Breast Cancer Res Treat. 2014;146(3):627–36.

199. Indraccolo S, Stievano L, Minuzzo S, Tosello V, Esposito G, Piovan E, et al. Interruption of tumor dormancy by a transient angiogenic burst within the tumor microenvironment. Proc Natl Acad Sci USA. 2006;103(11):4216–21.

200. Perego M, Tyurin VA, Tyurina YY, Yellets J, Nacarelli T, Lin C, et al. Reactivation of dormant tumor cells by modified lipids derived from stress-activated neutrophils. Sci Transl Med 2020;12(572).

201. Lan Q, Peyvandi S, Duffey N, Huang YT, Barras D, Held W, et al. Type I interferon/IRF7 axis instigates chemotherapy-induced immunological dormancy in breast cancer. Oncogene. 2019;38(15):2814–29.

202. Straume O, Shimamura T, Lampa MJ, Carretero J, Oyan AM, Jia D, et al. Suppression of heat shock protein 27 induces long-term dormancy in human breast cancer. Proc Natl Acad Sci USA 2012.

203. Persi E, Wolf YI, Horn D, Ruppin E, Demichelis F, Gatenby RA, et al. Mutation-selection balance and compensatory mechanisms in tumour evolution. Nat Rev Genet. 2021;22(4):251–62.

Sarah Wang and Andrew C. Dudley

Abstract

Vascular co-option is a non-angiogenic process whereby cancer cells use the preexisting vasculature for survival and motility. The structure and function of co-opted vasculature is typically preserved in contrast to angiogenic vasculature which grows chaotically and is highly permeable. The ability of cancer cells to co-opt preexisting vessels, or to switch between neo-angiogenesis and vessel co-option, is proposed as a mechanism for intrinsic or acquired resistance to anti-angiogenic therapies. Additionally, vessel co-option may impact other treatment modalities such as chemotherapy, radiation, surgery, and immunotherapy; for example, vessel co-option has been associated with a highly invasive cancer phenotype that underlies residual disease and recurrence after treatments including surgery or radiation. Although multiple cancer types appear "competent" to co-opt preexisting vasculature, cancers within the brain microenvironment such as glioma or brain metastases from lung, breast, and skin, frequently demonstrate vessel co-optive growth patterns. The presence of vessel co-option, by itself, has the potential to be a useful biomarker to stratify patient responses to anti-angiogenic therapy and targeting vessel co-option (e.g., via inhibition of perivascular adhesion, chemotaxis, and spreading) could help to prevent the colonization of cancer cells in the brain and other organ microenvironments.

Take-Home Lessons

- Vessel co-option is the utilization of preexisting vasculature that is less destructive to the surrounding tissue architecture than angiogenesis and is found in primary and metastatic sites of various cancer types.
- Vessel co-option contributes to resistance to anti-angiogenic therapy, perivascular invasion, dormancy, and cancer recurrence, and is essential during the colonization of the brain and other organ microenvironments.
- A deeper mechanistic understanding of vessel co-option may provide new therapeutic targets that could be considered for use in combinatorial strategies alongside anti-angiogenic therapy.
- Developing biomarkers and assays to determine why certain tumors "prefer" angiogenesis versus vessel co-option is an underexplored area that needs further study.

The Emerging Field of Vessel Co-option: A Non-angiogenic Mode of Tumor Vascularization

It is long known that cancer cells interact with and stimulate the formation of new vasculature; without access to the endothelium, solid tumors lack the ability to receive essential nutrients and oxygen and have an impaired ability to remove metabolic waste products. Most tumors that fail to establish a new blood supply will become dormant and remain at a diameter of approximately 2–3 mm^3. In 1971, Judah Folkman described the ability of tumors to actively promote the growth of new blood vessels, a process termed angiogenesis, as a means for tumors to overcome this limitation. He proposed that blocking angiogenesis would starve a tumor and be an effective means to induce dormancy or prevent metastasis [1]. Several studies in

S. Wang
Department of Microbiology, Immunology, and Cancer Biology, The University of Virginia, Charlottesville, VA, USA

A. C. Dudley (✉)
Department of Microbiology, Immunology, and Cancer Biology, The University of Virginia, Charlottesville, VA, USA

Emily Couric Cancer Center, The University of Virginia, Charlottesville, VA, USA
e-mail: acd2g@virginia.edu

© The Author(s), under exclusive license to Springer Nature Switzerland AG 2022
L. A. Akslen, R. S. Watnick (eds.), *Biomarkers of the Tumor Microenvironment*, https://doi.org/10.1007/978-3-030-98950-7_32

the following years have supported the concept that cancer is dependent on the vasculature and the promotion of angiogenesis has been included as a hallmark of cancer since 2000 [2]. However, while sprouting angiogenesis has been described as the predominant mode of tumor neovascularization, there has been a growing appreciation that tumors do not rely solely on the growth of new blood vessels via sprouting. So-called non-angiogenic forms of tumor vascularization include vasculogenic mimicry (the ability for tumor cells to differentiate and form vascular-like structures) and vessel co-option (utilization of the preexisting vasculature) [3]. Vessel co-option appears to be a common mechanism for tumor growth and invasion, particularly in highly vascularized organs such as the brain, liver, and lung. This chapter provides an overview of vessel co-option followed by an in-depth review of vessel co-option specifically in the brain microenvironment.

Vessel co-option is used to describe tumors that utilize the preexisting vasculature without inducing angiogenesis. Unlike chaotic and leaky angiogenic vessels, co-opted vessels often preserve the vascular scaffold and architecture of the surrounding tissue. Vessel co-opting cells can be found either invading the stroma around blood vessels or replacing the normal epithelium that directly attaches to endothelial cells [4]. While there are several historical reports describing tumors that do not disrupt the normal architecture of their microenvironments including the vasculature [5–7], it was not until 1999 that the term vessel co-option was formally used in the literature [8]. In addition to vessel co-option several other terms can be used to describe this non-angiogenic mode of vascularization [e.g., vascular co-option, angiotropism, pericyte mimicry, extravascular migratory metastasis, perivascular invasion/migration/satellitosis, alveolar filling or lepidic growth (in lung), replacement or trabecular growth (liver)]. At present, a large body of literature has accumulated and continues to provide evidence of tumor cells co-opting the vasculature in non-angiogenic growth patterns in a spectrum of primary and metastatic cancers of the lung, liver, brain, skin, lymph nodes, and other tissues [9]. For clarity, this chapter uses the term vessel co-option as synonymous for the additional terminology found in the literature and listed above.

The chosen mode of tumor vascularization is a multifactorial, complex process, and it is still unknown why some tumors "prefer" an angiogenic versus vessel co-optive pattern. As could be expected, some of the most frequently described microenvironments for vessel co-option include the lung, liver, and brain since these highly vascularized organs may be areas where cancer cells are less dependent on angiogenesis. Moreover, the tumor microenvironment may affect the vascularization of cells from similar origins as is observed by differences in the vascular status between primary and metastatic sites. For example, renal cell carcinoma (RCC) is known to rely predominantly on angiogenesis at the primary site but can demonstrate vessel co-option in RCC-to-lung metastases [10, 11]. Similarly, primary angiogenic breast cancers can switch to vessel co-opting lung metastases in preclinical models [11–14] and in human

patients [15]. However, the tumor microenvironment is not an obligate determinant of the mode of vascular dependencies. For instance, there are times where there are no reported differences in vascular status between primary and metastatic sites; this has been observed in patients with primary breast cancer that metastasized to the skin [16] and primary melanoma that disseminated to the brain [17]. Additionally, not all tumors in the lung, liver, and brain grow in a vessel co-optive pattern. To further add to the complexity of vascular dependencies, intratumoral heterogeneity is often observed where there are regions of vessel co-option and regions of angiogenesis within the same lesion. This has been demonstrated in a variety of patient settings including glioblastoma (GBM) [18], lung adenocarcinoma [19, 20], lung squamous cell carcinoma [20], hepatocellular carcinoma (HCC) [21–23], colorectal cancer (CRC) [11], breast cancer [11], lung-metastatic RCC [11], and CRC liver metastases [24, 25]. Furthermore, vascular status is a dynamic process and there can be switching between non-angiogenic and angiogenic growth patterns. This has most commonly been observed as the selection for non-angiogenic forms of tumor growth following resistance to anti-angiogenic therapy [26], which may be reversible upon drug withdrawal [27].

Vessel Co-option Is a Resistance Mechanism to Anti-angiogenic Therapy

Interest and attention to vessel co-option has been in part spurred by the disappointing clinical efficacy of anti-angiogenic therapies. Following the discovery that vascular endothelial growth factor-A (VEGF) is overexpressed in many solid tumors which drives sprouting angiogenesis, inhibitors against VEGF signaling were rationally developed [28, 29]. Bevacizumab, a monoclonal antibody against VEGF, was first approved in 2004, and additional agents have subsequently been clinically approved as anti-angiogenic therapies (e.g., sorafenib, aflibercept, axitinib, nintedanib, ramucirumab, regorafenib, sunitinib, and vatalanib). These agents have been used in several tumor types including breast cancer, non-small cell lung cancer (NSCLC), CRC, GBM, RCC, HCC, pancreatic neuroendocrine tumors (PNET), gastro-esophageal, thyroid, cervical, and ovarian cancers [30–32]. While improved progression-free survival (PFS) and overall survival (OS) has been observed in advanced RCC, HCC, and CRC, no significant improvement has been found in pancreatic ductal carcinoma (PDAC), prostate cancer, breast cancer, or melanoma. Efficacy in NSCLC is mixed in terms of OS, and in GBM, the benefits of anti-angiogenic therapy are linked to improved quality of life and not OS. Additionally, responses to anti-angiogenic therapy are not durable and often extend survival by only weeks or a few months. Furthermore, even when these agents appear to have moderate efficacy in advanced stage cancers, they fail to improve disease-free survival (DFS) in the postsurgical adjuvant setting [26, 32, 33]. Nevertheless, recent studies have shown a marked improvement in the efficacy of anti-angiogenic therapies when used in combination with chemotherapy, targeted therapies, or immune checkpoint blockade [34, 35]. For example, the IMbrave150 trial has demonstrated significantly improved PFS and OS with atezolizumab (checkpoint inhibitor) plus bevacizumab versus sorafenib in patients with unresectable, treatment-naïve HCC [36].

Though not the only proposed mechanism of resistance (e.g., redundancy in pro-angiogenic growth factors, metabolic adaptations, stromal and immune cell contributions), vessel co-option provides a rational explanation for both intrinsic and acquired resistance to anti-angiogenic therapy. Even before results from clinical trials, some investigators speculated that non-angiogenic growth patterns would be a barrier to efficacy [20]. In the brain, several studies using orthotopic models of glioma demonstrate that treatment with anti-angiogenic therapy induces cancer cells to become invasive and migrate along the pre-existing vasculature [37–46]. Similar patterns of infiltrative growth after anti-angiogenic therapy have been observed in human autopsy and resected specimens of glioma [41, 47]. In the lungs, a model using Lewis lung carcinoma demonstrated residual cancer cells growing in a vessel co-optive pattern after treatment with angiostatin (an anti-angiogenic agent) [48]. Primary HCC and liver-metastatic CRC also display strong evidence of vessel co-option in intrinsic and acquired resistance to anti-angiogenic therapies [24, 49–51]. Additionally, human samples of breast cancer metastases to the lungs, liver, lymph nodes, skin, and brain show a high prevalence of vessel co-option, and this is a compelling explanation for the lack of improvement in OS in metastatic breast cancer patients [7, 30, 52]. Preclinical models give support to this premise where the growth of angiogenic primary breast tumors was inhibited by anti-angiogenic agents, but metastases, which utilized vessel co-option as a means of survival, persisted despite treatment [11, 14, 53].

Vessel Co-option as a Prognostic Marker and Potential Interplay with Cancer Therapeutics

Associations between a vessel co-optive growth pattern and patient prognosis can be difficult to assess due to limitations related to sample acquisition and preparation (i.e., biopsies are a snapshot in space and time that cannot account for spatial or temporal intratumoral heterogeneity). Additionally, there is a discrepancy in the criteria used to define vessel co-option between different studies. Despite these limitations, there appears to be a trend toward poorer prognosis when co-option is present, suggesting that vessel co-option may play an important role in tumor recurrence and overall patient survival. Most prognostic studies comparing vessel co-option-dependent versus angiogenesis-dependent forms of tumor growth relate to lung and liver cancers. While there are some studies in lung cancer that show a greater percentage of vessel co-option asso-

ciated with a lower risk of recurrence [19, 54, 55] and longer OS [56, 57], studies that include a more diverse spectrum of NSCLC histological subtypes associate vessel co-option with a poorer prognosis (an increased risk of recurrence [20, 58–60] and shorter OS [60–64]). In CRC liver metastases, a retrospective meta-analysis of 2,432 patients (data from 23 studies) demonstrated that a majority of studies associated an unfavorable outcome with vessel co-option (also called "replacement" growth pattern) [65]. Recently, guidelines have been established for scoring of histopathological growth patterns in the liver [66, 67], and a study using these guidelines in a cohort of 732 patients similarly demonstrated worse OS and PFS in vessel co-optive CRC liver metastases [68]. Another study observed that patients with CRC-liver metastases and a vessel co-optive growth pattern were more likely to have multi-organ recurrences [69]. Similarly, when vessel co-option was determined to be present, patients with liver-metastatic uveal melanoma and primary cutaneous melanoma had shorter OS [70] and an increased risk of metastasis [71–73], respectively.

The association of vessel co-option with a poor prognosis may be due to the more invasive properties of cancer cells that are "competent" to co-opt blood vessels, or due to a survival advantage conferred by the perivascular niche. In addition to a role for anti-angiogenic therapy resistance, vessel co-option is also likely to impact other treatments including surgery, radiation, chemotherapy, and immunotherapy. As described in further detail below, vessel co-optive cancer cells grow in a highly infiltrative pattern that may impede the ability to establish clean margins on surgical or radiation fields and therefore increase the risk of recurrence. Studies in early-stage lung cancer [20, 59, 60] or liver-metastatic CRC [74] have shown an association with higher recurrence rates after surgery. The perivascular niche and endothelial cell-derived factors may also play a role in promoting chemoresistance [75–77]. On the other hand, vessel co-opting cancer cells have better access to oxygen compared to non-vessel co-opting counterparts; thus, closer association with the vasculature could reduce hypoxia and increase exposure to chemotherapy or other targeted therapies within the circulation [78]. Additionally, due to the dependence on O_2, it is possible that vessel co-opting cancer cells would be more sensitive to radiotherapies that are often ineffective in more hypoxic tumors [79]. Thus, further studies are warranted to assess how vessel co-option impacts the success or failure of these different treatment modalities.

With the emergence of immunotherapies such as checkpoint inhibitors, the immune landscape in co-opted versus angiogenic tumors is another area of interest. Low-dose anti-angiogenic therapies are being studied as a way to normalize angiogenic vessels in order to improve T-cell infiltration and the efficacy of immunotherapy [78]. Thus, it could be hypothesized that areas of vessel co-option may have more "normal-like" vessels and therefore are more responsive to immunotherapy. However, studies of liver metastases show a trend toward lower immune infiltration in vessel co-opted tumors compared to angiogenic tumors [25, 80–83], which could possibly reduce responses to immunotherapy. Therefore, there remain many open areas of study to determine how vessel co-option as a mode of tumor vascularization could be targeted to improve anti-cancer therapies.

Evidence of Vessel Co-option in Human Brain Tissue

Observations of vessel co-option originate from histopathological samples of cancer patients, many of which were detected in brain malignancies. Early estimates suggested that 35% of gliomas form highly proliferative "cuffs" around capillaries as reported by Scherer, and this was termed "perivascular satellitosis" [84, 85]. These malignant cells around the vasculature were found both in early and late stages of disease, as well as at some distance away from the bulk tumor. Glioblastoma co-opting vessels have also been noted to have similar vascular density and morphology when compared to normal brain [18]. Additionally, studies have suggested that these co-opted vessels appear similar to preexisting brain vessels and can express brain-organotypic factors including those important for maintenance of the blood–brain barrier (BBB) [86, 87]. In a recent cohort of 37 paired melanoma metastases, a lower microvascular density was found in intracranial versus extracranial sites [88]. More mature non-angiogenic vessels are also found at greater proportions in matched brain metastases compared to the primary non-small cell lung carcinoma [89].

Vessel co-opting low-grade gliomas are predominantly found infiltrating the brain parenchyma as single cells in close proximity to the vasculature with minimal disruption to the BBB [86]. In contrast, high-grade gliomas can disrupt BBB function during vessel co-option by displacing astrocytes and pericytes, though some degree of coverage may still be retained [8, 90–96]. Brain metastases originating from melanoma, breast, lung, or CRC can also be found in a perivascular growth pattern similar to high-grade gliomas and show direct contact with endothelial cells [97–100] or they behave similarly to low-grade gliomas by surrounding preexisting vasculature without stripping away astrocytes and pericytes [98, 99]. While these studies have demonstrated the existence of vessel co-option in the brain, the relative incidence between vessel co-option and angiogenesis has not been well-established [7, 101]. Additionally, while vessel co-option is often observed following resistance to anti-angiogenic therapy, it has also been observed in treatment-naïve brain tumors [26].

Preclinical Models of Vessel Co-option in the Brain

Preclinical models have similarly demonstrated evidence of vessel co-option in a variety of brain tumors including primary GBM and brain metastases from lung, breast, CRC, and melanoma. When studying vessel co-option, it is impor-

tant to utilize physiologically relevant model systems that preserve the preexisting vasculature of the organ or tissue. Genetically engineered mouse models (GEMMs) can be used to faithfully mimic human cancers, and they avoid artifacts of experimental surgeries. However, these mice can take longer to develop tumors compared to transplantation models. Additionally, while GEMMs may be useful for studying primary brain cancer, there are very few models of spontaneous brain metastases and most studies using brain metastatic GEMMs [102–104] typically do not report vessel co-option status. Orthotopic transplantation and the development of spontaneous brain metastases is another method to recapitulate host–tumor interactions, but these can also take significant time to complete the metastatic process [105] and are more commonly used to study lung or liver metastases [11, 24, 51, 73, 106, 107]. Intracardiac injection of cancer cells is one method that enables the study of circulating metastatic cells, but this is also inefficient for establishing brain metastases unless brain tropic cells are generated first (by collecting subpopulations after multiple rounds of intracardiac injection) [108]. Intracarotid injection of tumor cells into the circulation is a model that more efficiently and consistently develops brain metastases [38, 96, 109]. However, ligation of the carotid artery during surgery can potentially cause brain injury and affect the growth, survival, and vessel co-option abilities of cancer cells. Intracranial transplantation using stereotactic coordinates is another widely used method to form brain tumors [8, 39, 42, 90, 93, 97, 105, 110–113]. However, this model is best used as an "established" metastasis model because it does not recapitulate the earlier stages of the metastatic process. In addition to these *in vivo* models, *ex vivo* brain slices can be grown for short periods of time on tissue culture inserts and co-cultured with cancer cells. Dynamic interactions between cancer cells and the brain vasculature can be monitored with real-time video microscopy to visualize and quantify perivascular motility following cancer cell seeding [90, 105, 108, 113–115].

Adhesion to the Vasculature Is Essential for Early Brain Colonization

Multiple studies have demonstrated that vessel co-option is necessary for cancer cells to thrive in the brain microenvironment and form metastatic outgrowths. Imaging of serially excised tissues of GBM [37, 94] or brain metastases [116] demonstrates a close association between cancer cells and the brain vasculature in early stages of tumor progression. More sophisticated intravital imaging has also provided evidence for cancer cell-to-vascular cell adherence followed by perivascular migration over time [96, 110, 112]. In a study using intracarotid injection of melanoma or lung cancer cells, Kienast et al. demonstrated that only those cancer cells that adhered to the abluminal surface of the vasculature formed metastases while those not in a perivascular position regressed or underwent cell death [96]. However, attachment to blood vessels did not necessarily equate to proliferation because some cancer cells which had attached to the vasculature exited the cell cycle and remained dormant. Interestingly, co-opted melanoma cells were still motile along the vasculature even when in a dormant state [96].

Several adhesion molecules including integrins and L1CAM were shown to be important for adherence to the vasculature and thus subsequent tumor progression. For example, it was demonstrated that β1-integrin was important for cell adhesion to the basal lamina components (fibronectin, laminin, vitronectin, and collagen I and IV) of brain capillaries [105]. β1-integrins can also activate focal adhesion kinase (FAK) and ERK1/2 phosphorylation to regulate proliferation. Loss of β1-integrin in intracardiac or intracranially injected breast and melanoma lines resulted in reduced adhesion to the vascular basal lamina and reduced proliferation [105]. Breast cancer cells also bind to the basal lamina using β4-integrin to activate receptor tyrosine kinases such as ErbB2 [117]. Interestingly, even "liquid tumors" show evidence of vessel co-option as acute lymphoblastic leukemia uses α6-integrin to migrate into the CNS on arachnoid vessels and bypass the BBB [118].

In addition to integrins, engagement of the adhesion molecule L1CAM was shown to be an important mechanism for metastatic colonization and spreading along the vasculature. In the brain, one of the first defenses against metastatic cells is the activation of plasmin (e.g., astrocytes release plasminogen activators, PA). Plasmin in the brain microenvironment leads to FasL-dependent death of cancer cells and inactivates the axon pathfinding molecule L1CAM that metastatic cells use to spread along the brain endothelium. In order to evade this defense mechanism and enable vessel co-option, brain metastatic cells from breast and lung cancers upregulate serpins that inhibit PA. Neuroserpin (SERPINI1) is normally expressed in the brain and was one of the most frequently upregulated anti-PA serpins alongside SERPINB2, in brain metastatic lesions [108]. A follow-up study demonstrated that L1CAM-dependent activation of the mechanosensitive YAP pathway was involved in metastatic colonization and pericyte-like spreading at multiple organ sites (brain, lung, and bone). In this study, aggressive cancer cells used vessel co-option immediately after extravasation or after cells were released from dormancy [106]. Thus, targeting the molecular mechanisms that impair the adhesion of cancer cells to the vasculature may be a potential therapeutic strategy that exploits a unique vulnerability of metastatic cells.

Vessel Co-option Associates with an Invasive Growth Pattern

While adherence to the preexisting vasculature is necessary for early formation of brain tumors [8, 96, 116], the significance of vessel co-option compared to sprouting angiogenesis in later stages of tumor progression is less clear. Some tumors switch to angiogenesis as a tumor progresses, while others predominantly rely on vessel co-option for their survival. Originally, it was thought that the angiogenic switch may be size dependent and activated only when tumors were deprived of essential nutrients and oxygen. Support for this hypothesis includes work from Holash et al. who used animal models of primary astrocytic brain tumors and brain metastases to demonstrate that vessel co-option can be transient with tumor size-dependent activation of angiopoetin-2 (Ang2) and vascular endothelial growth factor (VEGF) leading to sprouting angiogenesis [8]. However, other studies contradict this size-dependent hypothesis and demonstrate that macroscopic tumors do not have an obligate requirement for angiogenesis [11, 20–22, 24, 25, 37, 82, 119–121]. For example, in the brain microenvironment, a recent study of eight autopsy cases of melanoma brain metastases showed a vessel co-optive growth pattern with no evidence of angiogenesis irrespective of tumor size [122]. Additionally, upregulation of VEGF does not always lead to an angiogenic switch as studies by Kusters et al. and Leenders et al. found that constitutive overexpression of VEGF isoforms only promoted dilation of co-opted blood vessels in infiltrative brain tumors that grew in the Virchow-Robin space. Absent or minimal necrosis was found in these co-opting tumors suggesting a sufficient blood supply without hypoxia-induced angiogenesis [38, 109].

Notably, the invasive properties of cancer cells have been highly associated with the presence of vessel co-option. In a study investigating growth patterns in 247 brain metastasis patients who underwent neurosurgical resection, specimens with a more brain invasive growth pattern (as opposed to well-delineated) showed reduced peritumoral edema, hypoxia, and angiogenesis [123]. Histologically, non-angiogenic brain tumors appear to have a more irregular interface with normal adjacent tissue compared to angiogenic tumors [98, 123]. The preference for vessel co-option as an invasive strategy has also been demonstrated in GBM cell lines [37], and there appears to be a predominance for vessel co-option to occur at the tumor–brain interface [113]. Furthermore, imaging studies have demonstrated that malignant cells use the vasculature as a "highway" for invasion. For example, melanoma cells can travel ~580 μm in just four weeks along the abluminal surface of preexisting brain blood vessels [97] and glioblastoma cells use blood vessels to spread in a directional manner [110, 112].

While the vasculature can clearly be used as a pathway for cancer cell dispersal, there are also differing patterns of vessel co-option where cancer cells can migrate either as single cells or as a collective group. In gliomas, collective migration disrupts the BBB and is a more inflammatory process that can promote angiogenesis. Griveau et al. demonstrated that Olig2+ glioma that signaled through Wnt7 were more likely to undergo single-cell migration similar to the spread of oligodendrocyte precursor cells during development.

These Olig2+ cells were also enriched after anti-VEGF therapy, suggesting that anti-angiogenic therapies may select for cancer cells with the ability to co-opt the vasculature. Single-cell vessel co-option also has important implications for BBB integrity and immune evasion. For example, preservation of the BBB has important consequences for therapeutic targeting of cancer cells, namely that inhibiting Wnt7-driven perivascular invasion enhanced the efficacy of temozolomide (TMZ) [113]. Loss of BBB integrity is also known to play a role in increased macrophage infiltration [124], as well as migration and activation of resident microglia [125]. In the context of gliomas, both Olig2+ and Olig2- cancers increased the number of microglia present compared to normal brain tissue; however, microglia in Oligo2- (more angiogenic) tumors had a more activated (ameboid) morphology and an increased number of cells expressing genes related to macrophage infiltration [113]. Finally, compared to clusters of glioma cells, solitary vessel co-opting glioma cells are less detectable by MRI which may allow these cells to invade beyond a field of radiation or surgical resection [94, 113].

Embryonic Programs Contribute to Perivascular Migration and Dormancy

Cancer cells have been long known to reactivate dormant embryonically derived programs or hijack developmental pathways that are typically important for tissue/organ morphogenesis or wound healing [75, 126]. For example, it is hypothesized that the neural crest lineage of melanoma cells may underlie their vessel co-optive properties and preference for metastasis to the brain [126]. Neural crest-lineage cells undergo extensive extravascular migration along the abluminal surface of the vasculature during development as they differentiate to form multiple cell types including melanocytes, glial, and neuronal cells [127, 128]. Studies have shown that several genes related to neural crest migration or embryonic-like features are differentially expressed in vessel co-opting versus non-co-opting melanoma cells [129, 130]. Additionally, melanoma cells have the capability to migrate along neural crest tracks in the chick embryo [131]. Gliomas are also known to migrate along the vasculature similar to the migratory patterns of oligodendrocyte precursor cells in the developing nervous system [132].

Vascular niches have been implicated in the maintenance of cancer stem-like cells [133]. In the brain, the perivascular niche plays a crucial role in normal neurogenesis and the functions of neural stem or progenitor cells [134]. Cancer stem-like cells likely exploit similar mechanisms. Dormancy is a feature related to cancer stemness, and it has been observed that subpopulations of melanoma, lung, and breast cancer cells can remain dormant in the perivascular niche [96]. Another study showed that dormancy in brain metastatic breast cancer in the perivascular niche was maintained by thrombospondin-1 (TSP-1) released from resting endothelium. In contrast, activated endothelium downregulates TSP-1 and increases transforming growth factor beta (TGFβ) and periostin to spark the outgrowth of tumors that are angiogenesis dependent [135].

Additional Molecular Mechanisms of Vessel Co-option

The use of *ex vivo* brain slices has shown that cancer cells will adhere and migrate along the brain vasculature. Since these brain slices are not perfused and lack a gradient of nutrients and oxygen, this suggests that blood vessels may secrete chemoattractants that recruit nearby cancer cells. Factors that have demonstrated a role in the chemotaxis of cancer cells toward the brain vasculature include bradykinin, SDF1α, and IL-8. Vessel co-opting GBM cells express high levels of bradykinin receptor 2 (B2R), and bradykinin can induce their chemotaxis and invasion [114, 136]. Stromal cell-derived factor (SDF1α) and its receptor CXCR4 have also been implicated in the chemotaxis of co-opting brain tumors. CXCR4 is overexpressed on invasive GBM cells, and sequestered VEGF at the tumor–brain interface upregulates SFD1α in neurons and endothelial cells [137]. In vitro, CXCR4+ GBM cells migrate toward an SDF1α gradient; consequently, inhibition of CXCR4 can reduce migration, invasion, and survival in GBM [111]. CXCR4 inhibition also radiosensitized tumors leading to increased apoptosis and survival after radiation treatment [111]. Additionally, the SDF1α/CXCR4 pathway can be upregulated in GBM following anti-angiogenic treatment [138]. IL-8 and its receptors CXCR1 and CXCR2 can also play a role in GBM proliferation, invasion, and vasculogenic mimicry [139]. Co-culture of patient-derived GBM and endothelial cells demonstrates that EC-derived IL-8 stimulated chemotaxis and invasion of GBM [140, 141]. Another motility factor that has been described in vessel co-option of GBM is CDC42. Inhibition of CDC42 impaired vessel co-option; however, this was not a vessel co-option-specific phenotype as all migratory and infiltrative strategies were affected [90].

While adhesion, motility, and chemotaxis factors are strongly implicated in the molecular mechanisms that drive vessel co-option, there have been additional studies that link vessel co-option to secondary survival pathways. For example, EGFRvIII expression is upregulated in vessel co-optive, highly infiltrative, and aggressive GBM (brain slice and

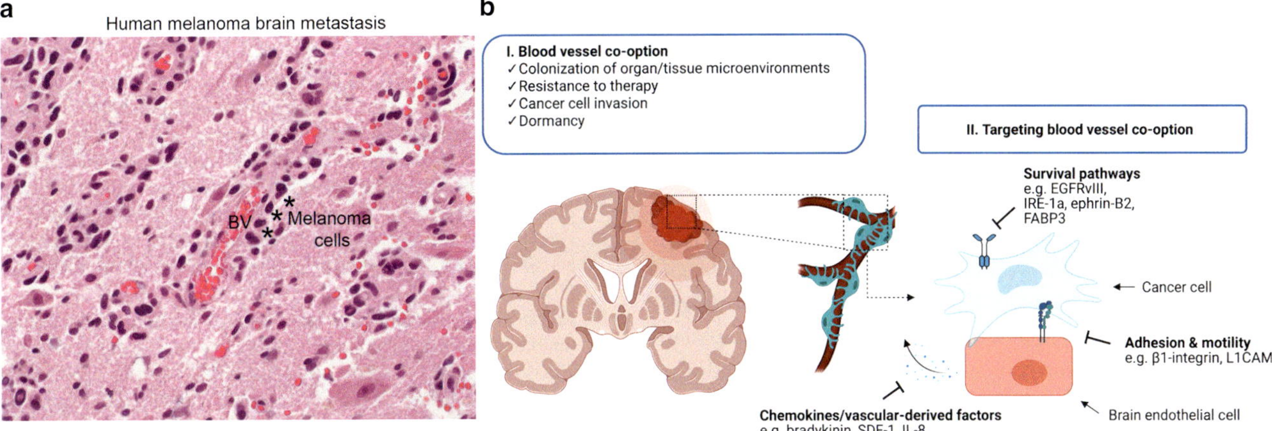

Fig. 32.1 Cancer cells utilize the preexisting vasculature in a process called vessel co-option to aid in the colonization of tumor microenvironments, particularly in the brain. (**a**) A human melanoma brain metastasis specimen stained with H&E shows "cuffs" of abundant melanoma cells at the blood vessel margins (BV = blood vessels and several melanoma cells have been marked with asterisks). Image used with permission of Dr. James Mandell, University of Virginia Department of Pathology. (**b**) Cancer cell occupation of the perivascular niche also plays an important role in resistance to anti-cancer therapies, survival, dormancy, and invasion. Potential avenues to therapeutically target vessel co-option include adhesion and motility factors, chemokines and other EC-derived molecules, and various survival pathways that control the growth, spreading, and motility of vessel-associated cancer cells. Images were created using BioRender

orthotopic models), but further molecular mechanisms are unclear [142]. IRE-1α is an ER transmembrane protein and cellular stress signal. IRE-1α decreases pathways for angiogenesis [143], and inactivation of IRE-1α in GBM cells induces vessel co-option in a U87 tumor model and increases migration in vitro [144]. Upregulation of ephrin-B2 in GBM was also shown to provide a role in anchorage-independent growth as downregulation of ephrin-B2 impairs vessel co-option and improves in vivo survival [145]. The brain is also a lipid-rich environment, and the fatty acid binding protein [FABP3; also called mammary-derived growth factor (MDGI)] has been implicated in vessel co-option. Targeting the FABP3/MDGI pathway with the antihistamine clemastine inhibited perivascular migration and invasive growth of GBM [146]. A summary of the various pathways that may contribute to vessel co-option is shown in Fig. 32.1.

Biomarkers of Tumor Vascularization

There are currently few or no clinically robust predictive biomarkers to identify patients that will respond well to anti-angiogenic therapy other than, in some cases, treatment-induced hypertension. VEGF expression itself has failed to be a good biomarker [147] likely because many non-angiogenic processes also utilize VEGF signaling. Microvascular density (MVD) was another biomarker of interest and has shown some associations with anti-angiogenic treatment outcomes in retrospective studies, but this has not been demonstrated to be a reliable marker overall [148, 149]. Histopathology is the current gold standard to differentiate between vessel co-option and angiogenesis and should be used to determine if the presence of vessel co-option can stratify patient response to anti-angiogenic therapy when pretreatment biopsy samples are available. However, given that pretreatment samples are often not available, noninvasive surrogate biomarkers of blood vessel co-option are warranted. Liquid biopsies and the use of circulating tumor cells, ctDNA, or exosomes [150] are a potential candidate to use for noninvasive biomarkers but have not yet been explored in the context of blood vessel co-option in cancer. The field of radiomics to quantify medical images to categorize tumor phenotypes is another emerging field [151], and there are some promising studies that demonstrate CT or MRI scans may be able to distinguish vessel co-option versus angiogenic tumors on imaging [7]. Recently, Cheng et al. demonstrated that radiomics-based analysis of liver CT scans could predict histopathological growth patterns (i.e., could be used to distinguish vessel co-option from angiogenesis) in CRC liver metastases [152] and prospective studies to validate this radiomics signature in patient stratification for anti-angiogenic therapy are of interest.

Conclusions

Vessel co-option is an emerging field of study in tumor vascular biology that has complemented decades of research on tumor angiogenesis. While knowledge of vessel co-option is still in its infancy, histological or molecular signatures to stratify the extent of co-option versus angiogenesis could be invaluable for predicting patient outcomes or responses to different therapies. Additionally, areas for exploration include (1) why and when do cancers prefer vessel co-option versus angiogenesis? (2) What molecular mechanisms promote or differentiate between non-angiogenic and angiogenic patterns of tumor growth? (3) Can detection of co-option be used as a biomarker for selection of patients who will not respond well to anti-angiogenic therapy? (4) Will targeting mechanisms of vessel co-option act synergistically with anti-angiogenic therapies to improve patient outcomes? Do cancer cells also co-opt lymphatic endothelium in different tissue/organ microenvironments? (5) How does vessel co-option impact cancer treatments such as surgery, chemotherapy, radiation, and immunotherapy? With these important questions in mind, it is paramount that we continue to collect data on the prevalence of vessel co-option versus angiogenesis and continue to use preclinical models that mimic physiologically relevant tumor microenvironments. It is also clear that the cancer hallmark "tumor angiogenesis" may require modification to include a broader definition of vascularization that recognizes the importance of non-angiogenic processes such as vessel co-option.

Conflicts of Interest There are no conflicts of interest to disclose.

Acknowledgments ACD is supported by grants from the American Cancer Society (129755-RSG-16-176-01-DDC), the National Institutes of Health/National Cancer Institute (2RO1 CA177875 and RO1 CA2558451), the Melanoma Research Alliance (ID612638), and funds from the Emily Couric Cancer Center at the University of Virginia. SW is supported by a pilot award from the Melanoma Research Foundation and an F30 award from the National Institutes of Health (1F30CA268842-01).

References

1. Folkman J. Tumor angiogenesis: therapeutic implications. N Engl J Med. 1971;285(21):1182–6.
2. Hanahan D, Weinberg RA. The hallmarks of cancer. Cell. 2000;100(1):57–70.
3. Donnem T, et al. Non-angiogenic tumours and their influence on cancer biology. Nat Rev Cancer. 2018;18(5):323–36.
4. Latacz E, et al. Pathological features of vessel co-option versus sprouting angiogenesis. Angiogenesis. 2020;23(1):43–54.
5. Erichsen J. Zwei falle von carcinosis acuta miliaris. Virchows Arch. 1861;21:465–79.
6. Moxon W. Case of transplantation of epithelial cancer from the trachea to the pulmonary tissue, probably by desecent of cancer germs down the bronchial tubes. Trans Pathol Soc. 1869;20:28–9.
7. Kuczynski EA, et al. Vessel co-option in cancer. Nat Rev Clin Oncol. 2019;16(8):469–93.
8. Holash J, et al. Vessel cooption, regression, and growth in tumors mediated by angiopoietins and VEGF. Science. 1999;284(5422):1994–8.
9. Zhang Y, Wang S, Dudley AC. Models and molecular mechanisms of blood vessel co-option by cancer cells. Angiogenesis. 2020;23(1):17–25.
10. Sardari Nia P, et al. Distinct angiogenic and non-angiogenic growth patterns of lung metastases from renal cell carcinoma. Histopathology. 2007;51(3):354–61.
11. Bridgeman VL, et al. Vessel co-option is common in human lung metastases and mediates resistance to anti-angiogenic therapy in preclinical lung metastasis models. J Pathol. 2017;241(3):362–74.
12. Bugyik E, et al. Mechanisms of vascularization in murine models of primary and metastatic tumor growth. Chin J Cancer. 2016;35:19.
13. Milne EN, et al. Histologic type-specific vascular patterns in rat tumors. Cancer. 1967;20(10):1635–46.
14. Guerin E, et al. A model of postsurgical advanced metastatic breast cancer more accurately replicates the clinical efficacy of antiangiogenic drugs. Cancer Res. 2013;73(9):2743–8.
15. Evidence for novel non-angiogenic pathway in breast-cancer metastasis. Breast Cancer Progression Working Party. Lancet. 2000;355(9217):1787–8.
16. Colpaert CG, et al. Cutaneous breast cancer deposits show distinct growth patterns with different degrees of angiogenesis, hypoxia and fibrin deposition. Histopathology. 2003;42(6):530–40.
17. Lugassy C, et al. Angiotropism, pericytic mimicry and extravascular migratory metastasis in melanoma: an alternative to intravascular cancer dissemination. Cancer Microenviron. 2014;7(3):139–52.
18. Wesseling P, et al. Quantitative immunohistological analysis of the microvasculature in untreated human glioblastoma multiforme. Computer-assisted image analysis of whole-tumor sections. J Neurosurg. 1994;81(6):902–9.
19. Strand TE, et al. The percentage of lepidic growth is an independent prognostic factor in invasive adenocarcinoma of the lung. Diagn Pathol. 2015;10:94.
20. Pezzella F, et al. Non-small-cell lung carcinoma tumor growth without morphological evidence of neo-angiogenesis. Am J Pathol. 1997;151(5):1417–23.
21. Kanai T, et al. Pathology of small hepatocellular carcinoma. A proposal for a new gross classification. Cancer. 1987;60(4):810–9.
22. Kojiro M. 'Nodule-in-nodule' appearance in hepatocellular carcinoma: its significance as a morphologic marker of dedifferentiation. Intervirology. 2004;47(3–5):179–83.
23. Sugihara S, Kojiro M, Nakashima T. Ultrastructural study of hepatocellular carcinoma with replacing growth pattern. Acta Pathol Jpn. 1985;35(3):549–59.
24. Frentzas S, et al. Vessel co-option mediates resistance to anti-angiogenic therapy in liver metastases. Nat Med. 2016;22(11):1294–302.
25. Nielsen K, et al. The morphological growth patterns of colorectal liver metastases are prognostic for overall survival. Mod Pathol. 2014;27(12):1641–8.
26. Kuczynski EA, Reynolds AR. Vessel co-option and resistance to anti-angiogenic therapy. Angiogenesis. 2020;23(1):55–74.
27. Kuczynski EA, Kerbel RS. Implications of vessel co-option in sorafenib-resistant hepatocellular carcinoma. Chin J Cancer. 2016;35(1):97.
28. Ferrara N, Gerber HP, LeCouter J. The biology of VEGF and its receptors. Nat Med. 2003;9(6):669–76.
29. Ferrara N, et al. Discovery and development of bevacizumab, an anti-VEGF antibody for treating cancer. Nat Rev Drug Discov. 2004;3(5):391–400.
30. Vasudev NS, Reynolds AR. Anti-angiogenic therapy for cancer: current progress, unresolved questions and future directions. Angiogenesis. 2014;17(3):471–94.

31. Ebos JM, Kerbel RS. Antiangiogenic therapy: impact on invasion, disease progression, and metastasis. Nat Rev Clin Oncol. 2011;8(4):210–21.

32. Jayson GC, et al. Antiangiogenic therapy in oncology: current status and future directions. Lancet. 2016;388(10043):518–29.

33. Roviello G, et al. The role of bevacizumab in solid tumours: a literature based meta-analysis of randomised trials. Eur J Cancer. 2017;75:245–58.

34. Ramjiawan RR, Griffioen AW, Duda DG. Anti-angiogenesis for cancer revisited: is there a role for combinations with immunotherapy? Angiogenesis. 2017;20(2):185–204.

35. Qiang H, et al. New advances in antiangiogenic combination therapeutic strategies for advanced non-small cell lung cancer. J Cancer Res Clin Oncol. 2020;146(3):631–45.

36. Finn RS, et al. Atezolizumab plus Bevacizumab in Unresectable Hepatocellular Carcinoma. N Engl J Med. 2020;382(20):1894–905.

37. Baker GJ, et al. Mechanisms of glioma formation: iterative perivascular glioma growth and invasion leads to tumor progression, VEGF-independent vascularization, and resistance to antiangiogenic therapy. Neoplasia. 2014;16(7):543–61.

38. Leenders WP, et al. Antiangiogenic therapy of cerebral melanoma metastases results in sustained tumor progression via vessel co-option. Clin Cancer Res. 2004;10(18 Pt 1):6222–30.

39. Rubenstein JL, et al. Anti-VEGF antibody treatment of glioblastoma prolongs survival but results in increased vascular cooption. Neoplasia. 2000;2(4):306–14.

40. Keunen O, et al. Anti-VEGF treatment reduces blood supply and increases tumor cell invasion in glioblastoma. Proc Natl Acad Sci USA. 2011;108(9):3749–54.

41. de Groot JF, et al. Tumor invasion after treatment of glioblastoma with bevacizumab: radiographic and pathologic correlation in humans and mice. Neuro-Oncology. 2010;12(3):233–42.

42. Kunkel P, et al. Inhibition of glioma angiogenesis and growth in vivo by systemic treatment with a monoclonal antibody against vascular endothelial growth factor receptor-2. Cancer Res. 2001;61(18):6624–8.

43. Paez-Ribes M, et al. Antiangiogenic therapy elicits malignant progression of tumors to increased local invasion and distant metastasis. Cancer Cell. 2009;15(3):220–31.

44. Lucio-Eterovic AK, Piao Y, de Groot JF. Mediators of glioblastoma resistance and invasion during antivascular endothelial growth factor therapy. Clin Cancer Res. 2009;15(14):4589–99.

45. Lu KV, et al. VEGF inhibits tumor cell invasion and mesenchymal transition through a MET/VEGFR2 complex. Cancer Cell. 2012;22(1):21–35.

46. Navis AC, et al. Effects of dual targeting of tumor cells and stroma in human glioblastoma xenografts with a tyrosine kinase inhibitor against c-MET and VEGFR2. PLoS One. 2013;8(3):e58262.

47. di Tomaso E, et al. Glioblastoma recurrence after cediranib therapy in patients: lack of "rebound" revascularization as mode of escape. Cancer Res. 2011;71(1):19–28.

48. O'Reilly MS, et al. Angiostatin: a novel angiogenesis inhibitor that mediates the suppression of metastases by a Lewis lung carcinoma. Cell. 1994;79(2):315–28.

49. Lazaris A, et al. Vascularization of colorectal carcinoma liver metastasis: insight into stratification of patients for anti-angiogenic therapies. J Pathol Clin Res. 2018;4(3):184–92.

50. Vlachogiannis G, et al. Patient-derived organoids model treatment response of metastatic gastrointestinal cancers. Science. 2018;359(6378):920–6.

51. Kuczynski EA, et al. Co-option of liver vessels and not sprouting angiogenesis drives acquired sorafenib resistance in hepatocellular carcinoma. J Natl Cancer Inst 2016;108(8).

52. Kerbel RS. Reappraising antiangiogenic therapy for breast cancer. Breast. 2011;20(Suppl 3):S56–60.

53. Ebos JM, et al. Accelerated metastasis after short-term treatment with a potent inhibitor of tumor angiogenesis. Cancer Cell. 2009;15(3):232–9.

54. Carretta A, et al. Evaluation of radiological and pathological prognostic factors in surgically-treated patients with bronchoalveolar carcinoma. Eur J Cardiothorac Surg. 2001;20(2):367–71.

55. Higashiyama M, et al. Prognostic value of bronchiolo-alveolar carcinoma component of small lung adenocarcinoma. Ann Thorac Surg. 1999;68(6):2069–73.

56. Offersen BV, et al. Patterns of angiogenesis in nonsmall-cell lung carcinoma. Cancer. 2001;91(8):1500–9.

57. Reinmuth N, et al. Prognostic significance of vessel architecture and vascular stability in non-small cell lung cancer. Lung Cancer. 2007;55(1):53–60.

58. Lu S, et al. Spread through Air Spaces (STAS) is an independent predictor of recurrence and lung cancer-specific death in squamous cell carcinoma. J Thorac Oncol. 2017;12(2):223–34.

59. Kadota K, et al. Tumor spread through air spaces is an important pattern of invasion and impacts the frequency and location of recurrences after limited resection for small stage I lung adenocarcinomas. J Thorac Oncol. 2015;10(5):806–14.

60. Pastorino U, et al. Immunocytochemical markers in stage I lung cancer: relevance to prognosis. J Clin Oncol. 1997;15(8):2858–65.

61. Sardari Nia P, et al. Different growth patterns of non-small cell lung cancer represent distinct biologic subtypes. Ann Thorac Surg. 2008;85(2):395–405.

62. Warth A, et al. Prognostic impact of intra-alveolar tumor spread in pulmonary adenocarcinoma. Am J Surg Pathol. 2015;39(6):793–801.

63. Renyi-Vamos F, et al. Lymphangiogenesis correlates with lymph node metastasis, prognosis, and angiogenic phenotype in human non-small cell lung cancer. Clin Cancer Res. 2005;11(20):7344–53.

64. Sardari Nia P, et al. Prognostic value of nonangiogenic and angiogenic growth patterns in non-small-cell lung cancer. Br J Cancer. 2004;91(7):1293–300.

65. Fernandez Moro C, Bozoky B, Gerling M. Growth patterns of colorectal cancer liver metastases and their impact on prognosis: a systematic review. BMJ Open Gastroenterol. 2018;5(1):e000217.

66. van Dam PJ, et al. International consensus guidelines for scoring the histopathological growth patterns of liver metastasis. Br J Cancer. 2017;117(10):1427–41.

67. Hoppener DJ, et al. Histopathological growth patterns of colorectal liver metastasis exhibit little heterogeneity and can be determined with a high diagnostic accuracy. Clin Exp Metastasis. 2019;36(4):311–9.

68. Galjart B, et al. Angiogenic desmoplastic histopathological growth pattern as a prognostic marker of good outcome in patients with colorectal liver metastases. Angiogenesis. 2019;22(2):355–68.

69. Nierop PMH, et al. Salvage treatment for recurrences after first resection of colorectal liver metastases: the impact of histopathological growth patterns. Clin Exp Metastasis. 2019;36(2):109–18.

70. Barnhill R, et al. Replacement and desmoplastic histopathological growth patterns: a pilot study of prediction of outcome in patients with uveal melanoma liver metastases. J Pathol Clin Res. 2018;4(4):227–40.

71. Wilmott J, et al. Angiotropism is an independent predictor of microscopic satellites in primary cutaneous melanoma. Histopathology. 2012;61(5):889–98.

72. Barnhill R, Dy K, Lugassy C. Angiotropism in cutaneous melanoma: a prognostic factor strongly predicting risk for metastasis. J Invest Dermatol. 2002;119(3):705–6.

73. Bald T, et al. Ultraviolet-radiation-induced inflammation promotes angiotropism and metastasis in melanoma. Nature. 2014;507(7490):109–13.

74. Eefsen RL, et al. Growth pattern of colorectal liver metastasis as a marker of recurrence risk. Clin Exp Metastasis. 2015;32(4):369–81.

75. Winkler F. Hostile takeover: how tumours hijack pre-existing vascular environments to thrive. J Pathol. 2017;242(3):267–72.

76. Lu J, et al. Endothelial cells promote the colorectal cancer stem cell phenotype through a soluble form of Jagged-1. Cancer Cell. 2013;23(2):171–85.

77. Gilbert LA, Hemann MT. DNA damage-mediated induction of a chemoresistant niche. Cell. 2010;143(3):355–66.

78. Jain RK. Normalizing tumor microenvironment to treat cancer: bench to bedside to biomarkers. J Clin Oncol. 2013;31(17):2205–18.

79. Rockwell S, et al. Hypoxia and radiation therapy: past history, ongoing research, and future promise. Curr Mol Med. 2009;9(4):442–58.

80. Donnem T, et al. Vessel co-option in primary human tumors and metastases: an obstacle to effective anti-angiogenic treatment? Cancer Med. 2013;2(4):427–36.

81. Vermeulen PB, et al. Liver metastases from colorectal adenocarcinomas grow in three patterns with different angiogenesis and desmoplasia. J Pathol. 2001;195(3):336–42.

82. Van den Eynden GG, et al. The histological growth pattern of colorectal cancer liver metastases has prognostic value. Clin Exp Metastasis. 2012;29(6):541–9.

83. Brunner SM, et al. Prognosis according to histochemical analysis of liver metastases removed at liver resection. Br J Surg. 2014;101(13):1681–91.

84. Scherer HJ. Structural development in gliomas. Am J Cancer Res 1938.

85. Scherer HJ. The forms of growth in gliomas and their practical significance. Brain 1940.

86. Bernsen H, et al. Gliomatosis cerebri: quantitative proof of vessel recruitment by cooptation instead of angiogenesis. J Neurosurg. 2005;103(4):702–6.

87. Claes A, Idema AJ, Wesseling P. Diffuse glioma growth: a guerilla war. Acta Neuropathol. 2007;114(5):443–58.

88. Weiss SA, et al. Melanoma brain metastases have lower T-cell content and microvessel density compared to matched extracranial metastases. J Neuro-Oncol 2020.

89. Jubb AM, et al. Vascular phenotypes in primary non-small cell lung carcinomas and matched brain metastases. Br J Cancer. 2011;104(12):1877–81.

90. Caspani EM, et al. Glioblastoma: a pathogenic crosstalk between tumor cells and pericytes. PLoS One. 2014;9(7):e101402.

91. Lyle LT, et al. Alterations in pericyte subpopulations are associated with elevated blood-tumor barrier permeability in experimental brain metastasis of breast cancer. Clin Cancer Res. 2016;22(21):5287–99.

92. Nagano N, et al. Invasion of experimental rat brain tumor: early morphological changes following microinjection of C6 glioma cells. Acta Neuropathol. 1993;86(2):117–25.

93. Lugassy C, et al. Pericytic-like angiotropism of glioma and melanoma cells. Am J Dermatopathol. 2002;24(6):473–8.

94. Watkins S, et al. Disruption of astrocyte-vascular coupling and the blood-brain barrier by invading glioma cells. Nat Commun. 2014;5:4196.

95. Cheng L, et al. Glioblastoma stem cells generate vascular pericytes to support vessel function and tumor growth. Cell. 2013;153(1):139–52.

96. Kienast Y, et al. Real-time imaging reveals the single steps of brain metastasis formation. Nat Med. 2010;16(1):116–22.

97. Bentolila LA, et al. Imaging of angiotropism/vascular co-option in a murine model of brain melanoma: implications for melanoma progression along extravascular pathways. Sci Rep. 2016;6:23834.

98. Berghoff AS, et al. Invasion patterns in brain metastases of solid cancers. Neuro-Oncology. 2013;15(12):1664–72.

99. Siam L, et al. The metastatic infiltration at the metastasis/brain parenchyma-interface is very heterogeneous and has a significant impact on survival in a prospective study. Oncotarget. 2015;6(30):29254–67.

100. Hung T, et al. Angiotropism in primary cutaneous melanoma with brain metastasis: a study of 20 cases. Am J Dermatopathol. 2013;35(6):650–4.

101. Gerstner ER, et al. VEGF inhibitors in the treatment of cerebral edema in patients with brain cancer. Nat Rev Clin Oncol. 2009;6(4):229–36.

102. Cho JH, et al. AKT1 activation promotes development of melanoma metastases. Cell Rep. 2015;13(5):898–905.

103. Kato M, et al. Transgenic mouse model for skin malignant melanoma. Oncogene. 1998;17(14):1885–8.

104. Meuwissen R, et al. Induction of small cell lung cancer by somatic inactivation of both Trp53 and Rb1 in a conditional mouse model. Cancer Cell. 2003;4(3):181–9.

105. Carbonell WS, et al. The vascular basement membrane as "soil" in brain metastasis. PLoS One. 2009;4(6):e5857.

106. Er EE, et al. Pericyte-like spreading by disseminated cancer cells activates YAP and MRTF for metastatic colonization. Nat Cell Biol. 2018;20(8):966–78.

107. Bentolila NY, et al. Intravital imaging of human melanoma cells in the mouse ear skin by two-photon excitation microscopy. Methods Mol Biol. 2018;1755:223–32.

108. Valiente M, et al. Serpins promote cancer cell survival and vascular co-option in brain metastasis. Cell. 2014;156(5):1002–16.

109. Kusters B, et al. Vascular endothelial growth factor-A(165) induces progression of melanoma brain metastases without induction of sprouting angiogenesis. Cancer Res. 2002;62(2):341–5.

110. Winkler F, et al. Imaging glioma cell invasion in vivo reveals mechanisms of dissemination and peritumoral angiogenesis. Glia. 2009;57(12):1306–15.

111. Yadav VN, et al. CXCR4 increases in-vivo glioma perivascular invasion, and reduces radiation induced apoptosis: a genetic knockdown study. Oncotarget. 2016;7(50):83701–19.

112. Voutouri C, et al. Experimental and computational analyses reveal dynamics of tumor vessel cooption and optimal treatment strategies. Proc Natl Acad Sci USA. 2019;116(7):2662–71.

113. Griveau A, et al. A glial signature and Wnt7 signaling regulate glioma-vascular interactions and tumor microenvironment. Cancer Cell. 2018;33(5):874–889 e7.

114. Montana V, Sontheimer H. Bradykinin promotes the chemotactic invasion of primary brain tumors. J Neurosci. 2011;31(13):4858–67.

115. Wang S, et al. JAK2-binding long noncoding RNA promotes breast cancer brain metastasis. J Clin Invest. 2017;127(12):4498–515.

116. Lorger M, Felding-Habermann B. Capturing changes in the brain microenvironment during initial steps of breast cancer brain metastasis. Am J Pathol. 2010;176(6):2958–71.

117. Fan J, et al. Integrin beta4 signaling promotes mammary tumor cell adhesion to brain microvascular endothelium by inducing ErbB2-mediated secretion of VEGF. Ann Biomed Eng. 2011;39(8):2223–41.

118. Yao H, et al. Leukaemia hijacks a neural mechanism to invade the central nervous system. Nature. 2018;560(7716):55–60.

119. Szabo V, et al. Mechanism of tumour vascularization in experimental lung metastases. J Pathol. 2015;235(3):384–96.

120. International Consensus Group for Hepatocellular NeoplasiaThe International Consensus Group for Hepatocellular, N., Pathologic diagnosis of early hepatocellular carcinoma: a report of the international consensus group for hepatocellular neoplasia. Hepatology. 2009;49(2):658–64.

121. Terayama N, Terada T, Nakanuma Y. Histologic growth patterns of metastatic carcinomas of the liver. Jpn J Clin Oncol. 1996;26(1):24–9.

122. Rodewald AK, et al. Eight autopsy cases of melanoma brain metastases showing angiotropism and pericytic mimicry. Implications for extravascular migratory metastasis. J Cutan Pathol. 2019;46(8):570–8.

123. Spanberger T, et al. Extent of peritumoral brain edema correlates with prognosis, tumoral growth pattern, HIF1a expression and angiogenic activity in patients with single brain metastases. Clin Exp Metastasis. 2013;30(4):357–68.

124. Bardehle S, Rafalski VA, Akassoglou K. Breaking boundaries-coagulation and fibrinolysis at the neurovascular interface. Front Cell Neurosci. 2015;9:354.

125. Kozlowski C, Weimer RM. An automated method to quantify microglia morphology and application to monitor activation state longitudinally in vivo. PLoS One. 2012;7(2):e31814.

126. Lugassy C, et al. Angiotropism, pericytic mimicry and extravascular migratory metastasis: an embryogenesis-derived program of tumor spread. Angiogenesis. 2020;23(1):27–41.

127. Lugassy C, et al. Could pericytic mimicry represent another type of melanoma cell plasticity with embryonic properties? Pigment Cell Melanoma Res. 2013;26(5):746–54.

128. Bailey CM, Morrison JA, Kulesa PM. Melanoma revives an embryonic migration program to promote plasticity and invasion. Pigment Cell Melanoma Res. 2012;25(5):573–83.

129. Lugassy C, et al. Gene expression profiling of human angiotropic primary melanoma: selection of 15 differentially expressed genes potentially involved in extravascular migratory metastasis. Eur J Cancer. 2011;47(8):1267–75.

130. Lugassy C, et al. Pilot study on "pericytic mimicry" and potential embryonic/stem cell properties of angiotropic melanoma cells interacting with the abluminal vascular surface. Cancer Microenviron. 2013;6(1):19–29.

131. Kulesa PM, et al. Reprogramming metastatic melanoma cells to assume a neural crest cell-like phenotype in an embryonic microenvironment. Proc Natl Acad Sci USA. 2006;103(10):3752–7.

132. Tsai HH, et al. Oligodendrocyte precursors migrate along vasculature in the developing nervous system. Science. 2016;351(6271):379–84.

133. Calabrese C, et al. A perivascular niche for brain tumor stem cells. Cancer Cell. 2007;11(1):69–82.

134. Goldman SA, Chen Z. Perivascular instruction of cell genesis and fate in the adult brain. Nat Neurosci. 2011;14(11):1382–9.

135. Ghajar CM, et al. The perivascular niche regulates breast tumour dormancy. Nat Cell Biol. 2013;15(7):807–17.

136. Seifert S, Sontheimer H. Bradykinin enhances invasion of malignant glioma into the brain parenchyma by inducing cells to undergo amoeboid migration. J Physiol. 2014;592(22):5109–27.

137. Zagzag D, et al. Hypoxia- and vascular endothelial growth factor-induced stromal cell-derived factor-1alpha/CXCR4 expression in glioblastomas: one plausible explanation of Scherer's structures. Am J Pathol. 2008;173(2):545–60.

138. Pham K, et al. VEGFR inhibitors upregulate CXCR4 in VEGF receptor-expressing glioblastoma in a TGFbetaR signaling-dependent manner. Cancer Lett. 2015;360(1):60–7.

139. Sharma I, et al. IL-8/CXCR1/2 signalling promotes tumor cell proliferation, invasion and vascular mimicry in glioblastoma. J Biomed Sci. 2018;25(1):62.

140. McCoy MG, et al. Endothelial cells promote 3D invasion of GBM by IL-8-dependent induction of cancer stem cell properties. Sci Rep. 2019;9(1):9069.

141. Infanger DW, et al. Glioblastoma stem cells are regulated by inter-leukin-8 signaling in a tumoral perivascular niche. Cancer Res. 2013;73(23):7079–89.

142. Lindberg OR, et al. GBM heterogeneity as a function of variable epidermal growth factor receptor variant III activity. Oncotarget. 2016;7(48):79101–16.

143. Auf G, et al. Inositol-requiring enzyme 1alpha is a key regulator of angiogenesis and invasion in malignant glioma. Proc Natl Acad Sci USA. 2010;107(35):15553–8.

144. Jabouille A, et al. Glioblastoma invasion and cooption depend on IRE1alpha endoribonuclease activity. Oncotarget. 2015;6(28):24922–34.

145. Krusche B, et al. EphrinB2 drives perivascular invasion and proliferation of glioblastoma stem-like cells. elife 2016;5.

146. Le Joncour V, et al. Vulnerability of invasive glioblastoma cells to lysosomal membrane destabilization. EMBO Mol Med 2019;11(6).

147. Miles D, et al. Bevacizumab plus paclitaxel versus placebo plus paclitaxel as first-line therapy for HER2-negative metastatic breast cancer (MERiDiAN): a double-blind placebo-controlled randomised phase III trial with prospective biomarker evaluation. Eur J Cancer. 2017;70:146–55.

148. Bais C, et al. Tumor microvessel density as a potential predictive marker for bevacizumab benefit: GOG-0218 biomarker analyses. J Natl Cancer Inst 2017;109(11).

149. Tolaney SM, et al. Role of vascular density and normalization in response to neoadjuvant bevacizumab and chemotherapy in breast cancer patients. Proc Natl Acad Sci USA. 2015;112(46):14325–30.

150. Perakis S, Speicher MR. Emerging concepts in liquid biopsies. BMC Med. 2017;15(1):75.

151. Lambin P, et al. Radiomics: the bridge between medical imaging and personalized medicine. Nat Rev Clin Oncol. 2017;14(12):749–62.

152. Cheng J, et al. Prediction of histopathologic growth patterns of colorectal liver metastases with a noninvasive imaging method. Ann Surg Oncol. 2019;26(13):4587–98.

Biomarker Panels and Contemporary Practice in Clinical Trials of Personalized Medicine

33

Nina Louise Jebsen, Irini Ktoridou-Valen, and Bjørn Tore Gjertsen

Abstract

Development of cancer therapy follows three main pathways: mutation-driven drug development, immunomodulatory therapy, and evolution of conventional chemo- and radiotherapy. All these therapeutic modalities require more precise biomarkers, not only for increasing accuracy and enhancing efficiency but also to avoid unnecessary toxicity for the patients and societal costs. In clinical trials, there is an increasing use of biomarker panels for risk stratification and therapy guidance. Heterogeneity in tumor biology leads to specific clinical manifestations and may provide guidance on the direction of future biomarker-tailored therapy. Here, we will use acute leukemia and sarcoma as examples, tumors originating from progenitors of hematopoietic or mesenchymal origin, respectively.

Single biomarkers, in particular genetic mutations, have been tested to optimize therapy with only limited success. Combining biomarkers of different nature may provide clinically relevant and robust panels that can be used in clinical trials in acute leukemia and soft tissue sarcoma, and hopefully other tumors. For simplifying biomarker approaches, functional subdivision of cancers into defined subsets may be the most promising path to provide molecular personalized therapy that optimally benefits the patient. We will exemplify the use of biomarkers in late- and early-phase clinical trials and illustrate how biomarker panels may assist in pivotal decision-making.

Take-Home Lessons

- Exploitation of comprehensive biomarker panels in early-phase clinical trials utilizing adaptive study designs may facilitate real-time decision-making during therapy.
- In leukemia, panels of markers including assessment of minimal residual disease are used to select intermediate-risk patients between allogeneic and autologous hematopoietic stem cell transplantation.
- An ongoing national study of Norwegian sarcoma patients applying a panel of 900 gene aberrations will provide insight into molecular mechanism which may be further exploited as targets for new therapeutic drugs.
- Improved understanding of the complex interplay between cancer cells and the microenvironment provides better characterization of the multistep development and progression of malignant tumors.
- Molecular biomarkers reflecting tumor progression or response to therapy serve as surrogate endpoints in assessment of clinical outcomes of personalized cancer therapy.
- The tumor microenvironment has been attributed an increasingly important role in understanding radiobiological effects, which are investigated in novel treatment designs applying targeted drugs and immunotherapy in order to augment radiation effects.

N. L. Jebsen · I. Ktoridou-Valen
University of Bergen, Bergen, Norway
e-mail: nina.louise.jebsen@helse-bergen.no;
irini.ktoridou-valen@helse-bergen.no

B. T. Gjertsen (✉)
Haukeland University Hospital, Bergen, Norway
e-mail: bjorn.gjertsen@uib.no

Introduction

Molecularly targeted therapeutics are less likely to be successful in large disease populations. Rather, a tailored approach is required [1]. This is a reality for the three main fields of cancer therapy development: (1) mutation-driven drug design, (2) immunomodulatory therapy, and (3) further improvement of conventional cancer surgery and chemo- and radiotherapy [2, 3]. Meta-analysis of selected oncology trials has indicated that a personalized, targeted therapy approach to treatment has better outcomes than non-personalized and cytotoxic agent regimes [3]. We see indications that advanced pathway analyses with identification of master regulators or functional genomics may represent alternative avenues for therapy individualization [4]. However, these methodologies need to be more mature and robust before they can be applied on a larger scale [5–7]. In parallel with the emerging precision medicine development, we also see improvement of conventional therapy principles including novel chemotherapeutics, antimetabolites, and improved radiation therapy [8, 9]. The experience with responders of conventional therapy, sometimes extraordinary responders [10], indicate that there may be molecular features that may be used as biomarkers for response [11]. The incentives for the development of such biomarkers for conventional therapy are limited [12].

It is clear that the molecular heterogeneity of human cancers and the ability to characterize this heterogeneity through next-generation sequencing techniques present new opportunities for the development of more effective treatments as well as challenges for the design and analysis of clinical trials. Simultaneously, understanding the importance of the tumor microenvironment has been accelerating. The microenvironment must be considered an intrinsic part of a malignant tumor [13]. Stromal fibroblasts and leukocytes are manipulated by cancer cells to facilitate critical steps in infiltration and metastasis by degrading extracellular matrix and providing a nurturing environment as well as to avoid attacks from the immune defense [14, 15]. There are indications that stromal cells activate embryologic transcription factors in cancer cells resulting in production of secretory proteins necessary for adhesion, motility, intercellular communication, angiogenesis, and invasion [13]. Moreover, release of microvesicles (containing both proteins and nucleic acids) plays an important role in cell-to-cell communication necessary for oncogenic transformation [16]. Improved knowledge about the fine-tuned cross talk between cancer cells and the microenvironment may provide better characterization of the multistep disease progression. Stromal cell chemokines involved in differentiation and tumor proliferation may serve as novel targets for oncologic treatment. Similar to the multiclonality of cancer, there are dramatic dynamic variations throughout the landscape of the tumor microenvironment. The abundance of stromal cells or proteinases has been shown to correlate with tumor aggressiveness [17]. Variations in the tumor vasculature and immune suppression contribute to this topographic heterogeneity and may explain differences in response or resistance to cancer therapy.

The use of biomarkers in oncology trial design has been well documented [18–20]. In this chapter, we will present selected examples from acute leukemia and sarcoma, which are two rare and aggressive malignancies characterized by distinct molecular and biological heterogeneity. In addition, we will exemplify adaptive basket design in tumor agnostic trials of immune modulating therapy in rare cancer types. Awareness of the significance of the interplay between cancer cells and tumor microenvironment has led to a paradigm shift also in understanding radiobiology. Hence, it is reasonable to reflect efforts to remodel radiation treatment by targeting the tumor microenvironment.

Based on these examples, we will discuss the use of multiple biomarkers, or biomarker panels, in the development of targeted cancer therapy. The question that remains unanswered is whether the perfect methodology exists on how to deploy biomarker panels in clinical trials.

Design of Biomarker Panels

A biomarker represents characteristics that are objectively measured and evaluated as an indicator of normal biological processes, pathogenic processes, or pharmacological responses to therapeutic intervention [21]. In addition to risk biomarkers foreseeing potential disease, there are at least three types of biomarkers relevant in clinical trials: diagnostic, prognostic, and predictive biomarkers. Diagnostic biomarkers assess the absence or presence of a disease. Prognostic biomarkers predict the natural progress of a disease and can be used to decide whether a patient should be treated or not. Predictive biomarkers are used to identify a treatment regime that is effective for a subgroup of patients [22]. This chapter will focus on predictive biomarkers and surrogate endpoints.

A clinically significant biomarker is associated with treatment of a patient subpopulation that has historically shown a differential and substantial clinical response, e.g., based on epidemiologic, pathophysiologic, therapeutic, or molecular evidence. Biomarkers include chromosomal aberrations and genomic alterations, such as deletions, insertions, mutations, or polymorphisms of DNA, as well as proteins, metabolomic patterns, histology, imaging, clinical observations, or even self-reported patient surveys. In some cases, a biomarker represents a bridge between understanding the mechanisms of preclinical findings and the observed clinical findings.

An important implication of the human genome project followed by the genomics projects in cancer is the mapping of recurrent mutations in cancer, where maybe 50% of the patients may comprise actionable mutations in their tumor

[19, 23]. Enrolment in clinical trials may reduce this to 20%, and as few as 5% may respond to a genomic approach to targeted therapy [19, 24]. However, some of the most important discoveries following next-generation sequencing are not necessarily identifying targeted therapy but provide an improved understanding of cancer development, e.g., germ line mutations and genetic susceptibility to pediatric cancer [25], mutations associated with external exposures, such as smoking [26], and, most importantly, the clonal evolution seen in cancers [27, 28]. However, a tempting clinical use of knowledge about these mutations is to direct experimental therapy. Unfortunately, several reports indicate that this has been of limited success in solid cancer, with therapy responses below 10% [19, 24]. Use of molecularly targeted agents outside their indications in patients with solid cancer failed to improve progression-free survival compared with standard treatment regimes.

Biomarker panels may consist of clinical parameters only [29], mutations [24], gene expression profiles [30], or protein expression panels [31]. In cases where the therapeutic impact implies treatment-related mortality or reduced overall survival such as in pediatric leukemia and in the decision-making of allogeneic hematopoietic stem cell transplantation (HSCT), the panel is composed of a mix of clinical and molecular markers. Similarly, categorizing the mesenchymal-derived gastrointestinal stromal tumors (GIST) into different risk groups to determine adjuvant treatment with tyrosine kinase inhibitors depends on macroscopic, morphologic, immunohistochemical, and molecular tumor features [32]. In soft tissue sarcoma, the Scandinavian Sarcoma Group (SSG) has pursued a pathway of biomarker-dependent risk stratification in two clinical studies of adjuvant chemotherapy (SSG XIII and SSG XX; see www.ssg-org.net). In order to meticulously select patient to undergo toxic treatment, prognostic tumor characteristics such as size, growth pattern, pleomorphic appearance, vascular invasion, mitotic count, and tumor necrosis have been systematically recorded since 1998 [33, 34]. An important feature of these panels is that they are developed carefully, stepwise, and over many years. This lengthy development is frustrating for the patients and for the physicians treating advanced cancer. However, attempts to shorten this development phase have so far shown limited success [24].

Biomarkers in Cancer Research

Biomarkers are biological features that can be used as diagnostic indicators and predictors for disease trajectory and therapy response [35]. Typical biomarkers used in cancer research are genetic alterations or proteins expressed by the tumor itself or in peripheral blood circulation. An emerging field of research is the investigation of biomarkers in the peripheral blood, including cell-free nucleic acids (eventually enveloped in cellular-derived microvesicles). Such liquid biopsies also include circulating tumor cells and endothelial cells derived from the tumor locations [36]. Designated biomarkers that assess the effect of a treatment by substituting clinical endpoints are called surrogate endpoints.

Survival rates are used as a measure of success in cancer therapy development. Overall survival is the final endpoint, with event-free survival as the most successful surrogate endpoint. In cancer with superior survival, overall survival may be a largely irrelevant endpoint and may not provide information about possible detrimental adverse events due to high dose or particular toxic susceptibility of the patients. This is exemplified in chronic-phase chronic myeloid leukemia (CML), where 5-year survival (after diagnosis) is more than 90% after the introduction of targeted kinase inhibitor (TKI) therapy in contrast to 50% 5-year survival before the imatinib era. In CML, quantitative PCR of the pathognomonic fused gene product *BCR-ABL1* is measured in the peripheral blood as a surrogate endpoint and used to accurately determine response and tumor load under therapy. PCR determination allows monitoring of persistent deep or complete molecular response in TKI-treated CML and could facilitate stopping treatment of patients with potentially toxic TKI therapy.

In GIST, the detection of a driving mutation in the c-*KIT* or *PDGFRA* proto-oncogene, which could be effectively targeted with imatinib, has improved the overall survival dramatically since introduced in 2001 [37]. However, wild-type GIST or tumors that harbor *PDGFRA* substitution mutation D842V do not respond to the same extent to imatinib [38]. These cases may demonstrate genetic alterations in downstream intracellular pathways such as *BRAF* and *RAS* or defects in the succinate dehydrogenase (SDH) complex and should be treated accordingly. Extended panels including potential prognostic and predictive genetic markers are therefore crucial in research trials. GIST may respond to sequential treatment with different TKIs, with each drug potentially adding months to the overall survival time. The clinical relevant endpoint to evaluate the efficacy of either one of the drugs is progression-free survival. Detection of molecular markers predicting resistance to a drug has become increasingly important to prevent overtreating cancer patients with toxic compounds. Likewise, overcoming acquired resistance against initially effective treatment remains a challenge. A new strategy to prevent drug-related induction of resilient cancer cells is to predefine alternating treatment targeting different molecular aberrations within the kinase receptors and related signaling pathway. This was investigated in the randomized ALT GIST trial, in which first-line imatinib monotherapy in advanced GIST is compared with imatinib alternating with regorafenib (ClinicalTrials.gov

Identifier: NCT02365441). The primary outcome (progression-free survival) did not reveal any meaningful difference between the groups [39]; however, more information is awaited from analyses of other endpoints.

Proteins involving the tumor microenvironment (TME) may serve as other biomarkers. Osteosarcoma is a rare mesenchymal bone tumor arising in young adults, where tumor development and growth prerequisite degradation of the tumor-hostile bone environment. It has recently been demonstrated that human osteosarcoma cells harbor strong expression of an endocytic collagen receptor (uPARAP/Endo 180), enabling tumor cells to directly mediate bone degradation [40]. Blocking uPARAP/Endo 180 in a murine model using a monoclonal antibody significantly reduced bone destruction, indicating a promising target for improved neoadjuvant therapy.

In some metastatic cancers, there has been limited improvement in survival until the emergence of immunological checkpoint inhibitors [2, 41]. In these cases, a rapid estimation of therapy response by surrogate endpoints may be needed for stratification of responders versus non-responders.

Similar molecular features of different cancers experience a wide range of clinical responses to targeted therapy. Therefore, it is increasingly clear that the tumor cells are highly dependent on their contextual setting [13, 42–44].

Among the most complex environments of a tumor may be the involvement of the gut microbiota, identified as an important co-player in the development of colon cancer [45]. In allogeneic hematopoietic stem cell transplantation, the gut microbiota regulates graft-versus-host reactions of the immune system [46], indicating a role in immunological graft-versus-tumor mechanisms. Along the same line, gut microbiota modulate responses to immunological checkpoint inhibitors in cancer patients and therefore may provide an explanation for some responders and non-responders [47]. Novel biomarkers will increasingly focus on tumor context for therapy selection.

Design of Clinical Trials in Cancer Research

Traditionally, cancer clinical trials are divided into phase I, II, III, and IV (Fig. 33.1). The focus of phase I trials is usually on safety, and the primary objective is to find a maximum tolerated dose for use in subsequent trials. In phase II trials, the primary objective is usually to quickly determine whether the new treatment regime has sufficient efficacy. The use of biomarkers (surrogate endpoints) is important for making early treatment decisions. Phase III trials are designed for establishing definitive clinical benefit, and survival is often used as a primary endpoint. Despite the divi-

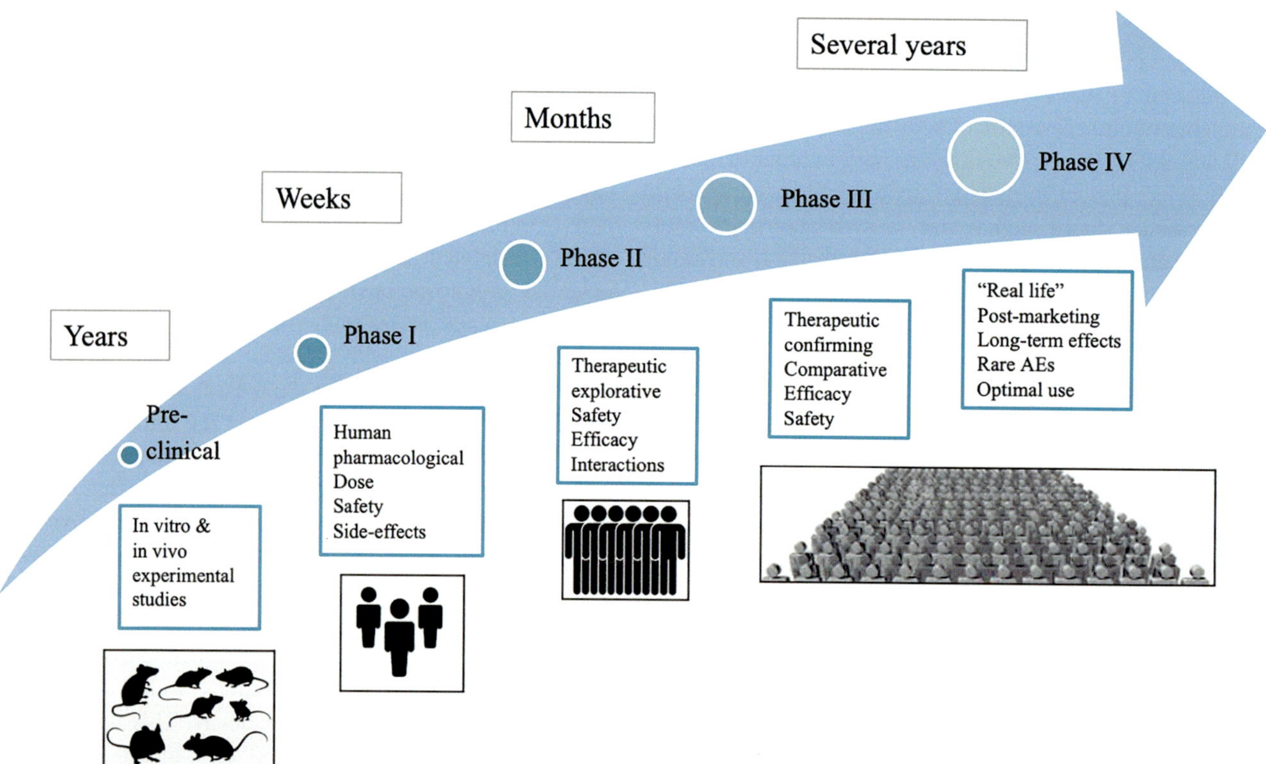

Fig. 33.1 Advancement through different phases in clinical trials

sion of trials into different phases, clinical trials should not be seen as distinct entities. Due to the failure rate of approximately 20% in phase III for approval of new cancer therapies, trial design and the strict trial phase design have been challenged [48]. There are now examples of phase Ib studies with expansion cohorts of patients numbering more than 1000 patients and where the US Food and Drug Administration (FDA) has used these data for a fast-track approval. It is important to design trials in the context of an extended scientific process that starts first with human trials and, if the process is not discontinued due to lack of sustained efficacy or safety problems, ends with a new treatment or medicine on the market. At the same time, a new therapeutic molecule may represent only a modest incremental improvement in one group of patients, while others may have an outstanding response. This is observed in the use of kinase inhibitors in sarcoma versus CML [49–51] and the use of immunological checkpoint inhibitors in non-small cell lung carcinoma versus Hodgkin's disease [52, 53]. Use of various trial designs will be needed to develop the full potential of a therapeutic molecule.

Clinical trial design for oncology studies can broadly be categorized into rule-based and model-based designs. Rule-based designs are often used in early-phase (I/II) cancer trials. A small number of patients start with an initial dose, and the occurrence of unacceptable dose-limiting toxicity (DLT) determines, based on prespecified rules, the dose for the next group of patients. Commonly used designs are the single- and two-stage up-and-down designs and optimal/flexible multiple-stage designs; see Chow and Liu [54]. The use of rule-based designs in early trials is appealing since they allow minimized exposure of patients to doses with unacceptable DLT. These designs can however be suboptimal from a statistical standpoint resulting in low efficiency. Model-based designs are usually more efficient. They employ statistical dose-response models to guide the dose-finding process and for estimating the effect (safety or efficacy) at different doses of the new investigational drug.

Clinical Trials for Targeted Therapy

The altered focus from cytotoxic agents to targeted therapy and predictive biomarkers has called for a shift from the classical paradigm in phase I studies where the primary focus is on safety (MTD) and phase II studies with primary focus on efficacy (see Mandrekar et al. [55]). Within the new targeted therapy paradigm, the focus is on identifying molecularly defined subgroups of patients who will benefit from the targeted therapy and on understanding the drug activity for these patients. Novel designs have been developed, in which predictive biomarkers play a central role. Among these are

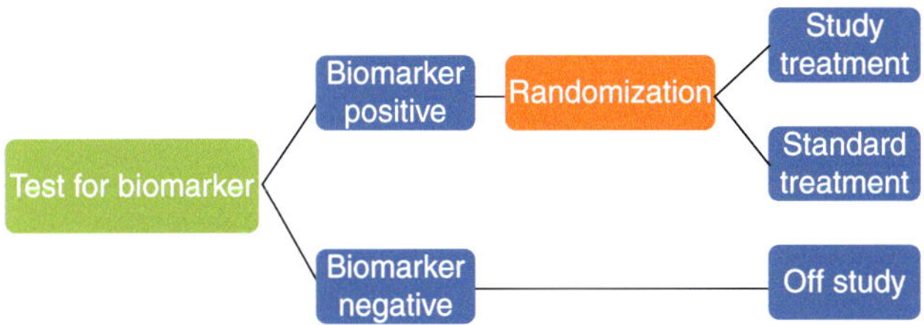

Fig. 33.2 Enrichment design, i.e., only biomarker positive patients are recruited into the clinical trial to receive experimental treatment

enrichment, adaptive, umbrella, and basket designs. Brief descriptions of these designs are given below.

Enrichment Designs

Enrichment designs involve diagnostic tests that are used to identify which patients are positive for a biomarker and thereby eligible for the trial (Fig. 33.2). The eligible patients are then randomized to either a test group or a control group. Obviously, enrichment designs are most appropriate when patients who are biomarker negative are unlikely to benefit from the new treatment. Non-eligible patients are spared from adverse events, and overall safety of the trial is increased. Moreover, because the focus is on a targeted subgroup of patients, enrichment designs have high efficiency meaning smaller patient groups, faster trials, and hence overall cost reduction [56]. Sometimes the biomarker negative patients can be included in a later separate study for the same treatment, but this is only meaningful if the treatment has proven to be successful for the targeted patients and if there is a reason to believe that biomarker negative patients could benefit as well. Before enrichment designs are employed, it is important that the mechanism of the predictive biomarker is well understood. Enrichment designs are hence most appropriate in late phases of cancer drug development.

Umbrella Designs

Umbrella designs consist of two or more cohorts or substudies, e.g., two enrichment designs connected through a uniform initial screening procedure. Patients are screened for predictive biomarkers and allocated into different cohorts (Fig. 33.3). Patients in cohort 1 are positive with respect to biomarker 1, patients in cohort 2 are positive with respect to biomarker 2, etc. Patients that are negative for all of the defined biomarkers may be allocated to a separate cohort. Within each of the biomarker positive cohorts, patients are randomized to a targeted agent or a control group. Umbrella

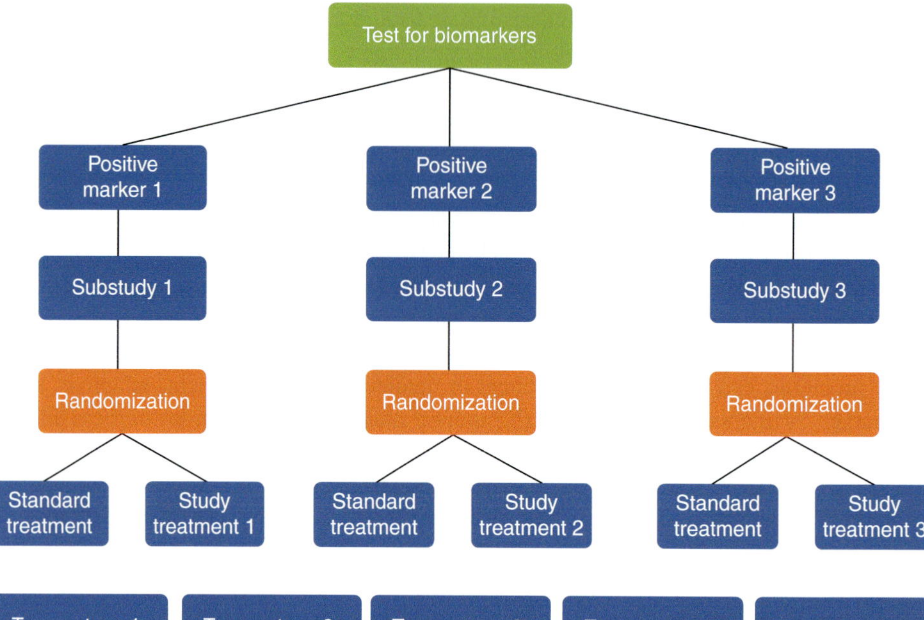

Fig. 33.3 Umbrella design, i.e., patients are screened for biomarkers and allocated into different marker-dependent substudies (different treatments) with subsequent randomization (study drug versus standard treatment)

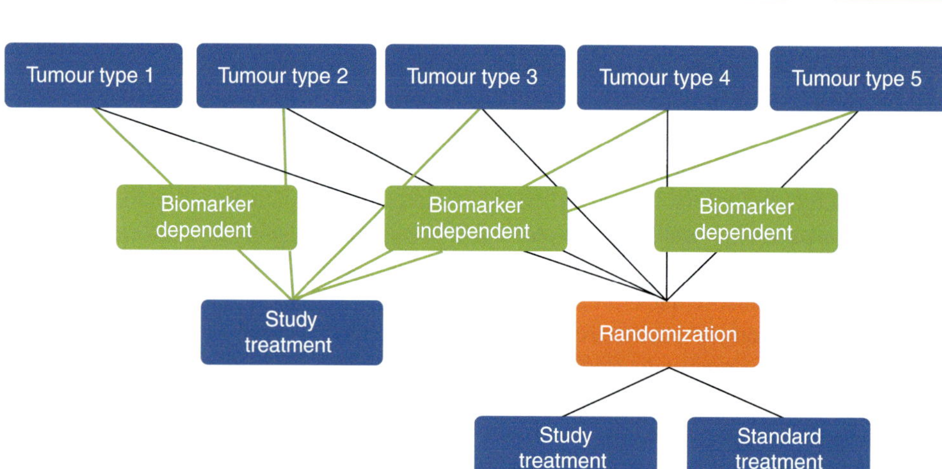

Fig. 33.4 Basket design, i.e., multiple cohorts based on different tumor types or biomarker status are given the same experimental treatment, with or without randomization

designs can be very useful, in particular, when a large number of patients are screened for low-prevalence biomarkers. As with enrichment designs, it is important that there is a strong rationale for using predictive biomarkers. These studies can be exploratory and have been used in different phases of drug development. The umbrella designs usually focus on a single histology or tumor subtype.

Basket Designs

Different from umbrella designs, the basket designs are often used when several tumors or histological types are under investigation. Basket designs are of an explorative nature and can be appropriate for phase I targeted therapy studies.

Patients are first screened and then allocated to cohorts depending on cancer type and molecular profile (Fig. 33.4). All patients within a cohort are then given the same targeted treatment.

Adaptive and Optimal Designs

Clinical trials are sequential in nature, and as a trial progresses, increasing amounts of data and information become available. The FDA has published guidance on adaptive design both for drugs and medical device clinical studies [57]. Adaptive designs allow a flexible approach to clinical trials enabling study teams to modify the design during the recruitment phase. Bayesian decision rules enable optimiza-

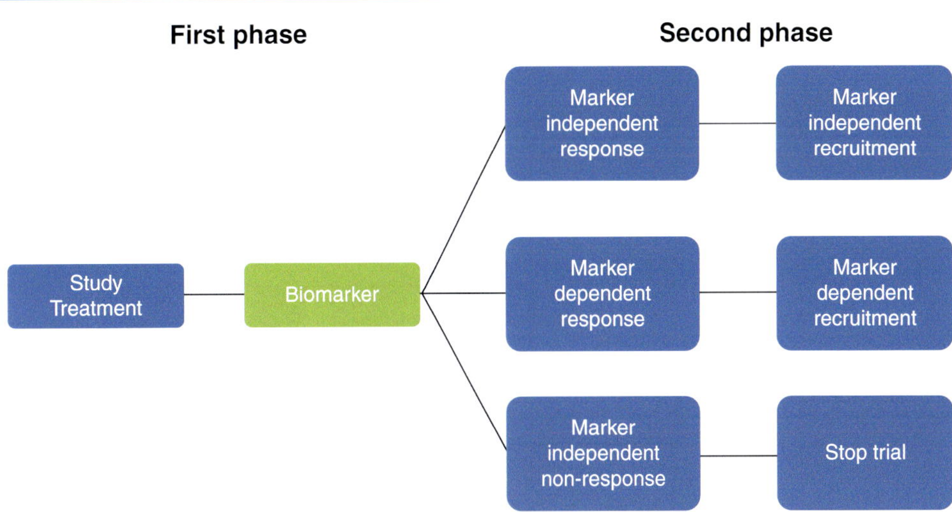

Fig. 33.5 Adaptive design, i.e., modifying the design during the recruitment phase by optimizing trial parameters based on interim analyses of treatment outcomes up-to-date cumulative knowledge, and the use of surrogate endpoints together with early stopping rules can shorten the study period [59, 60]

tion of trial parameters based on real-time data at defined intervals to determine patient pathways in a "learn-as-you-go" principle [58]. The hope is that the FDA guidance will encourage the proper use of adaptive designs, reducing resource requirements and increasing the chance of study success and regulatory compliance. Optimal design theory can be used to find the most efficient designs. Adaptive designs and Bayesian analysis (Fig. 33.5) are employed to utilize the most up-to-date cumulative knowledge, and the use of surrogate endpoints together with early stopping rules can shorten the study period.

Combining Clinical Trial Designs in Immunotherapy

The intratumoral heterogeneity remains a considerable obstacle to the implementation of efficient anticancer therapies. The quantity and quality of immune cells within the tumor microenvironment (TME) has been positively correlated to prognosis, for example, abundance of tumor-infiltrating lymphocytes (TILs), and especially CD8+ T cells, has been recognized as a predictive marker.

Immunoscoring in colorectal cancer was recently established by a collaborative group [61]. Infiltration of T cells in the TME represents "hot tumors," implying that tumor development is antagonized by the host immune response, as opposed to "cold" and non-immunogenic tumors in which T cell infiltration is absent. Antibodies targeting the inhibitory receptors CTLA4 and PD1 (checkpoint inhibitors) have shown promising efficacy in several but not all types of cancer and only subsets of patients experience clinical benefit where *preexistence* of TILs is considered to contribute to clinical response [62]. Patients lacking TILs may therefore require therapeutic interventions to prime the T cell response to enable clinical benefit of checkpoint inhibitor therapy.

Immune-modulatory approaches such as intratumoral injections of oncolytic peptides hold the potential to enhance immune-mediated anticancer activity [63] and can lead to even more effective treatment combined with immune checkpoint inhibitors (ICIs). Preclinical data has demonstrated marked impact of the membranolytic peptide LTX-315 on the TME by exposure of danger-associated molecular pattern molecules (DAMPs) subsequently inducing immunogenic cell death [64].

A dose-escalating phase I study of the oncolytic peptide LTX-315 (Clinical trial NCT01986426) illustrates an adaptive, multi-arm basket design comprising a broad panel of biomarkers in both blood and tissue samples [65]. In the initial stage multiple cohorts of different tumor types, non-biomarker dependent, received LTX-315 either sequentially or concurrently. Posttreatment biopsies demonstrated necrosis and increased CD8+ cell infiltration of the TME in 86% of the cases supervened by expansion of tumor-associated T cell clones in peripheral blood. Tumor volume regression was evident in 29% of the patients. The first patient with desmoid tumor treated with intratumoral injections of LTX-315 resulted in tumor regression of the thoracic wall lesion. A marked increase of CD8+ TILs in the lesion was accompanied by upregulation of immune gene signature (including effector T cell, T-helper type 1 cell, chemokine, and cytokine genes). These changes were followed by gradual symptom relief and long-term disease stabilization, indicating clinical benefit [66]. The second stage comprised three arms (A, B, C); arm A representing continuation of monotherapy in various histologically indifferent subtypes; arm B recruiting patients with melanoma receiving combination therapy of LTX-315 with intravenous ipilimumab; and arm C recruiting patients with triple negative breast cancer receiving LTX-315 in combination with intravenous pembrolizumab (Fig. 33.6). This two-stage adaptive trial scheme nicely integrates basket design and enrichment design subcohorts, also

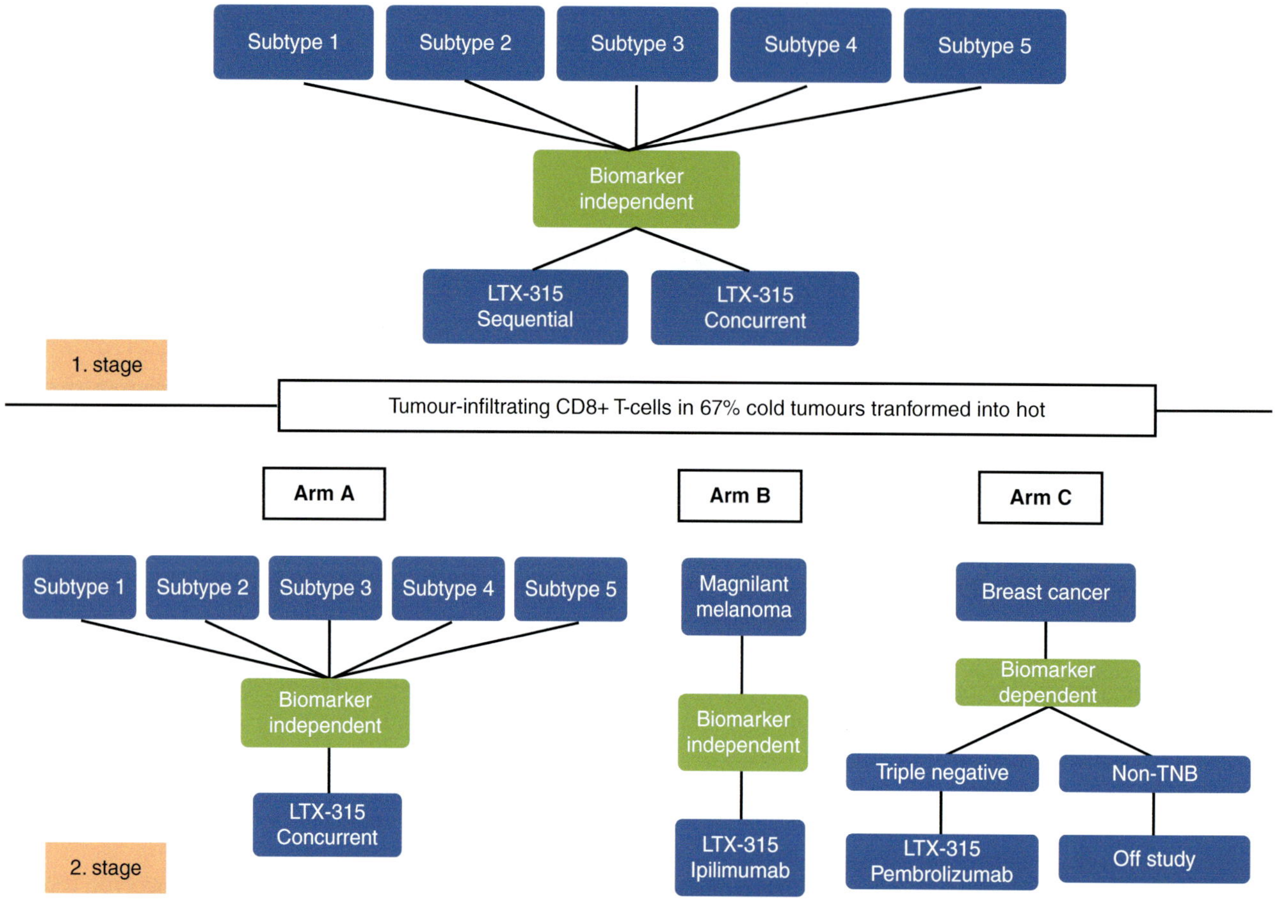

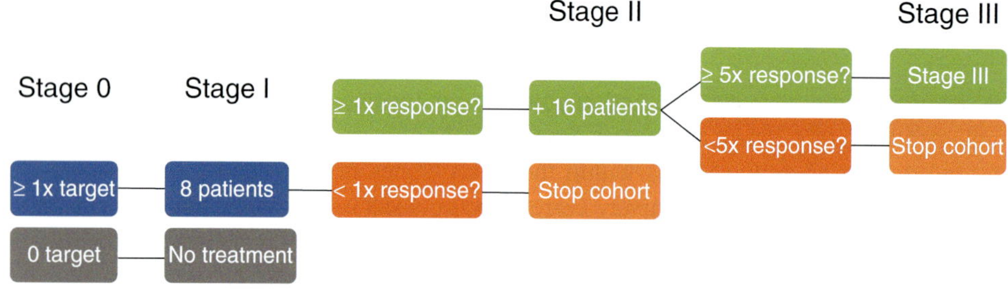

Fig. 33.6 Adaptive design in a phase I basket-trial of intratumoral LTX-315 monotherapy (stage I) refined to a triple arm trial integrating different combination therapies in two restricted cohorts (stage II) following real-time data analyses of biomarker predictabilities

Fig. 33.7 IMPRESS study design. Simon's two-stage model of expanding cohorts integrates basket design (within every cohort) in an overall umbrella design (multiple parallel cohorts). Given that a minimum 1 of 8 patients in a stage I cohort respond, the cohort is extended with another 16 patients (stage II). Five or more responses in total 24 patients (stage I + stage II) suggest further investigation (stage III) in an expansion cohort in order to confirm clinical benefit. Inadequate numbers of meaningful responses lead to cohort cessation

embodying a shift towards marker-dependent recruitment delineated from real-time biomarker-investigations.

Another example of combining study designs in clinical trials is the Drug Rediscovery protocol study [67], designed to effectively test a set of existing drugs using a precision medicine algorithm while minimizing the number of patients required. Efficacy of approved drugs outside indication is tested in patients with advanced cancer. Each tumor type/variant/drug treatment defines a separate cohort. This is a prospective, open-label, non-randomized combined basket, and umbrella trial. Patients will be enrolled into multiple parallel cohorts, each defined by one tumor type, one tumor profile, and one study drug. Patients will be treated with commercially available targeted anticancer drugs and can be included in treatment cohorts defined by a mutation, gene-fusion, a molecular profile (i.e., BRCA-ness), protein expression, or larger genomic alterations. Several similar projects have been initiated, including IMPRESS-Norway (Fig. 33.7).

Biomarker Panels in Late-phase Trials of Hematopoietic-derived Blood Cancer: Acute Lymphoblastic and Acute Myeloid Leukemia

The Nordic pediatric trial of acute lymphoblastic leukemia (ALL; NOPHO ALL 2008) represents the standard therapy for patients in the age group 1–45 years in Iceland, Finland, Denmark, Lithuania, Norway, and Sweden. Patients are stratified into three categories: normal, intermediate, and high risk for relapse. Therapy intensity is adjusted according to risk stratification [68]. This risk stratification is guided by a panel of markers, including white blood cell counts [69] and advanced flow cytometric determination of leukemic cell remnants, so-called minimal residual disease (MRD), after treatment. The impact of the biomarker panel in this trial is significant due to the increased toxicity experienced in the high-risk arm of therapy.

The Dutch hemato-oncology network (HOVON) has, in collaboration with the Swiss oncology society (SAKK), been running larger randomized phase III trials in acute myeloid leukemia (AML) patients 18–65 years of age [70]. The latter trials have incorporated an increasing number of molecular markers [71]. Not only have the presence of such markers been used but also have exclusion of high-risk markers, e.g., the length mutation or internal tandem repeat in the juxta-membranous domain of the receptor tyrosine kinase FLT3. Like for NOPHO, a panel of markers has been formed to guide therapy, using flow cytometry-based minimal residual disease assessment (MRD) or NPM1 mutation-specific quantitative PCR. MRD is used to select intermediate-risk patients between allogeneic and autologous hematopoietic stem cell transplantation. For the patients, this implicates careful selection between two cellular immunotherapies with large differences in mortality. Therapy-related mortality is below 5% in autologous HSCT, while approximates 20% in allogeneic HSCT [72].

The use of single-gene mutations has been used in adult and older AML to guide therapy. The molecular target FLT3 has been explored since 2000 but the results of FLT3-targeted therapy have been limited or even detrimental for the experimental group [73]. The third-generation FLT3 targeting agent quizartinib (AC-220) has been shown to have effect both in FLT3-mutated patients and to a certain degree in FLT3 wild-type AML cases. A phosphoproteomics panel examining proteins in AML cells has indicated a distinction between responders and non-responders independent of the FLT3-ITD status [74].

Based on the heterogeneity of most aggressive cancers, it is maybe a surprise that single biomarkers are able to predict therapy responses. Failure of FLT3-ITD to determine successful inhibitor therapy is likely from a biological perspective, even before we examine the quality and efficiency of the inhibitors. One of the important questions that arise is how an ideal biomarker panel could be constructed.

Biomarker Panels in Early-phase Trials of Mesenchymal-derived Cancer: Sarcoma

Mesenchymal stem cells or progenitor cells of connective tissues represent the origin of sarcomas, a rare heterogeneous group of diseases often with a specific morphology and a clearly defined macro- and microanatomical location [75, 76]. Many of the various subtypes of sarcoma are characterized by defined chromosome translocations, recurrent gene amplifications, and mutations.

Clinical trials have taken advantage of the defined genetic features and are testing targeted therapy based on the signaling pathways involved. Multidimensional analysis of biomarkers for future prognostic classifiers that reflect inter- and intra-tumor heterogeneity is in development [77], but such patient-stratifying tools have not been employed in clinical trials so far. GIST is the most common subset of sarcoma with high expression of the receptor tyrosine kinase c-*KIT*, and most patients with inoperable or recurrent GIST obtain temporary and often long-term disease control with kinase inhibitor therapy [50]. Like most oncogene-driven tumors that are sensitive to small-molecule inhibitors, relapse or disease progression due to secondary mutations of the kinase is a clinical problem in these sarcomas. Acquired imatinib resistance is typically associated with substitutions between the first and second receptor kinase domains, rarely found in untreated tumors. A likely mechanism explaining secondary clonal evolution is gatekeeper mutations interfering with binding of imatinib at the receptor site [78]. The oncogene activations in c-*KIT* are however still the driving force and the main target for therapy. In lack of secondary mutations, feedback mechanisms may be responsible for reactivation of c-*KIT*. Another explanation suggested is a morphologic shift with altered immune phenotyping insensitive to imatinib emerging as a result of the targeted therapy [79]. Novel multi-target TKIs, either alone or in combination, may be effective in imatinib-resistant GIST; again, genotype biomarkers may predict the likelihood of response. Hence, design of clinical research protocols must take into account the impact of these molecular hallmarks.

Within the field of sarcoma, there is an ongoing search for effective targeted therapy related to pathway aberrancies detected by mutational biomarker analyses. In Norway, a population-based recording of mutational status in all new cases of sarcoma has been initiated. This Norwegian Sarcoma Consortium (NoSarC) project assesses frozen tumor tissue according to a panel of approximately 900 mutations described in various types of cancers [80]. The project aims at increasing insight into molecular mechanism in sarcoma development as well as identifying aberrations which may be further exploited as targets for new therapeutic drugs. Potential targets will be validated in preclinical studies prior to further investigations in small-scale academic studies. The accumulation of functional information emerging from systematic genome sequencing may facilitate the development of second-line personalized medicine in orphan cancer types for which the rarity hampers large-scale clinical trials.

One interesting trial design is the EORTC trial, "CREATE," testing the ALK kinase inhibitor crizotinib in six defined rare diagnoses including three rare sarcoma subtypes (ClinicalTrials.gov Identifier: NCT01524926). However, specific *ALK* and/or *MET* pathway alterations in tumor tissue are not mandatory for patient registration thereby allowing control patients for pathway-targeted therapy. Furthermore, substantial tumor material should be available for central review and molecular diagnostics, and previous therapy is permitted. Trials have previously demonstrated the timely use of biomarkers in targeted therapy of rare diagnoses, including therapeutic antibodies against IGF-1R as well as the tyrosine kinase inhibitor pazopanib in soft tissue sarcomas [81, 82].

The Tumor Microenvironment and Radiotherapy: Mechanisms of Response and Resistance

High-energy ionizing radiation therapy plays a major role in curative treatment in approximately 40% of cancer cases, in addition to serving as a major instrument to control cancer-related symptoms in patients with advanced disease [83]. Radiotherapy is targeted towards tumor cell DNA, exerting effects directly by cluster damage of double strands, or indirectly by producing intracellular free radicals, which in turn results in impairment of the DNA. Consequently, tumor cells are eradicated instantly (apoptosis), or, proliferation is hampered by the event of a mitotic catastrophe during cell division.

Radiobiological research has typically focused on radiation effects and fractionation sensitivity in various tumor cells. The therapeutic window has been explained by the difference between cancer cells' and normal cells' ability to repair injury caused by ionizing radiation. Emphasis on side effects has been fundamental in order to balance normal tissue damage against dose-dependent biological effects on the tumor. The recognition that the TME, as a promoter of cancer cell growth, also plays a role in radioresistance, is currently changing the paradigm towards investigating the influence of radiotherapy on the stroma cells [83–85]. This change of understanding goes hand-in-hand with the mounting evidence that drugs targeting the TME, and in particular immune cells, completely transformed the prognosis in subgroups of previously drug-resistant cancer types. Consequently, concomitant chemotherapeuticals, targeted drugs, and immunotherapy are increasingly utilized to enhance radiation effects [86–89].

Retaining interactions with stroma cells is pivotal for sustaining tumor growth. Resilient network signaling between cancer cells, endothelial cells, fibroblasts, and immune cells may explain resistance to various cancer therapies as well as metastasis development. These interactions are modified during radiotherapy, and concern has been raised that such changes may promote invasive features [90]. Understanding how ionizing radiation influence the cross talk between tumor cells and stroma will enable us to remodel radiotherapy dose delivery in order to overcome paradoxical responses as well as augmenting efficacy by targeting the TME.

Microvascular damage plays a major role in explaining tumor response to radiotherapy (RT) [91]. Ionizing radiation destroys vulnerable endothelial cells, which results in obstructed tumor circulation and deprived oxygenation. Simultaneously, inflammatory responses lead to upregulating of integrins improving endothelial cell survival [85]. This dichotomy is also reflected in tumor hypoxia, which on one hand slows down cell growth in poorly oxygenated areas of the tumor, but on the other hand induces resilience and radioresistance of the tumor stem cell population—and possibly also in immune cells which are deranged to support tumor growth and evasion of immune attacks [90]. Activation of cancer cell genes associated with homeostasis and stress seems to promote adaption to the hostile TME [85]. Furthermore, the conditions of the TME induce mutagenesis and serves as a source of genetic instability in the tumor [92].

It has been shown that anti-angiogenetic (anti-VEGF) targeted therapy may sensitize tumor cells to radiation by reducing hypoxia through normalization of vessels [86, 93]. Radiation modulations targeting hypoxic stem cells may represent a key to further improve RT efficacy. Advanced dynamic molecular imaging utilizing PET or MRI has the potential to identify hypoxic areas [94, 95] Intensity modulated RT allows for redistribution of RT dose, with the potential to selectively magnify dosage to hypoxic areas in order to overcome radioresistance in tumor stem cells as well as repressed immune cells. Radiolabeled tracers have been utilized in the measurement of dynamic changes in intratumoral hypoxia, and may help to predict radiotherapy outcome, e.g., in models of head and neck cancer [94]. Refinement of personalized radiation dose distribution would require novel adaptive study designs [89]. Dynamic evaluation of tumor morphology during the course of fractionated radiotherapy may enable adjustment of dose distribution accordingly [85, 95]. Mediators of intratumoral cross talk may promote or interfere with progression, angiogenesis, and immunomodulation. Which factors that come into play are difficult to predict. This reflects a need for developing biomarker panels sensitive to radiation-induced changes in molecular and cellular profiles, enabling an increased understanding of therapeutic effects and counterproductive reactions in both tumor cells and TME.

Discussion and Summary

Biomarker panels are an increasingly integrated part of clinical trials, used for pivotal decision-making. It is likely that combinations of biomarkers that involve tumor environment and stromal features will increase prognostic precision with immunotherapy and targeted therapy. Adaptive designs and Bayesian designs are used to utilize the most up-to-date cumulative knowledge, and the use of surrogate endpoints together with early stopping rules can shorten the study period. Ethical perspectives need to be taken into account when designing a cancer study, for example, will the patients benefit from taking part in the trial?

FDA guides the process of obtaining an approved biomarker program in a clinical trial [20, 96]. This secures the quality of the biomarker assays but has also likely limited the use of biomarker assays in many US trials.

Even if genomics alone as guidance for therapy is unlikely to prove relevant for all types of cancer, the proportion of actionable mutations is likely to be so high that cancer genetics may provide significant clinical benefit [23]. Genomic profiling will not be sufficient to direct therapy in all patients, and alternative molecular profiling or drug sensitivity assays is needed. Development of functional biomarker assays are emerging and prepared for use in clinical trials such as single-cell immune and signaling profiling or in vitro cancer sensitivity assays for the selection of optimal therapy. AML patients responding to the combination of vitamin A, theophylline, and valproic acid displayed a low signaling signature of phospho-signaling proteins [96]. Functionality through in vitro testing of therapy response has been employed in single patients and with promising responses [7, 97, 98]. Limitations of this in vitro drug sensitivity assay include the absence of combination testing and novel therapy availability.

Studies in AML and ALL as well as in soft tissue sarcoma illustrate a robust use of biomarker panels. A combination of various modalities, from clinical data including cancer cell numbers via karyotype, gene expression, and mutational analyses, seems to guide therapy intensity at a higher accuracy. Similarly, surrogate markers for therapy effect need to be selected based on the nature of the disease, e.g., minimal residual disease determination by quantitative PCR in the presence of reliable markers or protein expression of the malignant clone by immunophenotype. The complexity of the decision tools for the physician seems to be increasing, and the future challenge will be to create a comprehensible and not too simplified diagnostic system that provides precision medicine to the heterogeneous tumor diseases of our patients.

References

1. Simon R. Biomarker based clinical trial design. Chin Clin Oncol. 2014;3(3):39. https://doi.org/10.3978/j.issn.2304-3865.2014.02.03.
2. DeVita VT Jr, Eggermont AM, Hellman S, Kerr DJ. Clinical cancer research: the past, present and the future. Nat Rev Clin Oncol. 2014;11(11):663–9. https://doi.org/10.1038/nrclinonc.2014.
3. Schwaederle M, Zhao M, et al. Impact of precision medicine in diverse cancers: a meta-analysis of phase II clinical trials. J Clin Oncol. 2015;33(32):3817–25. https://doi.org/10.1200/JCO.2015.61.5997.
4. Henry N, Hayes D. Cancer biomarkers. Mol Oncol. 2012;6:140–6. https://doi.org/10.1016/j.molonc.2012.01.010.
5. Boussemart L, Malka-Mahieu H, et al. eIF4F is a nexus of resistance to anti-BRAF and anti-MEK cancer therapies. Nature. 2014;513(7516):105–9. https://doi.org/10.1038/nature13572.
6. Behbehani GK, Samusik N, et al. Mass cytometric functional profiling of acute myeloid leukemia defines cell-cycle and immunophenotypic properties that correlate with known responses to therapy. Cancer Discov. 2015;5(9):988–1003. https://doi.org/10.1158/2159-8290.CD-15-0298.
7. Pemovska T, Kontro M, et al. Individualized systems medicine strategy to tailor treatments for patients with chemorefractory acute myeloid leukemia. Cancer Discov. 2013;3(12):1416–29. https://doi.org/10.1158/2159-8290.CD-13-0350.
8. Helleday T. Poisoning cancer cells with oxidized nucleosides. N Engl J Med. 2015;373(16):1570–1. https://doi.org/10.1056/NEJMcibr1510335.
9. Barker HE, Paget JT, et al. The tumour microenvironment after radiotherapy: mechanisms of resistance and recurrence. Nat Rev Cancer. 2015;15(7):409–25. https://doi.org/10.1038/nrc3958.
10. Conley BA, Staudt L, et al. The exceptional responders initiative: feasibility of a national cancer institute pilot study. J Natl Cancer Inst. 2021;113(1):27–37. https://doi.org/10.1093/jnci/djaa061.
11. Bilusic M, Girardi D, Zhou Y, Jung K, Pei J, Slifker M, Chen Q, Meerzaman D, Alpaugh K, Young D, Flieder D, Gray P, Plimack E. Molecular profiling of exceptional responders to cancer therapy. Oncologist 2020 Nov 19. https://doi.org/10.1002/onco.13600.
12. Kurtz DM, Esfahani MS, et al. Dynamic risk profiling using serial tumor biomarkers for personalized outcome prediction. Cell. 2019;178(3):699–713.e19. https://doi.org/10.1016/j.cell.2019.06.011.
13. Mbeunkui F, Johann DJ Jr. Cancer and the tumor microenvironment: a review of an essential relationship. Cancer Chemother Pharmacol. 2009;63(4):571–82. https://doi.org/10.1007/s00280-008-0881-9.

14. Choi SY, Collins CC, et al. Cancer-generated lactic acid: a regulatory, immunosuppressive metabolite? J Pathol. 2013;230(4):350–5. https://doi.org/10.1002/path.4218.

15. Balkwill FR, Capasso M, et al. The tumor microenvironment at a glance. Cell Sci. 2012;125(Pt 23):5591–6. https://doi.org/10.1242/jcs.116392.

16. Antonyak MA, Cerione RA. Microvesicles as mediators of intercellular communication in cancer. Methods Mol Biol. 2014;1165:147–73. https://doi.org/10.1007/978-1-4939-0856-1_11.

17. Junttila MR, de Sauvage FJ. Influence of tumour microenvironment heterogeneity on therapeutic response. Nature. 2013;501(7467):346–54. https://doi.org/10.1038/nature12626.

18. Mehta C, Schäfer H. Biomarker driven population enrichment for adaptive oncology trials with time to event endpoints. Stat Med. 2014;33:4515–31. https://doi.org/10.1002/sim.6272.

19. Ong M, Carreira S, et al. Validation and utilisation of high-coverage next-generation sequencing to deliver the pharmacological audit trail. Br J Cancer. 2012;111(5):828–36. https://doi.org/10.1038/bjc.2014.350.

20. Fontes Jardim DL, Schwaederle M, et al. Impact of a biomarker-based strategy on oncology drug development: a meta-analysis of clinical trials leading to FDA approval. J Natl Cancer Inst. 2015;107(11) https://doi.org/10.1093/jnci/djv253.

21. Trusheim MR, Berndt ER. The clinical benefits, ethics, and economics of stratified medicine and companion diagnostics. Drug Discov Today. 2015;20(12):1439–50. https://doi.org/10.1016/j.drudis.2015.10.017.

22. Sargent DJ, Mandrekar SJ. Statistical issues in the validation of prognostic, predictive, and surrogate biomarkers. Clin Trials. 2013;10:647–52. https://doi.org/10.1177/1740774513497125.

23. Garraway LA. Genomics-driven oncology: framework for an emerging paradigm. J Clin Oncol. 2013;31(15):1806–14. https://doi.org/10.1200/JCO.2012.46.8934.

24. Le Tourneau C, Delord JP, et al. Molecularly targeted therapy based on tumour molecular profiling versus conventional therapy for advanced cancer (SHIVA): a multicentre, open-label, proof-of-concept, randomised, controlled phase 2 trial. Lancet Oncol. 2015;16(13):1324–34. https://doi.org/10.1016/S1470-2045(15)00188-6.

25. Zhang J, Walsh MF, et al. Germline mutations in predisposition genes in pediatric cancer. N Engl J Med. 2015;373(24):2336–46. https://doi.org/10.1056/NEJMoa1508054.

26. Le Calvez F, Mukeria A, et al. TP53 and KRAS mutation load and types in lung cancers in relation to tobacco smoke: distinct patterns in never, former, and current smokers. Cancer Res. 2005;65:5076–83. https://doi.org/10.1158/0008-5472.CAN-05-0551.

27. Gerlinger M, Rowan AJ, Horswell S, et al. Intratumor heterogeneity and branched evolution revealed by multiregion sequencing. N Engl J Med. 2012;366:883–92. https://doi.org/10.1056/NEJMoa1113205.

28. Landau DA, Tausch E, et al. Mutations driving CLL and their evolution in progression and relapse. Nature. 2015;526(7574):525–30. https://doi.org/10.1038/nature15395.

29. Wheatley K, Burnett AK, et al. A simple, robust, validated and highly predictive index for the determination of risk-directed therapy in acute myeloid leukaemia derived from the MRC AML 10 trial. United Kingdom Medical Research Council's Adult and Childhood Leukaemia Working Parties. Br J Haematol. 1999;107(1):69–79.

30. Sparano JA, Robert MD, et al. Prospective validation of a 21-gene expression assay in breast cancer. N Engl J Med. 2015;373:2005. https://doi.org/10.1056/NEJMoa1510764.

31. Akbani R, Ng PK, et al. A pan-cancer proteomic perspective on The Cancer Genome Atlas. Nat Commun. 2014;5:3887. https://doi.org/10.1038/ncomms4887.

32. Joensuu H, Hohenberger P, et al. Gastrointestinal stromal tumour. Lancet. 2013;382(9896):973–83. https://doi.org/10.1016/S0140-6736(13)60106-3.

33. Engellau J, et al. Improved prognostication in soft tissue sarcoma: independent information from vascular invasion, necrosis, growth pattern, and immunostaining using whole-tumor sections and tissue microarrays. Hum Pathol. 2005;36(9):994–1002. https://doi.org/10.1016/j.humpath.2005.07.008.

34. Jebsen NL, et al. Five-year results from a Scandinavian sarcoma group study (SSG XIII) of adjuvant chemotherapy combined with accelerated radiotherapy in high-risk soft tissue sarcoma of extremities and trunk wall. Int J Radiat Oncol Biol Phys. 2011;81(5):1359–66. https://doi.org/10.1016/j.ijrobp.2010.07.037.

35. Lønning PE. Breast cancer prognostication and prediction: are we making progress? Ann Oncol. 2007;18(Suppl 8):viii3–7. https://doi.org/10.1093/annonc/mdm260.

36. Pantel K, Alix-Panabières C. Real-time liquid biopsy in cancer patients: fact or fiction? Cancer Res. 2013;73(21):6384–8. https://doi.org/10.1158/0008-5472.

37. Le Cesne A, et al. Optimizing tyrosine kinase inhibitor therapy in gastrointestinal stromal tumors: exploring the benefits of continuous kinase suppression. Oncologist. 2013;18(11):1192–9. https://doi.org/10.1634/theoncologist.2012-0361.

38. Joensuu H. Adjuvant therapy for high-risk gastrointestinal stromal tumour: considerations for optimal management. Drugs. 2012;72(15):1953–63. https://doi.org/10.2165/11635590-000000000-00000.

39. Yip et al. ALT-GIST: Randomized phase II trial of imatinib alternating with regorafenib versus imatinib alone for the first-line treatment of metastatic gastrointestinal stromal tumor (GIST). Sarcoma, J Clin Oncol 2019; 37, no. 15_suppl:11023. https://doi.org/10.1200/JCO.2019.37.15_suppl.11023.

40. Engelholm LH, Melander MC, et al. Targeting a novel bone degradation pathway in primary bone cancer by inactivation of the collagen receptor uPARAP/Endo180. J Pathol. 2015;238(1):120–33. https://doi.org/10.1002/path.4661.

41. Galluzzi L, Vacchelli E, Bravo-San Pedro JM, et al. Classification of current anticancer immunotherapies. Oncotarget. 2014;5(24):12472–508. https://doi.org/10.18632/oncotarget.2998.

42. Naumov GN, Folkman J, Straume O, Akslen LA. Tumor-vascular interactions and tumor dormancy. APMIS. 2008;116(7–8):569–85. https://doi.org/10.1111/j.1600-0463.2008.01213.x.

43. Labarge MA, Parvin B, et al. Molecular deconstruction, detection, and computational prediction of microenvironment-modulated cellular responses to cancer therapeutics. Adv Drug Deliv Rev. 2014;69-70:123–31. https://doi.org/10.1016/j.addr.2014.02.009.

44. Hellesøy M, Lorens JB. Cellular context-mediated Akt dynamics regulates MAP kinase signaling thresholds during angiogenesis. Mol Biol Cell. 2015;26(14):2698–711. https://doi.org/10.1091/mbc.E14-09-1378.

45. Mima K, Sukawa Y, et al. *Fusobacterium nucleatum* and T cells in colorectal carcinoma. JAMA Oncol. 2015;1(5):653–61. https://doi.org/10.1001/jamaoncol.2015.1377.

46. Eriguchi Y, Takashima S, et al. Graft-versus-host disease disrupts intestinal microbial ecology by inhibiting Paneth cell production of α-defensins. Blood. 2012;120(1):223–31. https://doi.org/10.1182/blood-2011-12-401166.

47. Vétizou M, Pitt JM, et al. Anticancer immunotherapy by CTLA-4 blockade relies on the gut microbiota. Science. 2015;350(6264):1079–84. https://doi.org/10.1126/science.aad1329.

48. Bates SE, Berry DA, Balasubramaniam S, Bailey S, LoRusso PM, Rubin EH. Advancing clinical trials to streamline drug development. Clin Cancer Res. 2015;21(20):4527–35. https://doi.org/10.1158/1078-0432.CCR-15-0039.

49. Krause DS, Van Etten RA. Tyrosine kinases as targets for cancer therapy. N Engl J Med. 2005;353(2):172–87. https://doi.org/10.1056/NEJMra044389.

50. Casali PG, Le Cesne A, et al. Time to definitive failure to the first tyrosine kinase inhibitor in localized GI stromal tumors treated with imatinib as an adjuvant: a European Organisation for Research and Treatment of Cancer Soft Tissue and Bone Sarcoma Group Intergroup Randomized Trial in Collaboration With the Australasian Gastro-Intestinal Trials Group, UNICANCER, French Sarcoma Group, Italian Sarcoma Group, and Spanish Group for Research on Sarcomas. J Clin Oncol. 2015;33(36):4276–83. https://doi.org/10.1200/JCO.2015.62.4304.

51. Hanfstein B, Müller MC, et al. Response-related predictors of survival in CML. Ann Hematol. 2015;94(Suppl 2):S227–39. https://doi.org/10.1007/s00277-015-2327-x.

52. Ansell SM, Lesokhin AM, Borrello I, et al. PD-1 blockade with nivolumab in relapsed or refractory Hodgkin's lymphoma. N Engl J Med. 2015;372:311–9. https://doi.org/10.1056/NEJMoa1411087.

53. Brahmer J, Reckamp KL, Baas P, et al. Nivolumab versus docetaxel in advanced squamous-cell non-small-cell lung cancer. N Engl J Med. 2015;373:123–35. https://doi.org/10.1056/NEJMoa1504627.

54. Chow SC, Liu JP. Design and analysis of clinical trials: concepts and methodologies. 3rd ed. London: Wiley; 2014.

55. Mandrekar SJ, Dahlberg SE, et al. Improving clinical trial efficiency: thinking outside the box. Am Soc Clin Oncol 2015:e141–7. https://doi.org/10.14694/EdBook_AM.2015.35.e141.

56. Boessen R, Heerspink HJ, et al. Improving clinical trial efficiency by biomarker-guided patient selection. Trials. 2014;15:103. https://doi.org/10.1186/1745-6215-15-103.

57. http://www.fda.gov

58. Thall F. Bayesian models and decision algorithms for complex early phase clinical trials. Stat Sci. 2010;25(2):227–44. https://doi.org/10.1214/09-STS315.

59. Burman CF, Miller F, Wong KW, editors. Improving dose-finding: a philosophic view. In: Handbook of adaptive designs in pharmaceutical and clinical development. Boca Raton: CRC, pp. 10.1–10.23; 2010.

60. Atkinson AC, Biswas A. Bayesian adaptive biased-coin designs for clinical trials with normal responses. Biometrics. 2005;61(1):118–25. https://doi.org/10.1111/j.0006-341X.2005.031002.x.

61. Angell HK, Bruni D, Barrett JC, Herbst R, Galon J. The immunoscore: colon cancer and beyond. Clin Cancer Res. 2020;26(2):332–9. https://doi.org/10.1158/1078-0432.CCR-18-1851.

62. Yost KE, Satpathy AT, Wells DK, Qi Y, Wang C, Kageyama R, McNamara KL, Granja JM, Sarin KY, Brown RA, Gupta RK, Curtis C, Bucktrout SL, Davis MM, Chang ALS, Chang HY. Clonal replacement of tumor-specific T cells following PD-1 blockade. Nat Med. 2019;25(8):1251–9. https://doi.org/10.1038/s41591-019-0522-3.

63. Zhou H, Mondragón L, Xie W, et al. Oncolysis with DTT-205 and DTT-304 generates immunological memory in cured animals. Cell Death Dis. 2018;9(11):1086. https://doi.org/10.1038/s41419-018-1127-3.

64. Vitale I, Yamazaki T, et al. Targeting cancer heterogeneity with immune responses driven by oncolytic peptides. Trends Cancer 2021:S2405-8033(20)30339–3. https://doi.org/10.1016/j.trecan.2020.12.012.

65. Spicer J, Marabelle A, et al. Safety, anti-tumor activity and T-cell responses in a dose-ranging phase 1 trial of the oncolytic peptide LTX-315 in patients with solid tumors. Clin Cancer Res 2021:clincanres.3435.2020. https://doi.org/10.1158/1078-0432.CCR-20-3435.

66. Jebsen NL, et al. Enhanced T-lymphocyte infiltration in a desmoid tumor of the thoracic wall in a young woman treated with intratumoral injections of the oncolytic peptide LTX-315: a case report. J Med Case Rep. 2019;13:177.

67. van der Velden DL, Hoes LR, van der Wijngaart H, van Berge Henegouwen JM, van Werkhoven E, Roepman P, et al. The Drug Rediscovery protocol facilitates the expanded use of existing anti-cancer drugs. Nature. 2019;574(7776):127–31.

68. Toft N, Birgens H, et al. Risk group assignment differs for children and adults 1-45 yr with acute lymphoblastic leukemia treated by the NOPHO ALL-2008 protocol. Eur J Haematol. 2013;90(5):404–12. https://doi.org/10.1111/ejh.12097.

69. Vaitkevičienė G, Forestier E, et al. Nordic Society of Paediatric Haematology and Oncologyv (NOPHO) High white blood cell count at diagnosis of childhood acute lymphoblastic leukaemia: biological background and prognostic impact. Results from the NOPHO ALL-92 and ALL- 2000 studies. Eur J Haematol. 2011;86(1):38–46. https://doi.org/10.1111/j.1600-0609.2010.01522.x.

70. Terwijn M, van Putten WL, et al. High prognostic impact of flow cytometric minimal residual disease detection in acute myeloid leukemia: data from the HOVON/SAKK AML 42A study. J Clin Oncol. 2013;31(31):3889–97. https://doi.org/10.1200/JCO.2012.45.9628.

71. Walter RB, Othus M, et al. Resistance prediction in AML: analysis of 4601 patients from MRC/NCRI, HOVON/SAKK, SWOG and MD Anderson Cancer Center. Leukemia. 2015;29(2):312–20. https://doi.org/10.1038/leu.2014.242.

72. Cornelissen JJ, Versluis J, et al. Comparative therapeutic value of post-remission approaches in patients with acute myeloid leukemia aged 40–60 years. Leukemia. 2015;29(5):1041–50. https://doi.org/10.1038/leu.2014.332.

73. Serve H, Krug U, et al. Sorafenib in combination with intensive chemotherapy in elderly patients with acute myeloid leukemia: results from a randomized, placebo-controlled trial. J Clin Oncol. 2013;31(25):3110–8. https://doi.org/10.1200/JCO.2012.46.4990.

74. Oellerich T, Mohr S, et al. FLT3-ITD and TLR9 use Bruton tyrosine kinase to activate distinct transcriptional programs mediating AML cell survival and proliferation. Blood. 2015;125(12):1936–47. https://doi.org/10.1182/blood-2014-06-585216.

75. Smith SM, Coleman J, et al. Molecular diagnostics in soft tissue sarcomas and gastrointestinal stromal tumors. J Surg Oncol. 2015;111(5):520–31. https://doi.org/10.1002/jso.23882.

76. Schöffski P, Cornillie J, Wozniak A, Li H, Hompes D. Soft tissue sarcoma: an update on systemic treatment options for patients with advanced disease. Oncol Res Treat. 2014;37(6):355–62. https://doi.org/10.1159/000362631.

77. Bühnemann C, Li S, et al. Quantification of the heterogeneity of prognostic cellular biomarkers in Ewing sarcoma using automated image and random survival forest analysis. PLoS One. 2014;9(9):e107105. https://doi.org/10.1371/journal.pone.0107105.

78. Antonescu CR, DeMatteo RP. CCR 20th anniversary commentary: a genetic mechanism of imatinib resistance in gastrointestinal stromal tumor-where are we a decade later? Clin Cancer Res. 2015;21(15):3363–5. https://doi.org/10.1158/1078-0432.CCR-14-3120.

79. Canzonieri V, et al. Morphologic shift associated with aberrant cytokeratin expression in a GIST patient after tyrosine kinase inhibitors therapy. A case report with a brief review of the literature. Pathol Res Pract. 2015;212(1):63–7. https://doi.org/10.1016/j.prp.2015.11.004.

80. http://kreftgenomikk.no/en/sarkom/

81. Schöffski P, Adkins D, et al. An open-label, phase 2 study evaluating the efficacy and safety of the anti-IGF-1R antibody cixutumumab in patients with previously treated advanced or metastatic soft-tissue sarcoma or Ewing family of tumours. Eur J Cancer. 2013;49(15):3219–28. https://doi.org/10.1016/j.ejca.2013.06.010.

82. Amur SG, Sanyal S, et al. Building a roadmap to biomarker qualification: challenges and opportunities. Biomark Med. 2015;9(11):1095–105. https://doi.org/10.2217/bmm.15.90.

83. Barker HE, Paget JT, Khan AA, Harrington KJ. The tumour microenvironment after radiotherapy: mechanisms of resistance

and recurrence. Nat Rev Cancer. 2015;15(7):409–25. https://doi.org/10.1038/nrc3958.

84. Barcellos-Hoff MH, Park C, Wright EG. Radiation and the microenvironment – tumorigenesis and therapy. Nat Rev Cancer. 2005;5(11):867–75. https://doi.org/10.1038/nrc1735.

85. Wang JJ, Lei KF, Han F. Tumor microenvironment: recent advances in various cancer treatments. Eur Rev Med Pharmacol Sci. 2018 Jun;22(12):3855–64. https://doi.org/10.26355/eurrev_201806_15270.

86. Jain RK. Normalization of tumor vasculature: an emerging concept in antiangiogenic therapy. Science. 2005;307:58–62.

87. Postow MA, Callahan MK, et al. Immunologic correlates of the abscopal effect in a patient with melanoma. N Engl J Med. 2012 Mar 8;366(10):925–31. https://doi.org/10.1056/NEJMoa1112824.

88. Demaria S, Bhardwaj N, McBride WH, Formenti SC. Combining radiotherapy and immunotherapy: a revived partnership. Int J Radiat Oncol Biol Phys. 2005;63(3):655–66. https://doi.org/10.1016/j.ijrobp.2005.06.032.

89. Ree AH, Redalen KR. Personalized radiotherapy: concepts, biomarkers and trial design. Br J Radiol. 2015;88(1051):20150009. https://doi.org/10.1259/bjr.20150009.

90. Barcellos-Hoff MH, Ravani SA. Irradiated mammary gland stroma promotes the expression of tumorigenic potential by unirradiated epithelial cells. Cancer Res. 2000 Mar 1;60(5):1254–60. Published March 2000.

91. Truman JP, García-Barros M, et al. Endothelial membrane remodeling is obligate for anti-angiogenic radiosensitization during tumor radiosurgery. PLoS One 2010;5(9). https://doi.org/10.1371/annotation/6e222ad5-b175-4a00-9d04-4d120568a897.

92. Bindra RS, Glazer PM, et al. Genetic instability and the tumor microenvironment: towards the concept of microenvironment-induced mutagenesis. Mutat Res. 2005;569(1–2):75–85. https://doi.org/10.1016/j.mrfmmm.2004.03.013.

93. Yoshimura M, Itasaka S, Harada H, Hiraoka M. Microenvironment and radiation therapy. Biomed Res Int. 2013;2013:685308. https://doi.org/10.1155/2013/685308.

94. Fatema CN, Zhao S, et al. Dual tracer evaluation of dynamic changes in intratumoral hypoxic and proliferative states after radiotherapy of human head and neck cancer xenografts using radio-labeled FMISO and FLT. BMC Cancer. 2014;14:692. https://doi.org/10.1186/1471-2407-14-692.

95. Lyng H, Malinen E. Hypoxia in cervical cancer: from biology to imaging. Clin Transl Imaging. 2017;5(4):373–88. https://doi.org/10.1007/s40336-017-0238-7.

96. Skavland J, Jørgensen KM, et al. Specific cellular signal-transduction responses to in vivo combination therapy with ATRA, valproic acid and theophylline in acute myeloid leukemia. Blood Cancer J. 2011;1(2):e4. https://doi.org/10.1038/bcj.2011.2.

97. Pemovska T, Johnson E, et al. Axitinib effectively inhibits BCR-ABL1(T315I) with a distinct binding conformation. Nature. 2015;519(7541):102–5. https://doi.org/10.1038/nature14119.

98. Malani D, Kumar A, et al. Implementing a functional precision medicine tumor board for acute myeloid leukemia. Cancer Discov. 2022;12(2):388–401. https://doi.org/10.1158/2159-8290.CD-21-0410.

Cancer Biomarkers: A Long and Tortuous Journey

34

Wen Jing Sim, Kian Chung Lee, and Jean Paul Thiery

Abstract

Cancer biomarkers are biomolecules released either by cancer cells or other cells from cancer patients in response to the tumorigenic process. Identification of cancer biomarkers is obtained principally through multi-omics while their detection can also require imaging. Reliance on a single biomarker or a single technology for diagnosis and disease management remains useful but does not permit understanding the complexity and evolution of the disease. Evolving technologies and strategies in building signature profiles and multi-omic data allow deepening our understanding in real time of the complex biology of the disease and permits to apply precision medicine. Each data point provided by each technology serves as a piece of the puzzle, which once combined shapes the way we perceive this disease and impact strategies designed for drug target development and disease management.

Take-Home Lessons
- Development of valuable diagnostics is time-consuming and cannot often be achieved.
- Single tissue biomarkers are progressively replaced by biomarker profiling from liquid biopsy.
- Combination of mutational profiles, post-translational modifications, spatial locations, and altered signaling pathways offer a much greater diagnostic power as compared to dysregulation of a single biomarker.
- Real-time assessment of cancer biomarkers enables better disease management.

Historical Perspective on Cancer Biomarkers

Cancer biomarker research began in 1847 with the discovery of large quantities of a particular protein in the urine of a patient with multiple myeloma, by Henry Bence-Jones; at the time, multiple myeloma was designated mollities ossium [1, 2]. The Bence-Jones Protein (BJP) was later definitively identified as the light chain of immunoglobulin (Ig)G, which is secreted by multiple myeloma cells [3]. Over 140 years later, BJP was also identified in the serum samples of myeloma patients [4] and, in 1998, a routine immunodiagnostic test was approved by the Food and Drug Administration (FDA) for the detection of BJP in the diagnosis of multiple myeloma and Waldenstrom's macroglobulinemia.

Over 100 years after BJP was identified, another biomarker, carcinoembryonic antigen (CEA), was identified by Dr Joseph Gold [5], and shown to be prevalent in blood samples from patients with colon cancer. Later, other biomarkers were discovered, including carbohydrate antigen (CA) 19-9 as a biomarker for colorectal and pancreatic cancer, CA15-3 for breast cancer, CA-125 for ovarian cancer, and prostate-specific antigen (PSA [KLK3]) for prostate cancer. These

W. J. Sim (✉)
Olink Proteomics, APAC, SG National University of Singapore S9, Singapore, Singapore
e-mail: wen.jing@olink.com

K. C. Lee
Institute of Molecular Cell Biology, Singapore, Singapore

BioCheetah Pte Ltd, Singapore, Singapore
e-mail: kclee@biocheetah.com

J. P. Thiery
Institute of Molecular Cell Biology, Singapore, Singapore

BioCheetah Pte Ltd, Singapore, Singapore

Guangzhou Laboratory, Guangzhou Laboratory International Biological Island, Guangzhou, China

Centre for Cancer Biomarkers CCBIO, Klinisk Institutt, Bergen, Norway
e-mail: tjp@gzlab.ac.cn

© The Author(s), under exclusive license to Springer Nature Switzerland AG 2022
L. A. Akslen, R. S. Watnick (eds.), *Biomarkers of the Tumor Microenvironment*, https://doi.org/10.1007/978-3-030-98950-7_34

early discoveries of biomarkers relied on empirical observations and substantially high levels of the biomarker in large tumors. Unfortunately, for the most part, these biomarkers have since been shown to be not specific to a particular type of cancer as originally thought, and as such, cannot be used to stratify disease states; indeed, CEA is elevated in both breast cancer and lung cancer, and CA-125 is also elevated in women with noncancerous gynecological conditions as well as those with cancer [6].

A biomarker is generally defined as any molecular, biochemical, physiological, or anatomical marker that can be measured as an indicator of a normal or abnormal condition or disease. In cancer research, a cancer biomarker often refers to a tumor-secreted molecule or a molecule that forms part of a specific response by the body to the tumor. Cancer biomarkers may include genetic, epigenetic, proteomic, metabolomic or imaging markers that are useful in cancer diagnosis and prognosis but also in predicting treatment response. When the term "biomarker" is used in the translational research context, it often alludes to a marker that can be used to provide insight into personalized medicine and one that can be used to accelerate or aid in the diagnosis, prognosis or monitoring of a disease. An ideal biomarker is one that can be detected in body fluids or harvested from easily accessible tissues, and one that can differentiate—with high specificity and sensitivity—malignant from benign tumors and aggressive from non-aggressive tumors. Such clinical specificity and sensitivity are vital attributes: high clinical specificity is key to reducing the frequency of false-negative results, and high clinical sensitivity aids in increasing the rate of detection. Table 34.1 shows the conventional FDA-approved clinically relevant biomarkers for various cancer types. Table 34.2 highlights the candidate biomarkers that have been identified through various studies.

Precision medicine—a new benchmark in medical care—aims to deliver the *right* treatment at the *right* dose to the *right* patient at the *right* time. Biomarkers identified through conventional means tend to be overexpressed in disease; this makes it difficult to distinguish a causal protein from a by-product of malignant transformation. Indeed, such conventional biomarkers lack information associated with disease risk or susceptibility, either at the early stage or during tumor progression. Consequently, additional biomarkers are required to assess risk, predict, detect, diagnose, and prognose cancer. Biomarkers for precision medicine should also offer clinical utility, and be able to predict treatment response and monitor outcome and recurrence [62]. There are several ways to classify biomarkers for their clinical utility. Mishra and Verma [63] suggested using DNA molecules for prediction, RNA molecules for detection, protein for diagnosis, and glycoproteins for prognosis. Another strategy suggested incorporating multi-omics to capture the complex regulatory

Table 34.1 Conventional FDA-approved clinically relevant biomarkers for various cancer types

Cancer biomarker	Cancer type	Application	References
Carbohydrate antigen 15.3 (CA 15-3)	Breast	Monitoring	[7, 8]
Estrogen, progesterone receptors (ER and PgR)	Breast	Stratification	[9, 10]
HER2	Breast	Monitoring	[11–13]
Carbohydrate antigen 27.29 (CA27.29)	Breast	Monitoring	[14]
Nuclear matrix protein 22 (NMP-22)	Bladder	Screening Monitoring Prognosis	[15]
Carcinoembryonic antigen (CEA)	Colorectal/hepatic	Monitoring Prognosis Recurrence	[16]
Alfa-fetoprotein	Hepatocellular carcinoma	Diagnosis Monitoring Recurrence	[17]
Calcitonin	Medullary carcinoma of thyroid	Diagnosis Monitoring	[21, 21]
Carbohydrate antigen 125 (CA125)	Ovarian	Diagnosis Prognosis Monitoring Recurrence	[22, 23]
Carbohydrate antigen 19-9 (CA 19-9)	Pancreatic	Monitoring	[24, 25]
Prostate cancer antigen 3 (PCA3)	Prostate	Prognosis	[26, 27]
Prostate-specific antigen (PSA)	Prostate/BPH	Screening Diagnosis Monitoring	[28, 29]
Human chorionic gonadotropin-β (HCG-β)	Testicular	Diagnosis Monitoring Recurrence	[30, 31]
Thyroglobulin	Thyroid	Monitoring	[32–34]

Table 34.2 Candidate biomarkers that identified for certain cancer type through various studies

Cancer biomarker	Cancer type	References
DNA mismatch repair (MMR) deficiency (dMMR)	Colorectal cancer	[35–37]
DNA polymerase gene epsilon/delta 1 (POLE/POLD1)	Colorectal cancer	[38–40]
PD-1/PD-L1	Non-small cell lung cancer	[41, 42]
T cell immunoglobulin-3 (TIM-3)	Breast, colorectal, hepatocellular, prostate cancer	{Qin, 2020, Prognostic Values of TIM-3 Expression in Patients With Solid Tumors: A Meta-Analysis and Database Evaluation; Solinas, 2019, Significance of TIM3 expression in cancer: From biology to the clinic; Wolf, 2020, TIM3 comes of age as an inhibitory receptor}
lymphocyte activation gene-3 (LAG-3)	Colorectal cancer, Hepatocellular cancer, Melanoma, Glioma	[43–45]
V-domain Ig suppressor of T-cell activation (VISTA)	Acute myeloid leukemia, Colorectal, glioma, melanoma, non-small cell lung cancer, pancreatic, prostate, kidney cancer.	[46–48]
interferon (IFN)-γ	Melanoma	[49, 50]
Indoleamine 2, 3-dioxygenase 1 (IDO1)	Breast cancer	[51, 52]
CD45RO+/CD8+T cells	Melanoma, endometrial cancer	[53, 54]
FoxP3+ Treg cells	Breast, cervical, gastric, lung, oropharyngeal, ovarian cancer	[55, 56]
Lactate dehydrogenase (LDH)	Melanoma, prostate cancer	[57]
STK11/LKB1 co-mutation	Non-small cell lung cancer	[58, 59]
EBV	Gastric cancer	[60, 61]

PD-1/PD-L1 Programmed cell death protein 1/ Programmed death Ligand 1, *CD45RO-* splice variant of Cluster of differentiation 45 (CD45) also known as protein-tyrosine phosphatase, receptor-type C, lacking the A, B, and C determinant, *CD8* Cluster of differentiation 8, *FoxP3* Forkhead box P3, *Treg* Regulatory T cells, *STK11* Serine/threonine kinase 11, *LKB1* Liver kinase B1, *EBV* Epstein–Barr Virus

network among DNA, micro-RNA, and proteins within different disease states. Clinically potentially useful biomarkers currently evaluated include numerous regulatory microRNAs, methylation profiles, single-nucleotide polymorphisms (SNPs), gene mutations, and expression levels in specific genes, peptides, proteins, lipids, metabolites, and other small molecules.

Risk Assessment

Biomarkers offer a quantitative means to identify individuals who are predisposed to certain types of cancer. Such biomarkers include BReast CAncer gene 1 and -2 (BRCA1 and BRCA2) for breast and ovarian cancers; epidermal growth factor receptor (EGFR), ERBB2 (HER2), Kirsten Rat Sarcoma (KRAS), and p53 for colorectal, esophageal, lung, liver, and pancreatic cancers; hypermethylation of myogenic differentiation 1 (MYOD1), cadherin 1 (CDH1), and cadherin 13 (CDH13) for cervical cancers; hypermethylation of p14, p16 and retinoblastoma 1 (RB1) for oral cancers; deregulated methylation of tumor suppressor genes p16, cyclin-dependent kinase inhibitor 2B (CDKN2B), and p14ARF for brain cancers.

Early Detection

Early detection and early intervention lead to much better outcomes for patients with cancer than later-stage detection; for example, the 5-year survival rate for breast cancer decreases from 90% when detected early to 30% at the late stage [64]. Early detection typically arises because of annual or periodic screening by physicians by way of mammograms, prostate exams, and Pap smears, among various other modes of screening. The goal of screening is to detect the presence of disease when subjects are asymptomatic, with screening tests ideally carried out in a non-invasive and inexpensive manner. There are several biomarkers used for screening: CA125 for ovarian cancer, PSA for prostate cancer, alpha-fetoprotein (AFP) for hepatocellular cancer in high-risk subjects; fecal occult blood testing (FOBT) for colorectal cancer; and vanillymandelic acid (VMA) for neuroblastoma in newborns [65]. Although PSA has been FDA-approved as a screening biomarker for prostate cancer, its contribution to mortality reduction is still controversial [66, 67]. Indeed, elevated PSA levels are found in individuals with benign prostatic hyperplasia and prostatitis [68]; these are false-positives for cancer screening. Biomarkers used for screening need to be specific to reduce the frequency of these false-positives and to prevent unnecessary psychological burden and costs to the patient.

Diagnosis

Diagnostic biomarkers are used to confirm a particular medical condition. Diagnostic biomarkers for cancer can be determined via radiological, anatomical, physiological, or molecular means, or through a combination of these methods. For example, PSA is used in combination with digital rectal examination (DRE) for the diagnosis of prostate cancer [69], and CA125 is used in combination with ultrasonography to improve diagnostic sensitivity in ovarian carcinoma. Nevertheless, cancer biomarkers used in combination with a panel of other markers in the absence of imaging tools can be equally effective in confirming a diagnosis. In 2005, Mor and colleagues [70] reported a 95% detection rate of ovarian carcinoma—with high specificity and sensitivity—using a biomarker panel comprising insulin-like growth factor 2, leptin, osteopontin, and prolactin. Recently, Gyllensten and his team proposed a protein biomarker signature for ovarian cancer alongside CA125 that could detect ovarian cancer stages I-IV with high specificity and sensitivity and improve diagnosis for women presenting with adrenal ovarian masses [71]. In another instance, Kumar and colleagues [72] identified and characterized a novel panel of five urinary biomarkers that showed more than 93% sensitivity with an almost 100% specificity for detection of transitional bladder carcinoma via immunoblot-based assay. Subsequent revalidation work using an ELISA-based assay on the same panel of urinary biomarkers from three different cohorts of transitional bladder carcinoma patients produced an overall sensitivity and specificity of 91.7% and 92.2%, respectively [73]. Yet, there remain a number of cancers, like head and neck cancer [74], for which there are no clinically useful diagnostic biomarkers. Furthermore, whereas X-ray remains the primary tool for a clinical diagnosis of lung cancer, the search for a biomarker for an accurate diagnosis of lung cancer is still needed. In 2018, Fang and colleagues reported a panel of prolactin (PRL), CEA and a C-terminal fragment of cytokeratin-19 (CYFRA21) as potential serum biomarkers for the diagnosis of non-small cell lung cancer (NSCLC), exhibiting 90% sensitivity and 95% specificity [75].

Prognosis

Prognosis is the likely outcome or the course of a disease; i.e., the probability of cure or recurrence. A prognostic biomarker can either be used to provide information about the disease outcome or predict the response to different therapeutic modalities. For prognosis of disease outcome, cancer biomarker levels and imaging results can reflect tumor burden: elevated expression and larger tumor masses tend to translate to poor prognosis while lower expression and smaller masses reflect the likelihood of a better outcome. With good correlation to tumor burden, biomarkers can be used during cancer staging using the tumor-node-metastasis (TNM) classification, with numerous biomarkers currently proving to be of value. For instance, lactate dehydrogenase (LDH) has been used for lymphoma staging [76]. In breast cancer, elevated HER2 serum levels are correlated with poorer prognosis [77], whereas high estrogen receptor (ER) expression is indicative of a good prognosis and tends to indicate those patients most likely to respond favorably to hormonal therapy (e.g., selective aromatase inhibitors or ER modulators; [78]. KRAS, a biomarker for numerous cancer types (colorectal, esophageal, lung, liver, and pancreatic), is predictive for treatment response in patients with colorectal cancer, with somatic KRAS mutations linked with poor response to anti-EGFR therapies [79].

Treatment Modalities

The classical treatments for cancers have been and remain to include surgery preceded or more often followed by radiotherapy and chemotherapy. However, over the last two decades the discovery of mutations activating kinases have prompted the synthesis of inhibitors targeting relatively specifically their catalytic domain. Tyrosine kinases (TKs) have progressively become major targets for cancer treatment [80, 81] albeit patients are still today also receiving conventional treatments. TK dysregulations in cell signaling through mutations, translocations or amplifications have been linked with tumorigenesis, tumor progression, invasion, and metastasis. Indeed, tyrosine kinase inhibitors (TKI) have been developed against a range of TKs, including ALK, EGFR, FGF, HER2, KIT, MEK, MET, NTRK, PDGFR, RET, and VEGFR [82]. Nonetheless these treatments are also facing the same issue as radiotherapy and chemotherapy namely the acquisition of resistance to these targeted therapies. These observations have elicited a regain of interest in the potential to leverage the immune system of patients. However, the immune system is rarely able to cope with the development of tumors which are not spontaneously regressing. The lack of recognition was initially attributed to the downregulation of major histocompatibility complex (MHC) class 1. The remarkable discovery of immune checkpoints has shed light on how the immune system fails to recognize cancer cells as foreign cells. Programmed death (PD)-1 is a checkpoint protein expressed on T cells that helps to limit or shut-down an immune response to prevent damage to healthy tissues.

However, this dampened response is detrimental when T cells bind to cancer cells since a functional immunological synapse cannot be established. The binding of PD-1 to PD-L1 activates a phosphatase which annihilates TCR signaling through a set of tyrosine kinases thereby allowing cancer cells to evade immune surveillance.

Different immune checkpoint inhibitors, such as antibodies against PD-1 and PD-L1, have been developed and tested for the treatment of various cancers, including bladder, colorectal, hepatocellular, lung, and renal cancers, as well as Hodgkin's lymphoma and melanoma [83]. Antibodies that target PD-1 or PD-L1 inhibit their interaction and provide the opportunity for an immune response to be elicited against the cancer cells. Currently, approved antibodies against PD-L1 (atezolizumab, avelumab, and durvalumab) and PD-1 (pembrolizumab, nivolumab) enhance antitumor immunity and improve clinical responses in the treatment of different cancer types [84].

Treatment modalities have also recently sought to incorporate cell-based immunotherapies. In this regime, T lymphocytes from the patient are modified ex vivo via two main strategies to render them able to recognize cognate peptides or epitopes on cancer cells before they are reintroduced into the patient. In the first strategy, a TCR—identified by its specificity for recognizing a peptide presented by an HLA protein—is transduced into peripheral blood monocytes, which are then cultured in vitro under conditions that aim to enrich the T cell population. This approach is currently used for virally induced cancers, such hepatitis B virus (HBV) in hepatocarcinoma [85, 86], Epstein–Barr Virus (EBV) in naso-pharyngeal carcinoma, some gastric cancers [87, 88] and human papilloma virus (HPV) in cervical and pharyngeal cancers [89, 90]. Solid tumors are now targeted by oncofetal cell-surface markers, such as NY-ESO-1, MAGE C2, and MAGE A3-6 [91, 92]. The second strategy is based on the transduction of a chimeric antigen receptor-modified T cell (CAR-T cell). This chimeric molecule is composed of a single chain antibody that specifically recognizes a cell-surface epitope expressed by cancer cells. Upon ligation to its epitope, the chimeric molecule activates an immune response through its cytoplasmic domain containing CD3*zeta* together with co-stimulatory cytoplasmic domains of other receptors localized in the immunological synapse. There are now many different versions of these chimeric molecules to optimize activation of the immune response; indeed, CAR-T cells are increasingly used for the treatment of hematological malignancies [93–95] and the FDA has recently approved Bristol Myers Squibb's lisocabtagene maraleucel, a CD19-directed CAR-T cell, for relapsed or refractory large B cell lymphoma. CAR-T cells with single chain antibody recognition of other surface markers in solid tumors are now entering clinical trials. These biomarkers include MUC1, EGFR, NKG2D, Mesothelin, and GD2 (https://clinicaltrials.gov).

Based on this principle, CAR-NK cells engage in a similar killing mechanism but recognize a different target. NK cells operate without TCRs and this strongly reduces the risk of rejection, suggesting the potential of using allogeneic CAR-NK cells for cell therapies [96, 97]. Indeed, CAR-NK cell therapies have been recently evaluated in B cell malignancies (NCT03056339) and glioblastoma (NCT03383978).

Monitoring Therapeutic Response and Recurrence

Biomarkers that fluctuate according to tumor burden can play a role in therapeutic monitoring. Such biomarkers are required to increase with progressive disease, decrease or be undetectable with remission, and remain unchanged when the disease is stable. Consequently, not all screening markers can be used as monitoring markers (and vice versa). For example, CA19-9 was approved by the FDA in 2002 as a monitoring marker for pancreatic cancer but is not recommended as a screening biomarker.

Monitoring biomarkers can also be used to assess the effectiveness of a therapeutic regime. They are clinically useful in identifying patients who do not respond or gain resistance to administered therapeutics, thereby allowing effective clinical decision-making as to whether an alternative therapy should be employed. Particular types of monitoring biomarkers can be used to evaluate therapeutics and to monitor recurrence; for example, CA125 in ovarian cancer [98], CEA in colorectal cancer [16, 99], and PSA in prostate cancer [100].

Biomarkers that reflect immunomodulation during immunotherapy are indicative of efficacy and toxicity. For instance, the infusion of CAR-T cells into a patient results in the release of a series of cytokines by T cells, which, in turn, elicits the release of a repertoire of cytokines by other immune cells. Such release profiles can help to indicate the efficacy of the regime: there is an inherent risk of triggering a cytokine storm, which can cause massive side effects in patients [101]. Finally, monitoring biomarkers can also be indicative of graft vs host disease, and this benefit is essential when allogenic CAR-T is employed as a treatment option [102].

Clinical Trials

Clinical trials follow a carefully controlled and typical path, with various phases of trials undertaken at different stages and with different cohorts to test drug efficacy prior to its release globally. Consequently, different biomarkers are required across these different phases. Phase I clinical trials require a set of biomarkers that can reflect toxicity and efficacy: Toxicity is assessed via the presence of organ-damage markers as well as caspase-related and immune markers, whereas efficacy is assessed using biomarker profiles in pharmacodynamics as well as at surrogate endpoints. A surrogate endpoint measures the effect of a treatment at a particular juncture that may correlate with a real clinical endpoint.

Clinical trials are held in accordance with one of the primary aims of precision medicine: i.e., to deliver the *right* dose to the *right* patient at the *right* time. Dose selection relies on an understanding of the complex relationship between a drug dosage and response. To that end, a set of biomarkers are identified that correlate with these pharmacodynamics to help to determine the appropriate dosages required for Phase II trials. Guttman and coworkers have successfully demonstrated that biomarkers that correlate well with pharmacodynamics help to establish the "maximum effective dose" instead of the more common practice of using the "maximum tolerated dose" for Phase II trials [103]. Indeed, there has been an increasing number of trials using biomarkers as a measurement outcome concomitant with the standard measures of side-effect symptoms, blood pressure, and imaging.

Another utility of biomarkers in clinical trials is patient stratification: comparing responders with non-responders [104]. Multi-time-point assessment of patients—baseline, during treatment, and after treatment—aid in establishing which biomarker signatures can differentiate among various groups. An upcoming strategy to improve the success rates of clinical trials is patient enrichment [105], which involves the enrollment of patients into trials based on their biomarker profile. Through retrospective studies, matching responders with their baseline biomarker profiles (i.e., prior to treatment) can help to identify those patients who are likely to respond to treatment. Thus, the further recruitment of new patients with similar baseline profiles helps to increase the success rate of these subsequent trials [106].

Post-Market

One of the key avenues for identifying effective drugs is through repurposing: i.e., drugs previously designed for "purpose A" but later tested and approved for "purpose B."

Rapamycin approved as an immunosuppressant for preventing kidney transplant rejection, was repurposed for oncology treatment in recent years due to an improved understanding of the role of mTOR and associated signaling network in cancer [107, 108]. Such label extension and repurposing can only be effective if we have a deeper understanding of the mechanism of action of drugs in specific diseases [109]. Biomarker profiling of treated samples in the laboratory can help to provide information on immunomodulation and the pathways that are targeted by each drug. For example, Metformin approved by FDA for treating obese type 2 diabetes has been reported to activate 5' adenosine monophosphate-activated protein, AMPK, a key sensor in cellular metabolism, thereby inhibiting mTOR signaling involved in tumor survival [110]. A protein fingerprint can be generated for each drug to provide a rationale for combination therapy. This is demonstrated in the use of Itraconazole for clinical cancer therapy in combination with other drugs. Itraconazole induced mTOR inhibition and cholesterol trafficking pathway, thereby inhibiting angiogenesis in cancer treatment. Itraconazole when used in combination with chemotherapy, pemetrexed, enhanced both progression-free and overall survival of lung cancer patients [111]. However, when in combination with rituximab, Itraconazole impaired rituximab's efficacy on lymphoma [111, 112]. Rituximab's mode of action requires the recruitment of CD20 to lipid rafts while Itraconazole inhibition on trafficking pathways interferes with rituximab function [111]. Biomarkers can also be used for post-market surveillance to understand adverse events or risks as they arise during real-world usage of the drug, serves as a means of comparison between new drugs, existing options, standard of care, and long-term monitoring of the efficacy of the drugs or combinations of drugs to ensure that treatment continues to be safe for patients.

Technology

The era of relying on a single disease biomarker has evolved to one of a "molecular signature," which depends on the identification of multiple biomarkers that can be used to distinguish patterns in and across multiple disease states. This paradigm shift was brought about by modern technologies that not only offered substantial throughput but empowered researchers to perform parallel and serial analyses. Indeed, these large-scale studies led to the identification of a range of clinically useful biomarkers that have been since included as a standard of care within clinical diagnostic tests. With such improvements in technology, many molecular biomarkers are now routinely identified, including mutations in driver genes, gene rearrangements, fusions or other alterations, copy number changes, methylation changes, and hyperphosphorylation.

Genomics

Next-generation sequencing (NGS) enables sequencing with a very high depth of coverage. As the number of gene alterations and biomarkers increases in oncology, more researchers are now opting for NGS technologies over conventional ones such as single gene testing and targeted panel testing. The dynamic range of NGS stretches from whole-genome sequencing to the limited sequencing of a pre-specified panel of genes. The choice of application depends on several factors, such as ease of analysis, technical efficiency, and cost.

Recent years have seen an increase in the commercial availability of various multi-gene panels designed to interrogate specific tumors or genes, with panel gene numbers ranging from 20 to 30 genes to 400–500 genes. These panels provide flexibility in terms of the numbers of samples analyzed in each run, thereby increasing efficiency and reducing cost [113]. Targeted gene panels are preferentially used in the clinical setting because of their greater depth of coverage in regions of interest as well as their faster turnover rate as compared with whole-genome (WGS) and whole-exome sequencing (WES) [114]. However, there remains some controversy as to the actual benefits of using a multi-gene panels over single gene testing. A recent retrospective study showed no survival gain among patients with NSCLC for whom genomic profiling was undertaken using targeted multi-gene panels versus patients for whom only single-gene testing of *EGFR* and *ALK* genes was performed [115]. However, the additional information delivered by multi-gene testing and the low cost of adding additional biomarkers to the panel potentially justify undertaking a more comprehensive genomic profiling. Indeed, targeted panels consisting of gene mutations (e.g., EGFR mutation T790M) can be used to inform on the development of acquired resistance against first-generation TKIs in samples from NSCLC [116]. In contrast, targeted panels that offer information about the downstream activation of certain pathways provide a rationale for combinatorial therapy and new treatment options; this has been shown for patients with melanoma and NSCLC [117–122]. Collectively, such findings have changed the standard of care for patients with NSCLC and have significantly improved survival.

WGS and WES are widely used in the research space to provide a huge reservoir of genomic information for translational research applications and to improve our understanding of cancer biology. A recent study utilized WGS to analyze 2,520 metastatic tumor samples. The study identified genetic events in the metastases of 22 solid tumors, 62% of which were identified with at least one actionable alteration [123]. The challenge of implementing the findings of WGS or WES in therapy, however, lies in the identification of mutations and alterations that are unable to be matched to a specific drug. This is evident in many genotype-matched trials: even though 40% of patients are reported to have actionable mutations, only 10% to 15% of these patients can be subsequently treated with genotype-matched drugs [114, 124–127].

WGS and WES are used not only identify SNVs but to study coding mRNA and non-coding RNA, such as miRNA and long non-coding RNA. Long-read RNA sequencing in tumors has been used to identify novel spliced isoforms and gene fusions associated with tumor progression and, often times, to determine acquired resistance to treatment [128–131]. In addition, long-read sequencing techniques have helped to detect SNVs, CNVs, and changes in the methylation profiles of genomic DNA from patients with brain cancer [132]. In another study on renal cancer, RNA sequencing analysis led to the identification of significant differential gene expression of 652 protein-coding genes and 92 long non-coding RNA genes in carcinoma cell lines derived from primary and metastatic sites [133].

Two sequencing techniques are used to analyze the different populations of immune cells in a tumor biopsy: single-cell RNA sequencing and CITE (Cellular Indexing of Transcriptomes and Epitopes) sequencing. These methods are used on known biomarkers to assess whether a tumor is colonized (hot) or not (cold) by immune cells. These techniques can also assess treatment response. Recently, Perturb-CITE-seq was used to identify mechanisms of resistance to immune checkpoint inhibitors (ICIs) among models from melanoma patient samples [134]. Perturb-CITE-seq combines CRISPR-based perturbation screens and massively parallel single-cell RNA sequencing to provide both RNA and protein readouts (epitopes of cell-surface proteins).

Proteomics

Compared with genomics technologies, proteomics technologies are less well established in terms of the throughput and depth of data attained [135]. Modern proteomics workflows that include prefractionation and multienzyme digestion strategies are now able to cover deep cellular proteomes. The sample types for proteomics have expanded in recent years from tissue (biopsy, tumoral, peritumoral, and nontumoral), blood (serum and plasma), and cerebrospinal fluid to include circulating tumor cells (CTCs) and exosomes [136–138].

Spatial Proteomics

Conventional tests such as immunohistochemistry (IHC) and fluorescence in situ hybridization (FISH) are currently used to detect biomarkers in tumors. IHC is used to detect changes at the protein level as a result of gene aberrations like that found in the androgen receptor in patients with prostate cancer [139, 140], as well as specific DNA rearrangements [141, 142] and point mutations like isocitrate dehydrogenase 1 and 2 isoforms in acute myeloid leukemia [143]. FISH has been the gold standard for assessing DNA rearrangements and is used to confirm IHC results in gene amplifications. In the last decade, IHC has been used to determine PD-L1 expression in certain tumor types, and this is used to select specific patients for treatment with anti-PD-1/PD-L1 therapies [144, 145].

Nanostring technology is a more recent tool that enables the analysis of up to 40 proteins in a single formalin-fixed paraffin-embedded sample while being able to retain information on spatial biology and cell–cell interactions; such information is useful, particularly in the study of cancer cell-immune cell interactions [146]. In nanostring technology, the digital spatial profiling probes are tagged with unique photocleavable DNA oligos, which are released after guided UV exposure and quantification at specific regions of interest (ROIs). Van and coworkers described the use of GeoMx digital spatial profiling for the analysis of immune cell abundance in breast cancer tumor sections [147].

Untargeted Proteomics

Mass spectrometry (MS)-based assays have improved over the past decade, now offering higher mass accuracy, higher detection capabilities, and shorter cycling times, with increased throughput and more reliable data. Furthermore, in addition to determining the identification and abundance of proteins, MS can now be used for protein localization and interactions, for establishing interaction networks and post-translational modifications (phosphorylation, ubiquitination, glycosylation), and for determining differences in various disease stages as compared with that of healthy tissues [148–150]. A study by Liu and colleagues [151] used matrix-assisted laser desorption ionization-time of flight (MALDI-TOF) MS to analyze the N-glycome of IgG in normal individuals and patients with benign and colorectal cancers. The team identified nine IgG N-glycans that were differentially expressed in colorectal patients, five of which correlated with the progression of colorectal cancer. These findings suggest that further studies investigating aspects of glycan chemistry (e.g., fucosylation and sialylation) might

help to reveal the mechanisms associated with the development of colorectal cancer.

Biomarker quantification using MS often depends on the use of stable isotopic labels that give rise to covalently derivatized peptides. Initially, such quantifications were mostly applicable to cell line-based studies; for example, a study by Hu et al., using stable isotope labeling by amino acids in cell culture (SILAC) technology, identified Cdc42–Cdc42 binding protein A (Cdc42BPA) signaling as a prognostic biomarker for colon carcinoma invasion [152]. The authors used two cell line models, HCT 116-I8 and HCT 116, grown in either light (Arg 0, Lys 0) or heavy (Arg 10, Lys 8) medium for 7 days, and analyzed the samples using an LTQ-Orbitrap hybrid MS. More recently, similar analyses rely on isobaric tags for relative and absolute quantitation (iTRAQ) or tandem mass tags (TMT) [153]. The advantage of using TMT in clinical proteomics is the high degree of multiplexing—up to 16plex—to significantly reduce the liquid chromatography (LC)-MS time requirements for the analysis of increasingly large patient cohorts. TMT was also recently used to identify biomarkers that could predict the efficacy of trastuzumab-based treatment in HER2-positive breast cancer patients [154]. The team identified 18 differentially expressed serum biomarkers in resistant patients at baseline before trastuzumab-based therapy, with 3 of these proteins (CST3, LDHA, SRGN) validated by LC-MS/MS multiple reaction monitoring (MRM) quantification.

Although iTRAQ and TMT remain conventional methods and are widely used, much effort has been made to develop label-free methods. Miyauchi and colleagues used sequential window acquisition of all fragment ion spectra (SWATH) MS in combination with LC-MS/MS on a triple TOF 5600 to develop quantitative targeted absolute proteomics (QTAP). The authors used this technique to identify upregulated plasma biomarkers in glioblastoma tumor specimens and cystic fluid [155], identifying an upregulation in APOB, CRP, C9, LRG1, and SERPINA3, and a downregulation in APOA4, GSN, IGHA1 in glioblastoma tumors. Furthermore, aside from CRP, the authors also detected all candidate proteins.

MS is also used in metabolomics to identify metabolites as markers for certain carcinoma [156, 157]. A study by Wang and colleagues utilized MS metabolic analyses to identify 21 differentially expressed metabolites in the blood, which were then developed into a panel. This panel showed 84.4% specificity and 92.2% sensitivity on validation breast carcinoma and non-breast carcinoma set [158]. In addition, Holmes et al. [159] showed the feasibility of MS to detect cancer volatile organic compounds in breath samples: this insight holds significant promise for biomarker discovery in gastric- and respiratory-related cancers [160–163].

Targeted Proteomics

Targeted proteomics platforms range from single-plex to multiplex formats in basic research, and these platforms are then applied to diagnostics. Enzyme-linked immunosorbent assay (ELISA) is a quantitative analytical method that measures antigen–antibody interactions via an enzyme-linked conjugate and enzyme substrate, using a color or fluorescent signal for detection. With the development of multiplex technologies, ELISA can now be used to measure multiple biomarkers in a single run. The challenges with multiplex assays lie in improving the specificity, sensitivity and throughput of the assay: a lower throughput will increase the specificity and sensitivity, and vice versa. For example, a low-plex multiplex, consisting of single molecule array technology (SiMoa)—regarded as an ultrasensitive 4-10 plex immunoassay—has been used for the detection of low-abundance biomarkers [164, 165]. Schubert et al. demonstrated the feasibility of measuring incremental changes in PSA levels in mice using SiMoa [165]. Later, Wei et al. used SiMoa technology to develop an extracellular vesicle (EV) marker assay to profile EVs directly from cell culture supernatants or the plasma of patients with cancer [166]. The team showed that colorectal cancer correlated with higher measures of CD9-CD63 and EpCAM-CD63; thresholding allowed patients with colorectal cancer to be distinguished from healthy patients and patients with benign tumors. SiMoa technology can also be used to distinguish among prognostic biomarkers for overall survival. Darlix et al. applied SiMoa technology to measure Tau serum levels in patients with metastatic breast cancer (MBC), which allowed for the successful stratification of MBC patients with brain metastases from those without metastases [167].

Another low-plex technology is Meso Scale Discovery (MSD) technology, which combines electrochemiluminescence and planar bead-based arrays to measure multiple analytes in a single sample. Recently, this technology was used to analyze 14 different proinflammatory protein biomarkers of which serum amyloid A (SAA) and IL-18 were identified as prognostic markers for breast cancer recurrence [168].

Midplex multiplex assays are largely represented by Luminex technology (40–60 plex per panel; best suited for testing 3–500 targets) and Proximity Extension Assay (PEA) technology (48–96 plex per panel; best suited for testing 48–1164 targets). Liu et al. developed a Luminex-based assay to measure the production of cytokines, chemokines, checkpoint-related proteins, and growth factors as an avenue to evaluate treatment efficacy. They found that response to treatment correlated with lower baseline levels of HGF or IL-8; patients with decreased levels of IL-8 or increased levels of CTLA-4 (CD152) during treatment were better responders [169]. PEA was also recently used to measure over 300 proteins simultaneously. The authors reported a protein signature of 19 serum proteins that increased diagnostic capacity in TNM I-II stage gastric cancer patients, distinguishing patients from control patients with high diagnostic sensitivity (93%), specificity (100%) and area under receiver operating characteristic curve (AUC) (0.99) [170].

Lower throughput approaches are often used to measure known and relevant biomarkers or to validate findings and observations. Contrastingly, higher throughput approaches are used for target discovery and to investigate mechanisms of action or signaling pathways. Such high-throughput, targeted approaches are largely represented by targeted MS, SOMAScan, and PEA technology.

MS data acquisition is represented by three modes: data-dependent acquisition (DDA), data-independent acquisition (DIA), and targeted data acquisition (TDA). In DDA, a defined number of precursor ions from the full scan are selected for fragmentation. DIA, on the other hand, acquires a full MS spectrum followed by sequential MS/MS isolation, whereas TDA selects a list of precursors for fragmentation before moving on to detect major product ions [171, 172]. DIA has been used for ovarian cancer biomarker discovery and validation using parallel reaction monitoring (PRM) MS, with four biomarkers identified: apolipoprotein (APO) A-IV, C-reactive protein (CRP), transthyretin (TTR), and transferrin (TF) [172]. Another study used DIA for the detection of highly complex clinical plasma biomarkers in pancreatic cancer paired with the use of a spectral library of over 14,000 peptides [173]. Validation of the technique on a cohort clinical sample suggested the robustness and advantages of this targeted approach for biomarker development.

Different aptamer-based technologies have been developed to facilitate biomarker discovery, including CELL-SELEX technology for the identification of cell-surface biomarkers and SOMAScan for the unbiased detection of thousands of proteins in biological samples [174, 175]. Studies suggest that SomaScan has a specificity in the range of 73% to 86% [176, 177]. These technologies have been used for malignant pleural mesothelioma [178] and for the detection of biomarkers in NSCLC, where 44 protein biomarkers were identified. From this data, the authors developed a 12-protein panel that could distinguish NSCLC samples from control samples with 83% specificity and 89% sensitivity in the validation set [178]. Another study using the technology identified 300 protein biomarkers with unknown associations to prostate cancer exosomes [179].

PEA technology is a multiplex assay that combines high-affinity antibody binding and DNA amplification to deliver a high throughput assay with high specificity and sensitivity. PEA technology overcomes the issues associated with non-specific antibody binding that is typical of multiplex assays by using DNA-tagged paired antibodies. Each antibody in the pair is designed with a DNA tail that has a complimentary sequence to that of the other and will hybridize when in proximity. When there is non-specific antibody binding, the DNA tails do not hybridize and the non-specific complex cannot be not detected by the assay, thereby delivering high specificity and close to zero cross reactivity [180]. Correctly hybridized regions are extended by a polymerase to form a DNA barcode, which is amplified and detected via qPCR or NGS, delivering high sensitivity and protein detection in the femtomolar range. PEA technology has been used for the development of a protein biomarker signature for ovarian cancer. The authors measured 593 proteins across 3 cohorts of patients with ovarian cancer and benign tumors, and validated an 11-protein biomarker signature (AUC of 94%, sensitivity of 85%, and specificity of 93%) using an independent cohort [71]. Other recent large-scale plasma profiling studies have shown the feasibility of establishing stable protein fingerprints for each healthy individual among patient cohorts, with changes in the proteome profile potentially useful for early disease diagnosis [181, 182].

Multi-Omics

The basic research community and numerous diagnostics-based companies have shifted their focus to search for biomarkers that can be used to complement studies on drug target identification and validation as a way to improve treatment modalities and diminish the impact of cancer and its treatment on patient quality of life. The current strategy for immunotherapy intervention explores the possibility of turning a "cold" into a "hot" tumor to improve immunotherapy response [183]. A study by Sade-Fieldman et al. demonstrated the utility of combining deep tumor-based scRNASeq data and plasma proteomics to provide insights into the tumor microenvironment among those with melanoma [184]. Another study by Villani et al. demonstrated the use of scRNA and proteomics to characterize and identify six dendritic cell and four monocyte subtypes in human blood; such knowledge could further improve immune monitoring in disease [185].

We now know that a single technology, like sequencing, for the assessment of risk and for the identification of new causal biomarkers for certain cancers, cannot easily determine whether mutations are driver mutations [186]. Indeed, many somatic "hotspot" mutations labeled as "drivers" might be passenger mutations occurring in highly mutable hotspots [187]. One of the newer strategies employed by pharmaceutical companies to search for causal protein biomarkers is protein quantitative trait loci (pQTL). This method requires a combination of GWAS data and proteomics data to identify *cis* and *trans* pQTL: *cis* pQTLs are the direct effect of a gene locus on the protein, whereas *trans* pQTLs refer to regulatory regions. Using the "Mendelian randomization" algorithm provides the opportunity to identify proteins that are causal to disease with up to 99% accuracy: drugs designed against these causal proteins have a four-times higher chance of FDA approval [188].

Concluding Remarks/Summary

The complexity of diagnosis, prognosis, and treatment lies in the heterogeneity of the tumor: the complex assembly of malignant and stromal cells along with inflammatory and immune cells within the tumor microenvironment (TME). Extensive efforts have been made to understand the mechanisms of intrinsic and extrinsic tumor escape, studying the expression of various molecules in the TME and the dynamic plasma proteome. Recently, suggestions have been made to profile both fluids extracted from tumor blood lakes and the TME with the plasma of patients to assess the feasibility of using liquid biopsies to predict the immune status in the TME. Predictive markers of ICIs have been expanded from single markers to multifactorial markers and include both expressed molecules and circulating effector cell ratios, such as central memory/effector T-cell ratio and neutrophil-to-lymphocyte ratio. Because of the exponential improvement in technologies, biomarker discovery has also increased, along with the ability to embark on large-scale prospective studies. However, all new biomarkers require time for assessment and validation for their diagnostic, prognostic, or predictive value before they can be used routinely in clinical practice. Overall, the ideal biomarker or biomarker signature should be convenient to use in the clinical setting and accurately diagnose, monitor, or inform about a patient's clinical response (Fig. 34.1). The gap between bench and bedside is brought closer by these evolving technologies and data processing efforts, providing us with a better understanding of the complex biology associated with cancer progression, and bestowing upon us the opportunity to refine our strategy for personalized and precise cancer treatment.

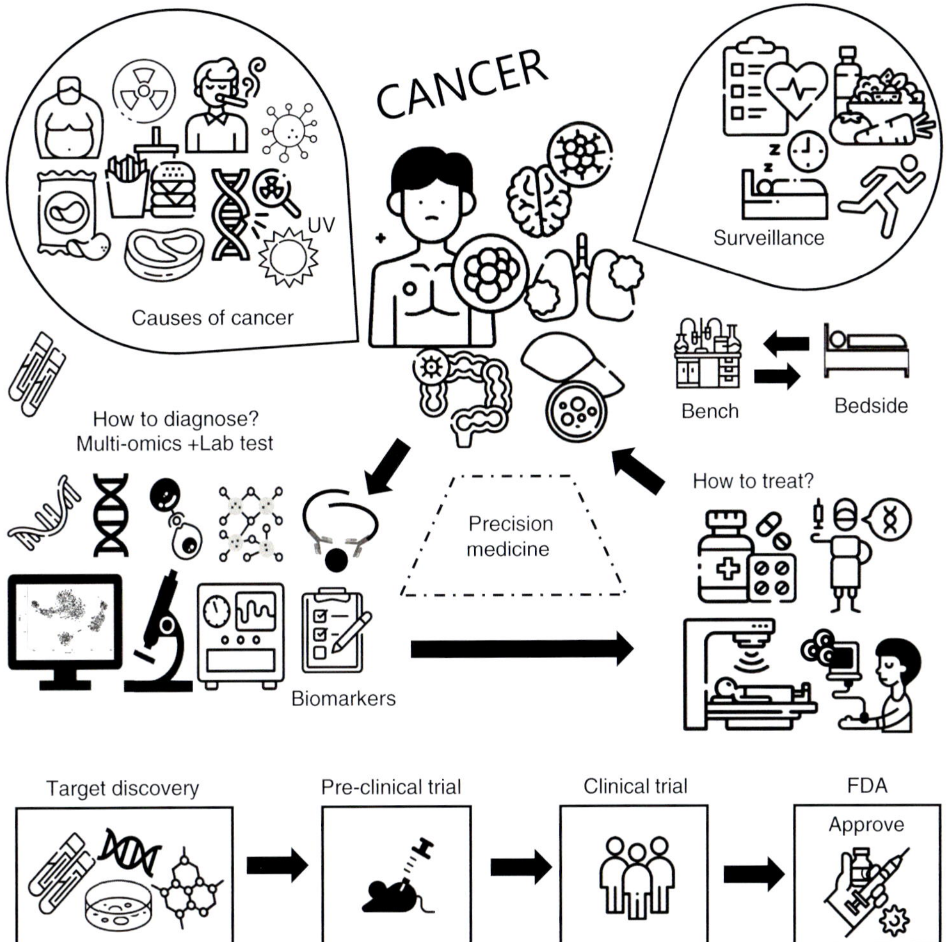

Fig. 34.1 An ideal biomarker or a biomarker signature should be convenient to use in the clinical setting and accurately diagnose, monitor, or inform about a patient's clinical response. The use of biomarkers can provide information on how lifestyle habits such as intake of processed food, soda, red meat, smoking, exercise affects the body in terms of inflammation and susceptibility to cancer. Sets of combination biomarkers identified through lab tests and multi-omics studies can help stratifying patients and predict their response to drugs. Biomarkers can be used to provide real-time biology of patients' response toward the treatment. The earlier non-responsive signatures can be detected in patients, the faster an adaptive therapy can be applied for a potentially better outcome. Biomarkers can also be used for relapse surveillance. To obtain an ideal biomarker signature for use in clinical setting not only requires adequate scientific rigor but also the need to address the missing links between Research use only (RUO) biomarker discovery and in vitro diagnostics (IVD) reagents, Clinical Laboratory Improvement Amendments (CLIA) vs Food and Drug Administration (FDA) regulations

Acknowledgments Jean Paul Thiery is supported by a core funding from The Bioland and Guangzhou Laboratory, Bioisland Guangzhou. Graphics were created using Icons from www.flaticon.com. We are much indebted to Dr. Rebecca Jackson for careful editing of the manuscript.

References

1. Jones HB. Some account of a new animal substance occurring in the urine of a patient labouring under mollities Ossium. Edinb Med Surg J. 1850;74:357–68.
2. Kyle RA. Multiple myeloma: how did it begin? Mayo Clin Proc. 1994;69:680–3. https://doi.org/10.1016/s0025-6196(12)61349-4.
3. Edelman GM, Gally JA. The nature of Bence-Jones proteins. Chemical similarities to polypetide chains of myeloma globulins and normal gamma-globulins. J Exp Med. 1962;116:207–27. https://doi.org/10.1084/jem.116.2.207.
4. Sinclair D, Dagg JH, Smith JG, Stott DI. The incidence and possible relevance of Bence-Jones protein in the sera of patients with multiple myeloma. Br J Haematol. 1986;62:689–94. https://doi.org/10.1111/j.1365-2141.1986.tb04092.x.
5. Gold P, Freedman SO. Demonstration of tumor-specific antigens in human colonic carcinomata by immunological tolerance and absorption techniques. J Exp Med. 1965;121:439–62. https://doi.org/10.1084/jem.121.3.439.
6. Yilmaz A, Ece F, Bayramgürler B, Akkaya E, Baran R. The value of Ca 125 in the evaluation of tuberculosis activity. Respir Med. 2001;95:666–9. https://doi.org/10.1053/rmed.2001.1121.
7. Bast RC, Ravdin P, Hayes DF, Bates S, Fritsche H, Jessup JM, Kemeny N, Locker GY, Mennel RG, Somerfield MR, Panel A.S.o.C.O.T.M.E. 2000 update of recommendations for the use of tumor markers in breast and colorectal cancer: clinical prac-

tice guidelines of the American Society of Clinical Oncology. J Clin Oncol. 2001;19:1865–78. https://doi.org/10.1200/JCO.2001.19.6.1865.

8. Molina R, Barak V, van Dalen A, Duffy MJ, Einarsson R, Gion M, Goike H, Lamerz R, Nap M, Sölétormos G, Stieber P. Tumor markers in breast cancer- European Group on tumor markers recommendations. Tumour Biol. 2005;26:281–93. https://doi.org/10.1159/000089260.

9. Colleoni M, Viale G, Zahrieh D, Pruneri G, Gentilini O, Veronesi P, Gelber RD, Curigliano G, Torrisi R, Luini A, et al. Chemotherapy is more effective in patients with breast cancer not expressing steroid hormone receptors: a study of preoperative treatment. Clin Cancer Res. 2004;10:6622–8. https://doi.org/10.1158/1078-0432.CCR-04-0380.

10. Paik S, Tang G, Shak S, Kim C, Baker J, Kim W, Cronin M, Baehner FL, Watson D, Bryant J, et al. Gene expression and benefit of chemotherapy in women with node-negative, estrogen receptor-positive breast cancer. J Clin Oncol. 2006;24:3726–34. https://doi.org/10.1200/JCO.2005.04.7985.

11. Bhatt AN, Mathur R, Farooque A, Verma A, Dwarakanath BS. Cancer biomarkers - current perspectives. Indian J Med Res. 2010;132:129–49.

12. Gutierrez C, Schiff R. HER2: biology, detection, and clinical implications. Arch Pathol Lab Med. 2011;135:55–62. https://doi.org/10.1043/2010-0454-RAR.1.

13. Ross JS, Slodkowska EA, Symmans WF, Pusztai L, Ravdin PM, Hortobagyi GN. The HER-2 receptor and breast cancer: ten years of targeted anti-HER-2 therapy and personalized medicine. Oncologist. 2009;14:320–68. https://doi.org/10.1634/theoncologist.2008-0230.

14. Jensen JL, Maclean GD, Suresh MR, Almeida A, Jette D, Lloyd S, Bodnar D, Krantz M, Longenecker BM. Possible utility of serum determinations of CA 125 and CA 27.29 in breast cancer management. Int J Biol Markers. 1991;6:1–6.

15. Kibar Y, Goktas S, Kilic S, Yaman H, Onguru O, Peker AF. Prognostic value of cytology, nuclear matrix protein 22 (NMP22) test, and urinary bladder cancer II (UBC II) test in early recurrent transitional cell carcinoma of the bladder. Ann Clin Lab Sci. 2006;36:31–8.

16. Koizumi F, Odagiri H, Fujimoto H, Kawamura T, Ishimori A. Clinical evaluation of four tumor markers (CEA, TPA, CA50 and CA72-4) in colorectal cancer. Rinsho Byori. 1992;40:523–8.

17. Chen L, Ho DW, Lee NP, Sun S, Lam B, Wong KF, Yi X, Lau GK, Ng EW, Poon TC, et al. Enhanced detection of early hepatocellular carcinoma by serum SELDI-TOF proteomic signature combined with alpha-fetoprotein marker. Ann Surg Oncol. 2010;17:2518–25. https://doi.org/10.1245/s10434-010-1038-8.

18. Johnson PJ, Williams R. Serum alpha-fetoprotein estimations and doubling time in hepatocellular carcinoma: influence of therapy and possible value in early detection. J Natl Cancer Inst. 1980;64:1329–32. https://doi.org/10.1093/jnci/64.6.1329.

19. Minami T, Tateishi R, Kondo M, Nakagomi R, Fujiwara N, Sato M, Uchino K, Enooku K, Nakagawa H, Asaoka Y, et al. Serum alpha-fetoprotein has high specificity for the early detection of hepatocellular carcinoma after hepatitis c virus eradication in patients. Medicine (Baltimore). 2015;94:e901. https://doi.org/10.1097/MD.0000000000000901.

20. Bae YJ, Schaab M, Kratzsch J. Calcitonin as biomarker for the medullary thyroid Carcinoma. Recent Results Cancer Res. 2015;204:117–37. https://doi.org/10.1007/978-3-319-22542-5_5.

21. van Veelen W, de Groot JW, Acton DS, Hofstra RM, Höppener JW, Links TP, Lips CJ. Medullary thyroid carcinoma and biomarkers: past, present and future. J Int Med. 2009;266:126–40. https://doi.org/10.1111/j.1365-2796.2009.02106.x.

22. Charkhchi P, Cybulski C, Gronwald J, Wong FO, Narod SA, Akbari MR. CA125 and ovarian cancer: a comprehensive review. Cancers (Basel). 2020;12 https://doi.org/10.3390/cancers12123730.

23. Funston G, Hamilton W, Abel G, Crosbie EJ, Rous B, Walter FM. The diagnostic performance of CA125 for the detection of ovarian and non-ovarian cancer in primary care: A population-based cohort study. PLoS Med. 2020;17:e1003295. https://doi.org/10.1371/journal.pmed.1003295.

24. Dong Q, Yang XH, Zhang Y, Jing W, Zheng LQ, Liu YP, Qu XJ. Elevated serum CA19-9 level is a promising predictor for poor prognosis in patients with resectable pancreatic ductal adenocarcinoma: a pilot study. World J Surg Oncol. 2014;12:171. https://doi.org/10.1186/1477-7819-12-171.

25. Poruk KE, Gay DZ, Brown K, Mulvihill JD, Boucher KM, Scaife CL, Firpo MA, Mulvihill SJ. The clinical utility of CA 19-9 in pancreatic adenocarcinoma: diagnostic and prognostic updates. Curr Mol Med. 2013;13:340–51. https://doi.org/10.2174/1566652 4011313030003.

26. Loeb S, Partin AW. Review of the literature: PCA3 for prostate cancer risk assessment and prognostication. Rev Urol. 2011;13:e191–5.

27. Marks LS, Bostwick DG. Prostate cancer specificity of PCA3 gene testing: examples from clinical practice. Rev Urol. 2008;10:175–81.

28. Matoso A, Epstein JI. Defining clinically significant prostate cancer on the basis of pathological findings. Histopathology. 2019;74:135–45. https://doi.org/10.1111/his.13712.

29. Yusim I, Krenawi M, Mazor E, Novack V, Mabjeesh NJ. The use of prostate specific antigen density to predict clinically significant prostate cancer. Sci Rep. 2020;10:20015. https://doi.org/10.1038/s41598-020-76786-9.

30. Fowler JE, Sesterhenn IA, Mostofi FK. Detection of AFP and HCG in metastatic testicular cancer after treatment with chemotherapy or radiation therapy. Urology. 1989;33:74–7. https://doi.org/10.1016/0090-4295(89)90074-5.

31. Milose JC, Filson CP, Weizer AZ, Hafez KS, Montgomery JS. Role of biochemical markers in testicular cancer: diagnosis, staging, and surveillance. Open Access J Urol. 2011;4:1–8. https://doi.org/10.2147/OAJU.S15063.

32. Gianoukakis AG. Thyroglobulin antibody status and differentiated thyroid cancer: what does it mean for prognosis and surveillance? Curr Opin Oncol. 2015;27:26–32. https://doi.org/10.1097/CCO.0000000000000149.

33. Mazzaferri EL, Robbins RJ, Spencer CA, Braverman LE, Pacini F, Wartofsky L, Haugen BR, Sherman SI, Cooper DS, Braunstein GD, et al. A consensus report of the role of serum thyroglobulin as a monitoring method for low-risk patients with papillary thyroid carcinoma. J Clin Endocrinol Metab. 2003;88:1433–41. https://doi.org/10.1210/jc.2002-021702.

34. Prpić M, Franceschi M, Romić M, Jukić T, Kusić Z. Thyroglobulin as a tumor marker in differentiated thyroid cancer - clinical considerations. Acta Clin Croat. 2018;57:518–27. https://doi.org/10.20471/acc.2018.57.03.16.

35. Marmorino F, Boccaccino A, Germani MM, Falcone A, Cremolini C. Immune checkpoint inhibitors in pMMR metastatic colorectal cancer: a tough challenge. Cancers (Basel). 2020;12 https://doi.org/10.3390/cancers12082317.

36. Overman MJ, Lonardi S, Wong KYM, Lenz HJ, Gelsomino F, Aglietta M, Morse MA, Van Cutsem E, McDermott R, Hill A, et al. Durable clinical benefit with nivolumab plus ipilimumab in DNA mismatch repair-deficient/microsatellite instability-high metastatic colorectal cancer. J Clin Oncol. 2018;36:773–9. https://doi.org/10.1200/JCO.2017.76.9901.

37. Zhang Y, Sun Z, Mao X, Wu H, Luo F, Wu X, Zhou L, Qin J, Zhao L, Bai C. Impact of mismatch-repair deficiency on the colorectal

cancer immune microenvironment. Oncotarget. 2017;8:85526–36. https://doi.org/10.18632/oncotarget.20241.

38. Domingo E, Freeman-Mills L, Rayner E, Glaire M, Briggs S, Vermeulen L, Fessler E, Medema JP, Boot A, Morreau H, et al. Somatic POLE proofreading domain mutation, immune response, and prognosis in colorectal cancer: a retrospective, pooled biomarker study. Lancet Gastroenterol Hepatol. 2016;1:207–16. https://doi.org/10.1016/S2468-1253(16)30014-0.

39. Gong J, Wang C, Lee PP, Chu P, Fakih M. Response to PD-1 blockade in microsatellite stable metastatic colorectal cancer harboring a. J Natl Compr Canc Netw. 2017;15:142–7. https://doi.org/10.6004/jnccn.2017.0016.

40. Song Z, Cheng G, Xu C, Wang W, Shao Y, Zhang Y. Clinicopathological characteristics of POLE mutation in patients with non-small-cell lung cancer. Lung Cancer. 2018;118:57–61. https://doi.org/10.1016/j.lungcan.2018.02.004.

41. Gandhi L, Rodríguez-Abreu D, Gadgeel S, Esteban E, Felip E, De Angelis F, Domine M, Clingan P, Hochmair MJ, Powell SF, et al. Pembrolizumab plus chemotherapy in metastatic non-small-cell lung cancer. N Engl J Med. 2018;378:2078–92. https://doi.org/10.1056/NEJMoa1801005.

42. Rouquette I, Taranchon-Clermont E, Gilhodes J, Bluthgen MV, Perallon R, Chalabreysse L, De Muret A, Hofman V, Marx A, Parrens M, et al. Immune biomarkers in thymic epithelial tumors: expression patterns, prognostic value and comparison of diagnostic tests for PD-L1. Biomark Res. 2019;7:28. https://doi.org/10.1186/s40364-019-0177-8.

43. Fröhlich A, Sirokay J, Fietz S, Vogt TJ, Dietrich J, Zarbl R, Florin M, Kuster P, Saavedra G, Valladolid SR, et al. Molecular, clinicopathological, and immune correlates of LAG3 promoter DNA methylation in melanoma. EBioMedicine. 2020;59:102962. https://doi.org/10.1016/j.ebiom.2020.102962.

44. Guo M, Yuan F, Qi F, Sun J, Rao Q, Zhao Z, Huang P, Fang T, Yang B, Xia J. Expression and clinical significance of LAG-3, FGL1, PD-L1 and CD8. J Transl Med. 2020;18:306. https://doi.org/10.1186/s12967-020-02469-8.

45. Mair MJ, Kiesel B, Feldmann K, Widhalm G, Dieckmann K, Wöhrer A, Müllauer L, Preusser M, Berghoff AS. LAG-3 expression in the inflammatory microenvironment of glioma. J Neurooncol. 2021;152:533–9. https://doi.org/10.1007/s11060-021-03721-x.

46. Choi JW, Kim YJ, Yun KA, Won CH, Lee MW, Choi JH, Chang SE, Lee WJ. The prognostic significance of VISTA and CD33-positive myeloid cells in cutaneous melanoma and their relationship with PD-1 expression. Sci Rep. 2020;10:14372. https://doi.org/10.1038/s41598-020-71216-2.

47. Hou Z, Pan Y, Fei Q, Lin Y, Zhou Y, Liu Y, Guan H, Yu X, Lin X, Lu F, Huang H. Prognostic significance and therapeutic potential of the immune checkpoint VISTA in pancreatic cancer. J Cancer Res Clin Oncol. 2021;147:517–31. https://doi.org/10.1007/s00432-020-03463-9.

48. Huang X, Zhang X, Li E, Zhang G, Wang X, Tang T, Bai X, Liang T. VISTA: an immune regulatory protein checking tumor and immune cells in cancer immunotherapy. J Hematol Oncol. 2020b;13:83. https://doi.org/10.1186/s13045-020-00917-y.

49. Cui C, Xu C, Yang W, Chi Z, Sheng X, Si L, Xie Y, Yu J, Wang S, Yu R, et al. Ratio of the interferon-γ signature to the immunosuppression signature predicts anti-PD-1 therapy response in melanoma. NPJ Genom Med. 2021;6:7. https://doi.org/10.1038/s41525-021-00169-w.

50. Rodig SJ, Gusenleitner D, Jackson DG, Gjini E, Giobbie-Hurder A, Jin C, Chang H, Lovitch SB, Horak C, Weber JS, et al. MHC proteins confer differential sensitivity to CTLA-4 and PD-1 blockade in untreated metastatic melanoma. Sci Transl Med. 2018;10 https://doi.org/10.1126/scitranslmed.aar3342.

51. Wang S, Wu J, Shen H, Wang J. The prognostic value of IDO expression in solid tumors: a systematic review and meta-analysis. BMC Cancer. 2020a;20:471. https://doi.org/10.1186/s12885-020-06956-5.

52. Wang W, Huang L, Jin JY, Pi W, Ellsworth SG, Jolly S, Mellor AL, Machtay M, Kong FS. A validation study on IDO immune biomarkers for survival prediction in non-small cell lung cancer: radiation dose fractionation effect in early-stage disease. Clin Cancer Res. 2020b;26:282–9. https://doi.org/10.1158/1078-0432.CCR-19-1202.

53. Tietze JK, Angelova D, Heppt MV, Reinholz M, Murphy WJ, Spannagl M, Ruzicka T, Berking C. The proportion of circulating CD45RO. Eur J Cancer. 2017;75:268–79. https://doi.org/10.1016/j.ejca.2016.12.031.

54. Zhou WJ, Zhang J, Xie F, Wu JN, Ye JF, Wang J, Wu K, Li MQ. CD45RO. Theranostics. 2021;11:5330–45. https://doi.org/10.7150/thno.58337.

55. Saleh R, Elkord E. FoxP3. Cancer Lett. 2020;490:174–85. https://doi.org/10.1016/j.canlet.2020.07.022.

56. Santegoets SJ, Duurland CL, Jordanova ES, van Ham JJ, Ehsan I, van Egmond SL, Welters MJP, van der Burg SH. Tbet-positive regulatory T cells accumulate in oropharyngeal cancers with ongoing tumor-specific type 1 T cell responses. J Immunother Cancer. 2019;7:14. https://doi.org/10.1186/s40425-019-0497-0.

57. Knispel S, Gassenmaier M, Menzies AM, Loquai C, Johnson DB, Franklin C, Gutzmer R, Hassel JC, Weishaupt C, Eigentler T, et al. Outcome of melanoma patients with elevated LDH treated with first-line targeted therapy or PD-1-based immune checkpoint inhibition. Eur J Cancer. 2021;148:61–75. https://doi.org/10.1016/j.ejca.2021.01.034.

58. Burdett N, Desai J. New biomarkers for checkpoint inhibitor therapy. ESMO Open. 2020;5:e000597. https://doi.org/10.1136/esmoopen-2019-000597.

59. Shire NJ, Klein AB, Golozar A, Collins JM, Fraeman KH, Nordstrom BL, McEwen R, Hembrough T, Rizvi NA. STK11 (LKB1) mutations in metastatic NSCLC: prognostic value in the real world. PLoS One. 2020;15:e0238358. https://doi.org/10.1371/journal.pone.0238358.

60. Sun K, Jia K, Lv H, Wang SQ, Wu Y, Lei H, Chen X. EBV-positive gastric cancer: current knowledge and future perspectives. Front Oncol. 2020;10:583463. https://doi.org/10.3389/fonc.2020.583463.

61. Xie T, Liu Y, Zhang Z, Zhang X, Gong J, Qi C, Li J, Shen L, Peng Z. Positive status of epstein-barr virus as a biomarker for gastric cancer immunotherapy: a prospective observational study. J Immunother. 2020;43:139–44. https://doi.org/10.1097/CJI.0000000000000316.

62. Schrohl AS, Holten-Andersen M, Sweep F, Schmitt M, Harbeck N, Foekens J, Brünner N, Group, E.O.f.R., Treatment of Cancer, R., and Biomarker. Tumor markers: from laboratory to clinical utility. Mol Cell Proteomics. 2003;2:378–87. https://doi.org/10.1074/mcp.R300006-MCP200.

63. Mishra A, Verma M. Cancer biomarkers: are we ready for the prime time? Cancers (Basel). 2010;2:190–208. https://doi.org/10.3390/cancers2010190.

64. Weigelt B, Peterse JL, van 't Veer LJ. Breast cancer metastasis: markers and models. Nat Rev Cancer. 2005;5:591–602. https://doi.org/10.1038/nrc1670.

65. Duffy MJ. Use of biomarkers in screening for cancer. Adv Exp Med Biol. 2015;867:27–39. https://doi.org/10.1007/978-94-017-7215-0_3.

66. Jimenez PA, Teliska M, Liu B, Antonaccio MJ. Urokinase-type plasminogen activator stimulates wound healing in the diabetic mouse. Inflamm Res. 1997;46(Suppl 2):S169–70. https://doi.org/10.1007/s000110050164.

67. Yang Q, Kawaguchi T, Battistini B, Sirois P. Neutral endopeptidase degrades endothelins in guinea pig tracheal epithelial cells. Inflamm Res. 1997;46(Suppl 2):S171–2. https://doi.org/10.1007/s000110050165.

68. Catalona WJ, Smith DS, Ratliff TL, Dodds KM, Coplen DE, Yuan JJ, Petros JA, Andriole GL. Measurement of prostate-specific antigen in serum as a screening test for prostate cancer. N Engl J Med. 1991;324:1156–61. https://doi.org/10.1056/NEJM199104253241702.

69. Heidenreich A, Bellmunt J, Bolla M, Joniau S, Mason M, Matveev V, Mottet N, Schmid HP, van der Kwast T, Wiegel T, Zattoni F. EAU guidelines on prostate cancer. Part I: screening, diagnosis, and treatment of clinically localised disease. Actas Urol Esp. 2011;35:501–14. https://doi.org/10.1016/j.acuro.2011.04.004.

70. Mor G, Visintin I, Lai Y, Zhao H, Schwartz P, Rutherford T, Yue L, Bray-Ward P, Ward DC. Serum protein markers for early detection of ovarian cancer. Proc Natl Acad Sci U S A. 2005;102:7677–82. https://doi.org/10.1073/pnas.0502178102.

71. Enroth S, Berggrund M, Lycke M, Broberg J, Lundberg M, Assarsson E, Olovsson M, Stålberg K, Sundfeldt K, Gyllensten U. High throughput proteomics identifies a high-accuracy 11 plasma protein biomarker signature for ovarian cancer. Commun Biol. 2019;2:221. https://doi.org/10.1038/s42003-019-0464-9.

72. Kumar P, Nandi S, Tan TZ, Ler SG, Chia KS, Lim WY, Butow Z, Vordos D, De la Taille A, Al-Haddawi M, et al. Highly sensitive and specific novel biomarkers for the diagnosis of transitional bladder carcinoma. Oncotarget. 2015;6:13539–49. https://doi.org/10.18632/oncotarget.3841.

73. Lim JC, Lee TW, Thiery KC, J.P. Novel panel of urinary biomarkers for urothelial cancer. International Journal of Urology. 2018;25(Supplement s1):323.

74. Konings H, Stappers S, Geens M, De Winter BY, Lamote K, van Meerbeeck JP, Specenier P, Vanderveken OM, Ledeganck KJ. A literature review of the potential diagnostic biomarkers of head and neck neoplasms. Front Oncol. 2020;10:1020. https://doi.org/10.3389/fonc.2020.01020.

75. Fang R, Zhu Y, Khadka VS, Zhang F, Jiang B, Deng Y. The evaluation of serum biomarkers for non-small cell lung cancer (NSCLC) diagnosis. Front Physiol. 2018;9:1710. https://doi.org/10.3389/fphys.2018.01710.

76. Swan F, Velasquez WS, Tucker S, Redman JR, Rodriguez MA, McLaughlin P, Hagemeister FB, Cabanillas F. A new serologic staging system for large-cell lymphomas based on initial beta 2-microglobulin and lactate dehydrogenase levels. J Clin Oncol. 1989;7:1518–27. https://doi.org/10.1200/JCO.1989.7.10.1518.

77. Molina R, Jo J, Filella X, Zanon G, Pahisa J, Muñoz M, Farrus B, Latre ML, Gimenez N, Hage M, et al. C-erbB-2 oncoprotein in the sera and tissue of patients with breast cancer. Utility in prognosis. Anticancer Res. 1996;16:2295–300.

78. Duffy MJ. Predictive markers in breast and other cancers: a review. Clin Chem. 2005;51:494–503. https://doi.org/10.1373/clinchem.2004.046227.

79. Allegra CJ, Jessup JM, Somerfield MR, Hamilton SR, Hammond EH, Hayes DF, McAllister PK, Morton RF, Schilsky RL. American Society of Clinical Oncology provisional clinical opinion: testing for KRAS gene mutations in patients with metastatic colorectal carcinoma to predict response to anti-epidermal growth factor receptor monoclonal antibody therapy. J Clin Oncol. 2009;27:2091–6. https://doi.org/10.1200/JCO.2009.21.9170.

80. Drake JM, Lee JK, Witte ON. Clinical targeting of mutated and wild-type protein tyrosine kinases in cancer. Mol Cell Biol. 2014;34:1722–32. https://doi.org/10.1128/MCB.01592-13.

81. Jiao Q, Bi L, Ren Y, Song S, Wang Q, Wang YS. Advances in studies of tyrosine kinase inhibitors and their acquired resistance. Mol Cancer. 2018;17:36. https://doi.org/10.1186/s12943-018-0801-5.

82. Huang L, Jiang S, Shi Y. Tyrosine kinase inhibitors for solid tumors in the past 20 years (2001-2020). J Hematol Oncol. 2020a;13:143. https://doi.org/10.1186/s13045-020-00977-0.

83. Wu X, Gu Z, Chen Y, Chen B, Chen W, Weng L, Liu X. Application of PD-1 blockade in cancer immunotherapy. Comput Struct Biotechnol J. 2019;17:661–74. https://doi.org/10.1016/j.csbj.2019.03.006.

84. Sharpe AH. Introduction to checkpoint inhibitors and cancer immunotherapy. Immunol Rev. 2017;276:5–8. https://doi.org/10.1111/imr.12531.

85. Festag MM, Festag J, Fräßle SP, Asen T, Sacherl J, Schreiber S, Mück-Häusl MA, Busch DH, Wisskirchen K, Protzer U. Evaluation of a fully human, Hepatitis B Virus-specific chimeric antigen receptor in an immunocompetent mouse model. Mol Ther. 2019;27:947–59. https://doi.org/10.1016/j.ymthe.2019.02.001.

86. Krebs K, Böttinger N, Huang LR, Chmielewski M, Arzberger S, Gasteiger G, Jäger C, Schmitt E, Bohne F, Aichler M, et al. T cells expressing a chimeric antigen receptor that binds hepatitis B virus envelope proteins control virus replication in mice. Gastroenterology. 2013;145:456–65. https://doi.org/10.1053/j.gastro.2013.04.047.

87. Basso S, Zecca M, Merli P, Gurrado A, Secondino S, Quartuccio G, Guido I, Guerini P, Ottonello G, Zavras N, et al. T cell therapy for nasopharyngeal carcinoma. J Cancer. 2011;2:341–6. https://doi.org/10.7150/jca.2.341.

88. Slabik C, Kalbarczyk M, Danisch S, Zeidler R, Klawonn F, Volk V, Krönke N, Feuerhake F, Ferreira de Figueiredo C, Blasczyk R, et al. CAR-T cells targeting epstein-barr virus gp350 validated in a humanized mouse model of EBV infection and lymphoproliferative disease. Mol Ther Oncolytics. 2020;18:504–24. https://doi.org/10.1016/j.omto.2020.08.005.

89. Doran SL, Stevanović S, Adhikary S, Gartner JJ, Jia L, Kwong MLM, Faquin WC, Hewitt SM, Sherry RM, Yang JC, et al. T-cell receptor gene therapy for human papillomavirus-associated epithelial cancers: a first-in-human, Phase I/II study. J Clin Oncol. 2019;37:2759–68. https://doi.org/10.1200/JCO.18.02424.

90. Zhang Y, Li X, Zhang J, Mao L. Novel cellular immunotherapy using NKG2D CAR-T for the treatment of cervical cancer. Biomed Pharmacother. 2020;131:110562. https://doi.org/10.1016/j.biopha.2020.110562.

91. Kim SH, Lee S, Lee CH, Lee MK, Kim YD, Shin DH, Choi KU, Kim JY, Park DY, Sol MY. Expression of cancer-testis antigens MAGE-A3/6 and NY-ESO-1 in non-small-cell lung carcinomas and their relationship with immune cell infiltration. Lung. 2009;187:401–11. https://doi.org/10.1007/s00408-009-9181-3.

92. Thomas R, Al-Khadairi G, Roelands J, Hendrickx W, Dermime S, Bedognetti D, Decock J. NY-ESO-1 based immunotherapy of cancer: current perspectives. Front Immunol. 2018;9:947. https://doi.org/10.3389/fimmu.2018.00947.

93. Grupp SA, Kalos M, Barrett D, Aplenc R, Porter DL, Rheingold SR, Teachey DT, Chew A, Hauck B, Wright JF, et al. Chimeric antigen receptor-modified T cells for acute lymphoid leukemia. N Engl J Med. 2013;368:1509–18. https://doi.org/10.1056/NEJMoa1215134.

94. Lee DW, Kochenderfer JN, Stetler-Stevenson M, Cui YK, Delbrook C, Feldman SA, Fry TJ, Orentas R, Sabatino M, Shah NN, et al. T cells expressing CD19 chimeric antigen receptors for acute lymphoblastic leukaemia in children and young adults: a phase 1 dose-escalation trial. Lancet. 2015;385:517–28. https://doi.org/10.1016/S0140-6736(14)61403-3.

95. Neelapu SS, Locke FL, Bartlett NL, Lekakis LJ, Miklos DB, Jacobson CA, Braunschweig I, Oluwole OO, Siddiqi T, Lin Y, et al. Axicabtagene ciloleucel CAR T-cell therapy in refractory large B-Cell lymphoma. N Engl J Med. 2017;377:2531–44. https://doi.org/10.1056/NEJMoa1707447.

96. Liu S, Galat V, Galat Y, Lee YKA, Wainwright D, Wu J. NK cell-based cancer immunotherapy: from basic biology to clinical development. J Hematol Oncol. 2021b;14:7. https://doi.org/10.1186/s13045-020-01014-w.

97. Simonetta F, Alvarez M, Negrin RS. Natural killer cells in graft-versus-host-disease after allogeneic hematopoietic cell transplantation. Front Immunol. 2017;8:465. https://doi.org/10.3389/fimmu.2017.00465.

98. van Nagell JR, DePriest PD, Reedy MB, Gallion HH, Ueland FR, Pavlik EJ, Kryscio RJ. The efficacy of transvaginal sonographic screening in asymptomatic women at risk for ovarian cancer. Gynecol Oncol. 2000;77:350–6. https://doi.org/10.1006/gyno.2000.5816.

99. von Kleist S. The clinical value of the tumor markers CA 19/9 and carcinoembryonic antigen (CEA) in colorectal carcinomas: a critical comparison. Int J Biol Markers. 1986;1:3–8.

100. Evans CW. Program to correct inappropriate prescribing. Am J Hosp Pharm. 1989;46:69–70.

101. Brudno JN, Kochenderfer JN. Toxicities of chimeric antigen receptor T cells: recognition and management. Blood. 2016;127:3321–30. https://doi.org/10.1182/blood-2016-04-703751.

102. Liu P, Liu M, Lyu C, Lu W, Cui R, Wang J, Li Q, Mou N, Deng Q, Yang D. Acute graft-versus-host disease after humanized anti-CD19-CAR T therapy in relapsed B-ALL patients after allogeneic hematopoietic stem cell transplant. Front Oncol. 2020;10:573822. https://doi.org/10.3389/fonc.2020.573822.

103. Bissonnette R, Maari C, Forman S, Bhatia N, Lee M, Fowler J, Tyring S, Pariser D, Sofen H, Dhawan S, et al. The oral Janus kinase/spleen tyrosine kinase inhibitor ASN002 demonstrates efficacy and improves associated systemic inflammation in patients with moderate-to-severe atopic dermatitis: results from a randomized double-blind placebo-controlled study. Br J Dermatol. 2019;181:733–42. https://doi.org/10.1111/bjd.17932.

104. El Bairi K, Atanasov AG, Amrani M, Afqir S. The arrival of predictive biomarkers for monitoring therapy response to natural compounds in cancer drug discovery. Biomed Pharmacother. 2019;109:2492–8. https://doi.org/10.1016/j.biopha.2018.11.097.

105. Wang X, Zhou J, Wang T, George SL. On enrichment strategies for biomarker stratified clinical trials. J Biopharm Stat. 2018;28:292–308. https://doi.org/10.1080/10543406.2017.1379532.

106. Matsui S, Crowley J. Biomarker-stratified Phase III clinical trials: enhancement with a subgroup-focused sequential design. Clin Cancer Res. 2018;24:994–1001. https://doi.org/10.1158/1078-0432.CCR-17-1552.

107. Benjamin D, Colombi M, Moroni C, Hall MN. Rapamycin passes the torch: a new generation of mTOR inhibitors. Nat Rev Drug Discov. 2011;10:868–80. https://doi.org/10.1038/nrd3531.

108. Dancey J. mTOR signaling and drug development in cancer. Nat Rev Clin Oncol. 2010;7:209–19. https://doi.org/10.1038/nrclinonc.2010.21.

109. Verbaanderd C, Meheus L, Huys I, Pantziarka P. Repurposing drugs in oncology: next steps. Trends Cancer. 2017;3:543–6. https://doi.org/10.1016/j.trecan.2017.06.007.

110. Howell JJ, Hellberg K, Turner M, Talbott G, Kolar MJ, Ross DS, Hoxhaj G, Saghatelian A, Shaw RJ, Manning BD. Metformin inhibits hepatic mTORC1 signaling via dose-dependent mechanisms involving AMPK and the TSC complex. Cell Metab. 2017;25:463–71. https://doi.org/10.1016/j.cmet.2016.12.009.

111. Ringshausen I, Feuerstacke Y, Krainz P, den Hollander J, Hermann K, Buck A, Peschel C, Bueschenfelde MZ, C. Antifungal therapy with itraconazole impairs the anti-lymphoma effects of rituximab by inhibiting recruitment of CD20 to cell surface lipid rafts. Cancer Res. 2010;70:4292–6. https://doi.org/10.1158/0008-5472.CAN-10-0259.

112. Yang BR, Seong JM, Choi NK, Shin JY, Lee J, Kim YJ, Kim MS, Park S, Song HJ, Park BJ. Co-medication of statins with contraindicated drugs. PLoS One. 2015;10:e0125180. https://doi.org/10.1371/journal.pone.0125180.

113. Moorcraft SY, Gonzalez D, Walker BA. Understanding next generation sequencing in oncology: a guide for oncologists. Crit Rev Oncol Hematol. 2015;96:463–74. https://doi.org/10.1016/j.critrevonc.2015.06.007.

114. Hartmaier RJ, Charo J, Fabrizio D, Goldberg ME, Albacker LA, Pao W, Chmielecki J. Genomic analysis of 63,220 tumors reveals insights into tumor uniqueness and targeted cancer immunotherapy strategies. Genome Med. 2017;9:16. https://doi.org/10.1186/s13073-017-0408-2.

115. Presley CJ, Tang D, Soulos PR, Chiang AC, Longtine JA, Adelson KB, Herbst RS, Zhu W, Nussbaum NC, Sorg RA, et al. Association of broad-based genomic sequencing with survival among patients with advanced non-small cell lung cancer in the community oncology setting. JAMA. 2018;320:469–77. https://doi.org/10.1001/jama.2018.9824.

116. Bollinger MK, Agnew AS, Mascara GP. Osimertinib: a third-generation tyrosine kinase inhibitor for treatment of epidermal growth factor receptor-mutated non-small cell lung cancer with the acquired Thr790Met mutation. J Oncol Pharm Pract. 2018;24:379–88. https://doi.org/10.1177/1078155217712401.

117. Coit DG, Thompson JA, Algazi A, Andtbacka R, Bichakjian CK, Carson WE, Daniels GA, DiMaio D, Fields RC, Fleming MD, et al. NCCN guidelines insights: melanoma, version 3.2016. J Natl Compr Canc Netw. 2016;14:945–58. https://doi.org/10.6004/jnccn.2016.0101.

118. Ettinger DS, Aisner DL, Wood DE, Akerley W, Bauman J, Chang JY, Chirieac LR, D'Amico TA, Dilling TJ, Dobelbower M, et al. NCCN guidelines insights: non-small cell lung cancer, version 5.2018. J Natl Compr Canc Netw. 2018;16:807–21. https://doi.org/10.6004/jnccn.2018.0062.

119. Mok TS, Wu YL, Ahn MJ, Garassino MC, Kim HR, Ramalingam SS, Shepherd FA, He Y, Akamatsu H, Theelen WS, et al. Osimertinib or platinum-pemetrexed in EGFR T790M-positive lung cancer. N Engl J Med. 2017;376:629–40. https://doi.org/10.1056/NEJMoa1612674.

120. Planchard D, Smit EF, Groen HJM, Mazieres J, Besse B, Helland Å, Giannone V, D'Amelio AM, Zhang P, Mookerjee B, Johnson BE. Dabrafenib plus trametinib in patients with previously untreated BRAF. Lancet Oncol. 2017;18:1307–16. https://doi.org/10.1016/S1470-2045(17)30679-4.

121. Robert C, Karaszewska B, Schachter J, Rutkowski P, Mackiewicz A, Stroiakovski D, Lichinitser M, Dummer R, Grange F, Mortier L, et al. Improved overall survival in melanoma with combined dabrafenib and trametinib. N Engl J Med. 2015;372:30–9. https://doi.org/10.1056/NEJMoa1412690.

122. Soria JC, Ohe Y, Vansteenkiste J, Reungwetwattana T, Chewaskulyong B, Lee KH, Dechaphunkul A, Imamura F, Nogami N, Kurata T, et al. Osimertinib in untreated EGFR-mutated advanced non-small-cell lung cancer. N Engl J Med. 2018;378:113–25. https://doi.org/10.1056/NEJMoa1713137.

123. Priestley P, Baber J, Lolkema MP, Steeghs N, de Bruijn E, Shale C, Duyvesteyn K, Haidari S, van Hoeck A, Onstenk W, et al. Pan-cancer whole-genome analyses of metastatic solid tumours. Nature. 2019;575:210–6. https://doi.org/10.1038/s41586-019-1689-y.

124. Bo X, Burnstock G. Triphosphate, the key structure of the ATP molecule responsible for interaction with P2X-purinoceptors. Gen Pharmacol. 1993;24:637–40. https://doi.org/10.1016/0306-3623(93)90223-k.

125. Meric-Bernstam F, Brusco L, Shaw K, Horombe C, Kopetz S, Davies MA, Routbort M, Piha-Paul SA, Janku F, Ueno N, et al. Feasibility of large-scale genomic testing to facilitate enrollment onto genomically matched clinical trials. J Clin Oncol. 2015;33:2753–62. https://doi.org/10.1200/JCO.2014.60.4165.

126. Mertens WC, Bramwell VH, Banerjee D, Gwadry-Sridhar F, Lala PK. Sustained indomethacin and ranitidine with intermittent continuous infusion interleukin-2 in advanced malignant melanoma: a phase II study. Clin Oncol (R Coll Radiol). 1993;5:107–13. https://doi.org/10.1016/s0936-6555(05)80858-1.

127. Stockley TL, Oza AM, Berman HK, Leighl NB, Knox JJ, Shepherd FA, Chen EX, Krzyzanowska MK, Dhani N, Joshua AM, et al. Molecular profiling of advanced solid tumors and patient outcomes with genotype-matched clinical trials: the princess margaret IMPACT/COMPACT trial. Genome Med. 2016;8:109. https://doi.org/10.1186/s13073-016-0364-2.

128. Cavelier L, Ameur A, Häggqvist S, Höijer I, Cahill N, Olsson-Strömberg U, Hermanson M. Clonal distribution of BCR-ABL1 mutations and splice isoforms by single-molecule long-read RNA sequencing. BMC Cancer. 2015;15:45. https://doi.org/10.1186/s12885-015-1046-y.

129. Kohli M, Ho Y, Hillman DW, Van Etten JL, Henzler C, Yang R, Sperger JM, Li Y, Tseng E, Hon T, et al. Androgen receptor variant AR-V9 Is coexpressed with AR-V7 in prostate cancer metastases and predicts abiraterone resistance. Clin Cancer Res. 2017;23:4704–15. https://doi.org/10.1158/1078-0432.CCR-17-0017.

130. Nattestad M, Goodwin S, Ng K, Baslan T, Sedlazeck FJ, Rescheneder P, Garvin T, Fang H, Gurtowski J, Hutton E, et al. Complex rearrangements and oncogene amplifications revealed by long-read DNA and RNA sequencing of a breast cancer cell line. Genome Res. 2018;28:1126–35. https://doi.org/10.1101/gr.231100.117.

131. Tevz G, McGrath S, Demeter R, Magrini V, Jeet V, Rockstroh A, McPherson S, Lai J, Bartonicek N, An J, et al. Identification of a novel fusion transcript between human relaxin-1 (RLN1) and human relaxin-2 (RLN2) in prostate cancer. Mol Cell Endocrinol. 2016;420:159–68. https://doi.org/10.1016/j.mce.2015.10.011.

132. Euskirchen P, Bielle F, Labreche K, Kloosterman WP, Rosenberg S, Daniau M, Schmitt C, Masliah-Planchon J, Bourdeaut F, Dehais C, et al. Same-day genomic and epigenomic diagnosis of brain tumors using real-time nanopore sequencing. Acta Neuropathol. 2017;134:691–703. https://doi.org/10.1007/s00401-017-1743-5.

133. Yeh IJ, Liu KT, Shen JH, Wu YH, Liu YH, Yen MC, Kuo PL. Identification of the potential prognostic markers from the miRNA-lncRNA-mRNA interactions for metastatic renal cancer via next-generation sequencing and bioinformatics. Diagnostics (Basel). 2020;10 https://doi.org/10.3390/diagnostics10040228.

134. Frangieh CJ, Melms JC, Thakore PI, Geiger-Schuller KR, Ho P, Luoma AM, Cleary B, Jerby-Arnon L, Malu S, Cuoco MS, et al. Multimodal pooled Perturb-CITE-seq screens in patient models define mechanisms of cancer immune evasion. Nat Genet. 2021;53:332–41. https://doi.org/10.1038/s41588-021-00779-1.

135. Davies JA, Tindall H, Paton RC, Menys VC, Doig RL, Kester RC, McNicol GP. Platelet survival in patients treated with ticlopidine following reconstructive arterial surgery. Thromb Res. 1982;27:365–9. https://doi.org/10.1016/0049-3848(82)90083-4.

136. Amelio I, Bertolo R, Bove P, Buonomo OC, Candi E, Chiocchi M, Cipriani C, Di Daniele N, Ganini C, Juhl H, et al. Liquid biopsies and cancer omics. Cell Death Discov. 2020;6:131. https://doi.org/10.1038/s41420-020-00373-0.

137. Kim Y, Jeon J, Mejia S, Yao CQ, Ignatchenko V, Nyalwidhe JO, Gramolini AO, Lance RS, Troyer DA, Drake RR, et al. Targeted proteomics identifies liquid-biopsy signatures for extracapsular prostate cancer. Nat Commun. 2016;7:11906. https://doi.org/10.1038/ncomms11906.

138. Mader S, Pantel K. Liquid biopsy: current status and future perspectives. Oncol Res Treat. 2017;40:404–8. https://doi.org/10.1159/000478018.

139. Gupta S, Vanderbilt C, Abida W, Fine SW, Tickoo SK, Al-Ahmadie HA, Chen YB, Sirintrapun SJ, Chadalavada K, Nanjangud GJ, et al. Immunohistochemistry-based assessment of androgen receptor status and the AR-null phenotype in metastatic castrate resistant prostate cancer. Prostate Cancer Prostatic Dis. 2020;23:507–16. https://doi.org/10.1038/s41391-020-0214-6.

140. Waltering KK, Urbanucci A, Visakorpi T. Androgen receptor (AR) aberrations in castration-resistant prostate cancer. Mol Cell Endocrinol. 2012;360:38–43. https://doi.org/10.1016/j.mce.2011.12.019.

141. McLeer-Florin A, Moro-Sibilot D, Melis A, Salameire D, Lefebvre C, Ceccaldi F, de Fraipont F, Brambilla E, Lantuejoul S. Dual IHC and FISH testing for ALK gene rearrangement in lung adenocarcinomas in a routine practice: a French study. J Thorac Oncol. 2012;7:348–54. https://doi.org/10.1097/JTO.0b013e3182381535.

142. Yoshida A, Tsuta K, Wakai S, Arai Y, Asamura H, Shibata T, Furuta K, Kohno T, Kushima R. Immunohistochemical detection of ROS1 is useful for identifying ROS1 rearrangements in lung cancers. Mod Pathol. 2014;27:711–20. https://doi.org/10.1038/modpathol.2013.192.

143. Byers R, Hornick JL, Tholouli E, Kutok J, Rodig SJ. Detection of IDH1 R132H mutation in acute myeloid leukemia by mutation-specific immunohistochemistry. Appl Immunohistochem Mol Morphol. 2012;20:37–40. https://doi.org/10.1097/PAI.0b013e31822c132e.

144. Patel SP, Kurzrock R. PD-L1 expression as a predictive biomarker in cancer immunotherapy. Mol Cancer Ther. 2015;14:847–56. https://doi.org/10.1158/1535-7163.MCT-14-0983.

145. Scheel AH, Schäfer SC. Current PD-L1 immunohistochemistry for non-small cell lung cancer. J Thorac Dis. 2018;10:1217–9. https://doi.org/10.21037/jtd.2018.02.38.

146. Merritt CR, Ong GT, Church SE, Barker K, Danaher P, Geiss G, Hoang M, Jung J, Liang Y, McKay-Fleisch J, et al. Multiplex digital spatial profiling of proteins and RNA in fixed tissue. Nat Biotechnol. 2020;38:586–99. https://doi.org/10.1038/s41587-020-0472-9.

147. McCart Reed AE, Bennett J, Kutasovic JR, Kalaw E, Ferguson K, Yeong J, Simpson PT, Lakhani SR. Digital spatial profiling application in breast cancer: a user's perspective. Virchows Arch. 2020;477:885–90. https://doi.org/10.1007/s00428-020-02821-9.

148. Doll S, Gnad F, Mann M. The case for proteomics and phospho-proteomics in personalized cancer medicine. Proteomics Clin Appl. 2019;13:e1800113. https://doi.org/10.1002/prca.201800113.

149. Käll L, Vitek O. Computational mass spectrometry-based proteomics. PLoS Comput Biol. 2011;7:e1002277. https://doi.org/10.1371/journal.pcbi.1002277.

150. Tyanova S, Albrechtsen R, Kronqvist P, Cox J, Mann M, Geiger T. Proteomic maps of breast cancer subtypes. Nat Commun. 2016;7:10259. https://doi.org/10.1038/ncomms10259.

151. Liu X, Zheng W, Wang W, Shen H, Liu L, Lou W, Wang X, Yang P. A new panel of pancreatic cancer biomarkers discovered using a mass spectrometry-based pipeline. Br J Cancer. 2017;117:1846–54. https://doi.org/10.1038/bjc.2017.365.

152. Hu HF, Xu WW, Wang Y, Zheng CC, Zhang WX, Li B, He QY. Comparative proteomics analysis identifies Cdc42-Cdc42BPA signaling as prognostic biomarker and therapeutic target for colon cancer invasion. J Proteome Res. 2018;17:265–75. https://doi.org/10.1021/acs.jproteome.7b00550.

153. Bąchor R, Waliczek M, Stefanowicz P, Szewczuk Z. Trends in the design of new isobaric labeling reagents for quantitative proteomics. Molecules. 2019;24 https://doi.org/10.3390/molecules24040701.

154. Yang T, Fu Z, Zhang Y, Wang M, Mao C, Ge W. Serum proteomics analysis of candidate predictive biomarker panel for the diagnosis of trastuzumab-based therapy resistant breast cancer. Biomed Pharmacother. 2020;129:110465. https://doi.org/10.1016/j.biopha.2020.110465.

155. Miyauchi E, Furuta T, Ohtsuki S, Tachikawa M, Uchida Y, Sabit H, Obuchi W, Baba T, Watanabe M, Terasaki T, Nakada M. Identification of blood biomarkers in glioblastoma by SWATH mass spectrometry and quantitative targeted absolute proteomics. PLoS One. 2018;13:e0193799. https://doi.org/10.1371/journal.pone.0193799.

156. Chen Z, Li Z, Li H, Jiang Y. Metabolomics: a promising diagnostic and therapeutic implement for breast cancer. Onco Targets Ther. 2019;12:6797–811. https://doi.org/10.2147/OTT.S215628.

157. Dalal N, Jalandra R, Sharma M, Prakash H, Makharia GK, Solanki PR, Singh R, Kumar A. Omics technologies for improved diagnosis and treatment of colorectal cancer: technical advancement and major perspectives. Biomed Pharmacother. 2020;131:110648. https://doi.org/10.1016/j.biopha.2020.110648.

158. Wang Q, Sun T, Cao Y, Gao P, Dong J, Fang Y, Fang Z, Sun X, Zhu Z. A dried blood spot mass spectrometry metabolomic approach for rapid breast cancer detection. Onco Targets Ther. 2016;9:1389–98. https://doi.org/10.2147/OTT.S95862.

159. Holmes E, Wilson ID, Nicholson JK. Metabolic phenotyping in health and disease. Cell. 2008;134:714–7. https://doi.org/10.1016/j.cell.2008.08.026.

160. Abderrahman B. Exhaled breath biopsy: a new cancer detection paradigm. Future Oncol. 2019;15:1679–82. https://doi.org/10.2217/fon-2019-0091.

161. Durán-Acevedo CM, Jaimes-Mogollón AL, Gualdrón-Guerrero OE, Welearegay TG, Martinez-Marín JD, Caceres-Tarazona JM, Sánchez-Acevedo ZC, Beleño-Saenz KJ, Cindemir U, Österlund L, Ionescu R. Exhaled breath analysis for gastric cancer diagnosis in Colombian patients. Oncotarget. 2018;9:28805–17. https://doi.org/10.18632/oncotarget.25331.

162. Li M, Yang D, Brock G, Knipp RJ, Bousamra M, Nantz MH, Fu XA. Breath carbonyl compounds as biomarkers of lung cancer. Lung Cancer. 2015;90:92–7. https://doi.org/10.1016/j.lungcan.2015.07.005.

163. Mochalski P, Leja M, Gasenko E, Skapars R, Santare D, Sivins A, Aronsson DE, Ager C, Jaeschke C, Shani G, et al. Ex vivo emission of volatile organic compounds from gastric cancer and non-cancerous tissue. J Breath Res. 2018;12:046005. https://doi.org/10.1088/1752-7163/aacbfb.

164. Rissin DM, Kan CW, Campbell TG, Howes SC, Fournier DR, Song L, Piech T, Patel PP, Chang L, Rivnak AJ, et al. Single-molecule enzyme-linked immunosorbent assay detects serum proteins at subfemtomolar concentrations. Nat Biotechnol. 2010;28:595–9. https://doi.org/10.1038/nbt.1641.

165. Schubert SM, Arendt LM, Zhou W, Baig S, Walter SR, Buchsbaum RJ, Kuperwasser C, Walt DR. Ultra-sensitive protein detection via single molecule arrays towards early stage cancer monitoring. Sci Rep. 2015;5:11034. https://doi.org/10.1038/srep11034.

166. Wei P, Wu F, Kang B, Sun X, Heskia F, Pachot A, Liang J, Li D. Plasma extracellular vesicles detected by single molecule array technology as a liquid biopsy for colorectal cancer. J Extracell Vesicles. 2020;9:1809765. https://doi.org/10.1080/20013078.2020.1809765.

167. Darlix A, Hirtz C, Thezenas S, Maceski A, Gabelle A, Lopez-Crapez E, De Forges H, Firmin N, Guiu S, Jacot W, Lehmann S. The prognostic value of the Tau protein serum level in metastatic breast cancer patients and its correlation with brain metastases. BMC Cancer. 2019;19:110. https://doi.org/10.1186/s12885-019-5287-z.

168. Bera A, Russ E, Manoharan MS, Eidelman O, Eklund M, Hueman M, Pollard HB, Hu H, Shriver CD, Srivastava M. Proteomic analysis of inflammatory biomarkers associated with breast cancer recurrence. Mil Med. 2020;185:669–75. https://doi.org/10.1093/milmed/usz254.

169. Liu J, Li Y, Li Q, Liang D, Wang Q, Liu Q. Biomarkers of response to camrelizumab combined with apatinib: an analysis from a phase II trial in advanced triple-negative breast cancer patients. Breast Cancer Res Treat. 2021a;186:687–97. https://doi.org/10.1007/s10549-021-06128-4.

170. Shen Q, Polom K, Williams C, de Oliveira FMS, Guergova-Kuras M, Lisacek F, Karlsson NG, Roviello F, Kamali-Moghaddam M. A targeted proteomics approach reveals a serum protein signature as diagnostic biomarker for resectable gastric cancer. EBioMedicine. 2019;44:322–33. https://doi.org/10.1016/j.ebiom.2019.05.044.

171. Guo J, Huan T. Comparison of full-scan, data-dependent, and data-independent acquisition modes in liquid chromatography-mass spectrometry based untargeted metabolomics. Anal Chem. 2020;92:8072–80. https://doi.org/10.1021/acs.analchem.9b05135.

172. Rauniyar N, Peng G, Lam TT, Zhao H, Mor G, Williams KR. Data-independent acquisition and parallel reaction monitoring mass spectrometry identification of serum biomarkers for ovarian cancer. Biomark Insights. 2017;12:1177271917710948. https://doi.org/10.1177/1177271917710948.

173. Nigjeh EN, Chen R, Brand RE, Petersen GM, Chari ST, von Haller PD, Eng JK, Feng Z, Yan Q, Brentnall TA, Pan S. Quantitative proteomics based on optimized data-independent acquisition in plasma analysis. J Proteome Res. 2017;16:665–76. https://doi.org/10.1021/acs.jproteome.6b00727.

174. Gold L, Ayers D, Bertino J, Bock C, Bock A, Brody EN, Carter J, Dalby AB, Eaton BE, Fitzwater T, et al. Aptamer-based multiplexed proteomic technology for biomarker discovery. PLoS One. 2010;5:e15004. https://doi.org/10.1371/journal.pone.0015004.

175. Huang J, Chen X, Fu X, Li Z, Huang Y, Liang C. Advances in aptamer-based biomarker discovery. Front Cell Dev Biol. 2021;9:659760. https://doi.org/10.3389/fcell.2021.659760.

176. Suhre K, McCarthy MI, Schwenk JM. Genetics meets proteomics: perspectives for large population-based studies. Nat Rev Genet. 2021;22:19–37. https://doi.org/10.1038/s41576-020-0268-2.

177. Sun BB, Maranville JC, Peters JE, Stacey D, Staley JR, Blackshaw J, Burgess S, Jiang T, Paige E, Surendran P, et al. Genomic atlas of the human plasma proteome. Nature. 2018;558:73–9. https://doi.org/10.1038/s41586-018-0175-2.

178. Ostroff RM, Mehan MR, Stewart A, Ayers D, Brody EN, Williams SA, Levin S, Black B, Harbut M, Carbone M, et al. Early detection of malignant pleural mesothelioma in asbestos-exposed individuals with a noninvasive proteomics-based surveillance tool. PLoS One. 2012;7:e46091. https://doi.org/10.1371/journal.pone.0046091.

179. Webber J, Stone TC, Katilius E, Smith BC, Gordon B, Mason MD, Tabi Z, Brewis IA, Clayton A. Proteomics analysis of cancer exosomes using a novel modified aptamer-based array (SOMAscan™) platform. Mol Cell Proteomics. 2014;13:1050–64. https://doi.org/10.1074/mcp.M113.032136.

180. Assarsson E, Lundberg M, Holmquist G, Björkesten J, Thorsen SB, Ekman D, Eriksson A, Rennel Dickens E, Ohlsson S, Edfeldt G, et al. Homogenous 96-plex PEA immunoassay exhibiting high sensitivity, specificity, and excellent scalability. PLoS One. 2014;9:e95192. https://doi.org/10.1371/journal.pone.0095192.

181. Price ND, Magis AT, Earls JC, Glusman G, Levy R, Lausted C, McDonald DT, Kusebauch U, Moss CL, Zhou Y, et al. A wellness study of 108 individuals using personal, dense, dynamic data clouds. Nat Biotechnol. 2017;35:747–56. https://doi.org/10.1038/nbt.3870.

182. Zhong W, Edfors F, Gummesson A, Bergström G, Fagerberg L, Uhlén M. Next generation plasma proteome profiling to monitor health and disease. Nat Commun. 2021;12:2493. https://doi.org/10.1038/s41467-021-22767-z.

183. Duan Q, Zhang H, Zheng J, Zhang L. Turning cold into hot: firing up the tumor microenvironment. Trends Cancer. 2020;6:605–18. https://doi.org/10.1016/j.trecan.2020.02.022.

184. Sade-Feldman M, Yizhak K, Bjorgaard SL, Ray JP, de Boer CG, Jenkins RW, Lieb DJ, Chen JH, Frederick DT, Barzily-Rokni M,

et al. Defining T cell states associated with response to checkpoint immunotherapy in melanoma. Cell. 2018;175:998–1013.e1020. https://doi.org/10.1016/j.cell.2018.10.038.

185. Villani AC, Satija R, Reynolds G, Sarkizova S, Shekhar K, Fletcher J, Griesbeck M, Butler A, Zheng S, Lazo S, et al. Single-cell RNA-seq reveals new types of human blood dendritic cells, monocytes, and progenitors. Science. 2017;356 https://doi.org/10.1126/science.aah4573.

186. Le Tourneau C, Kamal M, Tsimberidou AM, Bedard P, Pierron G, Callens C, Rouleau E, Vincent-Salomon A, Servant N, Alt M, et al. Treatment algorithms based on tumor molecular profil-ing: the essence of precision medicine trials. J Natl Cancer Inst. 2016;108 https://doi.org/10.1093/jnci/djv362.

187. Hess JM, Bernards A, Kim J, Miller M, Taylor-Weiner A, Haradhvala NJ, Lawrence MS, Getz G. Passenger hotspot muta-tions in cancer. Cancer Cell. 2019;36:288–301.e214. https://doi.org/10.1016/j.ccell.2019.08.002.

188. Folkersen L, Gustafsson S, Wang Q, Hansen DH, Hedman Å, Schork A, Page K, Zhernakova DV, Wu Y, Peters J, et al. Genomic and drug target evaluation of 90 cardiovascular proteins in 30,931 individuals. Nat Metab. 2020;2:1135–48. https://doi.org/10.1038/s42255-020-00287-2.

Index

Benign prostatic hyperplasia associated PSA (BPSA), 470
Beta adrenergic signaling, 524
ß-arrestin, 524
Bevacizumab (Avastin®), 20, 412, 503, 513, 538
    in metastatic breast cancer, 412
    treatment, 392
Biglycan, 79
Biological conversation, 110
Biological processes, 415
Biomarker, 522, 564
    discovery and validation, 379
    medicine, 379
    panels
        adaptive and optimal designs, 554–556
        antibodies targeting, 555
        basket design, 554, 555
        biological features, 551, 552
        cancer therapy fields, 550
        clinical parameters, 551
        clinical trials, 552, 553
        targeted therapy, 553
        design of, 550, 551
        enrichment design, 555
        enrichment designs, 553
        FLT3-targeted therapy, 557
        functional genomics, 550
        heterogeneity, 557
        immune-modulatory approaches, 555
        impact of, 557
        IMPRESS study design, 556
        intratumoral heterogeneity, 555
        mesenchymal-derived cancer, 557, 558
        multidimensional analysis, 557
        post-treatment biopsies, 555
        quantity and quality of immune cells, 555
        radiotherapy, 558, 559
        targeted anticancer drugs, 557
        tumor microenvironment, 550
        umbrella designs, 553, 554
        use of, 550
        for pediatric brain cancer, 392, 393
    profiling, 568
Biomarker-based stratification of stage II or III GC patients, 390
Blood brain barrier (BBB), 511, 540
Blood flow, 33
Blood pressure, 33
Blood vascular invasion (BVI), 24
Blood vessel invasion, 502
Blood vessels, 24
Blood–brain barrier (BBB), 40
Blood-oxygen-level dependent (BOLD) MRI, 434
Bodenmiller laboratory, 360
Bombina variegata peptide 8 (Bv8), 249
Bone marrow (BM), 333
Bone marrow aspiration, 522
Bone marrow derived cell
    macrophages, 9
    mast cells, 10
    mesenchymal stem cells, 10
    neutrophils, 9
Bone morphogenic protein 30 (BMP), 522
Bone remodeling, 273
BRAF inhibitor, 317
Brain and central nervous system (CNS) cancers, 391, 392
Brain cancer, 392
Brain tumor

angiogenesis, 512–513
immunity, 513–515
BRCA1 and BRCA2 gene, 471
Breast cancer (BC), 289, 382, 384
    metastases, 411
    subtype classification, 407
Brownian motion, 429

C
CAF-associated genes, 408
Cancer, 93, 98, 126, 520–523
    biology, 402, 407
    molecular basis, 309
Cancer associated fibroblasts (CAF), 286, 370
Cancer biomarker
    clinical trials, 568
    diagnosis, 566
    early detection, 565, 566
    genomics, 569
    history of, 563, 564
    multi-omics, 572
    post-market, 568
    precision medicine, 564, 568
    prognosis, 566
    proteomics, 569, 570
    risk assessment, 565
    targeted proteomics, 571, 572
    technology, 568, 569
    therapeutic monitoring, 567
    treatment modalities, 566, 567
    types, 564, 565
    untargeted proteomics, 570
Cancer immunity, 160, 161
    CD4+ T cells, 161–165
    CD8+ T cells, 166, 167
    gamma delta T cells, 170, 171
    invariant NKT cells, 170
    MAIT cells, 170
    regulatory T cells, 169
    Tcells, 161
    tumor infiltrating lymphocytes, 171, 172
    unconventional T cells, 170
Cancer immunoediting, 163
Cancer immunotherapy, 461
Cancer metabolism, 432, 433
Cancer neuroscience, 291
Cancer stem cells (CSC), 38, 188, 443
Cancer-associated fibroblast (CAF), 54, 65, 100, 248, 381
Cancer-immune system interaction, 523
Carcinoembryonic antigen (CEA), 563
Carcinoma associated fibroblasts (CAF), 8, 113, 116
CAR-NK cell, 567
Castration resistant prostate cancer (CRPC), 454
CD3$^+$CD8$^+$ cytotoxic T cells (CTLs), 183
CD4$^+$ regulatory T cells (T$_{reg}$), 183
CD4+T cells to tumor promoting biology, 415
CD4+ Th2 cells, 163, 164
CD4+ Th9 cells, 165
CD4+ Th17 cells, 164, 165
CD4+ Th22 cells, 165, 166
CD4+Th cell, 163
CD8+ T lymphocytes, 231
CD10+ stroma signature, 407
CEA cell adhesion molecule 6 (CECAM6), 385
Cell adhesion, 406, 409

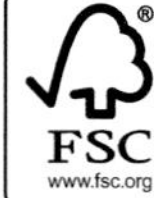

If you have any concerns about our products,
you can contact us on
ProductSafety@springernature.com

In case Publisher is established outside the EU,
the EU authorized representative is:
Springer Nature Customer Service Center GmbH
Europaplatz 3, 69115 Heidelberg, Germany

Printed by Libri Plureos GmbH
in Hamburg, Germany